Understanding
YOUR
Health

Understanding YOUR Health

sixth edition

Wayne A. Payne, Ed.D.

Ball State University, Muncie, Indiana

Dale B. Hahn, Ph.D.

Ball State University, Muncie, Indiana

Boston   Burr Ridge, IL   Dubuque, IA   Madison, WI   New York   San Francisco   St. Louis
Bangkok   Bogotá   Caracas   Lisbon   London   Madrid
Mexico City   Milan   New Delhi   Seoul   Singapore   Sydney   Taipei   Toronto

To our wives
Ruth and Ellen
and
Our children
Andrew and Ellen
Leslie and Laura

McGraw-Hill Higher Education

A Division of The **McGraw-Hill** *Companies*

UNDERSTANDING YOUR HEALTH, SIXTH EDITION

 This book is printed on recycled acid-free paper containing 10% postconsumer waste.

1 2 3 4 5 6 7 8 9 0 QPD/QPD 0 9 8 7 6 5 4 3 2 1 0

ISBN 0–07–039235–8

Vice president and editorial director: *Kevin T. Kane*
Publisher: *Edward E. Bartell*
Executive editor: *Vicki Malinee*
Senior developmental editor: *Melissa Martin*
Senior marketing manager: *Pamela S. Cooper*
Senior project manager: *Peggy J. Selle*
Senior production supervisor: *Mary E. Haas*
Coordinator of freelance design: *Michelle D. Whitaker*
Photo research coordinator: *John C. Leland*
Supplement coordinator: *Sandra M. Schnee*
Compositor: *Shepherd, Inc.*
Typeface: *10/12 Palatino*
Printer: *Quebecor Printing Book Group/Dubuque, IA*

Freelance cover designer: *Jamie O'Neal*
Cover image: © *Leland Bobbe/Tony Stone Images*

The credits section for this book begins on page 731 and is considered an extension of the copyright page.

Library of Congress Cataloging-in-Publication Data

Payne, Wayne A.
    Understanding your health / Wayne A. Payne, Dale B. Hahn.—6th ed.
      p.   cm.
    ISBN 0–07–039235–8
    1. Health.   2. College students—Health and hygiene.   I. Hahn,
Dale B.   II. Title.
RA777.3.P39   2000
613'.0434—dc21

                                       99–26520
                                        CIP

sererg
eryhsrtyh
zsdfed

www.mhhe.com

brief contents

We're talking to you!

You are our key customer. You've bought this McGraw-Hill textbook, and you expect it to play an integral role in your Personal Health course. We think you won't be disappointed. But only you can tell us whether our books are giving you the right information in the right format at the right price.

That's why McGraw-Hill is leading student focus groups across the U.S. and Canada. We are continually looking for ways to make our texts more accessible and more in tune with the needs of today's students.

We want to thank the students from Colorado State University, Southwestern College (Chula Vista, California), East Carolina University, and Florida A&M University who participated in our first nationwide focus groups.

Our thanks also go to the sponsoring instructors who helped make these initial brainstorming sessions a success: Karen Casey, Janna West Kolawski, Tom Brun, Sharon Knight, and Joseph P. Ramsey.

We want to hear from you. Contact any of our editorial or marketing team members at *www.mhhe.com/hper/health/personalhealth/teaminfo.mhtml*. Let us know how we can make our products better suit your educational needs. We assure you that we're listening.

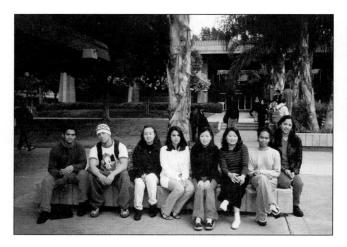 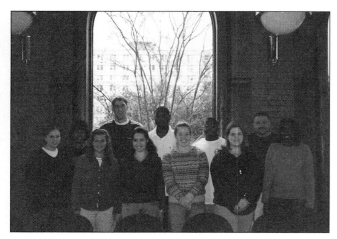

It's you and students like these at Southwestern College (left) and East Carolina University (right) who are helping to shape the future of McGraw-Hill's Health and Human Performance books and technology products.

contents

unit one

The Mind

2 Achieving Psychological Wellness

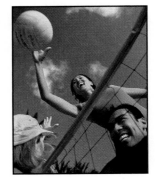

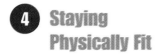

unit two

The Body

4 Staying Physically Fit

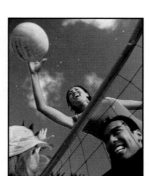

5 Understanding Nutrition and Your Diet

6 Maintaining a Healthy Weight

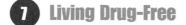

unit three

Addictive Substances

⑨ Rejecting Tobacco Use

unit four

Preventing Diseases

⑩ Reducing Your Risk of Cardiovascular Disease

11 Living with Cancer

12 Managing Chronic Conditions

13 Preventing Infectious Disease Transmission

unit five

Sexuality

14 Exploring the Origins of Sexuality

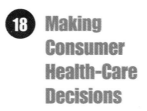

unit six

Consumerism and Environment

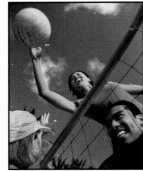

19 Caring for Our Environment

20   Protecting Your Safety

unit seven

The Life Cycle

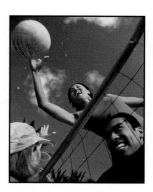

21   Accepting Dying and Death

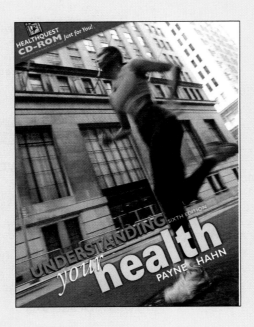

MCGRAW-HILL IS PROUD TO OFFER AN EXCITING NEW SUITE OF MULTIMEDIA PRODUCTS AND SERVICES CALLED COURSE SOLUTIONS.

Designed specifically to help you with your individual course needs, **Course Solutions** will help you integrate your syllabus with our premier titles and the state-of-the-art new media tools that support them.

AT THE HEART OF COURSE SOLUTIONS YOU'LL FIND:

- Fully integrated multimedia
- A full-scale Online Learning Center
- A Course Integration Guide

AS WELL AS THESE UNPARALLELED SERVICES:

- McGraw-Hill learning architecture
- McGraw-Hill course consultant service
- Visual Resource Library (VRL) image licensing
- McGraw-Hill student tutorial service
- McGraw-Hill instructor syllabus service
- PageOut: The Course Web Site Development Center
- PageOut Lite
- Other delivery options

COURSE SOLUTIONS truly has the solutions to your every teaching need. Read on to learn how we can specifically help you with your classroom challenges.

As a health educator, you already know that personal health is one of the most exciting courses a college student will take. Today's media-oriented college students are aware of the critical health issues of the new millennium. They hear about environmental issues, substance abuse, sexually transmitted diseases, fitness, and nutrition virtually every day. The value of the personal health course is its potential to expand students' knowledge of these and other health topics. Students will then be able to examine their attitudes toward health issues and modify their behavior to improve their health and perhaps even prevent or delay the onset of certain health conditions.

Understanding Your Health accomplishes this task with a carefully composed, well-documented manuscript written by two health educators who teach a personal health course to nearly 1,000 students each year. We understand the teaching issues you face daily in the classroom and have written this text with your concerns in mind.

This book is written for college students in a wide variety of settings, from community colleges to large four-year universities. The content is carefully constructed to be meaningful to both traditional- and nontraditional-age students. We have paid special attention to the increasing numbers of nontraditional students (those over age 25) who have decided to pursue a college education. The topics covered in the text often address the particular needs of these nontraditional students. *Understanding Your Health* continues to encourage students of all ages and backgrounds to achieve their goals.

Features of This Edition

Updated Content

As experienced health educators and authors, we know how important it is to provide students with the most current information available. Throughout each chapter we have included the very latest information and statistics, and the "As we go to press . . ." feature has allowed us to comment on breaking news right up to press time. In addition, we have introduced many timely topics and issues that are sure to pique students' interest and stimulate class discussion.

Comprehensive Health Assessment

The Comprehensive Health Assessment at the beginning of the book allows students to take a close look at their own current state of health, typical health behavior, and risk factors. Using this assessment, students can pinpoint trouble spots in their own health behavior and find out what they can do to reduce their risk of disease or other health conditions. For example, a student may discover a pattern of irresponsible alcohol use that puts him or her at risk of alcohol dependence, alcohol-related diseases, drunk driving, low academic performance, and social problems. The student can then turn to Chapter 8, "Using Alcohol Responsibly," to learn more about these risks and how to control them. At the end of the semester, students can take a look at their previous answers to see how their behavior changed as they learned more about health and wellness issues.

Healthy People: Looking Ahead to 2010

Each chapter begins with a discussion of the Healthy People 2010 national health goals now being drafted. We look at current trends and research data in key health areas, and we explore the steps we can take individually and collectively to reach these crucial goals. Students will thus be motivated to evaluate their individual contributions to these trends and take proactive steps to modify their health habits and behavior.

Behavior Change

Chapter 1 includes a useful section on behavior change strategies, including determining areas for improvement, setting specific goals, making a personal contract, devising a plan of action, charting progress, preparing for obstacles, and rewarding achievements. Other suggestions for improving health-related behavior are presented throughout the book.

Integrated Presentation of Aging

Topics of interest to midlife and elderly adults no longer appear in the chapter on dying and death, thus sending a more positive message about aging. Instead, the material has been integrated into appropriate chapters according to subject. For example,

Alzheimer's disease is now discussed in Chapter 12, "Managing Chronic Conditions." This reorganization allows both traditional and nontraditional students to learn about the physical and emotional changes that take place as we age.

Separate Coverage of Cancer and Chronic Conditions

Many students are close to someone who is living with a chronic condition—a grandparent with Alzheimer's or Parkinson's disease, a brother with cystic fibrosis, or a child with Down syndrome. They want and need basic, accurate information about these and other chronic diseases and conditions. Accordingly, *Understanding Your Health* features a separate chapter in which more than twenty of the most common chronic conditions are presented. In addition, rapid developments in cancer prevention, diagnosis, and treatment warrant a separate, more comprehensive chapter on cancer, in which we present the latest research and information.

Wellness and Disease Prevention

Throughout this new edition, you will notice that students are continually urged to be proactive in shaping their future health. For example, Chapter 5, "Understanding Nutrition and Your Diet," explains the health benefits of following a semivegetarian or other low-fat diet. Chapter 10, "Reducing Your Risk of Cardiovascular Disease," opens with a discussion of the major risk factors for heart disease and emphasizes that prevention must begin early. Even the chapter titles themselves invite students to take control of their own health behavior.

Topics for Today Articles

Topics for Today articles examine current issues that students are hearing about in today's news, such as volunteerism, extreme sports, alcohol advertising, and road rage. These often controversial health-related topics are a perfect starting point for class or group discussions. Because these essays are placed at the end of each chapter, they can be covered or not at the instructor's option.

Learning from Our Diversity Boxes

These new boxes expose students to alternative viewpoints and highlight what we can learn from the differences that make each of us unique. For example, what are the benefits and rewards for the athletes who participate in the Special Olympics? How do women with multiple sclerosis cope with the disease and continue to lead rich, fulfilling lives? What steps can inner-city minority youths take now to reduce their risk of heart disease later in life? Looking at these topics helps students realize that each of us makes important contributions and faces special challenges.

Personal Applications Questions

Personal Applications questions throughout each chapter ask students to think critically about what they have just read and apply the information to their own lives: What have I done in the last week to improve my cardiovascular health? Have I ever considered becoming a vegetarian? Do I know and observe safety guidelines for the recreational activities in which I participate? Questions like these invite students to reconsider their health behavior and make positive changes when necessary.

InfoLinks

InfoLinks boxes placed at the end of each Health Action Guide and Topics for Today article give students a starting point for exploring health information on the Internet. Log into the MADD website to learn how to host a party responsibly. Get tips on the most healthful menu choices at ethnic restaurants. Or check out helpful advice for preparing for exams and coping with test anxiety. A corresponding section at the end of the book provides descriptions of the websites so that students can see what each has to offer before logging on. InfoLinks will get students plugged in to the possibilities for learning about health on-line.

Exam Prep Guide

A perforated exam preparation section is included in the back of the book. The multiple-choice questions test students' retention of the material they have read. The critical-thinking questions allow them to integrate the concepts introduced in the text with the information presented in class lectures and discussions.

Vegetarian Food Pyramid

Many students now follow or are considering a vegetarian diet. To help them understand how such a diet meets nutrient needs, we have printed a vegetarian food pyramid with the USDA Food Guide Pyramid. For students who want to significantly reduce but not eliminate meat consumption, a Topics for Today article about the health benefits of following a semivegetarian diet is included in Chapter 5.

New or Expanded Topics

We are committed to making *Understanding Your Health* the most up-to-date health textbook available. Following is a sampling of topics that are either completely new to this edition or covered in greater depth than in the previous edition:

Chapter 1: Shaping Your Health
Updated morbidity and mortality statistics

Updated information on part-time students

New Health Action Guide on risk reduction

Chapter 2: Achieving Psychological Wellness
New Star Box on learning to cry

New Star Box on forgiveness as an emotionally healthy response

New Health Action Guide on understanding your mental health rights

Chapter 3: Coping with Stress
New coverage of psychoneuroimmunology

New information on non-ergot compounds (e.g., Midrin, Imitrex) for headaches

New Health Action Guide on dealing with work-related stress

New Star Box on how stress can trigger flare-ups of chronic diseases, such as asthma, lupus, and arthritis

Chapter 4: Staying Physically Fit
New information on fitness for the elderly

New information on creatine

Updated information on exercise across the life span, particularly during middle age

New coverage on how fitness saves companies money

Chapter 5: Understanding Nutrition and Your Diet
New information on fast foods, including prices, flavor ratings, and saturated fat content

New information on the pros and cons of using vitamin supplements

Surgeon general's definition of moderate alcohol consumption

Updated information on fat replacements

Updated information on Americans' eating habits

Chapter 6: Maintaining a Healthy Weight
Updated information on diet drugs, including Redux, phen-fen, and Meridia

Revised coverage of infant feeding

New height and weight chart

Updated information of the advantages and disadvantages of selected diets

New coverage of methods of determining body composition

Chapter 7: Living Drug-Free
Updated drug use statistics

New information on over-the-counter drugs

New information on methamphetamine abuse

Chapter 8: Using Alcohol Responsibly
New section on alcohol and the family

New section on alcoholism among elderly adults

New information on thrill-seeking genes

Updated statistics on college drinking

New information on SADD (Students Against Destructive Decisions)

Chapter 9: Rejecting Tobacco Use
Updated information on the tobacco settlement

New information on the increased incidence of smoking among adolescents

Latest statistics on tobacco production, sales, and per capita consumption

Updated statistics on tobacco-related cancer

New information on the EPA's risk assessment report on smokeless tobacco

Chapter 10: Reducing Your Risk of Cardiovascular Disease
New information on Ritalin and sudden cardiac death

New coverage of the link between CVD risk factors and mental decline

Updated CVD death and prevalence statistics

New discussion of the AHA's reclassification of diabetes and obesity as major CVD risk factors

Chapter 11: Living with Cancer
New information on cancer incidence

New Star Box on the power of the mind to help heal cancer patients

Latest information on management of breast cancer, including Herceptin, tamoxifen, and sentinel node biopsy

Updated information on calcium, folic acid, and arsenic in cancer treatment

Chapter 12: Managing Chronic Conditions
New information on the spiritual care of Alzheimer's patients

New description of the two types of multiple sclerosis

Revised discussion of spina bifida, including the importance of folic acid intake for prevention

New discussion of fibromyalgia

Chapter 13: Preventing Infectious Disease Transmission
New information on innovative immunization methods

New coverage of cord blood and stem cell therapies

Updated information on chronic fatigue syndrome

Expanded discussion of hepatitis

Updated coverage of drug treatments for HIV/AIDS

Updated and expanded coverage of STD treatments

Chapter 14: Exploring the Origins of Sexuality
New Health Action Guide on dysmenorrhea

Updated information on the most recent tampon scare

New section in the Topics for Today article on well-known men and women who have broken sex-role stereotypes

Chapter 15: Understanding Sexual Behavior and Relationships
New Health Action Guide on communicating with your partner

New Star Box on "secondary virginity"

New discussion of office romances

Chapter 16: Managing Your Fertility
New information on talking to your partner about birth control

Updated information on emergency contraception

Updated information on the cost of different methods of birth control

New discussion of abstinence

Updated information on abortion

Chapter 17: Becoming a Parent
New Learning from Our Diversity box on pregnancy and parenting after 40

New Health Action Guide on dealing with emotions during pregnancy and after giving birth, including the father's role

New coverage of the stages of parenting

Revised coverage of fetal distress, amniocentesis, survival past the fourth month of gestation, and morning sickness

Chapter 18: Making Consumer Health-Care Decisions
New Star Box on whether doctors or HMOs should determine which treatments patients receive

New discussion of whether insurance companies should pay for Viagra

New section on herbal medicines sold as dietary supplements

Chapter 19: Caring for Our Environment
New Learning from Our Diversity Box on the traditional Native American view of the environment

New Star Box on protecting North America's national parks

Expanded coverage of overpopulation

Chapter 20: Protecting Your Safety
New information on school shootings

New coverage of the safety of sport utility vehicles for both SUV drivers and other motorists

New information on workplace violence

New discussion of cell phones and driving safety

Updated crime statistics

New examples of road rage

Chapter 21: Accepting Dying and Death
New information on physician-assisted suicide, including Dr. Jack Kevorkian's recent use of active euthanasia

New sample living will for the state of Florida

New discussion of millennialist apocalyptic suicides

Updated estimated funeral costs

Successful Features

Along with its new features, *Understanding Your Health* has the following unique existing features that enhance student learning.

Two Central Themes

Two central themes—the multiple dimensions of health and the developmental tasks—are presented in Chapter 1. These give students a foundation for understanding their own health and achieving positive behavior change. A helpful illustration (Figure 1-1) depicts the completion of the developmental tasks within the dimensions of health.

Flexibility of Chapter Organization

The sixth edition of *Understanding Your Health* has twenty-one chapters. The first stands alone as an introductory chapter that explains the focus of the book. The arrangement of the remaining chapters follows the recommendations of both the users of previous editions of the book and reviewers for this edition. Of course, professors can choose to cover the chapters in any sequence that suits the needs of their courses.

Health Reference Guide

The Health Reference Guide found at the back of the book lists many of the most commonly used health resources. In this edition, we have included several Internet addresses as well as phone numbers and mailing addresses of various organizations and government agencies. The guide is perforated and laminated, making it durable enough for students to keep for later use.

Pedagogical Aids

In addition to the new pedagogical features listed previously, the following teaching aids proved to be successful in the first five editions of this book and have been included in this new edition.

Star Boxes

In each chapter, special material in Star Boxes encourages students to delve into a particular topic or closely examine an important health issue.

Personal Assessment Inventories

Each chapter contains at least one Personal Assessment inventory. These self-assessment exercises serve three important functions: They capture students' attention, serve as a basis for introspection and behavior change, and provide suggestions for carrying the applications further.

Health Action Guides

These unique boxes provide step-by-step guidelines for achieving health behavior change. They allow students to apply their knowledge in practical and life-enhancing ways.

Definition Boxes

Key terms are set in boldface type and defined in corresponding boxes. Pronunciation guides are provided where appropriate. Other important terms in the text are set in italics for emphasis. Both approaches facilitate student vocabulary comprehension.

Comprehensive Glossary

At the end of the text, all terms defined in boxes, as well as pertinent italicized terms, are merged into a comprehensive glossary.

Chapter Summaries

Each chapter concludes with a bulleted summary of key concepts and their significance or application. The student can then return to any topic in the chapter for clarification or study.

Review Questions

A set of questions appears at the end of each chapter to aid the student in review and analysis of chapter content.

Suggested Readings

Because some students want to know more about a particular topic, a list of annotated readings is given at the end of each chapter. These suggested readings are readily available at bookstores or public libraries. This edition contains more than fifty new annotated readings.

Appendices

Understanding Your Health includes four appendices that are valuable resources for the student:

- **First Aid.** This appendix outlines important general first-aid measures, such as what to do when someone is choking, bleeding, or in shock. It includes a special section on recognition and first-aid treatment of epileptic seizures.
- **Body Systems.** The systems of the human body have been clearly and accurately rendered in this appendix to make difficult anatomical concepts easier for students to understand.
- **Canadian Health.** Written by Canadian health educator Don Morrow, this section provides a comprehensive overview of the health promotion movement in Canada. It begins by presenting the historical background of the movement, including an explanation of important documents such as *A New Perspective on the Health of Canadians,* the *Ottawa Charter for Health Promotion,* and the theoretical model *A Framework for Health Promotion.* The section then introduces the *Action Statement for Health Promotion in Canada* and discusses current provincial perspectives, recent initiatives, and future directions.
- **InfoLinks Guide.** All of the new InfoLinks boxes, which appear within each Health Action Guide and Topics for Today article in the text, are listed and annotated in this useful appendix. Students can read concise descriptions of the

websites that interest them, and then choose which web pages to visit for more information.

Ancillaries

An extensive ancillary package is available to qualified adopters to enhance the teaching-learning process. We have made a concerted effort to produce supplements of extraordinary utility and quality. This package has been carefully planned and developed to help instructors derive the greatest benefit from the text. We encourage instructors to examine them carefully. Many of the products can be packaged with the text at a discounted price. Beyond the following brief descriptions, additional information about these ancillaries is available from your McGraw-Hill sales representative.

Instructor's Resource Materials

Instructor's Manual and Test Bank

The Instructor's Manual features chapter overviews, learning objectives, suggested lecture outlines with notes and recommended activities for teaching each chapter, Debating the Issues boxes, individual and community activities sections, suggestions for guest lectures, a list of current media resources, including software and on-line resources, and sixty-five full-page transparency masters of helpful illustrations and charts. In addition, the Personal Assessment inventories in the textbook and fifty others are combined into a single section of the instructor's manual. These assessments can be easily photocopied and given to each student as a single packet. The 2,000-item test bank contains multiple-choice, true or false, matching, and critical-thinking exam questions. It also includes questions to test students' knowledge of the new supplemental Topics for Today articles that appear at the end of each chapter in the text. The manual is perforated and three-hole punched for convenience of use.

Computerized Test Bank

The test bank software provides a unique combination of user-friendly aids that enable the instructor to select, edit, delete, or add questions, as well as construct and print tests and answer keys. The computerized test bank package is available for IBM Windows and Macintosh computers.

Visual Resources

Visual Resource Library

The Visual Resource Library is a CD-ROM containing about 200 carefully selected images that can be imported into any graphics or multimedia application. You can also use the images to make overhead transparencies. The photos and illustrations are organized by title, subject, and key word. This valuable tool is available to qualified adopters.

Overhead Transparency Acetates

Seventy-two key illustrations and graphics are available as transparency acetates. Attractively printed in full color, these useful tools facilitate learning and classroom discussion. They were chosen specifically to help explain complex concepts.

Health and Wellness Videodiscs

These videodiscs allow you to use images to enhance your classroom lectures and discussions in health and wellness courses. The photographs, tables, graphics, and other illustrations on the discs have been selected from McGraw-Hill Higher Education publications.

Video Library

Choose from the McGraw-Hill videotape library, which contains many quality videotapes, including selected Films for Humanities and all videos from the award-winning series *Healthy Living: Road to Wellness.* Digitized video clips are also available.

Student Self-Assessment Materials

TestWell: Making Wellness Work for You

This is a self-scoring, pencil-and-paper wellness assessment booklet developed by the National Wellness Institute in Stevens Point, Wisconsin, and distributed exclusively by McGraw-Hill. It adds flexibility to any personal health or wellness course by allowing adopters to offer pre- and post-assessments at the beginning and end of the course, or at any time during the semester.

FitSolve II Software

This software encourages students to evaluate their fitness behaviors and learn problem-solving skills by designing and implementing their own fitness programs. The colorful graphics and easy point-and-click data entry system allows students to focus on content and important concepts. The software provides many assessment activities students can use to evaluate their fitness level, such as the 1.5-mile run; the Rockport Fitness Walking Test; muscle, endurance, and flexibility tests; and body measurement analyses.

Internet Resources

Personal Health Supersite

www.mhhe.com/hper/health/personalhealth

At our Personal Health Supersite, you can find information about our books and telecourse, learn what conventions we plan to attend, and get updates to *Health Net* and *The AIDS Booklet.* The password-protected section of the site includes health news, downloadable personal assessments and lab activities, digitized still images, and a PowerPoint presentation created especially for *Understanding Your Health.*

McGraw-Hill Online Learning Center

The website for *Understanding Your Health* is a great resource for you and your students. It offers downloadable ancillaries, such as a PowerPoint presentation that corresponds to each chapter in the book. Students can take online quizzes, find updated health information, and log on to interactive web links.

McGraw-Hill Learning Architecture

MHLA is a sophisticated web-based course management tool allows you to bring technology into the classroom. If offers instructor and student e-mail capabilities, a test bank, a study guide, lecture outlines, web links, key terms, activities for HealthQuest, NutriQuest, and FitSolve, personal assessment software, video clips, and a PowerPoint presentation.

McGraw-Hill Course Solutions

McGraw-Hill is proud to offer an exciting new suite of multimedia products and services called Course Solutions. Designed specifically to meet your individual course needs, Course Solutions will help you integrate your syllabus with *Understanding Your Health* and the state-of-the-art new media tools that support it. At the heart of Course Solutions you'll find fully integrated multimedia tools, a full-scale Online Learning Center, McGraw-Hill Learning Architecture, McGraw-Hill Course Consultant Integrator Service, Visual Resource Library image licensing, a syllabus service, PageOut: The Course Web Site Development Center, PageOut Lite, and other delivery options. In addition, Course Solutions offers a unique Course Integrator Guide that ties together these tools. Written by a health expert, this printed manual will show you how to integrate *Understanding Your Health* with its available new media resources, including the Online Learning Center. Course Solutions truly meets your every teaching need. Contact your McGraw-Hill sales representative for more information.

McGraw-Hill PageOut: The Course Web Site Development Center

PageOut is a program that enables you to easily develop a website for your course. The site includes a course home page, an instructor home page, a customizable syllabus, web links, discussion areas, an online grade book, student web pages, and sixteen design templates. This program is now available to registered adopters of *Understanding Your Health.* If you adopt 200 or more copies per year of a McGraw-Hill text, our technology experts will create your website for you in 30 minutes or less. And even novices can turn a syllabus into a Web site in just a few minutes using PageOut Lite. For more information, log on to *www.pageout.net/pageout.html.*

Health Net: A Health & Wellness Guide to the Internet

This valuable new booklet is your navigational tool for exploring the vast array of health resources available on the Internet. A helpful introduction provides general information about the Internet. Each of the following sections in the booklet contains an annotated list of websites to supplement those listed in the text.

Interactive CD-ROMs

HealthQuest CD-ROM

by Robert Gold, Nancy Atkinson, Kathleen Mullen, and Robert McDermott
This interactive CD-ROM contains many assessment activities with customized feedback, activities to assess readiness for behavior change, a risk-analysis component, many articles from journals and other sources, and video and animation. An accompanying Instructor's Manual assists you in using this program in your course.

NutriQuest 2.0 CD-ROM

This user-friendly nutrition-analysis program can be used in a wide variety of courses. NutriQuest helps your students understand and apply key nutritional concepts. Users enter their food intake and energy expenditure, compare recommended servings, calories, and nutrients, and use this information to implement an appropriate weight loss (or gain) plan. Data can be stored for a specific food group, a meal, or a one- to three-day average.

Print Publications

Taking Sides: Clashing Views on Controversial Issues in Health and Society

This effective resource consists of previously published essays from conflicting viewpoints on a variety of topics, including health care, mind-body issues, substance abuse, sexuality, fitness, nutrition, the environment, and consumer health.

Annual Editions: Health

These books contain an array of previously published contemporary articles on topics your students want to know more about, such as stress, drug use, diseases, and sexuality. For more information about Annual Editions and Taking Sides, go to www.dushkin.com.

Primis Library of Personal Health

Primis is a new and evolving publishing program that provides a wide range of individualized, preselected, permission-precleared material for classroom use. Organized by the instructor and printed for each specific class, Primis features more than 230 high-quality selections to choose from, including public press articles and Taking Sides issues. In addition, an overview and summary, key concepts, and multiple-choice, true or false, and discussion questions are available for each selection. Visit the Primis website (www.mhhe.com/payne) for a regularly updated menu of articles.

The AIDS Booklet, *Fifth Edition*

This booklet, by Frank D. Cox, offers current, accurate information about HIV and AIDS: what it is, how the virus is transmitted, how the disease progresses, its prevalence among various population groups, symptoms of HIV infection, and strategies for prevention. Also included are discussions of the legal, social, medical, and ethical issues related to AIDS and HIV. Updated semiannually, this short booklet makes AIDS and HIV understandable to your students and ensures that they have the most current information possible.

UC–Berkeley Wellness Letter

Available to qualified adopters, this highly regarded health newsletter keeps you informed of the latest developments in the field.

Diet and Fitness Log

This logbook helps students track their diet and exercise programs. Since a computer is not always available, this booklet allows students to keep a handwritten record that's handy and portable.

Acknowledgments

The publisher's reviewers made excellent comments and suggestions that were very useful to us in writing and revising this book. Their contributions are present in every chapter. We would like to express our sincere appreciation for both their critical and comparative readings.

For the sixth edition:
Srijana Bajracharya
University of Maine-Presque Isle

Gary Chandler
Gardner-Webb University

Patricia Cost
Weber State University

John Downey
Long Beach City College

Emogene Fox
University of Central Arkansas

Jolynn Gardner
Anoka Ramsey Community College

Ann Wertz Garvin
University of Wisconsin-Whitewater

Patricia Gordon
Arkansas Tech University

Rene Gratz
University of Wisconsin-Milwaukee

Loretta Herrin
Benedict College

Norm Hoffman
Bakersfield College

Carol Johnson
University of Richmond

Susan MacLaury
Kean University

Lori Marti
Mankato State University

Randy McGuire
Eastern Kentucky University

Phyllis Murray
Eastern Kentucky University

Carol Parker
University of Central Oklahoma

Alan Peterson
Gordon College

Kerry Redican
Gordon College

McKay Rollins
Brigham Young University

For the fifth edition:
Lori Dewald
Shippensburg University

Chester A. Halterman
Northern Virginia Community College

Richard Hurley
Brigham Young University

John Janowiak
Appalachian State University

Jacquelynn K. Lott
Antelope Valley College

Rosalie D. Marinelli
University of Nevada

For the fourth edition:
Rosemary C. Clark
City College of San Francisco

Marianne Frauenknecht
Western Michigan University

Nancy Geha
Eastern Kentucky University

Jeffrey Hallam
Ohio State University

Dawn Larsen
Mankato State University

Loretta M. Liptak
Youngstown State University

Bruce M. Ragon
Indiana University

For the third edition:
Charles A. Bish
Slippery Rock University

G. Robert Bowers
Tallahassee Community College

Donald L. Calitri
Eastern Kentucky University

Shae L. Donham
Northeastern Oklahoma State University

P. Tish K. Doyle
University of Calgary

Judy C. Drolet
Southern Illinois University–Carbondale

Dalen Duitsman
Iowa State University

Mary A. Glascoff
East Carolina University

Sonja S. Glassmeyer
California Polytechnic State University–San Luis Obispo

Health Education Faculty
Cerritos College

Norm Hoffman
Bakersfield College

C. Jessie Jones
University of New Orleans

Jean M. Kirsch
Mankato State University

Duane Knudson
Baylor University

Doris McLittle-Marino
University of Akron

Juli Lawrence Miller
Ohio University

Victor Schramske
Normandale Community College

Janet M. Sermon
Florida A&M University

Myra Sternlieb
DeAnza College

Mark G. Wilson
University of Georgia

Focus group participants:
Danny Ballard
Texas A&M University

Robert C. Barnes
East Carolina University

Jacki Benedik
University of Southwestern Louisiana

Kathie C. Garbe
Youngstown State University

Virginia Peters
University of Central Oklahoma

Les Ramsdel
Eastern Kentucky University

James Robinson III
University of Northern Colorado

Linda Schiller-Moening
North Hennepin Community College

For the second edition:
Dan Adame
Emory University

Judith Boone Alexander
Evergreen Valley College

Judy B. Baker
East Carolina University

Robert C. Barnes
East Carolina University

Loren Bensley
Central Michigan University

Ernst Bleichart
Vanier College

Shirley F. B. Carter
Springfield College

Vivien C. Carver
Youngstown State University

Cynthia Chubb
University of Oregon

Janine Cox
University of Kansas

Dick Dalton
Lincoln University

Sharron K. Deny
East Los Angeles College

Emogene Fox
University of Central Arkansas

George Gerrodette
San Diego Mesa College

Ray Johnson
Central Michigan University

James W. Lochner
Weber State College

Linda S. Myers
Slippery Rock University

Virginia Peters
University of Central Oklahoma

James Robinson III
University of Northern Colorado

Merwin S. Roeder
Kearney State College

James H. Rothenberger
University of Minnesota

Ronald E. Sevier
El Camino Community College

Reza Shahrokh
Montclair State College

Albert Simon
University of Southwestern Louisiana

Dennis W. Smith
University of North Carolina–Greensboro

Loretta R. Taylor
Southwestern College

For the first edition:
Stephen E. Bohnenblust
Mankato State University

Neil Richard Boyd, Jr.
University of Southern Mississippi

William B. Cissell
East Tennessee State University

Victor A. Corroll
University of Manitoba

Donna Kasari Ellison
University of Oregon Umpqua Community College

Neil E. Gallagher
Towson State University

Susan C. Girratano
California State University–Northridge

Raymond Goldberg
State University of New York College at Cortland

Marsha Hoagland
Modesto Junior College

Carol Ann Holcomb
Kansas State University

Sharon S. Jones
Orange Coast College

Daniel Klein
Northern Illinois University

Susan Cross Lipnickey
Miami University of Ohio

Gerald W. Matheson
University of Wisconsin–La Crosse

Hollis N. Matson
San Francisco State University

David E. Mills
University of Waterloo

Peggy Pederson
Montana State University

Valerie Pinhas
Nassau Community College

Jacy Showers
Formerly of Ohio State University

Parris Watts
University of Missouri–Columbia

Wayne E. Wylie
Texas A&M University

Special Acknowledgments

Authors do not exist in isolation. To publish successful textbooks, an entire team of professionals must work together for an extended time. During the last fifteen years we have worked with many talented people to publish thirteen successful textbooks.

We would like to recognize these people for their outstanding contributions to this sixth edition of *Understanding Your Health.* Melissa Martin, our developmental editor, has done a wonderful job with the many elements related to this revision. Through her research efforts, Melissa has developed an exceptional ability to determine what college professors want to see in a textbook. (And we thought only professors could know this!) Furthermore, Melissa has a pleasant way of motivating authors to keep focused on the writing schedule. She is comfortable to work with and remains calm during the most difficult times. In fact, her calm demeanor belies the fact that she is doggedly determined to produce the best textbook in the market.

We have worked closely with our executive editor, Vicki Malinee, for the last seven book projects. Vicki keeps close tabs on the progress of our revisions. She is a "hands-on" editor who has a broad understanding of both the business and editorial sides of college publishing. Vicki has worked her way to the top of the profession by her careful attention to detail and ability to work well with a variety of constituencies.

Additional people deserve special recognition. Ed Bartell, our publisher, has impressed us with his knowledge of the discipline about which we write. He seems quite comfortable with our working relationship, and this bodes well for future projects. Pam Cooper, senior marketing manager, is as energetic a person as we have seen in college publishing. We are confident that her experience and enthusiasm will allow this book to reach many of our teaching colleagues.

Many people in the production end of this project deserve recognition. Their expertise and dedication have made *Understanding Your Health* well presented and visually appealing for today's college students. Peggy Selle's leadership as the project manager was once again superb. She made sure every manuscript detail was clear and every deadline met. Michelle Whitaker, who supervised the creation of the design, worked patiently with the editorial staff to craft an exciting and inviting appearance for the book.

Finally, we would like to thank our families for the continued support and love they have given us. More than anyone else, they know the energy and dedication it takes to write and revise textbooks. To them we continue to offer our sincere admiration and loving appreciation.

Wayne A. Payne
Dale B. Hahn

Comprehensive Health Assessment

Social and Occupational Health

	Not true/ rarely	Somewhat true/ sometimes	Mostly true/ usually	Very true/ always
1. I feel loved and supported by my family.	1	2	3	4
2. I establish friendships with ease and enjoyment.	1	2	3	4
3. I establish friendships with people of both genders and all ages.	1	2	3	4
4. I sustain relationships by communicating with and caring about my family and friends.	1	2	3	4
5. I feel comfortable and confident when meeting people for the first time.	1	2	3	4
6. I practice social skills to facilitate the process of forming new relationships.	1	2	3	4
7. I seek opportunities to meet and interact with new people.	1	2	3	4
8. I talk with, rather than at, people.	1	2	3	4
9. I am open to developing or sustaining intimate relationships.	1	2	3	4
10. I appreciate the importance of parenting the next generation and am committed to supporting it in ways that reflect my own resources.	1	2	3	4
11. I recognize the strengths and weaknesses of my parents' childrearing skills and feel comfortable modifying them if I choose to become a parent.	1	2	3	4
12. I attempt to be tolerant of others whether or not I approve of their behavior or beliefs.	1	2	3	4
13. I understand and appreciate the contribution that cultural diversity makes to the quality of living.	1	2	3	4
14. I understand and appreciate the difference between being educated and being trained.	1	2	3	4

	Not true/ rarely	Somewhat true/ sometimes	Mostly true/ usually	Very true/ always
	1	2	3	4
15. My work gives me a sense of self-sufficiency and an opportunity to contribute.	1	2	3	4
16. I have equal respect for the roles of leader and subordinate within the workplace.	1	2	3	4
17. I have chosen an occupation that suits my interests and temperament.	1	2	3	4
18. I have chosen an occupation that does not compromise my physical or psychological health.	1	2	3	4
19. I get along well with my coworkers most of the time.	1	2	3	4
20. When I have a disagreement with a coworker, I try to resolve it directly and constructively.	1	2	3	4

Points _____

Spiritual and Psychological Health

	Not true/ rarely	Somewhat true/ sometimes	Mostly true/ usually	Very true/ always
1. I have a deeply held belief system or personal theology.	1	2	3	4
2. I recognize the contribution that membership in a community of faith can make to a person's overall quality of life.	1	2	3	4
3. I seek experiences with nature and reflect on nature's contribution to my quality of life.	1	2	3	4
4. My spirituality is a resource that helps me remain calm and strong during times of stress.	1	2	3	4
5. I have found appropriate ways to express my spirituality.	1	2	3	4
6. I respect the diversity of spiritual expression and am tolerant of those whose beliefs differ from my own.	1	2	3	4
7. I take adequate time to reflect on my own life and my relationships with others and the institutions of society.	1	2	3	4
8. I routinely undertake new experiences.	1	2	3	4
9. I receive adequate support from others.	1	2	3	4
10. I look for opportunities to support others, even occasionally at the expense of my own goals and aspirations.	1	2	3	4
11. I recognize that emotional and psychological health are as important as physical health.	1	2	3	4

	Not true/ rarely	Somewhat true/ sometimes	Mostly true/ usually	Very true/ always
12. I express my feelings and opinions comfortably, yet am capable of keeping them to myself when appropriate.	1	2	3	4
13. I see myself as a person of worth and feel comfortable with my own strengths and limitations.	1	2	3	4
14. I establish realistic goals and work to achieve them.	1	2	3	4
15. I understand the differences between the normal range of emotions and the signs of clinical depression.	1	2	3	4
16. I know how to recognize signs of suicidal thoughts and am willing to intervene.	1	2	3	4
17. I regularly assess my own behavior patterns and beliefs and would seek professional assistance for any emotional dysfunction.	1	2	3	4
18. I accept the reality of aging and view it as an opportunity for positive change.	1	2	3	4
19. I accept the reality of death and view it as a normal and inevitable part of life.	1	2	3	4
20. I have made decisions about my own death to ensure that I die with dignity when the time comes.	1	2	3	4

Points _____

Stress-Management

	Not true/ rarely	Somewhat true/ sometimes	Mostly true/ usually	Very true/ always
1. I accept the reality of change while maintaining the necessary stability in my daily activities.	1	2	3	4
2. I seek change when it is necessary or desirable to do so.	1	2	3	4
3. I know what stress-management services are offered on campus, through my employer, or in my community.	1	2	3	4
4. When necessary, I use the stress-management services to which I have access.	1	2	3	4
5. I employ stress-reduction practices in anticipation of stressful events, such as job interviews and final examinations.	1	2	3	4
6. I reevaluate the way in which I handled stressful events so that I can better cope with similar events in the future.	1	2	3	4

	Not true/ rarely	Somewhat true/ sometimes	Mostly true/ usually	Very true/ always
7. I turn to relatives and friends during periods of disruption in my life.	1	2	3	4
8. I avoid using alcohol or other drugs during periods of stress.	1	2	3	4
9. I refrain from behaving aggressively or abusively during periods of stress.	1	2	3	4
10. I sleep enough to maintain a high level of health and cope successfully with daily challenges.	1	2	3	4
11. I avoid sleeping excessively as a response to stressful change.	1	2	3	4
12. My diet is conducive to good health and stress management.	1	2	3	4
13. I participate in physical activity to relieve stress.	1	2	3	4
14. I practice stress-management skills, such as diaphragmatic breathing and yoga.	1	2	3	4
15. I manage my time effectively.	1	2	3	4

Points _____

Fitness

	Not true/ rarely	Somewhat true/ sometimes	Mostly true/ usually	Very true/ always
1. I participate in recreational and fitness activities both to minimize stress and to improve or maintain my level of physical fitness.	1	2	3	4
2. I select some recreational activities that are strenuous rather than sedentary in nature.	1	2	3	4
3. I include various types of aerobic conditioning activities among the wider array of recreational and fitness activities in which I engage.	1	2	3	4
4. I engage in aerobic activities with appropriate frequency, intensity, and duration to provide a training effect for my heart and lungs.	1	2	3	4
5. I routinely include strength-training activities among the wider array of fitness activities in which I engage.	1	2	3	4
6. I routinely vary the types of strength-training activities in which I participate in order to minimize injury and strengthen all of the important muscle groups.	1	2	3	4
7. I do exercises specifically designed to maintain joint range of motion.	1	2	3	4

	Not true/ rarely	Somewhat true/ sometimes	Mostly true/ usually	Very true/ always
8. I believe that recreational and fitness activities can help me improve my physical health and my emotional and social well-being.	1	2	3	4
9. I include a variety of fitness activities in my overall plan for physical fitness.	1	2	3	4
10. I take appropriate steps to avoid injuries when participating in recreational and fitness activities.	1	2	3	4
11. I seek appropriate treatment for all injuries that result from fitness activities.	1	2	3	4
12. I believe that older adults should undertake appropriately chosen fitness activities.	1	2	3	4
13. My body composition is consistent with a high level of health.	1	2	3	4
14. I warm up before beginning vigorous activity, and I cool down afterward.	1	2	3	4
15. I select properly designed and well-maintained equipment and clothing for each activity.	1	2	3	4
16. I avoid using performance-enhancing substances that are known to be dangerous and those whose influence on the body is not fully understood.	1	2	3	4
17. I sleep seven to eight hours daily.	1	2	3	4
18. I refrain from using over-the-counter sleep-inducing aids.	1	2	3	4
19. I follow sound dietary practices as an important adjunct to a health-enhancing physical activity program.	1	2	3	4
20. My current level of fitness allows me to participate fully and effortlessly in my daily activities.	1	2	3	4

Points _____

Nutrition and Weight Management

	Not true/ rarely	Somewhat true/ sometimes	Mostly true/ usually	Very true/ always
1. I balance my caloric intake with my caloric expenditure.	1	2	3	4
2. I obtain the recommended number of servings from each of the food groups.	1	2	3	4
3. I select a wide variety of foods chosen from each of the food groups.	1	2	3	4
4. I understand the amount of a particular food that constitutes a single serving.	1	2	3	4

	Not true/ rarely	Somewhat true/ sometimes	Mostly true/ usually	Very true/ always
5. I often try new foods, particularly when I know them to be healthful.	1	2	3	4
6. I select breads, cereals, fresh fruits, and vegetables in preference to pastries, candies, sodas, and fruits canned in heavy syrup.	1	2	3	4
7. I limit the amount of sugar that I add to foods during preparation and at the table.	1	2	3	4
8. I consume an appropriate percentage of my total daily calories from carbohydrates.	1	2	3	4
9. I select primarily nonmeat sources of protein, such as peas, beans, and peanut butter, while limiting my consumption of red meat and high-fat dairy products.	1	2	3	4
10. I consume an appropriate percentage of my total daily calories from protein.	1	2	3	4
11. I select foods prepared with unsaturated vegetable oils while reducing my consumption of red meat, high-fat dairy products, and foods prepared with lard (animal fat) or butter.	1	2	3	4
12. I carefully limit the amount of fast food that I consume during a typical week.	1	2	3	4
13. I consume an appropriate percentage of my total daily calories from fat.	1	2	3	4
14. I select nutritious foods when I snack.	1	2	3	4
15. I limit my use of salt during food preparation and at the table.	1	2	3	4
16. I consume adequate amounts of fiber.	1	2	3	4
17. I routinely consider the nutrient density of individual food items when choosing foods.	1	2	3	4
18. I maintain my weight without reliance on over-the-counter or prescription diet pills.	1	2	3	4
19. I maintain my weight without reliance on fad diets or liquid weight loss beverages.	1	2	3	4
20. I exercise regularly to help maintain my weight.	1	2	3	4

Points _____

Alcohol, Tobacco, and Other Drug Use

	Not true/ rarely	Somewhat true/ sometimes	Mostly true/ usually	Very true/ always
1. I abstain or drink in moderation when offered alcoholic beverages.	1	2	3	4
2. I abstain from using illegal psychoactive (mind-altering) drugs.	1	2	3	4
3. I do not consume alcoholic beverages or psychoactive drugs rapidly or in large quantities.	1	2	3	4
4. I do not use alcohol or psychoactive drugs in a way that causes me to behave inappropriately.	1	2	3	4
5. My use of alcohol or other drugs does not compromise my academic performance.	1	2	3	4
6. I refrain from drinking alcoholic beverages or using psychoactive drugs when engaging in recreational activities that require strength, speed, or coordination.	1	2	3	4
7. I refrain from drinking alcoholic beverages while participating in occupational activities, regardless of the nature of those activities.	1	2	3	4
8. My use of alcohol or other drugs does not generate financial concerns for myself or for others.	1	2	3	4
9. I refrain from drinking alcohol or using psychoactive drugs when driving a motor vehicle or operating heavy equipment.	1	2	3	4
10. I do not drink alcohol or use psychoactive drugs when I am alone.	1	2	3	4
11. I avoid riding with people who have been drinking alcohol or using psychoactive drugs.	1	2	3	4
12. My use of alcohol or other drugs does not cause family dysfunction.	1	2	3	4
13. I do not use marijuana.	1	2	3	4
14. I do not use hallucinogens.	1	2	3	4
15. I do not use heroin or other illegal intravenous drugs.	1	2	3	4
16. I do not experience blackouts when I drink alcohol.	1	2	3	4
17. I do not become abusive or violent when I drink alcohol or use psychoactive drugs.	1	2	3	4

	Not true/ rarely	Somewhat true/ sometimes	Mostly true/ usually	Very true/ always
	1	2	3	4
18. I use potentially addictive prescription medication in complete compliance with my physician's directions.	1	2	3	4
19. I do not smoke cigarettes.	1	2	3	4
20. I do not use tobacco products in any other form.	1	2	3	4
21. I minimize my exposure to secondhand smoke.	1	2	3	4
22. I am concerned about the effect that alcohol, tobacco, and other drug use is known to have on developing fetuses.	1	2	3	4
23. I am concerned about the effect that alcohol, tobacco, and other drug use is known to have on the health of other people.	1	2	3	4
24. I seek natural, health-enhancing highs rather than relying on alcohol, tobacco, and illegal drugs.	1	2	3	4
25. I take prescription medication only as instructed, and I use over-the-counter medication in accordance with directions.	1	2	3	4

Points _____

Disease Prevention

	Not true/ rarely	Somewhat true/ sometimes	Mostly true/ usually	Very true/ always
1. My diet includes foods rich in phytochemicals.	1	2	3	4
2. My diet includes foods rich in folic acid.	1	2	3	4
3. My diet includes foods that are good sources of dietary fiber.	1	2	3	4
4. My diet is low in dietary cholesterol.	1	2	3	4
5. I follow food preparation practices that minimize the risk of food-borne illness.	1	2	3	4
6. I engage in regular physical activity and am able to control my weight effectively.	1	2	3	4
7. I do not use tobacco products.	1	2	3	4
8. I abstain from alcohol or drink only in moderation.	1	2	3	4
9. I do not use intravenously administered illegal drugs.	1	2	3	4
10. I use safer sex practices intended to minimize my risk of exposure to sexually transmitted diseases, including HIV and HPV.	1	2	3	4

	Not true/ rarely	Somewhat true/ sometimes	Mostly true/ usually	Very true/ always
11. I take steps to limit my risk of exposure to the bacterium that causes Lyme disease and to the virus that causes hantavirus pulmonary syndrome.	1	2	3	4
12. I control my blood pressure with weight management and physical fitness activities.	1	2	3	4
13. I minimize my exposure to allergens, including those that trigger asthma attacks.	1	2	3	4
14. I wash my hands frequently and thoroughly.	1	2	3	4
15. I use preventive medical care services appropriately.	1	2	3	4
16. I use appropriate cancer self-screening practices, such as breast self-examination and testicular self-examination.	1	2	3	4
17. I know which chronic illnesses and diseases are part of my family history.	1	2	3	4
18. I know which inherited conditions are part of my family history and will seek preconceptional counseling regarding these conditions.	1	2	3	4
19. I am fully immunized against infectious diseases.	1	2	3	4
20. I take prescribed medications, particularly antibiotics, exactly as instructed by my physician.	1	2	3	4

Points _____

Sexual Health

	Not true/ rarely	Somewhat true/ sometimes	Mostly true/ usually	Very true/ always
1. I know how sexually transmitted diseases are spread.	1	2	3	4
2. I can recognize the symptoms of sexually transmitted diseases.	1	2	3	4
3. I know how sexually transmitted disease transmission can be prevented.	1	2	3	4
4. I know how safer sex practices reduce the risk of contracting sexually transmitted diseases.	1	2	3	4
5. I follow safer sex practices.	1	2	3	4
6. I recognize the symptoms of premenstrual syndrome and understand how it is prevented and treated.	1	2	3	4
7. I recognize the symptoms of endometriosis and understand the relationship of its symptoms to hormonal cycles.	1	2	3	4

	Not true/ rarely	Somewhat true/ sometimes	Mostly true/ usually	Very true/ always
	1	2	3	4
8. I understand the physiological basis of menopause and recognize that it is a normal part of the aging process in women.	1	2	3	4
9. I understand and accept the range of human sexual orientations.	1	2	3	4
10. I encourage the development of flexible sex roles (androgyny) in children.	1	2	3	4
11. I take a mature approach to dating and mate selection.	1	2	3	4
12. I recognize that marriage and other types of long-term relationships can be satisfying.	1	2	3	4
13. I recognize that a celibate lifestyle is appropriate and satisfying for some people.	1	2	3	4
14. I affirm the sexuality of older adults and am comfortable with its expression.	1	2	3	4
15. I am familiar with the advantages and disadvantages of a wide range of birth control methods.	1	2	3	4
16. I understand how each birth control method works and how effective it is.	1	2	3	4
17. I use my birth control method consistently and appropriately.	1	2	3	4
18. I am familiar with the wide range of procedures now available to treat infertility.	1	2	3	4
19. I accept that others may disagree with my feelings about pregnancy termination.	1	2	3	4
20. I am familiar with alternatives available to infertile couples, including adoption.	1	2	3	4

Points _____

Safety Practices and Violence Prevention

	Not true/ rarely	Somewhat true/ sometimes	Mostly true/ usually	Very true/ always
1. I attempt to identify sources of risk or danger in each new setting or activity.	1	2	3	4
2. I learn proper procedures and precautions before undertaking new recreational or occupational activities.	1	2	3	4
3. I select appropriate clothing and equipment for all activities and maintain equipment in good working order.	1	2	3	4

	Not true/ rarely	Somewhat true/ sometimes	Mostly true/ usually	Very true/ always
4. I curtail my participation in activities when I am not feeling well or am distracted by other demands.	1	2	3	4
5. I repair dangerous conditions or report them to those responsible for maintenance.	1	2	3	4
6. I use common sense and observe the laws governing nonmotorized vehicles when I ride a bicycle.	1	2	3	4
7. I operate all motor vehicles as safely as possible, including using seat belts and other safety equipment.	1	2	3	4
8. I refrain from driving an automobile or boat when I have been drinking alcohol or taking drugs or medications.	1	2	3	4
9. I try to anticipate the risk of falling and maintain my environment to minimize this risk.	1	2	3	4
10. I maintain my environment to minimize the risk of fire, and I have a well-rehearsed plan to exit my residence in case of fire.	1	2	3	4
11. I am a competent swimmer and could save myself or rescue someone who was drowning.	1	2	3	4
12. I refrain from sexually aggressive behavior toward my partner or others.	1	2	3	4
13. I would report an incident of sexual harassment or date rape whether or not I was the victim.	1	2	3	4
14. I would seek help from others if I were the victim or perpetrator of domestic violence.	1	2	3	4
15. I practice gun safety and encourage other gun owners to do so.	1	2	3	4
16. I drive at all times in a way that will minimize my risk of being carjacked.	1	2	3	4
17. I have taken steps to protect my home from intruders.	1	2	3	4
18. I use campus security services as much as possible when they are available.	1	2	3	4
19. I know what to do if I am being stalked.	1	2	3	4
20. I have a well-rehearsed plan to protect myself from the aggressive behavior of other people in my place of residence.	1	2	3	4

Points _____

Health Care Consumerism

	Not true/ rarely	Somewhat true/ sometimes	Mostly true/ usually	Very true/ always
1. I know how to obtain valid health information.	1	2	3	4
2. I accept health information that has been deemed valid by the established scientific community.	1	2	3	4
3. I am skeptical of claims that guarantee the effectiveness of a particular health-care service or product.	1	2	3	4
4. I am skeptical of practitioners or clinics who advertise or offer services at rates substantially lower than those charged by reputable providers.	1	2	3	4
5. I am not swayed by advertisements that present unhealthy behavior in an attractive manner.	1	2	3	4
6. I can afford proper medical care, including hospitalization.	1	2	3	4
7. I can afford adequate health insurance.	1	2	3	4
8. I understand the role of government health-care plans in providing health care to people who qualify for coverage.	1	2	3	4
9. I know how to select health-care providers who are highly qualified and appropriate for my current health-care needs.	1	2	3	4
10. I seek a second or third opinion when surgery or other costly therapies are recommended.	1	2	3	4
11. I have told my physician which hospital I would prefer to use should the need arise.	1	2	3	4
12. I understand my rights and responsibilities as a patient when admitted to a hospital.	1	2	3	4
13. I practice adequate self-care to reduce my health-care expenditures and my reliance on health-care providers.	1	2	3	4
14. I am open-minded about alternative health-care practices and support current efforts to determine their appropriate role in effective health care.	1	2	3	4
15. I have a well-established relationship with a pharmacist and have transmitted all necessary information regarding medication and use.	1	2	3	4
16. I carefully follow labels and directions when using health-care products, such as over-the-counter medications.	1	2	3	4

	Not true/ rarely	Somewhat true/ sometimes	Mostly true/ usually	Very true/ always
17. I finish all prescription medications as directed, rather than stopping use when symptoms subside.	1	2	3	4
18. I report to the appropriate agencies any providers of health-care services, information, or products that use deceptive advertising or fraudulent methods of operation.	1	2	3	4
19. I pursue my rights as fully as possible in matters of misrepresentation or consumer dissatisfaction.	1	2	3	4
20. I follow current health-care issues in the news and voice my opinion to my elected representatives.	1	2	3	4

Points _____

Environmental Health

	Not true/ rarely	Somewhat true/ sometimes	Mostly true/ usually	Very true/ always
1. I avoid use of and exposure to pesticides as much as possible.	1	2	3	4
2. I avoid use of and exposure to herbicides as much as possible.	1	2	3	4
3. I am willing to spend the extra money and time required to obtain organically grown produce.	1	2	3	4
4. I reduce environmental pollutants by minimizing my use of the automobile.	1	2	3	4
5. I avoid the use of products that contribute to indoor air pollution.	1	2	3	4
6. I limit my exposure to ultraviolet radiation by avoiding excessive sun exposure.	1	2	3	4
7. I limit my exposure to radon gas by using a radon gas detector.	1	2	3	4
8. I limit my exposure to radiation by promptly eliminating radon gas within my home.	1	2	3	4
9. I limit my exposure to radiation by agreeing to undergo medical radiation procedures only when absolutely necessary for the diagnosis and treatment of an illness or disease.	1	2	3	4
10. I avoid the use of potentially unsafe water, particularly when traveling in a foreign country or when a municipal water supply or bottled water is unavailable.	1	2	3	4
11. I avoid noise pollution by limiting my exposure to loud noise or by using ear protection.	1	2	3	4
12. I avoid air pollution by carefully selecting the environments in which I live, work, and recreate.	1	2	3	4

	Not true/ rarely	Somewhat true/ sometimes	Mostly true/ usually	Very true/ always
	1	2	3	4
13. I do not knowingly use or improperly dispose of personal care products that can harm the environment.	1	2	3	4
14. I reuse as many products as possible so that they can avoid the recycling bins for as long as possible.	1	2	3	4
15. I participate fully in my community's recycling efforts.	1	2	3	4
16. I encourage the increased use of recycled materials in the design and manufacturing of new products.	1	2	3	4
17. I dispose of residential toxic substances safely and properly.	1	2	3	4
18. I follow environmental issues in the news and voice my opinion to my elected representatives.	1	2	3	4
19. I am aware of and involved in environmental issues in my local area.	1	2	3	4
20. I perceive myself as a steward of the environment for the generations to come, rather than as a person with a right to use (and misuse) the environment to meet my immediate needs.	1	2	3	4

Points _____

TOTAL POINTS _____

Interpretation

715–800 points

Congratulations! Your health behavior is very supportive of high-level health. Continue to practice your positive health habits, and look for areas in which you can become even stronger. Encourage others to follow your example, and support their efforts in any way you can.

550–714 points

Good job! Your health behavior is relatively supportive of high-level health. You scored well in several areas; however, you can improve in some ways. Identify your weak areas and chart a plan for behavior change, as explained at the end of Chapter 1. Then pay close attention as you learn more about health in the weeks ahead.

385–549 points

Caution! Your relatively low score indicates that your behavior may be compromising your health. Review your responses to this assessment carefully, noting the areas in which you scored poorly. Then chart a detailed plan for behavior change, as outlined at the end of Chapter 1. Be sure to set realistic goals that you can work toward steadily as you complete this course.

Below 385

Red flag! Your low score suggests that your health behavior is destructive. Immediate changes in your behavior are needed to put you back on track. Review your responses to this assessment carefully. Then begin to make changes in the most critical areas, such as harmful alcohol or other drug use patterns. Seek help promptly for any difficulties that you are not prepared to deal with alone, such as domestic violence or suicidal thoughts. The information you read in this textbook and learn in this course could have a significant effect on your future health. Remember, it's not too late to improve your health!

To Carry This Further . . .

Most of us can improve our health behavior in a number of ways. We hope this assessment will help you identify areas in which you can make positive changes and serve as a motivator as you implement your plan for behavior change (see Chapter 1). If you scored well, give yourself a pat on the back. If your score was not as high as you would have liked, take heart. This textbook and your instructor can help you get started on the road to wellness. Good luck!

Understanding
YOUR
Health

chapter
one

Shaping Your Health

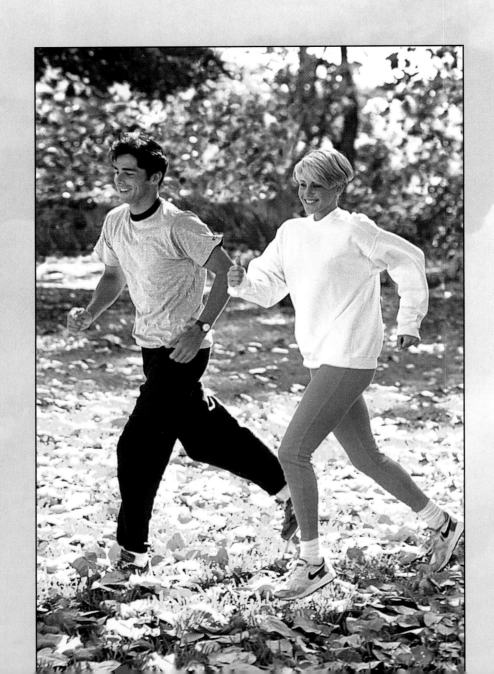

"**T**ake care of your health, because you'll miss it when it's gone." Younger people hear this advice often from their elders. Many younger adults haven't given their health a second thought. But older people understand that the resources that comprise good health make possible the very activities that give our lives meaning—fulfilling relationships, gainful employment, effective parenting. Clearly, these important areas of adult involvement will be difficult to undertake in the absence of good health. As you read this book, ask yourself this question: "Will I be healthy enough to do the things I need and want to do as I move through each stage of my life?"

HEALTHY PEOPLE: LOOKING AHEAD TO 2010

In 1990 a document titled *Healthy People 2000: National Health Promotion and Disease Prevention Objectives*[1] outlined a strategic plan for promoting the health of the American public. The plan included 300 health objectives in 22 priority areas. Forty-seven of the 300 were identified as "sentinel" objectives—particularly significant goals that could quickly indicate the progress of 1990s health promotion efforts.

Progress toward achieving the objectives was assessed near the middle of the decade and reported in a document titled *Healthy People 2000: Midcourse Review and 1995 Revisions*.[2] Progress was reported in many areas, but little or no headway had been made in others. In particular, few gains were made toward achieving the three broadest objectives: (1) increasing the span of healthy life; (2) reducing health disparities (differences) among Americans; and (3) gaining access to preventive services.

A new plan for improving the health of Americans, called *Healthy People 2010*[3] (see p. 5), is now being formulated and will be completed by January 2000. We will refer to this new plan within each chapter where appropriate.

Real Life
Real choices

- Name: Tim Castleman
- Age: 20
- Occupation: University student

"You're the man of the family now." The last time Tim Castleman was home on break from his university, he was browsing through his father's bookshelves and found that line in an old novel about a boy whose farmer father had died and who had to leave school to help care for his family. The story, with its dramatic overtones of duty and sacrifice, seemed quaintly remote to Tim, whose father, at 47, was a successful executive pursuing a healthy lifestyle and whose death was a possibility Tim had never even thought about.

A few months later, those all-but-forgotten words played an endless refrain in Tim's mind as he stood alone in his father's study, numb with shock and grief. Just three nights earlier, Tim's uncle had called him at school to choke out the story about a rainy highway, a speeding truck, a disregarded red light—and his father's instant death in a side-impact collision.

Tim's family lives in an affluent suburb, not on a farm. His father was well insured and left his family comfortably provided for, so Tim hasn't had to quit school to support his mother and younger sisters.

Financial security eases many burdens, but the once bright landscape of Tim's life now seems more like a harsh desert to him. Unable to accept his father's sudden death and the end of their warm, trusting relationship, Tim let his schoolwork slide and is now at home, taking a semester off to "get himself together." A track star at college, he's abandoned his daily workout and has gained seventeen pounds eating snack foods and drinking beer. He goes to church each Sunday with his family but derives no comfort from the rituals; he believes that the loving God of his childhood has first punished and then deserted him. College friends call Tim to find out how he's doing and when he'll be back at school; his uncle tries hard to fill his father's place; his mother urges him to seek counseling or talk to the family's pastor.

Lonely, frightened, and bitter, Tim won't talk—or listen—to anyone. He spends most of his time alone, his mood swinging between rage and despair.

As you study this chapter, think about some positive steps Tim could take to deal with his feelings, and prepare yourself to answer the questions in **Your Turn** at the end of the chapter.

Health Concerns of the Coming Century

It is evident that, in spite of astonishing progress on many fronts, we continue to face a number of serious health challenges. Heart disease, cancer, accidents, drug use, and mental illness all are important concerns for each of us, even if we are not directly affected by them. Also becoming increasingly troublesome are the complex problems of environmental pollution, violence, health care costs, and AIDS and other sexually transmitted diseases. Table 1-1 lists the leading causes of death in the United States.[4] World hunger, over-population, and the threat of domestic and international terrorism are other health-related issues that will affect us, as well as the generations that follow.

The health concerns just mentioned are by no means unmanageable. Fortunately, we as individuals can reduce the likelihood of encountering many of these conditions by making choices in the way we live our lives. On a personal level, we can decide to pursue a plan of healthful living to minimize the incidence of illness and disease and to extend life.

Health: More Than the Absence of Illness?

What exactly is health? Is it simply the absence of disease and illness, as Western medicine has held for centuries—or does health embrace other elements we ought to consider as we move into the twenty-first century?

Recently a national news magazine produced a special issue detailing significant advances in medicine.[5] The articles described vividly in words and images the impressive progress being made in fields such as cancer treatment, gene manipulation, computer-aided surgery, and infectious disease control. Because of articles like this that relate health to medical care, most of us continue to hold to our traditional perception of health as (1) the virtual absence of disease and illness (low levels of *morbidity*) and (2) the ability to live a long life (reduced risk of *mortality*). In striving to be fully "health educated" in the new century, perhaps we need to consider a broader definition that more accurately reflects the many aspects of health that are gaining recognition in contemporary society. Look forward to an alternative definition of health near the end of the chapter.

Healthy People 2010

On page 3 we provided a brief review of the federal government's initiatives to promote health: *Healthy People 2000: National Health Promotion and Disease Prevention Objectives* (1990) and *Healthy People 2000: Midcourse Review and 1995 Revisions.* We also introduced the newest set of national health objectives, *Healthy People 2010,*[2] which is now being formulated.

Healthy People 2010 will be a health promotion program intended to complement a global initiative, *Health for All,* being launched by the World Health Organization. Although the goals of the two programs will be similar, *Healthy People 2010* focuses on the projected needs of *this* country as we begin the next century. The *Healthy People 2000* program is becoming outdated because of changing demographics since 1990, such as rapidly growing populations of elderly and nonwhite people. In addition, new preventive therapies, vaccines, and pharmaceuticals and new diagnostic and treatment technologies have changed the face of medical care and health promotion. Global forces, such as emerging infectious diseases, destruction of tropical rainforests, and environmental interdependence, have also influenced Americans' health needs.

Central to the design of *Healthy People 2010* are 20 areas in which health promotion activities are critically important, such as mental disability, chronic disease prevention and treatment, increased physical activity, improved nutrition, and more rigorous food and drug safety requirements. Making progress in these 20 areas of health promotion will allow the nation to reach four "enabling goals": (1) the promotion of healthy behavior; (2) the protection of health; (3) the assurance of access to quality health care; and (4) the strengthening of community prevention. When these goals have been achieved, the American public should anticipate two additional benefits: (1) increased years of healthy life; and (2) the elimination of health disparities between various segments of the population. These latter two accomplishments were also goals of the earlier programs.

Healthy People 2010 is not fully developed at this time. It is, however, possible to speculate about the program's relationship to the topical areas addressed in each chapter of your textbook. Yet to be decided is the focus of *Healthy People 2010,* an important factor that will influence its eventual content and implementation. Possible focuses of the program, referred to as "models," include:

Disparities model: In this model the indicators of needed health care are based on the differences in health status between a particular segment of the population and the population as a whole. For example, stroke reduction programs might be directed specifically toward the subpopulations most likely to be affected, such as smokers or people with known cardiovascular risks, rather than to the population as a whole.

Leading contributors model: In contrast to the disparities model, which focuses on differences among groups of Americans, the leading contributors model focuses on high-risk behaviors related to morbidity or mortality. For example, programs would be developed to address problem behaviors such as unprotected sex, alcohol misuse, and the unsupervised availability of firearms in homes with children.

Social indicators model: Both disparities among subpopulations (disparities model) and high-risk behavior patterns (leading contributors model) that contribute to morbidity or mortality may exist because of powerful societal forces that affect some people. The social indicators model would use these unique factors to shape program content and implementation. For example, subpopulations characterized by limited formal education, parenting by young single people, or homelessness each would be addressed differently by *Healthy People 2010.*

Sentinel model: When a profound environmental event occurs, the health of some people can be permanently harmed. For example, a single event such as contracting a food-borne infection, being exposed to high-level radiation in a workplace accident, or the use of an intentionally poisoned over-the-counter (OTC) product can undo a lifetime of healthful living. Events of this type are defined as sentinel events and could serve as the bases of health-related program development and implementation.

Prevention model: A familiar model with which to view indicators for program development and implementation is that of preventable illness, such as childhood infectious diseases, cardiovascular diseases, and adult-onset diabetes mellitus (type II). In this model, primary prevention (such as education and immunization), secondary prevention (such as routine screening to identify early those people at risk), and tertiary prevention (comprehensive treatment so conditions do not worsen) would form the basis for program development and implementation.

As noted earlier, no single approach (or combination of approaches) has been identified for use in *Healthy People 2010.* By the beginning of the millennium, however, the program should be in place and its direction clear.

Traditionally Defined Health Care

By the time they reach college age, most Americans are familiar with the many ways in which traditionally defined health care is provided. Here are some easily recognizable examples, all of which serve to reinforce our traditional definition of health.

Episodic Health Care

The vast majority of Americans use the services of professional health care providers during periods (episodes) of illness and injury, that is, when we are "unhealthy." We consult providers seeking a diagnosis that will explain why we are not feeling well. Once a problem is identified, we expect to receive effective treatment from the practitioners that will lead to our

| Table 1-1 | Top 10 Causes of Death in the United States as Reported in 1997[3] |

Cause of Death	Number of Cases
1. Heart disease	732,409
2. Cancers	534,310
3. Cerebrovascular disease (stroke)	153,306
4. Chronic obstructive pulmonary disease	101,628
5. Accidents	91,437
6. Pneumonia	81,473
7. Diabetes	56,692
8. HIV infection	42,114
9. Suicide	31,142
10. Homicide and legal intervention (males only)	19,707

Factors That Affect Well-Being

In anticipation of the new definition of health we will present later in the chapter, study this list of factors (shown below) that today's adults associated with the ability to feel good about their lives.[6] Note that virtually none makes direct reference to being free of illness and disease or to living long into the future. Rather, they are more aligned with a personally defined sense of being adequately independent, self-sufficient, responsible, respected by others, and nurturing.

- A sense of *personal satisfaction* (82%) was identified as the most important feeling that should be experienced during adulthood.
- A sense of *being in control* of one's life (80%) was the second most identified index of adult well-being.
- A sense that one was a partner in a *good marriage* (78%) appeared as the third most important component of living well as an adult.
- A sense that one was *competent at one's job* (69%) placed employment in fourth position—important, but clearly below the factors listed above. Also, note that *making a lot of money* was selected by only 25 percent as being of primary importance in defining adult life satisfaction.
- A sense that one's *children were (or would be) successful* was cited by 63 percent of the adults sampled as an important factor in feeling a sense of well-being.

Having studied these responses, you also may appreciate more fully the meaning we assign to having a sense of well-being and the role health plays in making it possible.

recovery (the absence of illness) and a return to health. If we are willing to be compliant with the care strategies prescribed by our practitioner, we should soon be able to define ourselves as "healthy" once again.

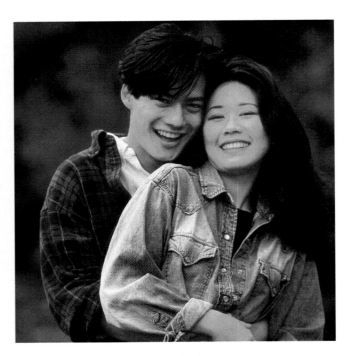

Sexual health concerns are ranked first among the top five key health issues facing college students in the 1990s.

Personal Applications

- To what extent are you a user of episodic health care? How would you describe your expectations upon entering the physician's office? Are you usually compliant with the physician's instructions?

Preventive Medicine

Simple logic suggests that it makes more sense to prevent illness than to deal with it through episodic health (medical) care. This philosophy characterizes **preventive medicine.** Unfortunately, however, many physicians say they have little time to practice preventive medicine because of the large number of episodically sick people who fill their offices every day.

When physicians do practice preventive medicine, they first attempt to determine their patient's level of risk for developing particular conditions. They make this assessment by identifying **risk factors** (and **high-risk health behaviors**) with a variety of observational techniques and screening tests, some of which may involve taking tissue samples from the body (invasive).

Once they have identified levels of risk in a patient, health practitioners try to lower those risk levels through patient education, lifestyle modification, and, when necessary, medical intervention. Continued compliance on the part of the patient will result in a lower level of risk that will continue over the years. Note that preventive medicine is guided by practi-

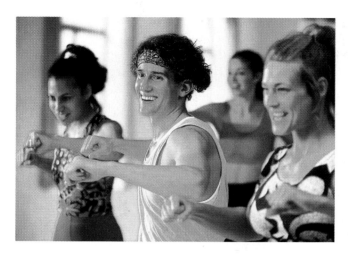

Risk reduction activities, such as fitness classes, are an important part of health promotion and a wellness lifestyle.

tioners, and patients are expected to be compliant with the direction they are given.

Although preventive medical care appears to be a much more sensible approach than episodic care in reducing morbidity and mortality, third-party payers (insurance plans) traditionally have not provided coverage for these services. Managed health care plans that earn a profit by preventing sickness, such as health maintenance organizations, or HMOs (see Chapter 18), are much more receptive to the concept and practice of preventive medicine.

Individual Health Promotion

Throughout the United States, YMCA/YWCA-sponsored wellness programs, commercial fitness clubs, and corporate fitness centers offer risk-reduction programs under the direction of qualified instructors, many of whom are university graduates in disciplines. Using approaches similar to those employed in preventive medicine, these nonphysician health professionals attempt to guide their clients toward activities and behaviors that will lower their risk of chronic illness. Unlike preventive medicine, with its sometimes invasive assessment procedures and medication-based therapies, wellness and fitness programs are not legally defined as medical practices and thus do not require the involvement of physicians. In addition, the fitness focus, social interaction, and healthy lifestyle orientation these programs provide tend to mask the emphasis on preventing chronic illness that would be the selling point of such efforts if they were undertaken as preventive medicine.

Community Health Promotion

In addition to the individual **health promotion** practice just described, a group-oriented form of health promotion is offered in many communities. This approach to improving health is directed at empowering individuals, organized in a variety of groups (such as church congregations), so they can develop programs that promote their own health and well-being.

The key to successful community-based health promotion is **empowerment.** In the context of health, empowerment refers to a process in which individuals or groups of people gain increasing control over their health. To take control over health matters, individuals and groups must learn to "liberate" themselves from a variety of barriers that tend to restrict health enhancement. In this sense, people learn to take charge of their lives, regardless of any current forces that discourage positive health changes. Empowered people and groups do not blame individuals or environmental realities for health conditions but focus on producing constructive change through dialogue and collaboration.[7]

Empowerment programs have produced positive health consequences for individuals and groups that traditionally have been underserved by the health care system, such as minority populations. Once such people are given needed information, inroads into the political process, and skills for accessing funding sources, they become better able to plan, implement, and operate programs tailored to their unique health needs. In many communities, empowered people have organized grassroots campaigns to

---

Personal Applications

• What community-based health promotion programs are you familiar with in your community? On your campus? How are the community members empowered to become responsible for promoting their own health?

---

preventive medicine physician-centered medical care in which areas of risk for chronic illnesses are identified that they might be lowered.

risk factor a biomedical index such as serum cholesterol level, or a behavioral pattern such as smoking, associated with a chronic illness.

high-risk health behavior a behavioral pattern, such as smoking, associated with a high risk of developing a chronic illness.

health promotion movement in which knowledge, practices, and values are transmitted to people for use in lengthening their lives, reducing the incidence of illness, and feeling better.

empowerment the nurturing of an individual's or group's ability to be responsible for their own health and well-being.

prevent neighborhood violence, improve childhood nutrition, promote healthy lifestyles, or prevent drug use among youth. When successful, these programs stand as excellent examples of the reality that people can make a difference when they become empowered.

Wellness

Perhaps the most visible form of health promotion seen today is **wellness.** In the minds of its practitioners, wellness is a *process* of determining risk factors through periodic assessment and the provision of information, behavior change strategies, and individual or group counseling that ultimately leads to the adoption of a *wellness lifestyle.* Once adopted, this wellness lifestyle (characterized by low-risk, health-enhancing behaviors) over time should produce a *sense of well-being* (also called wellness by some wellness practitioners).

We might ask how wellness differs from health promotion (at the individual level) or from preventive medicine, since both focus on risk reduction through prescribed changes in behavior. In response, wellness practitioners suggest that wellness is not driven by concerns about morbidity and mortality. Rather they suggest that wellness, leading to the adoption of a wellness lifestyle and ultimately a sense of well-being, is intended to unlock the full potential of individuals as they interact within a variety of life's arenas, including the workplace and the larger environment. The fact remains, however, that many wellness programs on college campuses, in local hospitals, and in the corporate world are engaged in the same risk-reduction activities that characterize health promotion and even preventive medicine. Most likely wellness professionals believe that the key to unlocking our fullest potential and experiencing a sense of well-being is not being burdened by chronic illness. Or perhaps wellness is something less tangible than the events scheduled in the wellness center at work or on campus.

Multidimensional Perceptions of Health

Despite the emphasis on the structure and function of the body that seems to characterize episodic health care, preventive medicine, individual and community health promotion, and even wellness, two multidimensional perceptions of health have coexisted with those focused primarily on risk reduction. These are the World Health Organization's call for an expanded view of health and the increasingly popular concept of holistic health.

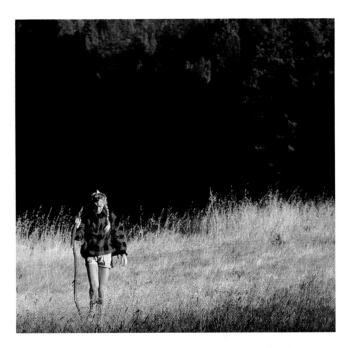

Nurturing your spirituality is an integral part of holistic health.

WHO's Three-Part Definition of Health

One of the most widely recognized and most frequently quoted definitions of health is that given by the Geneva-based World Health Organization: "Health is a state of complete physical, mental, and social well-being and not merely the absence of disease and infirmity."[8]

This is a multifaceted view of health that encompasses physical, mental, and social dimensions. The WHO definition indicates that health extends beyond the structure and function of our bodies to include feelings, values, and reasoning. It also embraces the nature of our interpersonal relationships and interactions.

Holistic Health

A currently popular description of health expands the definition supplied by the World Health Organization. **Holistic health** encompasses not only the physical, mental, and social aspects of the definition but also embraces two additional components: intellectual and spiritual dimensions.[9,10] The holistically healthy person functions as a *total person.*

Holistic health may be the broadest definition of health, although the wellness movement also uses these dimensions in addition to two other dimensions: occupational and environmental wellness. In any case, a holistic concept of health can help us better understand how a person whose lifestyle is characterized by high-risk behaviors or who has serious physical illnesses like cancer or heart disease can, on a given day, experience life in a satisfying and mean-

HEALTH ACTION GUIDE

The Importance of Risk Reduction

Prescriptions for good health usually place considerable importance on *risk reduction*. Health-care professionals stress the importance of identifying behavioral patterns and biomedical indexes that suggest the potential for illness or death. Each of us has the opportunity to receive information, counseling, behavior change strategies, and medical therapies designed to lower our risk. The extent to which we act on this opportunity is our degree of *compliance*. In most cases, compliant people do have lower levels of risk and can expect to have fewer illnesses, or have them later rather than earlier in life, and live longer lives.

What are the health-enhancing "rules" that are believed to lower the risk of poor health? Unfortunately, there is no universally agreed upon list. In fact, books related to risk reduction present lists with as many as 121 steps to good health and as few as six or eight. Accordingly, we will advance their list, to which you can add or subtract on the basis of your own experiences and study.

- *Refrain from using tobacco in any form.* This rule is so critically important that the surgeon general of the United States has identified smoking as the single most important reversible factor contributing to illness and early death.
- *If you drink alcohol, do so in moderation.* This is particularly important for people who must drive or operate machinery, women who are pregnant or planning to become pregnant, and people taking certain medications.
- *Engage in regular exercise designed to train the cardiorespiratory system as well as maintain muscle strength.* You can use a wide array of exercises as the basis of a fitness program, and you can develop specific programs around recommendations about frequency, duration, and intensity of activity.
- *Eat a balanced diet that includes a wide array of choices from each of the food groups.* Pay attention to the recommended amounts of carbohydrate, protein, and fat, as well as the specific food items that supply these three nutrients.

- *Develop effective coping techniques for use in moderating the effects of stress.* Effective coping can reduce the duration of physiological challenge the body faces during periods of unexpected change. Remember, however, that some forms of coping can themselves be sources of additional stress.
- *Maintain normal body weight.* Persons who are excessively overweight or underweight may experience abnormal structural or functional changes, predispose themselves to chronic illnesses, and unnecessarily shorten their lives. Lifelong weight management is preferable to intermittent periods of weight gain and loss.
- *Receive regular preventive health care from competent professionals.* This care should include routine screening and risk-reducing lifestyle management, early diagnosis, and effective treatment if needed.
- *Maintain an optimistic outlook.* Anger, cynicism, and a pessimistic outlook on life can erode the holistic basis on which high-level health is built. Several chronic conditions, including cardiovascular diseases and cancers, occur more frequently in persons who lack a positive outlook on their own lives and life in general.
- *Establish a personally meaningful belief system.* Over the course of long life the presence of such a system and the supportive faith community usually associated with it may prove to be the last effective health resource we will possess.

The risk reduction approaches detailed above are certainly not all inclusive. They are, however, representative of those found on the seemingly endless number of lists in circulation both within and outside the health-care community. You are, of course, free to add to or delete from this list.

InfoLinks
www.cdc.gov/nccdphp/nccdhome.htm

ingful manner. The physical dimension is an important part of health, but a high level of functioning in the other dimensions of health can sometimes offset the limitations of physical illness.

Today's College Students

In this text we explore health issues of interest to students of both traditional and nontraditional ages. We also recognize the diversity of today's college student population and address the health concerns of all students.

Students of Traditional College Age

Although many terms are used to describe the years between adolescence and adulthood, we will refer to these as the **young adult years.** For our purposes, this period spans the traditional undergraduate years, from ages eighteen to twenty-four.

Statistics indicate that more than 13 million students are enrolled in U.S. colleges today. Slightly more than half of these students are women. Minority students make up approximately 25 percent of American college students, foreign students total nearly 3 percent, and almost three out of five students (57 percent) attend college full time.[11]

wellness a broadly based term used to describe a highly developed level of health.

holistic health a view of health in terms of its physical, emotional, social, intellectual, and spiritual makeup.

young adult years segment of the life cycle from ages eighteen to twenty-four; a transitional period between adolescence and adulthood.

Learning
From Our Diversity

Back to the Future: Nontraditional-Age Students Enrich the College Experience

To anyone who's visited an American college campus in the last ten years, it's abundantly clear that the once typical college student—white, middle class, between the ages of eighteen and twenty-four—is no longer in a majority on campus. In most institutions of higher learning, today's student body is a rich tapestry of color, culture, language, ability, and age. Wheelchair-accessible campuses roll out the welcome mat for students with disabilities; the air is filled with the music of a dozen or more languages spoken by students from virtually every part of the world; students in their 60s chat animatedly with classmates young enough to be their grandchildren.

Of all the trends that are changing the face of college enrollment in the United States, perhaps the most significant is the increasing diversity in the age of students now on campus. No longer regarded as oddball exceptions, older students today are both a common and welcome sight in colleges and universities across the country. Many women cut short their undergraduate education—or defer graduate school—to marry and raise children. Divorcees, widows, and women whose children are grown often return to college, or enroll for the first time, to prepare for professional careers. And increasingly, both men

and women are finding it desirable, if not essential, to further their education as a means of either keeping their current job or qualifying for a higher position.

Just as children are enriched by the knowledge and experience of their grandparents and other older relatives, so too is today's college classroom a richer place when many of the seats are filled by students of nontraditional age. Without being didactic or preachy, older students can provide valuable guidance and direction to younger classmates who may be uncertain of their career path, or who may be wrestling with decisions about marriage and parenthood. Older students can also serve as role models for young people from unstable homes or disadvantaged backgrounds who may have grown up without consistent adult support. In doing so, nontraditional-age students can gain helpful insights about young people's feelings, attitudes, challenges, and aspirations.

Among the many important benefits of today's increasingly diverse college campus, surely one of the most significant is the enhanced opportunity for intergenerational communication and understanding made possible by the growing numbers of students of nontraditional age.

In your classes, how would you characterize the interactions between traditional-age students and those of nontraditional age? In what ways are they enriching each other's college experience?

More than half (56 percent) of all undergraduate college students are of traditional age. This book is directed first at these students. However, because of significant growth in the proportion of older students, we will also address a variety of life experiences and developmental tasks appropriate to these students. Unquestionably, the nontraditional students in our classes help our traditional-age students understand the wide and varied role that health plays throughout the life cycle.

Students of Nontraditional Age

In 1995, nearly 45 percent of American college students are classified as **nontraditional students.** Included in this vast overlapping group are part-time students (see the Star Box on this page), military veterans, students returning to college, single parents, older adults, and evening students. These students enter the classroom with a wide assortment of life experiences and observations. Most of these students are twenty-five to forty years old. Read the Learning from Our Diversity box above for a closer look at nontraditional students.

Many nontraditional students are trying to juggle an extremely demanding schedule. The responsibilities

Ages of Part-Time College Students[11]	
18–24	29%
25–34	33%
35–49	27%
50–64	5%
65+	1%
Remainder—age unknown	

of managing a job, a schedule of classes, and perhaps a family present formidable challenges. Performing these tasks on a limited budget compounds the difficulty. For nontraditional-age students, concerns over paying next month's rent, caring for aging parents, or finding affordable child care are as common as the challenges that confront students of traditional age.

For these reasons, we want to make this textbook meaningful for both traditional and nontraditional students. Much of the information we present applies to both categories of students. We ask nontraditional students to do two things as you read this book: (1) reflect on your own young adult years, and (2) examine your

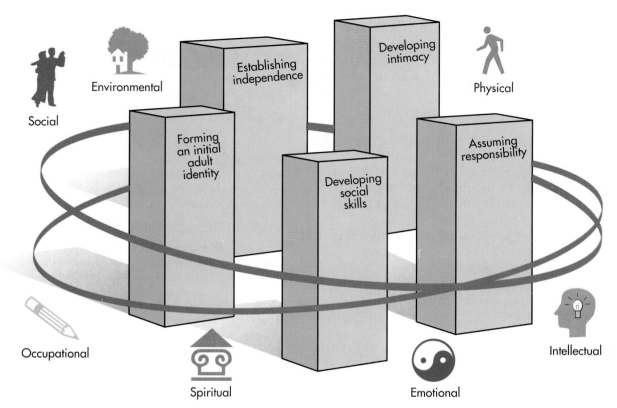

Figure 1-1 Mastery of the developmental tasks through a balanced involvement of the seven dimensions of health will lead to your enjoying a more productive and satisfying life.

current lifestyle to see how the decisions you made as a younger adult are affecting the quality of your life now. As a nontraditional student, you may have young adult children whose lives you can observe in light of the information you will find in this book.

Minority Students

Although enrollment patterns at colleges and universities vary, the overall number of minority students is increasing. In 1995, about one of four college students was a minority student, with African-Americans, Hispanic-Americans, Asian-Americans, and Native Americans representing the largest groups of minority students.[11] These students bring a rich variety of cultural influences and traditions to today's college environment.

Students with Disabilities

People with disabilities are another rapidly growing student population, currently comprising 5.4 percent of all undergraduates.[12] Improved diagnostic, medical, and rehabilitation procedures coupled with improved educational accommodations have opened up opportunities for these students at an increasing rate. In addition to students who have visible disabilities, such as blindness, deafness, or a physical disability requiring use of a wheelchair, a greater

number of students with "hidden" disabilities are appearing on campuses. Examples are students with learning disabilities (including attention deficit disorders), those with psychiatric and emotional problems, and those recovering from alcohol and substance abuse.

Developmental Tasks of Young Adulthood

Because most of today's undergraduate college students range between the ages of eighteen and perhaps forty, we will address several areas of growth and development (defined as *developmental tasks*) that characterize the lives of people in this age group (Figure 1-1). When people sense that they are making progress in some or all of these areas, they are likely to report a sense of life satisfaction or, as we describe it, a sense of well-being.

nontraditional students administrative term used by colleges and universities for students who, for whatever reason, are pursuing undergraduate work at an age other than that associated with the traditional college years (18–24).

Forming an Initial Adult Identity

For most of childhood and adolescence, young people are seen by adults in their neighborhood or community as someone's son or daughter. With the onset of young adulthood, that stage has almost passed; both young people and society are beginning to look at each other in new ways.

As emerging adults, most young people want to present a unique identity to society. Internally they are constructing perceptions of themselves as the adults they wish to be; externally they are formulating the behavioral patterns that will project this identity to others.

Completion of this first developmental task is necessary for young adults to enjoy a productive and satisfying life. As a result of their experiences in achieving an initial adult identity, they will become capable of answering the central question of young adulthood: "Who am I?" Interestingly, many nontraditional students are also asking themselves this question as they progress through college and anticipate the changes that will result from completing a high level of formal education.

Establishing Independence

In contemporary society the primary responsibility for socialization during childhood and adolescence is assigned to the family. For nearly two decades the family is the primary contributor to a young person's knowledge, values, and behaviors. By young adulthood, however, students of traditional college age should be demonstrating the desire to move away from the dependent relationship that has existed between themselves and their families.

Travel, peer relationships, marriage, military service, and, of course, college have been traditional avenues for disengagement from the family. Generally the ability and willingness to follow one or more of these paths will help a young adult establish independence. Success in these endeavors will depend on the willingness to use a variety of resources we will explore later.

Obtaining Entry-Level Employment

For at least the last sixty years students have pursued a college education in large part to gain entry into many occupations and professions. Students of today certainly anticipate that a college degree will open doors for what may be their first substantial employment—sometimes referred to as *entry-level employment*.

In many respects employment meets needs beyond those associated purely with money. Employment provides the opportunity to assume new responsibilities in which the skills learned in college can be applied and expanded. Employment also involves taking on new roles (such as colleague, mentor, partner) that may play an important part in the way we

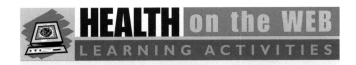

HEALTH on the WEB
LEARNING ACTIVITIES

Following a Healthy Lifestyle

Students taking a personal health course usually want to improve their health behavior in a specific area. You may know exactly which behavior you want to change, but it might also be helpful for you to complete a lifestyle inventory. Go to www.psychtests.com/lifestyl.html and complete the 25 statements. When you click *Send*, the inventory will be scored online and you will get your results on screen.

Practicing Preventive Behaviors

For a comprehensive health evaluation, visit the Wellness-Sources website at www.wellness-sources.com/eval/history.html. Complete the health history questionnaire by answering all the questions. It is important that your answers be thorough and complete. When you have finished, click the *Submit* button. Then click on the *Back* button of your browser to get to the test results page for your completed evaluation.

Learning the Creative Journal Method

The creative journal method was developed by Dr. Lucia Capacchione, a registered art therapist and respected lecturer. A pioneer in the field of creativity and healing, Dr. Capacchione promoted the healing power of writing and drawing. Creative journaling is a tool for personal growth, health and healing, creative development, and life planning. You can learn how to begin your creative journal at www.healthy.net/othersites/creativejournal/index.html. Select *Creative Journal Exercises and Activities* to get started.

For more activities, log on to our Online Learning Center at www.mhhe.com/hper/health/payne.

define ourselves for the remainder of our lives. In addition, employment provides a new and more independently oriented arena in which friendships (intimacy) can be pursued. By no means least important, entry-level employment provides the financial foundation on which we can establish independence.

Assuming Responsibility

The third developmental task in which students of traditional college age are expected to progress is the assumption of increasing levels of responsibility. Young adults have a variety of opportunities to assume responsibility. College-age young adults may accept responsibility voluntarily, such as when they join a campus organization or establish a new friendship. Other responsibilities are placed on them when professors assign term papers, when dating partners exert pressure on them to conform to their expectations, or when employers require consistently productive work. In other situations they may accept responsibility for doing a particular task not for themselves but for the benefit of others. As important and demanding as these areas of responsibility are, a more fundamental responsibility awaits young adults: the responsibility of maintaining and improving their health and the health of others.

Developing Parenting Skills

For most, but certainly not for all, young adulthood marks the entry to parenthood, one of the most important responsibilities anyone can choose to assume. The multitude of decisions associated with this twenty-year-plus commitment will literally shape the remainder of life. Examples are whether to parent or not (if so, when to begin, how many children to have, what interval between each child) and the role parenting will play in the context of overall adulthood. The ability to make sound decisions, and then to develop the skills and insight necessary to parent effectively, may be the most challenging aspect of growth and development that confronts young adults.

Developing Social Skills

The fourth developmental task of the young adult years is developing an expanded range of appropriate and dependable social skills. Adulthood ordinarily involves "membership" in a variety of groups that range in size from a marital pair to a national political party or international corporation. These memberships will require the ability to function in many different social settings and with a wide variety of people.

The college experience traditionally has prepared students very effectively in this regard, but interactions in friendships, work relationships, or parenting may require that they make an effort to grow and develop beyond levels they achieved by belonging to a peer group. Young adults will need to refine a variety of social skills, including communication, listening, and conflict management.

Developing Intimacy

The task of developing intimacy usually begins in young adulthood and continues through midlife. During this time it is developmentally important to establish one or more intimate relationships. Most people in this age group are viewing intimacy in its broadest sense as a deeply close, sharing relationship. Intimacy may unfold in the context of dating relationships, close friendships, and certainly mentoring relationships.

Involvement in intimate relationships varies, with some people having many relationships and others having only one or two. The number does not matter. From a developmental standpoint, what matters is that we have others with whom to share our most deeply held thoughts and feelings as we attempt to validate our own unique approach to living.

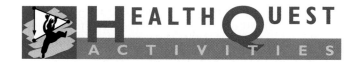

- Use the Wellboard to report your life score (number of years out of 114) and the score percentages for each of the eight health areas.
- Fill out the Wellboard using data from a fictional college student. On the first assessment screen, change the demographics to show how gender, ethnicity, age, marital status, and community affect average life expectancy.

Personal Applications

- If you are a student of traditional college age, how do you think completion of your college degree will give you opportunities for growth and development that otherwise would not exist?

Developmental Tasks of Midlife Adults

If you are a traditional-age student, have you wondered what it would be like to be twenty or thirty years older than you are now? What would you be doing, feeling, and thinking if you were the age of your parents? What are your parents thinking about and trying to accomplish as they move through their midlife years?

One thought that probably recurs all too often is the reality of their own eventual death. Their awareness that they will not live forever is a subtle but profoundly influential force that can cause them to be restless, to renew their religious faith, and to be more highly motivated to master the developmental tasks of midlife. This motivation and the awareness of the reality of death combine to produce the dynamic concept of being at "the prime of life"—a time when there seems to be a great deal to accomplish and less time in which to accomplish it.

Achieving Generativity

In a very real sense, midlife people are asked to do something they have not been expected to do previously. As a part of their development as unique people, they are expected to "pay back" society for the support it has given them. Most people in midlife begin to realize that the collective society, through its institutions (families, schools, churches), has been generous in its support of their own growth and development and that it is time to replenish these resources. Younger and older people may have needs that middle-aged people can best meet. By meeting the needs of others, midlife people can fulfill their own needs to grow and develop. *Generativity* reflects this process of contributing to the collective good.

The process of repaying society for its support is structured around familiar types of activities. Developmentally speaking, midlife people are able to select the activities that best use their abilities to contribute to the good of society.

The most traditional way in which midlife people repay society is through parenting. Children, with their potential for becoming valuable members of the next generation, need the support of people who recognize the contribution they can make. By supporting children, either directly through quality parenting or through institutions that function on behalf of children, middle-aged people repay society for the support they have themselves received. As they extend themselves outward on behalf of the next generation, they ensure their own growth and development. In similar fashion, their support of aging parents and institutions that serve the elderly provides another means to express generativity.

For people who possess artistic talent, generativity may be accomplished through the pleasure brought to others. Artists, craftspeople, and musicians have unique opportunities to speak directly to others through their talents. Volunteer work serves as another avenue for generativity. Most midlife people also express generativity through their jobs by providing quality products or services and thus contribute to the well-being of those who desire or need these goods and services.

Reassessing the Plans of Young Adulthood

Midlife people must also come to terms with the finality of their own deaths. Having done this, they often feel that it is time to think about their goals for adulthood they formulated twenty-five or more years previously. Their dreams must be revisited. This reassessment constitutes a second developmental task of midlife adults.

By carefully reviewing the aspirations they had as young adults, middle-aged people can more clearly study their short- and long-term goals. Specifically, strengths and limitations that were unrecognizable when they were young adults are now more clearly seen. The inexperience of youth is replaced by the insights gained through experience. A commitment to quality often replaces the desire for quantity during the second half of the life cycle. Time is valued more highly because it is now seen in a more realistic perspective. The dream for the future is more sharply focused, and the successes and failures of the past are more fully un-

derstood as this developmental task of reassessing earlier plans of young adulthood is accomplished.

Personal Applications

• If you are a nontraditional student, ask yourself how completing your college degree will allow you to redirect the developmental paths you took during young adulthood.

Developmental Tasks of Elderly Adults

In this section, we focus on the developmental tasks confronted by elderly people. Accepting the physical decline of aging, maintaining a high level of physical function, and establishing a sense of integrity are tasks of the elderly period.

Accepting the Decline of Aging

The general decline associated with the latter part of the life cycle is particularly serious between the seventh and eighth decades. Physically, emotionally, socially, intellectually, and occupationally, elderly people must accept at least some decline. For example, a person may no longer be able to drive a car, which could in turn limit participation in social activities. Even a spiritual loss may be encountered at those times when life seems less humane. Clearly, a developmental task to be accomplished by the elderly is to accept the nature and extent of these losses.

Maintaining a High Level of Physical Function

Because each segment of the life cycle should be approached with the fullest level of involvement possible, the second developmental task of the elderly is to maintain the highest level of physical function possible.

For areas of decline in which some measure of reversal is possible, the elderly are afforded an opportunity to seek *rehabilitation.* Whether through an individually designed program or through the aid of a skilled professional, the elderly can bring back some function to a previously high level.

The second approach, often used in combination with rehabilitation, is *remediation,* whereby an alternative to the area of loss is introduced. Examples of remediation include the use of hearing aids, audiocassettes, and prescription shoes. By using alternative resources, function can often be returned.

For a growing number of older adults, rehabilitation and remediation are rarely necessary because of the high level of physical fitness that they enjoy. For these older people, physical fitness has been maintained through regular physical conditioning activities (see Chapter 4). For most, only minor modifications are necessary to enjoy injury-free involvement.

Establishing a Sense of Integrity

The third major developmental task that awaits the elderly is to establish a sense of integrity, or a sense of wholeness, concerning the journey that may be nearly complete.[13] The elderly must look back over their lives to see the value in what they were able to accomplish. They must address the simple but critical questions, "Would I do it over again?" "Am I satisfied with what I managed to accomplish?" "Can I accept the fact that others will have experiences to which I can never return?"

If the elderly can answer these questions positively, then they will feel a sense of wholeness, personal value, and worth. Having established this sense of integrity, they will believe that their lives have had meaning and that they have helped society.

Since they have already experienced so much, many elderly people have no fear of death, even though they may fear the process of dying. Their ability to come to terms with death thus reinforces their sense of integrity.

Like all of the other developmental tasks, this critical area of growth and development is a personal experience. The elderly must assume this last developmental task with the same sense of purpose they used for earlier tasks. When elderly people can feel this sense of integrity, their reasons for having lived will be fully understood.

A New Definition of Health

At the beginning of the chapter we asked you to consider an alternative way to view health—a view that would be far less centered in morbidity and mortality. The definition we propose takes into account the difference between *what health is for* (its role) and *what it is* (its composition), instead of focusing on the traditional view of health as not being sick and living a long time.

The Role of Health

To understand the role of health in the context of our definition, we can use the analogy of an automobile. An automobile is designed to transport people safely, comfortably, and expediently to particular places where they need or want to be. The role of health is very similar to that of the car. We depend on our health to let us participate in the events that contribute to our growth and development in every

stage of our lives. Developmentally, the process of moving through young adulthood does not occur simply because of the passage of time, but because people of that age can participate in those experiences (developmental tasks) considered appropriate for that phase of life. Clearly, the absence of health would markedly impede their ability to complete those developmental tasks.

The Composition of Health

If we accept the role of health just described, we can define the composition of health in a manner that is more developmentally centered than would be the absence of illness and disease and the probability of living a long life. In fact, we might return to the analogy of the automobile and ask: Now that we know what an automobile is *for* (its role), what *is* an automobile (its composition or nature)? To answer this question with technical accuracy we would consult an automotive engineer. Understandably, however, most of us are more interested in the role of the automobile than its composition, yet each is defined by the other.

If the question regarding the composition of an automobile is stated in terms of health, we can define the composition of health as a collection of resources, both intrinsic (internal) and extrinsic (external) to the individual, needed to participate fully in the events that constitute growth and development. On the basis of this definition, the absence of appropriate and adequate resources would prevent one from carrying out the role of health as defined earlier.

In light of this statement of health's composition, we ask you to consider two important questions you must answer for yourself. First, is it possible even to be an adult (young adult, midlife adult, or older adult) without the resources necessary to participate in the events that constitute these stages of life? Second, how do we know what resources are necessary for successful involvement in each stage of adult life without first understanding the developmental tasks that make up each stage? Clearly, these questions are not raised with respect to the traditional definition of health.

The Multiple Dimensions of Health

As we learned earlier, health has been viewed for many decades as being multidimensional. In this section we present our interpretation of these dimensions to prepare you to see the relationship of each to our unique definition of health.

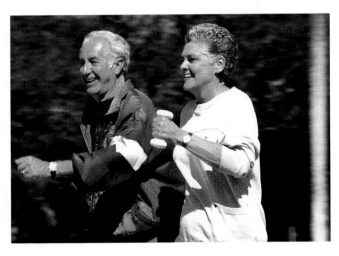

Traditional medicine has focused on improving the physical dimension of health.

Physical Dimension of Health

Most of us have a number of physiological and structural characteristics we can call on to aid us in accomplishing the developmental tasks described earlier. Among these physical characteristics are our body weight, visual ability, strength, coordination, level of endurance, level of susceptibility to disease, and powers of recuperation. In certain situations the physical dimension of health may be the most important. This almost certainly is why traditional medicine for centuries has equated health with the design and operation of the body.

Emotional Dimension of Health

We also possess certain emotional characteristics that can help us as we grow and develop. The emotional dimension of health encompasses our ability to cope with stress, remain flexible, and compromise to resolve conflict.

For young adults, growth and development often give rise to emotional vulnerability, which may lead to feelings of rejection and failure that can reduce productivity and satisfaction. To some extent we are all affected by feeling states, such as anger, happiness, fear, empathy, guilt, love, and hate. People who consistently try to improve their emotional health appear to enjoy life to a much greater extent than do those who let feelings of vulnerability overwhelm them or block their creativity.

Social Dimension of Health

A third dimension of health encompasses social skills and insights. Because most pre–young adult growth and development is undertaken in the presence of others, many experiences contribute to the enhancement of existing social skills. In adulthood, including young adulthood, the composition of the social world changes, principally because of our exposure to a wider array of people and the expanded roles associated with employment, parenting, and community involvement.

The social abilities of many nontraditional students may already be firmly established. Entering college may encourage them to develop new social skills that help them socialize with their traditional-age student colleagues. After being on campus for a while, nontraditional students are often able to interact comfortably with traditional students in such diverse places as the library, the student center, and the bookstore. This interaction enhances the social dimension of health for both types of students.

Intellectual Dimension of Health

The ability to process and act on information, clarify values and beliefs, and exercise decision-making capacity ranks among the most important aspects of total health. Coping skills, flexibility, and the knack of saying the right thing at the right time may not serve many young adults as well as their ability to use information and understand new ideas. Certainly one's unwillingness to grasp new information or to undertake an analysis of beliefs will hinder the degree of growth and development the college experience can provide.

Spiritual Dimension of Health

The fifth dimension of health is the spiritual dimension. Although certainly it includes religious beliefs and practices, many young adults would expand it to encompass more diverse belief systems, including relationships with other living things, the nature of human behavior, and the need and willingness to serve others. All are important components of spiritual health.

Through nurturing the spiritual dimension of our health, we may develop an expanded perception of the universe and better define our relationship to all that it contains, including other people. To achieve growth in the spiritual dimension of health, many people undertake a serious study of doctrine associated with established religious groups and will assume membership in a community of faith. For others, spiritual growth occurs as they open themselves to new experiences that involve nature, art, body movement, or music. Taking a walk in the woods, visiting an art museum, listening to classical music, talking with young children, writing poetry, caring for the environment, painting a picture, or pushing the body to its physical limits all are ways to nurture one's spiritual resources.

Occupational Dimension of Health

A significant contribution made by the currently popular wellness movement is that it defines for many people the importance of the workplace to their sense of well-being. In today's world, employment and productive efforts play an increasingly important role in

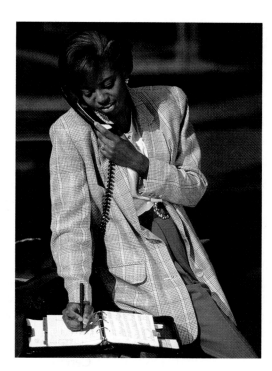

The occupational dimension of health is especially important to nontraditional-age students, who often have to balance school with work, parenting, and other responsibilities.

how we perceive ourselves and how we see the "goodness" of the world in which we live. In addition, the workplace serves as both a testing ground for and a source of life-enhancing skills. In our place of employment we gain not only the financial resources to meet our demands for both necessities and luxuries, but also an array of useful skills like conflict resolution, experiences in shared responsibility, and intellectual growth that can be used to facilitate a wide range of non-employment-related interactions. In turn, the workplace is enhanced by the healthfulness of the individuals who contribute to its endeavors.

Environmental Dimension of Health

Central to the definition of health we will offer in the next section is the contention that the world that lies outside the individual is a potential resource that can be used in meeting life's demands. In every dimension of health, we are affected by the air, water, land, and climate in ways that, ideally, enhance our growth and development as it has been described in this chapter. In this view we not only have access to that which the environment offers but also, and at least as important, we have a responsibility to be stewards of that environment. We cannot overemphasize the significance of our responsibility to care for the land and its animal and plant inhabitants.

Our Definition of Health

In addition to the more traditional focus on health in terms of the absence of illness and disease and the probability of a long life, both of which we believe are highly desirable, we now invite you to consider the alternative definition of health we promised at the beginning of this chapter. In essence, we propose to redefine health. By combining the role of health with the composition of health, we offer a new definition of health that we believe is unique to this book:

Health is a reflection of your ability to use the intrinsic and extrinsic resources within each dimension of health in order to participate fully in the activities that contribute to growth and development during each stage of the life cycle.

We believe it is essential to understand that the very ability to define and then recognize the existence of needed resources depends on an understanding of growth and development itself. It also requires the ability to determine whether needed resources exist or must be cultivated. The question *Are you healthy enough to (or for) . . . ?* will be raised throughout this textbook; at the same time, of course, we also will place appropriate emphasis on the more traditional perceptions of health.

Personal Applications

• Identify a situation in which you lacked particular resources that would have been helpful in becoming more independent, responsible, socially interactive, or occupationally competent.

Charting a Plan for Behavior Change

Students taking a personal health course usually decide to change their health behavior in one or more specific ways. We encourage our students to complete a "health behavior change project" as part of their course requirements. Sometimes students know exactly which behavior they want to alter. They may have found this behavior while completing the Comprehensive Health Assessment at the beginning of this book.

Other students browse through various chapters in the textbook to see what topics are of special interest to them. It might be helpful for you to examine the Personal Assessments in each chapter. For example, if you are interested in behavior change related to alcohol use, you might look at page 236 and complete the Personal Assessment entitled "How do you use alcoholic beverages?" If you are thinking about a behavior change concerning weight management, you could

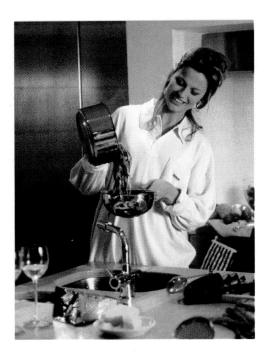

Many students want to change a specific health behavior, such as following a more nutritious diet.

complete the Personal Assessment titled "Should you consider a weight loss program?" on page 173.

Some of the health behaviors our students typically want to change are the following:

- To gain or lose weight
- To stop smoking
- To stop using smokeless tobacco
- To eliminate or reduce caffeine consumption
- To develop better sleeping patterns
- To reduce levels of stress
- To improve physical fitness
- To reduce alcohol consumption .
- To eat more nutritiously
- To develop more friendships
- To enhance the spiritual dimension of health

To change your behavior, you must now attempt to complete the following ten steps:

1. Establish some baseline data about your behavior. Baseline data is information about your current health and behavior that you can use later for comparison. This could take many forms, depending on your behavior. For example, you might weigh yourself for three consecutive days early in the morning. If you plan to stop smoking, keep track of your smoking patterns for a few days. If you are changing your diet, write down everything you eat for a three- or four-day period. We suggest keeping a journal and recording your activities and feelings related to the behavior.

2. Summarize your baseline data. Identify any patterns you see. Accept this information as an accurate indicator of your current health behavior. Use this textbook to find information about your behavior that could help you plan behavior-change strategies.

3. Establish some specific goals. Start with increments small enough to be within your grasp. For example, if you plan to lose weight, you might start out with a goal of one pound per week for the next three weeks. If you plan to stop smoking, you might start out by cutting down on your daily intake by five cigarettes. Think in terms of small, gradual progress toward your goals.

4. Make a personal contract to accomplish your goals. In this contract, you will want to indicate both starting and completion dates. Especially useful at this point are the Health Action Guides found in each chapter. These guides, such as the ones on page 143 (Dietary Recommendations) and page 348 (Eat to Lower Your Cancer Risk), will help you focus on specific activities to reach your goals. Identify any milestones along the way. Indicate the time, personal resources, and energy you will need to commit to this project.

5. Devise a plan of action and set specific goals. As you develop your strategy, try to control the environment in which you function so that you can replace old cues with new ones. For example, if you are trying to improve your sleep, you may wish to calm yourself before bed by reading rather than by listening to loud music or watching a television drama. If you are trying to improve your eating behavior, make a careful attempt to avoid walking by a place where donuts are available.

6. Chart your progress in your diary or journal. As you implement your behavior-change plan, keep a record of how you are doing. Making this chart visible also helps. For instance, posting an eating record on the refrigerator door is a good motivator for some people.

7. Encourage your family and friends to help you. Social support is important in any behavior-change attempt. Your friends may want to join you so that they can change their own behavior, and you can support each other. However, some friends or family members might be jealous of or misunderstand your efforts, and their behavior might discourage you. Avoid these people if at all possible . . . at least while your project is under way.

8. Set up a reward system. Rewards tend to motivate people and can serve to reinforce your positive changes. If you achieve success at a

Real Life
Real choices

- In which of the seven dimensions of health is Tim's life lacking since his father's death?
- What are some ways in which Tim can improve these aspects of his health?
- Can friends and family be helpful to Tim in this effort? If so, in what ways?

And Now, Your Choices . . .
- If a close friend of yours suddenly lost a parent, how would you try to help?
- If one of your parents died suddenly, how could your friends be most helpful to you?

---

particular point in your plan, reward yourself with a special meal, new clothes, or a weekend trip. Pat yourself on the back occasionally for your efforts. Relish your success.

9. Prepare for obstacles along the way. No one who achieved anything of importance did it without a few setbacks along the way. For example, you might neglect your fitness plan during a long holiday weekend. Prepare yourself mentally for an occasional obstacle. The key is to try to get back on course as soon as possible after a setback. Work through your setbacks with a forgive-and-forget attitude.

10. Revise your plan as necessary. Try to remain somewhat flexible in your approach to behavior change. A strategy that works for a while might not work as well after a month or two, so be prepared to reevaluate your goals and try new techniques when necessary.

Personal Applications

- Which of your health behaviors do you want to change? How will you accomplish your goals?

Summary

- When used to define health, morbidity and mortality relate to the prevalence of particular diseases and illnesses and to death resulting from those diseases and illnesses.
- A wide array of health problems (for example, cancer, cardiovascular disease, HIV/AIDS) persist despite today's highly sophisticated health care technology.
- When we seek the services of health care practitioners because of symptoms of illness or disease, we are said to be seeking episodic health care.
- Preventive medical care attempts to minimize the incidence of illness and disease by identifying early indicators of risk to bring them under control.
- Individual health promotion involves risk-reduction activities similar to those used in preventive medical care, except that the techniques cannot be invasive, such as some used in preventive medical care (Pap test, cholesterol profile, genetic screening, contrast media-based medical imaging), and are directed by professionals who are not physicians.
- Community health promotion involves the empowerment of individuals so that they can organize and participate in their own health promotion activities.

- Wellness pursuits often resemble risk-reduction activities undertaken in health promotion.
- Multidimensional perceptions of health, including holistic health, have existed for decades.
- Current multidimensional definitions of health may include many or all of the following dimensions: physical, emotional, social, intellectual, spiritual, occupational, and environmental.
- Today's college campus is a dynamic blend of students of both traditional and nontraditional ages and of diverse backgrounds, cultures, and attributes.
- Each phase of the life cycle involves a set of personal developmental tasks that are common to all, yet may be undertaken differently by each individual.
- Young adulthood is characterized by six key developmental tasks: forming an initial adult identity, establishing independence, assuming responsibility, developing social skills, developing parenting skills, and developing intimacy.
- The role of health is to enable individuals to participate in the activities that collectively constitute growth and development.
- The composition of health is the intrinsic and extrinsic resources on which individuals can draw to participate fully in their own growth and development.

Review Questions

1. What are morbidity and mortality, and how are they involved in the more traditional definitions of health?
2. As we approach the twenty-first century, what are some of the more pressing health-related concerns we must confront?
3. When and from whom do people seek episodic health care?
4. In preventive medical care, who determines a person's level of risk and determines what risk-reduction techniques might be applied?
5. In terms of professional personnel and the types of risk-reduction techniques used, how does individual health promotion differ from preventive medical care?
6. In community-based health promotion, who is ultimately responsible for organizing and implementing risk-reduction services?
7. In the view of a layperson, how do wellness-based activities differ from those associated with individual health promotion?
8. What are the dimensions of health included in the World Health Organization's definition of health? What dimensions have been added to formulate the current definition of holistic health?
9. In addition to chronological age, what other characteristics are encompassed in most definitions of the nontraditional student?
10. What is meant by the statement that life cycle stage growth and development is "predictable yet unique"?
11. How does your textbook's definition of health differ from traditional definitions? How does it differentiate between the role of health and the composition of health?
12. Why is it necessary to understand developmental expectations (developmental tasks) before we can answer the question, "Are you healthy enough to . . . ?"

References

1. *Healthy people 2000: national health promotion and disease prevention objectives* (full report, with commentary). DHHS publication; no. (PHS) 91-50212. Washington, DC: U.S. Department of Health and Human Services. Public Health Service.
2. *Healthy people 2000: midcourse review and 1995 revisions.* DHHS publication; no. (PHS). Washington, DC: U.S. Department of Health and Human Services. Public Health Service.
3. Healthy People 2010 Homepage. http://www.health.gov/healthypeople/
4. U.S. Bureau of the Census. *Statistical abstract of the United States: 1997.* 117th ed. Washington, DC: U.S. Government Printing Office, 1997.
5. The frontiers of medicine. *Time* 1996 Fall; 148 (Special Issue, 14):47–50.
6. *Yankelovich Monitor 1997,* as reported in What is success?, *USA Today* 1998 Jan 19:1A.
7. McKenzie JF, Smeltzer JL. *Planning, implementing and evaluating health promotion programs.* 2nd ed. Boston: Allyn & Bacon, 1997.
8. World Health Organization. Constitution of the World Health Organization. *Chronicle of the World Health Organization* 1947; 1:29–43.
9. Blonna R. *Coping with stress in a changing world.* St Louis: Mosby, 1996.
10. Ledermann EK. *Medicine for the whole person: a critique of scientific medicine.* Boston: Element Books, 1997.
11. U.S. Department of Education, National Center for Education Statistics. *Digest of education statistics, 1997.*
12. U.S. Department of Education, National Center for Education Statistics. *The 1995–96 national postsecondary student aid study,* October 1997.
13. Erikson EH. *Childhood and society* (reissue edition). New York: W.W. Norton, 1993.

Suggested Readings

Ledermann EK. *Medicine for the whole person: a critique of scientific medicine.* Boston: Element Books, 1997. As a physician Ledermann is well versed in the scientific basis of illness and disease. At the same time, however, he believes that a holistic approach to the management of illness is the only truly effective way to restore health. Numerous case studies support this contention. A spiritually satisfying life based on the formation of a personal conscience is seen as the basis for high-level health.

Justice B. *A different kind of health: finding well-being despite illness.* Houston: Peak Press, 1998. At some point in their lives, most people will be diagnosed with a life-threatening illness. At this point it is necessary to redefine health so that an individual can maintain a sense of well-being in spite of the presence of illness. This excellent book examines the process through which persons with serious and even terminal illness have nonetheless achieved high-level health and a sense of well-being.

Weil A. *8 weeks to optimum health.* New York: Fawcett Books, 1998. In the opinion of some critics, Dr. Weil's newest book is "one book too many" in terms of his commercially successful writings regarding a holistic approach to health. His supporters, however, contend that this third book is highly valuable because it extends beyond promoting a holistic approach to include an emphasis on spontaneous healing. Like Dr. Weil's other books, this title is based on a mix of emotional optimism and familiar information regarding diet, supplements, exercise, and mind-body interfacing.

Clinebell HJ. *Anchoring your well-being: Christian wholeness in a fractured world.* Nashville, TN: Upper Room Press, 1997. In recent years, books advocating a Christian-centered approach to dealing with a variety of health problems, including obesity, chemical dependency, and terminal illness, have gained popularity. This title extends this spiritually centered approach in the direction of broad-based healthful living. The author suggests that biblical text can provide significant direction in shaping our spiritual, physical, and emotional life, as well as influencing our work, play, and relationship to the environment.

Religious Diversity on Campus:
A Different Kind of School Spirit

Spirituality and the American university have a long history together. Many universities and colleges were founded for the dual purpose of advancement of knowledge and training of clergy. Although the university's mission has changed and broadened over the years, today there are more than two hundred colleges associated with the Roman Catholic Church, ninety with the United Methodist Church, and hundreds of others associated with one of sixty other religious organizations.[1] Of course, there are thousands of publicly sponsored institutions. How does this compare with the religious orientation of students? In a survey of college freshmen conducted for Northwestern Mutual Life Insurance Company during January 1998, over 2,000 students were asked if they believed in God. In response, 89 percent indicated that they did, while 9 percent responded that they did not. When asked if they attended religious services on a fairly regular basis, 57 percent reported that they did, 11 percent indicated occasional attendance, and 32 percent stated that they did not attend religious services at all. As to the role religion would play in their later lives, 42 percent stated that it would play a more important role in the future, 52 percent saw little change occurring from their current relationship to religion, and 3 percent thought it would become less important over time.[2]

You may have sought out your college because of its church ties or precisely because it lacked any. Or you may have chosen your college regardless of its affiliation, seeking to pursue a unique field of study, and then found yourself in a minority on campus. Whatever your situation, your school can remain true to its foundations while challenging and strengthening your personal beliefs by exposing you to the beliefs of others.

The Role of the University

One's religion is a personal characteristic in a world of variety. Religious diversity in America has its foundation in the U.S. Constitution in that no ties were established between the government and a state or favored church. Today we are even more diverse, coming from different ethnic backgrounds, religions, and socioeconomic levels and speaking different native languages. Every day we are exposed to positive and negative images and judgments of our differences from others. While some would argue that it is not within the university's scope to develop the student's spirituality, nevertheless the American Council on Education asserts that "a university that exposes its students to only one vision of culture places its students at excessive risk of accepting or even perpetuating intolerance, distortion, injustice and prejudice."[3] When a creationist guest lecturer comes to campus and tells an evolutionary biology student who is a Christian that she cannot be saved by Jesus if she continues to follow her program of study, she must be secure with her beliefs. When a fringe group arrives on campus spreading divisive and hateful messages, someone needs to stand up for fellowship and unification. When a cult comes to recruit members, students need not be susceptible to its tactics. Students who have had some experience with people of other religions are more likely to accept their own religious beliefs and practices and to resist these outside pressures.

Spirituality in Daily Life

People often display outward signs of their religious diversity. You or a classmate may wear a particular hat, head covering, dress, suit, or piece of jewelry that reflects a certain religious background. You may participate in customs of your faith that others are not familiar with, such as fasting, regimented prayer, dance, not working on important religious holidays, or marking yourself on a holy occasion. One example is the Catholic custom of marking the forehead with ash on Ash Wednesday. There may also be signs of your university's religious affiliation around your campus, such as religious statues and artwork or buildings named after religious figures. Religious symbolism on your campus may be inconspicuous or nonexistent, but the diversity still exists.

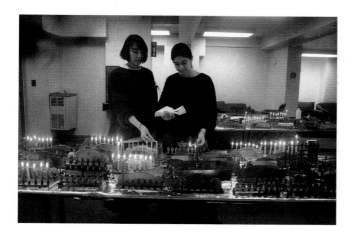

These Jewish students at Sterns College in New York are lighting menorahs in celebration of Chanukah.

Whether you attend church, temple, or synagogue weekly, monthly, occasionally, or never, your spiritual beliefs are probably reflected in your daily living. M. Scott Peck, in his now classic *The Road Less Traveled* (1978), defines religion more broadly than the organized denomination to which you belong.[4] He defines religion as a worldview—your understanding of the world and your place in it. On the basis of this definition, even the 9 percent of students who do not believe in God have a religious dimension to their lives in accordance with their emerging world view. The college years tend to be important in the evolution of your worldview. As your frame of reference is enlarged, your worldview becomes more realistic.[4] If you chose a college that is distant from your hometown, you may be encountering people really different from you for the first time. International students attending your university bring an even greater variety of perspectives to your campus. College is also the crucial time when you are choosing and preparing for your professional vocation, and being in touch with your spiritual side can increase the odds that you will find meaning and happiness in your chosen field of work.

Who Are You Going to Be?

Most college handbooks and catalogs speak of educating the whole person and preparing responsible citizens. Today they accomplish this not necessarily by en-

couraging a shared religious belief with each student, but by promoting the underlying values of a diverse and democratic society, which fosters a respect for the beliefs of others through understanding. This type of education may help to heal the religious conflicts of the past and present (Protestants vs. Catholics in Northern Ireland, Christians vs. Muslims in Bosnia, and Muslims vs. Jews in the Middle East, just to name a few religious conflicts familiar to today's students) by beginning a religious dialogue of the future.

As universities expose us to the beliefs of others, they initiate growth in our own spirituality and prepare us for life as well as for making a living. Just like learning, spiritual growth does not stop on graduation day: College is a foundation for future individual progress in both areas. Others may ask you what you plan to do when you graduate, but perhaps you should ask yourself "Who am I going to be?"

For Discussion . . .

Does your college have courses that explore religious diversity? Are your friends from similar or different religious backgrounds from yours? Have you ever been to a wedding or other religious celebration of another faith? What religions are represented in your health class?

References

1. Rodenhouse MP, Torregrosa CH, eds. *1998 higher education directory* (serial). Falls Church, VA: Higher Education Publications, 1998.
2. Generation 2001: *A survey of the first college graduating class of the new millennium*. Louis Harris & Associates for Northwestern Mutual Life, 1998. (http://www.northwesternmutual.com/2001)
3. American Council on Education. *American universities and colleges*. 15th ed. New York: Walter de Gruyter, 1997.
4. Peck MS. *The road less traveled, a new psychology of love, traditional values and spiritual growth*. New York: Simon & Schuster, 1978.

InfoLinks
www.firstthings.com
www.mcdc.org

u n i t One

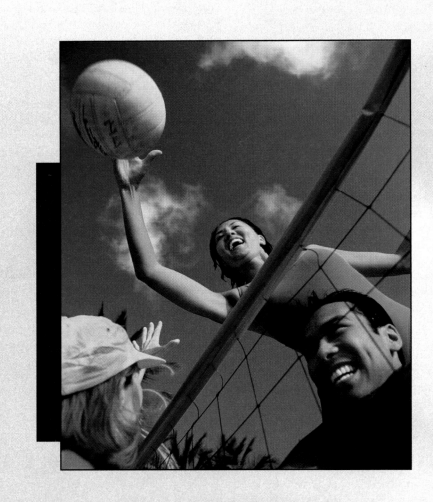

The Mind

The first unit in this textbook covers two topics that are closely linked to how we handle change in our lives. Chapter 2 discusses psychological wellness, and Chapter 3 deals with stress management. As explained below, your personal growth closely relates to each of the seven dimensions of your health.

1 Physical Dimension

The physical dimension of health is concerned with the structure and function of all body systems. Many of the experiences that will shape your feelings about yourself are made possible by good physical health. In addition, effective coping skills often require us to draw on the physical dimension of health.

2 Emotional Dimension

Our responses to stress are primarily emotional. Feelings of uneasiness arising from the demands of college, relationships, parenting, or work are the hallmarks of stress. Fortunately, you can cope with change by using the resources of your emotional dimension of health. Your sense of humor, capacity for empathy, and defense mechanisms will help you cope with demanding changes in your life.

3 Social Dimension

Growth and development are influenced by the people with whom you interact. When things go well with roommates, co-workers, or your spouse or children, you begin to feel capable as a social person. Occasional failures in social relationships can produce stress but can also remind you that emotional growth and coping skills take time to develop.

4 Intellectual Dimension

As you grow older, you will call on your intellectual resources with increasing frequency. These resources will help you enjoy life more fully and understand your emotional and spiritual growth. During difficult times, your mind may be your most dependable coping source. A book, concert, or art exhibit may be a refuge from the stress of the classroom, family, or office.

5 Spiritual Dimension

Many of today's students are searching for a deeper understanding of the meaning of life. Many students feel pressured to accept the spiritual beliefs of the majority. The uncertainties of exploring what to believe and how to express those beliefs can create stress. Your spirituality can be a valuable resource during periods of stress. Meditation, introspection, and prayer can free people from some of the stress of living in a fast-paced, sometimes uncaring world. To believe deeply in something and to act on that belief by serving others leads to personal growth.

6 Occupational Dimension

The vocation you choose will have a lasting effect on shaping the person you will become. Many people choose an occupation that allows them to serve others. However, work can be a primary source of life stress. Some of this stress is unwelcome and can be harmful. But occupational stress can also challenge you to perform at your peak, generating a sense of pride and accomplishment.

7 Environmental Dimension

Accepting responsibility to be a steward of our environment will enhance your emotional growth. A willingness to care for the environment in concrete ways, such as recycling or reducing water use, reflects your psychological wellness. In addition, minimizing environmental stressors, such as pollution, noise, and traffic, will help keep stress levels in check.

chapter

two

Achieving Psychological Wellness

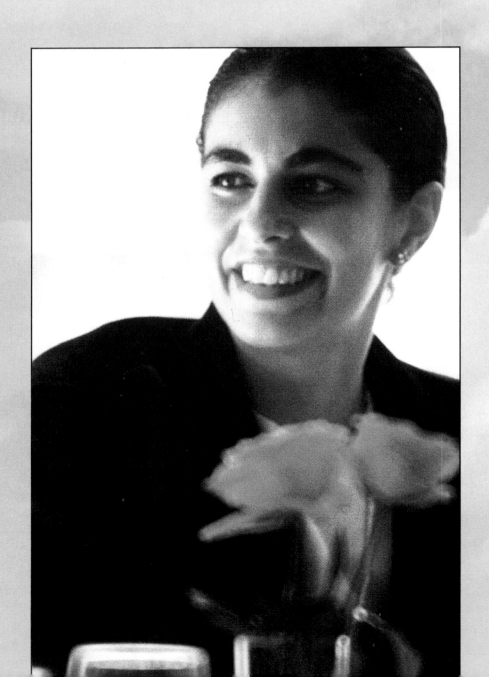

Have you recently been frustrated, angry, fearful, content, excited, or happy? Have you occasionally felt anticipation or anxiety about doing something new? These feelings are all part of the emotional dimension of health. Emotionally well people display a wide range of emotions in response to the experiences that make up their lives. Psychological wellness has a broader meaning than emotional wellness. A person who is psychologically well not only shows a normal range of emotions but also has a clear perception of reality and his or her place in the world. You will learn more about emotional and psychological wellness as you study this chapter.

HEALTHY PEOPLE: LOOKING AHEAD TO 2010

In the area of emotional, mental, and cognitive disorders, an important objective of the *Healthy People 2000* report was to reduce the prevalence of mental disorders within the general population. The *Midcourse Review*, however, did not address progress in reaching this objective.

Another important objective was to increase the use of community support services in the prevention and treatment of severe, persistent mental disorders. Data reported in the *Midcourse Review* clearly showed that substantial gains were made in the development of state-level clearinghouses to better identify existing resources. Unfortunately, adult patients of primary care providers, including family physicians, internal medicine specialists, and obstetricians and gynecologists, were unlikely to have received counseling or referral to these resources for treatment.

Healthy People 2010 will probably continue the focus on mental health and mental disorders that was established in 1990. Services will be offered to primary care physicians to help them recognize and refer patients with cognitive, emotional, and behavioral problems.

Real Life
Real choices

- Name: Keisha Saunders
- Age: 34
- Occupation: University student/single parent

It's a bright, crisp, blue and gold day—the first day of the fall term at the university—and Keisha Saunders has been awake since 5:30 A.M., excited and anxious as she prepares to return to school full time after fourteen years. She left her bachelor's program in nursing at the end of her sophomore year to get married, and the intervening years have been full of challenges: her husband's death in a construction accident, being a single parent to her two sons while holding down a full-time job, and painstakingly building up her back-to-school fund. Cheerful, energetic, determined, and hardworking, Keisha has handled these competing demands with confidence and grace. Now her goal is to complete her bachelor's degree and then go on for a master's so she can either teach or work as a clinical supervisor.

Keisha ticks off items on her mental list: breakfast dishes done, kittens fed, boys off to school—time to go. She glances

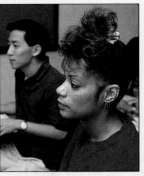

in the mirror near the front door, and what had been mild anxiety suddenly turns to doubt and fear. I'm too old, she thinks. I don't have anything in common with these kids—the freshmen are just a few years older than Jamal (her older boy, thirteen). Should I try to fit in, fade into the woodwork, be the class den mother? Will the other students ignore me, make fun of me, roll their eyes when I talk in class? Will I even be older than some of the instructors? Am I making the biggest mistake of my life?

As you study this chapter, think about the challenges Keisha faces as a nontraditional student returning to school, and prepare yourself to answer the questions in **Your Turn** at the end of the chapter.

Keys to Mental Health

How do you feel about yourself? When you apply resources from the multiple dimensions of health (see Chapter 1) in ways that allow you to direct your growth, assess deeply held values, deal effectively with change, and have satisfying interactions with others, you will be emotionally healthy. As such, you will develop and maintain a positive self-concept and a high level of self-esteem. *Self-concept* can be described as a perception, or mental picture, of yourself created by the interplay of beliefs, values, and experiences. Your self-concept is also balanced by information derived from your behavior. *Self-esteem* is a sense of self-acceptance that accompanies a valid self-concept. The existence of an adequate level of self-esteem is routinely reported to be the basis of our sense of emotional well-being. Note, however, that an overly high level of self-esteem, leading to excessive egotism, is related to violent behavior and the absence of self-control.[1,2]

Emotionally healthy people can become less emotionally healthy over time and may, in fact, develop a diagnosable psychological illness. Information about selected *psychopathological conditions*, also referred to as *emotional* or *mental disorders*, is given in a later section of the chapter. However, as you will see, psychological wellness is much more than just the absence of these conditions.

Do, Should, Can Real Men Cry?

Many (if not most) American men find it difficult, if not impossible, to shed tears, particularly in the presence of others. The effect of repressing tears, and the emotions with which they are associated, is thought to dispose men to unnecessarily high levels of physiological deterioration.

Why men find crying so difficult when, in fact, it would be healthier for them to do so is a difficult question to answer. Sociobiologists suggest that from the beginning of human existence, the male nervous system was programmed to produce less serotonin than the female system, thus rendering men less sensitive to the expressions of emotional needs of others, particularly women and the young.

A less biologically oriented reason why males are less inclined than women to cry might simply be "because that's the way they are brought up." In other words, men could "unlearn" the traditional expectation that they will not show their emotions.

Emotional and Psychological Wellness

Is there a difference between emotional and psychological wellness? Many people believe that there is little real difference between the terms. Accordingly, they use the terms *emotional, mental,* and *psychological wellness* (or health) interchangeably.

The Importance of Forgiveness

In an excellent video titled *Late Frost*[3] (often used in gerontology classes), an elderly gentleman muses the important lessons of life that are finally recognized by those who have lived to reach old age. A particularly poignant moment occurs when the man thanks God for having given him the ability to *forget*. On closer examination, however, we can see that forgetfulness is not a strange attribute for us to want or to be thankful for. This is because frequently our ability to forget harmful events reflects the fact that we have first been able to *forgive* those who have hurt us so deeply.

Experts in the field of mind-body connectedness suggest we can eventually forgive, but only when we truly want to do so. In other words, we must be willing to work in order to forgive and thus forget our pain. Accordingly, we must master a process involving these difficult but necessary steps:

The ability to embrace our anger. Although unpleasant and unhealthful, anger is a human attribute that is both natural and important in its ability to lead us toward positive change. Its initial strongly felt presence must be recognized and accepted as such.

The ability to look beyond our own pain. In spite of the fury that rages inside us, the person whose actions have caused us such unbearable pain is a person of value as well. We must at some point look for the redeeming qualities this person possesses.

The ability to refrain from speaking derogatorily. In spite of the hurt others have caused us, to continue speaking in demeaning ways about others negates our ability to see them as having redeeming value as people.

The ability to see a future free from anger. Much as athletes visualize their own "perfect" performance, when deeply injured we must stay focused on what life will be like when we have finally moved beyond our anger and hurt.

The ability to begin wishing well to those who have hurt us. Earlier we were told to see our offenders as people of value. Now we must internalize this attitude to the extent that we can begin to truly wish these people well.

The ability to persevere. Even though the offense against us may have taken only seconds, it may require months or even years for us to replace our pain and anger with a sense of forgiveness. We cannot rush the process, nor can we give up on it.

When we can forgive those who have hurt us, particularly those who have been close and dear, the debilitating effects of stress stemming from anger eventually will subside. Forgiving will then lead to a form of forgetting that spares the body, mind, and spirit.

We believe, however, that a difference does exist between these terms: Emotional wellness has a narrower, more focused meaning, while psychological wellness is a more global term. Emotional wellness relates to individuals' specific responses to changing situations within their environment. These responses are subjective and reflect the person's value orientation. Defense mechanisms, such as rationalism and denial, are routinely used to soften the more painful and less acceptable of these feelings. Indeed, responses to change reflecting a sense of joy, anger, compassion, sympathy, empathy, frustration, and disappointment are familiar, healthy emotions. Emotionally well people feel good about their responses to change, whereas those who are negative about their own feelings and their responses to change are less emotionally healthy.

In comparison to emotional health, psychological health relates to the unfolding of a wide array of psychological traits. The extent of these traits is far too broad to be discussed in this textbook but includes the development of language, memory, perceptual processes, awareness states, and, of course, the interfacing of the mind and body. Psychologically well people deal rationally with the world, display a fully functional personality, and resolve conflict in a constructive manner. Psychologically well people, who are also generally very emotionally healthy, use more aspects of the psyche than just their feeling states. Accordingly, of course, psychological dysfunction is more profound than emotional distress in that the former involves varying degrees of loss of contact with reality.

Characteristics of an Emotionally and Psychologically Well Person

The characteristics most people associate with being emotionally well (and very likely psychologically well also) are listed below.[4]

Emotionally well people:

- Feel comfortable about themselves
- Are capable of experiencing the full range of human emotions
- Are not overwhelmed by their emotions (either positive or negative emotions)
- Accept life's disappointments
- Feel comfortable with others
- Receive and give love easily
- Feel concern for others when appropriate
- Establish goals, both short term and long term
- Function autonomously where and when appropriate
- Generally trust others

Personal Applications

• How close do you come to meeting the characteristics of an emotionally well person?

Personality

Although difficult to define, *personality* is a familiar concept that we use to describe the emotional makeup of people, including ourselves. People routinely use adjectives such as *pleasing, destructive,* or *positive* to define the personality of someone in an attempt to describe how they believe the person feels about life and the approach he or she takes in living life. Think about instances when you have been asked by someone to describe the personality of a friend, spouse, employer, or neighbor. Isn't it likely that you associate another's "good" personality with the existence of emotional and psychological wellness?

Although there are many viewpoints concerning personality development, a general consensus is that two factors, *innate* and *environmental,* influence the shaping of personality.[5,6] Innate factors most likely relate to something called *temperament.* We all know people who are "by nature" quiet, outgoing, serious, or shy. Nothing, in our opinion, seems capable of changing these people in the opposite direction. Even though temperament appears to have a biological basis, it still seems to play a part in how we define the emotional health of others. Some would suggest that temperament is the best means we have of observing the innate basis of personality.

Environmental factors influence the more flexible aspects of personality—those that depend on basic temperament. The "up" or "down" moods that exist on a given day, or in a given situation, can be affected by factors as diverse as traffic congestion, weather, social relationships, family harmony, job concerns, and the financial resources that we possess. Understandably, then, the personality of another person may prove to be very different after you have had an opportunity to interact with him or her over the course of several days and in a variety of settings.

The Normal Range of Emotions

You probably know others who seem to be cheerful all the time. These people appear to be confident, happy, and full of good feelings twenty-four hours a day. Although some people like this may exist, they are truly the exceptions. For most people, emotions are more like a roller coaster ride. At times, they feel good about themselves and others; other times, nothing seems to be going right. Once you know them better, these same people may show that they feel happy, sad, pleased, uncertain, confident, excited, and afraid all in the same day or week. To outsiders, they might even appear to be moody. To the mental health professional, however, these same people would probably seem to be normal, since the feeling states that they are demonstrating all fall within a normal range of emotions.

Everyone, not only college students, experiences a range of emotions. This is normal and healthy. Experiencing a range of emotions is an important part of experiencing life. You should not expect to remain calm and rational every minute of the day. You also should not expect to adjust effectively to every situation with which you are confronted. Life has its ups and downs, and the concept of the *normal range of emotions* reflects this. If one concept is important for you to understand about being emotionally and psychologically well, it is this one.

Happiness and a Sense of Humor

Perhaps the most prized emotion to be experienced is a feeling of happiness about life—a feeling that is more likely to occur when day-to-day events are entered into with an underlying sense of humor.

Maintaining a sense of humor is now known to be a critically important component of the emotional dimension of health.[7] People who possess this resource understand that life is not meant to be one long, boring exercise. Part of the reason for living is to have fun. Life taken too seriously can be the most unhappy life imaginable.

Recognizing the humor in daily situations and occasionally being able to laugh at yourself will make you feel better not only about others but also, more importantly, about yourself. Others will enjoy being associated with you, and your ability to perform physically and to recover from injuries and illnesses will probably be enhanced.[8,9] For example, any student-athlete who has experienced a career-threatening injury can attest that a positive outlook and a sense of humor were key ingredients in relation to the speed and extent of recovery.

Self-Esteem

The key to overall emotional wellness may be connected to the existence of self-esteem. As discussed earlier in the chapter, we develop a sense of self-esteem as more and more information that supports our self-concept accumulates. Thus we feel capable and reflect a sense of control in a wide variety of situations in which we find ourselves. We are able to get along with others, cope in stressful situations, and make contributions when we work with others. Self-esteem gives us a sense of self-worth and may offset our self-defeating behavior patterns. As you will see when you complete the Personal Assessment on page 31, people with high levels of self-esteem find a comfortable balance between their idealized self and where they actually are.

Personal Assessment

How Does Your Self-Concept Compare with Your Idealized Self?

Below is a list of 15 personal attributes, each portrayed on a 9-point continuum. Mark with an X where you think you rank on each attribute. Try to be candid and accurate; these marks will collectively describe a portion of your sense of self-concept. When you are finished with the above task, go back and circle where you *wish* you could be on each dimension. These marks describe your idealized self. Finally, in the spaces on the right, indicate the difference between your self-concept and your idealized self for each attribute.

Decisive					**Indecisive**					_____
9	8	7	6	5	4	3	2	1		
Anxious					**Relaxed**					_____
9	8	7	6	5	4	3	2	1		
Easily influenced					**Independent thinker**					_____
9	8	7	6	5	4	3	2	1		
Very intelligent					**Less intelligent**					_____
9	8	7	6	5	4	3	2	1		
In good physical shape					**In poor physical shape**					_____
9	8	7	6	5	4	3	2	1		
Undependable					**Dependable**					_____
9	8	7	6	5	4	3	2	1		
Deceitful					**Honest**					_____
9	8	7	6	5	4	3	2	1		
A leader					**A follower**					_____
9	8	7	6	5	4	3	2	1		
Unambitious					**Ambitious**					_____
9	8	7	6	5	4	3	2	1		
Self-confident					**Insecure**					_____
9	8	7	6	5	4	3	2	1		
Conservative					**Adventurous**					_____
9	8	7	6	5	4	3	2	1		
Extroverted					**Introverted**					_____
9	8	7	6	5	4	3	2	1		
Physically attractive					**Physically unattractive**					_____
9	8	7	6	5	4	3	2	1		
Lazy					**Hardworking**					_____
9	8	7	6	5	4	3	2	1		
Funny					**Little sense of humor**					_____
9	8	7	6	5	4	3	2	1		

To Carry This Further . . .

1. Overall, how would you describe the difference between your self-concept and your idealized self (large, moderate, small, large on a few dimensions)?

2. How do sizable gaps for any of your attributes affect your sense of self-esteem?

3. Do you think that any of the gaps exist because you have had others' ideals imposed on you or because you have thoughtlessly accepted others' ideals?

4. Identify several attributes that you realistically believe can be changed to narrow the gap between your self-concept and your self-ideal and, thus, foster a well-developed sense of self-esteem.

The beginning of positive self-esteem can be traced back to childhood. For those nontraditional students who are also parents, there are many ways in which interactions with young children impart powerful messages about self-worth. Warm and supportive physical contact, verbal exchanges involving talking "with" rather than "to" children, and the gradual loosening of control so that more and more decisions become those of the child serve to inform children that they are competent and valued. Ultimately, however, we are responsible for developing our own sense of self-esteem. Recall from page 28 that an unhealthy sense of egotism may stem from excessive self-esteem. The following guidelines will help you nurture an appropriate level of this important trait:

Maintain satisfying group relationships. The best way to do this is to become affiliated with existing groups, such as social clubs, volunteer organizations, church groups, professional organizations, athletic groups, or any other group that you believe will help you feel a sense of "belonging."

Set and reach realistic goals. Achieving your goals allows you to feel power and control over your own life. In turn, this leads to improved self-confidence and further pride and motivation. The key is to make these goals realistic so that honest success can be achieved.

Recognize the uniqueness of yourself and others. Happy people understand and appreciate that people are indeed unique. By knowing other happy people you will enhance your own self-esteem. Enjoy the satisfaction of a compliment when it is given. Take time out each day to think about your special strengths and abilities and how they differ from (or are similar to) those possessed by others. Pat yourself on the back regularly and remind yourself that you are unique and special.

Form and maintain a relationship with a mentor. Happy people (or those who wish to be) look for certain key figures in life who have been helpful and who have inspired them. These role models serve as mentors. The importance of having a mentor should not be overlooked.

Personal Applications

• What goals can you set for yourself this year that will enhance your self-esteem once you have achieved them?

Developing Communication Skills

Shyness and loneliness, two of the more common conditions suggesting a less-than-optimal level of emotional wellness, will be described later in the chapter. Both of these conditions can be a consequence of feeling uncomfortable with others. When people find it difficult to initiate or even participate in conversations with others, it is likely that they have not developed some of the communication skills with which others feel comfortable. In this section of your textbook, we will investigate how speaking and listening can foster improved social relationships. We will also look at the use of unspoken communication as an aid to social interaction. Remember that how people see themselves (their self-concept) influences how they feel about themselves (their self-esteem).

Verbal Communication

Communication between people can be viewed in terms of a particular person's role as sender or receiver of the spoken language. You can enhance your effectiveness as a sender of verbal information by implementing several important steps:[10]

- Take the time to think before speaking. Effective communication requires that you know what you want to say.
- Focus your words on your most important thoughts and ideas. Not every idea is as important as the central ideas that you are attempting to communicate.
- Speak clearly and concisely. This will aid the listener, particularly when ideas are complex or new.
- Talk with, rather than at, the listener. Speaking with other people encourages listeners to share freely and comfortably with those speaking.
- Start on a positive note. Even when the message is negative, a more positive atmosphere is established when a conversation begins in this manner.
- Seek feedback from listeners. Provide frequent intervals between ideas to allow listeners to respond.
- Use other forms of communication to transmit important ideas when face-to-face conversation is not effective. Written communication or the use of a carefully selected third person is often highly effective.

Verbal communication requires that you function as skillfully as a listener, or receiver, as you do as a sender of spoken ideas. Certainly, there are skills for structuring the exchange of information. A variety of listening approaches appear below:

- Listen with attention. In many situations it will be important to hear and understand everything that is being said.
- When appropriate, listen selectively to what the speaker is saying. The best use of time and "listening energy" may be to filter out some of what is being said while continuing to concentrate on the main points or on interesting, new, or important information.
- On some occasions, it may be necessary to guide the speaker to ensure that excessive or confusing information is not being transferred. This is accomplished by asking carefully planned questions intended to clarify a continuing stream of information.

Nonverbal Communication

We often share information without saying a word. This is nonverbal communication. It is important that you recognize nonverbal communication techniques so that you can control the effects that your messages have on others.[11]

- Facial expressions often condition the receptiveness with which your messages will be met. Be aware of your facial expressions to be sure they are consistent with your message.
- Eye contact is an important component of positive nonverbal communication. Practice by looking in the mirror, at a face on television, or at a photograph.
- Learn to comfortably touch others, particularly when you would want to be touched in a similar situation or setting. Touching may be the most important component of nonverbal communication. Do so, however, with care and sensitivity.
- Learn the appropriate distance between you and another person. People have their own ideas of how close is too close and how far is too far, and these are strongly influenced by individual and cultural differences.
- Dress for success. You are often judged by the appropriateness of what you are wearing in a particular setting or at a particular time. The "wrong clothing" may quickly ruin the impression you are trying to make.

- Electronic mail has introduced a new form of "nonverbal" communication that may involve yourself and hundreds of others, most of whom you will never meet in person. Concern exists in some quarters regarding the extent to which chronic use of e-mail might erode other aspects of interpersonal communication.[12] (See www.netaddiction.com for a test of your Internet "addiction.")

As with verbal communication, when nonverbal components are recognized and controlled, communication is undertaken more effectively.

Maslow's Hierarchy of Needs

Abraham Maslow has been among the significant contributors to the understanding of personality and emotional growth. Central to Maslow's contribution to twentieth-century American psychological thought is his view of emotional growth in terms of the individual's attempt to meet inner needs, what he called *the hierarchy of needs.*[13] Maslow lists motivational requirements for fulfilling specific needs in the following order: physiological needs, safety needs, belonging and love needs, esteem needs, and self-actualization needs (Figure 2-1). He distinguishes between the lower *deficiency needs* (those that cannot be done without) and the higher *being needs*, those that are a part of the search for full humanism. In Maslow's model, people do not seek the higher needs until the lower demands have been reasonably satisfied.

The healthiest and most effective people in society are those whose lives embody *being values* such as truth, beauty, goodness, faith, wholeness, and love. Maslow labels these people as **transcenders. Self-actualization,** the highest level of self-development, and at the apex of the needs triangle, is clearly evident in the transcender's personality. Transcenders are those whose emotional and psychological development has reached its fullest level. They can be described as follows:[13]

- Transcenders have more peak or creative experiences and naturally speak the language of being values.
- Transcenders are more responsive to beauty, more holistic in their perceptions of humanity

---

transcenders   self-actualized people who have achieved a quality of being ordinarily associated with higher levels of spiritual growth.

self-actualization   the highest level of personality development; self-actualized people recognize their roles in life and use personal strengths to reach their fullest potential.

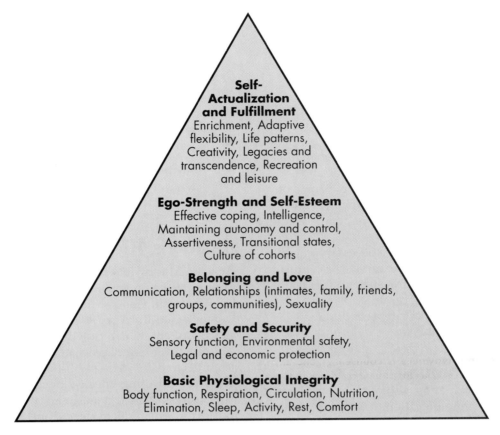

Figure 2-1   Maslow's hierarchy of needs.

and the cosmos, adjust well to conflict situations, and work toward goals and purposes.

- Transcenders are innovators who are attracted to mystery and the unknown and see themselves as instruments for the actualization of the transpersonal being values.
- Transcenders tend to fuse work and play. They are less attracted by the rewards of money and objects and more motivated by the satisfaction of being and service values.
- Transcenders are more likely to accept others with an unconditional positive regard, and are more oriented toward spiritual reality.

With some consideration, you will notice the similarity between transcenders and people with positive self-esteem. The Health Action Guide on page 35 will help you foster your emotional growth. In doing so, you may become more transcendent.

Creative Expression

Emotionally and psychologically well people have a free and open approach to life. They think and act positively. They also assess people and situations realistically and constructively. When others interact with emotionally healthy people, they quickly notice

their flexibility in solving problems. How did these individuals become so secure, competent, and constructive? Is it possible that others will also mature in this direction? What resources will you need to grow in a similar fashion?

The Institute of Personality Assessment at the University of California has identified traits that characterize creative people. Assuming that **creativity** is closely related to psychological health, these traits may help describe psychologically healthy people:

- Creative people are intuitive and open to new experiences. They are spontaneous and expressive and have the courage to reveal themselves. They are relatively free from fear and are not disturbed by the unknown, the mysterious, or the puzzling.
- Creative people are less interested in detail than in meaning and implications. They tend to be more theoretical than practical in their orientation. These people have the ability to unify, synthesize, and integrate materials and experiences.
- Creative people are independent, self-accepting, and autonomous, yet they are not authoritarian in their attitudes. They tend to function best when allowed to work independently.

HEALTH ACTION GUIDE

Fostering Your Emotional Growth

Emotional growth requires both knowing about yourself and learning from new experiences. The activities listed below can be used in support of these requirements:

Keep a daily journal. Writing down your thoughts and making note of experiences are effective tools in fostering greater self-understanding. Once written, the information that these accounts contain can be reprocessed for an even greater awareness of self.

Join a support group. Sharing experiences and feelings in the presence of people who can "stand in your shoes" creates an environment that will support your efforts to grow as a more interesting and self-directed person. Additionally, being an active participant in a support group also functions as a "new experience" through which new insights into your sense of self-worth can be gained.

Take an assertiveness course. Learning how to greet others, give and receive compliments, use "I" statements, express spontaneity, and state your feelings of disagreement are important tools in developing self-confidence. Very likely, an assertiveness course is or will be offered on your campus.

Seek counseling. Nowhere is counseling generally more available and affordable than on a college campus. Clearly, much can be learned about your sense of self and the psychological factors that have shaped it. Furthermore, growth-enhancing skills can be formulated and tested in both individual and group counseling sessions. Contact the campus health center or the psychological services center for referral to an experienced psychologist or counselor. What additional activities can you think of that would further your self-knowledge or serve as new experiences?

InfoLinks
www.mhsource.com/healthieryou.html

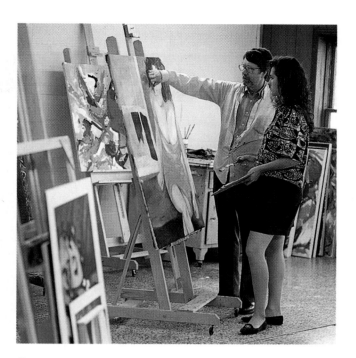
Creative expression can occur in a variety of forms.

Faith Development and Spiritual Resources

A fully developed sense of self-esteem may require that you be knowledgeable and accepting of yourself as a person of **faith.** Many older adults have little difficulty sharing that they believe in something or someone greater than themselves and that this belief brings them great comfort and a sense of support. Many report that because of their personal level of faith, they do not fear death because they know that their lives have had meaning within the context of a larger plan. Further, they would urge younger people to search for both the strength and direction in their lives that faith provides.[14]

As a resource in the spiritual dimension of health, the existence of faith provides a basis on which your belief system can mature and your expanding awareness of life's meaning can be fostered. In addition, the existence of faithfulness gives meaning (or additional meaning) to your vocation and assists you in better understanding the consequences of

- Creative people are flexible. They do not use all-or-none thinking but recognize that there are many ways to interpret the same situation.
- Creative people are governed by an internal set of values and are persistent in developing ideas and working toward goals.

Some people reviewing the preceding list may recognize many of these characteristics as being already well developed in their own personalities. Others may never have demonstrated some traits listed, and they may now appear far beyond their reach. Nevertheless, most people can increase their creativity by letting their high level of health help them face new challenges from which they gain greater knowledge of their strengths and limitations.

Personal Applications

• Which traits of creativity have you developed? How do you express your creativity?

creativity innovative ability; insightful capacity to solve problems; ability to move beyond analytical or logical approaches to experience.

faith the purposes and meaning that underlie an individual's hopes and dreams.

Learning
From Our Diversity

Celebration and Commemoration: Toward a Richer Sense of Community

In every culture around the globe, the bonds between people of different ages, sexes, interests, and occupations are strengthened by participation in shared rituals to celebrate everything from births, weddings—even deaths—to sports victories, religious events, and military triumphs. With costumes and masks, flags and banners, food and drink, song and dance, tears and laughter, we come together to mourn and rejoice, to look back and look ahead, to remember and renew.

As the "global village" expands and Americans are exposed to an ever-greater variety of cultures and traditions, we find ourselves increasingly joining in the rituals of many ethnic groups and nations. Perhaps the most obvious example is St. Patrick's Day. On every 17th of March, a sea of green engulfs the streets, offices, retail establishments, and bars of all fifty states—and many "wearers o' the green" have not a trace of Irish in their background.

Now coming into its own as a Mexican-American holiday is a celebration known as Cinco de Mayo ("the fifth of May"), which commemorates Mexico's defeat of the French in the battle of Puebla on that date in 1862. As Mexican-American writer Maudi Gomez Schneider explains, "The defeat of the larger, better equipped French army has come to symbolize national pride in the Mexican peoples who joined together to win the battle."[15]

For generations a persecuted minority in the United States, Mexican-Americans are winning increasing recognition and acceptance for their contributions to American life and culture—and their annual festivals to commemorate Cinco de Mayo are drawing ever-larger crowds of non-Hispanics who enjoy sharing traditional foods like tamales, roasted corn, and other ethnic specialties, and who love to sway to the beat of mariachi, ranchera, and banda music.[16] Street vendors can't keep up with the demand for spicy Mexican food—and the taps flow freely with Dos Equis, Corona, and other popular Mexican beers. Parades, complete with brightly decorated floats, Mexican horsemen, folk dancers, drill teams, and marching bands, draw crowds of thousands.

Rapidly moving toward the day when the members of so-called "minority groups" will outnumber Caucasians of northern European descent in the "great melting pot," Americans increasingly are learning about—and learning to enjoy—the dazzling array of celebrations offered by our country's rich and diverse ethnic populations. So, while the Battle of Puebla has little or no meaning for most Americans not of Hispanic descent, the increasing popularity of Cinco de Mayo shows a growing awareness of the many ways of celebrating events that are meaningful to people of other cultures.

Think about your favorite holidays. What are their ethnic roots? How does celebrating them enhance your psychological well-being?

your vocational efforts. Further, faith in something (or someone) influences many of the experiences that you will seek throughout life and tempers the emotional relationships that you have with these experiences.[17] In virtually all cultures, faith and its accompanying belief system provide individuals and groups with rituals and practices that foster the development of a sense of community. In turn, the community provides the authority and guidance that nurtures the emotional stability, confidence, and sense of competence needed for living life fully.[14] Interestingly, the positive influence of a community of faith in fostering the health of others was demonstrated when prayer directed toward HIV/AIDS patients, who were unaware

that they were being prayed for, was associated with clinical signs of improvement.[18]

Taking a Proactive Approach to Life

Beyond the several approaches to high-level emotional health already discussed, the plan that follows is intended to give you even greater control of enhancing your feelings of self-esteem. A key to emotional health is the ability to control the outcomes of experiences and thus to learn about your own emotional resources.

Constructing Mental Pictures

Actively taking charge of emotional growth begins when you construct a mental picture of what you are like. This mental picture or perception should be composed of the most recent and accurate information you have about yourself concerning the knowledge

Personal Applications

• In what or whom do you place your deepest trust? How could you enhance your spirituality or strengthen your religious beliefs?

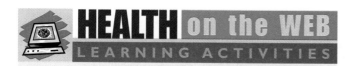

Rating Your Emotional Intelligence

To evaluate several aspects of your emotional intelligence, go to www.psychtests.com/emotionaliq.html and complete the inventory, which will evaluate your emotional intelligence and suggest ways to improve it. It is important that you be honest and answer according to what you really feel or believe, rather than what you think is considered a right answer on this test.

Determining Whether You're an Extrovert or an Introvert

"Learn to live comfortably with yourself." Regardless of the exact words used to convey this idea, you will eventually realize that to have a productive and satisfying life you must know who you are. However, what you see in yourself is often determined by what you wish to see. One important trait to evaluate is whether you are more oriented toward the outer world (extroversion) or the inner world (introversion). Go to www.psychtests.com/extraver.html and complete the 27-item inventory. Are you more extroverted or introverted? Are you happy with this trait?

Evaluating Your Anxiety Level

Excessive anxiety can be caused by the demands of work, school, or family, by relationship difficulties, financial concerns, or many other factors. The first step toward controlling anxiety is to recognize it. You can complete a 30-item inventory to measure your level of anxiety at www.psychtests.com/anxiety.html. Do you have a high anxiety level? If so, how can you begin to control it? Remember, a professional evaluation is in order if your anxiety is excessive and persistent.

For more activities, log on to our Online Learning Center at www.mhhe.com/hper/health/payne.

Communication Can Be Therapeutic

In the pages that follow you will read about selected emotional disorders and the forms of psychotherapy that are in place to help people deal with these conditions. Virtually all forms of therapy emphasize verbalization (largely by the client). It follows that verbal exchange between people who are experiencing emotional upheavals and other people is a common form of "therapy" in dealing with day-to-day distress.

In a recent survey for *Prevention Magazine*,[19] a large number of women (who are more inclined than men to verbalize their emotional concerns) were asked to identify the people to whom they turn to share the story of their emotional distress.

- *Husbands* (39%) and *friends* (38%) were the two sounding boards most frequently chosen by the women surveyed. Very likely, the friends chosen would have been described as the women's closest friends.
- *Children* (20%) and *mothers* (15%) represented the third and fourth choices of the women surveyed. Almost certainly, the children identified as being sounding boards were themselves adults or nearly so.
- Romantic partners (9%) and persons from within their *communities of faith* (6%) played some role as recipients of women's concerns, but clearly less so than might have been imagined. Perhaps romantic partners are too intimately connected to be seen as completely trusted listeners.
- The final two statistics are intriguing, if not surprising. *Fathers* (1%) were rarely seen as preferred listeners for their daughter's problems. *No one* (14%) was more frequently chosen than might have been expected. This finding seems disturbing in light of the stress-reducing role good friends and close family members can play during times of emotional distress. (see Chapter 3).

that is important to you, the values that you hold, and the activities in which you are competent.

Before continuing to the second step in the plan for emotional development, it is important that you construct, in addition to a mental picture about yourself, similar mental pictures about yourself in relation to other people and material objects, including your residence and college or work environment, to gain a clearer picture of these relationships.

For example, Clara moved to a large city to become a jewelry designer after graduating from college with a degree in fine arts. Two years later, Clara's business was thriving and she had been able to move to a loft apartment in which one room served as a studio. Nevertheless, Clara felt that something was missing. She constructed a mental picture in which she saw herself as a resourceful, creative, independent person who was comfortable in her new surroundings. However, Clara realized that she wanted a partner with whom to share her success and her life.

Accepting Mental Pictures

The second step of the plan involves an acceptance of these perceptions. Acceptance implies a willingness to honor the truthfulness of the perceptions that you have formed. For example, Clara should acknowledge her professional success and her artistic ability but must also accept that she has been unable to establish a long-term intimate relationship.

As in the first step of the plan, the second stage requires time and commitment. Controlling emotional development is rarely a passive process. You must be willing to be introspective (inwardly reflective) about yourself and the world around you.

Undertaking New Experiences

To mature emotionally, you must progress beyond the first two steps of the prescription and test the newly formed perceptions you have constructed. This testing is accomplished by undertaking a new experience or by reexperiencing something in a different way.

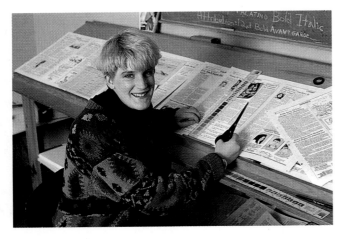

Completing an internship in a career field that interests you could be a challenging new experience.

For example, one of your authors traveled to London with 31 students, and most of them took advantage of every opportunity out of class to meet new people, see new places, and have new experiences. No part of the United Kingdom (or Europe, for that matter) seemed to be beyond their reach. Over the course of our fifteen weeks together, they became more confident and self-assured as the result of being independent and self-directed in taking risks. In retrospect, no combination of reading assignments, guest lectures, and field trips could have produced the emotionally fulfilling maturation that was accomplished away from their university's London Centre.

New experiences do not necessarily require high levels of risk, foreign travel, or money. They may be no more "new" than deciding to move from the dorm into an apartment, to change from one shift at work to another, or to pursue new friendships. The experience itself is not the end that you should be seeking; rather, it is a means of collecting a new pool of information about yourself, others, and the objects that form your material world. Volunteering to help an organization or cause you believe in is a great way to learn more about yourself and the world around you. To find out how becoming a volunteer can enhance your emotional wellness, turn to the Topics for Today article on page 49.

Clara, whom we described previously, volunteered to teach art therapy classes to chronically ill patients at a local hospital. This work was enjoyable and fulfilling for Clara, and she formed friendships with a few of the other hospital volunteers. Clara also met and began dating Marcel, a staff physical therapist.

Personal Applications

• What new experiences might you undertake to enhance your emotional wellness and growth?

Reframing Mental Pictures

When you have completed the first three steps in the plan for achieving emotional growth, the new information about yourself, others, and objects becomes the most current source of information available. Regardless of the type of new experience you have undertaken and its outcome, you are now in a position to modify the initial perceptions that were constructed during the first step of the plan. Once completed, you have new insights, knowledge, and perspectives.

Clara reframed her mental pictures in light of the changes that had taken place in her life. Her volunteer work gave her a new appreciation for art, and she discovered depths of caring in herself that she had not known existed. In addition, she now saw herself as part of a circle of friends and as a partner in a long-term relationship with Marcel. With her proactive approach to life, Clara had created challenges for herself from which she changed and grew.

Psychological Dysfunction and Its Management

On any given day, millions of Americans are limited in their ability to participate fully in life because they have dysfunctional feelings and a diminished sense of self-worth.[20] In the sections that follow, we will investigate selected disorders, identify professionals who are prepared to deal with such conditions, and take a look at the techniques they employ to help those who are afflicted.

Selected Forms of Emotional/ Psychological Dysfunction

How common are these disorders? Quite common! More than a dozen disorders affect more than 90 million people. In addition, the lives of millions of others are touched by their relationships to the affected people. Accordingly, we have selected six clinical conditions that are most likely to be recognized by readers: general anxiety disorders, depression (both bipolar and unipolar), suicide, obsessive-compulsive disorder, panic disorders, and schizophrenia.

General Anxiety Disorders

The familiar word *anxiety* refers to unfocused *worry* or excessive concern. In people with general anxiety disorder (GAD), this anxiety or concern is expressed more consistently and intensely than in most people. When general anxiety seems most closely related to concerns over health problems, the condition is referred to as *anxiety disorder due to general medical condition(s)*.[21]

People with GAD are characterized not only by having excessive levels of worry (anxiety) but also by having difficulty in controlling the expression of this excessive concern. To the observer, people with GAD often seem restless, unable to concentrate, and fa-

HEALTH ACTION GUIDE

Understanding Your Mental Health Rights

With the growth of managed health care during the 1990s, employees' health-care benefits underwent marked changes, including restrictions on the type, duration, and coverage of services provided. Perhaps the areas of care most negatively affected were mental health and chemical dependency treatment. Accordingly, individuals should be familiar with the specific nature of the mental health and chemical dependency coverage their health insurance provides and exercise fully their rights to access these services.

As a member of a group health insurance plan, you have the right to obtain needed information regarding the plan and should feel comfortable asking questions in each of the following areas:

What benefits are available through my plan? Ask for a copy of your plan. Study your plan to see the type of coverage it provides for mental health and chemical dependency treatment. Learn how you obtain these services, how you appeal restrictions, and what your financial obligations are regarding particular forms of treatment that might be considered nonstandard.

What types of professional treatment am I entitled to receive? Unless this is spelled out clearly in printed material, ask your plan representative about the type of professional you may see for the duration of treatment, and the availability of second opinions.

What, if any, are the contractual limitations between providers and my plan? Ask if your providers are receiving special incentives for restricting the duration of your treatment, limiting referrals to specialists, or limiting the treatment options to minimize costs to the plan.

What type of information regarding my diagnosis and treatment will be made available to others, and to what extent? Particularly, in regard to mental health and chemical dependency care, you may have understandable concerns about information passing from your health-care provider, through your plan, and eventually reaching people within or even outside your workplace.

What mechanisms exist to ensure nondiscrimination in other aspects of my benefit package? As a plan member seeking care for mental health concerns or chemical dependency, you may want to ask if your acceptance of care will adversely influence your ability to obtain or retain benefits such as life insurance, disability insurance, or insurance for long-term care.

How does my plan meet the federal requirement for equal coverage of bodily illness and disease and of mental health or chemical dependency-related conditions? In light of the recent enactment of these requirements, your plan may not yet have disseminated information regarding its compliance with the law. Your question may remind the plan administrators to fully explain this important factor.

The questions above are not all-inclusive, but they offer guidance in ensuring that you are receiving the most comprehensive mental health and chemical dependency care to which your health insurance plan entitles you.

InfoLinks
www.bazelon.org

---

tigued due to the lack of adequate sleep because of their chronic anxiety. In addition, they often appear tense, as if their muscles were chronically prepared for explosive action regardless of the circumstances.

The treatment of GAD is, like many emotional disorders, approached through multiple treatment modalities, including counseling and pharmacological agents. In counseling, the therapist and others try to reduce stimuli that might be associated with the source of the patient's unfocused anxiety. Other approaches are designed to reduce anxiety through empathetic recognition of the painful symptoms patients experience. In addition, psychotherapy attempts to establish constructive coping techniques through which patients can become increasingly competent in managing remaining feelings of anxiety.

In support of the psychotherapy, the use of medications, such as benzodiazepines, can reduce somatic symptoms and help patients feel better. When anxiety impairs the ability to think, a nonbenzodiazepine, buspirone, is used. Antidepressants are often effective when depression accompanies an anxiety disorder. Response to treatment is variable, but some patients do show significant improvement.

Mood Disorders

Mood disorders, particularly depression, may be one of the most frequently occurring conditions that physicians fail to recognize. This may happen because depressed (or manic) people do not seek evaluation or because symptoms of mood disorders may be masked or confused with symptoms associated with other conditions. Today this is particularly unfortunate, since mood disorders can be treated with both medications and psychotherapy. Upon learning the symptoms of mood disorders, most people report knowing others whose moods and behavior clearly suggest such conditions, particularly clinical depression.

Bipolar Disorder   An important mood disorder is **bipolar disorder,** the condition widely known as *manic-depression.* Bipolar disorders are characterized by alternating periods of mania, in which affected people are highly excited, easily distracted, and very confident, followed by periods of depression, during which they lack motivation, withdraw from interpersonal involvement, harbor negative feelings of self-worth, and may even consider suicide. Traditionally, bipolar disorders have been treated with lithium, a drug that tends to normalize mood swings.[22]

> **bipolar disorder**   emotional disorder in which the mood swings between highly excited and depressed periods—manic-depression.

Depression Depression, a mood disorder classified as a **unipolar disorder,** is far more common than bipolar disorder. Depression is often described as falling into one of two categories: major depression and dysthymic depression. The classification depends on the onset and duration of symptoms. Major depression is characterized by the sudden (within a two-week period) onset of the following symptoms. Major depression can be mild, moderate, or severe.

1. Depressed mood most of the day
2. Markedly diminished interest or pleasure in all, or almost all, activities
3. Significant weight gain or loss when not dieting
4. Insomnia or hypersomnia nearly every day
5. Psychomotor agitation or retardation nearly every day
6. Feelings of worthlessness or excessive guilt nearly every day
7. Diminished ability to think or act decisively

Major depression is sometimes referred to as *endogenous depression* or *primary depression* because it frequently occurs without warning and in the absence of any environmental event, such as divorce, loss of employment, or death of a friend, that could logically account for its appearance. Accordingly, the cause of major depression is now thought to be biological, focusing on altered neurotransmitter function (at the synaptic junctions of the central nervous system [CNS]). This leads to a lethargic mood until it subsides on its own or is reversed by the use of neurotransmitter-altering medications. This form of depression is primarily treated with antidepressant medications, with or without supportive psychotherapy. Improvement, in conjunction with sustained use of antidepressant medication and/or psychotherapy, is usually very good.

Currently, four major types of antidepressant medications are in use: monoamine oxidase (MAO) inhibitors, tricyclic antidepressants, selective serotonin reuptake inhibitors (SSRIs) such as Prozac, and the newer serotonin/norepinephrine reuptake inhibitors such as Serzone and Effexor.[23] The physician considers the specific advantages of each class of medication in determining appropriate treatment. The later two forms have proven to be highly effective with relatively few of the side effects and **contraindications** associated with the MAO inhibitors and tricyclic antidepressants.

The second form of clinical depression, dysthymic depression, is often referred to as *exogenous, secondary,* or *reactive depression* because its onset can generally be traced to one or more environmental events, such as marital instability, sexual repression, or the death of a spouse or child. Symptoms associated with this form of depression, such as low energy level, poor appetite, sleep difficulties, and low self-esteem, are gradual in their onset; the duration of this form of depression may extend over months or years in the absence of effective treatment.

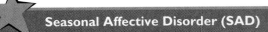

Seasonal Affective Disorder (SAD)

Recently, scientists have discovered that certain people may be especially vulnerable to depression on a seasonal basis. SAD is a form of depression that develops in certain people who live in cold climates. SAD affects four times as many women as men and is characterized by weight gain, excessive lethargy and sleep, social withdrawal, loss of sex drive, and mood swings, including feeling anxious and irritable. Although seen in adolescents, SAD more commonly begins in the young adult years.

SAD patients routinely feel much better with the coming of spring and summer, when the days are longer and the amount of sunlight increases. Fortunately, exposure to prescribed amounts of intense fluorescent light (phototherapy) helps many sufferers of SAD during the winter months. Anyone who suspects SAD or other forms of depression should seek professional assistance, perhaps through a counseling center or health center on campus.

In comparison to major depression, dysthymic depression is much more frequently treated with psychotherapy to address the more chronic, deep-seated causes. Antidepressant medication may also play a role in the treatment of this form of depression. A biological (or inherited) cause is less likely for this form of depression than for major depression. Interestingly, persons who are somewhat pessimistic by nature seem less likely than most people to experience depression. The Health Action Guide on page 41 lists resources for help with depression.

Personal Applications

• Have you ever been depressed? If so, what (if anything) seemed to trigger these feelings, and how did you resolve them?

Suicide One of the major tragedies of our time is the high incidence of suicide. In the last year for which statistics are available, 30,900 people in the United States killed themselves, including 5,300 under twenty-five years of age.[24] Among young people, suicides follow accidents as the second leading cause of death, although in certain segments of the young adult population deaths from homicide and HIV/AIDS now exceed those of accidents and suicide.

What separates the potentially suicidal person from the nonsuicidal person is the degree of despair and depression experienced and the inability to cope with it. Suicidal people tend to become overwhelmed with a range of destructive emotions, including anxiety, anger, loss of self-esteem, hopelessness, and loneliness (see the Star Box on p. 41). Suicidal people may feel that their death is a solution to all that is afflicting them. Rarely, however, does

HEALTH ACTION GUIDE

Resources for Help with Depression

If you or a friend had concerns about depression, would you know where to search for help? Regardless of where you are—large city, suburban community, or a rural area—a variety of resources are available.

- Seek help from your university health center, personal physician, or community health center.
- Try your university mental health counseling and treatment programs.
- Family and social service agencies can identify mental health specialists.
- Check the telephone book for private psychologists or psychiatric clinics.
- Talk with your professor.
- Contact one of the organizations listed below:
  The Depression/Awareness, Recognition and Treatment Program (operated by the National Institute of Mental Health) Room 15-C-05, 5600 Fishers Lane Rockville, MD 20857
  The National Foundation for Depressive Illness P.O. Box 2257 New York, NY 10016
  The National Mental Health Association 1021 Prince St. Alexandria, VA 22314
  The Manic-Depressive Illness Foundation 2723 P St. Washington, DC 20007

InfoLinks
http://depression.cmhc.com

Warning Signs of Suicidal Behavior

Change in appetite
Change in sleep pattern
Decreased concentration
Decreased interest in activities that were a source of pleasure
Sudden agitation or sudden slowing down in level of activity
Social withdrawal
Feelings of hopelessness, worthlessness, and self-reproach
Inappropriate or excessive guilt
Suicidal thoughts and/or talk
Making a suicide plan
Writing a suicide note
Giving away prized possessions
Recent humiliating life event
Lack of social support

suicide solve a problem. In fact, college students who use suicide to resolve academic failure, difficulties with relationships, or an inability to find employment leave far greater problems for others that dwarf the original concern.

Suicide Prevention Many communities are recognizing the need to provide or expand suicide preven-

Loneliness

Although not always associated with depression, signs of loneliness are displayed by many people who are depressed. People are said to be lonely if they desire close personal relationships but are unable to establish them. It is quite possible to feel isolated and without friends even when you are around many people in your everyday life. Feeling lonely is a common concern for many college students.

The difference between "being alone" and "feeling lonely" is important. Many people enjoy being alone occasionally to relax, to exercise, to read, to enjoy music, or just to think. These people can appreciate being alone, but they can also interact comfortably with others when they wish. However, when being alone or isolated is not an enjoyable experience and seeking close relationships is very difficult, then feeling lonely can produce serious feelings of rejection.

One unfortunate aspect of loneliness is that it tends to continue in people year after year, unless they take an active approach to change it. Chronically lonely people frequently cope with their loneliness by becoming consumed by their occupations or adopting habit-forming behaviors that make them feel even more lonely.

The positive side of loneliness is that successful techniques exist that can help most lonely people. Counseling can help change how these people think about themselves when they interact with others. Another way involves teaching people important social skills, such as starting a conversation, taking social risks, and introducing themselves. Through social skills training, people can also learn to talk comfortably on the telephone, give and receive compliments, and even learn how to enhance their appearance. If you need help in this area, contact your campus counseling center or health center.

tion services. Suicide prevention centers are already available in many communities. Most suicide prevention centers operate twenty-four-hour hot lines and are staffed through volunteer agencies, mental health centers, public health departments, and hospitals. Staff members in these centers have extensive training in counseling skills required to deal with suicidal people. Phone numbers for these services can be found in the telephone directory.

What signs and symptoms could indicate that a person might be considering suicide? It is recommended that we watch for the signs listed in the Star Box to the left. People need professional help when they show a clustering of these suicide warning signs for more than two weeks.

unipolar disorder depressed state during which people experience periods of lack of motivation and other symptoms—depression.

contraindication existing characteristic or condition whose presence makes the use of a particular medication or therapy inappropriate.

Obsessive-Compulsive Disorder Until recently, **obsessive-compulsive disorder (OCD)** was thought to be relatively rare, but today the condition is much more frequently seen due to the "unmasking" of its existence in terms of public awareness. Classified as an anxiety disorder, OCD appears to arise from a genetic predisposition, as the condition is known to run in families. The inherited biological basis for OCD is currently believed to involve the neurotransmitter serotonin as it functions in the locus ceruleus, an area in the fourth ventricle of the brain. The selective serotonin reuptake inhibitors used in treating depression, such as Prozac, Paxil, and Zoloft, are now used, often in combination with behavioral therapy.[25]

Obsessive-compulsive disorder presents itself as a combination of the following emotional and behavioral symptoms. The first four characteristics reflect the obsessive dimension of the condition, while the latter three reflect the compulsive dimension.[21]

Obsessive

1. Intrusive, recurrent, inappropriate thoughts, impulses, or images that are routinely felt to be uncomfortable
2. Unsuccessful attempts at offsetting these feelings by ignoring or neutralizing them through other actions
3. The obsessive feelings arise from within the individual
4. A lack of interest in problems that others would consider to be "real-life problems" as attention is focused on obsessive feelings

Compulsive

1. Repetitive behavior, such as counting, checking on doors, or handwashing, in response to the obsessive thoughts described above
2. The compulsive behaviors are unreasonable
3. The compulsive actions are time consuming and interfere with daily activities

When used in the absence of pharmacological support, behavioral therapy (see p. 45) may be beneficial for persons with OCD, but a combination approach appears most effective.

Panic Disorders (Panic Attack) A **panic attack** would be a difficult experience for most people to forget, since panic attacks generally have several unpleasant components. A partial listing of the more typical components of a panic attack follows.[21]

1. Rapid heart rate, chest pain, and palpitations that when combined may simulate the feelings of a myocardial infarction, or heart attack (see Chapter 10)
2. Sweating, chills, hot flashes, dizziness, and feelings of light-headedness
3. Choking, shortness of breath, and feelings of smothering
4. Nausea and vomiting
5. Feelings of numbness
6. Decentralization and depersonalization leading to feelings of loss of control, including "going crazy" and impending death

The distress of having a first attack and then having subsequent attacks, combined with worrying about the onset of the next, forms the basis of a panic disorder.

At this time the cause of panic disorder is thought to be an interplay of genetic predisposition to excessive cortical activity and triggering environmental events. Recent investigation has focused on specific brain areas that monitor internal and external stimuli going to the brain's cortex. These areas may contain faulty receptor sites for the neurotransmitters that produce cortical excitation. Accordingly, environmental events that have some potential to alter body function, such as caffeine consumption, strenuous activity, and breathing air with an excessive carbon dioxide content, can cause the brain to be overly aroused, thus producing a panic attack. An awareness of the cause of the attacks seems to be helpful in reducing the frequency of attacks.[26]

Today panic disorder can be successfully treated with a combination of medications, including benzodiazepines, clonazepam, monoamine oxidase inhibitors (MAOI), and antidepressants, particularly the selective serotonin reuptake inhibitors. These drugs work by blocking the excessive flow of excitatory signals reaching the surface (cortex) of the brain.[26]

Schizophrenia Schizophrenia, a label applied to a group of conditions associated with **personality deterioration,** is the most disabling illness that can be encountered by those afflicted and their families.[26] The characteristics associated with this disease attest to its debilitating nature.[21]

1. Delusions (false beliefs of importance)
2. Hallucinations (false sensory perceptions)
3. Disorganized speech
4. Catatonic behavior (immobility)
5. Negativism (motiveless response to all instruction)
6. Observable dysfunction in work, social, and self-care activities (in comparison to that in place prior to the onset of symptoms)

The preceding symptoms are generally continuous for a period of at least six months following onset and cannot be accounted for on the basis of any other general mood disorders. Various subtypes of schizophrenia, such as paranoid, disorganized, catatonic, and undifferentiated schizophrenia, are recognized by mental health professionals. Each form of the condition dictates the specific treatment employed, with some forms having a better prognosis than others. At this time, however, partial recovery is much more likely than is a complete return to high-level functioning.

The cause of schizophrenia (and other psychoses) has several contributing factors. The interplay of both biological and environmental factors seems necessary for the condition to express itself. Clearly, schizophrenia runs in families, has its clinical onset in late adolescence or early adulthood, and may be triggered by environmental stressors.

The biological basis of schizophrenia received significant attention in this decade after the discovery that genetically predisposed faulty functioning of receptor sites for the neurotransmitter dopamine is central to the onset of the condition. Clozapine (Clozarol), the current drug of choice in treating schizophrenia, and to a lesser degree chlorpromazine (Thorazine) and haloperidol (Haldol), has significantly improved management of the condition. Several clozapine-like agents are now being tested and are nearing market availability and should further improve the management of schizophrenia. Recent recognition of other neurotransmitters involved in schizophrenia, gamma-aminobutyric acid (GABA) and glutamate, requires further study and drug-related research. The presence of these additional pathways may explain the still-limited effectiveness of current treatment.[27]

Therapists Involved in the Management of Psychological Disorders

As in other areas of health care, a variety of practitioners, each of whom has unique training and uses specific therapies, treat and manage the mental health conditions just desribed. In the section that follows, we provide a brief description of the services rendered by psychiatrists, psychologists, counselors, and psychiatric social workers.

Psychiatrists

Psychiatry is the medical speciality concerned with diagnosis, treatment, and long-term management of the emotional and psychological disorders. Physicians who practice within this area of clinical medicine are, of course, **psychiatrists.** A variety of subspecialists, including child and adolescent psychiatrists, community psychiatrists, forensic psychiatrists, and neuropsychiatrists, can be found in major urban centers and in affiliation with large medical centers.

In comparison with other mental health practitioners, psychiatrists are unique in that they are medical practitioners holding the M.D. or D.O. degree (see

Chapter 18). On the basis of this medical licensing, psychiatrists are permitted to use diagnostic and treatment modalities unavailable to others. For example, psychiatrists may use medical imaging, invasive diagnostic tests, pharmacologic agents, electroconvulsive therapy, and surgery as components in the treatment of mental illness. Of course, like other practitioners, they also employ a variety of psychotherapies.

Psychologists

Unlike psychiatrists, **psychologists** are more limited in the treatment of mental illnesses because they do not possess the M.D. or D.O. degree. The academic preparation of psychologists involves graduate work in one or more fields of psychology, such as counseling, educational, industrial, or clinical psychology. The Ph.D., Ed.D., and M.S. degrees are most common among psychologists, although some practitioners, particularly those in the area of pastoral counseling, have completed degree work in divinity-related fields prior to their clinical training.

Atlhough psychologists may practice in a group setting with psychiatrists and thus have indirect access to medications and other treatment modalities, they are legally limited to the use of psychotherapy. The particular type of psychotherapy employed depends largely on the theoretical orientation of their university training. Selected forms of psychotherapy will be described later in the chapter (see pp. 44–45). Psychologists may also have special interest in particular client populations and thus have credentials in areas such as family, marriage, or sex therapy. Currently more than forty states have state-level certification for psychologists, based in part on standards developed by national (and even international) certification bodies.

---

obsessive-compulsive disorder emotional disorder in which inappropriate thoughts, impulses, or images are responded to with unreasonable repetitive behaviors.

panic attack sudden unanticipated onset of fearfulness, including physiological symptoms such as rapid heart rate, chest pain, and shortness of breath.

personality deterioration sudden or gradual change in personality, generally associated with the loss of functional abilities and an impaired quality of life.

psychiatrist physician trained in the diagnosis and medical treatment of emotional and psychological disorders.

psychologist non-physician practitioner trained in the diagnosis and treatment of emotional and psychological disorders through the use of psychotherapy.

Counselors

The mental health field of counseling is more broad-based than that of psychiatry and psychology in that a wider array of professionals, including psychiatrists and psychologists, engage in counseling others. For example, ministers, primary care physicians, guidance/counseling personnel in schools, chemical dependency counselors, employee assistance program counselors, and social workers supply counseling to selected groups. The word *counseling* describes both a field of practice and a form of practice directed toward certain patient populations.

Because of the range of settings in which some form of counseling occurs and the varying backgrounds of professionals who deliver counseling services, it is difficult to address specifically the education and certification that accompanies the practice of counseling. Certainly most states, professional associations, and mental health institutions have standards by which they judge the preparation of individual practitioners. However, with the existence of mail order college degrees, unaccredited storefront "colleges," and other means of securing transcripts and certificates of training, people most in need of professional assistance may be vulnerable to people who lack true professional counseling skills. Certainly, the consumer should be aware that it is still too easy in some areas of the country and on the Internet for almost anyone to claim counseling expertise.

Social Workers

As unrelated as it may initially appear, the field of social work is closely aligned with the current delivery of psychological health services. This relationship becomes more evident when the environmental aspects of various mental health disorders are considered. Clearly, the social environment within the family during a child's formative years provides much emotional resourcefulness. Conversely, often the social environment—in the form of peer group expectations, the demands of marriage and parenting, and the pressures of the workplace—eventually becomes the source of stress that triggers emotional distress. Who, then, would be better suited than the trained social worker to support ongoing therapy? The social worker can help define the problem, assist with modifying the family environment, and access and coordinate the many community services needed to support the patient's care.

An area of graduate-level specialization in the field of social work is that leading to certification as a psychiatric social worker. Those who hold this graduate degree are fully trained in psychotherapy and, thus, able to participate as therapists in the clinical setting. Psychiatric social workers, at least in some areas, engage in direct fee-for-service practices, much in the same manner of psychologists.

Cyberspace Psychotherapy: Treatment over the Internet

Is it possible to receive effective psychotherapy over the Internet? The answer is a qualified "yes." Although the trend is growing rapidly, concern exists over the lack of regulation and the effectiveness of the therapy received. Those who are interested in an on-line relationship with a psychotherapist should consider the following questions:

- What are the psychotherapist's academic/professional credentials?
- What fee structure is in place, and how are fees to be paid?
- How does the therapist protect confidential information?
- In what manner is a crisis situation managed, and under what circumstances is the therapist available for face-to-face counseling?
- Is the therapist able to refer and institutionalize if conditions warrant?

If all or most of these questions are answered satisfactorily, this new approach to psychotherapy may be appropriate. If not, traditional formats are generally available in most communities.

Forms of Psychotherapy

The current field of psychotherapy includes more than 200 approaches to the delivery of mental health services.[28] In spite of this apparent diversity, however, most specific approaches are based on only a few basic therapeutic approaches. In the section that follows, we look at psychoanalysis, psychodynamic therapy, behavioral therapy, cognitive therapy, and supportive therapy. In addition, the population to be served dictates the specific group composition and practice setting in which each is practiced. These include individual, small group, pair, and family configurations. In today's world, insurance companies strongly influence the type of therapy that a patient receives by deciding how much coverage will be assigned to each.

Psychoanalysis

Psychoanalysis is an extensive, intensive, and expensive form of therapy designed to identify the deepest unresolved conflicts of childhood that have shaped an individual's emotional makeup. By describing the events associated with these conflicts, patients are eventually able to more fully understand their own current emotional distress and move beyond their own past. This is accomplished by engaging in the uninterrupted expression (free association) of feelings and the detailed descriptions of past events within the context of trusting relationships with their therapists. This transference of previously unrecognized needs onto the therapist allows for clearer insights into the client's own makeup and a gradual setting aside of defense mechanisms though which the person formerly coped with guilt and anxiety. Because of the nature of its practice, psychoanalysis is the most individually centered form of therapy.

Because five to six weekly sessions are required, each lasting about an hour, and extending over years, psychoanalysis is the most expensive form of therapy within the mental health marketplace. Today, group health care plans will not approve this form of therapy, so its use has been restricted to the few who can afford it.

Psychodynamic Therapy

With the virtual unavailability of psychoanalysis, the basic tenets of psychoanalytical theory have been modified for use in a brief and more affordable format called *psychodynamic therapy.* In this form of insight-oriented therapy, people "associate" with their therapists much as is done in psychoanalysis, but only regarding conflicts and feelings of emotional distress that are occurring in the present. Therapists function as sounding boards so that patients can better understand their current distress and respond healthfully on a short-term basis, even when the origins of conflict are deeply buried in the past. Beyond the insights gained through this form of therapy, psychodynamic therapy can also provide a supportive environment and is, in this regard, well suited for people who are confronting the stressors associated with day-to-day activities (see Chapter 3).[28]

In recent years the tenets of psychodynamic therapy, and many other forms of psychotherapy, have been combined in a single supportive session called *brief counseling and therapy* or *single-session therapy.* In these single, intense, highly focused sessions, therapists attempt to help their clients understand the nature of a particularly emotionally stressful event, without attempting to uncover the deeper underlying conflicts that account for the current situation. The belief that such brief therapy does work is based on the observation that many people in more conventional therapy do not return after the first session, and that the underlying causes of deep, unresolved emotional conflict may never be resolved regardless of the amount of time and money spent. Thus, brief therapy is cheaper and probably as effective.

Behavioral Therapy

In somewhat the same way that brief counseling and therapy attempts to focus quickly and concisely on the most immediate problems being experienced by clients, behavioral therapy too is relatively brief and focused on behavioral approaches to resolving or living more comfortably with emotional distress.[28] By employing a variety of techniques, such as deep breathing, assertiveness training, systematic desensitization, and biofeedback, therapists assist clients in establishing control over their emotions during periods of conflict. Although generally done on a one-to-one basis with a therapist, behavioral therapy's various behavioral control techniques can also be introduced to individuals within group settings. Behavioral therapy has proven particularly successful when used with older adults, often in institutional settings.

Cognitive Therapy

As the name implies, *cognitive therapy* is based on developing an understanding of why conflict arises, how particular feelings and responses are counterproductive, what is likely to happen in the future, and which response patterns can be employed effectively in future settings. In particular, therapists try to help clients extinguish faulty thinking patterns that have relied on exaggeration, catastrophizing, overgeneralizing, or ignoring the causes of emotional conflict.[28]

Cognitive therapy can be undertaken individually or in group settings and is generally extended over ten to twenty sessions. This particular form of psychotherapy has proved to be effective in dealing with the depression experienced by those who are caring for the elderly.[28]

Supportive Therapy

Supportive therapy is often used in conjunction with other approaches to therapy already described. However, as a form of therapy in and of itself, supportive therapy employs empathetic communication by the therapist to undergird the constructive efforts being undertaken by clients. Encouragement and careful listening are the key skills employed by professionals who practice this focused form of therapy.

Group Therapy

Although many of the therapies described can be undertaken in groups, group therapy is a vehicle for resocialization of clients to offset the devastating effects of social isolation. In addition, the group setting allows a form of peer education to unfold in which clients learn from the successful efforts of others in resolving conflict or in gaining control of change. Because group therapy has been successful in the treatment of chemical dependency and eating disorders, it is a familiar form of psychotherapy in college counseling centers. In addition, it is cost effective in comparison to the expense of the one-to-one psychotherapy approaches described earlier.

Specialized Fields of Practice

One or more of these therapies are routinely used to treat people experiencing conflict arising from specific types of relationships or behavioral patterns.

Your Turn

- What kinds of risks is Keisha Saunders taking by returning to school after fourteen years?
- Of the challenges Keisha confronts as a nontraditional student, which do you think are real and which might she be imagining or exaggerating?
- In what ways can Keisha's life experiences and personal qualities contribute to her success as a nontraditional student?

And Now, Your Choices . . .
- If you're a nontraditional student, imagine you're in circumstances similar to Keisha's. What would be your concerns? How do you think you would behave?
- If you're a traditional student, have you ever been in class with one or more nontraditional students? If so, what did you like or dislike about the experience? Why?

For example, some therapists deal only with problems related to sexual dysfunction, and, thus, are specifically trained and certified as sex therapists. Accordingly, other therapists, on the basis of training, certification, and practice, see couples (or individuals) who are experiencing marital conflict. Thus, these therapists have practices that are focused or limited to marriage counseling. A third version of a trend toward greater specialization is that of family therapy. Again, using one or more approaches, family therapists deal with family members as a group, or with each member individually, as the course of therapy dictates. Specialized training and certification standards exist in this specialized area as they do for sex and marital therapists.

Specialization leads to greater expertise and more focused experience in a particular area for therapists, so it is likely that more restricted fields of practice will appear. However, we feel confident that the ultimate outcome of psychotherapy may relate as much to the relationships between clients and therapists as it does to the particular approaches used. Further, the ultimate success of therapy depends on the level of compliance that grows out of client-practitioner relationships.

Personal Applications

- If you were experiencing an emotional disorder, such as depression, would you consider consulting a therapist? Which form of treatment described would you feel most comfortable with?

Emotional and Psychological Wellness: A Final Thought

As discussed in the introduction to Chapter 2, psychological health is much more than the absence of mental illness. Rather, it is the resourcefulness that you are able to apply toward directing your own growth, assessing your beliefs and values, and dealing effectively with change, particularly when it is unexpected. Emotionally and psychologically healthy people possess a self-concept constructed on satisfying traits that can contribute to the well-being of others. Consequently, they experience an appropriately high level of self-esteem. The specific resources that each person draws from the emotional and spiritual dimensions of health to accomplish this will, of course, be unique.

Summary

- A positive self-concept fosters the development of self-esteem, which is the basis of emotional health and psychological well-being.
- Emotional wellness, reflecting familiar feeling states, is a component of a larger psychological wellness.
- Emotionally healthy people demonstrate an array of predictable emotional characteristics.
- Although biological factors may shape temperament, most mood states are influenced strongly by environmental factors.
- Emotionally healthy people display a normal range of emotions.
- Maintaining a sense of humor is a key to happiness and a healthy sense of well-being.
- People can nurture their self-esteem through the use of several effective techniques.
- Comfortable and effective verbal communication fosters enjoyable and self-enhancing social interaction.
- Nonverbal communication techniques often reinforce the effect of verbally communicated messages.
- Transcenders demonstrate characteristics associated with Maslow's highest level of need fulfillment, self-actualization.

- Creative people routinely demonstrate traits that are known to be associated with high levels of emotional well-being and psychological health.
- The existence of faith can form the foundation on which lifelong emotional well-being can be established.
- A four-step plan for creating the positive change that leads to an enhanced self-concept and self-esteem can be learned by everyone.
- General anxiety disorders (GAD) are common but respond well to both psychotherapy and appropriate medications.
- Mood disorders, including bipolar disorder, exogenous depression, and endogenous depression, often respond to appropriate therapy.

- Suicide has been described by some as a permanent solution to temporary problems.
- Obsessive-compulsive disorders and panic disorders are now effectively treated with medications in combination with psychotherapy.
- Schizophrenia is among the most limiting forms of psychological illness and may be caused by a genetically predisposed biological change in brain function.
- A wide range of health professionals treat emotional and psychological illnesses.
- Multiple forms of psychotherapy are available, ranging from in-depth psychoanalysis to short-term cognitive approaches.

Review Questions

1. What relationship is thought to exist between self-concept and self-esteem?
2. What is the difference between emotional wellness and psychological wellness? Which is the broader term?
3. What are the characteristics commonly demonstrated by emotionally well people?
4. Which component of your personality is most likely shaped by biological factors?
5. What is meant by the term "a normal range of emotions"?
6. What relationship is thought to exist between humor and a sense of emotional well-being?
7. What techniques have proved effective in helping people to nurture their own self-esteem?
8. What specific techniques are associated with effective verbal communications? What nonverbal communication techniques are useful in enhancing social interaction and supporting verbal communication?
9. How do transcenders appear and how does transcendence relate to need fulfillment?
10. What traits are associated with high levels of creativity?
11. How can faith form the foundation upon which a sense of well-being can develop?
12. What four steps can allow you to have some control over change and enhance your self-concept and self-esteem?
13. What behavioral and emotional characteristics are associated with a general anxiety disorder? What treatment approaches might prove effective?
14. How can one differentiate between the various forms of depression? What is the most effective treatment for each form?
15. How is suicide a "permanent solution to a temporary problem"?
16. What approaches are used today in the treatment of obsessive-compulsive disorder and panic disorders?
17. What physical and behavioral characteristics are frequently seen in persons with schizophrenia?
18. What professional titles are most frequently held by people engaged in the diagnosis, treatment, and management of emotional and psychological disorders?
19. What forms of psychotherapy are most frequently used today?

References

1. Baumeister RF, Smart L, Boden JM. Relation of threatened egotism to violence and aggression: the dark side of high self-esteem. *Psychol Rev* 1996 Jan; 103(1):5–33.
2. Bushman BJ, Baumeister RF. Threatened egotism, narcissism, self-esteem, and displaced aggression: does self-love or self-hate lead to violence? *J Pers Soc Psychol* 1998 July; 75(1):219–229.
3. *Late frost: reflections on aging.* Sherborn, MA: Aquarius Productions, 1993.
4. Sprunger MJ, PhD personal interview, April 1, 1997.
5. Grazino WG, Jensen-Campbell LA, Sullivan-Logan GM. Temperament, activity, and expectations for later personality development. *J Pers Soc Psychol* 1998 May; 74(5):1266–1277.

6. Caspi A, Silva PA. Temperamental qualities at age three predict personality traits in young adulthood: longitudinal evidence from a birth cohort. *Child Dev* 1995 April; 66(2):486–498.

7. Thorson JA et al. Psychological health and sense of humor. *J Clin Psychol* 1997 Oct; 53(6):605–619.

8. Yoshino S. Fujimori J. Kohda M. Effects of mirthful laughter on neuroendocrine and immune systems in patients with rheumatoid arthritis. *J Rheumatol* 1996 April; 23(4):793–794.

9. McGhee P. Rx: Laughter. *RN* 1998 July; 61(7):50–53.

10. Masters W, Johnson V, Kolodny R. *Human sexuality.* 5th ed. New York: HarperCollins, 1995.

11. Haas A, Haas K. *Understanding sexuality.* 3rd ed. St. Louis: Mosby, 1993.

12. Young K. *Caught in the Net: how to recognize the signs of Internet addiction and a winning strategy for recovery.* New York: John Wiley & Sons, 1998.

13. Maslow AH. *The farthest reaches of human nature.* Magnolia, MA: Peter Smith, 1983.

14. Hemenway JE, ed. *Assessing spiritual needs: a guide for caregivers.* Minneapolis: Augsburg Press, 1993.

15. Schneider M. Reflections on Cinco de Mayo: bridging two cultures. *Hispanic* 1996 May; 9(5):66.

16. Suryaraman M. San Jose, Calif., has one of nation's largest festivals for Cinco de Mayo. *Knight-Ridder/Tribune News Service* 1996 May 6: 506K7882.

17. Fowler J. *Faith development and pastoral care.* Philadelphia: Fortress Press, 1987.

18. Targ E, Thomson KS. Can prayer and intentionality be researched? Should they be? *Altern Ther Health Med* 1997 Nov; 3(6):92–96.

19. Hart Research Associates for *Prevention Magazine,* as reported in Can we talk?, as reported in *USA Today* 1997 March 18: 1D.

20. Regier DA et al. The U.S. mental and addictive disorders service systems: epidemiologic catchment area prospective 1-year prevalence rates of disorders and services. *Arch Gen Psychiatry* 1993; 50:85.

21. American Psychiatric Association. *Diagnostic and statistical manual of mental disorders.* 4th ed. Washington DC: American Psychiatric Association, 1994.

22. Jefferson JW. Lithium. Still effective despite its detractors. *Brit Med J* 1998 May; 316(7141):1330–1331.

23. *Physicians' desk reference.* 51st ed. Oradell, NJ: Medical Economics, 1998.

24. U.S. Bureau of the Census. *Statistical abstract of the United States: 1997.* 117th ed. Washington DC: U.S. Government Printing Office, 1997.

25. van Balkom et al. Cognitive and behavioral therapies alone versus in combination with fluvoxamine in the treatment of obsessive compulsive disorder. *J Nerv Ment Dis* 1998 Aug; 186(8):492–499.

26. Keltner NL, Schwecke LH, Bostrom CE. *Psychiatric nursing.* St. Louis: Mosby, 1995.

27. The frontiers of medicine. *Time* 1996 Fall; 148 (special issue, 14):47–50.

28. Teague ML, McGhee VL, Kearns D. *Health promotion: achieving high-level wellness in the later years.* 3rd ed. Madison, WI: Brown & Benchmark, 1997.

Suggested Readings

Caplan PJ. *They say your're crazy: how the world's most powerful psychiatrists decide who's normal.* Reading, MA: Addison-Wesley, 1996. This book, written by a mental health professional, is a highly critical look at the limitations of the *Diagnostic and Statistical Manual of Mental Disorders,* which is used throughout the field as the basis for diagnosing disorders. Once identified as dysfunctional by the content of the manual, the label often remains for a lifetime. The author is particularly critical of the weakness of the manual in regard to conditions seen in women and the emotional damage that exists until the end of life.

Gersten D, Dossey L. *Are you getting enlightened or losing your mind: how to master everyday and extraordinary spiritual experiences.* San Antonio, TX: Three Rivers Publishing, 1998. Where is the fine line that divides some profound psychological disorders, such as schizophrenia, and the equally unfamiliar and uncomfortable spiritual experiences some people report? Are near-death experiences, out-of-body experiences, visitations by angels, and cases of spontaneous healing the products of spiritual connectedness or illnesses to be diagnosed and treated? Dennis Gersten, MD, a practicing psychiatrist, attempts to help the reader discern between dysfunction and the occasional windows to spiritual transformation.

Lazarus AA, Lazarus CN. *The 60-second shrink: 101 strategies for staying sane in a crazy world.* San Luis Obispo, CA: Impact Publishing, 1997. This easy-to-read and easy-to-understand book is comprised of tightly compressed packets of information (about 60 seconds' worth) concerning the nature and resolution of virtually every problem faced in today's demanding world. Readers will learn about effective ways to control anger, improve marital relations, recognize depression, and counter anxiety. Those with a daily 60 seconds to spare may experience improved mental health while enjoying a morning cup of coffee.

Regush N. *The breaking point: understanding your potential for violence.* Buffalo, NY: Key Porter Books (Firefly Press), 1998. Can we learn to accept violent behavior as a natural component of people's psychological makeup? The author, a respected investigative reporter, contends that we can and must. In his view, so long as we place violent behavior in the category of "belonging to others," we will never address the changes in society needed to allow persons, including ourselves, to control this continuously present aspect of human nature.

topics for Today

Lending a Helping Hand: Becoming a Volunteer

From now on in America, any definition of a successful life must include serving others. —*Former President George Bush*

For a generation of Americans now in middle age, two federally funded voluntary agencies, Peace Corps[1] and VISTA[2] (Volunteers in Service to America), have provided new college graduates an opportunity to put their idealism into action by using their newly learned skills in service to others. Today hundreds (if not thousands) of programs at the local, state, national, and international levels provide a similar opportunity. Most recently, President Clinton committed renewed support of volunteerism for young adults by launching AmeriCorps, a paid service initiative, to help with college tuition. In April 1997 he joined forces with General Colin Powell to promote a "volunteer summit" held in Philadelphia. Volunteer service is what our leaders call for, but are we listening?

Americans traditionally have expended their time, talents, and energy more freely in support of others than have the citizens of many other highly industrialized nations. In fact, today 90 million Americans volunteer, and the monetary value of their volunteer time is estimated at $200 billion a year.[3] Many of these volunteers serve on committees, babysit, coach, and lead scout troops. Amigos de las Americas[4] (a program for teens to live and volunteer in Latin America), International Executive Service Corps[5] (a program for retired U.S. executives to help businesses in 122 foreign nations), and World Teach[6] (a program for college graduates to teach English in a foreign country) are examples of agencies that are using the skills of Americans to improve conditions in other parts of the world.

Helping Others and Improving Yourself

All major religions teach that it is more blessed to give than to receive. Of course, service benefits those in need, but volunteering is also good for the volunteer. It provides companionship, friendship, and fellowship in working toward a common goal. It allows us to use skills and talents that we normally don't use at our daily jobs. In this way, volunteering encourages us to branch out, learn new things, and become more well rounded. Volunteering can help someone have more power over his or her life. When working for a cause of deep personal concern, volunteers can be involved with information gathering and decision making that helps them to feel less helpless when facing that issue.

Other volunteers have different motivations. Some want to give back something to their neighborhood, hometown, or society at large. Some want to make the world a better place; they feel a strong sense of community and hurt when others hurt.[7] Some simply realize that action on an issue of importance to them requires their participation. A few volunteers are required to serve. In 1990, Southern University began requiring undergraduates to complete 60 clock hours of community service before graduation.[8]

More important than why or how people serve is that they *do* serve. Hungry people are fed, and trees are saved one by one—and it makes a difference. It also makes a difference in the lives of the volunteers. Providing service is good for the human psyche. It brings people from different backgrounds together, makes them feel useful, and raises the aspirations of all involved.

Helping others may also help your career. You can make business contacts as you meet other volunteers. Or becoming a volunteer might help your bosses identify you as someone with a balanced life who has unique ideas and displays strong leadership skills.[9] Volunteer work can even help your academic career. Most of the Southern University students mentioned above ended up enjoying their volunteer opportunities and improving their academic performance through the structure, planning, and discipline they learned while volunteering.[8]

Diversity among Volunteers

Volunteers are a very diverse group. Among recent American Institute of Public Service Jefferson Award recipients was Gustavo Reneria, a fourteen-year-old who teaches English to Latino immigrant children, and Billy Early, a 106-year-old woman who has logged more than 128,000 volunteer hours with the Red Cross.

That's equal to sixty-four years of forty-hour work weeks. She plans to volunteer for at least another ten years![10] The unsung volunteers who do not receive official recognition for their efforts are just as important. "Slowdog," for example, is a twenty-five-year-old college dropout who volunteers for the Center for Democracy and Technology, a group that fights for the preservation of free speech on the Internet. One group of volunteers is made up of college students who spend their summers at housing projects in Hartford, Connecticut, to counsel, tutor, and play with the children who live there. Elizabeth Wolff helps build schools and fight toxic waste with the Community Organization for Reform Now, ACORN. And Jacquette Johnson, whose picture appears at right, works with the Humane Society of Missouri to find loving homes for abused, neglected, and unwanted animals. Thankfully, the list goes on and on with the names of mothers, fathers, sisters, brothers, sons, daughters, neighbors, and friends whose gift of time and caring truly benefits us all.

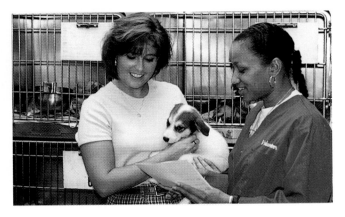

Jacquette Johnson helps both animals and their new owners by volunteering as an adoption counselor at the Humane Society of Missouri.

Ways to Volunteer

No matter what your interests, abilities, or time commitments, there is much you can do. Just a few of the many areas of volunteer opportunities are listed below:

AIDS	Literacy
Arts/cultural enrichment	Mental health
Business assistance	Nutrition
Citizenship	Physical environment
Civic affairs	Psychosocial support services
Consumer services/ legal rights	Recreation and sports
Day care/Head Start	Teen pregnancy prevention
Disaster response/ emergency preparedness	Parenting
Drug abuse/alcoholism	Transportation and safety
Education	
Employment	Animal welfare
Health issues	Women's crisis centers
Law enforcement/ crime prevention	

You can make a difference alone, with a few friends, or as part of an established organization. The Student Environmental Action Coalition has chapters at 2,200 high schools and colleges, VISTA (Volunteers in Service to America), and the Peace Corps, United Way, Salvation Army, and Red Cross are just a few of the national organizations in need of volunteers. To volunteer, you can contact one of these agencies or your local church, hospital, nursing home, city recreation department, or scout council directly or call the Nationwide Hotline on Volunteer Opportunities at 800-424-8867 or the Points of Light Foundation at 800-879-5400.

For Discussion . . .

Do you currently volunteer? Why or why not? If you decided to become a volunteer, what areas of work would most interest you? Can you think of a volunteer who has touched your life? How do you feel about compulsory volunteer service?

References

1. Peace Corps: *The toughest job you'll ever love.* October, 1998. (http://www.peacecorps.gov/home.html)
2. Catalog of Federal Domestic Assistance: *Volunteers in Service to America.* October, 1998. (http://aspc.os.dhhs.gov/cfda/p94013.htm)
3. Wofford H, Waldlman S, Bandow D. AmeriCorps the beautiful? *Policy Review* 1996; 79:28–36.
4. Amigos de las Americas. March, 1996. (info@amigoslink.org)
5. International Executive Service Corps. March, 1996. (62054816@eln.attmail.com)
6. World Teach. March, 1996. (worldteach@hiid.harvard.edu)
7. Morris T: Volunteerism & the community: a win-win situation. *Work & Learning Network News* 1998. 1(1):1–2.
8. Carpenter BW, Jacobs JS. Service learning: a new approach in higher education. *Education* 1994; 115(1):97–98.
9. Loeb M. The big payoff from public service. *Fortune* 1996; 133(5):135.
10. Meyerson A. Hundred-gallon heroes. *Policy Review* 1996; 75:7.

chapter
three

Coping with Stress

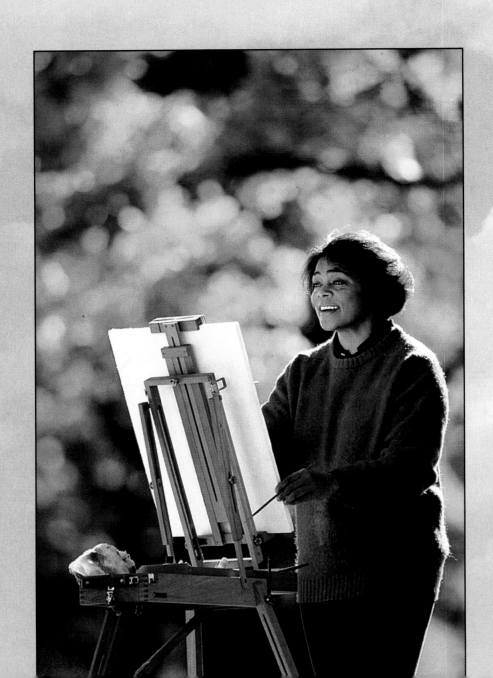

In the midwestern states, there is a familiar saying that if you don't like the weather, just wait a few minutes and it will change. Just as the weather is characterized by change, daily living is also influenced by change. Almost everything in the immediate environment holds the potential for being threatening because of its ability to change. Being able to control or adjust to this change can enrich life because change is often challenging, stimulating, and rewarding. When people handle change poorly, however, their responses result in a state of stress that can be both unpleasant and disruptive to wellness.

HEALTHY PEOPLE: LOOKING AHEAD TO 2010

An initial objective of the *Healthy People 2000* report was to reduce the proportion of people with stress-related health conditions. Progress in this area at mid-decade was most likely related to the development of worksite stress management programs. By 1995, nearly 40 percent more employees had access to stress management programs than in 1990.

However, the *Midcourse Review* also noted a lack of progress in reducing the number of people who were under stress but were unable to or uninterested in addressing this condition. For some people, community and worksite stress management programs continued to be unavailable. For others, the inability to master coping techniques or use them regularly reduced the effectiveness of the programs in which they enrolled.

Because stress significantly influences the development of illnesses such as cancer, cardiovascular disease, eating disorders, and infectious conditions, *Healthy People 2010* will continue to emphasize the importance of better and more widely available stress management programs. Several focus areas, including mental health services and community and educational programs, lend themselves to the further development of stress management programs.

Real Life
Real choices

- Name: Kate Sullivan
- Age: 21
- Occupation: Student/telemarketer/custodian

Four months from earning her bachelor's degree in social work, Kate Sullivan should be proud, happy, and excited. She'll graduate with honors from a state university, and she's already been awarded a fellowship to work on her master's degree.

Kate does feel happy about her accomplishments and her future—when she has time. That's not very often, because for the last four years she's done very little except study and work. Although she's on a tuition scholarship, Kate must work to pay for her living expenses, as well as making payments on the used car she needs to get to and from school and her two part-time jobs.

The oldest of seven children in a single-parent family, Kate sends home half of what she earns each month. When she was small, her father died in an automobile accident and left no money or insurance. After working for more than twenty years in a fertilizer processing plant, her mother is now on Social Security disability because of damage to her lungs and skin. Kate's younger brothers and sisters aren't old enough to earn much

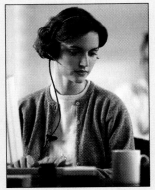

money, and Kate wants them to concentrate on their schoolwork, so she puts in as many extra hours as she can at her two jobs.

Parties, sports, clubs, vacations—these are foreign words to Kate. All her life she's worked hard and taken on adult responsibilities, and it's never occurred to her to feel sorry for herself. Recently, however, she's had trouble concentrating on her schoolwork, and more than once she's fallen asleep in a lecture. She averages about five hours of sleep a night and has been waking up feeling as tired as if she's run a marathon. Concerned friends and her academic adviser urge her to ease up and take some time off to relax, but Kate is afraid that if she lets up for a minute, she'll never catch up.

As you study this chapter, think about the stressors in Kate's life and prepare yourself to answer the questions in **Your Turn** at the end of the chapter.

Stress and Stressors

Late each summer, tens of thousands of students, both of traditional age and nontraditional age, begin a new academic year that is certain to confront them with change. New majors, courses, classmates, child care providers, living arrangements, practice schedules, and employment responsibilities arise within hours of arrival on campus and continue in various ways throughout the course of the semester. Whether these episodes of change serve as **stressors** and elicit the emotional and physiological change that we call **stress** depends largely on the interpretation made by the students.

For those who become distressed by the types of changes just described, the discomfort may relate closely to their fears of the unknown, failure, commitment, disapproval, and even success.[1] In comparison, those students who thrive in the face of change do so largely because of differences in their interpretation regarding the unpleasantness of change, the insights they have gained from past experiences dealing with change, and the array of effective coping skills they have developed by trial and error and by the careful observation of those who handle change well.

Although people often use the words *stressor* and *stress* interchangeably, they represent different concepts. Hans Selye,[2] the father of our current stress

theory, described stress as the nonspecific response of the body to any demand made on it. Stress can be viewed as a physiological and psychological response to exposure to some factor, agent, or event that forces us to change or adapt. Some experts categorize stressors as *acute* when caused by a single episode of stress, *episodic* when stress relates to a pattern of challenge (for example, the examinations given by a particular professor), and *chronic* when feelings of distress are ever present (for example, a work environment characterized by routine harassment by a supervisor or coworker). Regardless of their rate of occurrence, however, stressors are the cause; stress is the effect. The absence of change can also serve as a stressor, such as when a relationship is not maturing despite the effort you have put into it.

Variation in Response to Stressors

Because individuals are unique, a stressor for one person might not be a stressor for another. For example, if a babysitter must be found because the local public schools are closed for a teachers' in-service day, some people are more distressed than others. This variation results from the unique interpretation each person applies in making decisions about the disruptive nature and seriousness of the change.[3]

Learning
From Our Diversity

Stress in a Minor Key: Dealing with the Pressure of Discrimination

Throughout this chapter you will learn about the complex relationship between events defined as stressful and the mind-body response that results. You will read about the emotional discomfort that accompanies stressful events and, by the end of the chapter, will appreciate more fully the subtle but powerful physical responses of the body to stressors. These responses are of concern to health-care professionals because they affect the functioning of all body systems and are believed to play a role in medically diagnosable illness. People who are exposed to chronically high levels of stress appear to be at greater risk for potentially serious health problems than those exposed to less powerful stressors.

In contemporary American society, selected groups of people are exposed to powerful and frequent stressors because of their group affiliation. Minority status based on gender, race, ethnicity, sexual preference, disability, educational attainment, and a host of other characteristics subjects individuals to discrimination by majority segments of society. This in turn gives rise to a wide array of stressors, high levels of stress, and stress-induced illnesses. In fact, cross-sectional research that compares members of minority groups to their counterparts from majority groups frequently reports that minorities experience higher

levels of illness known to have stress-related components.[4] Hypertension in African-American males, for example, is frequently reported in magazine articles addressing minority health issues, accompanied by an explanation of the relationship between discrimination, anger, the stress response, elevated blood pressure, and the eventual risk of stroke and heart attack.

Experts suggest that perhaps the most effective tool for coping with racial discrimination is for African-Americans not to suppress anger or release it aggressively but to express it calmly, to be assertive, and to seek support—from friends, church, or a support group. Other ways to minimize the harmful effects of discrimination are to exercise regularly and to eat a diet low in fat and salt. Additional healing techniques are meditation and psychological counseling.

In a perfect world, no one would suffer the humiliation and rage induced by discrimination. In our less than perfect world, however, it's good to know that people subjected to such unfair treatment can take positive steps to minimize its effects on their health and well-being.

If you are a minority group member, how do you handle the discrimination you encounter? If you are not a minority, how do you think you would react if you were subjected to unfair treatment on the basis of your skin color, religion, ethnic heritage, or physical characteristics?

Personal Applications

- Thinking back to your most recent stressful experiences, what were the stressors responsible for the stress that you felt? Should similar situations arise again, would you be more or less likely to define them as stressors? Why?

Positive or Negative Stressors

Stressors produce the same generalized physical response whether individuals view these stressors as good or bad. Poor academic performance, loss of a friend, or being the only minority student on the dorm floor can cause stress (see the Learning from Our Diversity box above), just as giving birth, receiving a promotion, or starting a passionate romance can be a stressor. In each case, the effect on the body's physical function is relatively similar.

Selye coined the word **eustress** (in contrast to distress) for positive stress. Stressors that produce eustress can enhance longevity, productivity, and life satisfaction. Examples include the mild stress that helps you stay alert during a midterm examination, the anticipation you feel on the first day of a new job,

and the exhilarating stress you feel during vigorous exercise. In fact, some suggest that a personality type, type R (risk takers), may "require" the regular occurrence of high-risk activities.[5] Activities such as skydiving, roller coaster riding, and white-water rafting are undertaken frequently by those with type R personalities to generate an epinephrine (adrenaline) rush (see p. 64) and thus a sense of well-being. These people in particular demonstrate a strong sense of confidence, self-effectiveness, courage, creativity, and optimism that they use to plan to be stressed.

---

stressors   factors or events, real or imagined, that elicit a state of stress.

stress   the physiological and psychological state of disruption caused by the presence of an unanticipated, disruptive, or stimulating event.

eustress (**yoo** stress)   stress that adds a positive, enhancing dimension to the quality of life.

distress   stress that diminishes the quality of life; commonly associated with disease, illness, and maladaptation.

Selye calls harmful, unpleasant stress **distress.** Distress that is not controlled can result in a variety of illnesses (see below) and even death. For persons who have experienced profound distress, such as that associated with combat, the incidence of illness and illness-inducing behaviors clearly is higher.[6,7] Again, however, similar experiences may be more or less stressful, depending on the person's interpretation of the event's unpleasantness. Further, when distress becomes overwhelming, some people may attempt suicide.[8]

Personal Applications

• If the body's response to stressors is similar for distress and eustress, how do we learn to distinguish between the two?

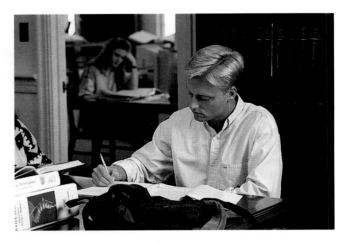

College life presents many stressors.

Inevitability of Stress

Only in death can stress be avoided. People live their lives trying to accommodate a variety of stressors, many of which they are unaware. Stress motivates and stimulates people to action. The key to lifelong satisfaction seems to lie in the ability to accommodate myriad positive and negative stressors. Mental health professionals encourage people to identify the stress levels at which they can best function as productive, contributing, happy people.

Uncontrolled Stress Related to Disease States

If the effect of a stressor is not minimized or resolved, the human body becomes exhausted, producing emotional and physical breakdown. This breakdown leads to stress-related diseases and disorders. Among the major diseases that have some origin in unresolved stress are hypertension, stroke, heart disease, kidney disease, depression, alcoholism, and gastrointestinal disorders (including irritable bowel syndrome and diverticulitis). Other stress-related disorders are migraine headaches, allergies, asthma, hay fever, anxiety, insomnia, impotence, and menstrual irregularities. The dependency-related behaviors of cigarette smoking, overeating and undereating, and underactivity relate in part to unresolved stress. Completing the Personal Assessment on page 57 will help you determine your risk for stress-related illness.

College-Centered Stressors

For some people who have not attempted college course work, the idea that college life could be stressful must seem strange. After all, even for non-

traditional students, isn't it the good life to be on an exciting campus with thousands of bright, interesting people?

For those of us who study or teach on college campuses, these perceptions are hard to understand.[9] We know all too well that the undergraduate experience is serious because of its role in preparation for life. For the part-time, nontraditional student who comes to campus for course work (often at night) and then returns to work, family, and community responsibilities, college classes can be especially stressful. Complete the Personal Assessment on page 58 to determine your level of vulnerability to stress.

In college and university settings, stressors can arise from any of the following areas.

Employment Expectations

For those students who believe that the main purpose of getting a college education is to prepare them for a job and a higher standard of living than that of their parents, the question of having chosen the "right" course of study is at times extremely stressful. Uncertainty about job opportunities, technical capabilities, starting salaries, and the need for a graduate degree becomes increasingly pressing when one begins to realize that college will soon end and that the world of employment (or nonemployment) awaits.

For the nontraditional-age student who is already working, employers' needs and expectations can create stress. Having a key presentation at work and an important examination at school on the same day, for example, can be overwhelming. Working students often feel torn between these demands. Some employers may even create difficulties for an employee who returns to school because they fear that he or she will move on to a better job after graduation.

Personal Assessment

Which of the following events have you experienced in the past 12 months?

Life event	Point value
_____ Death of a close family member	100
_____ Jail term	80
_____ Final year or first year in college	63
_____ Pregnancy (yours or your partner's)	60
_____ Serious illness or injury	53
_____ Marriage	50
_____ Any interpersonal problems	45
_____ Financial difficulties	40
_____ Death of a close friend	40
_____ Arguments with your roommate (more than every other day)	40
_____ Major disagreements with your family	40
_____ Major change in personal habits	30
_____ Change in living environment	30
_____ Beginning or ending a job	30
_____ Problems with your boss or professor	25
_____ Outstanding personal achievement	25
_____ Failure in a course	25
_____ Final examinations	20
_____ Increased or decreased amount of dating	20
_____ Change in working conditions	20
_____ Change in your major	20
_____ Change in your sleeping habits	18
_____ Vacation of several days	15
_____ Change in eating habits	15
_____ Family reunion	15
_____ Change in recreational activities	15
_____ Minor illness or injury	15
_____ Minor violations of the law	11

SCORE: _____

Interpretation

Life events can function as stressors that influence the body through activation of the stress response. An accumulation of 150 or more points (see point ranges below) in a 1-year period may lead to increased physical illness during the coming year. Of course, you must remember that, for a given person, certain events may be more or less stressful than the point values indicated.

Less than 100: limited likelihood of stress-related illness

101 to 200: moderate likelihood of stress-related illness

201 or above: high likelihood of stress-related illness

To Carry This Further . . .

Having completed this Personal Assessment and evaluated your responses based on the interpretation, were you surprised by the number of stress points that you generated? Are there stressors listed that you have not encountered either in your own experiences or in those of your close friends?

Personal Assessment

A wide variety of situations can function as stressors that influence us physically and psychologically. This assessment will help you to identify situations that could be stressful and to determine your overall vulnerability to stress. Use the following scoring system for each situation listed.

1 = Always (yes)
2 = Almost always
3 = Most of the time
4 = Some of the time
5 = Never (no)

Situation	Score
I get the appropriate amount of sleep my body needs to function.	_____
I exercise to the point of perspiring at least twice a week.	_____
I do not smoke, or I smoke less than half a pack of cigarettes a day.	_____
I regularly attend club or social activities.	_____
I have one or more friends to confide in about personal matters.	_____
I am able to vent my feelings when angry or worried.	_____
I am able to organize my time effectively.	_____
I drink fewer than three cups of coffee (or tea or cola drinks) a day.	_____
I take quiet time for myself during the day.	_____
I do not procrastinate; I get things done right away.	_____
Before a test, I go to bed at the same time I normally would.	_____
I live at home (with my family or spouse) while attending school.	_____
I try not to let other people's problems become my own.	_____
(If sexually active) I practice safe sex.	_____
The people closest to me are supportive of my goals.	_____
I have money to meet recreational expenses.	_____
I am attending college by choice.	_____
I rarely compare myself with my friends.	_____
I do not hold a job and go to school full time.	_____
My grade point average goal is set only for personal satisfaction.	_____
I do not plan to go on to higher levels of education.	_____

Scoring

Your Total Points _____ – 20 = _____ Final Score

Interpretation

30–49   Points = Vulnerable to stress
50–75   Points = Seriously vulnerable to stress
76–105   Points = Extremely vulnerable to stress

To Carry This Further . . .

Having completed this Personal Assessment and the interpretation based on your responses, is the "stress status" indicated by your score compatible with your feelings regarding your vulnerability to stress? Have you identified the specific types of behavior that need alteration to reduce your level of vulnerability to stress?

Institutional Expectations

For entry into the "community of educated people," college places demands of various types on students. Concerns centered on course selection, course withdrawal, admission to upper-division classes or graduate school, and performance on examinations (see the Health Action Guide below) are all potential stressors. For those who are just beginning the process of orchestrating a schedule of class work that will encompass eight semesters or twelve quarters or longer, the frustration arising from this responsibility can be quite stressful. Nontraditional students who are attempting to balance school with family and employment may find these expectations to be particularly demanding. (See the Health Action Guide on p. 68.)

Financial Support

How much does a college education cost? Is it worth the money, especially at a time when loans are difficult to find and expensive to repay? Should students consider ROTC as a source of assistance in light of the fact that a military obligation awaits after graduation? For some students these questions are not stressful, but for many students these are among the most pressing of all concerns. Each registration period,

each loan application, and each statement of need reintroduces these feelings of frustration and uncertainty for some college students.

Personal Expectations

While addressing the new freshmen during their orientation meeting, a college dean may tell students to shake the hands of the two people sitting next to them, because on the basis of the school's attrition (dropout) rate, one will not be in their class at the end of the year. As they extend their hands to the persons next to them, the reality strikes that hands are being extended toward them. Will they be among the students who will fail to complete the freshman year? Will they be among the nearly 47 percent of all college students who do not complete an undergraduate degree within five years of beginning college?[10]

Family Expectations

For many traditional-age students, college is an experiment in disengagement from the family. For nine months each year they are given a relatively free hand at structuring their lifestyle—being responsible for completing course requirements, establishing social relationships, and managing their own time.

If these responsibilities seem difficult, then they may be stressed by the feeling that they are not capable of doing what others expect. For many, this "disengagement shock" is the most pressing stressor that they will face. For some, the adjustment will be too great and they will return to their families or to work before making further educational decisions. For nontraditional students, family expectations may come from spouses or children who are counting on them to do well in school.

Time Management

As suggested above, the productive use of time is a significant problem for many college students either because of the poor use of "free time" associated with a typical school day or because of the added demands of marriage, employment, and parenting. Even the minutes you spend each day commuting, waiting in campus lines, attending athletic practice, or hanging out with friends can make quality time for schoolwork in short supply. Ultimately, however, it becomes an issue of priorities and the management of your time.

Although there is no single best approach to managing your time, most experts suggest that the following would be helpful:

- Keep a log of how you use your time for one week. Check about each half hour to see what you are doing at that time.
- Analyze these records, and eliminate those activities that take too much time relative to their importance.

HEALTH ACTION GUIDE

Coping with Test Anxiety

Examinations have always been a major part of student life. Consequently, many students develop an incapacitating anxiety when preparing to take tests. Compare your current test preparation activities with the following approach recommended by experts:

- Find a location conducive to study.
- Set a formal schedule for your test preparation.
- Keep complete resources, including class notes, background reading material, and reference texts, available.
- Create learning aids to help you, such as review questions, illustrations, outlines, definitions of technical terms, and sample test items.
- Be your own best friend by going to class, taking notes, joining and contributing to an ongoing study group, asking questions in class, and making appointments to visit with your professor to clarify material.
- Be kind to yourself by getting adequate sleep, eating balanced meals, exercising, taking time to be reflective, and staying sober.

On the basis of your comparisons, do you have any greater insight as to why you might be anxious about examinations? How do your study habits compare? Remember, most colleges and universities have counseling centers that can help you with study skills and test anxiety.

InfoLinks
www.collegeview.com/student/step1.html

- Once you have made these eliminations, divide your time into blocks so that related activities can be scheduled together. Examples might include academics, employment, recreation, and socializing.
- Schedule specific activities within each block of time. Attempt to conclude each activity you start.
- Reassess your activities occasionally and make adjustments when necessary.[11]

Cultural Conflicts

For many people, the culture of which they are a part does not assign great value to formal education, particularly a college education. Breaking away from a family that believes that little can be attained by more education or departing from a neighborhood characterized by poverty, gangs, crime, and drug abuse will challenge even the most resourceful person. Fortunately, as colleges and universities become more experienced in meeting the needs of these students, greater sensitivity on the part of faculty, staff, and fellow students, in combination with support programs, is making these transitions easier. It is necessary, however, for students to join the institution in searching out and finding each other so that these resources can be used effectively in reducing the stress of attaining a higher education.

Religious Faith

Consider this scenario: By the end of the first semester at college you no longer attend religious services. You become an agnostic by the middle of the second semester, and by the end of your first year in college you are a confirmed atheist.

As ridiculous as this scenario may sound, it could be the anticipated "falling from grace" imagined by some as they see young people leave the security of their homes for life on the "radical" college campus. Interfaith dating could be an even more common religion-oriented stressor. Questions about religion can become a part of the educational experience and be the source of uncertainty and stress. Higher education is designed to challenge your knowledge, values, and practices so that you may serve people better in the future. Many will find their religious beliefs challenged. Regardless, in a recent survey of young adults ages 18 to 30, 42 percent identified *religious involvement* as one of their highest priorities, up 4 percent since a similar survey in 1989.[12]

Faculty Expectations

Faculty members consider the college classroom a very real part of the world. It is an arena in which they experience success or failure. It is one of their major means of achieving a sense of contribution. Most professors take their teaching seriously, and they expect students to pursue their studies with

equal seriousness. Should students disregard this academic reality, stressors could occur in the form of poor grades or weak employment recommendations. Indeed, faculty expectations can be a major stressor for students.

Education in a college or university setting is never passive. It will nearly always demand active participation and effort and at times may demand more than students believe they are capable of giving. Not surprisingly, it is frequently the source of many stressors.

Personal Applications

- In comparison to the college-related situations that were stressful for you when you began college, are your most recent stressors different? If so, why? Which collegiate stressors are most likely to follow you from the college campus into your later life?

Life-Centered Stressors

For all of us, day-to-day living provides stressors that must be confronted and resolved. Although these stressors might differ from those associated with college, these life-centered stressors hold the same potential for causing physical and psychological distress.

When adults were asked to identify the causes of their stress, not surprisingly, many familiar factors surfaced.

Cost of Living

From necessities to luxury items, the cost of goods and services can easily exceed our financial resources. Particularly for nontraditional students with children, rent to pay, and a limited earning ability, the cost of living can be a powerful stressor.

Other Financial Concerns

On a nearly day-to-day basis most Americans have concerns regarding expenses that are less predictable than those associated with fixed expenses such as food and housing. Included among these are the costs associated with baby-sitting, entertainment, medical care costs, and home repairs. In regard to longer-term financial transactions, people are often confused and concerned about the complexity of contracts, retirement plans, taxes, loans, and investments.

Job Insecurity

Driven by corporate concerns over profit and competitiveness, the downsizing (or "rightsizing") of the American workforce has emerged as a principal stressor of the 1990s. Particularly for middle-age employees, the uncertainty of not knowing whether on a given day their job will be eliminated is a stressor of major proportions. When loss of health insurance and retirement benefits is added to the mix, the stress of the workplace may be greater than at any time since the Great Depression.

Loss of Property
When a home, business, or farm is lost, a sense of chronic stress may result. Each year, in all areas of the country, tornadoes, hurricanes, drought, floods, brush fires, arson, vandalism, and accidents destroy years of investment and effort. In too many cases the victims had inadequate insurance and limited financial ability to repair and rebuild, and ultimately the lack of strength and resolve to commit so much again.

Being Too Busy
People can often experience short and long periods of time during which more is asked of them than they have time to give. Single parents who are also college students find that the lack of time is constant. The day seems too short for all that needs to be done (see the Topics for Today article on p. 74).

Relaxation
At times people can be consciously aware that relaxation is in their best interest but are nevertheless unable to do so. Far too often they bring lists (both real and mental) of things that need to be done into those aspects of their lives that should be free from the demands of work, school, and parenting.

Family Illness
Many people eventually may experience family illnesses involving spouses, children, or aging parents. Middle-aged, nontraditional students who are part of

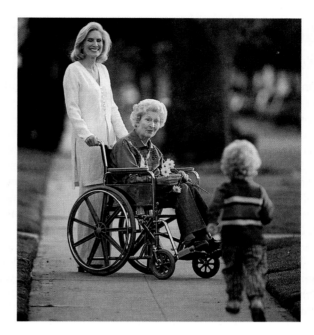

Midlife adults in the "sandwich generation" may have both children and aging parents to care for.

the "sandwich generation" may find that having children and older parents who both need care can be very stressful. When elderly parents become frail, they often live far from the homes of their adult children, thus complicating the orchestration of the services they need.

Personal Illness
Often without notice, people can be confronted by their own illnesses, leading to fear, apprehension, and inconvenience. In addition to the monetary costs, changes in role relationships, modifications of lifestyle, and challenges to self-esteem resulting from physical changes and the pain of recognizing our own mortality can make illness a major life stressor.

Personal Safety
Today, more than ever, concerns over personal safety introduce stress into many people's lives. As random, senseless killings escalate on the streets, at worksites, and in homes, many would claim this as a significant source of stress also.

Clearly, the college and lifestyle-related factors identified can result in stress that challenges the mind and insults the integrity of the body. (See HealthQuest Activities box.)

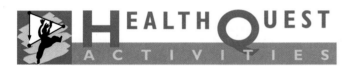

- The *How Stressed Are You?* activity in Module 1 allows you to look at several areas of your life (including money, school, relationships, and health) and identify stress caused by events and daily hassles. You can also rate your perceived stress level for each area. Use this feature to find out which area or areas generate the highest levels of stress for you.

- The *CyberStress* activity in Module 1 simulates a stress-filled day and can be used to help you assess your reactions to daily stressors. Choose the scenario that most closely matches your own. For example, if you work and go to school, you should check both on the preferences screen. As you are presented with stressful situations, choose the reaction that is closest to how you would react. At the feedback screen, print the screen showing your score. Then evaluate your experience by answering the questions in the *What do you think?* section.

Personal Applications

• Which life-centered stressors are most familiar to you already? Which do you anticipate being a part of your future? In what way might this anticipation work to your benefit?

Generalized Physiological Response to Stressors

Once under the influence of a stressor, people's bodies respond in remarkably similar, predictable ways. For example, on being asked to stand up in front of a group and talk, a person's heart rate increases, throat becomes dry, palms sweat, and he or she feels dizzy or lightheaded. The person may even become nauseated. Similar feelings would be felt if a person were told that she had lost her job or that her spouse wanted a divorce. It is clear that different stressors are able to elicit these common physical reactions.

Selye described the typical physical response to a stressor in his **general adaptation syndrome** model. Selye stated that the human body moves through three stages when confronted by stressors, as explained below.

Alarm Reaction Stage

Once exposed to any event that is seen as threatening, the body immediately prepares for difficulty. The involuntary changes described in Figure 3-1 are controlled by hormonal and nervous system functions and quickly prepare the body for the **fight-or-flight response**.[13]

Resistance Stage

The second stage of response to a stressor, the resistance stage, reflects the body's attempt to reestablish internal balance, or a state of homeostasis. The high level of energy seen in the initial alarm stage cannot be maintained very long. The body therefore attempts to reduce the intensity of the initial response to a more manageable level. This is accomplished by reducing the production of adrenocorticotropic hormone (ACTH) (see p. 64), thus allowing specificity of adaptation to occur. Specific organ systems become the focus of the body's response, such as the cardiovascular and digestive systems.[14]

Because of the ability to move from an alarm stage into a less damaging resistance stage, effective coping or a change in the status of the stressor will probably occur. As control over the stressful situation is gained, homeostasis is even more completely established and movement toward full recovery is seen. At the completion of this recovery, the body has returned to its prestressed state and there is minimal evidence of the stressor's existence.

Exhaustion Stage

Body adjustments required as a result of long-term exposure to a stressor often result in an overload. Specific organs and body systems that were called on during the resistance stage may not be able to resist a stressor indefinitely. Exhaustion results, and the stress-producing hormone levels again rise. In extreme or chronic cases, exhaustion can become so pronounced that emotional breakdown or death can occur.

The Stress Response

Why could something as familiar as a telephone ringing late at night cause a person to feel fear and near-panic? Why is it that your hands sweat, your muscles tense, and your appetite leaves as you wait in the hallway outside the classroom in which your final examination is to be held? These answers are simple and based on the body's primitive interpretation of reality. The body is looking for energy because it believes that all change is threatening and can be confronted by running, fighting, scaring the "adversary" away, or engaging it in sexual activity (the flight, fight, fright, or folly response). For these responses, the body simply needs energy for physical activity. In the sections that follow, Figure 3-1 will be explained.

Stressors

For a state of stress to exist, a person must first be confronted by change, real or imagined. Any change holds the potential for becoming a stressor and subsequently stimulating the stress response.

Sensory Modalities

Before a change event can be responded to as a stressor, however, the central nervous system must first sense the event. With the exception of stressors that are products of the imagination, a person must hear, smell, taste, feel, or see something changing so that it can be transformed into electrical impulses within the nervous system and thus become capable of eliciting the stress response.

Cerebral Cortex

Events become stressors when, on entering the cerebral cortex of the brain, they are perceived as stressors. By a person's own determination, some, but not all, events are stressors. Remember the phone ringing late at night? Should that very same phone have rung twelve hours earlier (during the afternoon), its ringing would probably not have been interpreted as stressful. Recall that in most cases the more accurately you interpret change, the less often you will experience stress.

---

general adaptation syndrome the sequenced physiological response to the presence of a stressor; the alarm, resistance, and exhaustion stages of the stress response.

fight-or-flight response the reaction to a stressor by confrontation or avoidance.

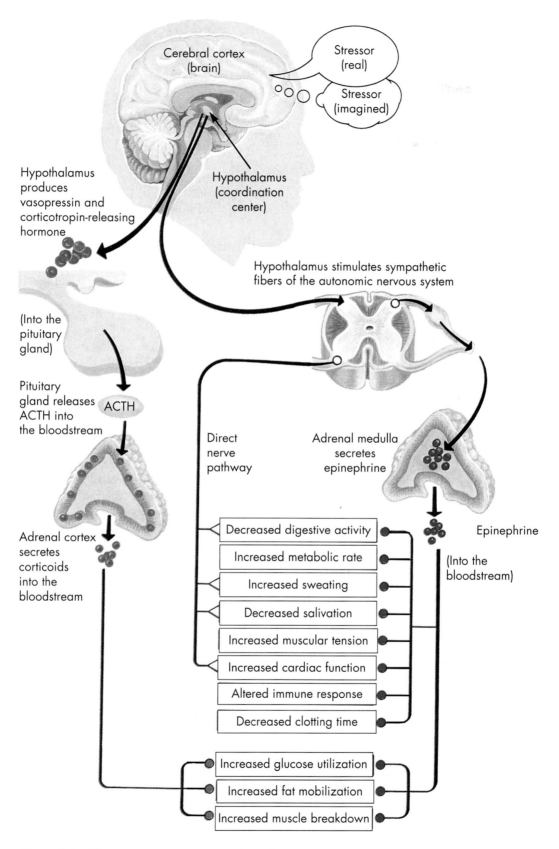

Figure 3-1 The stress response: physiological reactions to a stressor.

Endocrine System

The body's response to the presence of a stressor involves not only the brain and nervous system but also the *endocrine system.* The process of interconnecting the nervous system and the endocrine system is the task of the **hypothalamus,** a structure located deep within the brain. The hypothalamus is situated immediately above the gland that plays the most important role in regulating the endocrine system, the **pituitary gland.**[15]

During periods of stress, communication between the hypothalamus and the pituitary gland is accomplished by the release from the hypothalamus of chemical messengers into the blood flowing directly to the pituitary gland. Two of these, *vasopressin* (VP) and *corticotropin-releasing hormone* (CRH), influence the production of **adrenocorticotropic hormone (ACTH).**[16] ACTH is then released into the bloodstream, ultimately reaching the paired **adrenal glands**[15] of the endocrine system. ACTH stimulates the outer layer (cortex) of the adrenal glands to produce a family of chemical substances called **corticoids.** The mineralocorticoids principally influence blood volume and, thus, blood pressure by conserving water and salt, while glucocorticoids support the powerful hormone **epinephrine** (commonly known as **adrenaline**) in the release of energy.

The hypothalamus also activates the adrenal gland directly through a branch of the autonomic nervous system. This direct sympathetic stimulation of the adrenal gland is also responsible for the production of epinephrine. Epinephrine causes most of the changes that occur in the body to produce the rapid, short-term high energy levels required in the stress response.

Epinephrine-Influenced Responses

Once epinephrine has been released by the medulla of the adrenal gland, many of the following tissue responses can be expected.

Decreased Digestive Activity

Because the body needs energy when a stressor must be avoided or an adversary must be defeated, it cannot wait for digestion to change food into glucose. Rather, the body must turn to the glucose already circulating in the bloodstream or in a storage form within tissue. As a consequence, the entire digestive system slows down. It is not surprising, then, that many people who are under chronic stress report episodes of gastric distress, including constipation and irritable bowel syndrome.

Increased Metabolic Rate

Epinephrine increases the **metabolic rate.** Glucose already within the system is rushed by blood circulation to the muscle cells, where it is combined with oxygen (cellular respiration) for the release of energy.

Increased Sweating

To control the elevated temperature generated by the accelerated energy production, the body sweats. The accumulated fluid forms on the skin surface, where it evaporates, thus lowering the body's temperature.

Decreased Salivation

As a result of the overall shutdown of the digestive system, the production of saliva, which contains digestive enzymes, is also reduced. Thus people who are under the influence of any type of stressor may report a "cotton-mouth" sensation.

Increased Muscular Tension

Twitching and tautness of the arms and legs during times of stress reflect how close to the fully contracted state the body's skeletal muscles have become. By maintaining the muscles in this condition, the body is prepared for the fight-or-flight response. When muscle tension is continued for extended periods, however, headaches (see the Star Box on p. 65), a stiff neck, and temporomandibular joint (TMJ) dysfunction can result.

Increased Rate of Cardiac and Pulmonary Function

During periods of stress, heart and lung activity increases. Epinephrine helps increase the rate of *cardiac* and *pulmonary* function. An overall upsurge in heart output and blood pressure and the rate and depth of breathing ensure maximal oxygenation of tissue.

Altered Immune System Response

At the onset of the stress response, immune system cells are mobilized as if in anticipation of bodily injury. However, during periods of prolonged stress, elevated levels of adrenal hormones appear to have a destructive effect on important cells within the immune system.[16] The exact nature of the stressors (type versus duration) and the specific mechanisms of the stress responses that most influence immune function, however, are not fully established.[17,18]

Decreased Clotting Time

The body prepares for injury during the stress response. Blood clotting time decreases during stress. As a consequence, blood tends to clot more easily.

Influences of Corticoids and Epinephrine on Energy Release

Increased Glucose Use

Because glucose is the body's most basic source of energy, an early feature of the stress response is the

Preventing Headaches

An estimated 45 million Americans suffer from headaches. If you have chronic headache symptoms or symptoms that are especially bothersome, you should seek medical help. Headaches can result from many causes. The three most common categories follow:

Tension
Description: A dull constricting pain centered in the hatband region. Pain may be on both sides of the head and extend down the neck to the shoulders. Produced by stress, eye strain, muscle tension, sinus congestion, temporomandibular joint (TMJ) dysfunction, nasal congestion, or caffeine withdrawal.
   Treatment: Nonnarcotic pain relievers, muscle relaxants, relaxation exercises, massage.
   Prevention: Preventive relaxation exercises, certain antidepressant medications.

Migraine
Description: Throbbing pain on one side of the head, usually preceded by visual disturbances. Sensitivity to lights and sounds; nausea and dizziness. More common in women. May be triggered by a number of causes. Can last from a few hours to two days.
   Treatment: Rest in a quiet, dark place. Nonnarcotic pain relievers (such as Excedrin M). Ergot compounds (prescription medications). Non-ergot compounds (such as Midrin or Imitrex).
   Prevention: Avoidance of certain foods, perhaps including red wines, other alcoholic beverages, ripened cheeses, chocolate, cured meats, and MSG (monosodium glutamate). In some cases, prescription medications are recommended.

Cluster
Description: Focused, intense pain near one eye; often producing a red and teary eye, as well as a runny nose. Headaches occur daily for weeks or months. They mainly affect men and last up to two hours.
   Treatment: Oxygen and/or ergot compounds during the headache.
   Prevention: Avoidance of alcohol and nitrite-containing foods. Various prescription medications, including antidepressants, steroids, ergotlike compounds, or heart-regulating drugs.

release of glycogen (the storage form of glucose) from its deposit sites, particularly the liver.

Increased Fat Use

If a stressor is not eliminated promptly, the body's supply of glucose may become depleted. The body then turns to its two remaining energy reserves, fat deposits and muscle tissue. Fat breakdown will result in release of usable energy and the production of metabolic waste products that will eventually cause the body to use its most protected energy deposits, muscle tissue.

Muscle Tissue Breakdown and Use

If the stressor is unusually powerful, energy demands will continue to the point that muscle tissue becomes involved. Fortunately, most of today's stressors are resolved long before this occurs.

   Although in the short term all of the responses shown in Figure 3-1 are valuable when confronting a stressor, long-term exposure to these breakdown processes has a destructive effect on physical health. During the resistance phase of the stress response, the body will shift the efforts of a prolonged "fight" to specific body systems. When this shift occurs, the **psychosomatic disorders** associated with chronic stress begin.

hypothalamus (hype oh **thal** a muss)   the portion of the midbrain that provides a connection between the cerebral cortex and the pituitary gland.

pituitary gland (puh **too** it tary)   the master gland of the endocrine system; the wide variety of hormones produced by the pituitary are sent to structures throughout the body.

adrenocorticotropic hormone (ACTH) (uh **dreen** oh kore tick oh **trope** ick)   a hormone produced in the pituitary gland and transmitted to the cortex of the adrenal glands; stimulates production and release of corticoids.

adrenal glands   the paired triangular endocrine glands located on the top of each kidney; site of epinephrine and corticoid production.

corticoids   hormones generated by the adrenal cortex; corticoids influence the body's control of glucose, protein, and fat metabolism.

epinephrine (epp i **neff** rin)   a powerful adrenal hormone whose presence in the bloodstream prepares the body for maximal energy production and skeletal muscle response.

adrenaline   the common name for epinephrine.

metabolic rate (met uh **bol** ick)   the rate or intensity at which the body produces energy.

psychosomatic disorders   physical illnesses of the body generated by the effects of stress.

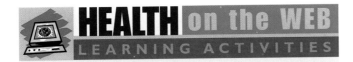

Exploring the Link Between Stress and Disease

Stress significantly influences the development of illnesses such as cancer, cardiovascular disease, and eating disorders, and uncontrolled stress is linked to an increased incidence of violence. Go to www.stressless.com/AboutSL/StressFacts.cfm to read a more detailed list of the negative effects of stress on people's health. What did you learn about stress and disease? What specific things could you do to reduce your own stress level?

Dealing with Stress

In our lives we must continually manage a variety of stressors, even some of which we are not aware. Mental health professionals encourage us to be aware of how much stress we can comfortably accommodate. The *Quick Stress Assessment* can help you decide how well you are dealing with your own stressors. Go to www.stressless.com/AboutSL/StressTest.cfm to complete the questionnaire. How could you improve your reactions to stress?

Mastering Stress

To fight and conquer stress, we must develop a realistic strategy to respond to today's fast-paced, demanding lifestyle. Develop your own stress strategy by mastering the techniques presented at www.coolware.com/health/medical_reporter/stress.html. Which techniques do you think may work best for you? Choose one or two of them to try today.

For more activities, log on to our Online Learning Center at www.mhhe.com/hper/health/payne.

Stress and Psychoneuroimmunology

In an earlier section of the chapter, the relationship of stress to both illness and the function of the immune system is briefly discussed (see p. 64). Additional information seems warranted in light of the growing interest in these topics within the scientific community.[19]

On the basis of clinical observation and laboratory studies, it is recognized that feelings associated with stress (depression and anxiety) and the disruption of social support systems relate to the weakening of the immune response and the development of some illnesses.[19] For example, a study involving self-assessment of stress levels and the occurrence of colds demonstrated that as levels of chronic stress increase, colds become more common.[20] In another study, immunizations were less effective in producing an immune response in students stressed by upcoming examinations than in those not scheduled to take examinations. What is not known, however, is which mechanisms certain stressors use in altering immune system function (nervous and endocrine systems versus nervous system

only), whether studies done with immune cells removed from the body reflect what occurs in the body, and whether studies done with animals can be applied to humans.

In spite of these limitations, theoretical explanations for a strong relationship between stress and the absence of social support and immune system function can be made. Accordingly, a growing number of studies are under way to further clarify which pathways are involved in the stress-immune system interplay, and the use of social support therapy is becoming a component in the treatment of serious illness, such as breast cancer and cardiovascular disease.

Personality Traits

Can personality play a role in making people more or less prone to stress? If so, what outlook on life is now considered to be the most stress-producing? The answer to the latter question has changed over the past two decades.

The initial, and still widely recognized, theory describing personality's role in fostering stress was that of type A and type B personalities, developed by cardiologists Friedman and Rosenman. In this model, time-dependence (hurry sickness) was related to high levels of stress and, eventually, to heart disease.

Today, the concept of time-dependence as being the most influential personality trait associated with high levels of stress has given way to concern over high levels of anger and cynicism. *Anger* is the intense feeling of rage and fury that accompanies unexpected change. For people who for whatever reasons seem to be always angry, the stress put on the body is detrimental to both physical and emotional health.[21] The term *angry heart* describes a condition frequently seen in people who have had a heart attack.

Closely akin to anger is *cynicism*, the second personality trait that fosters high levels of stress. This trait is associated with a deeply held dislike and distrust of others and their ideas. Cynics have nothing good to say about others. They are, perhaps, profoundly angry about their relationships with others and can only express this feeling by being very critical. Regardless, cynicism, like anger, places the body under chronic stress and erodes the physical and emotional well-being of the cynic. Perhaps the only effective treatment for chronically angry or cynical people is either a profoundly moving personal experience that truly changes their outlook on life, such as the birth of a child, or counseling to get in touch with the reasons underlying their negative outlook.

Intensity of Stressors

Not everyone reacts similarly to a given stressor. For example, for increasing numbers of people, cigarette smoke is a stressor, yet two nonsmokers may have different reactions to being near someone else's cigarette smoke. One person might feel only mild stress or annoyance, whereas another person could feel severe stress. Thus we might expect different behavioral responses by people exposed to the same stressor. Again, recall that each person's response to change depends on how he or she interprets defining events as stressors. This interpretation itself is conditioned by intrinsic and extrinsic factors that are largely unique to that person. Intrinsic factors relate to the dimensions of health discussed in Chapter 1, whereas extrinsic factors may include social support and culturally defined perceptions.

Coping: Reacting to Stressors

In some ways, developing appropriate and effective coping skills is more difficult today than in the past. No longer is it socially acceptable to escape stressors through negative dependency behavior, withdrawal, or aggressiveness. The emphasis now is on lifestyle management techniques, such as time management, that are not only effective but also supportive of overall wellness, social relationships, and the environment.

Stress-Management Techniques

Experts in stress management have proposed several effective techniques for coping with stress. Each of these techniques is described in the material that follows, with specific instructions for use provided for some. You will not know whether a particular coping technique is effective for you until you study the technique and then use it for an adequate period of time.

Self-Hypnosis

Techniques for increased awareness, mental relaxation, and enhanced self-directedness are taught by trained professionals to people capable of being hypnotized. These techniques, which can be learned in one lesson, are self-administered in daily sessions lasting ten to twenty minutes each. Beware of unqualified practitioners, who frequently sell their services through newspaper advertisements. Professional organizations, such as psychological or psychiatric societies, can recommend qualified therapists.

The Relaxation Response

The "relaxation response" is a relaxation technique developed by Herbert Benson, M.D., through which one learns to quiet the body and mind. Relaxation technique centers on exhalation and allowing the body to relax while sitting in a comfortable position. This technique can be learned in a single session but requires a commitment to making time to practice. Relatively effective for most people, the technique is described in Dr. Benson's book, *The Relaxation Response.*

Progressive Muscle Relaxation

Pioneered by the work of Edmund Johnson (author of *You Must Relax*), progressive muscle relaxation (PMR) is a procedure in which each of several muscle groups is systematically contracted and relaxed. By learning to recognize the difference between contracted and relaxed muscles, Johnson believed that people would be able to purposely place certain muscles into a controlled state of stress-reducing relaxation.

PMR is based on the appropriate use of positioning, breathing, and concentration. The position of choice is lying on the floor, with the hands at the sides and palms facing upward. Once a comfortable position has been assumed, alternating periods of inhalation and exhalation are begun. As a person inhales, the muscles are contracted, whereas during exhalation, muscle groups are relaxed. Concentration is focused on the "feelings" of relaxation that accompany the release of tension during each exhalation. Once mastered, the basics of participation can be carried out in almost every setting, including a moving car, at work at one's desk, and in a college classroom. Depending on a person's level of expertise, contractions last from a maximum of one hundred seconds, through fifty seconds, to a minimum of five seconds. The face, jaw, neck, shoulders, upper chest, hands and forearms, abdomen, lower back, buttocks, thighs, calves, and feet are tightened and then relaxed progressively. To the extent possible, each muscle group within the area is included.

Quieting

Quieting involves using a set of specific responses, such as striving for a positive mental state, an "inner smile," and a deep exhalation, with the tongue and the shoulders relaxed, immediately on sensing the onset of stress. This technique can be practiced at any time; it is easily learned and supplies immediate feelings of being "on top of stress." The technique can be learned by reading *QR: The Quieting Reflex*, by Charles Stroebel.

Yoga

An ancient exercise program for the mind and body, yoga can be learned from a qualified instructor in one to three months. Yoga is practiced daily in a quiet setting in sessions lasting fifteen to forty-five minutes. It can alter specific physiological functions, enhance flexibility, and free the mind from worry. Many good yoga books, classes, and videotapes are available.

Diaphragmatic Breathing

A coping technique with elements of both relaxation and quieting is diaphragmatic breathing. Aspects of this practice are seen in the Lamaze approach to childbirth, yoga, and tai chi. Although no single explanation for its

HEALTH ACTION GUIDE

Reducing Work-Related Stress

Regardless of how it is described—career, profession, job, or simply work—employment is at times a stressful experience for virtually everyone. Stressors in the workplace range from physically dangerous assignments and burdensome workloads to oppressive managerial styles and demeaning treatment by coworkers. Some of these stressors confront employees on their first day of work, whereas others occur with advancement or the changing nature of the organization and its objectives. Often, in fact, workplace stress results from stressors outside the workplace rather than the factors described above, but the impact of those stressors follows employees to their work every day.

Workplace stressors are so diverse that they are difficult, if not impossible, to anticipate and prevent. Nevertheless, a general game plan for managing workplace stress can help. In fact, many of the points listed below apply equally to the home, school, and community.

- Focus primarily on the present, for the past cannot be recaptured and the future at best can only be anticipated. Anticipation and reflection unquestionably are important, but it is our current situation that offers the greatest opportunity for control.
- Evaluate problems on an individual basis. Although it might be helpful to consider similar problems together, doing so at the start can make all of them seem insurmountable. Once isolated, individual stressors are often seen as less demanding than initially anticipated, and they can be rank ordered in terms of their urgency of resolution.
- Evaluate the time available to direct toward the most pressing stressors. Too much or too little time spent on

particular stressors can be less productive than placing those stressors on-hold until a more opportune time.

- Seek constructive criticism from valued others, both inside and outside the workplace. The experience and perspectives of others may prove to be the most valuable resources for managing stressors. A positive attitude in the face of stress often stimulates others to extend their assistance more quickly and effectively than does a defeatist attitude.
- Remain aware of the demands of work-related stressors without becoming overly focused on them. Coping effectively with such stressors depends on maintaining a balance between the time and energy directed toward stress reduction and that expended in other directions, such as hobbies and social interaction.
- Maintain fitness for the demands of employment. Physical, emotional, social, intellectual, spiritual, occupational, and environmental resourcefulness (see Chapter 1) are required for effective functioning in all areas of life, including those related to employment. Explore the availability of health-enhancing support within the workplace, as well as that which is accessible outside.

Once implemented, this proactive plan for the effective resolution of work-centered stress should enhance the satisfaction that can (but does not necessarily) accompany decades spent earning a living.

InfoLinks
www.hyperstress.com

---

effectiveness can be given, when practiced regularly, diaphragmatic breathing produces relaxation that buffers the powerful stress response. A description of the three-component approach to the practice of diaphragmatic breathing follows:

1. Assume a comfortable position. Lie on the floor with arms by your sides, eyes closed, back straight. Begin breathing from the diaphragm, rather than by the normal method of lifting the chest.
2. Concentrate. The ability to concentrate is important in diaphragmatic breathing. This can be difficult but is most easily mastered by following the flow of air as it enters the body and flows deeply into the lower levels of the lungs, followed by the rising of the stomach as the air leaves the lungs. Each ventilation can be fragmented into four distinct steps: (1) take air into your lungs through the nose and mouth, (2) pause slightly before exhaling, (3) release the air to flow out via the path from which it entered, and (4) pause slightly after exhalation before repeating step 1.

3. Visualize. Diaphragmatic breathing promotes relaxation most fully when it is practiced in conjunction with visualization. What is visualized varies from person to person, but many feel that envisioning the air or even clouds entering the body with each breath, traveling down the path taken by the air, and leaving through the nostrils is very effective. Extending the image of the air flowing through the entire body (energy breathing) rather than only into the lungs is even more effective.

Once mastered, diaphragmatic breathing will quiet the body. Experienced users of this technique can temporarily lower their breathing rate from a typical rate of fourteen to eighteen breaths per minute to as few as four breaths per minute. In doing so, the entire nervous system is slowed, in direct opposition to its role in the stress response.

Meditation

Meditation, in a wide variety of forms, allows the mind to transcend thought effortlessly when the person concentrates on a focal point. In transcendental meditation, a widely recognized approach to meditation, people re-cite a mantra, or a personal word, twice daily. TM is a seven-step program that is taught by trained profes-sionals. TM centers are listed in the telephone directory.

In other meditation approaches, alternative focal points are used to establish the depth of con-centration needed to free the mind from conscious thought.[3] Physical objects, such as a disk painted on a wall, can be used effectively. Music and relaxing environmental sounds, such as the sounds of ocean waves, can be focal points, as can bodily sounds such as breathing.

Regardless of the specific object used, once a technique is mastered, a variety of physiological changes, reflecting a relaxation of bodily function, can be observed. Changes within the electrical activ-ity of the brain also reflect a stress-reducing level of function.

Biofeedback

Biofeedback is a system for monitoring and subse-quently controlling specific physiological functions, such as heart rate, respiratory rate, and body tem-perature. Training with an experienced instructor and appropriate monitoring instruments requires weekly sessions that last one hour or longer over a period of twelve or more weeks. When used with other tension-reduction techniques, biofeedback pro-vides concrete reinforcement of stress-reduction goals. For more information, contact the Biofeedback Society of America, 4301 Owens Street, Wheat Ridge, Colorado 80033.

Exercise

A wide variety of movement activities are intended to reduce stress, expend energy, promote relaxation, provide enjoyment through social contact, and, possi-bly, promote the formation of biological opiates. Running, jogging, lap swimming, walking, rope skip-ping, biking, stair climbing, and aerobic dancing workouts are all excellent ways to burn the energy produced by the stress response (see Chapter 4). Equipment needs, facilities, and required skills vary. Three to four sessions per week lasting a half hour per session are sufficient for most people. Health and fitness clubs also offer enjoyable exercise programs.

Personal Applications

• Which of the suggested approaches to coping with stress could you most comfortably develop? When can you start to develop these skills?

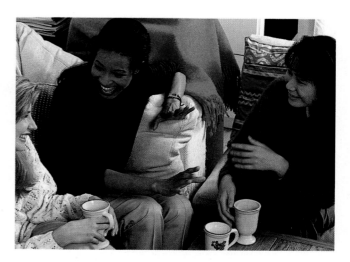

The fabric of our lives is woven from the pleasure of day-to-day activities.

A Realistic Perspective on Stress and Life

The development of a realistic approach to today's fast-paced demanding lifestyle may best be achieved by fostering many of the following perspectives:[22]

Do not be surprised by trouble. Anticipate problems and see yourself as a problem solver. Although each specific problem is unique, it is, nevertheless, most likely similar to past experiences. Use these past experiences to quickly recognize workable approaches to resolving new problems.

Search for solutions. Act on a partial solution, even when a complete solution seems distant. By resolving some aspects of a problem, you can gain time for more focused consideration of the remaining difficulties. In addition, some progress is a confidence builder that can help you remain committed to finding a complete solution.

Take control of your own future. Set out to accomplish all of the items on your agenda. Do not view yourself as a victim. Also, recall from Chapter 2 that being proactive in controlling change is an excellent way to learn more about yourself and recognize capabilities that you were previously unaware of.

Move away from negative thought patterns. Do not extend or generalize difficulties from one area into another. Further, negativity about yourself, in the form of self-doubt and self-blame, is certain to erode your feelings of success.

Rehearse success. Do not disregard the possibility of failure. Rather, focus on those things that are necessary and possible to ensure success. The

Dealing with Posttraumatic Stress Disorder

As diverse as they may seem, abused children, witnesses to fatal car crashes, natural disaster victims, rape victims, and combat veterans hold something in common: the possibility of developing *posttraumatic stress disorder (PTSD)*. In PTSD, victims experience again the emotions and physical discomfort associated with their initial traumatic experiences. The National Institutes of Health estimate that as many as 60 percent of all Americans have undergone a traumatic event of the type capable of generating PTSD, with from 3 percent to 8 percent eventually developing the disorder. Considerably higher levels of PTSD have been observed in combat veterans (30%) and in prisoners of war and concentration camp survivors (50%). Some experts, however, dispute these latter figures on the basis that the actual events may have been gradually "redefined" in the minds of the victims, making them more stressful later than they were at the time they occurred.[23]

The clinical diagnosis of PTSD is based on the persistent recurrence of dreams or flashbacks in which the traumatic event is occurring again; the persistent avoidance of activities, settings, or conversations related to the traumatic events; and the persistent display of signs of nervous system arousal, such as insomnia, outbursts of anger, and the inability to concentrate.[24] Victims of PTSD also appear hypervigilant and display startled responses to many stimuli associated with the original event.

Treatment of posttraumatic stress disorder is an evolving science whose specifics depend to a large degree on the clinical orientation of the psychotherapists involved. In general, however, all therapists want their patients to eventually feel comfortable confronting memories of the stressful events so they can understand their distressing symptoms. Reluctance to talk about the event in fear that therapists will not understand, or a fear of experiencing the event yet again, make initial treatment sessions difficult. In some instances people with PTSD project onto the therapist blame for the events themselves. Once past this period, however, therapy generally progresses as planned.

Regardless of the specific approaches taken, both during and after psychotherapy, people with PTSD are helped by supportive family, friends, employers, and neighbors in dealing with their initial needs for secretiveness and feelings of mistrust and isolation. In fact, in some PTSD groups, such as those composed of battered women and incest survivors, group support provided by fellow survivors and extended mutual aid provided by individuals or agencies has led to improvement, even without psychotherapy.

---

very act of "imaging," in which a person sees himself or herself performing skillfully, has proven beneficial in a variety of performance-oriented activities. Application of this technique may prove helpful in resolving stress, as it has in the fields in which it has been traditionally used, such as dance and gymnastics.

Accept the unchangeable. The direction your life takes is only in part the result of your own doing. Cope as effectively as possible with those events over which you have no direct control; beyond a certain point, however, you must let go of those things over which you have little control.

Live each day well. Combine activity, contemplation, and a sense of cheerfulness with the many things that must be done each day. Celebrate special occasions. Undertake new experiences. Learn from your mistakes. Recognize your accomplishments. Most importantly, however, remember that the fabric of our lives is far more heavily influenced by day-to-day events than it is by the occasional milestones of life.

Act on your capacity for growth. Undertake new experiences and then extract from them new information about your own interests and capacities. The multiple dimensions of health identified in Chapter 1 will, over the course of your lifetime, provide a wide array of resources that will allow growth to occur throughout your entire life.

Allow for renewal. Make time for yourself, and take advantage of opportunities to pursue new and fulfilling relationships. Foster growth in each of the multiple dimensions of health—physical, emotional, social, intellectual, spiritual, occupational, and environmental. Initial renewal in one dimension may serve as a springboard for renewal in others.

Tolerate mistakes. Both you and others will make mistakes. Recognize that these can cause anger, and learn to avoid feelings of hostility. Mistakes, carefully evaluated, can serve as the basis for even greater control and more likely success in those activities not yet undertaken.

With a realistic and positive outlook on life, you will need less coping time to live a satisfying and productive life. Change, in all aspects of life, is inevitable. In the presence of high-level wellness, change should be anticipated, nurtured, and then incorporated into your maturing sense of self.

Real Life
Real choices

- What are the sources of stress in Kate Sullivan's life?
- Does Kate have any choice about the structure and pace of her life?
- Do you agree or disagree with Kate that she can't afford to take time to relax?

And, Now, Your Choices . . .
- If you were in Kate's circumstances, what, if anything, would you do differently? The same? Why? What kinds of stresses are you under, and how do you deal with them?

Summary

- Stressors are real or imagined events capable of eliciting the emotional and physical stress response in people who feel threatened by the change associated with these events.
- The absence of adequate change may also function as a stressor for some people.
- Stress is the emotional and physical response of the body to the presence of a stressor.
- Not all people perceive the same event as being equally threatening; thus some people feel stressed by an event that others do not perceive as stressful.
- The term *eustress* is assigned to the stress response when its presence is interpreted as being positive (such as stress experienced when riding a roller coaster).
- The term *distress* is assigned to the stress response when its presence is interpreted as being uncomfortable, threatening, or frightening.
- Both eustress and distress elicit the predictable stress response—often referred to as the fight, flight, fright, or folly response, or more simply the fight-or-flight response.
- Many familiar physical conditions, such as hypertension, hay fever, and eating disorders, are caused or worsened by the presence of stress.
- The college experience is the source of a wide variety of stressors, including demands associated with difficulty in meeting individual and institutional expectations.
- Life in general is a constant source of stressors, including many arising from interpersonal, occupational, and financial concerns.
- The general adaptation syndrome occurs in three distinct phases—the alarm phase, the resistance

phase, and the exhaustion phase. However, recovery from the stressor usually takes place before exhaustion can occur.
- An intricate interplay involving the brain, the autonomic nervous system, and endocrine system results in a series of physiological changes that prepare the body to respond to stressors.
- Critical to the stress response are the sensory modalities, the cerebral cortex, the hypothalamus, the adrenal glands, the hormone ACTH, the corticoids, and epinephrine.
- The physiological changes seen in various organ systems, organs, and tissues can all be understood in terms of the body's need for readily available sources of energy.
- Stress is now recognized as being detrimental to the normal functioning of the immune system, thus depriving a person of the protection needed to resist infectious diseases and destroy cancerous cells.
- People whose personalities are characterized by chronic anger and cynicism may be more vulnerable to the damaging effects of stress than other people.
- A wide variety of coping techniques, including self-hypnosis, relaxation, quieting, yoga, diaphragmatic breathing, meditation, and exercise, can be employed in the effective resolution of stress.
- A realistic outlook on life may protect some people from the potentially damaging effects of stressors, thus enhancing health and generating a sense of well-being.

Review Questions

1. What is the difference between a stressor and stress?
2. What types of feelings are experienced in conjunction with periods of distress, and what feelings are experienced in conjunction with periods of eustress?
3. What accounts for the observation that a particular situation may prove stressful to one person but apparently not to another person?
4. What are several of the more familiar health conditions attributed to chronic unresolved stress?
5. In what way does the college experience contribute to the stress level of students?
6. What techniques can be applied toward more effective time management?
7. What life experiences do typical Americans report as being most stressful?
8. When stated in terms of the general adaptation syndrome, what are the three stages of the stress response and in what order do they occur? What usually occurs before the exhaustion stage is reached?
9. In what predictable manner does the stress response unfold? What is the role of the endocrine system? What portions of the nervous system play important roles in the unfolding of the stress response? How do the digestive and cardiovascular systems contribute to the fight-or-flight response?
10. In regard to the successful unfolding of the stress response, what specific roles are played by the sensory modalities, the cerebral cortex, the hypothalamus, the adrenal glands, the hormones vasopressin, CRH, and ACTH, the corticoids, and epinephrine?
11. What specific changes in organ systems, individual organs, and tissues can be accounted for on the basis of the body's search for readily available energy stores to deliver to the skeletal muscles?
12. What is pyschoneuroimmunology? To date, what has research found in regard to immune function and the occurrence of stress?
13. What is the role of anger and cynicism in the development of chronically high levels of stress?
14. How would you briefly describe each of the following: self-hypnosis, progressive muscle relaxation, quieting, yoga, diaphragmatic breathing, meditation, and exercise?
15. What traits characterize people with a realistic outlook on daily living?
16. Why are PTSD levels reported by combat veterans much higher than those of nonveterans who have witnessed life-end events?

References

1. O'Grady D. *Taking the fear out of change.* Reading, PA: Bob Adams, 1995.
2. Selye H. *Stress without distress.* New York: New American Library, 1975.
3. Blonna R. *Stress management.* St. Louis: Mosby, 1996.
4. Racial tension undermines the health of blacks. *APA Monitor,* American Psychological Association, 1998 Sept. (http://www.apa.org)
5. Seaward BL. *Managing stress: principles and strategies for health and well-being.* 2nd ed. Boston: Jones & Bartlett, 1996.
6. Havens JE et al. Reported physical health in Resistance veterans from World War II. *Psycho Rep* 1998; 82 (3 Part I):987–996.
7. Neylan TC et al. Sleep disturbances in the Vietnam generation from a nationally representative sample of Vietnam veterans. *Am J Psychiatry* 1998; 55(7):929–933.
8. Wunderlich U, Bronisch T, Wittchen HU. Comorbidity patterns and young adults with suicide attempts. *Eur Arch Psychiatry Clin Neurosci* 1998; 248(2):87–95.
9. Murry B. College youth haunted by increased pressure. *APA Monitor,* American Psychological Association, 1998 Sept. (http://www.apa.org)
10. U.S. Department of Education, National Center for Education Statistics. *Digest of Education Statistics, 1997,* NCES 98-015, Washington, DC: 1997.
11. Burchert W. A key to managing time: planning and discipline. *USA Today* 1990 April 16:9A.
12. Carey AR, Rechin K. Young adults' priorities. *USA Today* 1998 April 13:1A.
13. Girdano D, Everly G. *Controlling stress and tension: a holistic approach.* 5th ed. Englewood Cliffs, NJ: Prentice-Hall, 1996.
14. New England Deaconess Hospital & Harvard Medical School Mind-Body Institute Associates' Staff et al. *The wellness book: the comprehensive guide to maintaining health and treating stress-related illness.* New York: Birch Lane Press, 1993.
15. Saladin KS. *Anatomy & physiology: the unity of form and function.* Dubuque, IA: WCB/McGraw-Hill, 1998.
16. Scott LV, Dinan TG. Vasopressin and the regulation of hypothalamic-pituitary-adrenal axis function: implications for the pathophysiology of depression. *Life Sci* 1998; 62(22):1985–1998.
17. Cohen S, Herbert TB. Health psychology: psychological factors and physical disease from the perspective of

human psychoneuroimmunology. *Ann Rev Psychol* 1996; 47:113–142.

18. Cohen S et al. Types of stressors that increase susceptibility to the common cold in healthy adults. *Health Psychol* 1998; 17(3):214–223.

19. Vitkovic L, Koslow SH., eds. *Neuroimmunology and mental health.* NIH Pub No 94-3274. U.S. Department of Health and Human Services, Public Health Service, National Institutes of Health, National Institute of Mental Health, Rockville, MD: U.S. Government Printing Office, 1994.

20. Leventhal H, Patrick-Miller L, Leventhal EA. It's long-term stressors that take a toll: comment on Cohen et al (1998). *Health Psychol* 1998; 17(3):211–213.

21. Kawachi I et al. A prospective study of anger and coronary heart disease, The Normative Aging Study. *Circulation* 1996; 94(9):2090–2095.

22. McGinnis L. *The power of optimism.* New York: Harper & Row, 1990.

23. Posttraumatic stress disorder. *Harv Men Health Lett* 1996 June (Part I); 1996 July (Part II).

24. Long PW. Posttraumatic stress disorder, diagnostic criteria (American description). *Internet Mental Health* 1998 Sept 16. (http://www.mentalhealth.com)

Suggested Readings

Carlson R. *Don't sweat the small stuff with your family: simple ways to keep daily responsibility and household chaos from taking over your life.* New York: Hyperion, 1998. This book is highly recommended for family-centered reading, particularly by parents with their pre-teen children. The authors present 100 short stories about people and their lives to assist readers in recognizing the things in life that are truly important. The quality of relationships routinely wins out over the quantity of "things."

McLaughlin Jr P. *Catch fire: A seven-step program to ignite energy, defuse stress, and power boost your career.* New York: Fawcett Books, 1998. Ideal for young persons entering the world of work and for those already along the corporate road, this book blends scientific information and the personal experiences of individuals who have energized themselves to a higher level. The author emphasizes the importance of positive mind-sets, personalized "energy zones," high levels of health based on sound diet and exercise practices, and humorous, yet channeled, approaches to problem solving.

Vienne V, Lennard E (photographer). *Art of doing nothing: simple ways to make time for yourself.* New York: Clarkson Potter, 1998. Can "doing nothing" be the best thing you can do for yourself? The author believes so, and through essays and photographs enlightens readers on the value of "being" rather than "doing." Readers learn how to enhance sensory experiences and enjoy the peaceful passing of time.

Davis M, Eshelman ER, and Mckay M. *The relaxation and stress reduction workbook.* New York: Fine Communications, 1997. Now in its fourth edition, this popular how-to manual approaches stress reduction holistically, emphasizing mind-body-spirit homeostasis. Self-assessment exercises help readers identify the stressors in their lives, while information and illustrated instructions provide techniques for countering stress. The authors detail a variety of stress-reducing approaches, including meditation, visualization, biofeedback, progressive relaxation, and assertiveness training. Recommended for both lay persons and health-care professionals.

topics *for* Today

Going It Alone: Managing the Stress of Single Parenthood

No One to Help

"I've got too much to do and no one to help." Does this sound a lot like your life? Well, imagine having children depending solely on you. Then again, maybe you don't have to imagine. All too many people know the stresses of single parenting from experience. In 1996, nearly one-fourth of all families were single-parent families; 78 percent of these families were headed by women.[1] Single-parent families can be formed when parents separate or divorce or when a spouse dies. Single-parent families may also start out that way; the breakup rate of couples who agree to be together outside of marriage is well above the divorce rate. Increasingly, unmarried women over thirty are choosing to raise children without male partners. Rosie O'Donnell, Diane Keaton, and Madonna are three well-known examples. Other nontraditional families are headed by gay men, lesbians, or lesbian or gay couples.

From 1972 to 1996, the number of female-headed single-parent families more than tripled, reaching 12.5 million in 1996.[2] Of course, not all single-parent families or single parents themselves are the same, but the following generalizations have been observed: (1) Single parents tend to be younger than married parents and (2) single mothers tend to be younger than single fathers.[3] Since the vast majority of single parents are women and a large percentage of that group are young, it is not surprising that they're often in dire financial straits. Women still earn an average of only $0.76 to every dollar a man earns,[4] and women who become parents by the age of twenty have 37 percent lower incomes than women who become mothers after age twenty-seven.[2,5] The stress of single parenthood goes far beyond financial issues. Pressures of time, emotional strain, guilt, and social stereotyping weigh heavily on the parent going it alone.

The Financial Burden

Income tends to vary with family structure. In 1994 married parents made an average of $43,130/year, widows $22,790/year, divorced or separated mothers $18,580/year, and never-married mothers $9,820/year.[6] Even though these figures are alarming, what might not stand out is that today 36.5 percent of all female-headed single-parent families fall below the poverty line (close to 60% for minorities).[1] Under current guidelines, poverty levels are: $10,850 (2 persons), $13,659 (3 persons), and $16,450 (4 persons), with $2,800 added for each additional person.[7] Making life even more difficult, only one-third of single mothers are entitled to receive child support, and even for those lucky enough to get it, two-thirds of the payments are less than the court ordered.[2] Some states are redoubling their efforts to collect child support. In Illinois a person's driver's license can be revoked for being in default of child support payments, and in Indiana, wanted posters of the top offenders are posted at highway rest areas.

Many other government programs, however, such as welfare, AFDC (Aid to Families with Dependent Children), Medicaid, food stamps, education, training, and employment programs are inadequate or even counterproductive. On the other side of the equation, education can go a long way in fighting poverty. Socioeconomic contrasts of children of one- and two-parent families were not as dramatic when the parents had attended college or at least graduated from high school.[8]

Time to Learn

As the manufacturing jobs in this country are replaced by low and minimum wage service jobs, everyone, married and single alike, needs more and more education to earn an income that will support a family. Thus many single parents find themselves returning to school in order to improve their families' standard of living. At school, loans, scholarships, grants, subsidized day care, and on-campus housing may help ease the burden single parents feel—that is, *if* these services exist at their university. In exchange, there are bound to be extra time demands unique to the school setting. Much of what is expected of college students is to be done outside of class on "their own time," but single parents especially are always

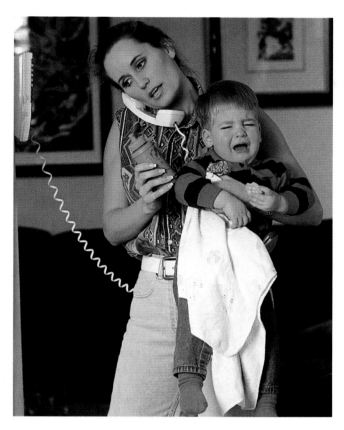

Single parents face many conflicting demands on their time and energy.

on call for their kids, so they don't have much, if any, of their own time. Reading textbooks, studying for tests, and writing papers must be done while fixing supper, helping with baths, and reading bedtime stories or put off to the precious few hours when everyone else is in bed. Group projects, papers, and study sessions require finding and paying for a sitter. In-class requirements may also create a conflict for single parents. What would you do if faced with a sick child on the day of the no-makeup midterm exam?

The divorced mother is more apt to be faced with balancing the pressures of education with working more hours at more than one job. There are time stresses for working parents as well. Seventy-nine percent of single parents with children ages six to seventeen work, and 59 percent of those with children under six are employed.[8] Balancing family and work is another type of problem for single fathers. Men are often taught to define themselves by their work and show their love of family by providing for them. The role of primary caregiver is most likely new to them, whereas women are often familiar with both worlds, having been torn between the two for quite a while.

Cultural expectations also influence the view of employers. Mothers don't catch much of a break at work, but many employers are even less sympathetic to adjusting a father's work schedule, since child and family issues tend to be viewed as women's issues. A single father may also run into conflicts between family and leisure time. When women get together they can usually involve the children in the activity, but activities such as golfing and going out with "the guys" often preclude bringing the children.

Child Care and Parenting

If single parents can find child care, it is often too costly. The expense of child care can consume 25 percent to 60 percent of the family income.[5] If the parent moves into his or her parents' house to cut costs and have grandparental child care readily available, there may be child-rearing conflicts, with the parent and grandparent(s) setting different rules, which leaves the children confused. Parental authority is weakened if the parent is viewed as a child again. A different blended household arises when a grandparent needs care and moves into the home of his or her child and grandchildren. Many women are finding themselves in the sandwich generation, nurturing both their children and elderly parents.

If the father is absent, the lack of a same-sex role model for male children can become a worry. The presence of a grandfather or uncle in the house eases this concern somewhat, but the involvement of playmates' or classmates' fathers in their children's lives may cause some sadness or at least wistfulness. When a father is occasionally present, he may turn into a "Disneyland Dad," only taking on the role of friend and entertainer, leaving Mom with all the day-to-day responsibility.

Emotional Stress

With reduced finances, excessive demands on their time, and reduced social supports, solo parents often experience emotional and parental isolation. It is common for single parents to experience responsibility overload from the tension, pressure, and confusion of their circumstances, task overload from social isolation, and emotional overload from having the sole responsibility of their children without anyone to step in to relieve them or simply worry with them.

Many times the family must relocate to adjust to their new situation, which is also a source of stress and isolation. In too many cases, domestic violence can intensify the sense of instability. Single-parent families also get negative messages from the outside. Society, as a whole, tends to blame and label single mothers. Those who are unwed are sometimes seen as immoral and destined to be poor, and those who are divorced are unfairly judged not to have measured up in some way in satisfying their ex-husband's needs. Many women are looked down upon simply because their last name is different from that of their children.

Tips to Reduce Stress

Despite these often overwhelming difficulties, many single parents have come up with creative ways to reduce their stress levels. A few suggestions are listed here:

- Join an organized group, such as Parents without Partners.
- Join or organize a group of neighborhood or workplace single parents.
- Trade child care time with other single parents.
- Arrange for a friend or relative to baby-sit sometime when you have nothing planned, and pamper yourself.
- Write about it, talk about it, sing about it, paint about it, or express yourself in some other positive way.
- Take a bubble bath.
- Drink a flavored tea.
- Light a candle for no reason.

Perhaps most important of all is to remind yourself often that you are doing the best you can with the resources you have.

The Outlook

Against the odds, women and men across this country are making single parenthood work. New insights into both the strengths and causes of stress within single-parent families could help give these families the support they need. We owe future generations that much.

For Discussion . . .

Are you a single parent? If so, what is the most important thing that you wish people would understand about single parenting? Were you raised in a single-parent household? How did this affect you? If you do not fall into the two categories above, what was your biggest misconception about single-parent families? What government policies on family issues need to be changed? How would you change them?

References

1. U.S. Bureau of the Census. *Statistical abstract of the United States, 1997.* 117th ed. Washington, DC: U.S. Government Printing Office, 1997.
2. Kissman K, Allen JA. *Single-parent families.* Newbury Park, CA: Sage, 1993.
3. Ginglas M, Weinraub M. The more things change . . . single parenting revisited. *Fam Iss* 1995; 16(1):29–52.
4. Bureau of Labor Statistics. Women's earnings as a percent of men's, 1979–1997. *NEWS,* Washington, DC., 1998. (http://www.dol.gov/dol/wb/public/stats/main.htm)
5. Leslie MR, ed. *The single mother's companion.* Seattle: Seal Press, 1994.
6. Lino M. Income and spending patterns of single-mother families. *Mon Labor Rev* 1994; 117(5):29–38.
7. *Federal Register* 63(46):9236. Washington, DC: U.S. Government Printing Office, 1998.
8. Mulroy EA. *The new uprooted.* Westport, CT: Auburn House, 1995.

InfoLinks
www.parentsplace.com
www.parenthoodweb.com

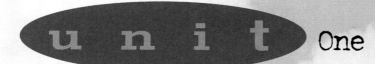
The information you have mastered in Unit One will be helpful to you as you work on the five developmental tasks this book addresses. Remember that the role of health is to assist you in completing the developmental tasks that will allow you to enjoy a sense of well-being.

Forming an Initial Adult Identity

You may have noticed that we have qualified the adult self-identity concept as initial, or tentative. This suggests an identity that is temporary—one that can evolve over time. The idea that further changes in your identity are possible and even probable can lead to feelings of uncertainty, confusion, and stress. However, we believe that as you increasingly come to grips with your evolving identity, you will find new opportunities for growth, creativity, and service. In many ways this personal growth and development can be an exciting experience. High-level emotional wellness encourages the formation of your emerging identity. Through healthful introspection and reflection, you learn a great deal about the person you are becoming. By exploring the ways you handle stressful situations, you learn even more about yourself. Indeed, interest in your emotional and spiritual makeup will serve you throughout life as you repeatedly ask "Who am I?"

Establishing Independence

This developmental task is represented by your steady movement away from a dependent relationship with family and friends. For nontraditional students, it may be represented by a similar pulling back from dependence on a spouse, limited employment opportunities, or parenting. Regardless, to progress toward independence you must be successful in dealing with people, institutions, programs, and yourself. Establishing independence is a developmental progression in which emotional health can play an extremely supportive role. Your emotional maturity is a primary factor in determining the rate at which you progress toward independence. Stress will probably be produced in those who progress too slowly or too rapidly in their search for independence. For those who move toward relative independence at a rate soundly based on their needs and health resources, this search will produce eustress. Enjoy the journey.

Assuming Responsibility

Although an adult of any age may lack an adequately developed sense of responsibility, it is in the young adult years that significant progress in that direction is expected. To whom is one most responsible? We take the position that primary responsibility during the young adult years must be to yourself. For example, mastery of all five of the developmental tasks is your responsibility. Parents, faculty, and friends cannot force you to take charge of your own development; your growth in confidence, self-respect, and insight gained through new experiences rests in your own hands. Fortunately, this is the way most students want it.

Developing Social Skills

Since the costs of making friends and keeping friendships can sometimes be high, we would like to introduce someone who can be helpful in your search for improved social interaction—a mentor. For the purposes of this book, a mentor is a person slightly older than you (eight to fifteen years older) who functions not as a peer nor as a parent substitute, but as an exemplar, counselor, and a person capable of sharing your aspirations. The process of identifying potential mentors within an occupational, educational, or recreational setting cannot be prescribed. Potential mentors need not be of your own sex, nor do they necessarily need to hold a position significantly higher than yours.

It is through mentor relationships that some will find the most pleasurable social, occupational, and professional rewards. With your mentor you will sense a more deeply focused relationship by which to evaluate initial successes and failures. Your mentor will listen, demand, share, critique, and counsel as you progress in this challenging period of life.

Developing Intimacy

To develop intimacy, you must be willing and able to extend your identity to others in an open manner. Intimacy is almost always accompanied by feelings of vulnerability as well as the possibility of rejection. Consequently, stress and intimacy usually go together. Effective coping skills are important resources to develop in any relationship, especially an intimate one. Think of intimate relationships as new experiences that will help to shape your life.

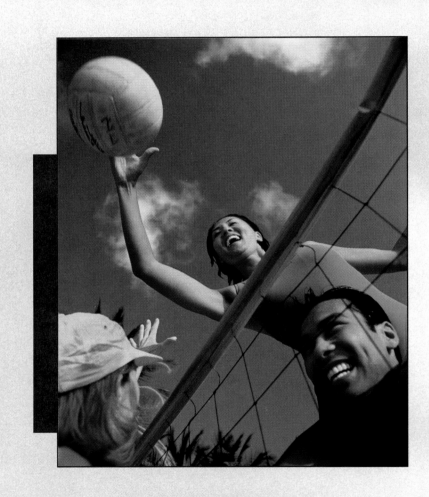

The Body

Unit Two comprises three chapters whose content is especially relevant to college students: fitness, nutrition, and weight management. This unit will help you learn how to improve your health in these areas.

1 Physical Dimension

Health experts believe that fitness, nutrition, and weight management are interrelated. How well our bodies work depends on what we eat and how we exercise. Healthy bodies allow us to participate in daily activities and recover more quickly from illness and injury.

2 Emotional Dimension

When you start a fitness program or begin to pay attention to your diet, you learn about your level of motivation and commitment. You will be challenged, but the emotional rewards for your efforts, such as an improved self-concept and greater confidence, can be substantial.

3 Social Dimension

The social dimension of health is closely related to fitness, nutrition, and weight management. Exercising with friends offers an opportunity for social interaction. Participation in most group fitness activities involves listening, sharing, and counseling. Food, like alcohol, can function as a "social lubricant" by bringing and holding people together. However, an excessive food intake and lack of exercise can hinder social relationships when a person is significantly above his or her desirable weight.

4 Intellectual Dimension

Some evidence suggests that people feel mentally sharper after they exercise. Many students report that they can study more efficiently after a workout. People deprived of adequate exercise and proper nutrition may suffer intellectual impairment. Regular physical acitivity, a sound diet, and effective weight management will allow you to enjoy a wide range of new experiences that can lead to improved intellectual functioning.

5 Spiritual Dimension

Throughout this text we emphasize that an important part of your spiritual growth is serving others. Staying physically fit, following a healthful diet, and managing your weight can enhance your ability to serve others. You can express your own faith and help others find meaning in their lives when you take proper care of your health.

6 Occupational Dimension

Just as you can better serve others when you feel your best, you can also pursue a career and carry out daily occupational tasks when you take care of your body. Some job functions, such as traveling and heavy lifting, require that you be in good physical condition. In addition, being fit can help you deal more effectively with the stress that inevitably accompanies employment. Taking care of your body can increase your self-esteem and improve your confidence—a definite plus when you are trying to land a job or earn a promotion.

7 Environmental Dimension

Participation in fitness activities offers you great opportunities for appreciating your role in protecting the environment—a hike through the woods or a day on the lake can renew your commitment to keeping our land unspoiled and our waterways clean. Even your choice of foods can indicate your respect for the environment when you select organic produce or follow a vegetarian diet.

chapter
four

Staying Physically Fit

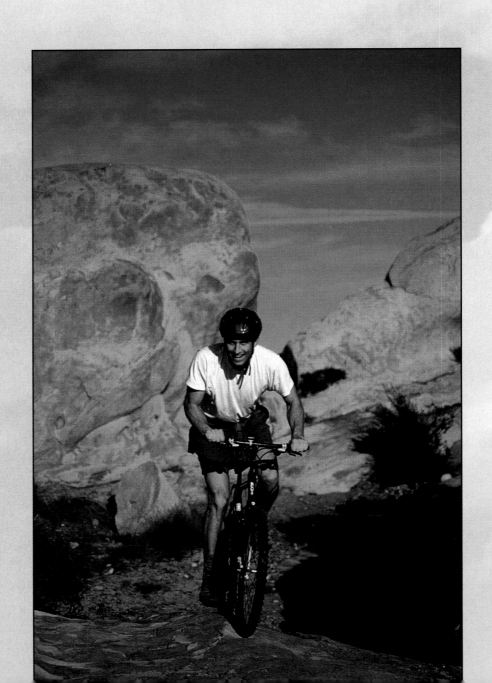

For many college students, the day begins early in the morning; continues with classes, research, study, a job, or family activities; and does not end until after midnight. This kind of pace demands that the student be physically fit. Even a highly motivated college student must have a conditioned, rested body to maintain such a schedule.

Of course, many college students do not look at fitness as a means to a more satisfying, exciting life. Instead, many students look for the cosmetic benefits of fitness. They want to look in the mirror and see the kind of body they see in the media: one with well-toned muscles, a trim waistline, and an absence of flabby tissue, especially on the arms, legs, abdomen, and hips. Thus, many students become motivated to start fitness programs because they hope that they can build a better body for themselves. Through their efforts to do so, students usually start to feel better, physically and mentally. They realize that physical fitness can improve every aspect of their lives, because they see it happening with each passing week.

Fortunately, you need not become a full-time athlete to enjoy the health benefits of fitness. Incorporating regular, moderate physical activity, such as brisk walking or dancing, into your life, can benefit your health and your overall quality of life.[1]

HEALTHY PEOPLE: LOOKING AHEAD TO 2010

Many of the *Healthy People 2000* objectives focused on getting Americans to increase their participation in activities that improve cardiorespiratory fitness. With an estimated 250,000 deaths per year in the United States attributable to the lack of physical activity, encouraging our sedentary society to become more active is clearly important.

The *Midcourse Review* concluded that progress toward achieving these objectives has been mixed. A somewhat higher percentage of adults now engage in moderate to vigorous physical activity. However, no progress has been made in reducing the percentage of

adults who do not participate in leisure-time physical activity. The objective of increasing the number of worksite fitness programs has been fully achieved.

Unfortunately, the nation has lost ground in several areas. For example, since 1990 the percentage of students in grades 9 through 12 involved in physical education courses has decreased. The proportion of time that students are physically active during these class periods has also dropped. The *Healthy People 2010* document is expected to address these serious concerns.

Real Life
Real choices

The Fitness Imperative: A Matter of Life and Health

- Name: Jack Wozniak
- Age: 44
- Occupation: sales representative
- Physical characteristics: 5′11″, 182 lb

No caffeine. No alcohol. No smoking. No red meat. No rich desserts. No road trips. Plenty of fruits and vegetables; plenty of rest; moderate daily exercise.

To Jack Wozniak, a hard-charging, fun-loving embodiment of the Type A personality, that list of restrictions sounded like the last chapter in the book of his life. A successful sales representative for a plastics manufacturer, Jack spent 8 months out of each year on the road. At his last annual checkup his blood pressure had risen to 175 over 85, and he grudgingly admitted to his concerned physician that 18 years of rushing for the red-

eye, wining and dining prospects, and sleeping in strange beds were taking their toll. Factor in no exercise, a two-pack-a-day smoking habit, and a passion for beer and corn chips, and you're looking at a disaster waiting to happen.

It did. One morning Jack was battling rush-hour traffic to the airport to catch a plane for Dallas. He never made it. When he woke up, he found himself in a cardiac-care unit, hooked up to more wires and flashing dials than the space shuttle. Not even 45, he'd suffered a massive heart attack, and his doctor was offering him a stark choice: maintain your lifestyle and die, or follow a new regimen and (maybe) live.

As you study this chapter, think about a healthy approach to exercise for someone of Jack's personality type and lifestyle, and prepare yourself to answer the questions in **Your Turn** at the end of the chapter.

Benefits of Fitness

Following a program of regular aerobic exercise improves the efficiency of your cardiovascular and respiratory systems. More specifically, regular aerobic exercise strengthens the muscles of your heart, enabling your heart to pump more blood with fewer strokes, meeting the demands you place on it. As a result, your resting heart rate may become slower than in the past, indicating that you have become more physically fit. At the same time, your respiratory system becomes stronger and more efficient in delivering oxygen to the tissues of your body.[1] This cardiorespiratory fitness enables you to deal with the routine and extraordinary demands of your daily life more easily.

Cardiorespiratory fitness is the foundation for whole-body fitness. This fitness increases your capacity to sustain a given level of energy for a prolonged period. Thus your body can work longer and at greater levels of intensity.

As you will see, cardiorespiratory fitness has important benefits for everyone, including children (p. 103), women (p. 96), and the elderly (p. 95).

In addition, improving your cardiorespiratory (aerobic) fitness has a variety of benefits that can improve nearly all parts of your life. Aerobic fitness can help you gain the following physical benefits:

- Reduce the proportion of low-density lipoproteins ("bad cholesterol") and increase the proportion of high-density lipoproteins ("good cholesterol") in your blood
- Increase the capillary network in your body
- Reduce your risk of heart disease
- Prevent hypertension

- Improve your blood lipid and lipoprotein profile
- Improve **collateral circulation**
- Strengthen your lungs
- Control your weight
- Stimulate bone growth
- Ward off infections
- Improve the efficiency of your other body systems
- Increase your longevity

Aerobic fitness also brings a variety of other benefits that, although not immediately obvious, are no less important. For example, the increased stamina that comes with cardiorespiratory fitness enables you to complete and better enjoy your daily activities. In addition, your improved fitness level may reduce the severity and shorten the duration of common illnesses. Likewise, you will find your ability to cope with stressors to be increased with your fitness level. As a result, you may find your sense of well-being and confidence to be improved.

Older adults will find that improving their cardiorespiratory fitness enables them to enjoy their later years to a greater extent, giving them the energy and ability to participate in activities that they might have delayed for many years, such as traveling, or even activities they might never have considered, such as joining a square dance club or learning how to line dance.

When you become aerobically fit, you may be able to achieve a long-held goal, such as hiking part of the Appalachian trail, climbing Mt. Rainier, or bicycling through Europe. Others might find that becoming physically fit reduces their dependence on substances such as alcohol, cigarettes, or other drugs and that they sleep more soundly.

Learning
From Our Diversity

A Different Kind of Fitness: Developmentally Disabled Athletes Are Always Winners in the Special Olympics

In America, as in many other countries around the world, physical fitness and athletic prowess carry a high degree of prestige, whereas lack of conditioning and poor sports performance often draw scorn and rejection. As anyone knows who's ever been picked last when sides were being chosen for a schoolyard game, few things are more damaging to youthful self-esteem than being the player nobody wants.

Some of these children blossom into accomplished athletes as they gain coordination or are inspired and guided by caring coaches. Others, lacking strong interest in sports, turn to less physical arenas in which they can excel—drama, debating, music, computers, science.

But what about people who want to be athletes at almost any cost, but who have no realistic hope of attaining the standards of athletic accomplishment set for those in top physical condition? The Joseph P. Kennedy Foundation created an arena in which these athletes could compete when it established the Special Olympics in 1968. Joseph Kennedy was the father of President John F. Kennedy, whose older sister Rosemary was virtually shut away from the world when her family discovered she was mentally retarded. Many people at that time shared the Kennedys' view that the kindest way to treat family members who were developmentally disabled was to "protect" them

from stares and whispers by keeping them at home or placing them in institutions or residential facilities. Spearheaded by President Kennedy's sister Eunice Kennedy Shriver, the Special Olympics was intended to change the old attitudes toward developmentally disabled people by giving them an opportunity to compete at their own level and to celebrate their victories publicly.[18,19]

Now, nearly thirty years later, the Special Olympics holds both winter and summer games and boasts participation of more than 1 million developmentally disabled athletes in 140 countries around the world. The contests are open to athletes between the ages of eight and sixty-three, some of whom have proved wrong the specialists who claimed they would never walk, let alone compete internationally. "Mainstream" Olympic champions like figure-skating silver medalist Brian Orser and a host of well-known entertainers have attended opening-day ceremonies to cheer and inspire the special athletes.

But medals aren't what the Special Olympics is all about. No matter where a Special Olympian finishes in a contest, he or she is applauded and celebrated for the accomplishment of playing the game and seeing it through. The oath taken by each participant in the Special Olympics aptly states the credo of this remarkable group of athletes: "Let me win. But if I cannot win, let me be brave in the attempt."

In what ways other than physical conditioning do you think a developmentally disabled person might benefit from participating in the Special Olympics? What can the rest of us learn from these athletes' courage and perseverance?

Finally, while you are pursuing your physical fitness activities, you probably will meet other healthy, active people and find that you are expanding your circle of friends. The Learning from Our Diversity box above takes a look at the physical and social benefits for disabled people who participate in the Special Olympics.

Personal Applications

• What are your attitudes toward physical fitness? Does your present level of fitness allow you to effectively carry out the activities your schedule demands?

Components of Physical Fitness

Physical fitness is achieved when "the organic systems of the body are healthy and function efficiently so as to resist disease, to enable the fit person to engage in vigorous tasks and leisure activities, and to

handle situations of emergency."[2] In the following sections, we discuss cardiorespiratory endurance, muscular strength, muscular endurance, flexibility, and body composition.

Cardiorespiratory Endurance

If you were limited to improving only one area of your physical fitness, which would you choose—muscular strength, muscular endurance, or flexibility? Which would a dancer choose? Which would a marathon runner select? Which would an expert recommend?

The experts, who are exercise physiologists, would say that another fitness dimension is of even greater importance than those just listed. These research scientists regard improvement of your heart, lung, and blood vessel function as the key focal point

collateral circulation   the ability of nearby blood vessels to enlarge and carry additional blood around a blocked blood vessel.

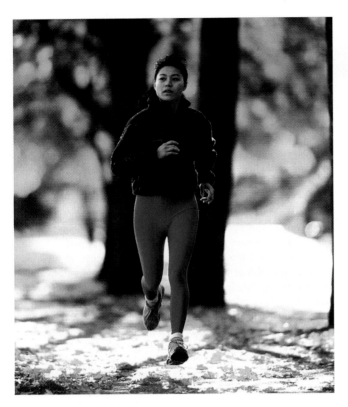

Cardiorespiratory fitness is essential for optimal heart, lung, and blood vessel function.

of a physical fitness program. **Cardiorespiratory endurance** forms the foundation for whole-body fitness.

Cardiorespiratory endurance increases your capacity to sustain a given level of energy production for a prolonged period. Development of cardiorespiratory endurance helps your body to work longer and at greater levels of intensity.

Occasionally your body cannot produce the energy it needs for long-term activity. Certain activities require performance at a level of intensity that outstrips your cardiorespiratory system's ability to transport oxygen efficiently to contracting muscle fibers. When the oxygen demands of the muscles cannot be met, **oxygen debt** occurs. Any activity that continues beyond the point at which oxygen debt begins requires a form of energy production that does not depend on oxygen.

This oxygen-deprived form of energy production is called **anaerobic** (without oxygen) **energy production,** the type that fuels many intense, short-duration activities. For example, rope climbing, weight lifting for strength, and sprinting are short-duration activities that quickly cause muscle fatigue; they are generally considered anaerobic activities. However, cardiovascular improvement has been seen among people who lift weights, especially those who use light weights repetitively.

Activities that are not generally associated with anaerobic energy production (walking, distance jogging, and bicycle touring) become anaerobic activities when they are either increased in intensity or continued for an extended period.

If you usually work or play at low intensity but for a long duration, you have developed an ability to maintain **aerobic** (with oxygen) **energy production.** As long as your body can meet its energy demands in this oxygen-rich mode, it will not convert to anaerobic energy production. Thus fatigue will not be an important factor in determining whether you can continue to participate. Marathon runners, serious joggers, distance swimmers, bicyclists, and aerobic dancers can perform because of their highly developed aerobic fitness. The cardiorespiratory systems of these aerobically fit people take in, transport, and use oxygen in the most efficient manner possible.

Besides allowing you to participate in activities such as those mentioned, aerobic conditioning (cardiorespiratory endurance conditioning) may also provide certain structural and functional benefits that affect other dimensions of your life. These recognized benefits have received considerable documented support. Some data, for example, strongly suggest that aerobic fitness can increase life expectancy[3] and reduce the risk of developing cancer of the colon, heart, uterus, cervix, and ovaries.[4]

Muscular Strength

Muscular strength is essential for your body to accomplish work. Your ability to maintain posture, walk, lift, push, and pull are familiar examples of the constant demands you make on your muscles to maintain or increase their level of contraction. The stronger you are, the greater your ability to contract muscles and maintain a level of contraction sufficient to complete tasks.

Muscular strength can best be improved by training activities that use the **overload principle.** By overloading, or gradually increasing the resistance (load, object, or weight) your muscles must move, you can increase your muscular strength. The following three types of training exercises are based on the overload principle.

In **isometric** (meaning "same measure") **exercises,** the resistance is so great that your contracting muscles cannot move the resistant object at all. Thus your muscles contract against immovable objects, usually with increasingly greater efforts. Because of the difficulty of precisely evaluating the training effects, isometric exercises are not usually used as a primary means of developing muscular strength and can be dangerous for people with hypertension.

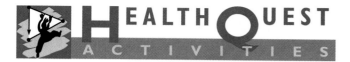

- The *How Fit Are You?* exercise in Module 2 will help you determine your current level of fitness in four major areas: body composition, cardiorespiratory capacity, muscular strength, and flexibility. Complete the series of questions about how much you exercise, what types of training you do, how intensely you exercise, and body size. After you complete the questions, *HealthQuest* will give you feedback in each of the four areas mentioned above. Then develop an individual plan for improving or maintaining your current fitness level.

- The *Exercise Interest Inventory* in Module 2 allows you to rate your feelings about certain aspects of exercise. *HealthQuest* provides feedback about the activities and exercises you would most enjoy, based on your individual needs and preferences. First, write down the five fitness activities that you like best or in which you most often participate. After each one, indicate your motivation for engaging in that particular activity. For example, you could list "enjoyment," "habit," or "convenience." When you have completed the *Exercise Interest Inventory*, compare the two lists. Are there any surprises? What factors had you not considered to be influential in your choice of exercise?

Progressive resistance exercises, also called isotonic or same-tension exercises, are currently the most popular type of strength-building exercises. Progressive resistance exercises include the use of traditional free weights (dumbbells and barbells), as well as Universal and Nautilus machines. People who perform progressive resistance exercises use various muscle groups to move (or lift) specific fixed resistances or weights. Although during a given repetitive exercise the weight remains the same, the muscular contraction effort required varies according to the joint angles in the range of motion.[2] The greatest effort is required at the start and finish of the movement.

Isokinetic (meaning "same motion") **exercises** use mechanical devices that provide resistances that consistently overload muscles throughout the entire range of motion. The resistance will move only at a preset speed regardless of the force applied to it. For the exercise to be effective, a user must apply maximal force. Isokinetic training requires elaborate, expensive equipment. Thus the use of isokinetic equipment may be limited to certain athletic teams, diagnostic centers, or rehabilitation clinics. The most common isokinetic machines are Cybex, Mini-Gym, Exergenie, KinCom, and Biodex.

Which type of strength-building exercise (machines or free weights) is most effective? Take your choice, since all will help develop muscular strength. Some people prefer machines because they are simple to use, do not require stacking the weights, and are already balanced and less likely to drop and cause injury.

Other people prefer free weights because they encourage the user to work harder to maintain balance during the lift. In addition, free weights can be used in a greater variety of exercises than weight machines. Workouts with free weights are also associated with visual images and specialized sounds, which some lifters prefer.

cardiorespiratory endurance the ability of the heart, lungs, and blood vessels to process and transport oxygen required by muscle cells so that they can contract over a period of time. Cardiorespiratory endurance is produced by physical activity that requires continuous, repetitive movements.

oxygen debt a physical state in which one's activity exceeds the body's ability to produce energy aerobically, causing the body to switch to anaerobic energy production. This produces an excess buildup of by-products, especially lactic acid, and a feeling of inability to "catch one's breath." Respiration and heart rate remain increased until the excess by-products are cleared and the body can return to aerobic energy production.

anaerobic energy production the body's alternative means of energy production, used when the available oxygen is insufficient for aerobic energy production. Anaerobic energy production is a much less efficient use of stored energy.

aerobic energy production the body's primary means of energy production, used when the respiratory and circulatory systems can process and transport sufficient oxygen to muscle cells to convert fuel to energy.

muscular strength the ability to contract skeletal muscles to engage in work; the force that a muscle can exert.

overload principle the principle whereby a person gradually increases the resistance load that must be moved or lifted; this principle also applies to other types of fitness training.

isometric exercises (eye so met rick) muscular strength-training exercises in which the resistance is so great that the object cannot be moved.

progressive resistance exercises muscular strength-training exercises in which traditional barbells and dumbbells with fixed resistances are used.

isokinetic exercises (eye so kin et ick) muscular strength-training exercises in which machines are used to provide variable resistances throughout the full range of motion.

Muscular Endurance

Muscular endurance is a component of physical fitness associated with strength. Muscles need energy to contract and to shorten their individual muscle fibers. Energy production requires that the circulatory system deliver oxygen and nutrients to the muscles. After these products are transformed into energy by individual muscle cells, the body must remove the potentially toxic waste by-products.

Amateur and professional athletes often wish to increase the endurance of specific muscle groups associated with their sports activities. This can be achieved by using exercises that gradually increase the number of repetitions of a given movement. However, muscular endurance is not the physiological equivalent of cardiorespiratory endurance. For example, a world-ranked distance runner with highly developed cardiorespiratory endurance and extensive muscular endurance of the legs may not have a corresponding level of muscular endurance of the abdominal muscles.

Flexibility

The ability of your joints to move through their natural range of motion is a measure of your **flexibility.** This fitness trait, like so many other aspects of structure and function, differs from point to point within your body and among different people. Not every joint in your body is equally flexible (by design), and over the course of time, use or disuse will alter the flexibility of a given joint. Certainly gender, age, genetically determined body build, and current level of physical fitness will affect your flexibility.

Inability to move easily during physical activity can be a constant reminder that aging and inactivity are the foes of flexibility. Failure to use joints regularly will quickly result in a loss of elasticity in the connective tissue and shortening of muscles associated with the joints. Benefits of flexibility include improved balance, posture, and athletic performance and reduced risk of low back pain.

As seen in young gymnasts, flexibility can be highly developed and maintained with a program of activity that includes regular stretching. Stretching also helps reduce the risk of injury. Athletic trainers generally prefer **static stretching** to **ballistic stretching** for people who wish to improve their range of motion, as ballistic stretching carries a higher risk of tears to soft tissue.

Body Composition

Body composition is the "makeup of the body in terms of muscle, bone, fat, and other elements."[2] Of particular interest to fitness experts are percentages of body fat and fat-free weight. Health experts are especially concerned about the large number of people in our society who are overweight and obese. Cardiorespiratory fitness trainers increasingly are recognizing the importance of body composition and are including strength-training exercises to help reduce body fat. (See Chapter 6 for further information about body composition, health effects of obesity, and weight management.)

Personal Applications

• Which component of fitness is most important to you, and why?

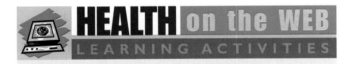

Rating Your Readiness for Physical Activity

Is a physician's examination really necessary before you begin an exercise program? Most exercise physiologists do not think so. However, if you are between the ages of 15 and 69, the PAR-Q can help you decide whether to check with a doctor before you start. Go to www.thriveonline.com/health/osteo/tools.parq1.html and answer the seven questions. If you're ready to get started, take the quiz below to decide which activities are best for you. Then let the workouts begin!

Determining Your Workout Personality

People who choose physical activities that they enjoy are much more likely to exercise regularly and stay fit. Charles Yokomoto, an educator who has studied personality type and sports, has created a personality test for exercise. Go to www.healthyideas.com/weight/quiz/personality and take the quiz he developed. Click the *Submit* button, and then read your results to find out which kind of aerobic workout is most likely to guarantee your fitness success.

Finding Your Target Heart Rate

Want to be sure you're training at an optimum level when you exercise? It's easy to calculate your target heart rate, and you can do it on-line! Go to www.healthchecksystems.com/heart.html and use the calculators provided. Simply enter your age and then click the *Calculate* button to see your results. Be sure to use this information during your next workout!

For more activities, log on to our Online Learning Center at www.mhhe.com/hper/health/payne.

Aging Physically

With aging, physical decline occurs and the components of physical fitness become more difficult to maintain. From the fourth decade onward, a gradual decline in vigor and resistance eventually gives way to various types of illnesses. In the opinion of many authorities, people do not die of old age. Rather, old age worsens specific conditions responsible for death. However, physical decline can be slowed and the onset of illness delayed by staying physically active. The process of aging can be described on the basis of predictable occurrences:[5]

- Change is gradual. In aging, gradual changes occur in body structure or function before specific health problems are identified.
- Individual differences occur. When two people of the same age are compared for the type and extent of change that has occurred with age, important differences can be noted. Even within the same person, different systems decline at differing rates and to varying extents.
- Greatest change is noted in areas of complex function. In physiological processes involving two or more major body systems, the most profound effects of physiological aging can be noted.
- Homeostatic decline occurs with age. Becoming older is associated with a growing difficulty in maintaining homeostasis (the dynamic balance among body systems). In the face of stressors, the older adult's system takes longer to respond, does not respond with the same magnitude, and may take longer to return to baseline.

Like growth and development, aging is predictable yet unique for each person.

Health Concerns of Midlife Adults

The period between forty-five and sixty-four years of age brings with it a variety of subtle changes in the body's structure and function. When life is busy and the mind is active, these changes are generally not evident. Even when they become evident, they are not usually the source of profound concern. Nevertheless, your parents, older students in your class, and people with whom you will be working are experiencing these changes:[5]

- Decrease in bone mass and density
- Increase in vertebral compression
- Degenerative changes in joint cartilage
- Increase in adipose tissue—loss of lean body mass
- Decrease in capacity to engage in physical work
- Decrease in visual acuity
- Decrease in basal energy requirements
- Decrease in fertility
- Decrease in sexual function

For some midlife adults these health concerns can be quite threatening, especially for those who view aging with apprehension and fear. Some middle-aged people reject these physical changes and convince themselves they are sick. Indeed, hypochondriasis is much more common among midlife people than among young people.

Osteoporosis

Osteoporosis is a condition frequently seen in late middle-aged women. However, it is not fully understood why white menopausal women are so susceptible to the increase in calcium loss that leads to fractures of the hip, wrist, and vertebral column. Well over 90 percent of all people with osteoporosis are white women.

The endocrine system plays a large role in the development of osteoporosis. At the time of menopause, a woman's ovaries begin a rapid decrease in the production of estrogen, one of two main hormones associated with the menstrual cycle. This lower level of estrogen may decrease the conversion of the precursors of vitamin D into the active form of vitamin D, the form necessary for absorbing calcium from the digestive tract. As a result, calcium may be drawn from the bones for use elsewhere in the body.

Additional explanations of osteoporosis focus on two other possibilities—hyperparathyroidism (another endocrine dysfunction) and the below-average degree of muscle development seen in osteoporotic women. In this latter explanation the reduced muscle mass is associated with decreased activity, which in turn deprives the body of the mechanical stimulation needed to facilitate bone growth.

muscular endurance the ability of a muscle or muscle group to function over time; supported by the respiratory and circulatory systems.

flexibility the ability of joints to function through an intended range of motion.

static stretching the slow lengthening of a muscle group to an extended stretch; followed by a holding of the extended position for a recommended period.

ballistic stretching a "bouncing" form of stretching in which a muscle group is lengthened repetitively to produce multiple quick, forceful stretches.

osteoporosis loss of calcium from the bone, seen primarily in postmenopausal women.

Premenopausal women have the opportunity to build and maintain a healthy skeleton through an appropriate intake of calcium. Current recommendations are for an intake of 1,200 mg of calcium per day. Three to four daily servings of low-fat dairy products should provide sufficient calcium. The diet also must contain adequate vitamin D because it aids in the absorption of calcium.

Many women do not consume an adequate amount of calcium. Calcium supplements, again in combination with vitamin D, can be used to achieve recommended calcium levels. It is now known that calcium carbonate, a highly advertised form of calcium, is no more easily absorbed by the body than are other forms of calcium salts. Consumers of calcium supplements should compare brands to determine which, if any, they should buy.

In premenopausal women, calcium deposition in bone is facilitated by exercise, particularly exercise that involves movement of the extremities. Today, women are encouraged to consume at least the recommended servings from the milk group and engage in regular physical activity that involves the weight-bearing muscles of the legs, such as aerobics, jogging, or walking.

Postmenopausal women who are not elderly can markedly slow the resorption of calcium from their bones through the use of estrogen replacement therapy. When combined with a daily intake of 1,500 mg of calcium, vitamin D, and regular exercise, estrogen therapy almost eliminates calcium loss. Of course, women will need to work closely with their physicians to monitor the use of estrogen because of continuing concern over the role of estrogen replacement therapy in the development of breast cancer.

Osteoarthritis

Arthritis is an umbrella term for more than one hundred forms of joint inflammation. The most common form is **osteoarthritis.** It is likely that as we age, all of us will develop osteoarthritis to some degree. Often called "wear and tear" arthritis, osteoarthritis occurs primarily in the weight-bearing joints of the knee, hip, and spine. In this form of arthritis, joint damage can occur to bone ends, cartilaginous cushions, and related structures as the years of constant friction and stress accumulate.

The object of current management of osteoarthritis (and other forms) is not to cure the disease but rather to reduce discomfort, limit joint destruction, and maximize joint mobility. Aspirin and non-steroidal anti-inflammatory agents are the drugs most frequently used to treat osteoarthritis.

It is now believed that osteoarthritis develops most commonly in people with a genetic predisposi-

tion for excessive damage to the weight-bearing joints. Thus the condition seems to run in families. Further, studies comparing the occurrence of osteoarthritis in those who exercise and those who do not demonstrate that regular movement may decrease the likelihood of developing this form of arthritis.

Health Concerns of Elderly Adults

In elderly people, it is frequently difficult to distinguish between changes caused by aging and those caused by disease. For virtually every body system, biomedical indexes for the old and young can overlap. In the respiratory system, for example, the oxygen uptake capacity of a man of seventy years may be no different from that of a man fifty-five years old who has a history of heavy cigarette smoking. Is the level in the elderly man to be considered an indicator of a disease, or should it be considered a reflection of normal old age? In dealing with the elderly, physicians frequently must make this kind of distinction.

In elderly people, as in midlife people, structural and physiological changes are routinely seen. In some cases, these are closely related to disease processes, but in most cases they reflect the gradual decline that is thought to be a result of the normal aging process. The most frequently seen changes include the following:

- Decrease in bone mass
- Changes in the structure of bone
- Decrease in muscle bulk and strength
- Decrease in oxygen uptake
- Loss of nonreproducing cells in the nervous system
- Decrease in hearing and vision abilities
- Decrease in all other sensory modalities, including the sense of body positioning
- Slower reaction time
- Gait and posture changes resulting from a weakening of the muscles of the trunk and legs

In addition to these changes, the most likely change seen in the elderly is the increased sensitivity of the body's homeostatic mechanism. Because of this sensitivity, a minor infection or superficial injury can be traumatic enough to decrease the body's ability to maintain its internal balance. An illness that would be easily controlled in a younger person could even prove fatal to a seemingly healthy seventy-five-year-old person.

Continuing to follow a physical fitness plan throughout midlife and older adulthood is essential to minimizing age-related health problems. The plan should be modified as necessary to accommodate changes in physical functioning (see the Star Box on p. 89 for an example).

Elderly Adults and Tai Chi Chuan

Continuing to follow a program of physical fitness is vital throughout midlife and older age. However, which types of exercise are most appropriate for older adults?

Many older adults choose gentle aerobic activities that put less stress and strain on joints, such as walking or water aerobics. Another option is the Chinese discipline tai chi chuan. Practitioners say that the slow, gentle movements of tai chi provide a variety of health benefits, such as improving physical strength and balance. Now a recent study[20] supports these beliefs, reporting that geriatric practitioners of tai chi enjoy greater flexibility, lower body fat, and greater peak oxygen uptake (an indication of cardiorespiratory fitness). The study concludes that tai chi may be prescribed as a suitable conditioning exercise for the elderly.

Personal Applications

• How do you plan to deal with the physical changes that will take place as you age? What can you do now to minimize the occurrence of health problems as you grow older?

Developing a Cardiorespiratory Fitness Program

For people of all ages, cardiorespiratory conditioning can be achieved through many activities. As long as the activity you choose places sufficient demand on the heart and lungs, improved fitness is possible. In addition to the familiar activities of swimming, running, cycling, and aerobic dance, many people today are participating in brisk walking, rollerblading, cross-country skiing, swimnastics, skating, rowing, and even weight training (often combined with some form of aerobic activity). Regardless of age or physical limitations, you can select from a variety of enjoyable activities that will condition the cardiorespiratory system. Complete the Personal Assessment on pages 90–91 to determine your level of fitness.

Many people think that any kind of physical activity will produce cardiorespiratory fitness. Many people consider golf, bowling, hunting, fishing, and archery to be forms of exercise. However, these activities generally fail to produce positive changes in your cardiorespiratory and overall muscular fitness; they may enhance your health, be enjoyable, and produce some fatigue after long participation, but they do not

meet the fitness standards recently established by the American College of Sports Medicine (ACSM), the nation's premier professional organization of exercise physiologists and sport physicians.[6]

The ACSM's most recent recommendations for achieving cardiorespiratory fitness were approved in 1990 and include five major areas: (1) mode of activity, (2) frequency of training, (3) intensity of training, (4) duration of training, and (5) resistance training. We summarize these recommendations. You may wish to compare your existing fitness program with these standards.

Mode of Activity

The ACSM recommends that the mode of activity be any continuous physical activity that uses large muscle groups and can be rhythmic and aerobic in nature. Among the activities that generally meet this requirement are continuous swimming, cycling, aerobics, basketball, cross-country skiing, rollerblading, step training (bench aerobics), hiking, walking, rowing, stair climbing, dancing, and running. Recently, water exercise (water or aqua aerobics) has become a popular fitness mode, because it is especially effective for pregnant women and elderly, injured, or disabled people.[7]

Endurance games and activities, such as tennis, racquetball, and handball, are fine as long as you and your partner are skilled enough to keep the ball in play; walking after the ball will do very little for you. Riding a bicycle is a good activity if you keep pedaling. Coasting will do little to improve fitness. Softball and football are generally less than sufficient continuous activities—especially the way they are played by weekend athletes.

Regardless of which continuous activity you select, it should also be enjoyable. Running, for example, is not for everyone—despite what some accomplished runners say! Find an activity you enjoy. If you need others around you to have a good time, corral a group of friends to join you. Vary your activities to keep from becoming bored. You might cycle in the summer, run in the fall, swim in the winter, and play racquetball in the spring. To help you maintain your fitness program, see the suggestions in the Health Action Guide on page 92. In addition, the Star Box on page 92 provides information on exercising in an urban environment.

osteoarthritis arthritis that develops with age; largely caused by weight bearing and deterioration of the joints.

Personal Assessment

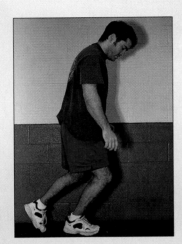

You can determine your level of fitness in 30 minutes or less by completing this short group of tests based on the National Fitness Test developed by the President's Council on Physical Fitness and Sports. If you are over 40 years old or have chronic medical disorders such as diabetes or obesity, check with your physician before taking this or any other fitness test. You will need another person to monitor your test and keep time.

Three-minute step test

Aerobic capacity. Equipment: 12-inch bench, crate, block, or step ladder; stopwatch. Procedure: face bench. Complete 24 full steps (both feet on the bench, both feet on the ground) per minute for 3 minutes. After finishing, sit down, have your partner find your pulse within 5 seconds, and take your pulse for 1 minute. Your score is your pulse rate for 1 full minute.

Scoring standards (heart rate for 1 minute)

Age	18–29		30–39		40–49		50–59		60+	
Gender	F	M	F	M	F	M	F	M	F	M
Excellent	<80	<75	<84	<78	<88	<80	<92	<85	<95	<90
Good	80–110	75–100	84–115	78–109	88–118	80–112	92–123	85–115	95–127	90–118
Average	>110	>100	>115	>109	>118	>112	>123	>115	>127	>118

Sit and reach

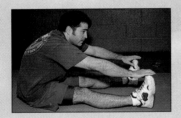

Hamstring flexibility. Equipment: yardstick; tape. Between your legs, tape the yardstick to the floor. Sit with legs straight and heels about 5 inches apart, heels even with the 15-inch mark on the yardstick. While in a sitting position, slowly stretch forward as far as possible. Your score is the number of inches reached.

Scoring standards (inches)

Age	18–29		30–39		40–49		50–59		60+	
Gender	F	M	F	M	F	M	F	M	F	M
Excellent	>22	>21	>22	>21	>21	>20	>20	>19	>20	>19
Good	17–22	13–21	17–22	13–21	15–21	13–20	14–20	12–19	14–20	12–19
Average	<17	<13	<17	<13	<15	<13	<14	<12	<14	<12

Arm hang

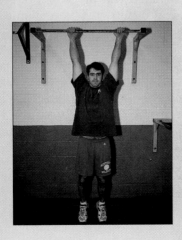
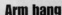

Upper body strength. Equipment: horizontal bar (high enough to prevent your feet from touching the floor); stopwatch. Procedure: hang with straight arms, palms facing forward. Start watch when subject is in position. Stop when subject lets go. Your score is the number of minutes and seconds spent hanging.

Scoring standards (heart rate for 1 minute)

Age	18–29		30–39		40–49		50–59		60+	
Gender	F	M	F	M	F	M	F	M	F	M
Excellent	>1:30	>2:00	>1:20	>1:50	>1:10	>1:35	>1:00	>1:20	>:50	>1:10
Good	:46–1:30	1:00–2:00	:40–1:20	:50–1:50	:30–1:10	:45–1:35	:30–1:00	:35–1:20	:21–:50	:30–1:10
Average	<:46	<1:00	<:40	<:50	<:30	<:45	<:30	<:35	<:21	<:30

Curl-ups

Abdominal and low back strength. Equipment: stopwatch. Procedure: Lie flat on upper back, knees bent, shoulders touching the floor, arms extended above your thighs or by your sides, palms down. Bend knees so that feet are flat and 12 inches from the buttocks. Curl up by lifting head and shoulders off the floor, sliding hands forward above your thighs or the floor. Curl down and repeat. Your score is the number of curl-ups in 1 minute.

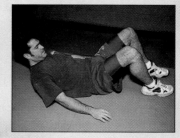

Scoring standards (number in 1 minute)

Age	18–29		30–39		40–49		50–59		60+	
Gender	F	M	F	M	F	M	F	M	F	M
Excellent	>45	>50	>40	>45	>35	>40	>30	>35	>25	>30
Good	25–45	30–50	20–40	22–45	16–35	21–40	12–30	18–35	11–25	15–30
Average	<25	<30	<20	<22	<16	<21	<12	<18	<11	<15

Push-ups (Men)

Upper body strength. Equipment: stopwatch. Assume a front-leaning position. Lower your body until chest touches the floor. Raise and repeat for 1 minute. Your score is the number of push-ups completed in 1 minute.

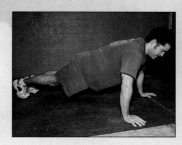

Scoring standards (number in 1 minute)

Age	18–29	30–39	40–49	50–59	60+
Excellent	>50	>45	>40	>35	>30
Good	25–50	22–45	19–40	15–35	10–30
Average	<25	<22	<19	<15	<10

Modified Push-ups (Women)

Upper body strength. Equipment: stopwatch. Assume a front-leaning position with knees bent up, hands under shoulders. Lower your chest to the floor, raise, and repeat. Your score is the number of push-ups completed in 1 minute.

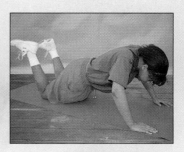

Scoring standards (number in 1 minute)

Age	18–29	30–39	40–49	50–59	60+
Excellent	>45	>40	>35	>30	>25
Good	17–45	12–40	8–35	6–30	5–25
Average	<17	<12	<8	<6	<5

To Carry This Further . . .

Note your areas of strengths and weaknesses. To improve your fitness, become involved in a fitness program that reflects the concepts discussed in this chapter. Talking with fitness experts on your campus might be a good first step.

Frequency of Training

Frequency of training refers to the number of times per week a person should exercise. The ACSM recommends three to five times per week. For most people, participation in fitness activities more than five times each week does not significantly improve their level

---

---

of conditioning. Likewise, an average of only two workouts each week does not seem to produce a measurable improvement in cardiorespiratory conditioning. Thus, although you may have a lot of fun cycling twice each week, do not expect to see a significant improvement in your cardiorespiratory fitness level.

Intensity of Training

How much effort should you put into an activity? Should you run quickly, jog slowly, or swim at a comfortable pace? Must a person sweat profusely to become fit? These questions all refer to **intensity** of effort.

The ACSM recommends that healthy adults exercise at an intensity level of between 60 percent and 90 percent of their maximum heart rate (calculated by subtracting your age from 220). This level of intensity is called the **target heart rate (THR)** (see the Health Action Guide on p. 93). This rate refers to the minimum number of times your heart needs to contract (beat) each minute to have a positive effect on your heart, lungs, and blood vessels. This improvement is called the training effect. Activity at an intensity below the THR will be insufficient to make a significant improvement in your fitness level. Although intensity below the THR will still help you expend calories and thus lose weight, it will probably do little to make you more

---

Exercising in an Urban Environment

People who live in large cities face special challenges as they pursue fitness activities. Some of these challenges are just annoying, but some challenges can be life-threatening. News reports occasionally tell of someone who was seriously injured or killed (accidentally or intentionally) while trying to exercise in an urban environment. Visitors to cities can also be confronted with these difficulties, and visitors may be less experienced adjusting to these challenges than those who live year-round in the city.

Among the obstacles are pollution, heavy vehicular and pedestrian traffic, and the possibility of criminal activity. These problems may also exist in small towns, but more likely they exist to a lesser degree. Resist the temptation to use "the city" as an excuse not to exercise. Fortunately, you can tailor a fitness program to fit the urban environment in numerous ways. Consider these strategies as you plan your fitness activities in the city.

- If you are unfamiliar with the environment, exercise indoors. It can be dangerous to jog, rollerblade, or cycle in a place where you could become lost. Exercise inside your home or apartment, a local health club or YMCA, or in your hotel. Many indoor exercise machines provide a good cardiorespiratory and strength-training workout. Some facilities also have swimming pools, indoor tracks, handball courts, and special fitness classes.

- If you plan to exercise outdoors, always do so with a partner. There is, indeed, safety in numbers. Exercising with a friend or two (or jogging with a large, leashed dog) can provide a

measure of protection. If you become injured, friends can help summon medical assistance.

- Try to avoid heavily congested areas. Cycling or jogging in heavy traffic is dangerous not only for you but also for other pedestrians and motorists. This is especially true during rush hours (7–9 A.M., noon, and 4–6 P.M.). Try to locate a relatively quiet place that also seems secure. If you are a visitor to an area, make certain you know whether a particular area is safe for walking, cycling, or jogging. Don't assume that every urban park is a safe haven for exercisers.

- Do not exercise outside at night. A city can take on an entirely different mood during the night. It is foolish to place yourself at risk by exercising outside when it is dark. Stick to the daylight hours.

- Be aware of pollution levels before you exercise. If there is a pollution warning, consider exercising indoors until the alert is over. If you are one who must exercise outside, you might wish to use a pollution mask; the mask will filter a significant amount of large particles. However, it may also serve to attract unnecessary attention.

- Consider carrying an alarm or protective spray device when exercising outdoors. This suggestion has both proponents and opponents. Carrying a protective spray device or alarm can be helpful, if you know how to use it in an emergency. Remember, some devices can be used against you, especially if an assailant surprises and overpowers you.

aerobically fit. On the other hand, intensity that is significantly above your THR will probably cause you to become so fatigued that you will be forced to stop the activity before the training effect can be achieved.

Choosing a particular THR between 60 percent and 90 percent of your maximum heart rate depends on your initial level of fitness. If you are already in relatively good physical shape, you might want to start exercising at 75 percent of your maximum heart rate. A well-conditioned person might select a higher THR for his or her intensity level, whereas a person with a low fitness level will still be able to achieve a training effect at the lower THR of 60 percent of maximum.

In the Health Action Guide below, the younger person would need to participate in a continuous activity for an extended period while working at a THR of 160 beats per minute. The older person would need to function at a THR of 117 beats per minute to achieve a positive training effect.

Determining your heart rate is not a complicated procedure. Find a location on your body where an artery passes near the surface of the skin. Pulse rates are difficult to determine by touching veins, which are more superficial than arteries. Two easily accessible sites for determining heart rate are the carotid artery (one on each side of the windpipe at the front of your neck) and the radial artery (on the inside of your wrist, just above the base of the thumb).

You should practice placing the front surface of your index and middle fingertips at either of these locations and feeling for a pulse. Once you have found a regular pulse, look at the second hand of a watch. Count the number of beats you feel in a ten-second period. Multiply this number by six. This number is your heart rate. With a little practice, you can become very proficient at determining your heart rate.

HEALTH ACTION GUIDE

How to Calculate Your Target Heart Rate

The target heart rate (THR) is the recommended rate for increasing cardiorespiratory endurance. To maintain a training effect, you must sustain activity at your THR. To find your THR, subtract your age from 220 (the maximum heart rate) and multiply by .60 to .90. Here are two examples:

For a 20-year-old person (wanting a THR of 80% of maximum)	For a 40-year-old person (wanting a THR of 65% of maximum)
Maximum heart rate: 220 − 20 = 200 200 × .80 = 160 THR = 160 beats per minute	Maximum heart rate: 220 − 40 = 180 180 × .65 = 117 THR = 117 beats per minute

InfoLinks
www.fitnesslink.com

Duration of Training

The ACSM recommends that the **duration** of training be between twenty and sixty minutes of continuous aerobic activity. Generally speaking, the duration can be on the shorter end of this range for athletic people whose activities use a high intensity of training (80% to 90% of maximum heart rate). Those who choose activities with a low range of intensity (60% to 70% of maximum heart rate) should maintain that activity for a longer time. Thus a fast jog and a moderate walk will require different amounts of time to accomplish the training effect. The fast jog might be maintained for twenty-five minutes, whereas the brisk walk should be kept up longer—perhaps for fifty minutes. Recently, however, some fitness experts have advocated a modified version of the ACSM's recommendations to accommodate less directed physical activity. See the Star Box on page 94 for a more detailed discussion.

Resistance Training

Recognizing the important fact that overall body fitness includes muscular fitness, the ACSM now recommends resistance training in its current standards. The ACSM suggests participation in strength training of moderate intensity at least two times a week. This training should help develop and maintain a healthy body composition—one with an emphasis on lean body mass. The goal of resistance training is not to improve cardiorespiratory endurance but to improve overall muscle strength and tone. For the average person, resistance training with heavy weights is not recommended because it can induce a sudden and dangerous increase in blood pressure.

The resistance training recommended by the ACSM includes one set of eight to twelve repetitions of eight to ten different exercises. These exercises should be geared to the body's major muscle groups (i.e., legs, arms, shoulders, trunk, and back) and should not focus on just one or two body areas. Isotonic (progressive resistance) or isokinetic exercises are recommended (see p. 85). For the average person, resistance training activities should be done at a moderate-to-slow speed, use the full range of motion, and not impair normal breathing. With just one set

frequency   the number of times per week one should exercise to achieve a training effect.

intensity   the level of effort put into an activity.

target heart rate (THR)   the number of times per minute the heart must contract to produce a training effect.

duration   the length of time one needs to exercise at the THR to produce a training effect.

Exercise Intensity: Regular or Lite?

You say you don't have the time or the inclination for regular, intense exercise? Then get your exercise by accumulating twenty to sixty minutes in short spurts, by weeding the garden, going dancing, climbing stairs, or painting the side of the house, say some researchers. Other researchers aren't sure of the benefits of such "exercise lite."

Several health professionals have recently begun to urge the American public to consider the health benefits of less directed physical activity than that prescribed by the American College of Sports Medicine. These fitness experts believe that people shy away from physical activity because they are afraid that a fitness program requires too much effort and commitment.

One key aspect of this revised approach is the belief that the twenty to sixty minutes of daily physical activity does not have to be accomplished all at once. People can accumulate their minutes in segments over the course of the day. For example, raking leaves for fifteen minutes, walking briskly for ten minutes at lunch, and dancing for ten minutes can produce health benefits if done on most days.

Of course, "exercise lite" does not mean simply getting up to change the channel rather than using the remote control. It means activities like a brisk walk, enough to speed up your breathing in a minute or two. A leisurely bike ride or working in the garden also qualifies. Consider these other possibilities:

- Get off the sofa during television commercials and walk around the house or in the yard.

- Whenever you can, take short, brisk walks. Brief extra walks around campus (e.g., taking the long way to class or your place of work) can consume calories and place some beneficial exertion on your cardiorespiratory system.

- Instead of phoning people in your apartment or residence hall, walk to their rooms. Rather than phoning a colleague in an office building, you can walk to his or her office.

- When possible, use stairs instead of elevators.

- Instead of parking as close to a building as you can, park your car farther away to increase your walking distance.

A study recently conducted in Dallas showed that volunteers in a "lifestyle group" enjoyed health benefits as great as those in a traditional, structured gym program. The lifestyle group lowered its average blood pressure and total cholesterol and improved its ratio of good to bad cholesterol. The lifestyle group gained about the same amount of muscle and lost the same amount of fat as the more intense gymnasium group. Finally, the lifestyle group burned the same number of calories from its activities, an average of 159 extra a day, as the more intense group.

Opponents of this "kinder, gentler" approach to fitness aren't sure of the benefits of this easy approach. One recent study reported that vigorous exercise such as jogging, walking quickly, or aerobics class will lengthen your life, but that lighter workouts will not. Experts are concerned that people who already exercise regularly may slack off and actually reduce their current fitness levels. Opponents also believe that, without a prescription for exercise, the public will fool itself into thinking it is much more active than it really is.

Which approach is better? Experts do not agree. If you already are following a regular, intense exercise program, by all means do not give it up. We know that the more aerobically fit you are, the better your odds of a long, healthy life. However, if you are doing little or nothing, whether because of your schedule, procrastination, or fear of intense exercise, easing into a program of exercise lite apparently can bring real benefits.

---

recommended for each exercise, resistance training is not very time consuming.

Warm-up, Workout, Cooldown

Each training session consists of three basic parts: the warm-up, the workout, and the cooldown.[2] The warm-up should last ten to fifteen minutes. During this period, you should begin slow, gradual, comfortable movements related to the upcoming activity, such as walking or slow jogging. All body segments and muscle groups should be exercised as you gradually increase your heart rate. Near the end of the warm-up period, the major muscle groups should be stretched. This preparation helps protect you from muscle strains and joint sprains.

The warm-up is a fine time to socialize. Furthermore, you can mentally prepare yourself for your activity or think about the beauty of the morning sky, the changing colors of the leaves, or the friends you will meet later in the day. Mental warm-ups can be as

beneficial for you psychologically as physical warm-ups are physiologically.

The second part of the training session is the workout, the part of the session that involves improving muscular strength and endurance, cardiorespiratory endurance, and flexibility. Workouts can be tailor-made, but they should follow the ACSM guidelines discussed previously in this chapter.

The third important part of each fitness session, the cooldown, consists of a five- to ten-minute session of relaxing exercises, such as slow jogging, walking, and stretching.[8] This activity allows your body to cool and return to a resting state. A cooldown period helps reduce muscle soreness.

Personal Applications

- Design a fitness program for yourself that includes each of the five components discussed in this chapter.

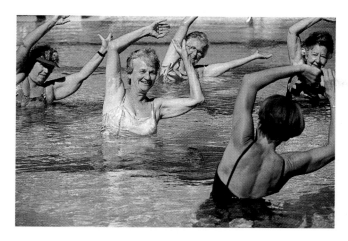

Well-designed fitness programs are beneficial to older adults.

Exercise for Older Adults

An exercise program designed for younger adults may be inappropriate for older people, particularly those over age fifty. Special attention must be paid to matching the program to the interests and abilities of the participants. The goals of the program should include both social interaction and physical conditioning.

Older adults, especially those with a personal or family history of heart problems, should have a physical examination before starting a fitness program. This examination should include a stress cardiogram, a blood pressure check, and an evaluation of joint functioning. Participants should learn how to monitor their own cardiorespiratory status during exercise.

Well-designed fitness programs for older adults will include activities that begin slowly, are monitored frequently, and are geared to the enjoyment of the participants.[9] The professional staff coordinating the program should be familiar with the signs of distress (excessively elevated heart rate, nausea, breathing difficulty, pallor, and pain) and must be able to perform CPR. Warm-up and cooldown periods should be included. Activities to increase flexibility are beneficial in the beginning and ending segments of the program. Participants should wear comfortable clothing and appropriate shoes and should be mentally prepared to enjoy the activities.

A program designed for older adults will largely conform to the ACSM criteria specified previously in this chapter. However, except for certain very fit older adults (such as runners and triathletes), the THR should not exceed 120 beats per minute. Also, because of possible joint, muscular, or skeletal problems, certain activities may have to be done in a sitting position. Pain or discomfort should be reported immediately to the fitness instructor.

Fortunately, properly screened older adults will rarely have health emergencies during a well-monitored fitness program. Many fit older adults can also safely exercise alone.

Low Back Pain

A common occurrence among adults is the sudden onset of low back pain.[10] Each year, 10 million adults develop this condition, which can be so uncomfortable that they miss work, lose sleep, and generally feel incapable of engaging in daily activities. Eighty percent of all adults who have this condition will experience these effects two to three times per year.

Although low back pain can reflect serious health problems, most low back pain is caused by mechanical (postural) problems. As unpleasant as low back pain is, the problem usually corrects itself within a week or two. The services of a physician, physical therapist, or chiropractor are generally not required after an initial visit.

By engaging in regular exercise, such as swimming, walking, and bicycling, and by paying attention to your back during bending, lifting, and sitting, you can minimize the occurrence of this uncomfortable and incapacitating condition.

Fitness Questions and Answers

Along with the five necessary elements to include in your fitness program, you should consider many additional issues when you start a fitness program.

Should I See My Doctor Before I Get Started?

This issue has probably kept thousands of people from ever beginning a fitness program. The hassle and expense of getting a comprehensive physical examination are excellent excuses for people who are not completely sold on the idea of exercise. A complete examination, including blood analysis, stress test, cardiogram, serum lipid analysis, and body fat analysis, is a valuable tool for developing some baseline physical data for your medical record.

Is this examination really necessary? Most exercise physiologists do not think so. The value of these measurements as safety predictors is questioned by many professionals. A good rule of thumb to follow is to undergo a physical examination if (1) you have an existing medical condition (such as diabetes, obesity, hypertension, heart abnormalities, or arthritis), (2) you are a man over age 40 or a woman over age 50.[11]

What Causes a "Runner's High"?

During or after exercise, a person occasionally experiences feelings of euphoria. Runners and joggers call these feelings the "runner's high." However, these positive feelings of relaxation, high self-esteem, and reduced stress are not limited to runners. Almost any fitness activity can leave participants with these intense positive feelings. Swimmers, aerobic exercisers, hikers, and cyclists all have reported exercise-induced highs.

Exercise May Ease Symptoms of PMS

Many women have long reported that exercise reduces the number and severity of symptoms that they suffer from premenstrual syndrome (PMS). Recent studies support those anecdotal reports.

In one study, 8,143 women were divided into four groups: competitive sportswomen, high exercisers, low exercisers, and sedentary women.[21] The study concluded that the high exercisers reported the greatest improvement in mood, and sedentary women the least. The results support the belief that women who exercise frequently may be protected from the deterioration of mood that occurs before and during menstruation.

The competitive sportswomen group did not enjoy this same level of benefit, possibly because of the extraordinary physical demands they place on their bodies.

Another study involving twenty-three premenopausal women found that those who engaged in regular aerobic exercise significantly improved their premenstrual symptoms, especially premenstrual depression, in addition to improving their aerobic capacity.[22]

Although these pleasurable feelings can be attributed in part to psychological causes, there is plenty of scientific evidence to suggest a physiological cause. During physical activity, the brain releases its own morphinelike (opiatelike) substances called *endorphins*. These chemicals are released by brain neurons and produce sensations that are pleasurable, and sometimes even numbing. Exercisers report that these episodes of euphoria are unpredictable. Sometimes they experience highs and sometimes they do not. However, endorphin highs are more likely to occur during or after a strenuous, challenging workout.

How Should "30-Somethings" Alter Their Exercise Programs?

People in their third decade of life need to make few if any significant adjustments in their fitness programs. Men and women can continue physical activities they have used since their twenties. If they feel mired in activities that now seem boring, "30-somethings" might try a new activity. However, any new activity (or increase in the intensity of a current activity) should be undertaken gradually.

Should Women Exercise During Pregnancy?

Pregnant women should continue to exercise.[12] During pregnancy a woman's entire body undergoes many physical changes. Muscles are stretched, joints are loosened, and tissues are subjected to stress. If a woman is in good physiological condition, she is more likely to handle these changes with few complications. The

baby may also benefit: Studies have shown that women who exercise moderately during pregnancy tend to give birth to healthier babies.[12]

Exercise during pregnancy can also increase a woman's muscle strength, making delivery of the baby easier and faster. Exercise can also help control her weight, improve her balance, and make it easier to get back to normal weight after delivery.

The types of exercises a woman should perform during pregnancy depend on the individual and the stage of pregnancy. Most pregnant women should perform general exercises that increase overall fitness and stamina, as well as exercises that strengthen specific muscle groups. Muscles of the pelvic floor, for example, should be exercised regularly, because these muscles will be supporting most of the extra weight of the baby.

A variety of exercises are appropriate, including walking, swimming, stretching, and strengthening exercises.[12] Yoga and tai chi are also good forms of exercise for pregnant women. The muscles of the pelvic floor, abdomen, and back are especially subject to stress and strain during pregnancy and delivery, so certain exercises can also be performed to strengthen these muscles. Exercises can also be performed to speed up recovery after delivery. Such postpartum exercises can be started in some cases within twenty-four hours after delivery. Exercises can even be started before conception if a pregnancy is anticipated.

Some types of exercise can put the fetus at risk. A pregnant woman should avoid any activity in which she becomes overheated, because her elevated body temperature will warm up the fetal environment. Thus pregnant women should not use saunas or hot tubs, nor should they exercise in a hot, humid environment. During the last trimester of pregnancy, women should also avoid any strenuous or high-impact exercise that involves bouncing, jumping, or jarring motions. Obviously, pregnant women should first consult with their obstetricians to develop a safe, productive exercise routine.

What Kinds of Aerobic Exercise Are Popular Today?

One of the most popular fitness approaches is aerobic exercise, including aerobic dancing. Many organizations sponsor classes in this form of continuous dancing and movement. The rise in popularity of televised and videotaped aerobic exercise programs reflects the enthusiasm for this form of exercise. Because extravagant claims are often made about the value of these programs, the wise consumer should observe at least one session of the activity before enrolling. Does the program meet the criteria outlined on pages 89–94?: mode of activity, frequency, intensity, duration, and resistance training.

Street dancing has become one of the most popular aerobic exercises. Popularized by rap music, classic funk, and the growth of vigorous "street jam" dancing in music videos, street dancing is an excellent way of having fun and developing cardiorespiratory fitness. Have you experienced this activity?

What Are Low-Impact Aerobic Activities?

Because long-term participation in some aerobic activities (for example, jogging, running, aerobic dancing, and rope skipping) may damage the hip, knee, and ankle joints, many fitness experts promote low-impact aerobic activities. Low-impact aerobic dancing, water aerobics, bench aerobics, and brisk walking are examples of this kind of fitness activity. Participants still conform to the principal components of a cardiorespiratory fitness program. THR levels are the same as in high-impact aerobic activities.

The main difference between low-impact and high-impact aerobic activities is the use of the legs. Low-impact aerobics do not require having both feet off the ground at the same time. Thus, weight transfer does not occur with the forcefulness seen in traditional, high-impact aerobic activities. In addition, low-impact activities may include exaggerated arm movements and the use of hand or wrist weights. All of these variations are designed to increase the heart rate to the THR without damaging the joints of the lower extremities. Low-impact aerobics are excellent for people of all ages, and they may be especially beneficial to older adults.

In-line skating (rollerblading) is one of the fastest-growing fitness activities. This low-impact activity has cardiorespiratory and muscular benefits similar to those of running without the pounding effect that running can produce. Rollerblading requires important safety equipment: sturdy skates, knee and elbow pads, wrist supports, and a helmet.

What Is the Most Effective Means of Fluid Replacement During Exercise?

Despite all the advertising hype associated with commercial fluid replacement products, for an average person involved in typical fitness activities, water is still the best fluid replacement. The availability and cost are unbeatable. However, when activity is prolonged and intense, commercial sport drinks may be preferred over water because they contain electrolytes (which replace lost sodium and potassium) and carbohydrates (which replace depleted energy stores). However, the carbohydrates in sports drinks are actually simple forms of sugar. Thus, sports drinks tend to be high in calories just like regular soft drinks. Regardless of the drink you choose, exercise physiologists recommend that you drink fluids before and at frequent intervals throughout the activity.

What Effect Does Alcohol Have on Sport Performance?

It probably comes as no surprise that alcohol use is generally detrimental to sport performance. Alcohol consumption, especially excessive intake the evening before an activity, consistently decreases the level of performance. Many research studies have documented the negative effects of alcohol on activities involving speed, strength, power, and endurance.[13]

Lowered performance appears to be related to a variety of factors, including impaired judgment, reduced coordination, depressed heart function, liver interference, and dehydration. Understandably, sports federations within the International Olympic Committee have banned the use of alcohol in conjunction with sports competition.

Only in the sports of precision shooting (pistol shooting, riflery, and archery) have studies shown that low-level alcohol use may improve performance, by reducing the shooter's anxiety and permitting steady hand movements. However, alcohol use has also been banned from these sports.[13]

Why Has Bodybuilding Become So Popular?

The popularity of bodybuilding has increased significantly in recent years for many reasons. Bodybuilders often start lifting weights to get into better shape—to improve muscle tone. They may just want to look healthier and feel stronger. When they realize that they can alter the shape of their bodies, they find that bodybuilding offers challenges that, through hard work, are attainable. Bodybuilders also report enjoying the physical sensations (the "pump") that result from a good workout. The results of their efforts are clearly visible and measurable. Some bodybuilders become involved in competitive events to test their advancements.

Perhaps we should dispel a few myths about bodybuilding. Are bodybuilders strong? The answer is emphatically—yes! Will muscle cells turn into fat cells if weight-lifting programs are discontinued? No, muscle cells are physiologically incapable of turning into fat cells. Will women develop bulky muscles through weight training? No, they can improve muscle size, strength, and tone, but unless they take steroids, their muscle mass cannot increase to the same degree as men's muscle mass. Is bodybuilding socially acceptable? Yes, for many people. Just observe all the health clubs and campus exercise rooms that cater to weight lifters and bodybuilders.

Can Anaerobic Exercise Provide Fitness Benefits?

Anaerobic exercise, such as strength training, can provide some of the same benefits as aerobic exercise, according to a recent study of law enforcement officers.[14] In this study, officers were assigned to either four months of circuit weight training or a nontraining control group. The study found that the weight trainers not only enjoyed a significant increase in strength and cardiovascular fitness but also significant improvements in mood, including decreases in anxiety, depression, and hostility. The circuit weight trainers also reported a decrease in physical complaints and an increase in their job satisfaction.

Where Can I Find Out About Proper Equipment?

College students are generally in an excellent setting to locate people who have the resources to provide helpful information about sports equipment. Contacting physical education or health education faculty members who have an interest in your chosen activity might be a good start. Most colleges also have a number of clubs that specialize in fitness interests—cycling, hiking, and jogging clubs, for example. Attend one of their upcoming meetings.

Sporting goods and specialty stores (for runners, tennis and racquetball players, and cyclists) are convenient places to obtain information. Employees of these stores are usually knowledgeable about sports and equipment. The Star Box on page 99 provides tips for choosing an athletic shoe, and the Star Box on page 101 discusses various popular types of home fitness equipment.

How Worthwhile Are Commercial Health and Fitness Clubs?

The health and fitness club business is booming. Fitness clubs offer activities ranging from free weights to weight machines to step walking to general aerobics. Some clubs have saunas and whirlpools and lots of frills. Others have course offerings that include wellness, smoking cessation, stress management, time management, dance, and yoga. The atmosphere at most clubs is friendly, and people are encouraged to have a good time while working out.

If your purpose in joining a fitness club is to improve your cardiorespiratory fitness, measure the program offered by the club against the ACSM standards. If your primary purpose in joining is to meet people and have fun, request a trial membership for a month or so to see whether you like the environment.

Before signing a contract at a health club or spa, do some careful questioning. Find out when the business was established, ask about the qualifications of the employees, contact some members for their observations, and request a thorough tour of the facilities. You might even consult your local Better Business Bureau for additional information. Finally, make certain that you read and understand every word of the contract.

What Is Crosstraining?

Crosstraining is the use of more than one aerobic activity to achieve cardiorespiratory fitness. For example, runners may use swimming, cycling, or rowing periodically to replace running in their training routines. Crosstraining allows certain muscle groups to rest and injuries to heal. In addition, crosstraining provides a refreshing change of pace for the participant. You will probably enjoy your fitness program more if you vary the activities. Further, your enjoyment will make it more likely that the *Healthy People 2010* objectives can be reached.

What Are Steroids and Why Do Some Athletes Use Them?

Steroids are drugs that physicians can legally prescribe for a variety of health conditions, including certain forms of anemia, inadequate growth patterns, and chronic debilitating diseases. Steroids can also be prescribed to aid recovery from surgery or burns. **Anabolic steroids** are drugs that function like the male sex hormone testosterone.[15] They can be taken orally or by injection.

Anabolic steroids are used by athletes who hope to gain weight, muscular size and strength, power, endurance, and aggressiveness. Over the last few decades, many bodybuilders, weight lifters, track athletes, and football players have chosen to ignore the serious health risks posed by illegal steroid use. More recently, steroid use among high school and college campuses has reached epidemic levels. The mass media has begun to focus attention on the dangers of steroid use, but many young athletes choose to ignore these warnings.

The use of steroids is highly dangerous because of serious, life-threatening side effects and adverse reactions. These effects include heart problems, certain

anabolic steroids (ann uh **bol** ick) drugs that function like testosterone to produce increases in weight, strength, endurance, and aggressiveness.

Choosing an Athletic Shoe

Aerobic Shoes

When selecting shoes for aerobic dancing, J. Lynn Reese, president of J. Lynn & Co. Endurance Sports, Washington, DC, advises the following:

- Check the width of the shoe at the widest part of your foot. The bottom of the shoe should be as wide as the bottom of your foot; the uppers shouldn't go over the sides.

- Look for leather or nylon uppers. Leather is durable and gives good support, but it can stretch. Nylon won't stretch and gives support, but it's not as durable. Canvas generally doesn't offer much support.

- Look for rubber rather than polyurethane or black carbon rubber soles. Treads should be fairly flat in the forefoot. If you dance on carpet, you can go with less tread; if you dance on gym floors, you may need more grab.

Basketball Shoes

What's most important when choosing a basketball shoe? John Burleson, of the Sports Authority, offers this advice:

- Cushioning. Cushioning is especially important in the forefoot area. Each shoe manufacturer has its own cushioning "system." For example, Nike has "Air," and Reebok promotes its "Hexalite" material, composed of hexagonal air chambers.

- Side support. Side support, also called lateral and medial support, is important for making quick directional changes.

- Fit of heel cup. Try on the shoe, and then put your little finger in behind the heel. It should fit snugly.

- Traction. Keep in mind the surface on which you play most often. More traction is needed on asphalt than on hardwood.

- Socks should be breathable and pull moisture away from the foot.

- "Rope" laces are more convenient than the more traditional flat laces because pulling on the ends will tighten up the laces on the whole shoe at once.

Running Shoes

Need new running shoes? Here's advice from Jeff Galloway, former Olympic runner and founder and president of Phidippides International aerobic sports stores, headquartered in Atlanta.

- Take time to shop, and find a knowledgeable salesperson. Good advice is crucial.

- Check the wear pattern on your old shoes to see whether you have floppy or rigid feet. Floppy-footed runners wear out their soles on the outside and inside edges; rigid-footed runners

wear out soles predominantly on the outside edges. Floppy-footed runners can sacrifice cushioning for support; rigid-footed runners can sacrifice support for cushioning.

- Know whether your feet are curved or straight and whether you have high arches or are flatfooted. The shoe should fit the shape of your foot.

Walking Shoes

Have you joined the millions of people who walk for fitness? If so, and if you are ready for a pair of athletic walking shoes, shoe manufacturer Nike has the following advice for you:

- Note where most of your weight falls on your foot when you walk. Are you landing mostly on the heel, or on the forefoot? This is where you will want cushioning.

- As with all other types of athletic shoes, take the time to find a knowledgeable salesperson who will provide good advice.

- Go for comfort. Stride in the different types of shoes at your typical walking pace and identify the shoes that are most comfortable.

- Choose shoes that are comfortable in the forefoot area, which will be carrying much of your weight.

- All-leather uppers are satisfactory for most walkers. If you are a serious walker, consider shoes with breathable uppers made of material such as mesh.

Crosstraining Shoes

Crosstraining shoes are a new hybrid, an all-purpose shoe for those who participate in a variety of fitness activities, such as basketball, weight lifting, or light trail hiking. If you tend to specialize in one type of activity (such as basketball), consider buying shoes designed specifically for that activity (for example, high-top basketball shoes for ankle support). To shop for an all-purpose crosstraining shoe, Nike recommends that you keep the following points in mind:

- Once again, comfort is paramount. Try to simulate the activity when you try on the shoe, such as rolling from side to side for court sports, fast movement for walking or running, or walking an incline for light hiking.

- If you tend toward one activity (such as running), look for crosstraining shoes that support that activity (for example, heel and forefoot cushioning for running).

- If you intend to use the shoes for activities with lots of lateral movement, such as court sports or aerobic classes, look for good lateral support.

continued

Choosing an Athletic Shoe—*Continued*

Aerobic Shoes

Flexibility: More at ball of foot than running shoes; less flexible than court shoes or running shoes; sole is firmer than running shoes. Uppers: Most are leather or leather-reinforced nylon. Heel: Little or no flare. Soles: Rubber if you dance on wood floors; polyurethane for other surfaces. Cushioning: More than court shoes; less than running shoes. Tread: Should be fairly flat, especially on forefoot; may also have "dot" on the ball of the foot for pivoting.

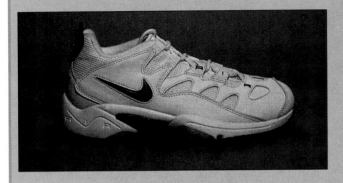

Basketball Shoes

Soles: Can be made from rubber for durability, EVA for lightweight cushioning, or polyurethane, which is both lightweight and durable. Flexibility: Should be most flexible in the forefoot, for making jump shots. Cushioning: Should absorb shock in the ball of the foot, for landing from jump shots. Heel: A snug-fitting heel cup is essential to keep the ankle in place; the shoe can be high-, mid-, or low-cut, depending on the amount of ankle support desired. Tread: For playing outdoors, the sole should be harder and the tread deeper; a smoother tread works well for playing on a court. Uppers: Can be made of leather for durability or nylon or other synthetics for breathability.

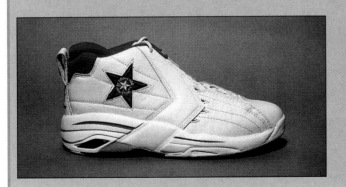

Running Shoes

Heel: Flare gives foot broader, more stable base. Soles: Usually carbon-based for longer wear. Cushioning: More than court shoes, especially at heel. Tread: "Waffle" or other deep-cut tread for grip on many surfaces.

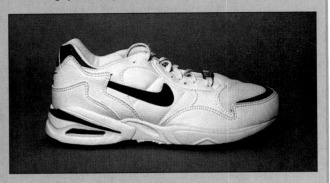

Walking Shoes

Cushioning: Can be forefoot and heel, or primarily forefoot or heel. Heel: May have some flare, similar to running shoes. Soles: Typically polyurethane for durability. Tread: Some tread for traction, but slightly flatter than running shoes.

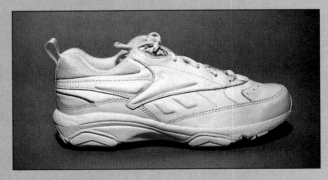

Crosstraining Shoes

Cushioning: Can be forefoot and heel, or primarily forefoot or heel. Tread: Can be moderate to aggressive.

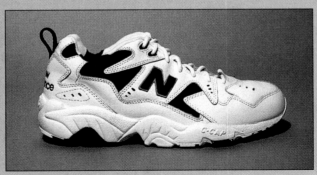

Home Fitness Equipment

In the past ten years, there has been an explosion in the purchase and use of home fitness equipment. This equipment is especially helpful for those who do not have access to health/fitness clubs, who prefer to exercise alone and at home, and who must exercise at irregular hours. Most forms of equipment can provide a good cardiorespiratory workout. However, few devices can also offer a balanced, whole-body strength workout. Thus, people looking for a complete workout may have to add some strength training, barbell work to their fitness program. A discussion of current popular devices follows.

Stationary Bicycles
Many models of stationary bikes are available, ranging in price from about $150 to $3,500 or more for a computerized exercise bike. Some upright bikes have a "dual action" component, whereby the user can "pump" extended handlebars for an upper-body workout. Other bikes allow the user to sit back while pedaling. These recumbent bikes take pressure off the lower back and permit the rider to exercise the hamstring muscles to a greater degree than upright bikes. Bike training stands that allow you to convert your regular bicycle into a stationary bike are also available.

Treadmills
Treadmills are relatively simple devices that consist of a moving belt stretched over two rollers. Two basic forms of treadmills are commonly used. The less expensive is the variety that is driven manually by the walking or running action of the user. Motorized treadmills are much more expensive and driven, of course, by an electric motor. The cost of a treadmill can range from several hundred dollars to nearly $15,000 for top-of-the-line models. Most electric models allow the user to change speeds and also the incline angle of the platform. Changing the incline angle can increase the intensity of the workout. First-time users are cautioned to start slowly and gradually become familiar with the motion of the motorized models. Getting on and off a moving belt can be a potentially dangerous task.

Stair Climbers
These devices allow the user to simulate climbing up a series of stair steps. This form of movement is much preferred to the actual, repetitive climbing of stairs that some people undertake in high-rise buildings. Stair climbers take much of the pressure off the knee joint. These machines vary in price from around $200 for the simplest lever model to $5,000 for a programmable model that varies the speed and amount of resistance. Some models come with an upper body component that allows the user to pump the arms while climbing.

Rowing Machines
Users of these machines exercise by simulating the movements involved in rowing a boat. Most brands have a sliding seat and movable handles that are similar to oars. Users push their feet against footplates while pulling back on the handles. The simplest models may cost around $300 and range up to more than $3,000 for health club models.

Ski Machines
Ski machines mimic the movements involved in cross-country skiing. Upper-body action involves alternating pulling movements of ropes or levers. Lower-body movements consist of large muscle back-and-forth movements of the legs. The exercisers feet move in fixed, parallel tracks and are held in place by pedal straps. The skiing movements take some practice to produce a smooth, coordinated motion. Costs range from several hundred to several thousand dollars.

Which Machine Is Best for You?
The machine that is best for you is the one that you will enjoy using. All too often, these machines are given as birthday or holiday gifts and used consistently for only a short time. (Notice all the ads for used fitness equipment in the classified ads section of your local paper.) Be certain to remember that machines can be somewhat specific in their focus. You may wish to broaden your workout with additional exercises or strength-building activities.

In terms of which device produces the greatest level of energy expenditure, a recent *Journal of the American Medical Association* article indicated that treadmill users walking or running "somewhat hard" expended (burned) more calories per hour than users of five other common home exercise machines. In this study, exercisers using a dual-action stationary bike and a regular stationary bike expended fewest calories per hour.[23]

---

forms of cancer, liver complications, and even psychological disturbances. The side effects on female steroid users are as dangerous as those on men. Figure 4-1 shows the adverse effects of steroid use.

Steroid users have developed a terminology of their own. Anabolic steroids are called "roids" or "juice." "Roid rage" is an aggressive, psychotic response to chronic steroid use. "Stacking" is a term that describes the use of multiple steroids at the same time.

Many organizations that control athletic competition (such as the National Collegiate Athletic Association [NCAA], The Athletics Congress, the National Football League, and the International Olympic Committee) have banned steroids and are testing athletes for illegal use. The death of professional football player Lyle Alzado highlighted the serious threat posed by steroid use. Fortunately, some athletes finally seem to be getting the message and are steering clear of steroids. (See As We Go to Press on p. 108.)

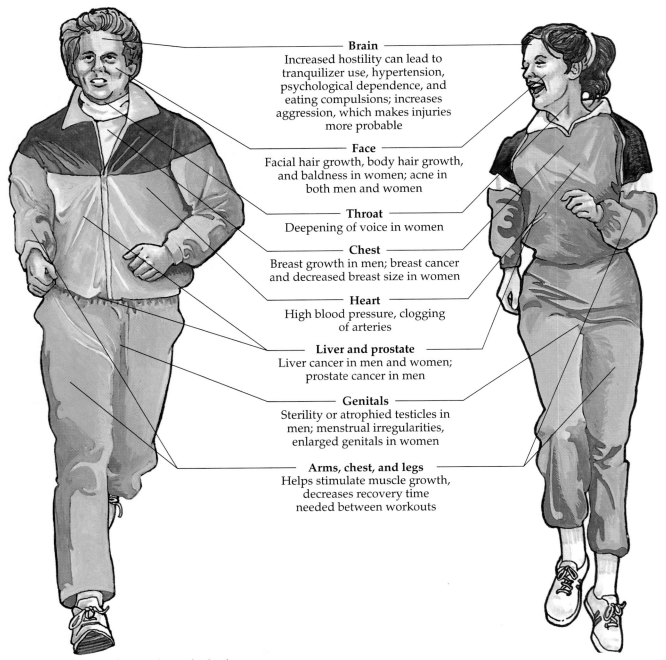

Brain
Increased hostility can lead to tranquilizer use, hypertension, psychological dependence, and eating compulsions; increases aggression, which makes injuries more probable

Face
Facial hair growth, body hair growth, and baldness in women; acne in both men and women

Throat
Deepening of voice in women

Chest
Breast growth in men; breast cancer and decreased breast size in women

Heart
High blood pressure, clogging of arteries

Liver and prostate
Liver cancer in men and women; prostate cancer in men

Genitals
Sterility or atrophied testicles in men; menstrual irregularities, enlarged genitals in women

Arms, chest, and legs
Helps stimulate muscle growth, decreases recovery time needed between workouts

Figure 4-1   Effects of steroids on the body.

Are Today's Children Physically Fit?

Major research studies published during the last ten years have indicated that U.S. children and teenagers lead very sedentary lives. Children ages six to seventeen score extremely poorly in the areas of strength, flexibility, and cardiorespiratory endurance. In many cases, parents are in better shape than their children.

This information presents a challenge to educators and parents to emphasize the need for strenuous play activity. Television watching and parental inactivity were implicated as major reasons in these stud-ies. For students reading this text who are parents or grandparents of young children, what can you do to encourage more physical activity and less sedentary activity? (See the Star Box on p. 103).

How Does Sleep Contribute to Overall Fitness?

Sleep is an important adjunct to a well-planned exercise program (see the Health Action Guide on p. 103). Sleep is so vital to health that people who are unable to sleep sufficiently (those with insomnia) or who are deprived of sleep experience deterioration in every dimension of their health. Fortunately, exercise is frequently associated with improvement in sleeping.

The value of sleep is apparent in a variety of positive changes in the body. Dreaming is thought to play an important role in supporting the emotional dimension of health. Problem-solving scenarios that occur during dreams seem to afford some carryover value in actual coping experiences. A variety of changes in physiological functioning, particularly a deceleration of the cardiovascular system, occur while you sleep. The feeling of being well rested is an expression of the mental and physiological rejuvenation you feel after a good night's sleep.

The amount of sleep needed varies among people. In fact, for any person, sleep needs vary according to activity level and overall state of health. As we age, the need for sleep appears to decrease from the six to eight hours young adults require. Elderly people routinely sleep less than they did when they were younger. This decrease may be offset by the short naps older people often take during the day. For all people, however, periods of relaxation, daydreaming, and even an occasional afternoon nap promote electrical activity patterns that help regenerate the mind and body.

What Exercise Danger Signs Should I Watch For?

The human body is an amazing piece of equipment. It functions well regardless of whether you are conscious of its processes. It also delivers clear signals when something goes wrong.

Kids, Go Outside and Play!

Unfortunately, children in the United States today are heavier, slower, and weaker than children in other countries.[16] We know that cardiovascular risk factors, such as obesity, tend to continue from childhood to adulthood. That is, patterns established in childhood, such as sedentary lifestyles, are difficult to break and can contribute to cardiovascular disease in adulthood.

By the same token, researchers have found that the children who perform better on standardized fitness tests have more favorable body composition and lipid profiles (a better ratio of good cholesterol to bad cholesterol, reducing the risk of cardiovascular disease).[17]

Organized fitness activities at school and at home can play an important role in helping your children become and stay fit. For example, comprehensive school-based health promotion and education programs can improve children's health and reduce their risk factors for diseases.

Playing video games with their friends might improve the eye-hand coordination of your children, but it is not a fitness activity!

You should monitor any sign that seems abnormal during or after your exercise. "Listen to your body" is a good rule for self-awareness. The Health Action Guide on page 104 lists some common warning signs to monitor.

However, such occurrences are extremely unusual. Fear of developing these difficulties should not deter you from starting a fitness program. These risks are minimal—and the benefits far outweigh the risks. Sports injuries are discussed further in the following section.

HEALTH ACTION GUIDE

Activities to Promote Sound Sleep

Can we work at being better sleepers? The answer is yes. Many activities, when done at the appropriate time, will aid you in your quest for sound sleep.

Activities for the Day

Schedule. Maintain a consistent schedule of daily activities; a disrupted day makes sleeping difficult.

Physical activity. Regular vigorous activity promotes sleep; exercising too near bedtime, however, can make you too energized to sleep soundly.

Eating. A large meal taken late in the evening interferes with sleeping; avoid heavy late-night snacks as well.

Alcohol use. A single drink in the evening may be relaxing, but too many drinks during the day can make sleeping difficult.

Central nervous system (CNS) stimulants. Coffee, tea, soft drinks with caffeine, and some medications can disrupt normal sleeping patterns.

Worry. Problems and concerns should be put behind you by the time you retire for the night; practice leaving your concerns at the office or in the classroom.

Rituals. A ritualistic "winding down" over the course of the evening promotes sleep; watching television, listening to music, and reading during the evening are excellent ways to prepare the body for sleep.

Activities for the End of the Day

Bathing. For many people, a warm bath immediately before retiring promotes sleep.

Yoga. The quiet, relaxing exercises of yoga promote sleep by slowing the body's activity level.

Snack or nightcap. A light snack of foods high in l-tryptophan (for example, eggs, tuna, and turkey) and a glass of milk will help you fall asleep.

Muscular relaxation. Alternating contraction and relaxation of the large muscles of the extremities aids the body in falling asleep.

Imaging. Quieting images can distract the mind, thus allowing you to fall asleep more easily.

Fantasies. Escaping into fantasies slows the mind and encourages the onset of sleep.

Breathing. Slow, deep breaths set a restful rhythm the body can "ride" into sleep.

Thinking. By envisioning yourself as sleeping soundly, you may actually fall asleep quicker.

InfoLinks
www.sleepnet.com

Sports Injuries

At any time during your participation in fitness or sport activities, it is possible that you will become injured, even if you carefully warm up before your exercise and cool down after your exercise. Hopefully, the injury will only be a minor one and you can rest and soon resume your fitness interests. Sometimes, however, an injury can be significant and require you to seek medical care and undergo extensive rehabilitation.

It is beyond the scope of this textbook to provide a comprehensive discussion of the prevention, care, and treatment of sports injuries. (You can find this information in an athletic training textbook, a fitness textbook, or a popular sports medicine book.) We will try to provide you with some general principles related to the prevention and care of sports injuries and a table that lists many common fitness injuries.[2]

Principle Number One: **A well-planned fitness program starts at a low level and progresses gradually and consistently.** This principle supports the concept of starting at a level of activity that can be handled comfortably. If the activity is a walking program, an unfit person should not begin with walks of five or six miles a day but should start with a shorter distance and gradually add additional distance in a consistent manner to avoid muscle, skeletal, or joint injuries.

Principle Number Two: **If you stop exercising for an extended time, do not restart the activity at the level at which you stopped.** Do not plan on returning to a high level of activity if you have been inactive for an extended time. Rather, reduce your activity significantly and gradually return to your earlier levels of activity.

HEALTH ACTION GUIDE

Exercise Danger Signs

- A delay of more than one hour in your body's return to a fully relaxed, comfortable state after exercise.
- A change in sleep patterns.
- Any noticeable breathing difficulties or chest pains. Exercise at your THR should not initiate these problems. You should consult a physician.
- Persistent joint or muscle pain. Any lingering joint or muscle pain might signal a problem. Seek the help of an athletic trainer, a physical therapist, or your physician.
- Unusual changes in urine composition or output. Marked color change in your urine could signal possible kidney or bladder difficulties. Drink plenty of water before, during, and after you participate in your activity.
- Anything unusual that you notice after starting your fitness program. Examples are headaches, nosebleeds, fainting, numbness in an extremity, and hemorrhoids.

InfoLinks
www.acsm.org/sportsmed/index.htm

Principle Number Three: **"Listen to your body."** Always be aware of the nature of your body as you are exercising. If you sense that something is wrong, stop the activity and assess the situation. For example, if you think you might be hurting your back or that a joint or muscle is becoming strained, stop and evaluate the situation. If you think something is wrong, by all means don't test your body by returning to the activity. (Have you ever seen a person with a suspected ankle injury "test" the ankle by hopping up and down on the injured leg? This makes no sense at all.) Pain indicates that something is wrong. If this is the case, seek a professional evaluation, perhaps from an athletic trainer or a physical therapist. A physician, especially one trained in sports medicine, can make an accurate diagnosis of the injury.

Principle Number Four: **Follow the rehabilitation instructions carefully.** Athletic trainers and physical therapists are trained to design effective rehabilitation programs. If you are injured, it is very important that you follow the advice of these professionals. This is especially true in cases where you start to feel better before the rehabilitation program is finished. Even though you feel better, your body may not be fully recovered. A return to activity too quickly may result in an even more serious injury that your original one. (This is especially true for adults over the age of forty.) The best advice is to resist the urge to return to your activity until you are given full clearance from your trainer or therapist.

Principle Number Five: **Develop a prevention approach.** After you recover from an injury, try to discover ways to prevent that injury from happening again. Learn about proper stretching exercises, effective strength-training activities, appropriate equipment, and the proper mechanics for your selected sports/fitness activities. Use this collective knowledge to prevent the injury from recurring.

For example, if you have injured your hamstring muscles while running, you will need to learn how to effectively stretch these muscles in the future. You will also need to learn how to strengthen these muscles through weight training. If your running shoes are old and worn, they may have to be replaced. Finally, if you are running too fast before warming up, you will want to start slowly and gradually increase your speed after the muscles are fully warmed up. Preventive actions like these will allow you to have a fitness program that is not regularly interrupted by a nagging injury.

For more information about specific sports injuries, look at Table 4-1 on pages 105–106.

Personal Applications

- What fitness injuries are most common in the activities in which you participate? What can you do to prevent such injuries?

Table 4-1 Common Injuries Associated with Physical Activity

Injury	Condition
Achilles tendinitis	A chronic tendinitis of the "heel cord" or muscle tendon located on the back of the lower leg just above the heel. It may result from any activity that involves forcefully pushing off with the foot and ankle, such as in running and jumping. This inflammation involves swelling, warmth, tenderness to touch, and pain during walking and especially running.
Ankle sprains	Stretching or tearing of one or several ligaments that provide stability to the ankle joint. Ligaments on the outside or lateral side of the ankle are more commonly injured by rolling the sole of the foot downward and toward the inside. Pain is intense immediately after injury, followed by considerable swelling, tenderness, loss of joint motion, and some discoloration over a 24- to 48-hour period.
Athlete's foot	A fungal infection that most often occurs between the toes or on the sole of the foot and that causes itching, redness, and pain. If the skin breaks down, a bacterial infection is possible. It may be prevented by keeping the area dry; using powder; and wearing clean, dry socks that do not hold moisture. It is best treated using over-the-counter medications that contain the active ingredient miconazole (MicaTin).
Blisters	Friction blisters can occur anywhere on the skin where there is friction or repetitive rubbing, but they most often occur on the hands or feet. The blister takes on a reddish color, becoming raised and filling with fluid. It can be quite painful, and if it occurs on the foot it may be disabling. Taking measures to reduce friction, such as wearing gloves, breaking in new footwear, and wearing appropriately fitting socks, is helpful in preventing blisters.
Groin pull	A muscle strain that occurs in the muscles located on the inside of the upper thigh just below the pubic area and that results from either an overstretch of the muscle or from a contraction of the muscle that meets excessive resistance. Pain will be produced by flexing the hip and leg across the body or by stretching the muscles in a groin-stretch position.
Hamstring pull	A strain of the muscles on the back of the upper thigh that most often occurs while sprinting. In most cases, severe pain is caused simply by walking or in any movement that involves knee flexion or stretch of the hamstring muscle. Some swelling, tenderness to touch, and possibly some discoloration extending down the back of the leg may occur in severe strains.
Patellofemoral knee pain	Nonspecific pain occurring around the knee, particularly the front part of the knee, or in the kneecap (patella). Pain can result from many causes, including improper movement of the kneecap in knee flexion and extension; tendinitis of the tendon just below the kneecap, which is caused by repetitive jumping; bursitis (swelling) either above or below the kneecap; and osteoarthritis (joint surface degeneration) between the kneecap and thigh bone. It may involve inflammation with swelling, tenderness, warmth, and pain associated with movement.
Plantar fasciitis or arch pain	Chronic inflammation and irritation of the broad ligament that runs from the heel to the base of the toes, forming part of the long arch on the bottom of the foot. It most often occurs in runners or walkers. It is frequently caused by wearing shoes that do not have adequate arch support. At first, pain is localized at the attachment on the heel; it then tends to move more onto the arch. It is most painful when you first get out of bed and in the evening when you have been on your feet for long periods.
Quadriceps contusion "charley horse"	A deep bruise of the muscles in the front part of the thigh caused by a forceful impact or by some object that results in severe pain, swelling, discoloration, and difficulty flexing the knee or extending the hip. Without adequate rest and protection from additional trauma, small calcium deposits may develop in the muscle.

continued

Table 4-1 *Continued*

Injury	Condition
Racquetball or golfer's elbow	Similar to tennis elbow, except the pain is located on the medial or inside surface of the arm just above the elbow at the attachment of the wrist and finger flexor muscles. It occurs in those activities that involve repeated, forceful flexion of the wrist, such as hitting a forehand stroke in racquetball. Golfers also develop this inflammation in the trailing arm from too much wrist flexion in a golf swing.
Shin splints	A "catch-all" term used to refer to any pain that occurs in the front part of the lower leg or shin, most often caused by excessive running on hard surfaces. Pain is usually caused by strain of the muscles that move the ankle and foot at their attachment points in the shin. It is usually worse during activity. In more severe cases it may be caused by stress fractures of the long bones in the lower leg, with the pain being worse after activity is stopped.
Shoulder impingement	Chronic irritation and inflammation of muscle tendons and a bursa underneath the tip of the shoulder, which results from repeated forceful overhead motions of the shoulder, such as in swimming, throwing, spiking a volleyball, or serving a tennis ball. Pain is felt when the arm is extended across the body above shoulder level.
Sunburn	An extremely common problem for anyone who exercises outside. Overexposure to the sun can ultimately cause certain types of skin cancer. It is critical to protect yourself from the sun by applying sunscreens and paying attention to the SPF (sun protection factor). Wearing a hat and other protective clothing to cover the skin can further help to minimize overexposure to ultraviolet light.
Tennis elbow	Chronic irritation and inflammation of the lateral or outside surface of the arm just above the elbow at the attachment of the muscles that extend the wrist and fingers. It results from any activity that requires forceful extension of the wrist. Typically occurs in tennis players who are using faulty techniques hitting backhand ground strokes. Pain is felt above the elbow after forcefully extending the wrist against resistance or applying pressure over the muscle attachment above the elbow.

Real Life
Real choices

Your Turn

- Would exercise have been beneficial to Jack in his pre–heart attack days? Why or why not?
- What kinds of exercise might Jack find enjoyable and healthful? What kinds of exercise do you think he should avoid?
- Before Jack begins a program of moderate exercise, what tests will his physician want him to undergo?

And Now, Your Choices . . .
- Do you exercise regularly? If so, how do you benefit from your exercise routine? What happens when you don't exercise?
- If you don't exercise regularly, what are your reasons? What forms of exercise do you think you would enjoy doing several times a week?

Summary

- Physical fitness allows one to avoid illness, perform routine activities, and respond to emergencies.
- The health benefits of exercise can be achieved through regular, moderate exercise.

- Fitness is composed of five components: cardiorespiratory endurance, muscular strength, muscular endurance, flexibility, and body composition.

- The American College of Sports Medicine's program for cardiorespiratory fitness has five components: mode of activity, frequency of training, intensity of training, duration of training, and resistance training.
- The target heart rate refers to the number of times per minute the heart must contract to produce a training effect.
- Training sessions should take place in three phases: warm-up, workout, and cooldown.

- Fitness experts are concerned about the lack of fitness in today's youth.
- Street dancing, step aerobics, and rollerblading are currently popular aerobic activities.
- College students who are interested in fitness should understand the important topics of steroid use, crosstraining, fluid replacement, body-building, and proper sleep.
- Following a few simple principles can help prevent many common sports injuries.

Review Questions

1. Identify the five components of fitness described in this chapter. How does each component relate to physical fitness?
2. What is the difference between anaerobic and aerobic energy production? What types of activities are associated with anaerobic energy production? With aerobic energy production?
3. List some of the benefits of aerobic fitness.
4. Describe the various methods used to promote muscular strength.
5. What does the principle of overload mean in regard to fitness training programs?
6. Identify the ACSM's five components of an effective cardiorespiratory fitness program. Explain the important aspects of each component.
7. Under what circumstances should you see a physician before starting a physical fitness program?
8. Identify and describe the three parts of a training session.
9. Describe some of the negative consequences of anabolic steroid use.
10. How can people improve their sleeping habits?
11. Discuss the five basic principles important in avoiding sports injuries.

References

1. Blair SN. C.H. McCloy research lecture: physical activity, physical fitness, and health. *Research Quarterly for Exercise and Sport* 1993; 64(4):365–76.
2. Prentice WE. *Fitness for college and life.* 4th ed. St. Louis: Mosby, 1994.
3. Prevention: keep on walking, keep on living. *Harvard Health Letter* 1998; 23(6):4.
4. Simon HB. Can you run away from cancer? *Harv Med Sch Health Lett* 1992; 17(5):5–7.
5. Ferrini AF, Ferrini RL. *Health in later years.* 2nd ed. Madison, WI: Brown & Benchmark, 1992.
6. American College of Sports Medicine. Position statement on the recommended quantity and quality of exercise for developing and maintaining fitness in healthy adults. *Med Sci Sports Exerc* 1990; 22(2):265–74.
7. White MD. *Water exercise.* Champaign, IL: Human Kinetics, 1995.
8. Arnheim DD, Prentice WE. *Principles of athletic training.* 8th ed. St. Louis: Mosby, 1993.
9. An exercise prescription for older people. *Harvard Health Letter.* 1998; 8(10):1–4.
10. National Institute of Arthritis and Musculoskeletal and Skin Diseases Clearinghouse. *Low back pain: information package.* National Institutes of Health (Public Health Service), Sept 1997.
11. U.S. Department of Health and Human Services. *Physical activity and health: a report of the Surgeon General.* Centers for Disease Control and Prevention, National Center for Chronic Disease Prevention and Health Promotion, 1996.
12. Marti J, Hine A. *The alternative health and medicine encyclopedia.* Cincinnati: Gale, 1995.
13. Williams MH. Alcohol and sport performance. *Sports Sci Exch* 1992; 4(40):1–4.
14. Norvell N, Belles D. Psychological and physical benefits of circuit weight training in law enforcement personnel. *J Consult Clin Psychol* 1993 June; 61(3):520–27.
15. Mishra R. Steroids and sports are a losing proposition. *FDA Consumer* 1991; 25(7):25–27.
16. DiNubile NA. Youth fitness—problems and solutions. *Prev Med* 1993 July; 22(4):589–94.
17. Harsha DW. The benefits of physical activity in childhood (review). *Am J Med Sci* 1995 Dec; 310 (Suppl 1):S109–S113.
18. Deacon J. The winning spirit. *Maclean's* 1997 Feb 3; 110(5):60.
19. Hawaleshka D. They are champions: winning isn't everything for Special Olympians. *Maclean's* 1997 Feb 17; 110(7):66.
20. Lan C et al. Cardiorespiratory function, flexibility, and body composition among geriatric tai chi chuan practitioners. *Arch Phys Med Rehabil* 1996 June; 77(6):612–16.

21. Choy PY, Salmon P. Symptom changes across the menstrual cycle in competitive sportswomen, exercisers, and sedentary women. *Br J Clin Psychol* 1995 Sept; 34 (pt 3):447–60.

22. Steege JF, Blumenthal JA. The effects of aerobic exercise on premenstrual symptoms in middle-age women: a preliminary study. *J Psychosom Res* 1993; 37(2):127–33.

23. Zeni AL et al. Energy expenditure with indoor exercise machines. *JAMA* 1996 May 8; 275(18).

Suggested Readings

Brown RL. *The 10-minute L.E.A.P.: lifetime exercise adherence plan.* New York: Regan Books, 1998. Richard Brown is a PhD-trained Olympic coach and trainer. He is certified as a "master coach" by the U.S. Olympic Track and Field governing body. His book guides people to achieve peak fitness performance without burnout or injuries. This book is appropriate for all people, regardless of their fitness level. Brown also provides information about staying focused and motivated, reducing stress, maintaining a healthful diet, and developing a training schedule. Over 100 charts and tables are included.

Brungardt K. *3-minute abs: achieving the look you've always wanted in only 3 minutes a day.* New York: HarperCollins, 1998. This is a small (96-page) book that completely covers specific training to strengthen the abdominal muscles. Brungardt, author of *The Complete Book of Abs*, teaches the reader how to train each of the three separate regions of the abdominal muscle—the upper, lower, and side regions. The author claims that with 3 minutes of exercise each day (and a very good diet!), a person can make a remarkable improvement in a short time.

Burleigh WB. *Fitness lite: a guide for those who have never taken exercise seriously.* Santa Barbara, CA: Capra Press, 1995. A short, easy-to-read, humorous look at fitness. Disguised in the humor is a solid sixteen-week fitness program that incorporates important elements, including nutrition, weight management, and aerobic exercise. Fun to read.

Kelder P, Siegel BS. *Ancient secrets of the fountain of youth.* New York: Doubleday, 1998. This short book (80 pages) describes the simple but effective series of exercises handed down through the ages by Tibetan monks. Users go through a series of "rites" or exercises that involve stretching, breathing properly, and focusing on one's thinking patterns. Followers of these rites report improved eating patterns, weight loss, increased stamina, and a deep sense of rejuvenation.

Newby-Fraser P. *Peak fitness for women.* Champaign, IL: Human Kinetics, 1995. You might think a seven-time Ironman Triathlon champion would aim a fitness book at only swimming, cycling, and running. However, Newby-Fraser elaborates on strength training, nutrition, crosstraining, flexibility training, and competition for women. Sound information, excellent photos, and beneficial workout sheets are included.

Peterson JA, Bryant CX, Peterson SC. *Strength training for women.* Champaign, IL: Human Kinetics, 1995. This is a comprehensive yet easy-to-read guide to strength training for women. Free weights, weight machines, and nonequipment options are explored. Many illustrations and the pros and cons of various approaches are presented so that the user can tailor a program for herself.

White MD. *Water exercise.* Champaign, IL: Human Kinetics, 1995. Written by a licensed occupational and massage therapist, this book focuses on fitness development and injury rehabilitation through water activities. Nearly eighty exercises are discussed and illustrated. Step-by-step programs are presented from beginner to advanced levels.

As We Go To PRESS

Androstenedione. Fall 1998 saw St. Louis Cardinals first baseman Mark McGwire hit 70 home runs, breaking Roger Maris's 37-year-old Major League home run record. Some skeptics speculated that McGwire's record could have been related to his use of legal, over-the-counter muscle-building supplement pills called androstenedione (or "andro"). Banned by the National Football League, the NCAA, and the Olympics, andro is not on the list of substances banned by baseball. Andro functions by raising the level of the male hormone testosterone. The drug also helps the body manufacture lean muscle mass and promotes recovery after injury. Interestingly, Chicago Cubs outfielder Sammy Sosa also broke Maris's record in 1998 by hitting 66 home runs. Reportedly, Sosa did not use androstenedione.

Creatine. A related story in 1998 was the emergence of the use of the performance aid creatine. Creatine is an amino acid (sold legally in pills, powders, liquids, and capsules) that seems to boost energy production, short-term muscle strength, and performance in activities involving short bursts of energy (anaerobic activities). Health consequences of high dosages and long-term use remain virtually unknown, since few scientific controlled studies have been performed on creatine.

topics for Today

Extreme Sports: Living on the Edge

What did you do last weekend? You say that you jumped out of an airplane while videotaping your buddy doing air acrobatics on a surfboard? Well, we've identified the skysurfers in the group. There are at least a couple of other variations on hurling oneself from a plane. Style skydivers perform six maneuvers as fast as possible (without the surfboard or cameraperson), while accuracy skydivers attempt to land on silver dollar-sized targets.[1] Bungee jumping is nothing extraordinary these days. People even get married while taking the plunge, but the new freestyle bungee jumping involves going over the edge while sitting in a recliner or dumpster.[2] Another extreme sport, the street luge, involves plummeting downhill feet first on a wheeled sled. In snow mountain bike racing, pedal speeds of 65 mph are reached before crashing into the padded speed trap at the end of the course—that is, *if* you don't fall off of your bike on the way downhill.[3]

If scaling a fifty-foot artificial frozen waterfall sounds like your thing, have somebody time you. After some practice, you may be the next Speed Ice Climbing Champion. If I haven't named your favorite sport yet, don't despair. Just a few of the other options are skateboarding, downhill or halfpipe snowboarding, indoor climbing, barefoot water ski jumping, aggressive in-line skating, supermodified shovel racing (likened to a soap box derby on snow) and the multisport endurance ecochallenge.[2,3,4,5] An ecochallenge involves 50 five-person teams that race twenty-four hours a day for seven days over 370 miles of rugged terrain. The team members take turns horseback riding and running alongside the horse for twenty-six miles, swimming with backpacks in cold mountain creeks, hiking a hundred miles across desert, navigating a 1,200-foot cliff face by rope, rafting over advanced-class rapids, and finishing with a twelve-hour, fifty-mile canoe paddle across a lake.

How did this extreme sports phenomenon arise? One sports writer puts it this way: "The world's always had daredevils; they're just more organized and obvious now."[2]

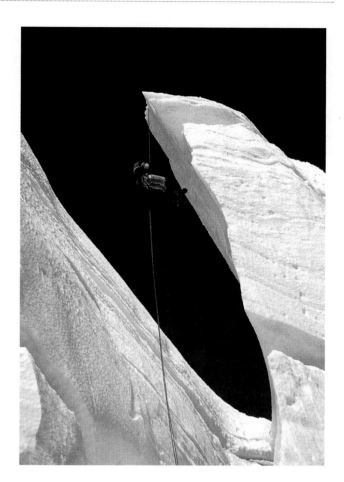

Origins and Growth

Extreme sports competition emerged in the mid-eighties as fun.[6] It was also about this time that in-line skates began replacing the old-style roller skates. Now nearly 25 million Americans in-line skate at least once a year, which makes the sport more popular than tennis and about as popular as golf.[7] In addition, over 6.5 million mountain bikes were sold in 1995 alone, and in the past five years 135 indoor climbing gyms have sprung up and 60 more are in the planning.[6] There are 2 million snowboarders, that many new rock and mountain climbers, thousands of extreme skiers, and over 25 percent more skydivers than a few years ago.[1] (Add seventy-two-year-old former president George Bush to the list of new skydivers.)

This rate of growth is phenomenal, and television is in the middle of it. In 1992 *MTV Sports* premiered to cover this new generation of sport.[1] Three years later, ESPN 1997 launched the X Games, billed as "not your father's Olympics." The Summer X Games, now a weeklong annual event, draw athletes from around the world. More than four hundred athletes competed in nine sports for over $375,000 in prize money in the Summer 1996 version.[8,9] Not to be outdone, *MTV Sports* coverage may expand, and the News Corp. and Fox networks also have extreme programming on the table.[5] A couple of the events have gone mainstream: mountain biking and halfpipe snowboarding were scheduled to be added to the Olympic Games.[1,3] The 1999 Summer X Games took place in San Francisco June 25–July 3.[10]

Who Pays

Where there is public interest and televised coverage, there is advertising. Being associated with extreme sports reinforces Pepsico's active and cutting-edge ad campaign for its Mountain Dew product. Taco Bell, a Pepsico subsidiary, markets the free-spirited, outdoor, energetic attitude to its core group of customers age eighteen to thirty-four. Some Chevy dealers offer trucks with X Game logos and include an extreme whitewater rafting trip or an extreme mountain bike with purchase.[4] Volkswagen offers K2 skis or a K2 snowboard with some of its car models.[11] Other sponsors include the U.S. Marines, Visa, Pringles, Snickers, AT&T, and Nike.[3] HealthSouth Corp., a rehabilitation care provider, is a sport climbing sponsor, and some equipment manufacturers sponsor competitions or individual athletes by providing free gear or small stipends.[6]

"Extremists take the money because it's there. They take the risks for reasons of their own."[2]

Who Plays

Although much of the marketing is directed at twenty-somethings, extreme sports attract participants from teens to athletes in their seventies. Neither is it strictly an American craze. Indoor climbing events in Europe routinely draw more than five thousand spectators, and just a quick glance at the roster of contestants at the 1997 Winter X Games revealed participants from the following countries: Austria, Switzerland, Norway, Finland, Italy, Canada, and the United States.[3,6]

At twenty-five, Tim Fairfield is one of the nation's top indoor sport climbers. He identifies with the "packaged radicalism" or what he sees as an "anti-establishment" sport.[6] Cheryl Stearns, world champion style and accuracy skydiver, sees her sport as fun, exciting, and different, building self-assurance and open-mindedness. Top U.S. in-line skater Anjie Walter, age twenty-eight, cites an addictive sense of accomplishment and empowerment, a feeling of heightened awareness, and a greater appreciation for living as benefits of the risks she takes.[1] Helen Klein, the seventy-two-year-old great-grandmother and ultramarathoner who finished the ecochallenge, put it this way: "I'd rather wear out than rust out."[2]

The Risks

Despite the physical fitness peak and mental rushes that these sports provide, they can be very expensive and involve serious risks. These sports require specialized equipment, safety gear, and clothing. A pair of in-line skates costs between $40 and $299.[7] That's only the beginning—if you get really into a sport, the costs skyrocket. Mia Azon, the 1994 number two women's sport climber, spent more than her $10,000 sponsorship and prize money training and competing in her sport in one year.[6] Extreme sports can also cost some athletes their health and even their life. People get hurt; injuries range from broken bones to dehydration to exertional rhabdomyolysis (the body's digestion of its own muscle tissue from overwork). Extreme athletes put not only themselves in danger by their activity; rescue workers who rescue extreme skiers from avalanches and medical workers called on to helicopter-lift athletes in trouble out of the rugged terrain are also put at risk.

More Than a Passing Fancy

Risky or not, extreme sports have caught on. As these events grow in popularity, though, they may lose some of their offbeat appeal. Extreme sports are not likely to get boring, however, as participants continue to add variety to their sports to keep the intensity of the experience fresh.

For those of you who want to check out the extreme scene from the safety of your computer, ICon CMT Corp. has a new on-line magazine, called *Charged*, for extreme sport enthusiasts.[12] You can check out any of four sections in *Charged*: Tar (street sports), Wet (water sports), Dirt (biking, etc.), and Frost (snow sports) at http://www.charged.com. So what are you doing this weekend?

For Discussion . . .

Have you ever tried an extreme sport? If so, would you recommend the experience to a friend? Why or why not? Do you think that the benefits of participation outweigh the risks? Were you surprised to learn of the level of popularity of these sports?

References

1. Bower J. Going over the top. *Women's Sports & Fitness* 1995; 17(7):21–23.
2. Hamilton K. Outer limits. *Newsweek* 1995; 125(25):78–81.
3. ESPN. Televised Coverage of Day 2 of Winter X Games, 1997.
4. Elliott S. The X Games: going to extremes in an effort to tap a growing segment of sports. *The New York Times* 1996; 145:D6.
5. Fitzgerald K. Extreme-ly hot: ESPN leads charge into new, daring sports targeted to young people. *Advertising Age* 1996; 67(26):44–45.
6. Fatsis S. Rad sports give sponsors cheap thrills. *The Wall Street Journal* 1995 May 12:B12.
7. Consumer Reports. The best deal on street wheels. *Consumer Reports* 1996; 61(7):20–25.
8. Brown R. X marks the spot for ESPN; extreme sports competition has lined up over a dozen sponsors. *Broadcasting & Cable* 1996; 126(15):53.
9. Hoffer R. Down and way out. *Sports Illustrated* 1995; 83(1):42–49.
10. Extreme Sports: X Games. (http://espnet.sportszone.com/extreme/xgames) Oct 5, 1998 (taken off the Web).
11. Volkswagen. Television commercial, 1996.
12. Wilson S. Electronically charged. *Folio: the Magazine for Magazine Management* 1996; 25(10):37.

InfoLinks
www.adventuresports.com
http://espn.go.com/extreme/
   index.html

Understanding Nutrition and Your Diet

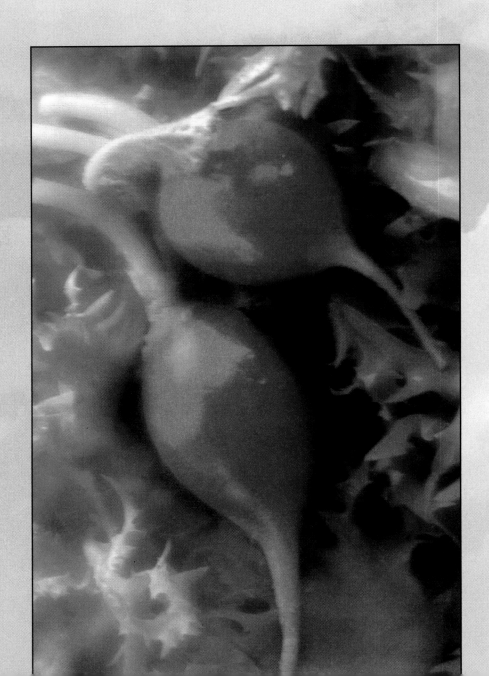

From the prenatal period throughout life, people must have adequate nutrition to prevent malnourishment and minimize the development of illnesses that may be worsened by poor dietary practices. Food supports growth and development by providing the body with the nutrients needed for production of energy, repair of damaged tissue, growth of new tissue, and regulation of physiological processes, all of which undergird full participation in the activities that constitute our days, weeks, months, and years of living. But our diets are more than that. Our food selections reflect personal, familial, and cultural traditions. The preparation and serving of food at regular mealtimes and during holiday gatherings and other special occasions enhances all of the dimensions of health. For example, taking bread and wine during Communion supports the spiritual dimension of health, sharing popcorn at the movies with your friends enhances the social dimension of health, and learning about the cuisine of another culture develops the intellectual dimension of health. As you read this chapter, keep in mind this balanced view of food as sustenance and food as a resource for the dimensions of health.

HEALTHY PEOPLE: LOOKING AHEAD TO 2010

Nutrition and dietary practices are closely related to many aspects of wellness, including fitness, weight management, cardiovascular health, and the prevention of diseases such as cancer, osteoporosis, and diabetes mellitus. Accordingly, several important nutrition-related objectives were included in the Healthy People 2000 report.

One objective was to reduce the percentage of total calories from fat, especially saturated fat, in Americans' diets. In 1995 the Midcourse Review reported that we were about one quarter of the way toward reaching these goals. Two related goals, introducing fat-reduced foods into supermarkets and

restaurants and limiting the sale of processed foods in stores and vending machines, had been reached at mid-decade.

The Healthy People 2010 goals in the area of nutrition will probably focus on two areas. The first is food safety, especially reducing bacterial contamination in processing and preparation. The second area is the refinement and expansion of food labeling, including the use of the term "organic" on food labels. The goals might also focus on countering the fast-food industry's aggressive marketing of supersize food items.

Real Life
Real choices

- Names: Vincent and Angela Martinelli
- Ages: 64 and 61
- Ethnic background: Italian
- Occupation: Restaurant owners
- Physical characteristics: Vincent: 5'9", 189 lb. Angela: 5'2", 143 lb.

Does anyone really know how many kinds of pasta there are in the world? If you want an expert opinion, the people to ask are Vincent and Angela Martinelli, the owners of a popular market and deli in their city's lively Italian neighborhood.

Martinelli's Fine Foods was started by Vincent's father in the 1920s, and Vincent began helping out when he was five years old. When his father died in the early 1950s, Vincent and Angela took over. Now in their sixties, they're beginning to talk about retiring and turning the business over to their daughter and her husband.

A family business like Martinelli's isn't a nine-to-five proposition. For more than forty years, Vincent and Angela have routinely worked twelve to fourteen hours a day, six days a week—at the same time raising five children and putting them through college. Their hectic, stressful schedule has left them little time for leisure, and they're looking forward to taking life easier when they retire.

Both Vincent and Angela enjoy cooking—and eating—the delicious dishes they offer for sale in the deli and for catered parties. Their favorite is fettucine carbonara, which features pasta in cream sauce with bacon. At a recent checkup, the Martinellis' physician found that Vincent's serum cholesterol level is elevated to the point where heart disease is a concern; and Angela, who has a family history of hypertension, is taking in as much as 3,000 milligrams of sodium per day.

As you study this chapter, think about some steps Vincent and Angela can take to adopt a healthier lifestyle, and prepare yourself to answer the questions in **Your Turn** at the end of the chapter.

Types and Sources of Nutrients

Your body relies on seven **nutrients** to carry out its physiological functions: carbohydrates, fats, protein, vitamins, minerals, dietary fiber, and water.* The first three—carbohydrates, fats, and protein—will be discussed together because they provide **calories.†** These calories are either used quickly by our bodies in energy metabolism or are stored in the form of glycogen or adipose tissue for delayed use as energy sources. The other nutrients—vitamins, minerals, dietary fiber, and water—are not sources of calories for the body. Their functions will be discussed later in the chapter.

Carbohydrates

Carbohydrates are various combinations of sugar units, or saccharides. The body uses carbohydrates primarily for energy. Each gram of carbohydrate contains *four* calories. Since the average person requires approximately 2,000 calories per day and about 60 percent of our calories come from carbohydrates, we obtain 1,200 calories per day from carbohydrates.[1]

Carbohydrates occur in three forms, depending on the number of saccharides (sugar) units that make

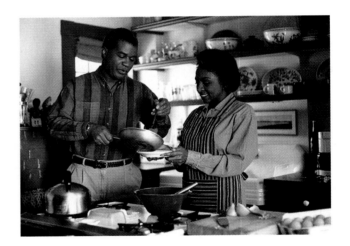

The shared preparation and serving of nourishing meals enhances your overall well-being.

up the molecule. Carbohydrates that contain only one saccharide unit are classified as monosaccharides, those with two units are disaccharides, and those with more than two are polysaccharides. Monosaccharides and disaccharides are more commonly called *sugars*, whereas polysaccharides are referred to as *starches*. Today it is recommended that about 58 percent to 60 percent of our total caloric intake come from carbohydrates, with starches supplying five times more carbohydrate calories than sugars.

Monosaccharides are the simplest sugar units. Four forms of monosaccharides exist: glucose, fruc-

---

*Since most of our water intake comes from beverages rather than from food, some nutritionists do not consider water a nutrient, even though it is essential for life.

†The term *calorie* is used here to refer to *kilocalorie* (1,000 calories), which is the accepted scientific expression of the energy value of a food.

tose, galactose, and an infrequently found form, mannose. Of these, *glucose* is the most important monosaccharide; it makes up the blood sugar used as the body's primary source of energy. It is almost the sole source of energy for the brain and nervous system. Glucose, also known as dextrose, is found in vegetables, honey, molasses, fruits, and syrup. *Fructose,* also called levulose, is another monosaccharide that provides a source of simple sugar. This simple sugar is most often derived from fruits and berries.

Disaccharides are sugars composed of two monosaccharides, one of which is always a glucose unit. *Sucrose* is perhaps the most widely recognized disaccharide source; it is better known as table sugar. Sucrose is a combination of a glucose and a fructose molecule. Other disaccharides include *maltose,* derived from germinating cereals, and *lactose,* the carbohydrate found in human and animal milk.

The average adult American now ingests approximately 125 pounds of sucrose each year—usually in colas, candies, and pastries, which offer few additional nutritional benefits.[2] For years excess sugar intake was implicated in a number of major health concerns, including obesity, micronutrient deficiencies, behavioral disorders, dental caries, diabetes mellitus, and cardiovascular disease. With the exception of dental caries, current scientific data fail to confirm that sugar per se directly causes any of these health problems. However, the inability of some people to digest milk sugar (lactose) is well documented. Lactose intolerance can be effectively managed.

Much of the sugar we consume is hidden; that is, sugar is a principal product we may overlook in a large number of food items. Foods such as ketchup, salad dressings, cured meat products, and canned vegetables and fruits frequently contain much hidden sugar. Corn syrup, frequently found in these items, is a highly concentrated sucrose solution. Whether it is overt or hidden, experts recommend that no more than 10 percent of our total calories come from sucrose and other sugars.

For a number of years sugar substitutes have been used in a wide array of foods, beverages, and other consumer products. Among the most familiar of these are saccharin and aspartame (Nutrasweet), both of which are several hundred times sweeter than sucrose. Two newer artificial sweeteners, acesulfame potassium (ace K), used in Pepsi One, and xylitol, found in some brands of chewing gum, have recently entered the marketplace. Xylitol, in syrup form, has antibacterial properties and could someday be used in treating ear infections.[3]

Polysaccharides are complex carbohydrates that are composed of long chains of glucose units. These long chains are better known as starches. They are among the most important sources of dietary carbo-

---

Personal Applications

• When you look at your current consumption of carbohydrates, how does it compare with the current recommendation in terms of percentage of total calories and ratio of simple to complex carbohydrates?

---

hydrates. Starches are found primarily in vegetables, fruits, and grains. Consumption of starches helps people receive much overall nutritional benefit, since most starch sources also contain significant portions of vitamins, minerals, protein, and water. Dietary fiber is also a polysaccharide (see p. 129). Starches are nutritional "good guys."

Fats

Fats (lipids, fatty acids) are an important nutrient in our diets. Fats provide a concentrated form of energy (*nine* calories per gram consumed versus four for carbohydrates and protein) and help give our foods high **satiety** value. Fats help to give our food its pleasing taste, or palatability. Fats also serve as carriers of fat-soluble vitamins A, D, E, and K. Without fat, these vitamins would quickly pass through the body. Fat insulates the body and helps it retain heat. Today it is recommended that no more than 25 percent to 30 percent of our calories come from fat. Complete the Personal Assessment on pages 118–119 to see whether you eat too many fatty foods. If so, the Health Action Guide on page 116 offers tips for reducing the amount of fat in your diet.

Dietary sources of fat are often difficult to identify. The visible fats in our diet, such as butter, salad oils, and the layer of fat on some cuts of meat, represent only about 40 percent of the fat we consume. Most of the fat we eat is "hidden" in food because it is incorporated into the food during preparation or used to fry the food, or it is in food that we have not learned to recognize as being high in fat, such as a candy bar.

---

nutrients elements in foods that are required for the growth, repair, and regulation of body processes.

calories units of heat (energy); specifically, one calorie (used here to mean *kilocalorie*) equals the heat required to raise the temperature of one kilogram of water one degree Celsius.

carbohydrates chemical compounds comprising sugar (or saccharide) units; the body's primary source of energy.

satiety (suh *tie* uh tee) a feeling of no longer being hungry; a diminished desire to eat.

When shopping, we often notice that the fat content of some foods is reported by its percentage of the product's weight. In selecting the type of milk we drink, for example, we see that milk ranges from skim milk (no fat) to low-fat milk (½%) through reduced-fat milk (1% to 2%) to whole milk (3% to 4%). The labeling term *reduced fat* for 1% and 2% milk was introduced in 1997 to reflect that these types of milk are no longer considered low fat.

It is important for parents of infants and toddlers to know that current medical opinion advises strongly against any limiting of fats in the diets of children younger than two years of age.[4] This recommendation is, of course, based on the demands for energy and the nutritional requirements that accompany the rapid growth that occurs during this formative stage of life.

Every type of dietary fat is made up of a combination of three forms of fat (saturated, monounsaturated, and polyunsaturated), based on chemical composition. Today, consumers need to pay attention to the amount of each type of fat in dietary fat because of the role that each form plays in heart disease (see Chapter 10). **Saturated fats,** including those found in animal sources and in vegetable oils to which hydrogen has been added (hydrogenated), becoming *trans-fatty acids,* need to be carefully limited in a modern healthy diet. The presence of trans-fatty acids (an altered form of normal vegetable oil molecule) is associated with changes in the cell membrane, including those cells lining the artery wall. This possibly prevents these vessel wall cells from freeing cholesterol from their surfaces.[5] The amount of trans-fatty acids in the diet can be reduced by using liquefied margarines rather than the solid stick forms.

Fortunately, the replacement of saturated fats with monounsaturated and polyunsaturated fats and oils appears to lower blood cholesterol levels and reduce the risk of heart disease.[4] Vegetable oils tend to be low in saturated fats, with the exception of the tropical oils (coconut, palm, and palm kernel oils). Monounsaturated fats are found in high quantities in olive oil, peanut oil, and sesame oil. Polyunsaturated fats are especially prevalent in safflower oil and corn oil (Table 5-1).

Tropical Oils

Although all cooking oils (and fats such as butter, lard, margarine, and shortening) have the same number of calories by weight (nine calories per gram), some oils contain high percentages of saturated fats. All oils and fats contain varying percentages of saturated, monounsaturated, and polyunsaturated fats. The tropical oils—coconut, palm, and palm kernel—contain much higher percentages of saturated fats than do other cooking oils. Coconut oil is 92 percent saturated fat (see Table 5-1). Tropical oils can still be found in some brands of snack foods, crackers, cookies, nondairy creamers, and breakfast cereals, although they have been removed from most national brands. Do you check for tropical oils on the ingredients labels of the food you select?

How Much Fat Is Enough?

How advisable is a diet in which fat intake is restricted to less than 25 percent to 30 percent of total calories? Controversy over this question was examined in a leading medical journal.[6] In the article cited, researchers reported that when fat intake was significantly restricted in men who had high cholesterol levels, a known risk factor for cardiovascular disease, the

---

Skimming Off Fat, Calories, and Cholesterol

Below is a comparison of calories, fat, and cholesterol in 1 cup of several types of milk:

- **Whole.** 150 calories, 8 grams of fat, 5 grams of saturated fat, 33 mg of cholesterol

- **2%.** 120 calories, 5 grams of fat, 3 grams of saturated fat, 18 mg of cholesterol

- **1%.** 100 calories, 2.5 grams of fat, 1.5 grams of saturated fat, 10 mg of cholesterol

- **Skim.** 80 calories, 0 fat, 0 saturated fat, 4 mg of cholesterol

---

HEALTH ACTION GUIDE

Tips for Reducing the Fat Contents of Meals

A combination of the following practices can be used to reduce the fat content of meals. Can you suggest additional ways to reduce fat in your diet?

- Become familiar with today's food labels, and use the information provided to reduce the fat content of meals.
- Cut away and discard skin from meats such as chicken.
- When eating out, do not order foods with cream-based sauces, such as fettuccine alfredo.
- Trim fat from cuts of meat, including both the fat interspersed within the cut and that along the edges.
- Layer vegetables over baked potatoes to reduce the tendency to add butter, margarine, or sour cream.
- Request salad dressing and other condiments on the side so that you can control the amount you use.
- Eat more vegetables, fruits, and breads in place of meats and cheeses.
- Use jelly and apple butter in place of butter and margarine on toast, bread, and bagels.

InfoLinks
www.cspinet.org

Table 5-1	Comparison of Dietary Fats*			
Oil	**Mono**	**Poly**	**Sat**	**Chol**
Canola oil	62	32	06	00
Safflower oil	13	77	10	00
Corn oil	25	62	13	00
Olive oil	77	09	14	00
Peanut oil	49	33	18	00
Vegetable shortening	44	28	28	00
Beef fat	44	04	52	14
Palm oil	38	09	53	00
Butter	30	04	66	33
Coconut oil	06	02	92	00

*Comparisons of the percentages of monosaturated fat (Mono), polyunsaturated fat (Poly), and saturated fat (Sat) comprising selected dietary fats, in addition to their cholesterol (Chol) content

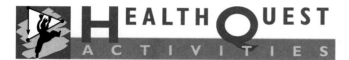

- One of the most valuable consumer skills you can acquire is the ability to read and interpret food labels. The *Food Labeling* activity in Module 3 demonstrates the purpose and importance of food labels. A tutorial outlines the steps in reading a food label, explains the terms used on food labels, and helps you evaluate health claims. The activity also gives you the opportunity to plan a meal and have it critiqued, using food labels as resources to guide you. Choose a food not listed in the activity and do a nutritional comparison of five different labels for that food. Compare the ingredients on each label to determine where the differences in nutrient content may be. Research the ingredients to find out their sources, other foods or substances that contain the ingredients, and the purpose for including each ingredient.

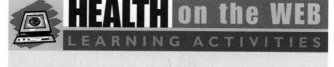

Taking the Fat or Fiction Quiz

Each of us should be aware of how much fat is in the foods we eat, whether we're concerned about our weight or not. Even in a slender person, too much dietary fat can lead to serious health problems. Fatty foods can be hard to recognize when the fat is used as an ingredient or during preparation. The Center for Science in Public Interest has been trying to raise the public's awareness of the dangers of too much dietary fat. Visit its website at www.cspinet.org/quiz and take the "Fat or Fiction: Nutrition Action Fat Quiz."[22] How much did you know about dietary fat? How can you limit your own fat intake?

Exploring the Food Guide Pyramid

The USDA Food Guide Pyramid is a terrific tool for deciding what to eat each day based on the Dietary Guidelines. The pyramid helps you choose a healthful diet that's best for you. Selecting more foods from the lower levels of the pyramid, known as "eating from the bottom," will help you get the nutrients you need while keeping calories under control. The USDA's on-line interactive Food Guide Pyramid will show you how to plan food selections that suit your tastes. Check it out at www.nal.usda.gov:8001/py/pmap.htm

Learning Your Vitamin ABCs

In spite of the abundance of vitamin-rich fruits, vegetables, grain products, and other healthful food selections, many people do not eat a balanced diet that contains a variety of foods. Go to www.thriveonline.com/shape/dyngames/gen/shape.vitamins.html and complete the quiz "Do You Know Your Vitamin ABCs?" How could you increase the variety of foods you eat? Think of a vitamin-rich food you've never tried, such as an unusual fruit or vegetable, and sample it at your next meal!

For more activities, log on to our Online Learning Center at www.mhhe.com/hper/health/payne.

men showed an unexpected decline in levels of high-density lipoprotein (HDL) cholesterol, the so-called "good" cholesterol thought to favor heart health (see Chapter 10).

Critics of the report contend that the researchers failed to consider the improved appearance of the arteries of people who restricted fat intake to as little as 10 percent of total calories. Resolution of the controversy will require studies in which both HDL levels and artery wall changes are considered in association with dietary modifications.

Cholesterol

A high level of **cholesterol** has also been reported to be a risk factor in the development of cardiovascular disease (see Chapter 10). Cholesterol is a necessary constituent of all animal tissue and is synthesized by our own bodies from carbohydrates and fats. Considerable evidence suggests that increased intake of saturated fats may increase serum (blood) cholesterol levels. However, after extensive investigation, the relationship between intake of dietary cholesterol and serum cholesterol levels remains unclear. Nevertheless, most doctors still recommend that people restrict their dietary

saturated fats fats that are difficult for the body to use; these are fats in solid form at room temperature; primarily animal fats.

cholesterol a primary form of fat found in the blood; lipid material manufactured within the body, as well as derived from dietary sources.

Personal Assessment

Fat has earned a bad reputation because of the health problems to which it contributes when we eat too much of it. The questionnaire below will help you think about the amounts and types of fat that you generally eat. For each general type of food or food habit, circle the response category that is most typical for you. If you never or almost never eat any items of a particular food type, just skip that type.

Food Type/Habit	High Fat	Medium Fat	Low Fat
Chicken	Fried with the skin	Baked, broiled, or barbecued with the skin	Baked, broiled, or barbecued without the skin
Fat present on meats	Usually eat	Sometimes eat	Never eat
Fat used in cooking	Butter, lard, bacon grease, chicken fat	Margarine, oil	Nonstick cooking spray or no fat used
Additions to rice, bread, potatoes, vegetables, etc.	Butter, lard, bacon grease, chicken fat, coconut oil, cream cheese	Margarine, oil, peanut butter	Butter-flavored granules or no fat used
Pizza toppings	Sausage, pepperoni, extra cheese, combination	Canadian bacon	Vegetable
Sandwich spreads	Mayonnaise or mayonnaise-type dressing	Light mayonnaise, oil and vinegar	Mustard, fat-free mayonnaise
Milk and milk products (e.g., yogurt)	Whole milk and whole-milk products	Low-fat milk and milk products	Skim milk and milk products
Sandwich side orders	Chips, potato salad, macaroni salad with creamy dressing	Coleslaw, pasta salad with clear dressing	Vegetable sticks, pretzels, pickle
Salad dressings	Blue cheese, ranch, Thousand Island, other creamy type	Oil and vinegar, clear-base dressing	Oil-free dressing, lemon juice, flavored vinegar
Typical meat portion eaten	6–8 ounces or more	4–5 ounces	2–3 ounces
Sandwich fillings	Beef or pork hot dogs, salami, bologna, pepperoni, cheese, tuna or chicken salad	Turkey hot dogs, 85% fat-free lunch meats, corned beef, peanut butter, hummus (chickpea paste)	95% fat-free lunch meats, roast turkey, roast beef, lean ham
Ground meats	Regular ground beef, sausage meat, ground meat, ground pork (about 30% fat)	Lean ground beef, ground chuck, turkey sausage meat (20%–25% fat)	Ground turkey, extra lean ground beef, ground round (about 15% fat)
Deep fried foods (e.g., french fries, onion rings, fish or chicken patties, egg rolls, tempura)	Eat every day	Eat once a week	Eat once a month or never

Food Type/Habit	High Fat	Medium Fat	Low Fat
Bread for sandwiches	Croissant	Biscuit	Whole wheat, French, tortilla, pita or pocket bread, bagel, sourdough, or English muffin
Cheeses	Hard cheeses (e.g., cheddar, Swiss, provolone, Jack, American, processed)	Part skim mozzarella, part skim ricotta, low-fat cheeses	Nonfat cheeses, nonfat cottage cheese, no cheese
Frozen desserts	Premium or regular ice cream	Ice milk or low-fat frozen yogurt	Sherbet, Italian water ice, nonfat frozen yogurt, frozen fruit whip
Coffee lighteners	Cream, liquid or powdered creamer	Whole milk	Low-fat or skim milk
Snacks	Chips, pies, cheese and crackers, nuts, donuts, microwave popcorn, chocolate, granola bars	Muffins, toaster pastries, unbuttered commercial popcorn	Pretzels, vegetable sticks, fresh or dried fruit, air-popped popcorn, bread sticks, jelly beans, hard candy
Cookies	Chocolate coated, chocolate chip, peanut butter, filled sandwich type	Oatmeal	Ginger snaps, vanilla wafers, graham crackers, animal crackers, fruit newtons

Scoring: (_____ × 2)   +   (_____ × 1)   +   (_____ × 0) =

TOTAL SCORE _____

Once you have completed the questionnaire, count the number of circles in each column and calculate your score as follows: multiply the number of choices in the left-hand (high-fat) column by 2 and multiply the number of choices in the middle by 1. Any number of choices in the right-hand column will equal 0.

Less than 10 = Excellent fat habits
10 to 20 = Good fat habits
20 to 30 = Need to trim some fat
Over 30 = Very high fat diet

If your score is 20 or above, try to substitute more foods from the middle (medium fat) column or, better still, the right (low fat) column for foods in the left-hand (high fat) column.

intake of cholesterol to 300 mg or less per day, reduce total fat and saturated fat intake, and exercise regularly. High-cholesterol foods include whole milk, shellfish, animal fat, and egg yolks. Only foods of animal origin can contain cholesterol. Thus, labels that appear on foods such as peanut butter and margarine trumpeting "cholesterol free" are overstating the obvious. It should be noted, however, that even foods high in cholesterol, such as shellfish, may provide other important nutrients and, therefore, could remain in a healthy diet but on a more modest basis.

Low-Fat Foods

Reflecting our growing concern about the role of dietary fats in many health problems has been the explosion of fat-free, low-fat, or reduced-fat food items appearing in stores and restaurants. Some nutritionists believe, however, that this trend could soon wane as the fast-food industry moves away from lower-fat items. Apparently, at least in terms of fast foods, the public favors familiar taste and super-sized portions over the longer-term benefits of weight maintenance and reduced incidence of heart disease.

Fat-Free Substitutes

Newly developed fat-free products containing fat substitutes (Simplesse, Simple Pleasures, Olestra, and Trailblazer) are available or soon to be available in the marketplace. At the time of this writing, products containing Olestra (marketed as Olean), such as WOW potato chips by Frito-Lay and Fat-free Pringles by Procter & Gamble are distributed nationwide. These products contain no cholesterol and have 80 percent fewer calories than similar products made with fat. Although Olestra-containing items appeared first in snack foods such as those just mentioned, they are or soon will be found in newer fat-free products such as ice cream, salad dressing, cheese spreads, yogurt, cakes, pies, and french fries.

The development of Olestra, as an example, required more than twenty-five years and $200 million on the part of Procter & Gamble, as an array of new technologies were required. In general, fat-free substitutes are made through processes called microparticulation, in which several fatty acids are bonded to a sugar molecule to create a triglyceride-like molecule that imparts all of the characteristics of fats but is incapable of being enzymatically broken down by the body as are the triglycerides.

In spite of the apparent desirability of the fat-free technology, concerns were voiced regarding the inability of these "nouveau fats" to carry fat-soluble vitamins (vitamins A, D, E, and K). Additional concern was raised over side effects in some people, such as abdominal cramping, loose stools, anal leakage, and an unpleasant aftertaste. Although these side effects have proved to affect only a small percentage of people who have eaten these products,[7,8] consumer acceptance of products made with fat-free substitutes is apparently disappointing to manufacturers. Lagging sales (some believe as much as 27 percent below projections) may reflect the relatively high prices of these products in comparison to their regular or reduced-fat shelf-mates. One consumer group, the Center for Science in the Public Interest, has requested that the FDA rescind its approval of Olestra. A member of the FDA's advisory panel also expressed concern about Olean's safety. At this time only a warning label describing the side effects must appear on products made with Olean.

Proteins

The term *protein* is derived from a word meaning "first importance." **Proteins** are manufactured in every living cell; they are composed of chains of amino acids. **Amino acids** are the "bricks" from which the body constructs its own protein. Twenty amino acids are used in various combinations to build the protein required for physiological processes to continue in a healthy manner.

The human body obtains amino acids from two sources—by breaking down protein from food (as if to take a brick wall apart for its bricks) or by manufacturing its own bricks (amino acids) within its cells. The latter process is less than fully successful because only eleven of the necessary twenty amino acids can be built by the body. The nine amino acids that *cannot* be built by the body are called *essential amino acids* (indispensable amino acids) because they must be obtained from outside the body through the protein in food. The eleven amino acids that the body itself can make are called *nonessential amino acids* (dispensable amino acids) because the body does not have to rely solely on food protein to obtain these bricks.[9]

In terms of food sources of amino acids, foods can be classified into one of two types, depending on whether they can supply the body with the essential amino acids or not. Complete protein foods contain all nine essential amino acids within their protein and are of animal origin (milk, meat, cheese, and eggs). The incomplete protein foods do not contain all of the essential amino acids and are of plant origin (vegetables, grains, and legumes [peas or beans, including chickpeas, butter beans, and tofu]). For some people, including vegan vegetarians (see pp. 146–147), people with limited access to animal-based food sources, or those who have significantly limited their meat, egg, and dairy product consumption, it is important to understand how essential amino acids can be obtained from incomplete protein sources. Fortunately, it is possible to combine various sources of incomplete protein foods to achieve complete sources. This requires the careful selection of plant foods in combinations that will provide all of the essential amino acids. The list below shows many usable combinations that include legumes and grains:

Sunflower seeds/green peas

Navy beans/barley

Green peas/corn

Red beans/rice

Sesame seeds/soybeans

Black-eyed peas/rice and peanuts

Green peas/rice

Corn/pinto beans

When even one essential amino acid is missing from the diet, deficiency can develop.

Protein serves primarily to promote growth and maintenance of body tissue. However, when calorie intake falls, protein will be broken down for glucose. This loss of protein can impede growth and repair of tissue. From this, it can be seen that adequate carbohydrate intake prevents protein from serving as an energy source.[9] Protein also is a primary component of enzyme and hormone structure; it helps maintain the *acid-base balance* of our bodies and serves as a source of energy (four calories per gram consumed). Nutritionists recommend that 12 to 15 percent of our caloric intake be from protein. Malnutrition in the world's underdeveloped countries is often seen in the protein deficiency disease called *kwashiorkor*. This disease is rarely seen in countries that have an abundant supply of protein.

Vitamins

Vitamins are organic compounds that are required in small amounts for normal growth, reproduction, and maintenance of health. Vitamins differ from carbohydrates, fats, and proteins because they do not provide calories or serve as structural elements for our bodies. Vitamins serve as *coenzymes*. By facilitating the action of **enzymes,** vitamins help initiate a wide variety of body responses, including energy production, use of minerals, and growth of healthy tissue.

Discovered just after the turn of the twentieth century, vitamins can be classified as *water soluble* (capable of being dissolved in water) or *fat soluble* (capable of being dissolved in fat or lipid tissue). Water-soluble vitamins include the B-complex vitamins and vitamin C. Most of the excess of these water-soluble vitamins is eliminated from the body during urination. The fat-soluble vitamins are A, D, E, and K. These vitamins are stored in the body in the adipose tissue or fat with excessive intake. It is therefore possible to consume

and retain too many of these vitamins, particularly A and D. Table 5-2 shows that all of the fat-soluble vitamins hold the potential for toxicity if taken in amounts that far exceed recommended dietary allowances (RDAs) (see Table 5-3A, B, and C). Most toxicity results from the use of supplements by adults or through excessive food intake of particular sources in very small children. When toxicity develops, the condition is referred to as **hypervitaminosis.**

The extent to which toxicity from water-soluble vitamins can occur is somewhat open to debate. As seen in Table 5-4, some of the water-soluble vitamins (niacin, B_6, and C) have been associated with toxic effects when taken in megadoses. For adults, intake of this level would occur only through the excessive use of supplements.

Because water-soluble vitamins dissolve rather quickly in water, you should be cautious in the preparation of fresh fruits and vegetables. One precaution is to avoid overcooking fresh vegetables. The longer fresh vegetables are steamed or boiled, the more water-soluble vitamins will be lost. Even soaking sliced fresh fruit or vegetables can result in the loss of vitamin C and B-complex vitamins.

To ensure an adequate vitamin intake, do not rely on bottled vitamins sold in grocery stores or health food stores. The best way is really the simplest and least expensive way: Eat a variety of foods. Unless there are special circumstances, such as pregnancy, infancy, or an existing health problem, virtually everyone in our society who eats a reasonably well-rounded diet consumes appropriate levels of all vitamins.

In spite of the availability of vitamin-rich foods, not all people eat a balanced diet based on a variety of foods. Also, recent studies suggest that a somewhat higher intake of vitamins A, C, and E for adults, and folacin (folic acid) before and during pregnancy, might have a positive effect in reducing the risk of developing colon cancer, atherosclerosis, birth defects, and depressed levels of HDL cholesterol (see Chapter 10).[10,11,12] In addition, consumption of an adequate

---

proteins compounds composed of chains of amino acids; primary components of muscle and connective tissue.

amino acids the building blocks of protein; manufactured by the body or obtained from dietary sources.

vitamins organic compounds that facilitate the action of enzymes.

enzymes organic substances that control the rate of physiological reactions but are not altered in the process.

hypervitaminosis excessive accumulation of vitamins within the body; associated with the fat-soluble vitamins.

Table 5-2   The Fat-Soluble Vitamins, Their Functions, Deficiency Conditions, and Food Sources

Vitamin	Major Functions	Deficiency Symptoms	People Most at Risk	Dietary Sources	RDA	Toxicity Symptoms
Vitamin A (retinoids) and provitamin A (carotenoids)	1. Vision, light, and color 2. Promotes growth 3. Prevents drying of skin and eyes 4. Promotes resistance to bacterial infection	1. Night blindness 2. Xerophthalmia 3. Poor growth 4. Dry skin (keratinization)	People in poverty, especially preschool children (still very rare)	Vitamin A Liver Fortified milk Provitamin A Sweet potatoes Spinach Greens Carrots Cantaloupe Apricots Broccoli	Women: 800 RE (4000 IU) Men: 1000 RE (5000 IU)	Fetal malformations, hair loss, skin changes, pain in bones
Vitamin D (cholecalciferol and ergocalciferol)	1. Facilitates absorption of calcium and phosphorus 2. Maintains optimum calcification of bone	1. Rickets 2. Osteomalacia	Breastfed infants, elderly shut-ins	Vitamin D-fortified milk Fish oils Tuna fish Salmon	5–10 micrograms (200–400 IU)	Growth retardation, kidney damage, calcium deposits in soft tissue
Vitamin E (tocopherols, tocotrienols)	1. Antioxidant: prevents breakdown of vitamin A and unsaturated fatty acids	1. Hemolysis of red blood cells 2. Nerve destruction	People with poor fat absorption (still very rare)	Vegetable oils Some greens Some fruits	Women: 8 α-tocopherol equivalents Men: 10 α-tocopherol equivalents	Muscle weakness, headaches, fatigue, nausea, inhibition of vitamin K metabolism
Vitamin K (phylloquinone and menaquinone)	1. Helps prothrombin and other factors for blood clotting	1. Hemorrhage	People taking antibiotics for months at a time	Green vegetables Liver	60–80 micrograms	Anemia and jaundice

RE, Retinol equivalents; IU, international units.

Table 5-3A   Adult Recommended Dietary Allowances,[1] Revised 1989

Category	Age (years)	Weight[2] (kg)	Weight[2] (lb)	Height[2] (cm)	Height[2] (in)	Protein (g)	Vitamin A (µg RE)[3]	Vitamin D (µg)[4]	Vitamin E (µg α-TE)[5]	Vitamin K (µg)
Males	15–18	66	145	176	69	59	1000	10	10	65
	19–24	72	160	177	70	58	1000	10	10	70
	25–50	79	174	176	70	63	1000	5	10	80
	51+	77	170	173	68	63	1000	5	10	80
Females	15–18	55	120	163	64	44	800	10	8	55
	19–24	58	128	164	65	46	800	10	8	60
	25–50	63	138	163	64	50	800	5	8	65
	51+	65	143	160	63	50	800	5	8	65
Pregnant						60	800	10	10	65
Lactating	1st 6 Months					65	1300	10	12	65
	2nd 6 Months					62	1200	10	11	65

[1]The allowances, expressed as average daily intakes over time, are intended to provide for individual variations among most normal people as they live in the United States under usual environmental stresses. Diets should be based on a variety of common foods to provide nutrients for which human requirements have been less well defined. See text for detailed discussion of allowances and of nutrients not tabulated.
[2]Weights and heights of reference adults are actual medians for the U.S. population of the designated age, as reported by NHANES II. The use of these figures does not imply that the height-to-weight ratios are ideal.

Table 5-3A   Continued

Vitamin C (mg)	Thia-min (mg)	Ribo-flavin (mg)	Niacin (mg NE)[6]	Vitamin B_6 (mg)	Folate (μ)	Vitamin B_{12} (μ)	Calcium (mg)	Phos-phorus (mg)	Mag-nesium (mg)	Iron (mg)	Zinc (mg)	Iodide (μ)	Sele-nium (μ)
			Water-Soluble Vitamins						**Minerals**				
60	1.5	1.8	20	2.0	200	2.0	1200	1200	400	12	15	150	50
60	1.5	1.7	19	2.0	200	2.0	1200	1200	350	10	15	150	70
60	1.5	1.7	19	2.0	200	2.0	800	800	350	10	15	150	70
60	1.2	1.4	15	2.0	200	2.0	800	800	350	10	15	150	70
60	1.1	1.3	15	1.5	180	2.0	1200	1200	300	15	12	150	50
60	1.1	1.3	15	1.6	180	2.0	1200	1200	280	15	12	150	55
60	1.1	1.3	15	1.6	180	2.0	800	800	280	15	12	150	55
60	1.0	1.2	13	1.6	180	2.0	800	800	280	10	12	150	55
70	1.5	1.6	17	2.2	400	2.2	1200	1200	320	30	15	175	65
95	1.6	1.8	20	2.1	280	2.6	1200	1200	355	15	19	200	75
95	1.6	1.7	20	2.1	260	2.6	1200	1200	340	15	16	200	75

[3]Retinol equivalents. 1 retinol = 1 μg retinol or 6 μg β-carotene.
[4]As cholecalciferol. 10 μg cholecalciferol = 400 IU of vitamin D.
[5]α-Tocopherol equivalents. 1 mg d-α tocopherol = 1 α-TE.
[6]1 NE (niacin equivalent) is equal to 1 mg of niacin or 60 mg of dietary tryptophan.

Table 5-3B   Estimated Safe and Adequate Daily Dietary Intakes (ESADDIs) of Selected Vitamins and Minerals for Adults*

Biotin (μg)	Pantothenic acid (mg)	Copper (mg)	Manganese (mg)	Fluoride (mg)	Chromium (mg)	Molybdenum (μg)
	Vitamins			**Trace Elements†**		
30–100	4–7	1.5–3.0	2.0–5.0	1.5–4.0	50–200	75–250

*Because there is less information on which to base allowances, these figures are not given in the main table of RDAs and are provided here in the form of ranges of recommended intakes.
†Because the toxic levels for many trace elements may be only several times the usual intake, the upper levels for the trace elements given in this table should not be habitually exceeded.

Table 5-3C   Estimated Minimum Sodium, Chloride, and Potassium Requirements of Healthy People*

Age	Weight (kg)*	Sodium (mg)*†	Chloride (mg)*†	Potassium (mg)‡
10–18	50.0	500	750	2000
>18§	70.0	500	750	2000

*No allowance has been included for large, prolonged losses from the skin through sweat.
†There is no evidence that higher intakes confer any health benefit.
‡Desirable intakes of potassium considerably exceed these values (~3500 mg for adults).
§No allowance included for growth. Values for those below 18 years assume a growth rate at the 50th percentile, reported by the National Center for Health Statistics and averaged for men and women.

Table 5-4 The Water-Soluble Vitamins, Their Functions, Deficiency Conditions, and Food Sources

Vitamin	Major Functions	Deficiency Symptoms	People Most at Risk	Dietary Sources	RDA or ESADDI	Toxicity
Thiamin	Coenzyme involved with enzymes in carbohydrate metabolism; nerve function	Beriberi, nervous tingling, poor coordination, edema, heart changes, weakness	People with alcoholism, people in poverty	Sunflower seeds, pork, whole and enriched grains, dried beans, peas, brewer's yeast	1.1–1.5 milligrams	None possible from food
Riboflavin	Coenzyme involved in energy metabolism	Inflammation of mouth and tongue, cracks at corners of the mouth, eye disorders	Possibly people on certain medications if no dairy products consumed	Milk, mushrooms, spinach, liver, enriched grains	1.2–1.7 milligrams	None reported
Niacin	Coenzyme involved in energy metabolism, fat synthesis, fat breakdown	Pellagra, diarrhea, dermatitis, dementia	People in severe poverty where corn is dominant food, people with alcoholism	Mushrooms, bran, tuna, salmon, chicken, beef, liver, peanuts, enriched grains	15–19 milligrams	Flushing of skin at >100 milligrams
Pantothenic acid	Coenzyme involved in energy metabolism, fat synthesis, fat breakdown	Using an antagonist causes tingling in hands, fatigue, headache, nausea	People with alcoholism	Mushrooms, liver, broccoli, eggs; most foods have some	4–7 milligrams	None
Biotin	Coenzyme involved in glucose production, fat synthesis	Dermatitis, tongue soreness, anemia, depression	People with alcoholism	Cheese, egg yolks, cauliflower, peanut butter, liver	30–100 micrograms	Unknown

amount of folic acid before and during pregnancy has been shown to reduce the incidence of neural tube birth defects.[13] Others who might benefit from a multivitamin/mineral supplement are vegans, people with limited milk intake and limited exposure to sunlight, people with lactose intolerance, and people on a severely restricted weight loss diet. To date, most of these findings have not been translated into specific recommendations, but they are drawing increased interest on the part of both the scientific community and the general public. Clearly, the antioxidation properties of vitamins A, C, and E interest health experts today.

Except for the people identified above, most Americans could go without supplementation. How would this occur? Today it is known that few Americans obtain 100 percent of the 14 RDAs on a daily basis, although the majority of people regularly obtain most (77%) of the RDAs every day. In fact, experts are confident that virtually all Americans would achieve the recommended RDAs on a daily basis by increasing their fruit and vegetable consumption to the recommended 5 to 6 servings daily. Therefore, in light of current eating patterns and the increase in fruit and vegetable consumption needed to achieve desired nutritional intake, the American Dietetic Association does not recommend the wide-scale use of vitamin and mineral supplements, particularly in amounts exceeding 100 percent of the current RDAs.[14] Physicians, however, routinely recommend supplementation to individual patients because of pregnancy, lactation, smoking, or recovery from specific conditions.

Minerals

Nearly 5 percent of the body is composed of inorganic materials, the *minerals*. Minerals function primarily as structural elements (in teeth, muscles, hemoglobin,

Table 5-4 *Continued*

Vitamin	Major Functions	Deficiency Symptoms	People Most at Risk	Dietary Sources	RDA or ESADDI	Toxicity
Vitamin B$_6$, pyridoxine, and other forms	Coenzyme involved in protein metabolism, neurotransmitter synthesis, hemoglobin synthesis, many other functions	Headache, anemia, convulsions, nausea, vomiting, flaky skin, sore tongue	Adolescent and adult women, people on certain medications, people with alcoholism	Animal protein foods, spinach, broccoli, bananas, salmon, sunflower seeds	1.8–2 milligrams	Nerve destruction at doses >100 milligrams
Folate (folic acid)	Coenzyme involved in DNA synthesis	Megaloblastic anemia, inflammation of tongue, diarrhea, poor growth, mental disorders	People with alcoholism, pregnant women, people taking certain medications	Green leafy vegetables, orange juice, organ meats, sprouts, sunflower seeds	180–200 micrograms	None, nonprescription vitamin dosage is controlled by FDA
Vitamin B$_{12}$ (cobalamins)	Coenzyme involved in folate metabolism, nerve function	Macrocytic anemia, poor nerve function	Elderly because of poor absorption, vegans	Animal foods, especially organ meats, oysters, clams (B$_{12}$ not naturally in plant foods)	2 micrograms	None
Vitamin C (ascorbic acid)	Collagen synthesis, hormone synthesis, neurotransmitter synthesis	Scurvy: poor wound healing, pinpoint hemorrhages, bleeding gums, edema	People with alcoholism, elderly men living alone	Citrus fruits, strawberries, broccoli, greens	60 milligrams	Doses >1–2 grams cause diarrhea and can alter some diagnostic tests

and thyroid hormones.) They are also critical in the regulation of a number of body processes, including muscle contraction, heart function, blood clotting, protein synthesis, and red blood cell synthesis. Approximately twenty-one minerals have been recognized as being essential for human health.[9]

Macronutrients (major minerals) are those minerals that are seen in relatively high amounts in our body tissues. Examples of macronutrients are calcium, phosphorus, sodium, potassium, and magnesium. Examples of *micronutrients*, minerals seen in relatively small amounts in body tissues, include zinc, iron, copper, selenium, and iodine. Although micro-nutrients **(trace elements)** are required only in small quantities, they are still essential. (See Tables 5-5 and 5-6 for listings of minerals and their functions.) As with vitamins, the safest, most appropriate way to receive a

sufficient amount of all necessary minerals is to eat a balanced diet.

Personal Applications

• Vitamins and other food supplements (such as amino acids, enzymes, and minerals) are readily available in most shopping mall health food stores. Do you use such supplements? If so, why? Are you confident that they are necessary and that they are safe to use in the quantities recommended on the containers?

trace elements   minerals whose presence in the body occurs in very small amounts; micronutrient elements.

Table 5-5   Key Trace Minerals

Mineral	Major Functions	Deficiency Symptoms	People Most at Risk	RDA or ESADDI	Nutrient-Dense Dietary Sources	Results of Toxicity
Iron	Part of hemoglobin and other key compounds used in respiration; used for immune function	Low serum iron levels, small, pale red blood cells, low blood hemoglobin values	Infants, preschool children, adolescents, women in childbearing years	Men: 10 milligrams Women: 15 milligrams	Meats, spinach, seafood, broccoli, peas, bran, enriched breads	Toxicity is seen in children who consume 200–400 milligrams in iron pills and in people with hemochromatosis; in this latter case, people over-absorb iron
Zinc	Over 200 enzymes need zinc, including enzymes involved in growth, immunity, alcohol metabolism, sexual development, and reproduction	Skin rash, diarrhea, decreased appetite and sense of taste, hair loss, poor growth and development, poor wound healing	Vegetarians, women in general, the elderly	Men: 15 milligrams Women: 12 milligrams	Seafood, meats, greens, whole grains	Reduces iron and copper absorption; can cause diarrhea, cramps, and depressed immune function
Selenium	Part of antioxidant system	Muscle pain, muscle weakness, heart disease	Unknown	55–70 micrograms	Meats, eggs, fish, seafood, whole grains	Nausea, vomiting, hair loss, weakness, liver disease
Iodide	Part of thyroid hormone	Goiter, poor growth in infancy when mother is deficient in pregnancy	None in America, since salt is usually fortified	150 micrograms	Iodized salt, white bread, saltwater fish, dairy products	Inhibition of function of the thyroid gland
Copper	Aids in iron metabolism; works with many enzymes, such as those involved in protein metabolism and hormone synthesis	Anemia, low white blood cell count, poor growth	Infants recovering from malnutrition, people who use overzealous supplementation of zinc	1.5–3 milligrams	Liver, cocoa, beans, nuts, whole grains, dried fruits	Vomiting, nervous system disorders

Table 5-5   Key Trace Minerals—*Continued*

Mineral	Major Functions	Deficiency Symptoms	People Most at Risk	RDA or ESADDI	Nutrient-Dense Dietary Sources	Results of Toxicity
Fluoride	Increases resistance of tooth enamel to dental caries	Increased risk of dental caries	Areas where water is not fluoridated and dental treatments do not make up for this lack of fluoride	1.5–4 milligrams	Fluoridated water, toothpaste, dental treatments, tea, seaweed	Stomach upset, mottling (staining) of teeth during development
Chromium	Enhances blood glucose levels	High blood glucose levels after eating	People on total parenteral nutrition and perhaps elderly people with non-insulin-dependent diabetes mellitus	50–200 micrograms	Egg yolks, whole grains, pork	Caused by industrial contamination, not dietary excess
Manganese	Aids action of some enzymes, such as those involved in carbohydrate metabolism	None in humans	Unknown	2–5 milligrams	Nuts, rice, oats, beans	Unknown in humans
Molybdenum	Aids in action of some enzymes	None in humans	Unknown	75–250 micrograms	Beans, grains, nuts	Unknown in humans

Table 5-6   Water and the Major Minerals

Name	Major Functions	Deficiency Symptoms	People Most at Risk	RDA or Minimum Requirement	Nutrient-Dense Dietary Sources	Results of Toxicity
Water	Medium for chemical reactions, removal of waste products, perspiration to cool the body	Thirst, muscle weakness, poor endurance	Infants with a fever, elderly in nursing homes	1 milliliter per calorie burned	As such and in foods	Probably occurs only in mental disorders: headache, blurred vision, convulsions
Sodium	A major ion of the extracellular fluid; nerve impulse transmission	Muscle cramps	People who severely restrict sodium to lower blood pressure (250–500 milligrams/day)	500 milligrams	Table salt, processed foods	High blood pressure in susceptible individuals

continued

Table 5-6   Water and the Major Minerals—*Continued*

Name	Major Functions	Deficiency Symptoms	People Most at Risk	RDA or Minimum Requirement	Nutrient-Dense Dietary Sources	Results of Toxicity
Potassium	A major ion of intracellular fluid; nerve impulse transmission	Irregular heartbeat, loss of appetite, muscle cramps	People who use potassium-wasting diuretics or have poor diets, as seen in poverty and with alcoholism	2000 milligrams	Spinach, squash, bananas, orange juice, other vegetables and fruits, milk	Slowing of the heartbeat; seen in kidney failure
Chloride	A major ion of the extracellular fluid; acid production in stomach; nerve transmission	Convulsions in infants	No one, probably, when infant formula manufacturers control product quality adequately	700 milligrams	Table salt, some vegetables	High blood pressure in susceptible people when combined with sodium
Calcium	Bone and tooth strength; blood clotting; nerve impulse transmission; muscle contractions; cell regulation	Poor intake increases the risk for osteoporosis	Women in general, especially those who constantly restrict their energy intake and consume few dairy products	800 milligrams (older than 24 years old)	Dairy products, canned fish, leafy vegetables, tofu, fortified orange juice	Very high intakes may cause kidney stones in susceptible people
Phosphorus	Bone and tooth strength; part of various metabolic compounds; major ion of intracellular fluid	Probably none; poor bone maintenance possible	Elderly consuming very nutrient-poor diets, possibly vegetarians and those with alcoholism	800 milligrams (older than 24 years)	Dairy products, processed foods, fish, soft drinks	Hampers bone health in people with kidney failure; poor bone mineralization if calcium intakes are low
Magnesium	Bone strength; enzyme function; nerve and heart function	Weakness, muscle pain, poor heart function	People on thiazide diuretics, women in general	Men: 350 milligrams Women: 280 milligrams	Wheat bran, green vegetables, nuts, chocolate	Causes weakness in people with kidney failure
Sulfur	Part of vitamins and amino acids; drug detoxification; acid-base balance	None	People who do not meet their protein needs	None	Protein food	None likely

Water

Water may well be our most essential nutrient, since without water most people would die from **dehydration** effects in less than a week. People could survive for weeks and even years without some of the essential minerals and vitamins. More than half the body's weight comes from water. Water provides the medium for nutrient and waste transport and temperature control and plays a key role in nearly all of the body's biochemical reactions. A common indication of inadequate fluid intake is strained, uncomfortable bowel movements.

Most people seldom think about the importance of an adequate intake of water and fluids. Adults require about six to ten glasses a day, depending on their exercise level and environment. However, because of the dehydrating effects of coffee, tea, and alcohol, the average American consumes the equivalent of only 4.6 glasses per day.[15] Of course, people also obtain needed fluids from fruits, vegetables, fruit and vegetable juices, milk, and noncaffeinated soft drinks. However, excessive water consumption by newborn infants dilutes sodium stores in the body, which may cause death.[16]

Fiber

Although not considered a nutrient by definition, **fiber** is an important component of sound nutrition. Fiber consists of plant material that is not digested but rather moves through the digestive tract and out of the body. Cereal, fruits, and vegetables all provide us with dietary fiber.

Fiber can be classified into two large groups on the basis of water solubility. *Insoluble* fibers are those that can absorb water from the intestinal tract. By absorbing water, the insoluble fibers give the stool bulk and decrease the time it takes the stool to move through the digestive tract. In contrast, *soluble* fiber turns to a "gel" within the intestinal tract and in so doing binds to liver bile, which has cholesterol attached. Thus, soluble fiber is valuable in removing (or lowering) blood cholesterol levels. Also, since foods high in soluble fiber are generally low in sugar and saturated fats, fiber may indirectly contribute to keeping blood sugar low and reduce the risk of colon cancer associated with diets high in saturated fats.

In recent years attention has been directed toward three forms of soluble fiber—oat bran, psyllium (from the weed plantain), and rice bran—for their ability to lower blood cholesterol levels. The sale of products containing oat bran, such as cereals and baked goods, has increased greatly since 1987. In fact, in 1997 oat fiber was deemed effective enough to alter packaging labels in a manner reflecting its supportive role in the prevention of heart disease.[17] To accomplish a five- to six-point lowering in cholesterol, a daily consumption of oat bran

equaling a large bowl of oat bran cold cereal or three or more packs of instant oatmeal would be necessary. Of course, oatmeal can be eaten as a cooked cereal or used in other foods, such as hamburgers, pancakes, or meatloaf. The role of psyllium and rice bran in lowering cholesterol levels is less well established. Psyllium can be obtained by using laxatives such as Metamucil, Citrucel, Konsyl, Fiberall fiber wafers, Mondame, and Perdiem fiber.

The Absorption of Nutrients

In a very real sense, food (as nutrients) is not "in the body" until it is digested and then absorbed into and through the walls of the gastrointestinal (GI) tract, into the bloodstream, and is distributed to the cell sites at which it will be used for energy, growth, repair, and regulation. Figure 5-1 depicts a highly diagrammatic representation of the GI tract showing specific absorption sites for several important nutrients. The first 18 inches of the small intestine is the most active site for absorption, surpassing the level of activity in the remainder of the small intestine, the large intestine, and stomach. It is also important to note that some portion of the alcohol contained in alcoholic drinks enters the body through the stomach wall (more in women than in men), although most is absorbed in the small intestine. Water and salts are principally regulated by the walls of the large intestine.

In light of the importance of the small intestine, any injury or disease in this location could seriously harm nutritional status by impairing the body's ability to obtain nutrients. In fact, in extreme cases of obesity (morbid obesity) a portion of small intestine is resected (cut away) in an attempt to restrict the movement of nutrients into the body. This drastic approach to weight loss is, of course, a double-edged sword in that many nutrients needed for overall health must then be supplemented, often for the rest of the person's life.

The Food Groups

As already mentioned, the most effective way to take in adequate amounts of nutrients is to eat a **balanced diet**, that is, to eat a diet that includes selections from different food groups (see Table 5-7). Today, the

---

dehydration abnormal depletion of fluids from the body; severe dehydration can lead to death.

fiber cellulose-based plant material that cannot be digested; found in cereal, fruits, and vegetables.

balanced diet a diet featuring food selections from each food group.

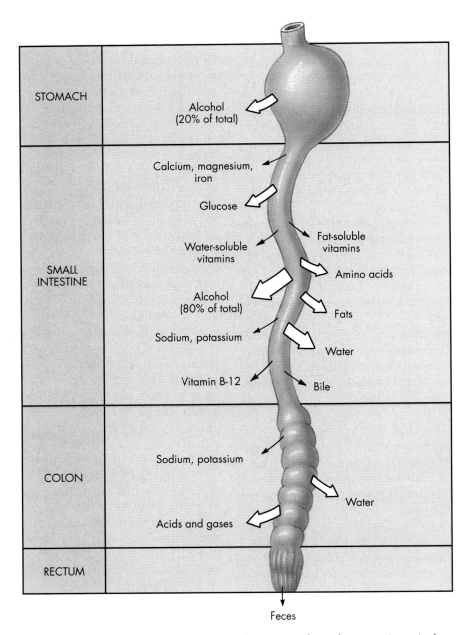

Figure 5-1   Important sites of nutrient absorption along the gastrointestinal tract. The size of the arrow indicates the relative amount of absorption at that site. (Note that this drawing depicts the GI tract as being "uncoiled" to simplify the presentation of its absorption sites.)

United States Department of Agriculture (USDA) Food Guide Pyramid outlines five groups for which recommendations have been established and an additional group (fats, oils, and sweets) for which no specific recommendations exist (Figure 5-2). Table 5-7 summarizes the major nutrients each food group supplies. To determine whether you are eating a healthful diet balanced with choices from each food group, complete the Personal Assessment on page 133.

Fruits

Two to four daily servings from the fruit group are recommended for an adult. The important function of this group is to provide vitamin A, vitamin C, complex carbohydrates, and fiber in our diets. The American Cancer Society indicates that this food group may play an important role in the prevention of certain forms of cancer. Included foods are citrus fruits and fruit juices. At least one serving high in vitamin C should be eaten

Table 5-7   Guide to Daily Food Choices

Food Group	Serving	Major Contributions	Foods and Serving Size*
Milk, yogurt, and cheese	2 (adult†) 3 (children, teens, young adults, and pregnant or lactating women)	Calcium Riboflavin Protein Potassium Zinc	1 cup milk 1½ oz cheese 2 oz processed cheese 1 cup yogurt 2 cups cottage cheese 1 cup custard/pudding 1½ cups ice cream
Meat, poultry, fish, dry beans, eggs, and nuts	2–3	Protein Niacin Iron Vitamin B_6 Zinc Thiamin Vitamin B_{12}‡	2–3 oz cooked meat, poultry, fish 1–1½ cups cooked dry beans 4 T peanut butter 2 eggs ½–1 cup nuts
Fruits	2–4	Vitamin C Fiber	¼ cup dried fruit ½ cup cooked fruit ¾ cup juice 1 whole piece fruit 1 melon wedge
Vegetables	3–5	Vitamin A Vitamin C Folate Magnesium Fiber	½ cup raw or cooked vegetables 1 cup raw leafy vegetables
Bread, cereals, rice, and pasta	6–11	Starch Thiamin Riboflavin§ Iron Niacin Folate Magnesium || Fiber || Zinc ||	1 slice of bread 1 oz ready-to-eat cereal ½–¾ cup cooked cereal, rice, or pasta
Fats, oils, and sweets		Foods from this group should not replace any from the other groups. Amounts consumed should be determined by individual energy needs.	

This is a practical way to turn the RDA into food choices. You can get all essential nutrients by eating a balanced variety of foods each day from the food groups listed here. Eat a variety of foods in each food group, and adjust serving sizes appropriately to reach and maintain desirable weight.

*May be reduced for children's servings.
†≥25 years of age.
‡Only in animal food choices.
\|\|Whole grains especially.
§If enriched.

daily. Two to four servings per day are recommended. One serving is equivalent to one medium apple, banana, or orange; ½ cup of chopped, cooked, or canned fruit; or ¾ cup of fruit juice.

Vegetables

Three to five servings from the vegetable group are recommended for an adult. As with the fruit group, the important function of this group is to provide vitamin A, vitamin C, complex carbohydrates, and fiber. Foods included in this group are dark green, yellow, and orange vegetables, canned or cooked vegetables, and tossed salads. At least one serving of a dark green, yellow, or orange vegetable containing fat-soluble vitamin A should be consumed every other day. **Cruciferous vegetables,** such as

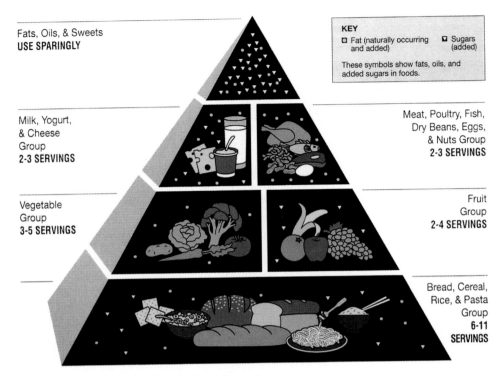

Figure 5-2   The USDA Food Guide Pyramid.

broccoli, cabbage, brussels sprouts, and cauliflower, may be especially helpful in the prevention of certain forms of cancer.[18]

On the basis of current recommendations, people should include three to five servings per day in their diets. One serving consists of 1 cup of raw, leafy vegetables, ½ cup of other vegetables, cooked or chopped raw, or ¾ cup of vegetable juice. Recently it has been determined that antioxidants in vegetables and fruits may slow age-related changes in cognitive function.[19] Additionally, recall the role that five to six daily servings of fruits and vegetables would have in relationship to 100 percent of the RDAs.

Milk, Cheese, and Yogurt

The milk, cheese, and yogurt group contributes two primary nutritional benefits: high-quality protein and calcium (required for bone and tooth development). Foods included in this group are whole milk, low-fat milk, yogurt, cheese, and ice cream. The adult recommendation is two to three cups of milk or two to three equivalent servings from this group each day. For teenagers the recommendation is four cups of milk each day. Recently, some physicians have begun recommending that premenopausal women consume three to four servings from this group to provide maximal protection from osteoporosis (see Chapter 4). One serving equals 1 cup of milk or yogurt, 1.5 ounces of natural cheese, or 2 ounces of processed cheese.

Because of the general concern over saturated fat, cholesterol, and additional calories, low-fat milk products are recommended in place of high-fat milk products. In November of 1996, the FDA released new, more consumer-friendly labels for some milk products. For example, 2 percent milk must now be labeled *reduced-fat milk* instead of low-fat milk, while skim milk may also be called *fat free, nonfat, no fat, zero fat, without fat, negligible source of fat,* or *insignificant source of fat.*

Meat, Poultry, Fish, Eggs, Dry Beans, and Nuts

Our need for daily selections from this protein-rich group is based on our daily need for protein, iron, and the B vitamins. Meats include all red meat (beef, pork, and game), fish, and poultry. Meat substitutes include cheese, dried peas and beans (legumes), and peanut butter. Eggs can also be used as meat substitutes; however, using only the separated egg whites provides an excellent source of protein without the accompanying fat, including cholesterol. The current recommendation for adults is four ounces total meat, poultry, or fish per day, preferably in two to three

cruciferous vegetables (crew **sif** er us)   vegetables that have flowers with four leaves in the pattern of a cross.

Personal Assessment

A primary requirement for good nutrition is a balanced diet. A variety of food selections forms the basis of this diet.

For a 7-day period, assign yourself the points indicated when each dietary requirement is met. Record your points in the appropriate column for each day. Total your daily and weekly points. Negative points for junk food consumption should be subtracted from your daily and weekly totals.

Food	Points	Maximum Score	Daily Score						
			M	T	W	T	F	S	S
Milk and milk products		30							
One cup of milk or equivalent	10								
Second cup of milk	10								
Third cup of milk	10								
Protein-rich foods		25							
One serving of eggs, meat, fish, poultry, cheese, dried beans, or peas	15								
One or two additional servings of eggs, meat, fish, poultry, or cheese	10 each								
Fruits and vegetables		30							
One serving of green or yellow vegetables	10								
One serving of citrus fruit, tomato, or cabbage	10								
Two or more servings of other fruits and vegetables, including potatoes	5 each								
Breads and cereals		15							
Four or more servings of whole-grain or enriched cereal or breads	5 each								
Junk foods (or negative point value foods)									
Sweet rolls	–5								
Fruit pies	–5								
Potato chips, corn chips, or cheese curls	–5								
Candy	–5								
Nondiet sodas	–5								
		100							

Point Record

Weekly point total _____

Negative point total _____

Adjusted weekly point total _____

Interpretation

600–700	Excellent dietary practices
450–599	Adequate dietary practices
300–449	Marginal dietary practices
Below 300	Poor dietary practices

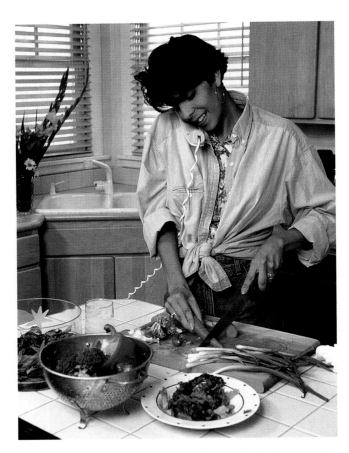

Vegetables provide vitamins, complex carbohydrates, and fiber and may help prevent some types of cancer. Are you eating three to five servings a day?

servings. However, some nutrition specialists suggest one serving per day (or every other day), with use of legumes as a protein supplement. One serving from this group consists of two to three ounces of cooked lean meat, poultry, or fish. One-half cup of cooked dry beans or one egg counts as one ounce of lean meat. Two tablespoons of peanut butter or one-third cup of nuts also counts as one ounce of meat.

If people select foods that fit into both the meat and the milk categories, they must be careful to include these foods in only one category for that particular day. Also, it is important that meat and fish are fresh, stored appropriately, and cooked adequately to reduce the likelihood of serious foodborne illnesses. The Health Action Guide on this page lists the USDA guidelines for safe handling of meat.

The fat content of meat varies considerably. Some forms of meat yield only 1 percent fat, whereas others may be as high as 40 percent fat. Poultry and fish are generally significantly lower in overall fat than are red meats. Interestingly, the higher the grade of red meat, the more fat will be marbled throughout the muscle fiber. Indeed, the higher grade steak usually tastes better, but that is because of its higher fat content.

Meats are generally excellent sources of iron. Iron is present in much greater amounts in red meats and organ meats (liver, kidney, and heart) than in poultry and fish. Iron plays a critically important role in hemoglobin synthesis on red blood cells and, thus, is an important contributor to physical fitness (see Chapter 4) and overall cardiovascular health (see Chapter 10).

Breads, Cereals, Rice, and Pasta

The nutritional benefit from the breads, cereals, rice, and pasta group lies in its contribution of B-complex vitamins and energy from its complex carbohydrates. Some nutritionists believe that the use of foods from this group promotes protein intake, since many foods in this group are prepared as complete-protein foods, such as macaroni and cheese, cereal and milk, and bread and meat sandwiches.

Six to eleven servings daily from this group are recommended. That may sound like a lot of food, but official serving sizes are small. For example, one slice of bread, one ounce of ready-to-eat cereal, or one-half cup of cooked cereal, rice, or pasta counts as a serving, so it's easy to eat several servings in a single meal. Several daily servings of any **enriched** or whole-grain bread or cereal are recommended. Milling of cereal grains into flour tends to deplete important nutrients, including fiber, vitamin B$_6$, vitamin E, magnesium, and various trace elements. The process of enrichment returns only four of these nutrients: thiamine, niacin, riboflavin (all B vitamins), and the mineral iron. Fortunately, whole-grain flour is a healthful alternative for most consumers, since few, if any, nutrients are lost in the milling process. The *cereal germ,* the fiber, and additional nutrients are not destroyed.

Fats, Oils, and Sweets

Where do such items as beer, butter, candy, colas, cookies, corn chips, and pastries fit into your diet? Today they are included under the label "fats, oils, and sweets." Most of the items mentioned contribute relatively little to healthful nutrition other than providing additional calories (generally from sucrose)

HEALTH ACTION GUIDE

USDA's Safety Tips for Proper Handling of Meat

- Keep meat refrigerated or frozen.
- Thaw meat in the refrigerator or microwave, not on the kitchen counter at room temperature.
- Keep raw meat separate from other foods.
- Wash working surfaces, utensils, and hands after use.
- Cook meat thoroughly.
- Refrigerate leftovers within two hours of cooking.

InfoLinks
www.usda.gov/cnpp/

and significant amounts of salt and fat. As you will see in Chapter 10, people who are salt-sensitive must reduce their salt intake as a step in preventing the development of high blood pressure. It is not surprising that many of these items are referred to collectively as *junk foods*. Of course, if particular food items, such as cookies, are made from high-quality flour and contain raisins and nuts, people can receive some nutritional benefit from consuming such goodies (see the discussion of nutrient density on pp. 144–145).

Understandably, the processed-food industry encourages this empty-calorie approach to eating. Many vending machines are filled with relatively expensive junk foods. Indeed, advertising for nonnutritious foods overwhelmingly exceeds advertising for nutritious foods. Although it is difficult to recall a television commercial for lettuce, broccoli, or green beans, we can all recite advertising slogans for our favorite soft drink, alcoholic beverage, breakfast snack, or candy bar. It takes a lot of willpower to say no to the foods in this group. Although they are of little nutritional value themselves, they can be part of a healthy diet if eaten only sparingly.

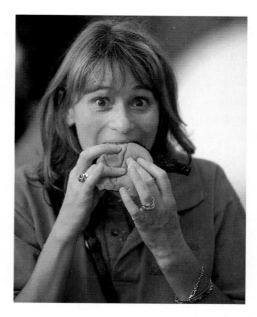

Most fast foods have a high fat density. Can you think of alternative foods you could eat on the go if you planned ahead?

Fast Foods

Fast foods are convenience foods usually prepared in walk-in or drive-through restaurants. In contrast to that of junk foods, the nutritional value of fast foods can vary considerably (see the Star Box on p. 136). As can be seen in the *calories from fat (%)* column, **fat density** remains a serious limitation of fast foods. In comparison to the recommended standard (25% to 30% of total calories from fat), 40 percent to 50 percent of the calories in fast foods are obtained from fats. A conversion some years ago from animal fat to vegetable oil for frying (to reduce cholesterol levels) did not alter the fat-dense nature of these food items. In fact, some nutritionists contend that the vegetable oil formula now used by the major fast-food companies is hydrogenated vegetable shortening and not liquid vegetable oil as advertised. If so, this shortening contributes fat in the form of trans-fatty acids, which are suspected contributors to arterial wall damage.

On the more positive side, fast-food restaurants have broadened their menus to include whole-wheat breads and rolls, salad bars, and low-fat milk products. Many provide nutritional information for consumers upon request or from well-stocked racks. The Health Action Guides on pages 138 and 143 provide suggestions for eating healthfully at fast-food restaurants and more formal restaurants.

Perhaps, however, the most regressive step taken by the fast-food industry has been the aggressive marketing of "combination" meals in which three

or four menu items are marketed for one price under a single numerical label . . . *"I'll take a number #1 with a diet drink."* Further, these already sizable meals are now being supersized at an "affordable" price for those who want maximum fat, salt, and calories in a single sitting. Of course, the driving force is profit. Extra cheese and more french fries, plus bacon to change the flavor of a meal, are inexpensive ways to raise profit margins. Earlier attempts to make fast food more health-enhancing seem to have taken a back seat to corporate earnings.

Personal Applications

• How often do you eat fast food and how likely are you to supersize your order? When having a fast-food meal, do you ever think about why you eat fast food and what alternatives you have? If so, what other options exist?

enriched the process of returning to foods some of the nutritional elements (B vitamins and iron) removed during processing.

fat density the percentage of a food's total calories that are derived from fat; above 30 percent reflects higher fat density.

Fast Food Ratings and Recommendations

Overall Ratings *Within types, listed in order of least to most fat*

Menu Item	Price	Weight	Fat TOTAL	Fat SATURATED	Calories from fat	Calories	Sodium	Flavor and texture score
CHICKEN SANDWICHES								
McDonald's Grilled Chicken Deluxe	$2.80	8 oz.	6 g.	1 g.	16%	330	970 mg.	○
Subway Roasted Chicken	3.20	9	6	1	16	348	978	◐
Wendy's Grilled Chicken	2.75	7	8	1.5	23	310	790	○
Jack in the Box Grilled Chicken Fillet	3.20	7	19	5	40	430	1070	○
Burger King BK Broiler	2.90	9	26	5	44	530	1060	○
Boston Market Boston Carver Chicken	4.30	12	32	11	38	760	1810	○
ROAST BEEF SANDWICHES								
Subway Roast Beef	2.95	8	5	1	15	303	939	○
Hardee's Big Roast Beef	2.50	6	24	9	47	460	1230	○
Arby's Giant Roast Beef	2.90	8	28	11	45	555	1561	○
CHICKEN NUGGETS/STRIPS/TENDERS *(number of pieces in order)*								
Wendy's Chicken Nuggets (5)	1.00	3	14	3	60	210	460	○
KFC Colonel's Crispy Strips (3)	2.65	3	16	3.7	54	261	658	○
McDonald's Chicken Nuggets (6)	1.90	4	17	3.5	53	290	510	○
Burger King Chicken Tenders (8)	2.50	4	22	7	57	350	940	○
Popeye's Chicken Tenderloins (5)	4.50	6	35	NA	57	550	800	◐
CHICKEN ENTREES [1]								
Boston Market (roasted)	5.25	5	17	4.5	46	330	530	○
KFC Tender Roast (roasted)	3.20	7	19	5.1	45	372	1161	○
Popeye's Louisiana Mild (fried)	3.50	5	27	NA	56	430	950	◐
KFC Original Recipe (fried)	3.25	7	34	8.5	57	540	1530	○
BURGERS								
Wendy's Single with Everything	2.10	8	20	7	43	420	920	○
Burger King Whopper Jr.	1.05	6	24	8	51	420	530	○
McDonald's Big Mac	2.20	8	28	10	48	530	880	○
Wendy's Big Bacon Classic	2.75	10	30	12	47	580	1460	◐
Hardee's The Works	2.05	8	30	12	51	530	1030	○
McDonald's Arch Deluxe with Bacon	2.65	9	34	12	50	610	1250	○
Burger King Double Cheeseburger with Bacon	2.55	8	39	18	55	640	1240	○
Jack in the Box Jumbo Jack with Cheese	1.50	9	40	14	55	650	1150	○
Burger King Big King	1.99	8	43	18	59	660	920	[2]
Burger King Whopper with Cheese	1.85	10	46	16	57	730	1350	○

[1] *Each item consists of a breast and wing; white meat*

[2] *Tested in only one city, where it scored ○.*

● Excellent   ◑ Very good   ○ Good   ◔ Fair   ● Poor

⭐ **Fast Food Ratings and Recommendations—cont'd**

Overall Ratings *Within types, listed in order of least to most fat*

Menu Item	Price	Weight	Fat TOTAL	SATURATED	Calories from fat	Calories	Sodium	Flavor and texture score
MASHED POTATOES WITH GRAVY								
KFC with Gravy	$ .95	5 oz.	6 g.	1 g.	45%	120	440 mg.	◐
Popeye's with Cajun Gravy	1.30	4	6	NA	54	100	460	○
Boston Market Homestyle and Gravy	1.55	7	9	5	41	200	560	◕
FRENCH FRIES (*size*)								
Hardee's (Large)	1.30	6	18	5	38	430	190	○
Jack in the Box (Jumbo)	1.35	4	19	5	43	400	220	○
McDonald's (Large)	1.33	5	22	4	44	450	290	◐
Wendy's (Biggie)	1.05	6	23	3.5	44	470	150	○
Burger King (Large)	1.35	5	25	7	48	470	300	○

Phytochemicals

In recent years a large group of physiologically active components thought to be able to deactivate carcinogens or function as antioxidants have been identified in a variety of fruits and vegetables. Among these are the carotenoids (from green vegetables), polyphenols (from onions and garlic), indoles (from cruciferous vegetables), and the allyl sulfides (from garlic, chives, and onions). These phytochemicals may play an important role in reducing the risk of cancer in people who consume a large quantity of foods (vegetarian or semivegetarian diets) from these two food groups.[20] So important are these several distinct classes of chemicals that they have been called "as essential as vitamins."[21] Whether the recommended minimum number of servings from the fruit and vegetable groups will be increased based on this new information remains to be seen.

Food Allergies

In the autumn of 1998 the public was reminded that foods enjoyed by the vast majority of people may be harmful to others because of their unique food allergies. For some people, peanuts, the familiar snack served on many plane flights, are such a food. At that time U.S. airlines were considering requests to provide "peanut-free" rows of seats to protect people known to be hypersensitive to peanuts and peanut-based products. Already many schools had established peanut-free tables in their lunchrooms for the same purpose.

The percentage of the population with food allergies is thought to be no greater than 1 percent to 3 percent.[22] For some members of this group, food-based hypersensitivities eventually may be serious or even life threatening. Because food allergies generally develop slowly, initial symptoms may not be fully recognized or even associated with food. Thus, burning in the mouth, a runny nose, and wheezing are disregarded and the allergy goes undiagnosed and untreated until a heightened level of sensitivity precipitates a more serious reaction.

Once a hypersensitivity to a food or group of foods is recognized, the following steps will help reduce the delay in accurately diagnosing and treating the condition:

1. On recognizing early symptoms, undertake a two-week dietary intake study, noting the occurrence of symptoms and the foods associated with each.
2. Submit food intake-related information to a physician for interpretation and subsequent evaluation.
3. Once a food-related allergy has been identified, learn the other names these foods may be called and the forms in which they may be marketed, prepared, and served.
4. Read labels carefully, realizing that ingredients in formerly well-tolerated foods may have been altered by the manufacturer.
5. When eating outside the home, ask about the ingredients and preparation of any food about which you have reservations. Make certain that fried foods have not been prepared in oils used to prepare other foods (for example, french fries prepared in oil initially used for deep-frying fish).
6. Once diagnosed, carry at all times and know how to self-inject the medications needed to

HEALTH ACTION GUIDE

Tips for Eating on the Run

- Limit deep-fried foods such as fish and chicken sandwiches and chicken nuggets, which are often higher in fat than plain burgers. If you are having fried chicken, remove some of the breading before eating.
- Order roast beef, turkey, or grilled chicken, where available, for a lower-fat alternative to most burgers.
- Choose a small order of fries with your meal rather than a large one, and request no salt. Add a small amount of salt yourself if desired. If you are ordering a deep-fat-fried sandwich or one that is made with cheese and sauce, skip the fries altogether and try a plain baked potato (add butter and salt sparingly), or a dinner roll instead of a biscuit; or, try a side salad to accompany your meal instead.
- Choose regular sandwiches instead of "double," "jumbo," "deluxe," or "ultimate." And order plain types rather than those with "the works," such as cheese, bacon, mayonnaise, and "special" sauce. Pickles, mustard, ketchup, and other condiments are high in sodium. Choose lettuce, tomatoes, and onions.
- At the salad bar, load up on fresh greens, fruits, and vegetables. Be careful of salad dressings, added toppings, and creamy salads (potato salad, macaroni salad, coleslaw). These can quickly push calories and fat to the level of other menu items or higher.
- Many fast-food items contain large amounts of sodium from salt and other ingredients. Try to balance the rest of your day's sodium choices after a fast-food meal.
- Alternate water, low-fat milk, or skim milk with a soda or a shake.
- For dessert, or a "sweet-on-the-run," choose low-fat frozen yogurt, where available.
- Remember to balance your fast-food choices with your food selections for the whole day.

InfoLinks
www.ag.uiuc.edu/~food-lab/nat

counter an allergic reaction. Prepare children to recognize their allergic symptoms and to respond appropriately.

Remember that although early allergic reactions may be subtle, they should never be disregarded.

Food Labels

Since 1973, food manufacturers have been required by the FDA to provide nutritional information (labels) on products to which one or more nutrients have been added or for which some nutritional claim has been made. Despite the presence of these labels, there was concern about whether the public could understand the labels as they appeared and whether additional information was required. Accordingly, the FDA, in consultation with individual states and public interest

HEALTH ACTION GUIDE

Making Healthful Restaurant Choices

The first thing to remember is that you are the customer, and it is permissible to make special requests. Restaurants may not be able to accommodate every request, but most will do their best to make reasonable changes or assist you in making a suitable choice. Here are some tips to keep in mind when dining out:

- Balance your choices. If you choose one dish that is higher in fat or sodium, balance the meal by choosing another that is lower.
- Plan ahead, and balance the remainder of your meals for the day.
- Resist the temptation to overload on bread (and especially the butter) that arrives when you are seated. You can request that the bread be served with the meal, and you can eat it without butter.
- Ask about preparations and ingredients. Order fish, chicken, or meat broiled without added fat. Ask if the vegetables are fresh or canned, and if they are served with sauce, butter, or cream. Whether for meat, vegetables, or salad, request sauce or dressing on the side, and use it sparingly.
- Ask about serving sizes. Many restaurants serve anywhere from 6- to 10-ounce servings of meat, fish, and poultry. Request a half-portion, or share a full one with your dining partner. Order an appetizer as your main course. These are often ample enough to serve as a meal.
- Be familiar with menu descriptions. *Breaded, fried, creamy, pan gravy, au gratin, scalloped,* and *rich* are all signals of higher-fat foods. *Poached, roasted, stir-fried,* and *steamed* are usually lower-fat selections. *Smoked, pickled, marinated, with soy sauce, mustard sauce,* and *Creole-style* usually signal high-sodium dishes.
- Read the menu completely. Pay attention to garnishes and accompaniments. Some restaurants will create an original main-course plate made up of an assortment of garnishes—like fruits or vegetables—if that appeals to you.
- Try ordering one course at a time rather than ordering all courses at the beginning and finishing everything, even though there is too much, and you're already full. Request a take-home bag and use leftovers for another meal.
- Request that salt be omitted during preparation, and then add it yourself if necessary.
- Ask for items that you do not see. Cream is usually offered with coffee, but low-fat milk or skim milk is usually available upon request. Light soups and fresh fruit are often staple items in the kitchen, even if they are not featured on the menu.
- Look for fresh fruit sorbets, poached fruits, or a simple plate of fresh seasonal fruit to top off your meal.

InfoLinks
www.navigator.tufts.edu

Learning
From Our Diversity

Eating Ethnic—The Healthy Way

If you're a traditional-age student, ask some older students what they ate when they were growing up. You're likely to hear a list that includes such quintessentially American favorites as meatloaf, mashed potatoes and gravy, chicken pot pie, hearty beef stew, and homemade fudge layer cake. If you're talking to older classmates whose heritage is largely western European, you probably won't find many exotic dishes on their childhood food list, because twenty-five or thirty years ago, ethnic food to most people of that background meant an occasional pizza or takeout chow mein. Big meals served "family style," featuring red meat and lots of side dishes—plus a rich dessert—were considered healthy, as well as essential for growing, active children. What's more, in many households, being able to put a big meal on the table was a sign of prosperity—a key consideration for anyone who suffered deprivation in the Great Depression of the 1930s.

Today, as we near the end of the twentieth century, our food focus is firmly on ethnic dishes, with their novel flavors and textures, their exotic spices, their alluringly foreign names. As we become increasingly familiar with the traditional favorites of a wide range of ethnic heritages, we incorporate them into our diet—sometimes because they're new to our jaded palates, sometimes because we want to be front and center with the current food fads, and sometimes because we read or hear that so-called ethnic foods are healthier for us than are the traditionally American dishes based on meat and potatoes.

It's true that many ethnic cuisines feature generous servings of vegetables, with just a bit of fish, meat, or poultry, plus spices, for flavor. Dishes are often cooked with heart-healthy olive oil instead of cholesterol-heavy butter, shortening, or lard. Protein is more likely to come from legumes than from meat, and dessert may be fruit with a small wedge of cheese instead of seven-layer fudge cake or rocky road ice cream. Good examples are the cuisines of China, the Mediterranean, and the Pacific Rim. Following such culinary traditions is indeed likely to provide us a far more healthful, balanced food intake than is the typically high-fat, high-calorie diet of most Americans.

But a word of caution is in order. Too many healthy ethnic favorites have crossed the ocean to America, only to be transformed into barely recognizable versions of themselves that are loaded with the sodium, sugar, and fat we seem to crave. In your favorite Italian *ristorante*, fresh vegetables and pasta are fine, but ladle on the heavy cream sauce and you're looking at a plateful of fatty calories. Ask for garlic and a little olive oil instead, and you'll save hundreds of calories and be able to savor the taste of every bite. In Chinese restaurants, watch out for big fat in little packages—crab Rangoon packed with cream cheese (Rangoon is in India, not China—doesn't that make you wonder?), butterfly shrimp (fried in batter), and potstickers (tasty but bursting with fat). Stick with fresh steamed vegetables—skip the sugary sweet and sour glaze—have a small amount of lean meat or fish, a serving of plain rice (not fried), and try eating with chopsticks. That way you'll have time to focus on what you're eating and savor some unusual textures and spices—which, after all, is what "eating ethnic" is all about!

What are your favorite ethnic foods? Why do you like them? In what ways might the ethnic foods you love have been modified to appeal to American tastes?

groups, developed new labeling regulations. Revised labels began appearing on food packages in May 1993. The newly adopted label is shown in Figure 5-3. Specific types of information contained on the new label are highlighted. Additionally, newly developed definitions for nutrition-related terms are shown in the Star Box on page 142.

Proposals for the labeling of raw foods, including fresh produce, meat, and seafood, are now being studied. Concern for consumer protection stems from recent disclosures regarding inadequate meat inspection, undercooking of hamburgers, and the risk of contaminated seafood. Currently, single-ingredient meat, fish, and poultry products are not required to have a label. In most areas of the country, however, the standard food label is being applied. Processed meat, fish, and poultry products, such as hot dogs, fish sticks, and chicken patties, must be labeled. Produce, such as vegetables and fruit, is not required to be labeled.[23]

Guidelines for Dietary Health

For decades the American public has received dietary guidelines from a variety of professional and government groups. In each case the intent has been to foster changes in dietary practices to reduce the risk of developing chronic diseases and enhance the overall nutritional health of the public. In most cases these guidelines have been generated by concerns over the actual dietary practices of the public as compared with those practices that should be followed on the basis of scientific understanding.

Although dietary guidelines of one type or another have been issued on many occasions, the *Dietary Guidelines for Americans* represent the most current and widely disseminated guidelines. The newest version appeared in 1995 as the fourth edition of *Nutrition and Your Health: Dietary Guidelines for Americans.*[24] As presently constructed, these guidelines are directed to healthy Americans two years of age and

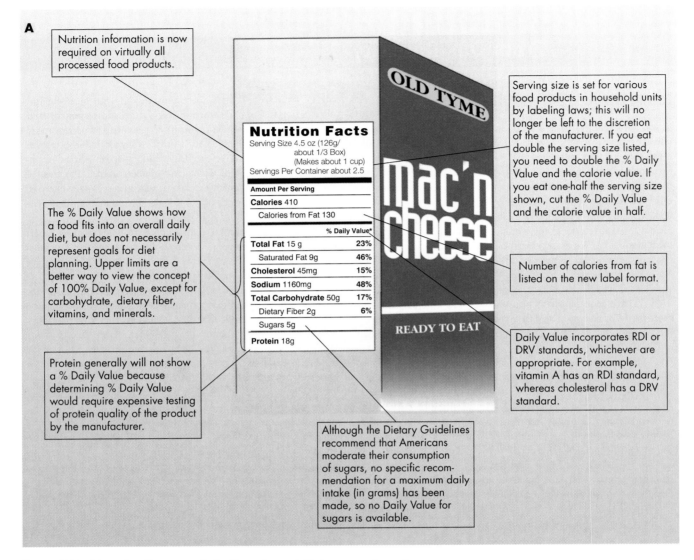

A

Nutrition information is now required on virtually all processed food products.

Serving size is set for various food products in household units by labeling laws; this will no longer be left to the discretion of the manufacturer. If you eat double the serving size listed, you need to double the % Daily Value and the calorie value. If you eat one-half the serving size shown, cut the % Daily Value and the calorie value in half.

The % Daily Value shows how a food fits into an overall daily diet, but does not necessarily represent goals for diet planning. Upper limits are a better way to view the concept of 100% Daily Value, except for carbohydrate, dietary fiber, vitamins, and minerals.

Number of calories from fat is listed on the new label format.

Protein generally will not show a % Daily Value because determining % Daily Value would require expensive testing of protein quality of the product by the manufacturer.

Daily Value incorporates RDI or DRV standards, whichever are appropriate. For example, vitamin A has an RDI standard, whereas cholesterol has a DRV standard.

Although the Dietary Guidelines recommend that Americans moderate their consumption of sugars, no specific recommendation for a maximum daily intake (in grams) has been made, so no Daily Value for sugars is available.

Nutrition Facts
Serving Size 4.5 oz (126g/ about 1/3 Box) (Makes about 1 cup)
Servings Per Container about 2.5

Amount Per Serving

Calories 410

Calories from Fat 130

	% Daily Value*
Total Fat 15 g	23%
Saturated Fat 9g	46%
Cholesterol 45mg	15%
Sodium 1160mg	48%
Total Carbohydrate 50g	17%
Dietary Fiber 2g	6%
Sugars 5g	
Protein 18g	

OLD TYME
mac'n cheese
READY TO EAT

Figure 5-3 Nutrition Facts panel. **A,** Top of panel; **B,** bottom of panel.

older and to health professionals who can influence the public's dietary practices. Information contained within these guidelines was extracted from a variety of sources, including the Surgeon General's Report on Nutrition and Health. The following discussion explains the specific guidelines.

Eat a variety of foods. At the very heart of these dietary guidelines, and virtually all others, is the contention that a wide variety of food from each food group (see p. 131) is necessary for people to achieve a truly balanced diet. When choices are limited to only a few selections from within each food group because of preference or traditional practice, the total representation of nutrients within each group can be lost, since no single selection is nutritionally complete.

Balance the food you eat with physical activity—maintain or improve your weight. The concept of energy balance (see Chapters 4 and 6), in which caloric intake is expended through regular physical activity rather than being placed into long-term storage as adipose tissue, is central to weight management. Additionally, in the absence of this balance, excessive weight gain will increase the likelihood of developing many of the chronic conditions that are detrimental to the health of middle-age and older adults.

Choose a diet with plenty of grain products, vegetables, and fruits. Complex carbohydrates, fiber, vitamins, and an array of minerals are critically important for sound nutritional health. Grain products, vegetables, and fruits are excellent sources of these important types of nutrients. These foods are also sources of the plant proteins whose consumption provides the body with needed amino acids.

Choose a diet low in fat, saturated fat, and cholesterol. Driven by several decades of research into the relationship of dietary fat, particularly saturated fat and cholesterol, to cardiovascular disease, this

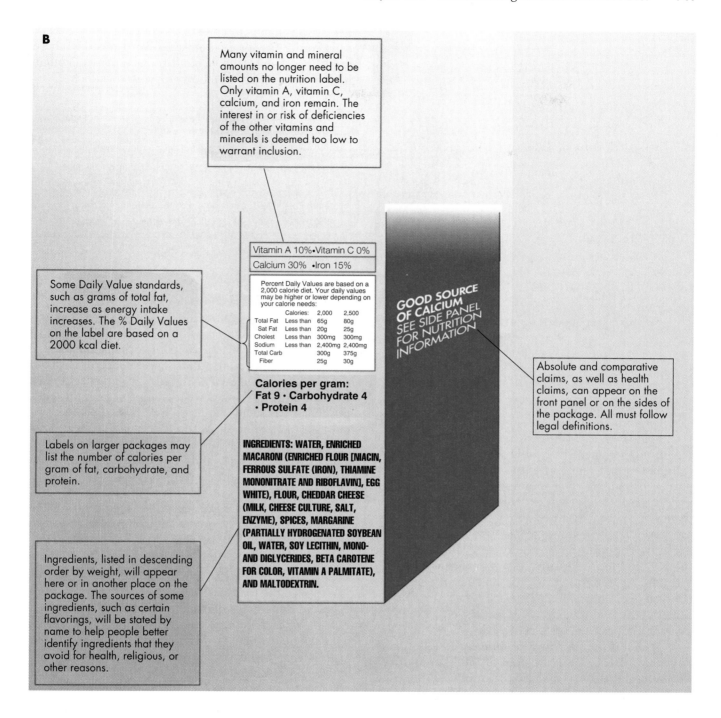

B

Many vitamin and mineral amounts no longer need to be listed on the nutrition label. Only vitamin A, vitamin C, calcium, and iron remain. The interest in or risk of deficiencies of the other vitamins and minerals is deemed too low to warrant inclusion.

Some Daily Value standards, such as grams of total fat, increase as energy intake increases. The % Daily Values on the label are based on a 2000 kcal diet.

| Vitamin A 10% •Vitamin C 0% |
| Calcium 30% •Iron 15% |

Percent Daily Values are based on a 2,000 calorie diet. Your daily values may be higher or lower depending on your calorie needs:		
	Calories: 2,000	2,500
Total Fat Less than	65g	80g
Sat Fat Less than	20g	25g
Cholest Less than	300mg	300mg
Sodium Less than	2,400mg	2,400mg
Total Carb	300g	375g
Fiber	25g	30g

Calories per gram:
Fat 9 · Carbohydrate 4
· Protein 4

Labels on larger packages may list the number of calories per gram of fat, carbohydrate, and protein.

INGREDIENTS: WATER, ENRICHED MACARONI (ENRICHED FLOUR [NIACIN, FERROUS SULFATE (IRON), THIAMINE MONONITRATE AND RIBOFLAVIN], EGG WHITE), FLOUR, CHEDDAR CHEESE (MILK, CHEESE CULTURE, SALT, ENZYME), SPICES, MARGARINE (PARTIALLY HYDROGENATED SOYBEAN OIL, WATER, SOY LECITHIN, MONO- AND DIGLYCERIDES, BETA CAROTENE FOR COLOR, VITAMIN A PALMITATE), AND MALTODEXTRIN.

Ingredients, listed in descending order by weight, will appear here or in another place on the package. The sources of some ingredients, such as certain flavorings, will be stated by name to help people better identify ingredients that they avoid for health, religious, or other reasons.

GOOD SOURCE OF CALCIUM SEE SIDE PANEL FOR NUTRITION INFORMATION

Absolute and comparative claims, as well as health claims, can appear on the front panel or on the sides of the package. All must follow legal definitions.

recommendation is of critical importance. As reported elsewhere in the chapter, careful monitoring of meat consumption and, particularly, following a vegetarian diet are excellent approaches to meeting this guideline.

Choose a diet moderate in sugars. Sugars are simple carbohydrates that provide the body with a readily available supply of calories, which provide energy to our working muscles. Unfortunately, however, they represent **empty calories** in that they carry little in the way of other important nutrients. Additionally, when consumed excessively, they can contribute to

energy imbalance, leading to weight gain. Alcoholic beverages and snack foods are principal sources of sugars and their empty calories for many college students. In contrast, the complex carbohydrates obtained by eating vegetables, fruits, and cereal grains are eventual sugar sources for the body and far more healthful than those derived directly from dietary sugars.

empty calories   calories obtained from foods that lack most other important nutrients.

★ **Definitions of Nutrition-Related Claims**

- *Free:* an amount that is "nutritionally trivial" and unlikely to have a physiological consequence
- *Calorie free:* fewer than 5 calories a serving
- *Sugar free:* less than 0.5 grams per serving
- *Sodium free* and *salt free:* less than 5 milligrams of sodium per serving
- *Fat free:* less than 0.5 grams of fat per serving, providing that it has no added fat or oil ingredient
- *Low fat:* 3 grams or less of fat per serving per 100 grams of the food
- *Low in saturated fat:* may be used to describe a food that contains 1 gram or less of saturated fat per serving and not more than 15 percent calories from saturated fat
- *Cholesterol free:* less than 2 milligrams of cholesterol per serving and 2 grams or less saturated fat per serving
- *Low in cholesterol:* 20 milligrams or less per serving and per 100 grams of food and 2 grams or less of saturated fat per serving

Choose a diet moderate in salt and sodium. In the 10 to 15 percent of people who possess a genetically based salt sensitivity, the dietary intake of salt (our principal source of sodium) should be monitored very carefully to prevent excessive fluid accumulation in the body leading to elevated blood pressure. For most people, however, normal kidney function clears excessive sodium from the body, thus minimizing the increase in blood pressure seen in salt-sensitive individuals. Although nutritionists generally see little concern over "normal" dietary salt intake for nonsalt-sensitive people, recommendations such as that appearing above continue to be made.

If you drink alcoholic beverages, do so in moderation. In light of the fact that alcohol barely qualifies as food (except as a source of empty calories), this dietary recommendation may seem out of place. As will be noted in Chapter 8, today moderation is defined as one drink for the average American woman and no more than two for her male counterpart. Unfortunately, for those who abuse it, perhaps no other "food" carries the same potential for both short-term and long-term health problems.

In addition to the guidelines just discussed, the most recent report also contains information for specific groups based on age, gender, and other factors. This appears in the Health Action Guide on page 143. Table 5-8 shows how healthful dietary changes can lower your risk of developing certain major diseases.

Whether the newest Dietary Guidelines for Americans will be more fully implemented than their pre-

decessors remains to be seen. Regardless, most Americans could move much closer toward meeting these guidelines. The Health Action Guide on page 143 offers helpful suggestions for modifying your own diet.

Personal Applications

- You were probably first taught a food group-based plan for healthy nutrition in elementary school, and again in middle school and high school. Do you feel comfortable with your ability to follow such a plan? If your current diet is unbalanced, when and how will you attempt to improve it?

Recommended Dietary Adjustments

Nutritionists are concerned about some of the dietary practices among young adults. These concerns exist because professionals realize that dietary practices established during the college years may continue throughout life. Of particular concern are those diets that are both unbalanced and lack the variety of food selections emphasized throughout this chapter, including many weight-reduction diets and those diets with an overreliance on *fast foods* and vending machine (snack) foods. The recommendations that follow are made with full knowledge that the demands of life, including college life, will continue to force some compromises in the adoption of healthful dietary patterns.

Additional Milk Consumption

Because of the tendency for older women to develop a loss in bone mass density, a condition called *osteoporosis,* it is recommended that adult women increase their dairy product intake to achieve the equivalent of four servings per day. This additional intake provides needed calcium, which may reduce the incidence of hip, wrist, and vertebral fractures in the elderly adult years. Excessive caloric and fat intake can be controlled by using skim milk or low-fat yogurt and by decreasing the daily intake of all fats. For people who do not like dairy products or who are allergic to milk, calcium supplements are an alternative. Of course, the other nutritional benefits from the milk group cannot be obtained through calcium supplements. (Osteoporosis is discussed further in Chapter 4.)

Additional Protein-Rich Sources

Premenopausal women often need to replace iron lost during menstruation. One way to do so is to eat three ounces of red meat three or four times per week. Iron obtained from red meat (called *heme iron*) is in its most *biologically available* form. A general lowering of fat intake will allow this small inclusion of red meat to be undertaken without increasing overall fat intake or adding calories.

Another way to maintain adequate iron stores is to include appropriate vegetables, fruits, and grain products in the diet. Some excellent vegetable sources of iron are lettuce, endive, beets, tomatoes, spinach, green peas, green beans, legumes, and broccoli. Good fruit sources of iron are apricots, cantaloupe, dates, prunes, and raisins. Enriched or whole-grain breads and breakfast cereals are also good iron sources. Milk products contain little iron. Vegetarians and others who eat little or no red meat should pay particular attention to their iron intake.

Iron supplements may help provide needed iron. However, it is a good idea to consult a physician before taking iron supplements. Supplements alone do not provide the additional benefits found in the protein-rich food group, and they may cause severe

HEALTH ACTION GUIDE

Dietary Recommendations

Issues for Most People: Your nutritional health could probably be enhanced if you implement the practices described here.

Fats and cholesterol: Reduce consumption of fat (especially saturated fat) and cholesterol. Choose foods relatively low in these substances, such as vegetables, fruits, whole-grain foods, fish, poultry, lean meats, and low-fat dairy products. Use food preparation methods that add little or no fat.

Energy and weight control: Achieve and maintain a desirable body weight. To do so, choose a dietary pattern in which energy (caloric) intake is consistent with energy expenditure. To reduce energy intake, limit consumption of foods relatively high in calories, fats, and sugars and minimize alcohol consumption. Increase energy expenditure through regular and sustained physical activity.

Complex carbohydrates and fiber: Increase consumption of whole-grain foods and cereal products, vegetables (including dried beans and peas), and fruits.

Sodium: Reduce intake of sodium by choosing foods relatively low in sodium and limiting the amount of salt added in food preparation and at the table.

Alcohol: To reduce the risk of chronic disease, drink alcohol only in moderation (no more than two drinks a day), if at all. Avoid drinking any alcohol before or while driving, operating machinery, taking medications, or engaging in any other activity requiring sound judgment. Avoid drinking alcohol while pregnant.

Issues for Some People: If your nutritional needs fall into one of the groups listed, you should implement the following recommendations.

Fluoride: Community water systems should contain fluoride at optimal levels for prevention of tooth decay. If such water is not available, use other appropriate sources of fluoride.

Sugars: Those who are particularly vulnerable to dental caries (cavities), especially children, should limit their consumption and frequency of use of foods high in sugars.

Calcium: Adolescent girls and adult women should increase consumption of foods high in calcium, including low-fat dairy products.

Iron: Children, adolescents, and women of childbearing age should be sure to consume foods that are good sources of iron, such as lean red meats, fish, certain beans, and iron-enriched cereals and whole grain products. This issue is of special concern for low-income families.

InfoLinks
www.nal.usda.gov/fnic/Dietary/dgreport.html

HEALTH ACTION GUIDE

Making Healthful Food Choices

It is very likely that you can improve your dietary health and reduce the risk of developing heart disease and cancer by implementing the following practices.

Eat More High-Fiber Foods
• Choose dried beans, peas, and lentils more often.
• Eat whole-grain breads, cereals, and crackers.
• Eat more vegetables—raw and cooked.
• Eat whole fruit in place of drinking fruit juice.
• Try other high-fiber foods, such as oat bran, barley, brown rice, or wild rice.

Eat Less Sugar
• Avoid regular soft drinks. One 12-ounce can has nine teaspoons of sugar!
• Avoid eating table sugar, honey, syrup, jam, jelly, candy, sweet rolls, fruit canned in syrup, regular gelatin desserts, cake with icing, pie, or other sweets.
• Choose fresh fruit or fruit canned in natural juice or water.
• If desired, use sweeteners that don't have any calories, such as saccharin or aspartame, instead of sugar.

Use Less Salt
• Reduce the amount of salt you use in cooking.
• Avoid adding salt to food at the table.
• Eat fewer high-salt foods, such as canned soups, ham, sauerkraut, hot dogs, pickles, and foods that taste salty.
• Eat fewer convenience and fast foods.

Eat Less Fat
• Eat smaller servings of meat. Eat fish, poultry, or vegetarian entrees more often.
• Choose only lean cuts of red meat.
• Prepare all meats by roasting, baking, or broiling. Trim off all fat. Limit addition of sauces or gravy. Remove skin from poultry.
• Avoid fried foods. Avoid adding fat when cooking.
• Eat fewer high-fat foods, such as cold cuts, bacon, sausage, hot dogs, butter, margarine, nuts, salad dressing, lard, and solid shortening.
• Drink skim or low-fat milk.
• Eat less ice cream, cheese, sour cream, cream, whole milk, and other high-fat dairy products.

InfoLinks
www.nal.usda.gov/fnic

Table 5-8   Recommended Dietary Changes to Reduce the Risk of Diseases and Their Complications

Change in Diet	Reduce Fats	Control Calories	Increase Starch* and Fiber	Reduce Sodium	Control Alcohol
Reduce risk of:					
Heart disease	✓	✓		✓	
Cancer	✓	✓	✓		✓
Stroke	✓	✓		✓	✓
Diabetes	✓	✓	✓		
Gastrointestinal disease†	✓	✓	✓		✓

*Starch refers to complex carbohydrates provided by fruits, vegetables, and whole-grain products.
†Primarily gallbladder disease (fat), diverticular disease (fiber), and cirrhosis (alcohol).

digestive complications. In addition, iron supplements must be stored carefully because they are a leading cause of death from accidental poisoning in young children.

Additional Vitamins C and A

Foods chosen from the fruit and vegetable groups on a regular basis should include those that are good sources of vitamins C and A. The inclusion of additional vitamin C in the diet will assist in the absorption of iron from bread, cereal, and eggs. For women of reproductive age, iron stores are an important consideration, since iron is a component of the hemoglobin found in red blood cells that are lost during menstruation.

In addition to the recommendation concerning vitamin C, larger servings of fruits and vegetables, particularly the dark green vegetables, are recommended. By increasing intake in this food group, desirable increases in **folacin** and vitamin A can be achieved. Folacin's role in intrauterine development and in preventing **macrocytic anemia** makes its increased presence in the diet of critical importance. High levels of carotenes found in dark green vegetables aid in the production of vitamin A, a necessary fat-soluble vitamin.

Additional Grain Product Consumption

The *Dietary Guidelines for Americans* recommend that 60 percent of our total calories come from carbohydrates. Increasing the quantity of whole-grain breads and cereals in the diet can make sure this recommendation is met. It should be noted, however, that cold cereal represents the principal source of complex carbohydrates in the diets of today's children. Caregivers therefore should include fruit when giving children a bowl of cereal and milk.

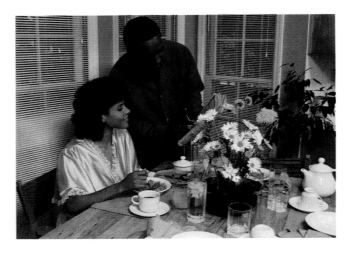

Eating more whole-grain cereals and breads can help you increase your carbohydrate and fiber intake.

Moderate Alcohol Consumption

Although moderation in alcohol consumption (see page 142) is not incompatible with good nutrition, too many Americans consume it in large amounts. Alcohol provides a significant amount of empty calories. This can be an important concern for alcohol users who wish to control their weight. Also, the overuse of alcohol can rob your body of its ability to absorb other nutrients successfully, may prevent you from consuming a healthy diet, and is associated with a wide variety of diseases, including cancer and liver complications. From a health standpoint, moderation in the use of alcohol makes a lot of sense.

Nutrient Density

For many college students, the consideration of nutrient density may prompt certain dietary adjustments. The *nutrient density* of a food item relates to its ability to

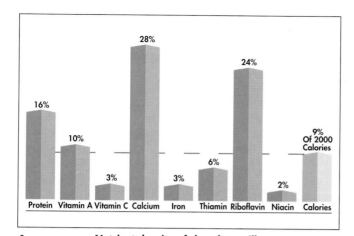

A   **Nutrient density of chocolate milk**

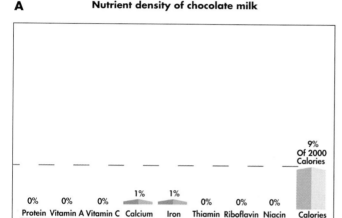

B   **Nutrient density of soda**

Figure 5-4 A comparison of the nutrient density of chocolate milk with that of soda. **A,** The bars that represent protein, vitamin A, calcium, and riboflavin are all taller than the calorie bar, showing that chocolate milk is nutrient dense for these nutrients. **B,** All of the nutrient bars are shorter than the calorie bar, illustrating that soda has a low nutrient density relative to the number of calories it supplies.

supply proportionally more of the RDA (for select vitamins and minerals) than it does daily calorie requirements. Foods with a high nutrient density are better choices than those that supply only empty calories. For example, a bag of potato chips or a bottle of beer has a much lower nutrient density than either a bean burrito or a slice of vegetable pizza. Choosing to eat foods with high nutrient density is especially important for people who are trying to limit caloric intake, either for weight management or to counter the decreased caloric needs of older adulthood. Figure 5-4 compares the nutrient density of chocolate milk to that of soda.

Vegetarian Diets

Vegetarian diets can be strongly recommended, particularly for people who are willing to be "good students"

of nutrition. In the sections that follow, various forms of vegetarianism will be addressed. Read carefully the Topics for Today article on pages 152 to 154, which describes **semivegetarianism,** a diet in which meat consumption is significantly reduced but not eliminated, and discusses the health benefits of vegetarianism in general. Figure 5-5 shows a vegetarian food guide pyramid modeled after the USDA Food Guide Pyramid.

A *vegetarian diet* relies on plant sources for most of the nutrients the body needs. Vegetarian diets encompass a continuum from diets that allow some animal sources of nutrients to those that not only exclude animal sources but also are restrictive even in terms of the plant sources of nutrients permitted. We will briefly describe three vegetarian diets, beginning with the least restrictive in terms of food sources.

Ovolactovegetarian Diet

Depending on the particular pattern of consuming eggs (*ovo*) and milk (*lacto*) or using one but not the other, ovolactovegetarianism can be an extremely sound approach to healthful eating during the entire course of the adult years. An **ovolactovegetarian diet** provides the body with the essential amino acids while limiting the high intake of fats seen in more conventional diets. The exclusion of meat as a protein source lowers the total fat intake, while the consumption of milk or eggs allows for an adequate amount of saturated fat to remain in the diet. The consistent use of vegetable products as the primary source of nutrients supports the current dietary recommendations for an increase in overall carbohydrates, an increase in complex carbohydrates, and an increase in fiber.

Meatlike products composed of textured vegetable protein are available in supermarkets. Nonmeat bacon strips, hamburger and chicken patties, and link sausage can be used by people who want to restrict their meat intake but still want a meatlike product. Soybeans are a primary source of this textured vegetable protein.

folacin (foe la sin)   folic acid; a vitamin of the B-complex group; used in the treatment of nutritional anemia.

macrocytic anemia (mac roe sit ick uh nee mee a)   form of anemia in which large red blood cells predominate, but in which total red blood cell count is depressed.

semivegetarianism   a diet that significantly reduces but does not eliminate meat consumption and allows consumption of dairy products and eggs.

ovolactovegetarian diet (oh voe lack toe veg a ter ee in)   a diet that excludes all meat but does allow the consumption of eggs and dairy products.

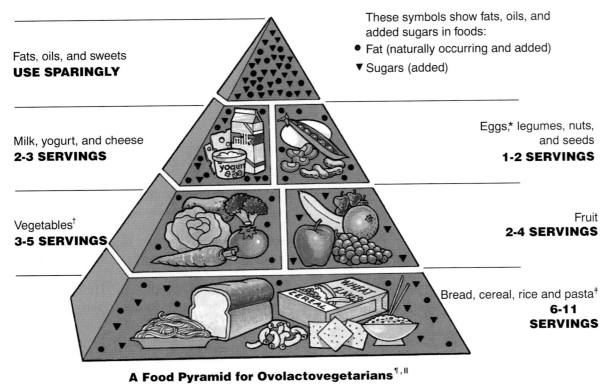

These symbols show fats, oils, and added sugars in foods:

● Fat (naturally occurring and added)

▼ Sugars (added)

Fats, oils, and sweets
USE SPARINGLY

Milk, yogurt, and cheese
2-3 SERVINGS

Eggs;* legumes, nuts, and seeds
1-2 SERVINGS

Vegetables†
3-5 SERVINGS

Fruit
2-4 SERVINGS

Bread, cereal, rice and pasta†
6-11 SERVINGS

A Food Pyramid for Ovolactovegetarians¶, ‖

*Lactovegetarians can omit eggs from this pyramid.

† Include one dark green or leafy variety daily.

‡ One serving of a vitamin- and mineral-enriched cereal is recommended.

¶ Contains about 75g of protein and 1650 calories.

‖ Base serving sizes on those listed for the Food Guide Pyramid.

Figure 5-5   A food pyramid for vegetarians.

Two relatively minor concerns associated with some ovolactovegetarian diets are those of zinc deficiency and the overuse of a wide variety of **food supplements.** Because of zinc's role in the body's use of iron, ovolactovegetarians may need to take this mineral in supplement form. However, the general use of large quantities of food supplements may be harmful or, at best, unnecessary.

Lactovegetarian and Ovovegetarian Diets

People who include dairy products in their diet but no other animal products, such as eggs and meat, are *lactovegetarians*. As with the ovolactovegetarian diet, little risk is associated with this dietary pattern. In contrast, people who exclude dairy products such as milk and cheese, yet consume eggs, are *ovovegetarians*. Both diets carry the advantages of ovolactovegetarianism but are a bit more demanding because of the elimination of one of the two nonmeat sources of animal products.

Vegan Vegetarian Diet

A **vegan vegetarian diet** is one in which not only meat but also other animal products, such as milk,

cheese, and eggs, are removed from the diet. When compared with the ovolactovegetarian diet, the vegan diet requires a higher level of nutritional understanding to avoid nutritional inadequacies.

One potential difficulty is that of obtaining all of the essential amino acids. Since a single plant source does not contain all the essential amino acids, the vegan must learn to consistently employ a complementary diet. By carefully combining various grains, seeds, and legumes, amino acid deficiency can be prevented.

In addition to the potential amino acid deficiency, the vegan could have some difficulty in maintaining the necessary intake of vitamin B_{12}. Possible ramifications of inadequate B_{12} intake include depression, anemia, back pain, and menstrual irregularity. Vegans often have difficulty maintaining adequate intakes of iron, zinc, and calcium.[1] Calcium intake must be monitored closely by the vegan. In addition, vitamin D deficiencies can occur. Supplements and daily exposure to sunshine will aid in maintaining adequate levels of this vitamin.

A final area of potential difficulty for the vegan is that of an insufficient caloric intake because of the satiation resulting from the voluminous nature of the diet. Early satiation caused by a large amount of fiber may lower carbohydrate intake to the point that protein stores (muscle mass) are used for energy.

When practiced knowledgeably, vegan vegetarianism is sound for virtually all people, including pregnant and **lactating** women, infants and children, non-frail older adults, and athletes. Of course, people in each of these groups must be sure their particular life cycle/lifestyle-related nutritional needs are met by vegan vegetarianism. However, because of the limitations discussed above, some nutritionists do not recommend the vegan vegetarian diet, even for adults. They suggest that unless followed for reasons closely related to ecological, philosophical, or animal rights beliefs, the total exclusion of animal products seems to accomplish little from a nutritional point of view that cannot be accomplished through ovolactovegetarianism or semivegetarianism.

Personal Applications

• If you have considered or tried a vegetarian diet, what was your primary reason for doing so? Many nutritionists view the semivegetarian diet as very sensible and more sustainable than other forms of vegetarianism. Do you agree? Could you move to semivegetarianism at this point in your life?

High-Risk Dietary Practices

Whereas the health benefits and relatively low risks of vegetarianism make those diets attractive, the diets in the following discussion hold the potential for serious health risks.

Unbalanced and Fad Diets

Nutritionists are particularly concerned about collegiate dietary patterns that are associated with an **unbalanced diet** to achieve or maintain weight loss. An unbalanced diet might consist of a single food (like pizza) or food selections from just one or two of the five main food groups. Whether you eat only grapefruit, bananas, avocados, or some other "special" foods, the point remains the same: A diet lacking variety and balance generally cannot provide you with all of the needed nutrients.

Nutritionists continue to inform us that college students, for some reason, tend to adopt these unbalanced diets more frequently than other adults. Noticing the poor dietary practices of a friend or roommate should prompt you to look carefully at your own dietary practices (see the Personal Assessment on p. 133). You should be certain that your own dietary pattern is not more unbalanced than you might have suspected.

Nutrition and the Older Adult

Nutritional needs change as adults age. Age-related alterations to the structure and function of the body are primarily responsible for this. Included among the changes that alter nutritional requirements and practices are changes in the teeth, salivary glands, taste buds, oral muscles, gastric acid production, and peristaltic action (movement of food through the gastrointestinal tract).[25] Older adults can find food less tasteful and harder to chew. Chronic constipation resulting from changes in gastrointestinal tract function can also decrease interest in eating.

The progressive lowering of the body's basal metabolism is another factor that eventually influences dietary patterns of older adults.[25] As energy requirements fall, the body gradually senses the need for less food. This gradual recognition of lower energy needs results in a lessened food intake and loss of appetite in many elderly people. Because of this decreased need for calories, nutrient density—the nutritional value of a food relative to the number of calories supplied—is an important factor for the elderly (see pp. 144–145).

Besides the physiological factors that influence dietary patterns among the elderly, several psychosocial factors alter the role of food in the lives of many older adults. Social isolation, depression, chronic alcohol consumption, loss of income, transportation limitations, and housing restrictions are factors in lifestyle patterns that can alter the ease and enjoyment associated with the preparation and consumption of food.[26]

International Nutritional Concerns

Whereas nutritional concerns in this country are centered on overnutrition, including fat density and excessive caloric intake, the main concern in many areas of the world is the limited quantity and quality of food. Reasons for these problems are many, including the limitations imposed by weather, the availability of arable land, religious practices, political unrest, war,

---

food supplements nutrients taken in addition to those obtained through the diet; includes powdered protein, vitamins, and mineral extracts.

vegan vegetarian diet (**vee** gun *or* **vay** gun) a vegetarian diet that excludes the consumption of all animal products, including eggs and dairy products.

lactating breastfeeding or nursing.

unbalanced diet a diet lacking adequate representation from each of the food groups.

Real Life
Real choices

- What is serum cholesterol? How can Vincent Martinelli modify his diet to lower his serum cholesterol level while still enjoying some tasty Italian specialties?
- What are some dietary sources of sodium? How can Angela Martinelli reduce her sodium intake?
- Can you design a nutritious, healthy meal featuring a popular Italian specialty like pizza or pasta?

And Now, Your Choices . . .
- What are your favorite specialty or ethnic foods? Do you consider them healthy or unhealthy? Why?
- How do you think your eating habits would change if you worked in a deli, bakery, or ice cream shop?

---

social infrastructure, and material and technical shortages. Underlying nearly all of these factors, however, is unabated population growth.

To increase the availability of food to the 82 countries and 840 million people[27] whose demand for food outweighs their ability to produce it, a number of steps have been suggested, including the following:

Increase the yield of land currently under cultivation.

Increase the amount of land under cultivation.

Increase animal production on land not suitable for cultivation.

Use water (seas, lakes, and ponds) more efficiently for the production of food.

Develop unconventional foods through the application of technology.

Improve nutritional practices through education.

In these countries, little progress is being made despite impressive technological breakthroughs in agriculture and food technology (such as "miracle" rice, disease-resistant high-yield corn, and soybean-enhanced infant foods), the efforts of governmental programs, and the support of the Food and Agricultural Organization of the United Nations and the USDA. In developing countries, where fertility rates are two to four times higher than those of the United States, annual food production would have to increase between 2.7 percent and 3.9 percent. If population growth and food production are not altered in these countries, basic needs will continue to be unmet.

As We Go To PRESS

Each year in this country we see a distressing increase in the incidence of foodborne infections. During the first eight months of 1998, 90 outbreaks of foodborne disease involving 8,700 people were reported to the FDA. Among these were *Cyclospora* infections from contaminated pesto sold in Washington, D.C., *E. coli* infections in Virginia traced to contaminated alfalfa sprouts, and cholera contracted by people who ate raw shrimp in Arizona. So alarming is the problem that some legislators recommend creating a "food czar" to oversee the nation's food supply, both domestic production and processing and the growing influx of foods from outside the United States. Additionally, calls for the widespread use of food irradiation are being debated.

Because of risks associated with foods contaminated with pathogenic microorganisms or their toxins, appropriate food preparation at home can do much to minimize the risk. Carefully following the recommendations listed (on the right) can significantly reduce the incidence of foodborne infections in the home.

1. Do not prepare food while ill or when you have cuts or sores on your hands.
2. Prepare working area by thoroughly cleaning surfaces with which food will have contact (countertops, etc.).
3. Wash hands thoroughly before beginning food preparation, and during the course of preparation whenever hands contact items or surfaces that have not been thoroughly cleaned. (Wash hands vigorously in hot running water, using soap, for 20 seconds or more.)
4. Wash hands properly after using the bathroom, touching pets, changing diapers, or touching your own hair or clothing.
5. Do not wipe or dry hands on apron or clothing.
6. Wash cuttingboards, knives, and other utensils after preparing each food item.
7. Before storing cuttingboards, knives, and other utensils, wash them, sanitize with a disinfectant, and allow to air dry.

8. When tasting food during preparation, cut or ladle a small amount into a separate dish or cup, thoroughly washing dish and utensil after each use.
9. Wipe spills on surfaces (including floors) immediately.
10. Wash hands thoroughly after disposing of trash.

In addition to these steps, it is important to maintain foods at appropriate temperatures during preparation, storage, and consumption.

Modified from: *Top Ten Tips to "Keep It Clean"—The First Step to Food Safety,* Food Safety Month, International Food Safety Council, September 1998.

Summary

- Carbohydrates, fats, and protein supply the body with calories.
- The molecular complexity of carbohydrates differs, with sugars being the least complex and starches the most complex.
- Fat plays important roles in nutritional health beyond serving as the body's primary site for the storage of excess calories.
- Dietary fats can be classified on the basis of their molecular makeup. Alteration of a fat's chemical bonding through hydrogenation may result in the formation of potentially harmful trans-fatty acids.
- Concern over tropical oils reflects a specific aspect of the role of dietary fats in sound nutrition.
- Cholesterol-free and low-fat foods play important roles in today's dietary practices.
- Fat-free foods made with Olestra (Olean) contain considerably fewer calories than their fat-containing counterparts, but they may be poorly tolerated by some people.
- Protein supplies the body with amino acids that subsequently provide the material needed by the body to construct its own protein.
- Protein of plant origin is incomplete protein in that any single source lacks one or more of the essential amino acids. Protein from animal sources is complete protein; however, it contributes to higher levels of saturated fat in the diet.
- Vitamins serve as catalysts for the body and are found in either water-soluble or fat-soluble forms.
- Minerals are incorporated into various tissues of the body and also participate in regulatory functions within the body.
- Adequate water and fluids are required by the body on a daily basis and are obtained from a variety of food sources, including beverages.
- Fiber is undigestible plant material and can be found in two forms, water-soluble and water-insoluble. Soluble fiber contributes to the removal of cholesterol from the blood, while insoluble fiber contributes to stool formation.
- Most nutrients are absorbed in the first 18 inches of the small intestine, at which point they enter into the venous blood for eventual distribution throughout the body.
- Six food groups are currently identified, although only five have been assigned a recommendation regarding number of daily servings. Each food group supplies specific nutrients to the diet.
- To follow a food group-based dietary plan, people must be able to classify each food, know the number of recommended servings from each food group, and recognize the amount of food that constitutes a single serving.
- For a well-balanced diet, a variety of foods from each group must be eaten, rather than relying on a single food or a few favorites.
- Fast foods should play a limited role in daily food intake because of their high fat density, as well as their high levels of sugar and sodium.
- Phytochemicals are food-based chemical compounds thought to give the body some protection against harmful chemical reactions, such as the formation of free radicals.
- Although affecting only a small percentage of the population, food allergies may be serious.
- New food labels provide considerably more information for the consumer than did labels used previously.
- The *Dietary Guidelines for Americans* focus on the role of fat, saturated fat, sugar, starch, sodium, alcohol, and weight management in health and disease.
- Additional dietary recommendations can be made for specific groups of people, such as increased calcium and red meat consumption for younger adult women.
- Ovolactovegetarian, lactovegetarian, vegan vegetarian, and semivegetarian diets represent different forms of vegetarianism.
- Older adults must consider the nutrient density of a particular food item because they need adequate levels of nutrients but require relatively fewer calories than young adults.
- A variety of factors contribute to malnourishment in many areas of the world.
- Improved food technology may not make it possible to feed the world's population in the absence of greater efforts to control population growth.

Review Questions

1. What unique contribution do carbohydrates, fats, and protein make to overall nutrition that is not made by the remaining nutrients?
2. Of the two forms of carbohydrate, which form has the most complex molecular structure and which has the simplest?
3. What roles does fat tissue play in nutritional health besides serving as the body's primary storage site for excess calories?
4. Of the three forms of fat, which is most closely associated with foods of animal origin?
5. What is the concern being voiced over the role of tropical oils and omega-3 fatty acids in sound dietary practices?
6. What large category of foods are by their very nature cholesterol-free? How might the consumption of low-fat foods serve as the basis of a nutritional problem?
7. What concerns do some nutrition experts have about the use of fat-replacement technology, such as Olestra?
8. What is the principal role of protein in the body?
9. What are the important nutritional differences between plant and animal sources of protein? Which food source supplies complete protein and which supplies incomplete protein?
10. Which vitamins are water soluble and which are fat soluble? What is the most current perception regarding the need for vitamin supplementation?
11. What roles do minerals play in the body? What is a trace element?
12. What is the current recommendation regarding daily fluid intake? Why is water considered an essential nutrient?
13. What are the two principal forms of fiber, and how does each of them contribute to health?
14. In terms of the entire length of the digestive tract, from which region are most nutrients absorbed into the circulatory system?
15. Identify each of the five food groups. What makes up the additional sixth group? Explain the nutritional benefit of each food group and the recommended daily adult serving minimums.
16. What must people know to consistently use a food group-based approach to sound nutrition? Why is "variety" an important concept underlying a food group-based approach to sound nutrition?
17. What is the principal concern regarding excessive fast-food consumption? How can food selection at a fast-food restaurant be made nutritionally healthier?
18. In the most general sense, what are phytochemicals and in which foods are they most abundant?
19. How prevalent are food allergies within the total population?
20. What are the specific areas of nutritional concern addressed by the current *Dietary Guidelines for Americans?*
21. Identify some general modifications recommended in the diets of young adults and the reasoning behind each.
22. Define a vegetarian diet. Explain the difference between an ovolactovegetarian, lactovegetarian, vegan vegetarian, and semivegetarian diet. Which one poses more potential nutritional problems? In what ways?
23. What is nutrient density, and how does it relate to the aging process?
24. What factors contribute to the shortages of food seen in many areas of the world? What one factor alone may offset all progress made in improving world food supply through improved food-growing technology?

References

1. Whitney EN, Cataldo CB, Rolfes SR. *Understanding normal and clinical nutrition.* 5th ed. Belmont, CA: West/Wadsworth, 1997.
2. Wardlaw GM. *Contemporary nutrition: issues and insights.* 3rd ed. St. Louis: Mosby, 1997.
3. Uhari M, Kontiokari T, Niemela M. A novel use of xylitol sugar in preventing acute otitis media. *Pediatrics* 1998 Oct; 102(4 Part 1):879–84.
4. U.S. Department of Health and Human Services. *Report of the expert panel on population strategies for blood cholesterol reduction.* NIH Pub No 9-3046. Washington, DC: U.S. Government Printing Office, 1990.
5. Willet WC, Ascherio A. Transfatty acids: are the effects only marginal? *Am J Public Health* 1994; 84:722.
6. Noop RH et al. Long-term cholesterol-lowering effects of 4 fat-restricted diets in hypercholesterolemic and combined hyperlipidemic men. The dietary alternatives study. *JAMA* 1997; 278(18):1509–25.
7. Cheskin LJ et al. Gastrointestinal symptoms following consumption of Olestra or regular triglyceride potato chips score. *JAMA* 1998; 279(2):150–52.
8. Hellmich N. Olestra has passed safety test, FDA says. *USA Today* 1998 June 18:1D.

9. Wardlaw GM, Insel PM. *Perspectives in nutrition.* 3rd ed. St. Louis: Mosby, 1996.

10. Rimm EB et al. Vitamin E consumption and the risk of coronary heart disease in men. *N Engl J Med* 1993; 328(20):1450–56.

11. Leary WE. Vitamins cut cancer in China study. *The New York Times* 1993 Sept 15.

12. Giovannucci E et al. Multivitamin use, folate, and colon cancer in women in the Nurses' Health Study. *Ann Intern Med* 1998; 129(7):517–24.

13. Czeizel AE, Dudas I. Prevention of the first occurrence of neural-tube defects by periconceptional vitamin supplementation. *N Engl J Med* 1992; 327(26):1832–35.

14. *Position of the American Dietetic Association: vitamin and mineral supplementation, 1998.* http://www.eatright.org/asupple.html

15. Yankelovich Partners for the Nutrition Information Center at The New York Hospital and the Bottled Water Association. As reported in *USA Today* 1998 Aug 25:1D.

16. Scariati PD et al. Water supplementation of infants in the first month of life. *Arch Pediatr Adolesc Med* 1997; 151(8):830–32.

17. FDA allows whole oat foods to make health claim on reducing the risk of heart disease. *FDA Talk Paper* 1997 Jan 21.

18. American Cancer Society. *Cancer facts and figures—1998.* Atlanta: The Association, 1998.

19. Joseph JA et al. Long-term dietary strawberry, spinach, or vitamin E supplementation retards the onset of age-related neuronal signal-transduction and cognitive behavioral deficits. *J Neurosci* 1998; 18(19):8047–55.

20. Phytochemicals in disease prevention. *Nutri-News.* St. Louis: Mosby, Jan 1995.

21. Schardt D. Phytochemicals: plants against cancer. *Nutri Action Health Lett* 1994 April.

22. How to spot and avoid food allergies. *Healthysigns.* Muncie, IN: Cardinal Health Systems, Fall 1998.

23. Office of the Federal Register National Archives and Research Administration. *Code of Federal Regulations: Food and Drugs* 1991; 21(Parts 170–199):417–20.

24. US Department of Agriculture, US Department of Health and Human Services: *Nutrition and your health: dietary guidelines for Americans,* ed 4, Home & Garden Bulletin No 323, Washington, DC, 1995, US Government Printing Office.

25. Hamptom JK, Craven RF, Heitkemper MM. *The biology of human aging.* 2nd ed. Dubuque, IA: Wm C. Brown, 1997.

26. Ferini AF, Ferrini RL. *Health in the later years.* 2nd ed. Madison, WI: Brown & Benchmark, 1992.

27. Winning the food race (special topics). *Population Reports* 1997 Dec; 25(4):1–23.

Suggested Readings

Reinhardt MW. *The perfectly contented meat-eater's guide to vegetarianism: a book for those who really don't want to be hassled about their diet.* Continuum Publishing Company, New York: Continuum Publishing Group 1998. Don't let the title fool you. This entertaining, informative, and humorous book presents the familiar contentions regarding the benefits of vegetarianism in a way that at first seems to reinforce the carnivore's belief that no one should turn away a good piece of beef when it is offered. However, by the time readers are finished with the book, the benefits of vegetarianism have been implanted in an effective manner.

Gastelu D, Hatfield F (contributor). *Dynamic nutrition for maximum performance: a complete nutritional guide for peak sports performance.* Garden City Park, NY: Avery Publishing Group, 1997. In light of the much-discussed role of dietary supplementation in baseball's record-breaking 1998 home run race, this book is an excellent source of information on the role of nutrition in athletic performance. Addressing athletes at all levels, as well as coaches, trainers, and nutritionists, the authors explore nutrition from the familiar foods through the most controversial dietary supplements.

McSwane D, Rue N, Linton R. *Essentials of food safety and sanitation.* Paramus, NJ: Prentice-Hall Press, 1998. In the world of commercial food services, poor food sanitation results in potentially large-scale outbreaks of illness, deaths, and great costs to the businesses or institutions that practice poor sanitation. The book's technical content is aligned with the 1997 FDA Food Code and the competencies needed to earn Food Manager Certification.

Nottingham S. *Eat your genes: how genetically modified food is entering our diet.* New York: St. Martin's Press, 1998. This well-researched and informative book investigates an array of issues associated with manipulation of our food supply through genetic engineering. The author presents the anticipated benefits of engineering animals and plants for human consumption, the potential undesirable consequences associated with these manipulated foods, and the ethical issues regarding raising animals for food consumption, including the cloning of animals. Also introduced is *pharming,* the use of agricultural products to deliver pharmacological agents.

topics for Today

Meals without Meat: Following a Semivegetarian Diet

People become vegetarians for many reasons. Some shun meat and animal products for ethical reasons. Others choose vegetarianism for health reasons. Often it seems that vegetarians are placed in opposition to those who eat meat, and that the two lifestyles are incompatible. In recent years, however, some people have found a middle ground between the two eating styles. These so-called semivegetarians are increasing their intake of vegetables and cutting back greatly on meat consumption but not necessarily eliminating meat entirely. According to a recent National Restaurant Association poll, one in five people choose to eat at restaurants that offer at least a few meatless entrees.[1]

There are several types of vegetarians. Vegans are the most restrictive with their diets, eating only fruits, grains, and vegetables. Lactovegetarians consume milk products along with fruits, vegetables, and grains, and ovolactovegetarians include both eggs and milk products in their diets. Semivegetarians add occasional servings of fish and poultry to the ovolactovegetarian diet, and some even eat red meat on occasion.

Benefits of Vegetarianism

It is currently estimated that in the United States about 12 million people identify themselves as vegetarians. Of these, an estimated one-third are semivegetarians, eating some fish and chicken, and sometimes, on a very limited basis, red meat. On the basis of studies conducted in the United Kingdom, semivegetarianism (or a somewhat less extreme *reduced meat eating*) may involve between 20 and 40 percent of the entire adult population.[2] Most of these people restrict meat consumption because of general health concerns. For adolescent and young adult females, however, the concern is largely centered on weight control. Needless to say, the meat industry has a keen interest in whether semivegetarianism and reduced meat-eating consumption patterns extend into a second generation.[3]

The health benefits of vegetarianism are many. Several of the leading causes of death in the United States are linked to red meat consumption. Cutting

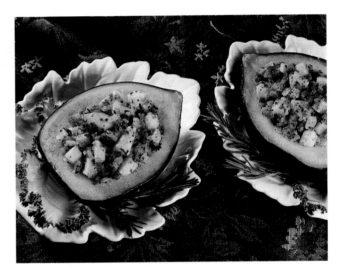

Vegetarian foods are often delicious as well as healthful.

meat consumption can decrease the risk of heart attacks, gallstones, high blood pressure, diabetes, and stroke,[4] and eating more vegetables in place of meat may decrease the risk of some types of cancer.[5] In addition, animals raised in factory farms are often given hormones to stimulate lean tissue (muscle) development and antibiotics to keep them healthy until they get to market. Constant exposure to antibiotics, however, may cause some bacteria to become resistant. A vegetarian diet can also aid in weight loss and prevention of obesity.

Some risks are associated with following a purely vegetarian diet, however. Protein in plants is generally of lower quality than protein found in animal products, so those on a vegetarian diet must be careful to eat a variety of plant foods to get all of the essential amino acids. Eliminating meat altogether may also lead to a deficiency of vitamin B_{12}, which can cause brain and nerve damage. Eating foods fortified with this vitamin, such as cereals, breads, and fruit juice, or taking vitamin supplements can ward off B_{12} deficiency. Vitamin D, which is needed for bone and tooth development, may be lacking in vegetarian diets. Vegans must make sure they get enough vitamin D by eating fortified foods or getting enough sunlight exposure to promote vitamin D production in the body. Vegetarians should eat plant foods high in iron, such as apricots, bran flakes, spinach, and turnip greens to prevent iron deficiency. Coupled with this, eating fruits and vegetables high in vitamin C helps the body to absorb more of the iron in the diet. Calcium supplements may also be necessary, since vegan diets may make calcium difficult to absorb.[6]

Is Semivegetarianism Really Vegetarian?

There is some controversy over whether the semivegetarian diet truly qualifies as "vegetarian." Many people on a strict vegetarian diet do not consider the semivegetarian diet to be vegetarian. To them, any consumption of meat products is considered a compromise to vegetarian principles. Likewise, there are debates over the appropriate use of dairy products and eggs among the various vegetarian groups. Some semivegetarians even acknowledge that they are not "real" vegetarians.

The use of the term *semivegetarian* may not be acceptable to some vegetarians, but there is little doubt that the semivegetarian diet is much healthier than the typical meat-laden Western diet. Semi (demi or quasi)[2] vegetarianism may be the smartest choice of all. A recent study revealed that "meat avoiders" had the lowest levels of fat intake per day (54 g) compared with both meat eaters (67 g) and vegetarians (61 g). This study concluded that when meat was totally eliminated from the diet, higher amounts of cheese and vegetable oils overcompensated for it.[1] Interest in the semivegetarian diet came about as a result of recommendations from several groups in the 1980s. The American Cancer Society, the American Heart Association, and the National Academy of Science all recommended dietary changes that were closely related to the typical semivegetarian diet. The health benefits of such a diet are well documented. The debate over whether semivegetarians should be categorized as vegetarians seems to revolve around ethical questions concerning treatment of animals. Many vegans especially denounce the eating of any meat or animal products, since they believe animals must be exploited to obtain these foods.[7] They are thus morally opposed to semivegetarianism. Cutting back, however, may at least cause a decrease in demand for meat and animal products, and some semivegetarians may see this as a moral justification for their dietary changes. Although the semivegetarian diet may not effectively address the ethical questions raised by animal rights activists, it has become an acceptable way of eating for many people who are looking for a way to eat more healthfully.

Becoming Semivegetarian

The semivegetarian diet may be desirable to some people because the limited consumption of meat products may help ward off some nutrient deficiencies, and such a diet can be healthier than that of the typical American. However, a person who wishes to adopt the semivegetarian diet should not make the change overnight. A sudden elimination of most meat and other animal products can be too drastic of a change to adhere to, so it is best to cut back on them gradually. Such a change should also be discussed first with a doctor, since dietary alterations can cause difficulty for people who are pregnant, nursing, or have health problems.

A gradual cutback in meat consumption can be accomplished by keeping track of how much meat you consume per day. Reduce meat consumption slowly until you have tapered off to about four ounces a day. Meat can be used as a condiment (such as chicken strips on a salad) instead of as a main course, and fish can be substituted for red meat. Try new vegetarian foods at each meal, and keep track of your likes and dislikes. Adding more fruit to your meals can increase the variety of your diet as well.

Using a vegetarian food pyramid can help non-meat eaters and semivegetarians to follow a healthful diet (see Figure 5-5, p. 146). This pyramid is similar to the USDA Food Guide Pyramid (see Figure 5-2, p. 132), but it replaces the meat, poultry, fish, dry beans, eggs, and nuts group with an eggs, legumes, nuts, and seeds group. (In 1996 the USDA confirmed that a vegetarian diet can fulfill the nutrient needs of Americans.[1]) Lactovegetarians can omit eggs from this group. The pyramid advises vegetarians of all types to eat six to eleven servings of bread, cereal, rice, and pasta; three to five servings of vegetables; two to four servings of fruit; and two to three servings of milk, yogurt, or cheese per day. Legumes can be used as a substitute for meats for obtaining iron, calcium, protein, and zinc, but keep in mind that vitamin B_{12} is not found in plant foods.[8] Semivegetarians can obtain some B_{12} from the limited meats they consume but should be careful not to decrease B_{12} intake too much. Also, the occasional fast-food meal is not forbidden. Fast food can provide a change of pace, and many healthy fast-food meals are available.

Children can also be involved in the change of diet (but consult your pediatrician first to be safe). Making dietary changes a family affair can make the adjustment easier. Getting kids involved in meal planning, cooking, and label reading can make things more interesting for them. Dietary changes can be a difficult adjustment for kids, however, so don't hold them to the same restrictions as the adults. This may help parents and children avoid arguments over meals and can make meals more enjoyable for the kids.

A semivegetarian diet may be an acceptable alternative for people who want to cut back significantly on meat consumption but who do not want to give up meat altogether. Reducing the amount of meat in the diet can have definite health benefits, while not eliminating meat can allow for variety in your diet and flexibility in social situations, such as banquets and receptions at which few or no meatless items are served.[1] Check with your doctor to see if such a diet could have advantages for you. Bon appétit!

For Discussion . . .

Is semivegetarianism more ethically sound than the typical Western diet, or is there no difference between eating meat occasionally and eating it often? Should semivegetarians be considered vegetarians? Is the ethical treatment of animals a consideration for you in the food choices you make? Is health a concern for you in your diet?

References

1. Jaret P. The new vegetarians. *Health* 1996 March; 10(3).
2. *Meat, meat eating, vegetarianism—introduction.* Jan 6, 1997. http://www.maf.govt.nz/mafnet/publications/9716/97160011.htm
3. *Meat, meat eating, vegetarianism—conclusion.* Jan 6, 1997. http://www.maf.govt.nz/mafnet/publications/9716/97160002.htm
4. *Position of the American Dietetic Association: vegetarian diets.* Nov 1997. http://www.eatright.org/adap1197.html
5. *Cancer facts and figures—1998.* Atlanta: The Society, 1998.
6. Whitney EN, Cataldo CD, Rolfes SR. *Understanding normal and clinical nutrition.* 5th ed. Belmont, CA: West/Wadsworth, 1997.
7. Singer P. *Animal liberation.* New York: Avon, 1975.
8. Nash J. The transition diet: from meat eater to vegetarian. *Essence* 1995 Jan; 25(9).

InfoLinks

www.vegsoc.org/index1.html
www.dol.net/~rave/cornellveg.html

chapter

six

Maintaining a Healthy Weight

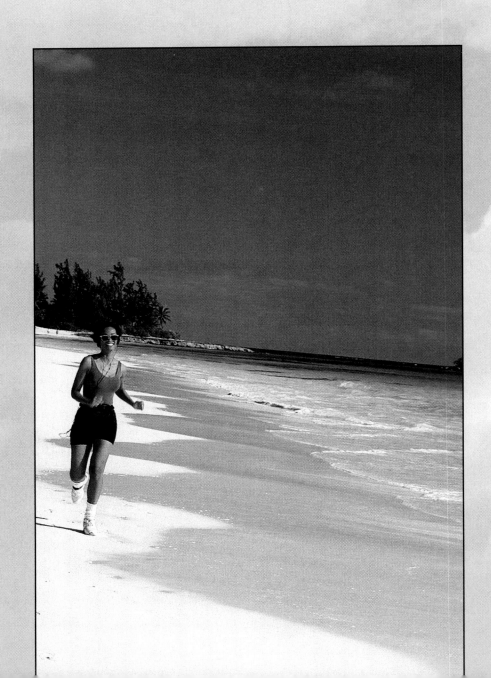

D ata collected from more than 20,000 people by the third National Health and Nutrition Examination Survey reveal a distressing picture of excessive weight and obesity in American society.[1] Principal among the findings of the study was the increase over 1980 levels in the percentage of people, including children, overweight enough to be considered unhealthy. At this time, 33 percent of men and 36 percent of women weigh 20 percent or more above the weight recommended by current height-weight tables. This is a 25 percent increase over 1980 levels. When the newest clinically oriented guidelines for defining and treating obesity (see p. 160) are applied, 97 million Americans, or 55 percent of the population, are considered overweight or obese.[2] These people face an increased risk of developing serious health problems, independent of other risk factors not directly related to weight.

What accounts for the high percentage of Americans defined as overweight or obese? Experts point to two salient factors: greater daily caloric consumption and a relatively low level of consistent physical activity. Today the average American man consumes 2,684 calories per day, compared with 2,457 calories in 1980, and the average woman consumes 1,805 calories per day, compared with 1,531 calories in 1980. Additionally, only 22 percent of adults engage in thirty minutes of moderately intense activity for the recommended number of days per week (see Chapter 4).

The increase in weight just reported occurs, of course, when the body is supplied with more energy than it can use and the excess energy is stored in the form of adipose tissue, or fat. This is called a positive caloric balance. The continuous buildup of **adipose tissue** leads to excess weight and eventually results in obesity. The prevailing opinion in the past has been that, in terms of medical risk, being only mildly overweight is not dangerous. Today, however, some information suggests otherwise. In fact, in a large study of thousands of nurses, researchers found that being of average or slightly below average weight relates to lower levels of premature death.[3]

Although the exact point at which excessive weight (resulting from excess adipose tissue) first becomes a health risk is not known with certainty, few experts question the real dangers to health and wellness from extreme obesity.[4] Among the health problems caused by or complicated by excess body fat are increased surgical risk, hypertension, various forms of heart disease, stroke, type II diabetes mellitus, several forms of cancer, deterioration of joints, complications during pregnancy, gallbladder disease, and an overall increased risk of mortality (see the Star Box on p. 158 and Table 6-1). So closely is obesity associated with chronic conditions, such as those just mentioned, that medical experts now recommend that obesity itself be defined and treated as a chronic disease.

HEALTHY PEOPLE: LOOKING AHEAD TO 2010

In the area of weight management, the *Healthy People 2000 Midcourse Review* indicated almost no progress. Obesity increased by over 100% among all adults ages 18 to 74. The lack of success in controlling weight among those under age 18 was particularly distressing. This failure was perhaps related to the demise of physical education classes in many school systems and to an increasingly sedentary lifestyle that revolves around watching television and playing electronic games.

Nevertheless, some positive programs were initiated during the 1990s. These included an increase in worksite physical fitness programs and nutrition programs that feature a weight management component. In addition, the percentage of adults who reported exercising regularly increased slightly.

Weight management goals will continue to receive significant attention in the *Healthy People 2010* objectives now being formulated. At least three of the target areas—chronic disease prevention, nutrition, and physical fitness—are clearly related to weight management. Reaching objectives in these areas will help to meet the broader goal of increasing years of healthy life among all Americans.

Real Life
Real choices

"Jeff, here's a drumstick—pass your plate down." Jeff's father, Ted, smiles affectionately at his son as he finishes severing the meaty drumstick from the huge, still steaming turkey in front of him.

"No, thanks, Dad—I'm really not that hungry," Jeff responds. "I'll just stick with what I've got and maybe have some turkey later."

"No turkey? But it's Thanksgiving—and there's hardly anything on your plate!" his Aunt Teresa exclaims from her place next to Jeff. "I'm fine, Aunt Terry," Jeff says patiently. "This is plenty."

The fact is, his plate *is* almost empty—just a spoonful of green beans, a dab of sweet potato, and some celery and radishes from the relish tray.

Jeff's sister, Alix, turns to Aunt Teresa. "Don't worry, he won't starve," she says with a teasing glance at her brother. "He's just temporarily lost his appetite over Kristi Martino in his algebra class."

Despite the jibe from his sister, Jeff welcomes the diversion created by her remark. He hadn't really thought about how he'd deal with his family's traditional Thanksgiving feast, in which he's always been an enthusiastic participant—until this year. Just a few months ago, at the beginning of his freshman year in high school, Jeff was encouraged by his best friend, Sean, to try out for junior varsity wrestling. Coach Horner liked Jeff's lean, compact build and his scrappy determination, and to his surprise, Jeff earned a slot as a welterweight on the JV team.

Since then, wrestling has been Jeff's passion. He never misses a practice, and he often goes to varsity practice to watch the skilled upperclassmen hone their moves. And so far he's won six out of eight matches—an impressive record for a newcomer, and a source of pride for Jeff and his teammates.

Everyone's noticed that wrestling has been a life-changing experience for Jeff. Always small for his age and shy, he's gained not only physical strength and coordination but also a quiet confidence that's helped him improve his social skills and take more of a leadership role in school activities.

But what people haven't noticed is something Jeff definitely doesn't want them to know about—the strict regimen he's developed to make sure he always makes his weight at pre-match weigh-ins. In wrestling, weight is measured not just in pounds but in ounces, and a few ounces too many can disqualify a wrestler from competing in his weight class. Jeff, who lives to wrestle, is determined always to be safely under the top weight for his class. Only vaguely aware of the principles of good nutrition, before a match Jeff opts to skip meals, instead substituting power bars and sports drinks. Sometimes this regimen leaves him feeling weak and lightheaded, and he's begun to have difficulty concentrating in class, but he's sure his method is the only way to ensure that he keeps his cherished place on the wrestling team.

As you study this chapter, think about Jeff's situation, and prepare yourself to answer the questions in **Your Turn** at the end of the chapter.

Body Image and Self-Concept

Although clinicians now have specific guidelines for the diagnosis and treatment of obesity, the general public has its own set of definitions and concerns regarding body weight. Principal among these is the issue of perceived physical attractiveness. This concern is caused (or reinforced) by the media, which tells people that being overweight does not conform to certain ideal **body images** (such as being tall, thin, and "cut" with muscular definition). The average actress and model, for example, is thinner than 95 percent of the female population and weighs 23 percent less than the average woman. Today's lean but muscular version of perfection is a very demanding standard for both women and men to meet.

In light of this challenge, people may become dissatisfied and concerned about their inability to resemble these ideals. The scope of this dissatisfaction is evident in a study of more than 800 women, which revealed that nearly half were unhappy with their weight, muscle tone, hips, thighs, buttocks, and legs (men may not be very different in this regard).[5] Not surprisingly, when this dissatisfaction exists, people

Health Risks of Obesity

Each of the diseases listed below is followed by the percentage of cases that are caused by obesity:

Colon cancer	10%
Breast cancer	11%
Hypertension	33%
Heart disease	70%
Diabetes (type II, non-insulin-dependent)	90%

As these statistics show, being obese greatly increases your risk of many serious and even life-threatening diseases.

can question their own attractiveness, and eventually, their self-concept and self-esteem declines. Only growing older lessens, but does not eliminate, this dissatisfaction.

In comparison with being overweight, little media attention has traditionally been paid to being underweight (see p. 185). However, the body image problems experienced by some extremely thin people can be equally distressing.

Table 6-1   Health Problems Associated with Excess Body Fat

Health Problems	Partially Attributed to:
Surgical risk	Increased anesthesia needs and greater risk of wound infections
Pulmonary disease	Excess weight over lungs
Type II diabetes mellitus (NIDDM)	Enlarged fat cells, which then poorly bind insulin and also poorly respond to the message insulin sends to the cell
Hypertension	Increased miles of blood vessels found in the fat tissue; however, no validated cause is yet known
Coronary heart disease	Increases in serum cholesterol and triglyceride levels, as well as a decrease in physical activity
Bone and joint disorders	Excess pressure put on knee, ankle, and hip joints
Gallbladder stones	An increase in cholesterol content of bile
Skin disorders	The trapping of moisture and microbes in fat folds
Various cancers	Estrogen production by fat cells; animal studies suggest excess energy intake encourages tumor development
Shorter stature (in some forms of obesity)	An earlier onset of puberty
Pregnancy risk	More difficult delivery and increased anesthesia needs (if used)
Early death	A variety of risk factors for diseases listed above

The greater the degree of obesity, the more likely and the more serious these health problems generally become. They are much more likely to appear in people who are greater than twice their desirable body weight.

Personal Applications

• Why, in your opinion, do we hold as attractive and fashionable a body type that is unrepresentative of the vast majority of American adults?

Defining Overweight and Obesity

The most prevalent forms of malnutrition in affluent countries are overweight and obesity. Most people think of malnourishment as a shortage of essential nutrients. In developing countries, food deprivation forms the basis of malnutrition. However, malnutrition can also be a disease of plenty. Because our food supply exceeds the needs of our population, people are able to eat more than is required for healthful living. They often consume more calories than they expend. They can then become overweight and may become obese.

How can people tell the difference between overweight and obesity? Nutritionists have traditionally said that obesity is apparent when fat accumulation produces a body weight that is more than 20 percent above an ideal or **desirable weight.** People are said to be **overweight** if their weight is between 1 percent and 19 percent above their desirable weight. The more people increase their weight above their desirable weight, the more likely they are to be

labeled obese. Of course, an exception to this relationship between overweight and obesity is excessive weight caused by extreme muscularity, such as that seen in many football players.

The term **obesity** requires further refinement. When people are between 20 percent and 40 percent above desirable weight, their obesity is described as *mild* (about 90% of all obese people), whereas excessive weight in the 41 percent to 99 percent above desirable range is defined as *moderate obesity* (about 9% of obese people), and weight of 100 percent or more above desirable is defined as *severe, gross,* or *morbid obesity* (less than 1% of obese people).

Being most familiar with the weight guidelines used in the past, most clinicians and the general

adipose tissue   tissue made up of fibrous strands around which specialized cells designed to store liquefied fat are arranged.

body image   our subjective perception of how our body appears.

desirable weight   the weight range deemed appropriate for people of a specific sex, age, and frame size.

overweight   a condition in which a person's excess fat accumulation results in a body weight that exceeds desirable weight by 1% to 19%.

obesity   a condition in which a person's excess fat accumulation results in a body weight that exceeds desirable weight by 20% or more.

public continue to use standard height/weight tables to determine the extent to which scale weight exceeds desirable weight and, thus, the existence of mild, moderate, or severe obesity. However, other techniques are now available that can be used to determine body composition. In the next section of this chapter, several of those techniques, including waist/hip ratio (*healthy body weight*), body mass index, hydrostatic weighing, skinfold measurements, and electrical impedance, are described.

Most recently the scientific community has issued guidelines for determining obesity for purposes of medical intervention. Specifically, an individual is overweight when BMI (body mass index) falls between 25 and 29.9, and one is obese when BMI is 30.0 or above. Aggressive medical intervention is necessary for people who, in addition to being obese, have a waist circumference of 40 or more inches (males) or 35 or more inches (females) and two or more of the following risk factors: diabetes, high blood pressure, high blood cholesterol and **sleep apnea.**[2] For obese people who demonstrate fewer risk factors, less aggressive treatment may suffice.

Obesity, although perhaps genetically and behaviorally determined early in life, often takes many years to develop fully. A daily caloric surplus of only ten calories yields ten unwanted pounds of fat in ten years; twenty or thirty years of consistent excess food intake or gradually declining activity can easily result in a **positive caloric balance** and, eventually, being overweight and even obese. Accordingly, to maintain a specific weight (as you will soon read) people must balance their energy intake with their energy expenditure. The key to losing weight and keeping it off is exercise and dietary control that is consistent with the current nutritional recommendations described in Chapter 5; in other words, eat healthfully and exercise regularly.

Determining Weight and Body Composition

A wide array of techniques exist to determine weight and body composition. Some techniques are, of course, much more accurate and more expensive than others. In the section that follows, a variety of these techniques are described.

Height/Weight Tables

The familiar 1983 Metropolitan Life Insurance Height and Weight Table can be the basis for determining whether your scale weight is below, at, or above desirable for your gender, height, and frame size. Some clinicians and most of the public turn to this table to assess body weight. However, the use of

this table and others like it is no longer considered the best way to determine whether body weight is acceptable. This has occurred because it is now recognized that this table excludes uninsurable people, disregards the influence of age, fails to consider other causes of mortality (such as smoking), and relies on subjective determinations of frame size to express the influence of body composition on weight. Fortunately, a new table intended for use with the guidelines describing BMI is now available and appears on page 161.

Healthy Body Weight

You can determine your healthy body weight by using the weight guidelines that are found in the *Dietary Guidelines for Americans* (Table 6-3).[6] This assessment involves converting two body measurements, the waist and the hip circumferences, into a waist-to-hip ratio (WHR) that can then be applied to weight ranges for people of particular ages and heights. Among people who have an acceptable WHR, female "healthy weight" is near the lower end of each weight range, whereas male "healthy weight" is at the higher end of each weight range.

To use these new weight ranges, the following procedure must be performed:

1. Measure around your waist near your navel while you stand relaxed, not pulling in your stomach.
2. Measure around your hips, over the buttocks where your hips are the largest.
3. Divide the waist measurement by the hip measurement.

Women with a WHR of less than .85 generally have a body weight that falls within the healthy range for their age and height; men with a WHR of less than 1.00 will also probably fall within the range that is considered healthy for their age and height. Any person whose WHR is equal to or greater than the recommended ratio should attempt to lose weight.

This assessment procedure was developed in response to the growing concern over the relationship between the amount of fat in the central abdominal cavity (upper body obesity) and the

---

sleep apnea a condition in which abnormalities in the structure of the airways lead to periods of greatly restricted air flow during sleeping, resulting in reduced levels of blood oxygen and placing greater strain on the heart to maintain adequate tissue oxygenation.

positive caloric balance caloric intake greater than caloric expenditure.

Table 6-2 Charting Weight

Height	100	105	110	115	120	125	130	135	140	145	150	155	160	165	170	175	180	185	190	195	200	205	210	215	220	225	230	235	240	245	250
5'0"	20	21	21	22	23	24	25	26	27	28	29	30	31	32	33	34	35	36	37	38	39	40	41	42	43	44	45	46	47	48	49
5'1"	19	20	21	22	23	24	25	26	26	27	28	29	30	31	32	33	34	35	36	37	38	39	40	41	42	43	43	44	45	46	47
5'2"	18	19	20	21	22	23	24	25	26	27	27	28	29	30	31	32	33	34	35	36	37	37	38	39	40	41	42	43	44	45	46
5'3"	18	19	20	20	21	22	23	24	25	26	27	27	28	29	30	31	32	33	34	35	35	36	37	38	39	40	41	42	43	43	44
5'4"	17	18	19	20	21	21	22	23	24	25	26	27	27	28	29	30	31	32	33	33	34	35	36	37	38	39	39	40	41	42	43
5'5"	17	17	18	19	20	21	22	22	23	24	25	26	27	27	28	29	30	31	32	32	33	34	35	36	37	37	38	39	40	41	42
5'6"	16	17	18	19	19	20	21	22	23	23	24	25	26	27	27	28	29	30	31	31	32	33	34	35	36	36	37	38	39	40	40
5'7"	16	16	17	18	19	20	20	21	22	23	23	24	25	26	27	27	28	29	30	31	31	32	33	34	34	35	36	37	38	38	39
5'8"	15	16	17	17	18	19	20	21	21	22	23	24	24	25	26	27	27	28	29	30	30	31	32	33	33	34	35	36	36	37	38
5'9"	15	15	16	17	18	18	19	20	21	21	22	23	24	24	25	26	27	27	28	29	30	30	31	32	32	33	34	35	35	36	37
5'10"	14	15	16	16	17	18	19	19	20	21	22	22	23	24	24	25	26	27	27	28	29	29	30	31	32	32	33	34	34	35	36
5'11"	14	15	15	16	17	17	18	19	20	20	21	22	22	23	24	24	25	26	26	27	28	29	29	30	31	31	32	33	33	34	35
6'0"	14	14	15	16	16	17	18	18	19	20	20	21	22	22	23	24	24	25	26	26	27	28	28	29	30	31	31	32	33	33	34
6'1"	13	14	15	15	16	16	17	18	18	19	20	20	21	22	22	23	24	24	25	26	26	27	28	28	29	30	30	31	32	32	33
6'2"	13	13	14	15	15	16	17	17	18	19	19	20	21	21	22	22	23	24	24	25	26	26	27	28	28	29	30	30	31	31	32
6'3"	12	13	14	14	15	16	16	17	17	18	19	19	20	21	21	22	22	23	24	24	25	26	26	27	27	28	29	29	30	31	31
6'4"	12	13	13	14	15	15	16	16	17	18	18	19	19	20	21	21	22	22	23	24	24	25	26	26	27	27	28	29	29	30	30

Weight

KEY: Healthy   Overweight   Obese

The starting point of what's considered overweight is now set at a body mass index of 25 to less than 30, say new guidelines from the National Institutes of Health. One previous definition set the starting point at a BMI of 27. The new and old guidelines define obese as a BMI of 30 or above.
Source: National Institutes of Health

Table 6-3	Healthy Weight: Recommended Guidelines	

| | Weight without Clothes | |
Height without Shoes	19–34 Years	35 Years and Over
5'	97–128	108–138
5'1"	101–132	111–143
5'2"	104–137	115–148
5'3"	107–141	119–152
5'4"	111–146	122–157
5'5"	114–150	126–162
5'6"	118–155	130–167
5'7"	121–160	134–172
5'8"	125–164	138–178
5'9"	129–169	142–183
5'10"	132–174	146–188
5'11"	136–179	151–194
6'0"	140–184	155–199
6'1"	144–189	159–205
6'2"	148–195	164–210
6'3"	152–200	168–216
6'4"	156–205	173–222
6'5"	160–211	177–228
6'6"	164–216	182–234

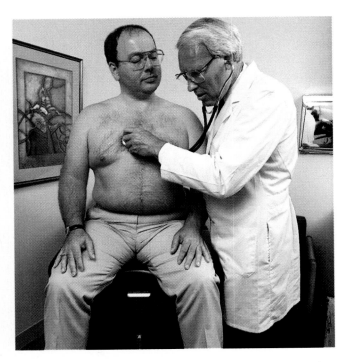

Accumulation of fat in the central abdominal cavity may be linked to the development of serious health problems.

development of several serious health problems. In addition to an unacceptably high waist-to-hip ratio, high blood pressure and/or a protruding stomach indicate a need to lose weight. Interestingly, the "spare tire" pattern of fat distribution is most frequently seen in men and most likely reflects the influence of testosterone.

In comparison with the upper body distribution seen in men, women more often demonstrate an excessive accumulation of fat in the hips and upper legs. This lower body obesity is less closely associated with chronic health problems such as cardiovascular disease and diabetes mellitus (type II).

As a point of interest, the guidelines noted on page 160 do not use WHR as a clinical marker for the treatment of obesity, but rather use only waist circumference (40 inches or more for men and 35 inches or more for women), believing it to be a better predictor of risk. Only time will tell about the continued use of healthy body weight in the diagnosis of overweight and obesity.

The *Dietary Guidelines for Americans* assessment procedure recognizes increasing age as a factor that influences body weight.[6] For people older than 35 years of age, this lifts some of the pressure to maintain a youthful appearance (including lower weight). Some nutritionists, however, believe that the same weight standards should apply to both older adults and younger adults.

Body Mass Index

Another means of assessing healthy body weight is the **body mass index (BMI).** The BMI indicates the relationship of body weight (expressed in kilograms) to height (expressed in meters) for both men and women.[7] The BMI does not reflect body composition (fat versus lean tissue) or consider the degree of fat accumulated within the central body cavity, nor is it adjusted for age. It is, nevertheless, widely used in determining obesity. As noted on page 160, a BMI of 25 to 29.9 indicates overweight, while a BMI of 30.0 or above represents obesity.

An alternative method of determining the BMI is to use a **nomogram** such as that in Figure 6-1. Like the BMI, the nomogram requires information about both weight and height. Once you have determined your BMI, its relationship to a desirable BMI can be evaluated using data found in Table 6-4.

Electrical Impedance

Electrical impedance is a relatively new method to determine body composition. This assessment procedure measures the electrical impedance (resistance) to a weak electrical flow directed through the body. Because adipose tissue resists the passage of the electrical current more than muscle tissue does, electrical impedance can be used to calculate the percentage of body fat. However, in addition to high cost and limited availability, psychological variables can reduce

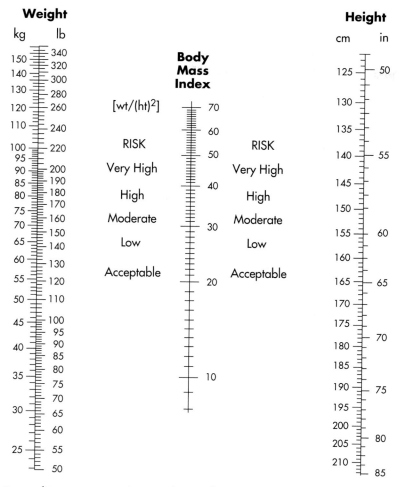

To use this nomogram, place a ruler or other straight edge between the body weight in kilograms or pounds (without clothes) located on the left-hand column and the height in centimeters or in inches (without shoes) located on the right-hand column. The BMI is read from the middle of the scale and is in metric units.

Figure 6-1 Using a nomogram is a simple way of finding your body mass index (BMI).

Table 6-4 Desirable Body Mass Index in Relation to Age

Age Group (years)	BMI (kg/m²)
19–24	19–24
25–34	20–25
35–44	21–26
45–54	22–27
55–65	23–28
>65	24–29

the practicality of electrical impedance. Additional techniques used to determine body composition include computerized axial tomography (CAT) scans, magnetic resonance imaging (MRI), infrared light transmission, and neutron activation. These tech-niques, like electrical impedance, have limited application because of cost and availability.

Skinfold Measurements

A **skinfold measurement** provides a relatively precise indicator of body fat percentage. Skinfold

body mass index (BMI) a numerical expression of body weight based on height and weight.

nomogram a graphic means of finding an unknown value.

electrical impedance a method used to measure the percentage of body fat using a harmless electrical current.

skinfold measurement a measurement to determine the thickness of the fat layer that lies immediately beneath the skin; this measurement is used to calculate body composition.

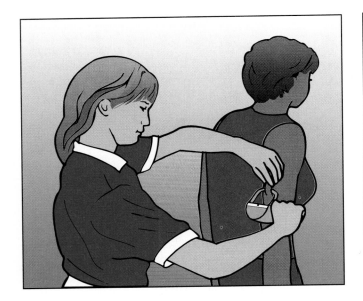

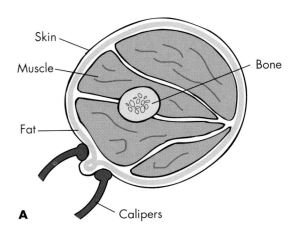

A

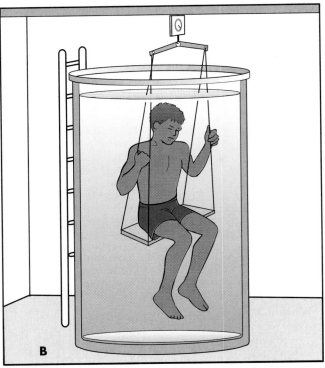

B

Figure 6-2 Two methods of determining body composition. **A,** Skinfold measurement using calipers. Skinfold measurements are used in equations that calculate body density and the percentage of body fat. **B,** Hydrostatic weighing. Percentage of body fat is determined by comparing a person's underwater body weight with his or her body weight out of the water.

measurements rely on constant-pressure **calipers** to measure the thickness of the layer of fat beneath the skin's surface. Skinfold measurements of subcutaneous fat are taken at several key places on the body (see Figure 6-2A). Measurements of skinfold thickness can then be used to establish the percentage of body fat. Once the percentage of body fat has been calculated, a relatively simple conversion can be made to determine desired body weight. It should be noted, however, that the skill of the person making the skinfold measurement is an important factor in the accuracy of this procedure.

Young adult men normally have a body fat percentage of between 10 percent and 15 percent. The normal range for young adult women is 20 percent to 25 percent.[8] When a man's body fat percentage exceeds 25 percent and a woman's body fat percentage exceeds 30 percent, they are classified as obese. The relatively higher percentage of fat found in women is related to the female's capacity for pregnancy and lactation.

Hydrostatic Weighing

Hydrostatic weighing (underwater weighing) is a precise method for determining the relative amounts of fat and lean body mass that make up body weight (Figure 6-2B). A person's percentage of body fat is determined by comparing the underwater body weight with the body weight out of the water. The necessity for expensive equipment and trained technicians make the use of this method impractical for the average person.

Appearance

Perhaps the simplest method of determining obesity may be to look in the mirror. The old saying "mirrors don't lie" speaks for itself. For most people, this method is fairly accurate and certainly inexpensive. Unless a person is very muscular or has retained an excessive amount of water, the reflection in the mirror should be a good indicator of whether one's weight is appropriate. Although this simple method does not allow a person to pinpoint a body fat percentage, the person should be able to visually determine whether he or she is excessively fat.

For some overweight and obese people, however, it can be difficult to be objective. They may not accurately judge their bodies. Their imagined (or desired) body image and their actual image are markedly different. For these people, disappointment and frustration are likely. The ability to accurately perceive one's own appearance (body image) is particularly difficult for people with anorexia nervosa (see p. 182).

For many people, it is important to appear physically attractive. This desired body image may or may not be compatible with their inherited body type or their ability to gain or lose weight. Nevertheless, they try to achieve the look that they have in mind.

In the body image that appears popular for today's women, hips, waist, and shoulders line up to suggest a vertical line. The once-popular emphasis on an "hourglass" figure has given way to a more angular, athletic appearance, somewhat similar to the body build of many young men. As is true for women, the weight and body composition of many men do not align with the body they wish to possess.

Whether the body image desired can reasonably be obtained seems unimportant to many people. Some spend hours each week in weight rooms and reduce or increase their food intake dramatically in a quest to attain the desired body image. For those who are ultimately unsuccessful, disappointment and frustration can result.

Personal Applications

• What methods have you used to determine whether you are underweight, desirable weight, overweight, or obese?

Origins of Obesity

Experts continue to question the origins of obesity. As you might expect, the many theories focus on factors within the individual, as well as from the environment. When a definitive cause is identified—and some interesting progress has been made toward this goal—it will comprise an interplay of genetic, metabolic, psychological, and environmental factors.[9] However, until a single all-inclusive discovery is made, if ever, it is safe to assume that obesity is a complex condition caused by a variety of factors. No two obese people will have gained their excessive weight in exactly the same way or for the same reasons.

Genetic Basis of Obesity

Based on studies involving both identical and fraternal (nonidentical) twins, raised together and separately, it has been demonstrated that both environ-ment and genetics influence obesity. In some cases the role of inherited tendencies toward excessive weight appears to be almost solely responsible for the amount and distribution of body fat.[10] For example, the "apple" shape associated with fat storage in males and the "pear" shape seen in females, which are associated with a greater likelihood of developing diabetes mellitus type II during middle adulthood, are strongly influenced by genetic factors.

Recently the role of a genetic contribution has been clarified somewhat by the discovery of "fat genes" in mice and, subsequently, an obesity gene in humans.[11] Initial speculation regarding the influence of these (or additional) genes centered on a protein that functions as a code that normally signals the body to terminate food consumption.[12] Research revealed that this protein, leptin, was present in lower levels in overweight mice than in normal mice. Researchers suspected that leptin would be found in lower levels in obese humans compared with those of average weight. Their results demonstrated, however, that obese humans actually have higher levels of leptin than those of average weight.[13] It is now speculated that faulty receptors for leptin might exist in some obese people, restricting the production of GLP-1, a protein that also plays an important role in the signaling of *satiety,* or fullness.[14] Recently a study reported significant weight loss in obese subjects who received synthetic leptin by injection.[15]

Appetite Center

Building on this new information about the genetic and neurophysiological basis of obesity, researchers have identified centers for the control of eating within the hypothalamus of the central nervous system (CNS). These centers, the *feeding center* for hunger and the *satiety center* for fullness, tell the body when it should begin consuming food and when food consumption should stop. These centers are thought to monitor continuously a variety of factors regarding food intake, including olfactory and visual cues, the body's stores of glucose, amino acids, and free fatty acids, the degree of stomach distention, information regarding basal metabolic rate, gastrointestinal hormone level, including leptin, and recently identified hormones, orexin A and orexin B, that influence hunger in rats.[16] As we acquire greater understanding of the hormones and neurotransmitters that influence hunger and satiety,

---

calipers a device used to measure the thickness of a skinfold from which percent body fat can be calculated.

hydrostatic weighing weighing the body while it is submerged in water.

drugs designed to influence their actions will appear. Some such drugs, in fact, already exist and are described later in the chapter.

Set Point Theory

Traditional theory has suggested that the energy expenditure and energy storage centers of the body possess a genetically programmed awareness of the body's most physiologically desirable weight. To maintain this so-called **set point** for desirable weight, the body adjusts its baseline use of energy, the basal metabolic rate (see pp. 170–171), upward or downward to accommodate an excessive intake of calories or an inadequate intake of calories, as the case may be. Thus, by burning more energy or storing more energy, the body maintains its "best" weight through the process of **adaptive thermogenesis.**

Using the set point theory to explain the difficulty of losing weight, it has been suggested that in the case of a person with a genetically conditioned tendency to store excessive energy (to gain weight easily), the body prevents planned weight loss from occurring easily by adjusting the set point to a lower level. In addition, according to the set point theory, to prevent further episodes of "starvation" from occurring, a new, higher set point is established and lost weight is regained to a level above that of the initial set point. Every time the dieter again attempts to lose weight, he or she will yo-yo between weight loss and subsequent weight gain.

Today, some researchers believe that the *yo-yo dieting* model, explained on the basis of set point readjustment, may not be accurate. Perhaps the weight gain that follows a period of dieting occurs merely because of the tendency for most people to gain fat and weight as they age. On the other hand, however, it may be a reflection of the difficulty of losing weight only through caloric restriction, without increasing caloric expenditure through physical activity.[17]

Related somewhat to set point and adaptive thermogenesis is the renewed interest in whether the small stores of brown fat (most fat is white fat) found in humans are involved in weight control. Located in small amounts in the upper back between the shoulder blades, this fat has the physiological ability to expend calories solely as heat without generating the high-energy units that are capable of being stored in fat cells.[18] In fact, a recently discovered "uncoupling protein" produced by the uncoupling protein 2 gene (*UCP2*) may somehow relate to the brown fat.[19]

Although considered dangerous by health experts, some people have experimented with the use of an enzyme called 2,4 Dinitrophenol (DNP), which is capable of "uncoupling" high-energy units in a manner similar to that done naturally by brown fat, thus preventing energy storage and weight gain.

Body Type

An inheritance basis for obesity could involve the interplay of somatotype (body build) and other unique energy-processing characteristics passed on from parents to their children.

The classic work of Sheldon is credited with establishing the now-familiar body types *ectomorph, mesomorph,* and *endomorph.* In the ectomorphic body type, a tall slender body seems to virtually protect individuals from difficulty with excessive weight. Ectomorphs usually have difficulty maintaining normal weight for their height.

The somewhat shorter, more heavily muscled, athletic body of the mesomorph represents a genetic middle ground in inherited body types. During childhood, adolescence, and adulthood, as long as activity levels are maintained, mesomorphic people will appear to be "solid" without appearing to be obese. For well-conditioned mesomorphs, scale weight may suggest obesity, but the excessive weight is more likely the result of heavy muscularity. Mesomorphs have their greatest difficulty with obesity during adulthood, when eating patterns fail to adjust to a decline in physical activity.

Endomorphs have body types that tend to be round and soft. Many endomorphs have excessively large abdomens and report having had weight problems since childhood.

Sheldon was interested in the personality traits and temperament of people with each body type. Today's scientists believe there is no connection between personality and physical characteristics. The relationship of body type to inheritance, body weight, and weight management cannot, however, go unnoticed. Sheldon's work simply gives the academic community labels with which to discuss its observations.

Infant and Adult Eating Patterns

Many **bariatricians** categorize obesity according to the way in which eating patterns seem to produce it. Two general eating patterns are related to two forms of obesity: hypercellular and hypertrophic obesity.

The first of these patterns involves infant feeding. Many researchers believe that the number of fat cells a person has will be initially determined during the first 2 years of life. Babies who are overfed will develop a greater number of fat cells than babies who receive a balanced diet of appropriate, infant-sized portions. Overfed babies, especially those with a family history of obesity, will tend to develop **hypercellular obesity.** When these children reach adulthood, they will have more fat cells. Many researchers now believe that these fat cells drive the body's metabolic processes in the direction of a positive caloric balance and a filling of these cells.

Armed with the knowledge that overfeeding can contribute to future obesity, parents of newborns and small children are faced with a potentially troubling problem: how to prevent excessive weight gain of a child without crossing the fine line into undernourishment or even malnourishment. Physicians recommend a balanced diet based on a variety of items from each food group, appropriate serving sizes, low-fat milk only after the age of two years, and regular physical activity. The use of these approaches is a good prescription for sound growth and development and the prevention of hypercellular obesity.

Late childhood and adolescence are also times during which excessive weight gain may result in the formation of hypercellular obesity. For adults, substantial weight gain (exceeding 75% above desirable weight) can stimulate an increase in the number of fat cells and thus move them toward this form of obesity.

A second type of obesity that has its origins in an eating pattern is called **hypertrophic obesity.** This form of obesity is related to a long-term positive caloric balance during adulthood. Over a period of years, existing fat cells increase in size to accommodate excess food intake.

Hypertrophic obesity is generally associated with excessive fat around the waist and is thought to contribute to conditions such as diabetes mellitus (type II, non-insulin-dependent diabetes), high levels of fat in the blood, high blood pressure, and heart disease. Hypertrophic obesity generally shows itself during middle age—a time when physical activity generally declines while food intake remains the same.

Externality

Studies have demonstrated that many obese people have highly developed levels of sensitivity to the outside world.[7] They can be said to have a high degree of *externality.* Thus in comparison with nonobese people, the eating behavior of some obese people may be more controlled by external stimuli, such as a clock, a food advertisement or commercial, or the smell of food, than by monitoring the body's internal environment. Consequently, high levels of externality can make it very difficult for an obese person to adjust to a controlled diet.

Endocrine Influence

For a number of years, people believed that obesity was the result of "glandular" problems. Often the thyroid gland was said to be underactive, thus preventing the person from "burning up" food. Obesity supposedly resulted from a condition over which the individual had no control.

Today it is known that only a few obese people have an endocrine dysfunction of the type that would result in obesity. Clinicians report that no more than 3 percent to 5 percent of the obesity they observe is the result of **hypothyroidism.**

Pregnancy

During a normal pregnancy, approximately 75,000 additional calories are required to support the development of the fetus and the formation of *maternal supportive tissues* and to fuel the elevated maternal metabolic rate. In addition, the woman will develop approximately nine extra pounds of adipose tissue, which will be used as an energy source during lactation. In total, the typical woman enters childbirth having gained approximately twenty-eight pounds over her prepregnancy weight. Early prenatal care should include specific information about both diet and fitness activities for the appropriate weight gain during pregnancy.

Ideally, after the birth of the baby, the mother will have a weight gain of only two to three pounds over her prepregnancy weight. This small amount of additional weight will normally be lost by the end of the sixth to eighth month after the birth of the baby. It should be noted, however, that for women with a history of weight cycling before pregnancy, weight gain during pregnancy may be greater. For most women, however, pregnancy and resultant obesity do not have to go hand in hand. In fact, on the basis of a study in Stockholm, postpregnancy weight retention was more closely related to lifestyle decisions than to any other factor.[20]

Decreasing Basal Metabolic Rate

The body's requirement for energy to maintain basic physiological processes decreases progressively with age. This change reflects the loss of muscle tissue with age in both men and women. This loss of muscle mass eventually alters the ratio of lean body tissue to fat. Thus, as the proportion of fat increases, the

---

set point   a genetically programmed range of body weight beyond which a person finds it difficult to gain or lose additional weight.

adaptive thermogenesis   the physiological response of the body to adjust its metabolic rate to the presence of food.

bariatrician   a physician who specializes in the study and treatment of obesity.

hypercellular obesity   a form of obesity seen in people who possess an abnormally large number of fat cells.

hypertrophic obesity   a form of obesity in which fat cells are enlarged, but not excessive in number.

hypothyroidism   a condition in which the thyroid gland produces an insufficient amount of its hormone, thyroxin.

energy needs of the body are more strongly influenced by the lower metabolic needs of fat cells.[21] This excess energy must then be stored in the fat cells of the body.

Although on a short-term basis little adjustment needs to be made to maintain weight, weight gain can be significant over time if adjustments are not made. A gradual decrease in caloric intake or a conscious effort to expend more calories can be effective in preventing the gradual onset of obesity.

Family Dietary Practices

The family subtly but effectively instructs children on many topics; information, values, and diverse skills are passed from one generation to the next. Food preferences and dietary practices are among the many areas of instruction for which the family assumes responsibility. In some families the lessons are taught as though they were outlined from a nutrition textbook, whereas for others the lessons taught are destined to lead to a life of malnourishment, including obesity. Between-meal snacking on unhealthful foods, large serving sizes, multiple servings, and high-calorie meals can lead to obesity. For busy families, the tendency to rely on fat-dense foods, including fast foods and other convenience foods, lays the foundation for excessive weight gain.

Not only do family behavioral practices contribute to obesity, but just as important, they can also play a constructive role in the weight loss achieved by obese children. Research suggests that when parents are trained to provide positive reinforcement to their children during the weight loss process, the children experience maximal success.

Inactivity

When weight management experts are asked to identify the single most important reason so much obesity exists in today's society, they are almost certain to point to inactivity. People of all ages tend to do less and therefore burn fewer calories than did their ancestors only a few generations ago. Automation in the workplace, labor-saving devices in the home, the inactivity associated with watching television, and a general dislike of exercising on a regular basis (see Chapter 4) are a few of the reasons that account for this inactivity.

As inactivity becomes the norm, not only does weight gain occur but the body is also progressively deprived of its most efficient way to reduce fat stores. Thus, inactivity is a double-edged sword that promotes the development of a weight problem while depriving individuals of a mechanism that would efficiently resolve the problem.

Caloric Balance

As previously mentioned, any calories consumed beyond those that are used by the body are converted to fat stores. People gain weight when their energy input exceeds their energy output. Conversely, they lose weight when their energy output exceeds their energy input (Figure 6-3). The basic formula is quite simple and can be analogous to a seesaw or lever with a fulcrum at the centerpoint. Weight remains constant when caloric input and caloric output are identical. In such a situation, our bodies are said to be in *caloric balance.*

Energy Needs of the Body

What are our energy needs? How many calories should we consume (or expend) to achieve a healthy weight? There is no single answer for everyone. Although there are some ballpark estimates for college-age men (2,500 to 3,300 calories) and women (approximately 2,500 calories), we all vary in our specific energy needs.[22] These needs are based on three factors: (1) the person's activity requirements, (2) the person's basal metabolism, and (3) the thermic effect of food.

Activity Requirements

Each person's caloric *activity requirements* vary directly according to the amount of daily physical work completed. For example, sedentary office workers will require a smaller daily caloric intake than will construction workers, letter carriers, or farm workers. Even within a given general job type, the amount of caloric expenditure will vary according to the physical effort required. A police officer who walks a neighborhood beat will usually expend many more calories than the typical police dispatcher or equestrian or motorcycle officer.

Physical activity that occurs outside the occupational setting also adds to caloric needs. Sedentary office workers may be quite active in their recreational pursuits. Or active employees may spend their off-hours lounging in front of the television. You must closely examine the total amount of work or activity you perform to accurately estimate your caloric requirements. Physical activity uses between 20 percent and 40 percent of caloric intake. See Table 6-5 for a breakdown of caloric expenditures for various recreational pursuits.

Pyramid Power—Mediterranean Style

In Chapter 5 we explored the components of the USDA Food Guide Pyramid, which is designed to help Americans make healthful food choices in appropriate quantities. As you'll recall, we're encouraged to enjoy relatively more servings of bread, cereal, rice, pasta, fruits, and vegetables (located on the first and second levels of the pyramid), while eating fewer servings of meat and dairy products and restricting our intake of fats, oils, and sweets (which occupy the narrower top levels of the pyramid).

Did you know there's another food pyramid that points the way to nutritious food selections that are essential to successful weight control? It's called the Mediterranean Pyramid, and some nutritionists believe it offers the best diet for good health (see the illustration below). Like the USDA Food Guide Pyramid, the Mediterranean Pyramid emphasizes a diet based on grains, fruits, and vegetables. The Mediterranean Pyramid recommends eating red meat just a few times a month and allows generous amounts of olive oil. The USDA Pyramid likewise calls for limited consumption of lean red meat, but it urges sparing consumption of all fats, including olive oil. Another important difference between these two pyramids is that the Mediterranean Pyramid calls for limited consumption of alcohol, which may reduce the risk of coronary heart disease; the USDA Pyramid makes no such recommendation.

Here are some of the other reasons many nutritionists advocate a diet based on Mediterranean favorites:

Greens: Dark leafy greens are rich in antioxidant vitamins, which may help guard against cancer and heart disease and possibly prevent damage to the eyes. Greens are also excellent sources of calcium, iron, and the B vitamin folic acid, which research shows can reduce the risk of neural tube (spinal cord) defects in fetuses. Folic acid may also reduce the risk of heart disease and stroke.

Legumes: Like dark leafy greens, legumes such as garbanzo beans (chick peas), cannellini beans, and red kidney beans are rich in folic acid and iron. What's more, they're high in protein, making them low-fat, no-cholesterol alternatives to meat. And they're great sources of soluble fiber, which can help reduce levels of blood cholesterol.

Garlic: Also shown to be effective in lowering blood cholesterol even when eaten in small quantities, garlic is a traditional staple of Mediterranean cuisine that adds flavor without contributing either fat or sugar.

Olive oil: For centuries, olive oil has been the fat of choice in Mediterranean cooking. Unlike butter and lard, animal products that are loaded with saturated fat, olive oil is a monounsaturated fat, which some studies suggest may reduce the risk of atherosclerosis.

Do you know any students of Mediterranean descent, such as those of Italian, Greek, or Turkish ancestry, who follow a diet based on the Mediterranean Pyramid? If so, what foods do they typically eat? Using the pyramid structure, make a diagram of your current food choices, with those you consume the most at the bottom and those you eat least at the top. How close is your diet to that recommended by the USDA Food Guide Pyramid? The Mediterranean Pyramid?

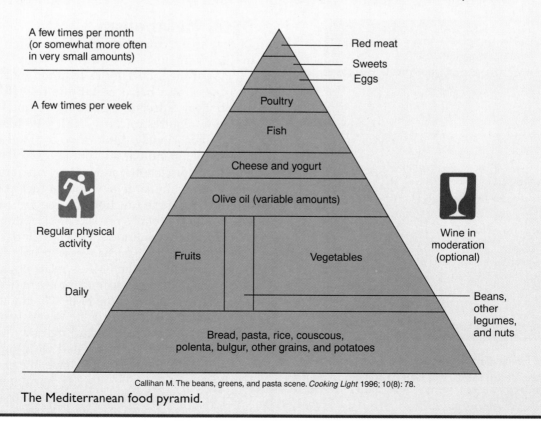

Callihan M. The beans, greens, and pasta scene. *Cooking Light* 1996; 10(8): 78.

The Mediterranean food pyramid.

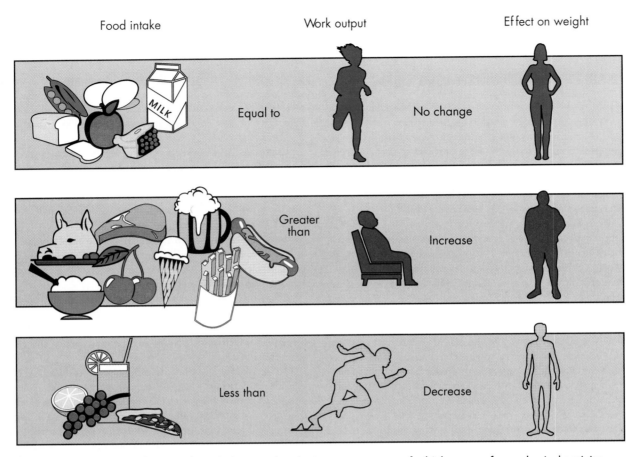

Food intake   Work output   Effect on weight

Equal to   No change

Greater than   Increase

Less than   Decrease

Figure 6-3   Caloric balance: caloric input equals caloric output, some of which comes from physical activity.

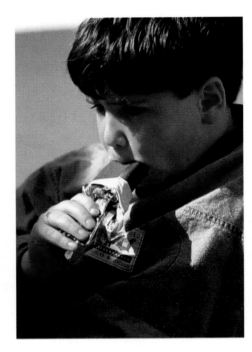

Unhealthful family dietary practices, such as reliance on fat-dense, calorie dense foods, can lead to childhood obesity.

Basal Metabolism

Of the three factors that determine caloric need, basal metabolism uses the highest proportion (50% to 70%) of the total calories required by each person. Expressed as a **basal metabolic rate (BMR),** basal metabolism reflects the minimum amount of energy the body requires to carry on all vital functions. You seldom consciously think of your blood circulation, respiration, glandular and brain activity, cellular metabolism, muscle tone, and body temperature as activities that require large amounts of fuel in the form of calories, but these functions do require energy. Even when you are totally relaxed or sleeping, these vital body functions continue to expend calories.

Basal metabolism changes as people age. For both males and females, the BMR is relatively high at birth and continues to increase until the age of two. Except for a slight rise at puberty, the BMR will gradually decline throughout the remainder of life. A variety of other variables also affect BMR, including body composition (muscular bodies are associated with higher BMRs), physical condition (fit people have higher BMRs), sex (males have 5% higher BMRs), hormone secretions (people with excessively active thyroid and adrenal glands have higher BMRs), sleep (BMRs are about 10%

Table 6-5   Calories Expended during Physical Activity

To determine the number of calories you have spent in an hour of activity, simply multiply the *calories per hour per pound* column by your weight (in pounds). For example, after an hour of archery, a 120-pound person will have expended 209 calories; a 160-pound person, 278 calories; and a 220-pound person, 383 calories.

Activity	Calories/Hour/Pound	Activity	Calories/Hour/Pound
Archery	1.74	Marching (rapid)	3.84
Baseball	1.86	Painting (outside)	2.10
Basketball	3.78	Playing music (sitting)	1.08
Boxing (sparring)	3.78	Racquetball	3.90
Canoeing (leisure)	1.20	Running (cross-country)	4.44
Cleaning	1.62	Running	
Climbing hills (no load)	3.30	11 min 30 sec per mile	3.66
Cooking	1.20	9 min per mile	5.28
Cycling		8 min per mile	5.64
5.5 mph	1.74	7 min per mile	6.24
9.4 mph	2.70	6 min per mile	6.84
Racing	4.62	5 min 30 sec per mile	7.86
Dance (modern)	2.28	Scrubbing floors	3.00
Eating (sitting)	0.60	Sailing	1.20
Field hockey	3.66	Skiing	
Fishing	1.68	Cross-country	4.43
Football	3.60	Snow, downhill	3.84
Gardening		Water	3.12
Digging	3.42	Skating (moderate)	2.28
Mowing	3.06	Soccer	3.54
Raking	1.44	Squash	5.76
Golf	2.34	Swimming	
Gymnastics	1.80	Backstroke	4.62
Handball	3.78	Breaststroke	4.44
Hiking	2.52	Free, fast	4.26
Horseback riding		Free, slow	3.48
Galloping	3.72	Butterfly	4.68
Trotting	3.00	Table tennis	1.86
Walking	1.14	Tennis	3.00
Ice hockey	5.70	Volleyball	1.32
Jogging	4.15	Walking (normal pace)	2.16
Judo	5.34	Weight training	1.90
Knitting (sewing)	0.60	Wrestling	5.10
Lacrosse	5.70	Writing (sitting)	0.78

lower during sleep), pregnancy (a 20% increase in BMR is typical, especially in the last trimester), body temperature (a 1° rise in body temperature increases BMR about 7%), and environmental temperature (deviations above and below 78° F result in increased BMRs).[7]

The most important variables related to BMR are aging, body composition, activity level, and caloric intake. For example, if people fail to recognize that BMR declines with aging, they might fail to adjust food intake accordingly and weight gain will occur. Also, for those who are thinner, the presence of lean tissue favors a higher basal metabolic rate with greater resistance to weight gain. Finally, an increase in physical activity will foster a faster BMR that will contribute to weight loss. In contrast, in those people with above-average levels of body fat, BMR rates are lower, thus providing the body with excess calories that will be stored as fat. If people restrict their caloric intake through dieting, their BMR will drop to a lower level, making weight loss increasingly harder to achieve. Use the formula in the Star Box on page 172 to determine your BMR and the approximate number of calories it requires.

basal metabolic rate (BMR)   the amount of energy (expressed in calories) the body requires to maintain basic functions.

Calculating Basal Metabolic Rate

The basal metabolic rate (BMR) reflects the amount of energy in calories (C) that your body requires to sustain basic functions. The formula below can be used to calculate your approximate basal metabolic rate.

$$\text{BMR per day} = 1\ C \times \frac{\text{body weight (lb)}}{2.2} \times 24$$

Example: 150-lb person

$$\text{BMR per day} = 1\ C \times \frac{150}{2.2} \times 24$$
$$= 1\ C \times 6.82 \times 24$$
$$= 1636.8\ C$$

This person would need approximately 1,637 calories to sustain the body at rest for an entire day. Activity of any kind, of course, elevates the requirement for calories.

NOTE: A woman's BMR would be approximately 5% lower than that of a man of the same age.

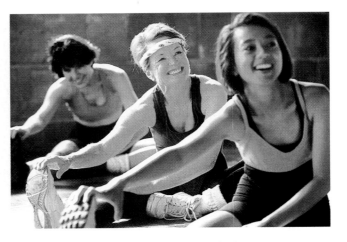

Engaging in regular physical activity is the key to maintaining optimal weight and body composition.

Thermic Effect of Food

Formerly called the *specific dynamic action of food,* or *dietary thermogenesis,* the thermic effect of food represents the energy our bodies require for the digestion, absorption, and transportation of food. This energy breaks the electrochemical bonds that hold complex food molecules together, resulting in smaller nutrient units that can be distributed throughout the body. This energy need is in addition to activity needs and basal metabolic needs. Researchers estimate that the thermic effect of food represents about 10 percent of our total energy needs.[7] Some nutritionists now consider the thermic effect of food merely a component of overall basal metabolism. This view is understandable, since the digestive process is a vital body function. Thus, some professionals categorize total energy needs into just two components: activity needs and basal metabolic needs.

Lifetime Weight Control

Obesity and frequent fluctuation in weight are clearly associated with higher levels of morbidity and mortality. Therefore, maintenance of weight and body composition at or near optimum levels is highly desirable. Although you may believe that this is a difficult goal to achieve, it is not unrealistic when begun early in life and from a starting point at or near optimum levels. You will need to draw on resources from each dimension of your health to maintain a lifestyle that fosters the maintenance of optimum weight and body composition. Keys to your success will include:

- **Exercise** Caloric expenditure through regular exercise, including cardiovascular exercise and strength training, is a key to maintaining optimum weight and body composition (see Chapter 4). For example, aerobic exercise is a particularly effective addition to a lifetime weight control program. This form of conditioning not only expends calories but also influences basal metabolic rate and trains the heart and lungs (see Chapter 4). The weight loss resulting from exercise, in comparison to dieting alone and dieting in combination with exercise, tends to be a smaller loss per unit of time, but more easily maintained. Clearly, dieting is not the most effective means of achieving and maintaining healthful weight loss.
- **Dietary modification** Meals planned around foods low in total fat and saturated fat and high in complex carbohydrates also play an important role in your ability to maintain optimum weight and body composition. Fresh fruits, vegetables, pastas, and, occasionally, lean meat such as skinless chicken and baked fish should be regular food choices (see the discussion of semivegetarianism in Chapter 5).
- **Lifestyle support** Not only must you be committed to a lifestyle featuring regular physical activity and careful food choices, but you must build a support group that will encourage you in these endeavors. Inform family, friends, classmates, and coworkers about your intent to rely on them for support and encouragement. Perhaps you will eventually serve as a role model for their involvement in a similar process.
- **Problem solving** Reevaluate your current approach to dealing with stressors. Replace any reliance on food as a coping mechanism with nonfood options, such as exercise or talking

Personal Assessment

Before undertaking a program, it is important to look at your past experiences and feelings about weight loss. Perhaps in doing so, you might decide that you would do better with other alternatives besides dieting.

Answer each of the following items with a "True" or "False" as it applies to you.

_____ 1. I am frustrated about my inability to stick to a diet.

_____ 2. I have less self-control than most dieters.

_____ 3. Most of the times I try to lose weight, I lose control and go off my diet.

_____ 4. When I try to develop a habit of regular exercise, something always interferes and I stop.

_____ 5. Exercise seems to be an ordeal to me.

_____ 6. I often feel tired during the day.

_____ 7. My weight has gone up and down several times when I go on and off diets.

_____ 8. My body seems to be getting thicker in the middle over the years.

_____ 9. My weight seems to be increasing over the years.

_____ 10. I find myself thinking about food more than I should.

_____ 11. I find myself thinking about my weight all through the day.

_____ 12. I feel there is probably no hope for my weight problem.

_____ 13. Sometimes I lose control and really binge on food.

_____ 14. I use food to make myself feel better when I am angry, nervous, or depressed.

_____ 15. Some people reject me as a friend because I am too heavy.

_____ 16. My social life is limited because of my weight.

_____ 17. My sex life is limited because of my weight.

_____ 18. Other people think I am unattractive because of my weight.

_____ 19. I put a lot of effort into choosing clothes that tend to cover up my weight problem.

To Carry This Further . . .

For those items that you answered as true, consider these recommendations:

Items 1, 2, and 3: Rather than going on a diet, why not try to reduce your fat intake by avoiding fried food and foods with added fat? Eat more low-fat foods, and make certain that your dairy products are low-fat and your meats are lean.

Items 4, 5, and 6: You need a gradual but regular exercise program. Check around your community, and identify a reputable program that has a proven success rate in helping others who have had a weight problem.

Items 7, 8, and 9: These items indicate the development of a weight problem that could truly be damaging your health. These are reasons for being serious about weight loss that go beyond appearance.

Items 10, 11, 12, 13, and 14: You may be into "living to eat" rather than "eating to live." Now is the time to give serious thought to what is important in your life, other than appearance-related needs.

Items 15, 16, and 17: Work at forming new relationships. Seek out people who are capable of looking beyond your physical appearance for those attributes that they will find to be attractive in you.

Items 18 and 19: As for 15 to 17, assess your current relationships. Put your efforts into relationships with people who seem capable of looking "inside" you, rather than only "at" you.

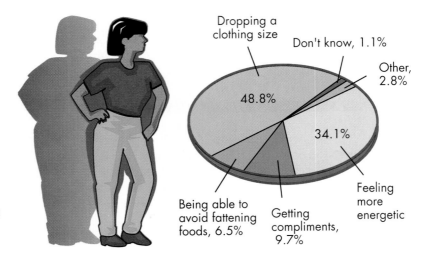

Figure 6-4   How do Americans measure success when it comes to losing weight? Most say dropping a clothing size is the best indicator that their diet is working.

with friends or family members. Additionally, your personal reward system may need to be reviewed to decrease the use of food as a reward for a job well done.

- **Redefinition of health**   You must develop the ability to think about health and wellness in a manner that recognizes the importance of proactivity (see Chapter 2) and involvement, rather than simply not becoming sick or incapacitated.

Assuming that you have an acceptable weight and body composition at this time, the lifestyle choices just suggested will make a significant contribution to the absence of a weight problem during your adult years. Aging will exert its effects to some degree on weight and body composition, but the damaging influences of poor dietary practices and a sedentary lifestyle will not be present.

Weight Management Techniques

For people who are already overweight, the need to reduce weight to attain their optimum weight and body composition will require intervention that in some ways may be different from the total lifestyle approach just described. However, upon reaching a more healthful weight and body composition, maintenance of that status will depend on adopting the lifestyle changes described. Remember that weight loss followed by weight gain may be less healthful (and certainly more frustrating) than maintaining body weight, even at levels above desirable. Complete the Personal Assessment on page 173 to determine whether you are a candidate for weight loss.

Weight loss occurs when energy taken into the body is less than that demanded by the body for physiological maintenance and voluntary activity. A number of approaches to weight loss can be pursued.

How do dieters know when they've succeeded? Figure 6-4 shows how Americans measure their progress at losing weight.

Dietary Alterations

A diet that reduces caloric intake is the most common approach to what seems to be a national obsession with weight loss. The choice of foods included in the diet and the amount of food that can be consumed are the two factors that distinguish the wide range of diets currently available. Unfortunately, dieting alone usually does not result in long-term weight loss. In fact, it is now recognized that weight lost through caloric restriction (dieting), regardless of the program format, is generally regained within 3 to 5 years and may foster binge eating in the process,[23] while weight lost through pharmacotherapy (see p. 178) is regained within 1 year of discontinuing medication. The Health Action Guide on page 175 provides suggestions for changing your eating patterns to increase your chances for long-term success.

Balanced Diets Supported by Portion Control

For nutritional health, a logical approach to weight loss and subsequent management of that loss is to establish a nutritionally sound balanced diet (low fat, low saturated fat, and high complex carbohydrate) that controls portions. This approach is best undertaken with nutritionists and physicians who are knowledgeable in diet management. After a study of your day-to-day energy needs, they can establish a diet designed to produce a gradual loss. A working understanding of portion size can be achieved using diet scales or through a nutrition education program in which realistic models of food servings are used. The Topics for Today article on page 190 takes a look at the "portion distortion" so prevalent in America. It also suggests ways you can control serving sizes.

A balanced diet–portion control approach to weight loss reflects a nutritionally sound program that offers some probability of success without the negative feature of forcing people to adapt to a restrictive approach to eating. People have extreme difficulty adjusting to a diet that presents them with uncommon foods. To people who need to lose weight, dieting is often bad enough without feeling that they must be deprived of foods that satisfy their emotional needs.

Fad Diets

People use a variety of fad diets in an attempt to achieve weight loss within a short time. These popular diets are often promoted in best-selling books written by celebrities or people who claim to be nutrition experts. With few exceptions, these approaches are both ineffective and potentially unhealthful. In addition, some require far greater expense than would be associated with weight loss or management techniques using portion control and regular physical activity. The pros and cons of a variety of popular diet plans are presented in Table 6-6.

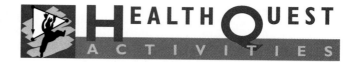

Low-Calorie Foods and Controlled Serving Sizes

Recently a variety of familiar foods have been developed in a reduced-calorie form. By lowering the carbohydrate content with the use of nonnutritive sweeteners, reducing the portion size, reducing the fat content of the original formulations, or removing fat entirely (see the discussion of Olestra in Chapter 5), manufacturers have produced "lite" versions of many food products. For example, many frozen entrees, such as Healthy Choice Oriental Beef with Vegetables (290 calories), Weight Watchers Lasagna Florentine (210 calories), and Healthy Choice Fettucine with Turkey and Vegetables (350 calories), are attractively low in calories. For some people who "lunch" on these entrees, satiety gives way to feelings of hunger by late afternoon, leading to snacking or, for some, even bingeing.

Controlled Fasting

In cases of extreme obesity, some patients are placed on a complete fast in a hospital setting. The patient is maintained on only water, electrolytes, and vitamins. Weight loss is profound because the body is quickly forced to begin **catabolizing** its fat and muscle tissue. Complete fasting is such an extreme approach to weight loss that it must be done in an institutional setting so that the patient can be closely monitored. Sodium loss, a negative nitrogen balance, and potassium loss are particular concerns.

Today some people regularly practice short periods of modified fasting. Solid foods are removed from

catabolizing the metabolic process of breaking down tissue for the purpose of converting it into energy.

Table 6-6 Advantages and Disadvantages of Selected Diets

Type of Diet	Advantages	Disadvantages	Examples
Limited food choice diets	Reduce the number of food choices made by the users Limited opportunity to make mistakes Almost certainly low in calories after the first few days	Deficient in many nutrients, depending on the foods allowed Monotonous—difficult to adhere to Eating out and eating socially are difficult Do not retrain dieters in acceptable eating habits Low long-term success rates No scientific basis for these diets	Banana and milk diet Fitonics for Life diet Kempner rice diet Lecithin, vinegar, kelp, and vitamin B_6 diet The New Beverly Hills Diet Fit for Life
Restricted-calorie, balanced food plans	Sufficiently low in calories to permit steady weight loss Nutritionally balanced Palatable Include readily available foods Reasonable in cost Can be adapted from family meals Permit eating out and social eating Promote a new set of eating habits	Do not appeal to people who want a "unique" diet Do not produce immediate and large weight losses	Weight Watchers Diet Prudent Diet (American Heart Association) Eating Thin for Life Lou Arrone's Weigh Less, Live Longer Fit or Fat Target Diet Take Off Pounds Sensibly (TOPS) Overeaters Anonymous
Fasting starvation diet	Rapid initial loss	Nutrient deficient Danger of ketosis >60% loss is muscle <40% loss is fat Low long-term success rate	ZIP Diet 5-Day Miracle Diet
High-carbohydrate diets	Emphasize grains, fruits, and vegetables High in bulk Low in cholesterol	Limit milk, meat Nutritionally very inadequate for calcium, iron, and protein	Quick Weight Loss Diet Pritikin Diet Hilton Head Metabolism Diet
High-protein, low-carbohydrate diets Usually include all the meat, fish, poultry, and eggs you can eat Occasionally permit milk and cheese in limited amounts Prohibit fruits, vegetables, and any bread or cereal products	Rapid initial weight loss because of diuretic effect Very little hunger Proponents contend that low carbohydrate intake prevents an exaggerated insulin response that fosters fat formation	Too low in carbohydrates Deficient in many nutrients—vitamin C, vitamin A (unless eggs are included), calcium, and several trace elements High in saturated fat, cholesterol, and total fat Extreme diets of this type could cause death Impossible to adhere to these diets long enough to lose any appreciable amount of weight Dangerous for people with kidney disease Weight lost, which is largely water, is rapidly regained Expensive Unpalatable after first few days Difficult for dieter to eat out	Dr. Stillman's Quick Weight Loss Diet Calories Don't Count by Dr. Taller Dr. Atkin's New Diet Revolution Scarsdale Diet Air Force Diet The Carbohydrate Addict's Life Span Program The Zone Mastering the Zone Diet Sugar Busters

Table 6-6 *Continued*

Type of Diet	Advantages	Disadvantages	Examples
Low-calorie, high-protein supplement diets			
Usually a premeasured powder to be reconstituted with water or a prepared liquid formula	Rapid initial weight loss Easy to prepare—already measured Palatable for first few days Usually fortified to provide recommended amount of micronutrients Must be labeled if >50% protein	Usually prescribed at dangerously low calorie intake of 300 to 500 cal Overpriced Low in fiber and bulk—constipating in short amount of time	Metracal Diet Cambridge Diet Liquid Protein Diet Last Chance Diet Oxford Diet
High-fiber, low-calorie diets			
	High satiety value Provide bulk	Irritating to the lower colon Decreases absorption of trace elements, especially iron Nutritionally deficient Low in protein	Pritikin Diet F Diet Zen Macrobiotic Diet
Protein-sparing modified fats			
<50% protein: 400 cal	Safe under supervision High-quality protein Minimize loss of lean body mass	Decreases BMR Monotonous Expensive	Optifast Medifast
Premeasured food plans			
	Provides prescribed portion sizes—little chance of too small or too large a portion Total food programs Some provide adequate calories (1,200) Nutritionally balanced or supplemented	Expensive Do not retrain dieters in acceptable eating habits Preclude eating out or social eating Often low in bulk Monotonous Low long-term success rates	Nutri-System Carnation Plan

the diet for a number of days. Fruit juices, water, supplements, and vitamins are used to minimize the risks associated with total fasting. However, unsupervised short-term fasting can be dangerous and is not generally recommended.

In addition to the controlled fasting just discussed, a somewhat different version of this practice is appearing with the long-term use of readily available, low-calorie, nutrient-dense food supplementation products such as Ensure, Boost, SlimFast, and Sustical. Regardless of whether they are marketed as nutrient-dense supplements for older adults or as adjuncts to weight loss diets, these drinks should not be viewed, or used, as meal replacements. Because these products contain no more than 400 calories (and the lite versions contain as few as 200 calories), their routine use as meal replacements could move even a young, healthy college student dangerously close to caloric inadequacy in a short time. Perhaps if used in place of a high-calorie snack or as a very occasional substitute for lunch, these supplements may not present the dangers that their routine use does.

Self-Help Weight Reduction Programs

In virtually every area of the country, at least one version of the popular commercial weight reduction programs, such as TOPS (Take Off Pounds Sensibly), Jenny Craig, and Nutri-System Weight Loss Centers, can be found. Popularized by Weight Watchers, these programs generally feature a format consisting of (1) a well-balanced diet emphasizing portion control and low-fat, low-saturated fat, and high–complex carbohydrate foods, (2) realistic weight loss goals to be attained over a reasonable period of time, (3) encouragement from supportive leaders and fellow group members, (4) emphasis on regular physical activity, and (5) a weight management program (follow-up program). The Health Action Guide on page 178 presents some guidelines for choosing a commercial weight loss program.

Although in theory these programs offer an opportunity to lose weight for people who cannot or will not participate in an activity program, their effectiveness is very limited. The minimal success of these

HEALTH ACTION GUIDE

Evaluating a Weight Loss Program

A reputable weight loss program will:

- Never promise or encourage quick weight loss
- Require a preenrollment physical examination
- Warn clients of the risk of developing health problems related to their weight loss, such as ketosis and diabetes-related complications
- Never promise a high level of success in achieving and maintaining weight loss

InfoLinks

www.shapeup.org

programs and the difficulty that working women have in attending meetings has resulted in falling enrollment and the development of home-based programs, such as those developed by hospital-based wellness programs, many YMCAs and YWCAs, and even Weight Watchers. Further, these programs are costly, especially when the program markets its own food products, when compared with self-directed approaches.

The Weight Loss Industry

In response to our nation's near obsession with thinness, a thriving weight loss industry exists to assist us in our attempts to lose weight. In 1990 a U.S. House of Representatives committee investigating questionable practices in the weight loss industry reported that Americans were spending $32 billion a year on various products and services in the quest for thinness.[24] A breakdown of this staggering sum indicated that $11.4 billion was spent on diet soft drinks alone. The weight loss industry, represented by a wide variety of programs and products, earned $9.9 billion, and health spas and exercise club memberships cost $8.5 billion. In addition to these expenditures, Americans spent $1.6 billion on luxury spas and $1 billion on artificial sweeteners. The most recent estimates (1995) suggest that Americans are spending in excess of $50 billion each year in an attempt to achieve and maintain weight loss.

The financial success of the weight loss industry in this country has in part been due to its effective television advertising. Skillfully produced commercials featuring successful program members suggest likely success for the viewer willing to sign on. Before 1994, these commercials were regular fare on daytime television. Today, however, commercials for diet programs such as Jenny Craig, Nutri-System, Weight Watchers, and others are considerably more restrained in their messages about success. Under directives issued by the FTC, today's advertisements can-

not misrepresent program performance. They must disclose that most weight loss is temporary, and they now inform the viewer that their loss will most likely not approximate that of the successful subjects featured in their commercials.

Most recently some nationally franchised weight loss programs have added a "medical" component to their format that involves prescribing medications. Consumers should be cautious in questioning the extent to which their medical supervision will be a regular component of the program rather than a brief, one-time physician visit involving little more than basic screening.

When people join these "enhanced" programs they should be certain that the medical evaluation and follow-up necessary for appropriate use of these prescription medications is of high quality. Time will tell, of course, whether this concern is justified.

Physical Intervention

A second approach to weight loss involves techniques and products designed to alter basic eating patterns.

Hunger/Satiety-Influencing Drugs

One of the fondest wishes of overweight people is to lose the desire to eat or to feel that they have had enough to eat. Today some OTC and prescription medications are being used or developed in an attempt to achieve these outcomes.

At this time, some appetite suppressants containing **phenylpropanolamine (PPA)** may still be sold in supermarkets and drugstores. The drug is clearly dangerous for some people. People with high blood pressure, thyroid problems, diabetes, depression, or glaucoma should not use PPA. In addition, PPA can interact with other medications to produce dangerous side effects.

The FDA has recently voiced concern about the use of the drug ephedrine (sometimes sold as *ma huong* and Chinese ephedra) in more than 200 over-the-counter (OTC) weight loss products, cold medicines, and energy-promoting products. Ephedrine has been associated with heart attacks and strokes. An FDA advisory panel is expected to recommend that no more than 24 mg of ephedrine per day (8 mg per dose) be taken.[25]

Through the 1980s and into the 1990s, two prescription medications, *fenfluramine* and *phentermine*, played an important role in the medical management of obesity. Both medications affect levels of serotonin, the neurotransmitter associated with satiety, thus producing feelings of fullness. Routinely used in combination as *fen-phen* (or phen-fen), these two medications were the "darlings" of physician-operated weight loss clinics until initial concerns centered on complications in people with angina, glaucoma, and hypertension were extended to include the rare but lethal condition known as *pulmonary hypertension.*

In the mid-1990s, a new serotonin-specific weight loss medication, *dexfenfluramine* (Redux), was approved for use in the United States. Results among patients who used the drug, in combination with dietary modification and exercise, seemed impressive. Unfortunately, a public primarily interested in only a pharmacotherapeutic approach to weight loss (without significant lifestyle changes) sought an even more effective "answer," and the weight loss clinics responded by combining dexfenfluramine (Redux) with fenfluramine. This combination, however, proved unexpectedly dangerous. In May 1997, the Mayo Clinic and other institutions reported they were seeing an increasing number of patients with serious heart valve damage who had no history of heart disease. In some cases the damage was so significant that the only alternative was heart valve replacement surgery. Epidemiological studies indicated that this damage was associated with the use of fenfluramine and dexfenfluramine, particularly in combination.[26] In September 1997 the FDA requested a voluntary recall of both medications by their manufacturers, and this request was honored.[27] Today neither drug is available.

At the time of this writing, weight loss clinics, including some nationally franchised programs that have adopted a "medical" component, have begun offering phentermine in combination with serotonin reuptake-inhibitory antidepressants, such as Prozac. Users of this combination should be aware that phentermine was never intended to be used for more than three months and that the use of antidepressants for weight loss is an "off-label" use, meaning that no specific research attesting to their appropriateness has been submitted to and approved by the FDA.

Nonhunger/Nonsatiety-Influencing Drugs

Although not approved by the FDA for general use, two interesting new pharmaceutical agents for reducing excessive weight and body fat have been identified. The first of these is Xenical (Orlistat). Unlike Redux (dexfenfluramine), which affects neurotransmitters that signal satiety, Xenical reduces fat absorption in the small intestine by about 30 percent. The drug is intended for people who are 20 percent or more above ideal weight and could cause a 10 percent loss of body weight without significant dietary restriction. Final FDA approval for Xenical is anticipated in 1999. In an attempt to build excitement about this drug on the part of practitioners and the public, its manufacturer began promotional activities even though the drug had received only a recommendation for approval by an FDA advisory committee. On dis-

covering this activity, the FDA ordered the manufacturer to cease all such promotional efforts.[28]

The second pharmaceutical agent for the medical management of obesity, sibutramine (brand name Meridia), gained FDA approval in November 1997. Sibutramine functions as a serotonin reuptake inhibitor, as did fenfluramine and dexfenfluramine, thus enhancing satiety. Unlike dexfenfluramine, however, sibutramine does not cause excessive production of serotonin in other areas of the nervous system. In addition, sibutramine retards the reuptake of norepinephrine, a second neurotransmitter that influences eating behavior. When combining Meridia with a reduced-calorie diet, a person with a BMI of 27 or greater should experience a weight loss of 10 to 15 pounds in 12 months, depending on dosage. Although Meridia may increase blood pressure in some users, it appears to be unrelated to the development of pulmonary hypertension or valvular heart disease, as was the case with fenfluramine and dexfenfluramine.[29]

Surgical Measures

When weight loss is imperative and the initial level of obesity is great, surgical intervention may be considered. A gastric resection is a major operation in which a portion of the small intestine is bypassed in an attempt to decrease the body's ability to absorb nutrients. Although the procedure can produce substantial loss of body weight, it is associated with many unpleasant and dangerous side effects (including diarrhea and liver damage) and various nutritional deficiencies. Not only is surgery required for this approach, but lifetime medical management is also necessary.

Gastroplasty (stomach stapling) is a surgical procedure that involves sealing off about half of the stomach with surgical staples. Once the procedure has been completed, the reduced capacity of the stomach decreases the amount of food that can be processed at any one time. As a result, patients feel full more quickly after eating a small meal. This procedure is reversible but carries the risks associated with surgery and the costs of a major surgical procedure.

Liposuction, or *lipoplasty,* is another form of surgical weight loss management. During this surgical procedure, a physician inserts a small tube through the skin and vacuums away adipose tissue. This procedure is generally used for stubborn, localized pockets of fat and is usually appropriate for people under the age of forty. Liposuction is more a cosmetic procedure than a general

phenylpropanolamine (PPA) (fen ill pro pan **ol** ah meen) the active chemical compound still found in some over-the-counter diet products.

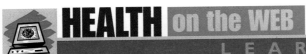

HEALTH on the **WEB**

L E A R N I N G   A C T I V I T I E S

Estimating Your Future Weight

Obesity and repeated weight loss and gain are linked to higher levels of disease. Thus it's important to maintain a healthy weight and body composition as you grow older. Remember, weight gain is not an inevitable part of aging! Go to www.healthyideas.com/weight/what_will_you to complete a quiz that tests your eating habits. The quiz will estimate how much you will weigh a year from today. If your results indicated unwanted weight gain, what can you do right now to prevent it?

Improving Your Body Image

In our image-conscious society, some people struggle continually with their weight and body image. Two serious disorders associated with such difficulties are anorexia nervosa and bulimia. In addition, compulsive exercising, compulsive eating, and other disorders are also cause for concern. Only a qualified professional can determine whether someone has a medically serious problem with body image. But Dr. Katharine Phillips has

developed a screening test that can help you understand your feelings about your appearance. Exploring your feelings is a good first step toward improving your body image. Go to www.homearts.com/depts/health/12bodqz1.htm and answer the nine questions on Dr. Phillips's questionnaire. Do you feel good about your body? What specific steps can you take to improve your body image?

Uncovering Diet and Exercise Myths

The more you know about diet and exercise, the more empowered you'll be to practice healthy behaviors in these areas. Sometimes, however, misconceptions about nutrition and physical activity can lead you down the wrong path. To see whether you're on the right track, go to www.nppc.org/CONS/HEALTH/mythquiz1.html and complete the "Dieting and Exercising Myths" quiz. Did anything surprise you?

For more activities, log on to our Online Learning Center at www.mhhe.com/hper/health/payne

---

approach to weight loss. Along with unrealistic expectations, the risks of infection, pain and discomfort, bruising, swelling, discoloration, abscesses, and unattractive changes in body contours are possible outcomes of liposuction. Consequently, people considering this procedure should carefully investigate all aspects of it, including the training and experience of the surgeon, to determine whether it is appropriate.

Acupuncture

Acupuncture is being used by an increasing number of American physicians as a treatment for obesity, as well as for a variety of other health problems. The appearance of acupuncture rings and earrings in drugstores, novelty shops, and in association with "one stop" weight loss/smoking abatement sessions advertised in the newspapers and held at local hotels suggests that the procedure has moved into the nonprofessional domain. Most people who receive acupuncture for the treatment of obesity are, fortunately, in the hands of fully trained practitioners. However, questions remain about its effectiveness, particularly in light of the difficulty of using **double-blind studies** to investigate techniques that employ the insertion of needles. At the time of this writing, the National Center for Complementary and Alternative Medicine, on the basis of a carefully controlled study, has found acupuncture effective for the discomfort associated with chemotherapy, surgical anesthesia, the pain associated with pregnancy and surgery, and several musculoskeletal conditions.[30] The effectiveness of acupuncture as a therapy for weight reduction has not yet been established.

Behavior Change Strategies

Several approaches designed to change learned eating patterns, such as *behavior modification,* aversive conditioning, and hypnosis, have been tried by people who want to lose weight. Because of the relatively small number of people involved in many of these approaches and the limited extent to which they have been scientifically studied, it is difficult to assess their long-term effectiveness. Nevertheless, they remain as alternatives to the approaches already described.

Personal Applications

• If you have ever tried to lose weight, what methods did you use? Were any of these methods potentially dangerous?

Weight Management: A Lifelong, Lifestyle-Based Approach

A recent study of weight loss conducted for the FDA showed that nearly 50 percent of American adults are attempting to lose weight through dieting. Most are able to lose weight, but very few are able to maintain their weight loss. Regardless of the weight loss method used, most people regain all of the lost weight within five years.[24] Further, in too many instances, the newly established weight is actually higher than the initial weight. This tendency for peo-

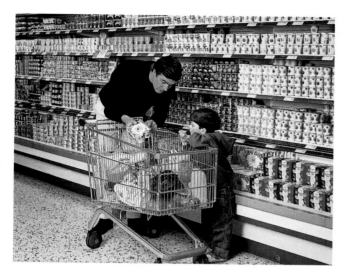

Successful lifelong weight management should involve the entire family in making food choices and participating in physical activity.

ple to lose weight only to end up heavier and then attempt to diet again is the yo-yo syndrome discussed earlier in the chapter. In addition, once widely used medications, fenfluramine and dexfenfluramine, are no longer available, whereas new medications are yet to be approved or have only very recently become available. Surgical intervention, of course, is limited to people with morbid obesity.

If we were to recommend a single approach to weight management that would, in theory, offer the maximum chance for success, we would suggest a program that combines healthful eating and aerobic exercise (as described in Chapter 4). Specifically, the program would have the following features:

- A varied, balanced approach to eating emphasizing portion control and low-fat, low-saturated fat, high-complex carbohydrate food items would be developed; with necessary modifications, the diet would be adopted by the entire family.
- Reasonable short-term weight loss goals and weight loss maintenance goals would be established at the beginning of the program and assessed regularly during its lifelong course.
- A well-planned (even professionally planned) aerobic fitness component would be developed and implemented as a part of this lifestyle-based undertaking. An appropriate weight training component would also be included. A familywide commitment to regular aerobic activity (walking, hiking, rollerblading, biking) would be even more helpful.
- The family would participate and serve as a source of encouragement for those members

who were having the most difficulty adapting to the lifestyle pattern required for success.

Physical Activity

The emphasis placed on a physical activity component in the model just described reflects our support of the many experts who now believe that the most important component of a weight-loss program is regular physical activity. Physical activity contributes to weight loss and the maintenance of weight loss because activity burns calories. It is important to remember that the need for calories decreases with age and with decreased activity.

At one time it was thought that physical activity could stimulate a twelve- to twenty-four-hour period of sustained elevation of the BMR. This elevated BMR was thought to result in more calories being burned, even after moderate exercise was completed. It is now thought that a more likely interval of BMR elevation after moderate exercise is two or three hours.[31] Regardless of the time factor, any period of elevation is a time of greater calorie expenditure.

An additional benefit derived from physical activity is that proportionately more fat is lost than is lost through dieting alone. Studies suggest that the weight loss achieved through physical activity is 95 percent fat and 5 percent lean tissue, such as muscle, in comparison with a loss of 75 percent fat and 25 percent lean tissue when dieting alone is used. Exercise also offers the benefits of increased heart and lung endurance, muscular strength, and flexibility.

Personal Applications

- If you have a weight problem, do you agree or disagree that you have a responsibility to yourself and to others to reduce your weight?

Eating Disorders

Perhaps it is not surprising that some people have medically identifiable, potentially serious difficulties with body image, body weight, and food selection.

acupuncture the insertion of fine needles into the body to alter electroenergy fields and cure disease.

double-blind study a scientific study in which both the researchers and the study participants are said to be "blind" because neither group knows the makeup of the test and control groups during the actual course of the experiment; this information is revealed only at the study's conclusion.

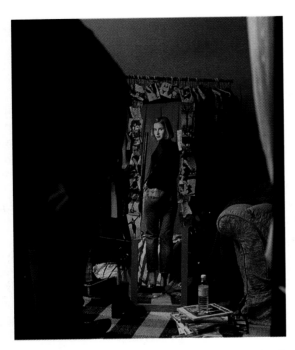

Poor body image and unmet emotional needs can lead to an eating disorder.

Among these disorders are two that are frequently seen among college students, anorexia nervosa and bulimia. In addition, compulsive exercising, compulsive eating, and disorders involving various combinations of anorexic and bulimic practices are also found in college populations. We have included these topics in the chapter on weight management because most eating disorders begin with dieting. However, most eating disorders also involve inappropriate food choices, as well as deep emotional needs. Those issues are discussed in Chapters 2 and 5.

Anorexia Nervosa

A young woman, competitive and perfectionistic by nature, determines that her weight (and appearance) is unacceptable. She begins to diet, often in conjunction with exercise, until she reaches a point at which she *appears* to be disregarding her appetite and her food consumption has virtually ceased.

The young woman in this description may be seen by her friends or roommates as active and intelligent and simply dieting and exercising with an unusual degree of commitment. Eventually, however, they observe that her food consumption has nearly stopped. Her weight loss has continued beyond the point that is pleasing—at least to others. Her growing frailness combined with noticeable changes in her hair and skin cause them to feel uncomfortable whenever they are around her. Nevertheless, her activity level remains high. When questioned about her weight loss, she says that she still needs to lose more weight.

This person is suffering from a medical condition called **anorexia nervosa** (see the Star Box on page 183). This self-induced starvation is life threatening in 5 percent to 20 percent of cases. The stunning amount of weight that some people with anorexia nervosa lose—up to 50 percent of their body weight—eventually leads to failure of the heart, lungs, and kidneys.

As weight loss-oriented as this condition seems, experts believe that the person with anorexia nervosa is attempting to meet a much deeper need for control. Specifically, in a family setting in which much is expected of the individual but little opportunity for self-directed behavior is provided, control over the body becomes a need-fulfilling tool.[32] Eventually, however, a normal body image is lost and the condition progresses as just described. Fortunately, psychological intervention in combination with medical and dietary support can return the person with anorexia nervosa to a more life-sustaining pattern of eating. Thus the person with anorexia needs to receive the care of professionals experienced in the treatment of anorexia nervosa. If others, including friends, coworkers, dorm mates, and parents, observe this condition, they should secure immediate assistance.

The prevalence of anorexia nervosa (and bulimia nervosa as well) has been very low in men as compared with women. Today, however, the incidence of both conditions is increasing in men as they begin to feel some of the same pressures that women feel to conform to the weight and body composition standards imposed by others. The "lean look" of young male models serves as a standard for more and more young men, whereas the requirements to "make weight" for various sports drives others. In the latter group, runners, wrestlers, jockies, and gymnasts frequently must lose weight quickly to meet particular standards for competition or the expectations of coaches and trainers. Life changes, such as the end of a relationship, the loss of employment, or the diagnosis of illness, can also stimulate the development of an eating disorder in men and women alike.

Researchers report that men are even less inclined than women to admit that they may have an eating disorder. Thus they are even less likely to seek treatment. In addition, physicians are still not as likely to suspect eating disorders in men as they are to suspect them in women.

Bulimia Nervosa

Bulimia nervosa reflects a dietary pattern in which people gorge themselves with food. When people practice a pattern of excessive eating followed by **purging,** they are said to suffer from *bulimarexia.* Most often, however, the term *bulimia* or *bulimia nervosa* is used to describe this binge/purge pattern. This condition, like anorexia nervosa, can lead to weight loss,

⭐ **Recognizing Anorexia Nervosa and Bulimia Nervosa**

The American Psychological Association uses the following diagnostic criteria to identify anorexia nervosa and bulimia.

Anorexia
- 15% or more below desirable weight
- Fear of weight gain
- Altered body image
- Three or more missed menstrual periods (younger women may never menstruate)

Bulimia
- Binge eating two or more times a week for three months
- A lack of control over bingeing
- Purging
- Concern about body image

Characteristic symptoms include the following. However, it is unlikely that all the symptoms will be evident in any one individual.

Anorexia
- Looks thin and keeps getting thinner
- Skips meals, cuts food into small pieces, moves food around plate to appear to have eaten

- Loss of menstrual periods
- Wears "layered look" in an attempt to disguise weight loss
- Loss of hair from the head
- Growth of fine hair on face, arms, and chest
- Extreme sensitivity to cold

Bulimia
- Bathroom use immediately after eating
- Inconspicuous eating
- Excessive time (and money) spent food shopping
- Shopping for food at several stores rather than one store
- Menstrual irregularities
- Excessive constipation
- Swollen and/or infected salivary glands, sore throat
- Bursting blood vessels in the eyes
- Damaged teeth and gums
- Dehydration and kidney dysfunction

but it differs in terms of the person's personality and specific behavioral patterns and the prospects for successful treatment. As with anorexics, most people with bulimia nervosa are young women, although the incidence in men is growing.

People with bulimia nervosa lose weight or maintain their weight not because they stop eating, but because they eat and then purge their digestive system by vomiting or using laxatives. Syrup of ipecac, a product used to help poisoning victims vomit, is so frequently abused by bulimics that efforts are under way to make this a prescription drug. In some situations, the "purge" does not occur by regurgitating undigested food, but rather takes the form of extensive exercise to expend calories or the use of diuretics (water pills) to lower scale weight through dehydration.

Compared with anorexics, bulimics tend to be extroverted, socially active, and less perfectionistic. A person's bulimia nervosa may be indicated to others primarily by the inconsistency between high food intake and concurrent weight loss. In the mid-1980s, medical experts estimated that as many as 19 percent of eighteen- to twenty-two-year-old women developed all the principal symptoms of bulimia as they were understood at the time. More recent estimates have dramatically lowered this estimate to less than 2 percent as more demanding clinical criteria were applied.

People with bulimia nervosa may gorge themselves with food (10,000 calories or more at a sitting) and then quietly disappear, only to return later seem-

ingly unaffected by the huge amount of food they recently ate. In all likelihood, they have quickly and quietly regurgitated the food. Like anorexics (although it is often unapparent to others), people with bulimia nervosa may demonstrate an extreme sensitivity to food. Thus they have many food likes and dislikes. This suggests that they have not managed to suppress their hunger. Bulimics feel hungry, overeat, and then resolve their guilt by vomiting or abusing laxatives.

Binge Eating

Although binge eating is only a component of bulimia nervosa, for some people binge eating, without a subsequent purge, constitutes their unique form of eating disorder. As the name implies, people who binge eat periodically consume large quantities of food in a short time. Whether called *bulimia,* "eating

---

anorexia nervosa   a disorder of emotional origin in which appetite and hunger are suppressed, and marked weight loss occurs.

bulimia nervosa   a disorder of emotional origin in which binge eating patterns are established; usually accompanied by purging.

purging   using vomiting or laxatives to remove undigested food from the body.

disorder not otherwise specified," or *binge-eating disorder,* this disorder also requires intervention and effective treatment.

The psychodynamic underlying binge eating may not differ greatly from those associated with other eating disorders. Feelings of fear, anxiety, depression, loss of control, and low self-esteem may cause people with this disorder to begin consuming food as a means of feeling in control over their current feeling state. The treatment of this eating disorder involves interventions similar to those described for bulimia nervosa.

Compulsive Exercise and Compulsive Eating

The compulsive nature of some people's exercising or eating patterns suggests a slightly different version of the two principal eating disorders. More than likely, a wide array of causes can account for both of these behavior patterns. In the case of compulsive exercise, in which a person may exercise several times daily for as many as six hours, a desire for control may exist much as it does in anorexia nervosa. In contrast, compulsive eating, in which people eat every time food is available, may be using food to reduce feelings of insecurity and stress. Again, concerns about body image and efforts at dieting may be the starting point for both of these behavior patterns. As in the more classic eating disorders, family members and friends should not fail to identify and respond to these conditions.

Treatment for Eating Disorders

The treatment of anorexia nervosa and bulimia nervosa is a complex and demanding undertaking. The components of therapy, drawn from medical and behavioral sciences, involve the cooperation of several health care providers. Each case of anorexia or bulimia must be approached from an individual perspective. The Star Box above lists resources for people with eating disorders.

The initial physical care for anorexia most often begins with hospitalization of the individual to stabilize the physical deterioration associated with starvation. Nasogastric tubes and intravenous feedings are sometimes necessary, particularly when the patient will not (or cannot) eat. In addition, medications, including serotonin reuptake-inhibiting antidepressants, such as Prozac, are often used to decrease obsessive-compulsive behavior, reduce anxiety, and improve mood. Medications can also be prescribed to improve appetite.

The psychological and familial components underlying anorexia nervosa require a variety of therapeutic approaches. Behavior modification, including eating contracts, is employed, as is psychotherapy in both individual and group formats. Nutritional counseling and family therapy counseling complete the therapy.[33]

Treatment for bulimia nervosa involves individual, family, and nutritional counseling. Unlike treatment for anorexia, however, bulimia treatment does not usually involve hospitalization. People with eating disorders need professional assistance. Unfortunately, the assistance available for treating bulimia appears to be somewhat less effective than that available to people with anorexia nervosa. This may relate to the difficulty of dealing effectively with the lack of control experienced by the bulimic.

Underweight

For some young adults, the lack of adequate body weight, called **underweight,** is a serious concern. Particularly for those who have inherited an ectomorphic body build (tall, narrow shoulders and hips, and a tendency toward thinness), attempts to gain weight are routinely undertaken, often with limited success.

HEALTH ACTION GUIDE

Weight Management Tips

Tips for Weight Loss

• You probably didn't gain your excessive weight eating alone. Seek the encouragement and support of family and friends in your weight loss efforts.

• Eat only at the table. Leave the table immediately after finishing your meal. And by all means never take your meal with you into other rooms of the house.

• Stop eating after one serving. A second helping may contribute more fat and calories than your diet can afford.

• If you must snack between meals, choose small, nutritious, low-fat snacks.

• Stay away from the kitchen. An innocent look into the refrigerator will almost certainly lead to a taste, a snack, or even a meal.

Tips for Weight Gain

• Make certain that there is no medical reason for your thinness.

• Have your current dietary practices evaluated so that appropriate modifications can be made.

• Begin a moderate exercise program to enhance your physical fitness.

• Incorporate the following recommendations into your dietary practice:

  • Substitute juice, soup, or hot chocolate for coffee.
  • Eat a healthy breakfast.
  • Learn appropriate portion sizes.
  • Replace junk foods with more healthy foods.

InfoLinks
www.weight.com

If these people are to be successful in gaining weight, they must discover an effective way to take in more calories than they burn (see the Health Action Guide on this page).

Nutritionists believe that the healthiest way to gain weight is to increase the intake of "calorie-dense" food. These foods are characterized by high fat density resulting from high levels of vegetable fats (polyunsaturated fats). Particularly good foods in this regard are dried fruits, bananas, nuts, granola, and cheeses made from low-fat milk. The current recommendation is to eat three calorie-dense meals of moderate size per day, interspersed with two or three substantial snacks. Using the Food Guide Pyramid shown on page 132, one should eat the higher number of recommended servings for each group.[34]

A second component of weight gain for those who are underweight is an exercise program that uses weight training activities intended to increase muscle mass. For all the reasons detailed in Chapter 4, the use of anabolic drugs in the absence of highly competent medical supervision has no role in healthful weight gain. In addition, carefully monitored aerobic activity should be undertaken in sessions adequate to maintain heart-lung health, while at the same time one should restrict unnecessary activity that expends calories.

For those who cannot gain weight in spite of having tried the preceding approaches, a medical evaluation could supply an explanation for being underweight. If no medical explanation can be found, the person must begin to accept the reality of his or her unique body type.

A Final Thought About Health and Weight Management

Recognizing the attention placed on physical attractiveness and its relationship to thinness, it is important to ask yourself if you are healthy enough to live comfortably with a body that probably does not (or will not always) compare favorably with the ideal. As you recall

---

underweight   a condition in which body weight is below desirable weight.

Real Life
Real choices

1. What are the hazards of controlling weight using Jeff's method?
2. How could Jeff change his eating patterns so he can maintain his wrestling weight without compromising his health?

3. What are the possible disadvantages of power bars, sports drinks, and other preparations that are designed for athletes in training?

from Chapter 1, your authors encourage the development of resourcefulness in every dimension of health, not simply the physical dimension. We hope that a high enough level of self-esteem grounded in your own respect for your feelings, beliefs, interpersonal skills, intellect, and sense of contribution and stewardship will more than offset the absence of perfect alignment with a body image that is obtainable by only a few.

Summary

- Recent studies confirm that Americans are becoming heavier and are more likely to be obese at all age levels. Changes in daily activity and caloric intake patterns have occurred since 1980.
- A variety of chronic health problems are caused or worsened by excessive weight.
- In a society that values thinness, body weight has a powerful effect on self-image and self-esteem. The physical characteristics of high fashion models clearly differ from those of the average American woman.
- Various standards (and names) can be used in defining types of obesity. All forms of obesity, however, relate to the existence of a positive caloric balance leading to an excessive accumulation of fat. Some people may be excessively heavy but not be overly fat.
- By midlife the majority of adults are overweight if not obese.
- Obesity and overweight can be measured (or determined) in a variety of ways, including height-weight tables, body mass index, waist-to-hip ratio, skinfold measurements, electrical impedance, and hydrostatic weighing.
- Theories regarding the cause of obesity focus on factors from within the individual and from the environment. Many complex theories exist regarding the role of inheritance, set point, body type, infant feeding patterns, pregnancy, aging, externality, family eating patterns, and inactivity.
- Current interest is high regarding obesity genes and the role of leptin in moderating caloric intake. The set point theory of energy regulation and its relationship to yo-yo dieting has been recently questioned. The role of brown fat remains of interest in current attempts to explain why some

people are more capable of expending calories while others quickly store extra calories.
- The body's energy needs arise from three functions: BMR, activity, and the thermic effect of food.
- A person's body type may play an important role in determining the extent to which excessive weight is gained. Infant feeding patterns may contribute to the development of excessive fat cells and hypercellular obesity. Moderate weight gain is closely associated with hypertrophic obesity.
- A well-managed pregnancy should not lead to excessive weight gain.
- A sense of externality may contribute to excessive caloric intake.
- Caloric balance influences weight gain, loss, and maintenance.
- Maintenance of weight and body composition is based on a lifetime commitment to a healthful diet, regular exercise, dietary modification, a support system, enhanced problem-solving abilities, and redefinition of the role of health in living.
- Weight management can be attempted through a variety of techniques, including dieting, dietary alteration, controlled fasting, and membership in a weight reduction program.
- Commercial weight reduction programs are highly visible players in a weight loss industry whose total earnings exceed $50 billion per year. Claims regarding success have been moderated by FTC directives.
- Although many people can lose some weight through dieting, very few who do so are able to maintain that weight loss.
- Physical intervention into weight loss and subsequent weight management may take the form

of surgery, new prescription medications, or complementary medical practices, such as acupuncture and hypnosis. The use of newly introduced prescription medications must be regarded as only one component of the long-term treatment of obesity as a chronic illness.

- Surgical approaches to weight reduction exist, but their use is limited to severe obesity and localized cosmetic changes.
- A combination approach involving low-fat, low-saturated fat, high-complex carbohydrate foods, portion-controlled dieting, and exercise may be the most effective way to lose weight. The effect of exercise on raising the body's basal metabolic rate may not be as extensive as once thought.
- Potentially serious eating disorders result, in part, from concerns about weight and body image. Eating disorders usually begin with dieting but are often sustained in an attempt to meet deeper needs.
- Although far less classic than anorexia nervosa and bulimia nervosa, binge eating and compulsive exercising are also forms of eating disorders.
- Calorie-dense foods, including some designed to be fat dense (from vegetable oils) as well, and careful restriction of activity can aid underweight people in gaining weight.

Review Questions

1. What trends regarding body weight changes have been noted among Americans in recent decades? How have daily caloric consumption patterns and activity patterns contributed to these changes?

2. In comparison to the bodies of most people, how do those of models compare? How might the body characteristics of high-visibility people adversely influence the self-image and sense of self-esteem of many young people?

3. In labeling various degrees of obesity, what percentage above desirable weight is categorized as mild, moderate, and severe (gross or morbid) obesity? Why is it possible to be overweight without being overfat?

4. By age 50, what percentage of people are not only overweight but obese as well?

5. In terms of assessing overweight and obesity, how are each of the following employed: height/weight tables, waist-to-hip ratio, body mass index, nomograms, electrical impedance, skinfold measurements, and hydrostatic weighing?

6. What is the most current thought regarding the role of genetics in the development of obesity? What was the anticipated role of leptin in moderating caloric intake?

7. Assuming the existence of appetite centers in the brain, where are these centers and what physiological signals do they monitor?

8. How can the theory of set point be described, and what is its relationship to yo-yo dieting? How does brown fat function and how does the functioning of the food supplement DNP resemble that of brown fat?

9. What are the three classic body types described by Sheldon, and what is the relationship of each to weight management concerns? How might early infant feeding patterns promote the development of obesity? How are hypertrophic and hypercellular obesity different?

10. What is externality and what role might it play in the development of obesity?

11. In a well-managed pregnancy, how much weight is gained during the pregnancy and how much remains immediately following childbirth?

12. In what ways might parents influence the eventual weight status of their children?

13. Explain the concept of caloric balance. What are the three areas of energy use associated with human functioning? How does BMR change with age? How has caloric expenditure through physical activity traditionally changed with age?

14. What are the principal components of lifetime weight control?

15. Of all of the forms of dietary alteration possible, why is a balanced diet with portion control the most strongly recommended? How might low-calorie, low-fat, and fat-free foods fit into a balanced diet with a portion-control approach to weight management?

16. In what conditions might controlled fasting be an appropriate adjunct to weight management? What format is generally followed by self-help weight reduction programs, such as Weight Watchers?

17. What requirement was recently imposed on weight reduction programs by the FTC? What new component have weight reduction programs added to their program format by incorporating the services of physicians?

18. What two effective weight loss medications were recalled by the FDA? What potentially serious problems were associated with their use? What new medications are (or soon will be) available for the medical management of obesity? In terms of medical management, why is obesity now regarded as a chronic illness?

19. What are the three general surgical approaches to weight reduction? Which is considered cosmetic? Which leads to a chronic need for nutritional supplementation?
20. What is the likely outcome of most weight reduction efforts? What combination of approaches do your authors recommend for long-term weight management, including initial loss and maintenance of that loss? What contributions does physical activity make to a long-term weight management program?
21. What are the diagnostic criteria used in defining anorexia nervosa and bulimia nervosa? What components characterize an effective treatment program for each of these eating disorders? In what ways do compulsive exercise and binge eating relate to anorexia and bulimia?
22. When choosing foods for use in treating underweight, what characteristics are considered desirable?

References

1. National Center for Health. *National health and nutrition examination survey (3)*. Ann Arbor, MI: Interuniversity Consortium for Political and Social Research, 1996.
2. *Clinical guidelines on the identification, evaluation, and treatment of overweight and obesity in adults*. As reported in *First federal obesity clinical guidelines* (NIH News Advisory): The National Institutes of Health, June 17, 1998.
3. Manson J et al. Body weight and mortality among women. *N Engl J Med* 1995; 333(11):677–85.
4. Crowley LV. *Introduction to human disease.* 4th ed. Boston: Jones & Bartlett, 1996.
5. Cash T, Henry P. Women's body images: the results of a national survey in the U.S.A. *Sex Role Res* 1995; 33(1):19–29.
6. U.S. Department of Agriculture/U.S. Department of Health and Human Services. Nutrition and your health: dietary guidelines for Americans. *Home and Garden Bulletin* 1995; 232.
7. Wardlaw GM, Insel PM. *Perspectives in nutrition.* 3rd ed. St. Louis: Mosby, 1996.
8. Prentice WE. *Fitness for college and life.* 5th ed. St. Louis: Mosby, 1997.
9. Cummings SM et al. *Position of The American Dietetic Association: weight management.* The American Dietetic Association, Oct 20, 1996. http://www.hod@eatright.org
10. Weighing the facts on obesity. *Worldview* 1992; Spring 4(1):1–4.
11. Clement K et al. Genetic variation in the B3-adrenergic receptors and an increased capacity to gain weight in patients with morbid obesity. *N Engl J Med* 1995; 333(6):352–54.
12. Halaas J et al. Weight-reducing effects on the plasma protein encoded by the obese gene. *Science* 1995; 269(5223):543–46.
13. Considine R et al. Serum immunoreactive-leptin concentrations in normal-weight and obese humans. *N Engl J Med* 1996; 334(5):292–95.
14. Is the obesity all in the genes? *Harv Health Lett* 1996 April; 21(6):1–3.
15. First report of successful weight loss in human with leptin. News Release. American Diabetes Association, June 14, 1998.
16. Sakurai T et al. Orexins and orexin receptors: a family of hypothalamic neuropeptides and G protein-coupled receptors that regulate feeding behavior. *Cell* 1998 Feb; 92(4):573–85.
17. National Task Force on the Prevention and Treatment of Obesity. Weight cycling. *JAMA* 1994; 272(15):1196–1202.
18. Ganong WF. *Review of medical physiology.* 7th ed. Norwalk, CT: Appleton & Lange, 1995.
19. Fleury C, Neverova M, Collins S. Uncoupling protein 2 gene. *Nat Gene* 1997; 15:269–72.
20. Ohlin A, Rossner S. Factors related to body weight changes during and after pregnancy: the Stockholm Pregnancy and Weight Study. *Obes Res* 4(3):271–76, 1996; May; 4(3) 271–76.
21. Vander A, Sherman J, Luciano D. *Human physiology: the mechanisms of body function* Dubuque, IA: WCB/McGraw-Hill, 1997.
22. Food and Nutrition Board. *Recommended dietary allowances.* Washington, DC: National Academy of Sciences, National Research Council, 1989.
23. Skender M et al: Comparison of 2-year weight loss trends in behavioral treatments of obesity: diet, exercise, and combination interventions. *Journal of The American Dietetic Association* 1996 April; 96(4):342–56.
24. Losing weight: what works and what doesn't work. *Consumer Reports* 1993; 58(6):347–52.
25. *Federal Register* 1997 June 4; 62(107):30677–30724. http://vm.cfsan.fda.gov/~lrd/fr970640a.html
26. Devereux RB. Appetite suppressants and valvular heart disease. *N Engl J Med* 1998 Sept 10; 339(11):765–66.
27. Food and Drug Administration. Public Health Service. FDA announces withdrawal of fenfluramine and dexfenfluramine. *HHS news.* U.S. Department of Health & Human Services, Sept 15, 1997.
28. Centers for Drug Evaluation and Research, Food and Drug Administration, Public Health Service. *Warning letters and notices of violation letters to pharmaceutical companies.* U.S. Department of Health & Human Services, May 22, 1998.
29. Food and Drug Administration. Public Health Service. FDA approves sibutramine to treat obesity. *FDA talk paper.* U.S. Department of Health & Human Services, Nov 24, 1997.

30. Acupuncture effective for certain medical conditions, panel says. *CAM Newsletter* 1998 Jan; 5(1):1–2.
31. Pearson D. Personal Interview. Ball State University Human Performance Laboratory, Aug 25, 1997.
32. Zerbe K. *The body betrayed.* Carlsbad, CA: Gurse Books, 1995.
33. Costin C. *The eating disorder sourcebook: a comprehensive guide to the causes, treatments, and prevention of eating disorders.* Los Angeles: Lowell House, 1996.
34. Gaining weight: a healthy plan for adding pounds. *Hot topics.* The American Dietetic Association, 1998. http://www.eatright.org/nfs10.html

Suggested Readings

Havey JG, White BI. *The easiest diet I never went on.* Mamaroneck, NY: The Health and Wellness Institute, 1997. The author, now regularly seen on television, recounts the struggles she experienced in her quest to reduce her weight by 125 pounds. A physician and a certified trainer use Julia's story to provide professional insights into the process. An inspiring and motivational story.

Mellin L. *The diet-free solution: 6 winning ways to permanent weight loss.* New York: Regan Books, 1998. A much-praised book by those who have tried "diet books" only to experience failure. The author takes her readers deep inside to the underlying emotional needs that have been routinely dulled (but not met) by compulsive eating. A workshop format then moves readers toward more nurturing relationships with themselves and others.

Nash JD. *The new maximize your body potential: lifetime skills for successful weight management.* Menlo Park, CA: Bull Publishing Company, 1997. Now in its second edition, this well-received book uses current scientific understanding as the foundation of a broad-based program to achieve and maintain a healthy body weight. Self-tests, exercises, and checklists help readers build a personalized program to change behavioral patterns associated with eating, exercise, stress reduction, and emotional management. Each chapter stands alone, thus allowing readers greater flexibility in reaching their own body potential.

Price D. *Healing the hungry self: the diet-free solution to lifelong weight management.* New York: Plume, 1998. Disturbances in the physical, emotional, mental, and spiritual "selves" that constitute each person are described as the basis for flawed relationships with food. The author, drawing on her expertise in the treatment of eating disorders, uses a workbook format to bring readers into contact with these "selves" in order to better understand each, thus enhancing their self-esteem and altering their relationship with food.

As We Go To PRESS

Study Looks at the Influence of Teen Fashion Magazines

Knowing that concerns regarding body image influences attempts to lose or gain weight, researchers sought clues to the factors that shape perceptions of attractiveness. A potential player in this process was thought to be fashion magazines such as *Seventeen* and *Glamour* read by large numbers of teenage girls. Over five hundred adolescent girls in grades 5 through 12 were asked to share their feelings regarding how the models used in these publications made them feel regarding their own physical attractiveness. The results proved disturbing to the researchers.

On the basis of the responses, given to the researchers by the young women interviewed, it was found that seven out of every ten readers reported that they were clearly influenced by the physical characteristics of models used in the magazines' photographs. Further, of this large majority of "influenced" readers, nearly one-half indicated the photographs made them feel they should attempt to lose weight through dieting or exercising. Interestingly, when the weight of the girls responding in this manner was assessed, it was found that only one-half were capable of being classified as overweight. The remaining one-half of the girls had no need to consider beginning a diet or exercising for purposes of lowering their already acceptable body weight.

In response to the concerns expressed by the researchers conducting this study, photo editors for both publications indicated they would attempt to find a more representative group of models for use in the future. It will, of course, be interesting to see if this evolution toward representation occurs.

Are You a Victim of Portion Distortion? Learning to Control Serving Sizes

Americans love to live large. According to social scientists, this is part of our national psyche, directly traceable to our wide-spaced national boundaries, ample open space, and rags-to-riches dreams. Buying into this myth is beneficial when it motivates people to stretch themselves in areas of personal growth and achievement. When it comes to eating, however, the living-large philosophy puts Americans on a collision course with a variety of health risks and hinders their weight control efforts.[1]

A Supersized Trend

The trend toward supersized food portions is nothing new. Restaurants have long used large portions to lure value-seeking customers. The trend reversed for a while during the health-conscious 1980s, when meat consumption was coincidentally at an all-time high. Large serving sizes are enjoying a revival, however, as part of the 1990s wellness backlash, which includes such risky behaviors as cigar smoking and increased consumption of hard liquor.

Bargain-hungry consumers weary of wellness warnings are just the clientele fast-food chains have been looking for. In an attempt to fend off competition within the industry as well as outside it, from new steak houses, ethnic eateries, full-service delis, and take-out restaurants, the fast-food industry is selling—and customers are buying—oversized portions of traditional favorites, such as burgers, fries, fried chicken, and pizza, in record numbers. Typically these supersized portions cost just pennies more than the standard-size serving. Another fattening sales strategy has been to offer combo meals—essentially the addition of a large order of fries and a giant drink to popular menu items for under fifty cents.[1,2,3]

Serving Size Recommendations

As with many health-related issues, portion control embodies many contradictions. The USDA has standardized food portions, which are used to develop la-

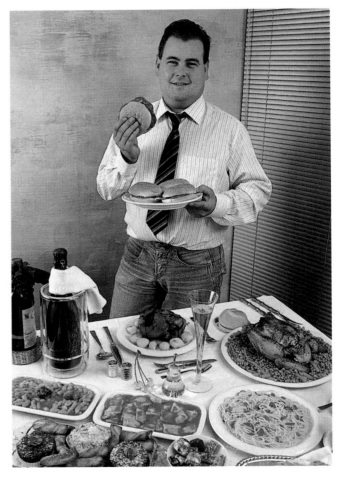

Consumers who are weary of wellness warnings have responded by consuming huge portions of fat-laden foods.

beling laws and the Food Guide Pyramid (FGP) serving size recommendations. The average American, accustomed to gigantic servings when dining out, finds serving sizes on food labels surprisingly puny and, on the other hand, the number of servings of produce and grains suggested on the FGP surprisingly high (see the table comparing typical with recommended

Typical Serving Sizes vs. USDA Food Guide Pyramid Official Serving Sizes

Food	Typical Serving Size and Number of Calories	Official Serving Size and Number of Calories
Popcorn	Movie theater serving (small) 7 cups—400 calories	3 cups—160 calories
Muffins	Restaurant serving ¼ lb. (4 oz)—430 calories	⅛ lb. (2 oz)—190 calories
French fries	McDonald's Super Size Fries 3 cups (6 oz)—540 calories	1½ cups (3 oz)—220 calories
Soft drinks	Can 1½ cups (12 oz)—140 calories 7-Eleven Double Gulp 8 cups (64 oz)—800 calories	1 cup (8 oz)—100 calories
Steak	Dinner house serving (Sirloin) About ½ lb, cooked 7 oz—410 calories Steak house serving (Porterhouse) About 1 lb, cooked 17 oz—1,150 calories	(Sirloin) About ⅓ lb, cooked 3 oz—170 calories

serving sizes).[4] Record numbers of low-fat and low-calorie foods are available, yet Americans are fatter than ever (average body weight has increased 7.5 pounds in the last decade).[1] Gourmets tend to favor small portions of fine food, whereas homestyle cooking enthusiasts prefer an abundance of food, especially meat and starch. Yet both groups are sporting wider waistlines.

Americans aren't entirely to blame for their ignorance of serving sizes. The USDA's standardization of serving sizes seems anything but standard to the average consumer. Food manufacturers and restaurant managers have been happy to ignore the USDA's advice and give cost-sensitive consumers the super-sized servings they desire. According to USDA standards, the amount of food that constitutes a serving varies. Some serving sizes are based on volume, and others on weight. For example, one-half of a three-inch-diameter bagel and one-half cup of cooked rice both constitute one serving from the grain, bread, and pasta group of the FGP. Three ounces of cooked chicken, one-half cup of cooked dried beans, or two tablespoons of peanut butter constitute one serving from the meat group. Even a single food, such as broccoli, can have different serving sizes depending on how it's prepared: According to the FGP, one serving of a fruit or vegetable equals one cup if eaten raw but only one-half cup if it's cooked.[4]

Despite pressure brought to bear by the Nutrition Labeling and Education Act of 1990, food manufacturers continue to package foods in nonstandard sizes. They have simultaneously been producing giant versions of trendy carbohydrate-rich foods, such as megamuffins, behemoth bagels, and miniature versions of favorite high-fat snacks like mini-cheese-filled Ritz crackers and bite-sized Oreos.

Food companies also persist in packaging multiple servings of certain foods, particularly snack foods, in what appear to be single-serving containers. Take a can of cola for instance. The USDA identifies a serving of soda as six ounces, but the typical soda can contains twelve ounces. This extra serving is inconsequential if you're drinking diet soda, but regular soda adds sixty-five calories, or roughly five teaspoons of sugar. Small packages of candy, chips, and cookies often exhibit this same deceptive packaging.[4]

The Portion-Distortion Trend Takes Shape

Well-meaning health care experts are partly to blame for this supersized servings trend. During the late 1980s and early 1990s, many of them urged people to eat less fat and more carbohydrates. The selling point for giving up favorite high-fat foods was that "you can eat more food for fewer calories." The underlying reasoning was sound—gram for gram, fat has twice as many calories as carbohydrates. Unfortunately, portion-ignorant Americans took this advice too literally and began devouring triple-sized tortillas, muffins, pretzels, bagels, and platters of pasta.

Letting someone else do the cooking doesn't make weight management any easier. Obesity experts identify dining out as a serious liability for diet-conscious diners. Because of the record numbers of women in the workforce, dining out is at an all-time high. In 1996 the average American ate out 4.1 times per week.[1,5] Chic restaurants, featuring small portions of artistically prepared food, are blossoming on every corner in large cities, but in the suburbs and the heartland, the trend is fast-food chains, take-out shops, casual restaurants, and convenience foods, including frozen meals, packaged mixes, and full-service deli items.[3]

Since many working women are also mothers, more than 80 percent of all dining-out dollars are spent at family-friendly eateries. Prices at these establishments are relatively low, but thanks to the supersized portions, calories tend to be high.[5]

Gourmets aren't faring any better when it comes to waist whittling. The small portions served in fine restaurants are no guarantee of low-calorie ingredients. Furthermore, just being in a restaurant, confronted with an overwhelming number of appealing food choices, causes many people to order more courses than they typically eat when dining at home. How often have you ordered an appetizer or felt overly full but still fallen prey to the dessert cart when it arrived at your table? Obesity experts believe this tendency to be seduced by the sight and smell of food partly explains the lack of healthy food choices on fast-food menus. Responding to consumer demand, McDonald's, Burger King, Taco Bell, and Kentucky Fried Chicken all added a variety of low-fat choices to their menus but found that, once on-site, their patrons were still ordering fries, burgers, full-fat burritos, or breaded and fried chicken. Paradoxically, the larger-portion items were selling better than the standard-sized versions of these foods. These chains have quietly been phasing out or significantly reducing their healthy menu options since early 1993.[6] For example, McDonald's replaced its McLean with a triple cheeseburger and the Arch Deluxe, both of which have significantly more calories than the Big Mac. Kentucky Fried Chicken's skinless roasted chicken was replaced by popcorn chicken, a breaded, deep-fried dish that has been breaking sales records.

Even diet-conscious diners who stick to heart-healthy menu choices can fall into calorie traps. A recent trip to an Olive Garden restaurant revealed that the pasta dishes on the heart healthy menu were large enough to feed three or four healthy hearts! Furthermore, they were accompanied by enough cheesy garlic breadsticks, plus soup or salad, to destroy anyone's best diet efforts. And Olive Garden is no exception. According to restaurant surveys conducted by the Center for Science in the Public Interest, most restaurants serve portions big enough for two to three people.[2]

Shrinking Your Serving Sizes

How can you dine defensively? Putting into practice the American Dietetic Association's 1997 National Nutrition Month campaign theme "All Foods Can Fit" is one option.[1,6] This slogan is predicated on the idea that a balanced lifestyle can lead to a balanced body weight. Educating yourself about dietary balance and serving sizes is a first step. The FGP provides a pattern for overall dietary balance and even allows you to include small amounts of sweets and fatty treats.[4] The FGP booklet supplies tables of food choices and serving size information. Learning to guesstimate sizes is also essential. You may need to use measuring cups and spoons and a food scale at home until you get the gist of it. A variety of mnemonic devices for estimating serving size are also available. The "Rule of Thumb for Serving Sizes" shown here is an easily learned, readily available approach. Other techniques include limiting meat servings to the size of a deck of cards or cassette tape, en-

---

A Rule of Thumb for Serving Sizes

Use the parts of your hand to estimate serving sizes when it's not possible or convenient to use a food scale or measuring cups and spoons.

1 thumb = 1 ounce of cheese

1 thumb tip = 1 teaspoon of foods such as mayonnaise, peanut butter, and sugar

3 thumb tips = 1 tablespoon

1 fist = 1 cup of pasta, rice, or vegetables

1 or 2 handfuls = 1 ounce of a snack food (1 handful of small foods, such as nuts, or 2 handfuls of larger foods, such as chips and pretzels)

1 palm (minus the fingers) = 3 ounces of meat, fish, or poultry

---

visioning a tennis ball to estimate one-cup servings, and thinking of a one-half cup serving as the size of two Ping-Pong balls. Books featuring attractive photographs are available to assist parents and teachers in teaching children to recognize the sizes of portions of various types of food.[7]

Additional lifestyle changes may also be necessary. Learning to eat more slowly will allow you to feel satisfied with a smaller portion of food because your brain will have time to receive the signal that you have eaten. You should avoid other activities while eating so that you're fully aware of what and how much you're consuming. Dining out less frequently or dividing all restaurant portions in two and packaging up half before beginning to eat can also help. Accepting the fact that planned activity is an essential element of weight control and learning how much activity it takes to burn off a slice of cake is also important. Remember, there are 3,500 calories in a pound of body fat. Each mile you walk expends about 100 calories, so you would need to walk thirty-five miles to lose one pound of fat.

In essence, Americans can have their cake and eat it too, but it takes practice and persistence to become adept at balancing it all.

For Discussion . . .

What foods do you often consume in supersized portions? Would you be satisfied with smaller servings? Do you tend to order more courses and eat past the point of satiation when you dine in a restaurant because you're treating yourself or because you want to be sure to get your money's worth? What factors do you think are driving the "wellness backlash"?

References

1. Califano J. Nation's "supersize" trend leading to supersized people. *The New York Times* 1996 Nov 24: F8.
2. Liebman B, Hurley J. One size doesn't fit all. *Nutrition Action Healthletter* 1996; 23(9):10–12.
3. Mowma P. What will customers want in 1996 and beyond? *Restaurants USA* 1995 December: P35.
4. The Food Guide Pyramid. U.S. Department of Agriculture. *Home & Garden Bulletin* 1992; 232.
5. National Restaurant Association. *Dining trends, 1996, quarterly reports.*
6. Woodburg R. The great fast-food pig-out. *Time* 1993; 141(26):51.
7. Hess MA. *Portion photos of popular foods.* Marketplace: The American Dietetic Association, 1997. http://www.eatright.org/catalog/cat162X.html

InfoLinks
http://recovery.hiwaay.net
www.caloriecontrol.org

MASTERING TASKS

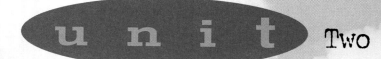

The Body

It is our hope that the information you have mastered in Unit Two will be helpful as you work on the five developmental tasks this book addresses. Of course, you must remember that all people work on these tasks in different ways and at varying speeds. However, it is through the completion of these developmental tasks that you will have a satisfying and productive life.

Forming an Initial Adult Identity

Developmentally speaking, traditional-age students have as one of their major responsibilities the establishment of an initial adult identity. Even nontraditional students (and professors) find that they are often working on their adult identities. In forming these identities, we are expected to blend those traits we currently have with those that we desire. What are the roles of fitness, nutrition, and weight management in forming and re-forming our identities? Your enhanced fitness level, interest in nutrition, and body weight will be evident to you and transmitted to others as a sense of personal self-acceptance. In a sense, you are telling the world, "I like what I am and I hope you like it, too." Your interest in these areas is also a commitment to the future as you plan for your adult years and as others plan theirs with you in mind. You are likely to become a person who is more capable of living a productive and satisfying life.

Establishing Independence

Independence, a much-desired freedom for those nearing the end of their formal education, is achieved by most adults regardless of whether they are interested in the health information presented in this unit. However, the quality of independence can be enhanced by a reasonable level of fitness and an interest in nutrition and weight management. Particularly in terms of your ability to cope with the new demands of independence, a well-developed state of fitness and a sound diet will help reduce stress and increase the level of alertness needed to master the demands of adulthood. For nontraditional students whose independence is already well established, continued interest and involvement in physical activity, nutrition, and weight management can add a measure of renewal to your demanding life as an employee, single person, spouse, or parent.

Assuming Responsibility

As people move through adulthood, to whom should they be most responsible? As we mentioned earlier, people should probably be most responsible to themselves. But the responsibility to oneself does not limit the need to be responsible to others. The reasons that compel you to appreciate health and to promote it to the fullest extent reach beyond yourself to include others with whom you come into contact. For this reason, your fitness level, nutritional status, and weight management can affect your ability to perform optimally. Beyond this rather philosophical connection be-

tween high-level health and responsibility is another, more concrete connection: Your motivation to maintain good cardiorespiratory fitness, nutrition, and weight management indicates your willingness and ability to assume responsibility. By being faithful to your fitness program and well-balanced diet, you help assure yourself that you are a responsible person.

Developing Social Skills

As your social interaction increases with entry into or movement through the adult years, the relationship between this unit's content and your developing social skills becomes evident. Much social contact with other adults centers on food and physical activity. Exercise classes, parties, cycling groups, cafeteria meals, outdoor cookouts, evenings with friends, reunions, and athletic teams represent some social groups that cater to our fitness or food desires. Through your participation in these common social groupings, you will have a great opportunity to practice and improve social skills. Cherish these opportunities. Indeed, social interactions will form a principal basis for a kind of personal enjoyment that will last a lifetime.

Developing Intimacy

To enjoy all that accompanies intimate relationships, a dependable level of physical health is necessary. Limited physical conditioning can reduce the scope of activities in which you can interact. The enjoyment of food and a commitment to fitness can be areas of common interest within an intimate relationship.

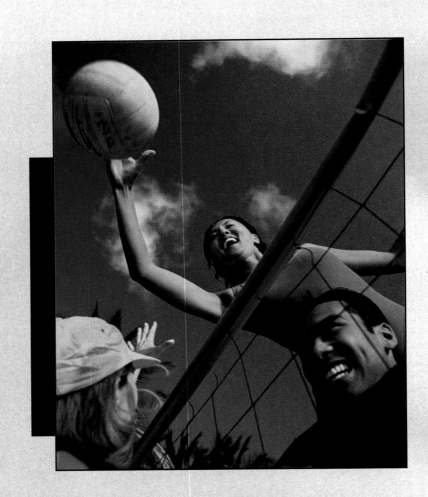

Addictive Substances

Health educators have no doubt that the use, misuse, and abuse of many drugs can impair health. These substances not only alter the functioning of the body and mind but also affect the other dimensions of health. In Unit Three, we take a look at addictive substances and their effects on the user.

1 Physical Dimension

The effects of substance use, especially the long-term use of tobacco and alcohol, are well understood. These substances clearly cause illness and death. Alcohol abuse can destroy the structure and function of many body systems. Tobacco use damages the cardiovascular system and the tissues of the respiratory tract and can cause cancer in many sites throughout the body. Chronic abuse of psychoactive drugs impairs many central nervous system functions. Even the experimental use of these drugs carries the danger of toxic overdose.

2 Emotional Dimension

Because psychoactive drugs alter nervous system functioning, many users experience depression and mood swings. For people who are predisposed to enter dependent relationships, drug use can become an unhealthy way of relieving stress. When psychological dependence combines with physical dependence, the addict may begin to lose touch with reality.

3 Social Dimension

Psychoactive drug use often takes place in social settings. For many people, drinking or using other drugs is a necessary first step toward enjoying the company of others. However, most people have little tolerance for inappropriate substance use, such as use of illegal drugs, excessive alcohol intake, and smoking in public places in which tobacco use in banned.

4 Intellectual Dimension

Intellectual impairment is one consequence of chemical abuse. People cannot perform well intellectually when they are feeling high or low or when their senses are dulled. Some people prefer to disregard information about the dangers of substance abuse, a choice that could prove extremely harmful to their health.

5 Spiritual Dimension

Although drug use has long played a role in the religious practices of people throughout the world, the nonceremonial use of drugs conflicts with the principles of service to others. Substance abuse can hinder spiritual growth by turning a person's focus inward, making it impossible to develop the other-directedness that is essential to a rich spiritual life.

6 Occupational Dimension

Use of both legal and illegal drugs clearly stands in the way of occupational health. Most workplaces are smoke-free, forcing smokers to stand outside or walk to the smoker's lounge to have a cigarette. These continual interruptions lower a worker's productivity. Illegal drug use can keep a job candidate from being hired, and use of illegal drugs or alcohol on the job can be dangerous and will certainly lower a worker's level of performance.

7 Environmental Dimension

As in the spiritual dimension of health, habitual drug use tends to turn a person's focus inward. When people attend to their own needs first and foremost, they are unlikely to become responsible stewards of our fragile environment.

chapter
seven

Living Drug-Free

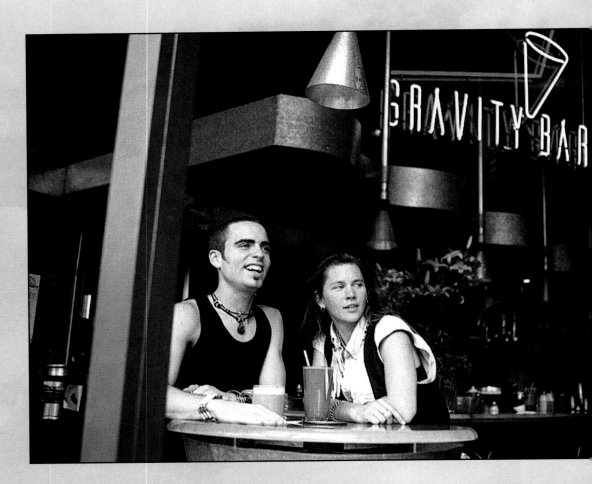

Many of today's young people are seeking healthy alternatives to illegal drug use. These students are enjoying good company and their favorite beverages at the Gravity Bar in Seattle, which serves non-alcoholic juice drinks and specialty coffees.

The use of psychoactive drugs can be tremendously disruptive in many people's lives, from tragic deaths to the loss of employment opportunities (most Fortune 500 companies use preemployment drug testing), to the deterioration of personal relationships, to babies born with profound birth defects. Perhaps realizing this, college students have generally moved away from using the most dangerous illegal drugs.

It is safe to say that in the late 1990s, however, drug use remains a significant problem for both college students and the general population. Alcohol is the most important problem drug for most college students (see Chapter 8), but other drugs pose risks for certain students (Figure 7-1). Additionally, many nontraditional students see the destructive effects of drug use on their neighborhoods and worry about their children being exploited by those who deal drugs.

HEALTHY PEOPLE: LOOKING AHEAD TO 2010

Achieving the *Healthy People 2000* objectives in the area of drug abuse is critically important for the nation. Substance abuse is directly responsible for 120,000 deaths each year in the United States, 100,000 of which are related to alcohol abuse and 20,000 to other drug use. In addition, substance abuse harms the emotional health of individuals, destroys families, and devastates communities.

For the first time in years, some headway was made in 1997 in preventing drug-related deaths and in reducing the number of drug-related hospital emergency visits.[1] However, there remains a group of hard-core drug users who are difficult to reach with anti–drug abuse messages. In addition, no progress appears to have been made in raising the age of first use of cigarettes, alcohol, or marijuana by children.[2]

The 1997 *Monitoring the Future study*[3] indicated that for the first time in the decade of the 1990s, marijuana and other drug use among eighth graders was declining. While tenth and twelfth graders' marijuana use was still rising, the use of other drugs among these groups was leveling off. Preventing initial and repeat drug abuse and providing adequate treatment for addicts will remain a high priority in the *Healthy People 2010* objectives now being drafted.

Real Life
Real choices

- Name: Barry Wolf
- Age: 44
- Occupation: architect

Anyone who grew up in the sixties can tell you it was quite a trip. Protest marches, communes, beads, beards, tie-dyeing, peace, love, harmony, drugs . . . and more drugs. In that tumultuous time, the door of a giant pharmaceutical cabinet swung open, and there it all was: acid (LSD), horse (heroin), speed, (amphetamines), 'ludes (Quaaludes, a barbiturate)—and everything in between, from airplane glue to hashish brownies.

Barry Wolf remembers. Before he started college in 1969, he'd already checked out some popular potions. He tried LSD and had the classic bad trip; took a turn with downers and slept through classes; and finally settled on good old garden-variety marijuana. Like countless other students, Barry loved to light up, mellow out, see the inner essence of wallpaper patterns, divine the true meaning of the lyrics of "Jumping Jack Flash" . . . and go on those freaked-out 2:00 A.M. convenience store raids in search of the world's biggest package of Ring-Dings.

Barry's 5-year architecture program was demanding and tough—no way to learn this exacting discipline while sleeping or stoned. He applied himself to his studies, smoked dope only on weekends, and graduated with a 3.5 GPA.

Today, more than 20 years later, Barry is a prosperous, sought-after architect. He has a solid marriage, two great daughters, and plenty of friends. And he still smokes dope. Never at work or in front of the kids; never while driving or drinking—just at gatherings of college friends, where they do *The Big Chill:* light up, listen to Jefferson Airplane, and reminisce about old wild times.

Barry's wife, Linda, smoked dope in college and quit when she graduated. She's disturbed about Barry's marijuana use and wants him to quit, for his own good and also because their pre-teen daughters need guidance from their parents on drug use. Barry says an occasional hit is no big deal, he's not hooked, and he'll quit when the kids are "older."

As you study this chapter, think about Barry's behavior and reasoning, and prepare yourself to answer the questions in **Your Turn** at the end of the chapter.

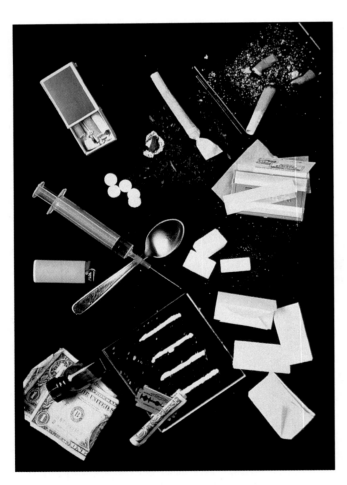

Drug use of all types remains a significant problem in the late 1990s.

Prevention: The Best Solution

We combat the drug problem in the United States on two fronts: the demand side and the supply side. The United States attempts to reduce the supply of illegal (illicit) drugs through drug interdiction efforts at our borders, through joint efforts with countries such as Mexico and Colombia, and through law-enforcement measures within our own borders.

However, the best way to avoid the immense costs of drug abuse is simply to reduce the demand. We do this by helping people develop the tools needed to avoid the use of illegal drugs (see the Health Action Guide on p. 201). Experts are currently mounting prevention efforts on three levels: primary, secondary, and tertiary. Take a look at each of these three levels. Which level is most familiar to you?

Primary Prevention

Primary prevention means reaching people who have not yet used illegal drugs and reducing their desire to try drugs. Primary prevention programs can target individuals, families, peer groups, neighborhoods, schools, workplaces, colleges, and the community.

A peer group prevention strategy would be training peers as leaders in an attempt to change the norms for drug use. Neighborhood prevention often includes efforts to create and maintain a safe neighborhood, promote a sense of loyalty to the community, and discourage drug traffickers. Schools educate

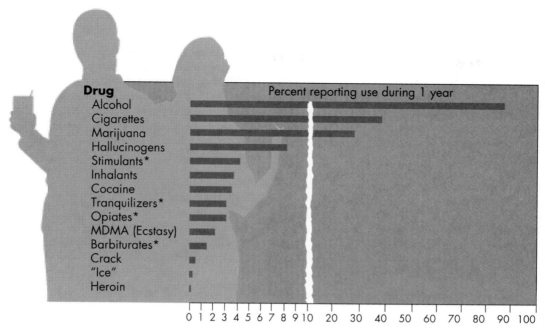

Drug	Percent reporting use during 1 year
Alcohol	
Cigarettes	
Marijuana	
Hallucinogens	
Stimulants*	
Inhalants	
Cocaine	
Tranquilizers*	
Opiates*	
MDMA (Ecstasy)	
Barbiturates*	
Crack	
"Ice"	
Heroin	

0 1 2 3 4 5 6 7 8 9 10 20 30 40 50 60 70 80 90 100

*Drug use was not under a doctor's orders.

Figure 7-1 Alcohol, cigarettes, marijuana, and hallucinogens are the four most common substances used by college students.

teachers in how to recognize high-risk youths, develop policies to involve parents, improve self-esteem in students, and implement student assistance programs (SAPs). SAPs are school-based intervention programs designed to reduce drug-related problems and prevent dependence among students. One well-known drug-education program is DARE, or Drug Abuse Resistance Education (see the Star Box on p. 202).

Workplace prevention methods include drug-testing policies and employee assistance programs (EAPs). EAPs are workplace-based programs that offer employees resources for dealing with mental and emotional problems, including drug-related problems. At colleges and universities, campus leaders work to reduce the availability of drugs on campus and limit the marketing of alcohol. Community strategies include drug-related policies, media campaigns, and comprehensive education, treatment, and law-enforcement services.

Some companies have begun marketing home drug-testing kits, targeted to parents who wish to prevent their children from beginning or continuing drug use. The kits allow the parent to send a vial of urine to a laboratory, then later call a telephone number for the test results. The tests can detect use of marijuana, PCP, cocaine, heroin, and other illicit drugs. Some experts recommend that such tests be used only as a last resort and say that they are no substitute for regular communication with one's children.

HEALTH ACTION GUIDE

Preventing Drug Use

In whatever capacity you interact with others, particularly children and adolescents, you can play a part in reducing drug use. To accomplish this:

- *Be informed.* Be aware of possible drug use by learning to recognize early involvement.
- *Be firm.* Communicate firmly and clearly your position on drug use and your concerns about the behavior you are observing.
- *Be consistent.* Follow through with the rules and consequences that you have established about appropriate behavior.
- *Be a good listener.* Take time to listen to other views, even when you are in total disagreement with them.
- *Be available.* Make yourself available to help or console others who might be involved with drug use.
- *Be loving.* Demonstrate love and concern, but say no when you mean it.
- *Be an example.* Never do what you do not want others to do.
- *Be involved.* Give as much support as possible to those who are also concerned about drug use.

InfoLinks
www.doorway.org

---

primary prevention measures intended to deter first-time drug use.

Daring to Reconsider Drug-Education Programs

You are probably familiar with the nation's most popular drug-education program, DARE (Drug Abuse Resistance Education). Depending on your age, you may have encountered this program yourself, as it is presented in nearly 80 percent of U.S. school districts. You may have seen celebrities such as Arsenio Hall publicizing the program. DARE sends police officers into schools to present seventeen sessions on resisting peer pressure to use specific drugs.

But community leaders no longer agree on the effectiveness of DARE. Spokane, Washington, officials recently dropped the program, and Seattle officials may follow. In addition, Richard Clayton, director of the Center for Prevention Research at the University of Kentucky in Lexington, reports that "DARE did not have any sustained effect on anything."[21]

Glenn Levant, head of DARE America, responded to the criticism: "Just because someone publishes a paper and calls it a study does not really mean anything, particularly when you're dealing with something as subjective as whether prevention works."

One new alternative program is called Life Skills Training.[21] Rather than use police officers, who represent authority to a group that is just beginning to challenge authority, Life Skills uses homeroom teachers and peers, leading fifteen sessions of improvisation and discussion designed to make students more confident, assertive, and able to analyze the messages they get from popular culture and from classmates. One study showed that seventh graders in a Life Skills program tracked through graduation used only half the drugs, alcohol, and tobacco of their peers. Which approach do you think would be more effective?

Personal Applications

• Have you encountered one of these primary prevention strategies yet? Did it change the way you think about illegal drugs? Did it discourage you from using drugs?

Secondary Prevention

Secondary prevention targets those who are beginning to experiment with drugs and uses detection, screening, intervention, and treatment of early drug abuse to help these people to avoid further use. These programs target high-risk individuals who are abusing drugs and who may be dependent and in need of treatment. These programs are considered secondary prevention because they do not prevent initial drug use but instead involve detection and treatment of drug problems before they become severe. Methods include crisis telephone hotlines, peer counseling, individual and family counseling, workplace training, and student and employee assistance programs (SAPs and EAPs).

A specific example of a secondary prevention technique is intervention, in which the drug-dependent individual is confronted about his or her behavior and urged to enter treatment as soon as possible.

Tertiary Prevention

Tertiary prevention (third-level prevention) targets drug-dependent individuals, such as crack or heroin addicts, and their families. These individuals require specialized, intensive help that includes rehabilitation and maintenance. Such intensive treatments may require temporary hospitalization. Additional treatment methods include intensive outpatient care, support groups, and after-care programs. Relapse prevention is designed to help people recovering from drug abuse maintain their drug-free lifestyles.

Some specific examples of tertiary prevention methods are counseling, drug therapy, educational and vocational services, urine testing, relapse prevention, and family, social, and community support. Currently, the number of people needing treatment is estimated to be three to four times the number receiving treatment.[4] Clearly we need to make drug treatment more available in the United States.

Personal Applications

• Do you know anyone who is dependent on drugs and needs help? What could you tell this person about assistance that is available in your community?

Addictive Behavior

This chapter explores the health consequences of drug use, misuse, and abuse. Before we talk about specific drugs, however, drug use should be put in the broader context of addictive behavior. Experts in human behavior view drug use and abuse as just one of the many forms of addictive behavior. Addictive behavior includes addictions to shopping, eating, gambling, sex, television, video games, and work, as well as addictions to alcohol or other drugs.

The Process of Addiction

The process of developing an addiction has been a much-studied topic. Addictive behavior seems to have three common aspects: exposure, compulsion, and loss of control.

Exposure

An addiction can begin after a person is exposed to a drug (such as alcohol) or a behavior (such as gambling) that he or she finds pleasurable. Perhaps this drug or behavior temporarily replaces an unpleasant feeling or sensation. This initial pleasure gradually (or in some cases quickly) becomes a focal point in the person's life.

Compulsion

Increasingly more energy, time, and money are spent pursuing the drug use or behavior. At this point in the addictive process, the person can be said to have a compulsion for the drug or behavior. Frequently, repeated exposure to the drug or behavior continues despite negative consequences, such as the gradual loss of family and friends, unpleasant physical symptoms after taking the drug, and problems at work.

During the compulsion phase of the addictive behavior, a person's "normal" life is likely to disintegrate while she or he searches for increased pleasures from the drug or the behavior. An addicted person's family life, circle of friends, work, or study patterns become less important than the search for more and better "highs." The development of tolerance and withdrawal are distinct possibilities. (These terms are discussed later in the chapter.)

Why some people develop compulsions and others do not is difficult to pinpoint, but addiction might be influenced by genetic makeup, family dynamics, physiological processes, personality type, peer groups, and available resources.

Loss of Control

Over time, the search for highs changes to a search to avoid the effects of withdrawal from the drug or behavior. Addicted people lose their ability to control their behavior. Despite overwhelming negative consequences (for example, deterioration of health, alienation of family and friends, or loss of all financial resources), addicted people continue to behave in ways that make their lives worse. The person addicted to alcohol continues to drink heavily, the person addicted to shopping continues to run up heavy debts, and the person addicted to food continues to eat indiscriminately. This behavior reflects a loss of control over one's life. Frequently, a person has addictions to more than one drug or behavior.

Intervention and Treatment

The good news for people with addictions is that help is available. Within the last two decades, much attention has been focused on intervention and treatment for addictive behavior. Many people can be helped through programs such as those described at the end of this chapter (see p. 223). These programs often include inpatient or outpatient treatment, family counseling, and long-term aftercare counseling.

It is common for people in aftercare treatment for addictive behavior to belong to a self-help support group, such as Alcoholics Anonymous, Gamblers Anonymous, or Sex Addicts Anonymous. These groups are often listed in the phone book or in the classified section of the newspaper.

Codependence

With all the focus placed on the person with a drug problem, often the families and loved ones of the addict do not receive the attention and help they need. You may already be familiar with the term *codependent,* but you might have assumed that this term applies only to those close to an alcoholic. In fact, this term can apply to anyone who is close to an individual addicted to any type of behavior, including addiction to drugs, sex, gambling, or other behaviors.

Codependent people typically become unaware of their own feelings, needs, and boundaries in their preoccupation with the addicted individual. They become focused on protecting or coping with the addict and often lose their own sense of identity. This stress often results in chaotic behaviors, addictions, and physical illnesses in the codependent person.

Private and public programs are also available to help the codependent person learn new behaviors. See Chapter 8 for more information about codependent behavior and resources.

Drug Terminology

Before examining drug actions or drug behavior, you must first be familiar with some basic terminology. Much of this terminology originates in the field of pharmacology, or the study of the interaction of chemical agents with living material.

What does the word **drug** mean? Each of us may have different ideas about what a drug is. Although a number of definitions are available, we will consider a drug to be "any substance, other than food, that by its chemical or physical nature alters structure or function in the living organism."[5] Included in this

---

secondary prevention measures aimed at early detection, intervention, and treatment of drug abuse before severe physical, psychological, emotional, or social consequences can occur.

tertiary prevention treatment and rehabilitation of drug-dependent people to limit physical, psychological, emotional, and social deterioration or prevent death.

drug any substance, other than food, that by its chemical or physical nature alters structure or function in the living organism.

broad definition is a variety of psychoactive drugs, medicines, and substances that many people do not usually consider to be drugs.

Psychoactive drugs alter the user's feelings, behavior, perceptions, or moods. Psychoactive drugs include stimulants, depressants, hallucinogens, opiates, and inhalants. Medicines function to heal unhealthy tissue. Medicines are also used to ease pain, prevent illness, and diagnose health conditions. Although some psychoactive drugs are used for medical reasons, as in the case of tranquilizers and some narcotics, the most commonly prescribed medicines are antibiotics, sulfa drugs, diuretics, oral contraceptives, and antihypertensive drugs. Legal substances not usually considered to be drugs (but that certainly are drugs) include caffeine, tobacco, alcohol, aspirin, and other over-the-counter (OTC) preparations (see the Star Box at right). These common substances are used so frequently in our society that they are rarely perceived as true drugs.

For organizational reasons, this chapter primarily deals with psychoactive drugs. Alcohol is covered in Chapter 8. The effects of tobacco are delineated in Chapter 9. Prescription and OTC drugs and medicines are discussed at length in Chapter 18. Environmental pollutants are covered in Chapter 19. Anabolic steroids, drugs used primarily for increasing muscle growth, are discussed in Chapter 4.

Dependence

Psychoactive drugs have a strong potential for the development of **dependence.** When users take a psychoactive drug, the patterns of nervous system function are altered. If these altered functions provide perceived benefits for the user, drug use may continue, perhaps at increasingly larger dosages. If persistent use continues, the user can develop a dependence on the drug. Pharmacologists have identified two types of dependences—physical and psychological.

A person can be said to have developed a physical dependence when the body cells have become reliant on a drug. Continued use of the drug is then required because body tissues have adapted to its presence.[6] The person's body needs the drug to maintain homeostasis, or dynamic balance. If the drug is not taken or is suddenly withdrawn, the user develops a characteristic **withdrawal illness.** The symptoms of withdrawal reflect the attempt by the body's cells to regain normality without the drug. Withdrawal symptoms are always unpleasant (ranging from mild to severe irritability, depression, nervousness, digestive difficulties, and abdominal pain) and can be life threatening, as in the case of abrupt withdrawal from barbiturates or alcohol. In this chapter the term **addiction** is used interchangeably with physical dependence.

Can Over-the-Counter Drugs Be Abused?

We all know that abuse of illegal drugs and prescription drugs is a serious problem in the United States. But many people also misuse and abuse over-the-counter drugs. Perhaps because these drugs can be purchased at a corner drug store without a prescription, we think that we can take them in any amount and for any purpose without risk, but this is not true. For example:[7]

- Students, athletes, and workers who must stay awake for long hours often misuse stimulants such as caffeine. High doses or use over a long time can lead to anxiety, hallucinations, severe depression, and physical or psychological dependence.
- Analgesics can have severe side effects. For example, aspirin can lead to Reye's syndrome if given to children with the flu or chicken pox. People with liver damage should also avoid aspirin. Acetaminophen is generally free of side effects, but large doses or overuse can cause rashes, fevers, or changes in blood composition. Ibuprofen also can cause side effects, and overuse can lead to confusion, tingling in the hands and feet, and vomiting.
- Laxatives are among the most widely misused and abused OTC medications. They should be restricted to short-term use, as chronic use leads to dependence.
- Antitussives and expectorants, both OTC preparations used to combat the symptoms of colds, may contain as much as 40 percent alcohol. Some young people abuse these medications for the effects of alcohol.
- Combining OTC drugs with prescription drugs can reduce or multiply the drug's effectiveness or cause other harmful reactions.

Many people misuse OTC drugs to increase their sense of well-being, to help them perform a task, or to treat unrelated illnesses or health problems. They often find themselves psychologically or physically dependent on the drug. With OTC drugs, we are responsible for treating ourselves safely. Follow these guidelines:

- Use OTC drugs primarily for the temporary relief of minor symptoms.
- Don't take OTC drugs longer than the label recommends. If your symptoms persist, or if new symptoms appear, see a doctor.
- If you are pregnant or nursing, check with your doctor before taking any medication—even herbal remedies.
- If you have allergies or chronic health problems, read the ingredient, warning, and caution statements carefully and check with your doctor or pharmacist if you have any questions about taking a product.
- Read the label on the drug container carefully before you start taking an OTC drug. Check it again each time you buy a new package, since the label could have changed.

Continued use of most drugs can lead to **tolerance.** Tolerance is an acquired reaction to a drug in which continued intake of the same dose has diminishing effects.[6] The user needs larger doses of the drug to receive previously felt sensations. The continued use of depressants, including alcohol, and opiates can cause users to quickly develop a tolerance to the drug.

Furthermore, tolerance developed for one drug may carry over to another drug within the same general category. This phenomenon is known as **cross-tolerance.** The heavy abuser of alcohol, for example, might require a larger dose of a preoperative sedative to become relaxed before surgery than the average person. The tolerance to alcohol "crosses over" to the other depressant drug.

A person who possesses a strong desire to continue using a particular drug is said to have developed psychological dependence. People who are psychologically dependent on a drug believe that they need to consume the drug to maintain a sense of well-being. They crave the drug for emotional reasons in spite of having persistent or recurrent physical, social, psychological, or occupational problems that are caused or worsened by the drug use. Abrupt withdrawal from a drug by such a person would not trigger the fully expressed withdrawal illness, although some unpleasant symptoms of withdrawal might be felt. The term *habituation* is often used interchangeably with psychological dependence.

Drugs whose continued use can quickly lead to both physical and psychological dependence are the depressants (barbiturates, tranquilizers, and alcohol), narcotics (the opiates, which are derivatives of the Oriental poppy: heroin, morphine, and codeine), and synthetic narcotics (Demerol and methadone). Drugs whose continued use can lead to various degrees of psychological dependence and occasionally to significant (but not life-threatening) physical dependence in some users are the stimulants (amphetamines, caffeine, and cocaine), hallucinogens (LSD, peyote, mescaline, and marijuana), and inhalants (glues, gases, and petroleum products).

Personal Applications

• Have you ever developed either a physical or psychological dependence on any drug? Do you find that you now require a larger dose of a particular drug to reach a high or low that you once felt with a smaller dose?

Drug Misuse and Abuse

So far in this chapter we have used the term *use* (or *user*) in association with the taking of psychoactive drugs. At this point, however, it is important to define *use* and to introduce the terms *misuse* and *abuse.*[5] By doing so, we can more accurately describe how drugs are used.

The term *use* is all-encompassing and describes drug-taking in the most general way. For example, Americans use drugs of many types. The term *use* can also refer more narrowly to misuse and abuse. We most often use the word in this latter regard.

The term **misuse** refers to the inappropriate use of legal drugs intended to be medications. Misuse may occur when a patient misunderstands the directions for use of a prescription or OTC drug or when a patient shares a prescription with a friend or family member for whom the drug was not prescribed. Misuse also occurs when a patient takes the prescription or OTC drug for a purpose or condition other than that for which it was intended or at a dosage other than that recommended.

The term **abuse** applies to any use of an illegal drug or any use of a legal drug when it is detrimental to health and well-being. The costs of drug abuse to the individual are extensive and include absenteeism and underachievement, loss of employment, marital instability, loss of self-esteem, serious illnesses, and even death. Complete the Personal Assessment on page 206 to determine whether you or someone you know may be abusing drugs.

Dynamics of the Addictive Personality

Many factors influence drug-taking behavior, including individual factors, immediate environmental factors, and more global factors. Specific aspects of each are discussed in the following sections.

---

psychoactive drug any substance capable of altering feelings, moods, or perceptions.

dependence a general term that refers to the need to continue using a drug for psychological or physical reasons or both.

withdrawal illness an uncomfortable, perhaps toxic response of the body as it attempts to maintain homeostasis in the absence of a drug; also called *abstinence syndrome.*

addiction compulsive, uncontrollable dependence on a substance, habit, or practice to such a degree that cessation causes severe emotional or physiological reactions.

tolerance an acquired reaction to a drug in which the continued intake of the same dose has diminished effects.

cross-tolerance transfer of tolerance from one drug to another within the same general category.

misuse the inappropriate use of legal drugs intended to be medications.

abuse any use of a legal or illegal drug in a way that is detrimental to health.

Personal Assessment

To assess whether you or someone you know may be abusing drugs circle Y for yes or N for no.

1. A sudden increase in or loss of appetite or sudden weight loss or gain   **Y N**

2. Moodiness, depression, irritability, or withdrawal   **Y N**

3. Disorientation, lack of concentration, or forgetfulness   **Y N**

4. Frequent use of eye drops or inappropriate wearing of sunglasses   **Y N**

5. Disruption or change in sleep patterns or a lack of energy   **Y N**

6. Borrowing money more and more, working excessive hours, selling personal items, or stealing or shoplifting   **Y N**

7. Persistent and frequent nosebleeds, sniffles, coughs, and other signs of upper respiratory infection   **Y N**

8. Change in speech patterns or vocabulary or a deterioration in academic performance   **Y N**

9. Feeling ill at ease with family members and other adults   **Y N**

10. Neglect of personal appearance   **Y N**

Interpretation

A yes response to more than three questions indicates that there may be drug dependence, and professional help should be obtained.

How to Intervene

If you find evidence that your family member or friend is abusing drugs, and he or she resists help or treatment, you may want to consider an *intervention*. An intervention is a planned confrontation by "significant others," including spouse, parents, children, boss, and friends, designed to break down drug abuse denial in a compassionate way.

Intervention is a serious step to help someone who may not want help, so it should be planned carefully. Many drug treatment centers have intervention experts on staff who can help plan and execute an intervention. Many bookstores also offer books on the subject. Following are some of the basic principles and techniques of intervention:[8]

- Individual intervention is often futile. Continued denial is much less likely in the face of a group. The number of people who should intervene depends on the severity of the drug use. Consider including the spouse, friends, counselors, neighbors, parents, and clergy; when the abuser is a child, also consider siblings, uncles, aunts, grandparents, teachers, coaches, and friends (who are not themselves using drugs).

- Get the help of a certified therapist experienced in drug and alcohol counseling. Look in the telephone book, ask at support group meetings, or talk to a probation officer.

- Gather information. Discuss the suspected drug abuse. Ask friends and family if they have pieces of the puzzle. Take notes. List all the incidents and evidence that point to drug abuse.

- In the case of children, designate someone to be available 24 hours a day to whom the child can call if the parents are unavailable or when the child does not feel comfortable going to the parents.

- Have a goal for the drug abuser. Some options are to start outpatient counseling, to enroll in inpatient treatment, or to take a drug and alcohol evaluation. For children, another option is a contract, with specific rules and consequences. If the drug abuser refuses to accept the goal, every member of the intervention should be ready to apply a consequence.

- Schedule the confrontation for two dates. If the abuser is unavailable or runs away from the first meeting, you have another date scheduled.

- Practice the intervention to identify gaps.

- Schedule the drug or alcohol evaluation or treatment immediately.

- Start with love. Be obvious about your caring for the individual before revealing your intention.

- Expect the worst. The drug abuser may scream, play the victim, lie, exaggerate, intimidate, flee, or become passive. The abuser may challenge anyone in the group who does not practice what he or she preaches.

Personal Assessment

- State the purpose of the meeting: "Everyone here cares about you and is concerned about you. Please share what's troubling you."
- Give the individual a chance to admit the drug abuse.
- Confront the individual with the drug-taking behavior. Use the notes.
- Focus on the behavior. Don't allow the abuser to sidetrack the group or raise other issues.
- Explain the intervention goals.
- Explain the consequences of refusing to comply with the goals.
- Leave the door open for further discussion or questions. Every member of the group should be available for support.
- Praise any cooperation, and end with hugs and other expressions of love.
- Document everything. Write down everything the abuser said and agreed to do.

To avoid these common mistakes:

- Do not conduct an intervention without the assistance of a drug treatment professional.

- Don't be caught unprepared. Know what you're talking about. Don't let any of the reactions surprise you. Be on time. Have the evaluation scheduled.
- Don't condemn the abuser or talk in broad generalities.
- Don't play the victim. Don't lose your temper. Don't negotiate.
- Don't assume the abuser will keep his or her word. Follow through with your consequences.
- Don't give up. If the individual runs away or refuses to cooperate, plan the next meeting.

To Carry This Further . . .

See the Star Box on page 226 and the Health Reference Guide at the back of this text for information about national groups and hot lines for drug use. They will help you find additional information about drug dependence and how to combat it.

Individual Factors That Influence Drug Abuse

Genetic predisposition, personality traits, attitudes and beliefs, interpersonal skills, and unmet developmental needs can lead to drug use.

Genetic Predisposition

The importance of genetic predisposition (inherited vulnerability) to drug use has not been fully determined. However, studies of alcoholics have demonstrated that genetic factors do play some role in the development of alcoholism. Research on genetic predisposition to the abuse of other drugs is much farther behind that for alcohol.

Personality Traits, Attitudes, and Beliefs

Although drug-taking behavior cannot be predicted strictly on the basis of personality type, correlations have been noted with certain aspects of personality (or temperament). For example, children who are easily bored and need continual activity and challenge are more likely to take drugs when they are older. A similar tendency is seen in children who are driven to avoid negative consequences for their actions and who crave immediate external reward for their efforts. Clusters of traits (as measured by personality inventories), including rebelliousness, rejection of behavioral norms, resistance to authority, and high tolerance for deviance, are also reported in drug abusers.

However, a cause-and-effect relationship between personality profile and drug abuse is difficult to prove. Perhaps the abuse of drugs actually creates the personality traits, rather than the other way around.

Interpersonal Skills and Self-Esteem

Drug abusers are usually deficient in interpersonal skills. They are likely to score lower on tests that measure well-being, tolerance of others, and achievement. They also often have lower self-esteem than those who do not abuse drugs. Again, the question of cause and effect must be raised.

Personal development results from success in daily living. When people lack positive experiences in school, employment, parenting, and varied aspects of community involvement, they may attempt to compensate through chronic heavy drug use. Of course, drug abuse removes them further from productive and satisfying growth and development, thus increasing compensatory use of drugs.

Environmental Factors That Influence Drug Abuse

Drug use can be fostered by factors within the immediate environment, which includes home and family, school, peers, and the community.

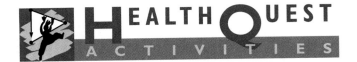

Home and Family

Drug abuse that begins in childhood is often associated with the home and family.[6] Children seem to be at greater risk when parents exhibit poor management skills, antisocial behavior, and even criminality. These families are often disorganized and have poorly defined roles for parenting and being a productive member of society. In many cases, adult family members abuse drugs themselves or tolerate those who do. As with tobacco use, parents can be the best or worst models children can have. The Star Box on page 209 explores the family environment in greater detail.

School

Children from disorganized or socially maladjusted families often have difficulty adjusting to the organized environment of the school. The following chain of events has been suggested to explain the relationship of a poor home environment and weak academic performance to drug abuse: An undesirable home environment contributes to poor school performance and poor social development; failure at school leads to loss of self-esteem, aggressive behavior, and loss of interest in school; these factors in turn may foster truancy and drug experimentation.

Peers

A clear relationship exists between peer group drug abuse and drug abuse among individual members. It is unusual for a student to remain an active member of a peer group in which the members abuse drugs and still abstain from drug use. Student athletes may compose one type of drug-using peer group.

Community

Drug availability, drug education, and drug treatment and rehabilitation vary among communities. As a result, drug abuse rates differ from one community to another. Students who are parents may be interested in the degree to which their communities foster or deter drug abuse.

Family Socialization and the Abuse of Drugs[6]

The family is one of the most important factors influencing drug-taking behavior. Adolescents who are likely to abuse drugs often come from families who foster the abuse of drugs. Listed below are contrasting patterns of child rearing.

"Traditional" or status-centered

- Each member's place in family is a function of age and sex status
- Father is defined as boss and, more important, as agent of discipline. He receives "respect" and deference from mother and children
- Emphasis on overt acts—what child does rather than why
- Valued qualities of child are obedience and cleanliness
- Emphasis on "direct" discipline: physical punishment, scolding, threats
- Social consensus and solidarity in communication; emphasis on "we"
- Emphasis on communication from parent to child
- Parent feels little need to justify demands to child; commands are followed with "because I say so"
- Emphasis on conforming to rules, respecting authority, maintaining conventional social order
- Child may attain a strong sense of social identity at the cost of loss of individuality and poor academic performance

"Modern" or person-centered

- Emphasis on selfhood and individuality of each member
- Father is more affectionate, less authoritative; mother becomes more important as agent of discipline
- Emphasis on motives and feelings—why child does what she or he does
- Valued qualities of child are happiness, achievement, consideration, curiosity, self-control
- Discipline based on reasoning, isolation, guilt, threat of loss of love
- Communication used to express individual experience and perspectives; emphasis on "I"
- Emphasis on two-way communication between parent and child; parent open to persuasion
- Parent gives good reasons for demands: not "Shut up" but "Please keep quiet or go into the other room; I'm trying to talk on the telephone"
- Emphasis on reasons for rules; particular rules can be criticized in the name of "higher" rational or ethical principles
- Child may attain strong sense of selfhood but may have identity problems and feel guilt, alienation

Which pattern do you think would contribute most effectively to minimizing the abuse of drugs? Would a combination of patterns be even more effective?

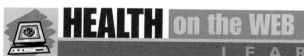

HEALTH on the WEB
LEARNING ACTIVITIES

Exploring Substance Use and Abuse

The National Center on Addiction and Substance Abuse (CASA), at Columbia University, takes an interdisciplinary approach (including health policy, medicine and nursing, communications, economics, sociology, anthropology, law enforcement, business, religion, and education) to studying all forms of substance abuse. CASA's mission is to raise awareness of the devastation caused by all forms of substance abuse. Visit CASA's website at www.casacolumbia.org/quiz/quiz3.htm and take the "New National Substance Abuse Quiz." What did you learn about substance abuse? How can you use your knowledge to help yourself or a friend or relative?

Learning About Marijuana Use

Many students who experiment with marijuana eventually become addicted to the drug. Marijuana addiction can cause or magnify problems in school, on the job, and with family and friends. Go to www.marijuana-anonymous.org/index.shtml and

click on "Am I An Addict?" The 12 questions related to marijuana use will help you decide whether you may have a problem with marijuana abuse.

Asking the Right Questions About Drug Use

The decision to seek treatment for a child or adolescent who is abusing drugs can be difficult. A professional drug abuse counselor can help parents, other family members, or friends determine whether treatment is necessary. When properly informed, relatives and close friends can be valuable partners in the treatment process. If you suspect that a child or teenager you know is abusing drugs, what questions should you ask? Go to www.aacap.org/factsFam/subabuse.htm and read through the list of 12 questions recommended by the American Academy of Child and Adolescent Psychiatry.

For more activities, log on to our Online Learning Center at www.mhhe.com/hper/health/payne

Societal Factors That Influence Drug Abuse

Factors such as the existence of a youth subculture, modeling and advertising, and the self-care movement affect drug use.

Youth Subculture

For many reasons, a distinctive youth subculture exists in the United States. It comprises people from twelve to seventeen years of age. This subculture has its own expectations, roles, and standards, and its own language, dress code, and behaviors.

Many people assume that the rate of drug abuse is higher in this group than in any other segment of American society. However, this belief is not supported by research. A recent study indicates that a higher rate of drug abuse occurs among eighteen- to thirty-four-year-olds.[9] Nevertheless, the drug abuse that does occur among those in the younger age group is of concern because patterns that are established at an early age can carry over into later life. In fact, during this period, experimentation with a **gateway drug** (alcohol, nicotine, or marijuana) often begins, which may lead to heavier drug use later. Specific *Healthy People 2010* objectives will be targeted toward this age group.

Modeling and Advertising

The influence others have on us by example of their own behavior is called *modeling*. Modeling of drug use within the peer group and family has already been presented. However, movie stars, musicians, and athletes also serve as models of behavior. Their example exerts a powerful influence on children and adolescents.

When models are employed by the media to sell products, advertising becomes an important factor in fostering drug use. The marketing of tobacco and alcohol products is perhaps the best example (see the Topics for Today article in Chapter 9). "Beautiful people" are depicted enjoying a social drug, such as alcohol, coffee, tea, or tobacco, in opulent surroundings that most viewers can only dream of being in. Celebrities participate in events sponsored by alcohol or tobacco companies. Company logos are shown on almost every item that appears on television, including the clothing and equipment of the participants, outfield walls, scoreboards, and race cars. Scenes of affluence and sexuality abound.

Personal Applications

• Can you recall a recent movie, television show, or music video in which drug use is glamorized? Do you believe that this modeling encourages children to begin using drugs?

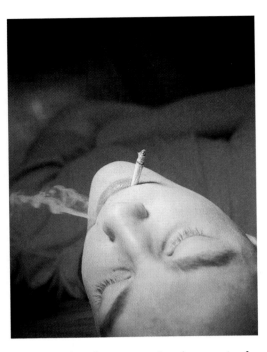

Marijuana is considered a gateway drug because it often leads the user to heavier drug use.

The Self-Care Movement

People's ability to engage in medical self-care makes drug use easier and more socially acceptable than in the past. In a society conditioned by the effectiveness and availability of OTC and prescription medications, the use of other drugs, both legal and illegal, to make ourselves feel better seems more reasonable than ever before. This attitude, then, fosters drug misuse and, for some, drug abuse.

Effects of Drugs on the Central Nervous System

To better understand the disruption caused by the actions of psychoactive drugs, a general knowledge of the normal functioning of the nervous system's basic unit, the **neuron**, is required.

First, stimuli from the internal or external environment are received by the appropriate sensory receptor, perhaps an organ such as an eye or an ear. Once sensed, these stimuli are converted into electrical impulses. These impulses are then directed along the neuron's **dendrite**, through the cell body, and along the **axon** toward the synaptic junction near an adjacent neuron. On arrival at the **synapse**, the electrical impulses stimulate the production and release of chemical messengers called **neurotransmitters.** These neurotransmitters transmit the electrical impulses from one neuron to the dendrites of adjoining neurons. Thus neurons function in a coordinated fashion

Effect of Drugs on the Central Nervous System

This illustration depicts the disruption caused by the action of a psychoactive drug on the central nervous system (1). Neurotransmitters are chemical messengers that transfer electrical impulses across the synapses between nerve cells (2). Psychoactive drugs interrupt this process, thus disrupting the coordinated functioning of the nervous system.

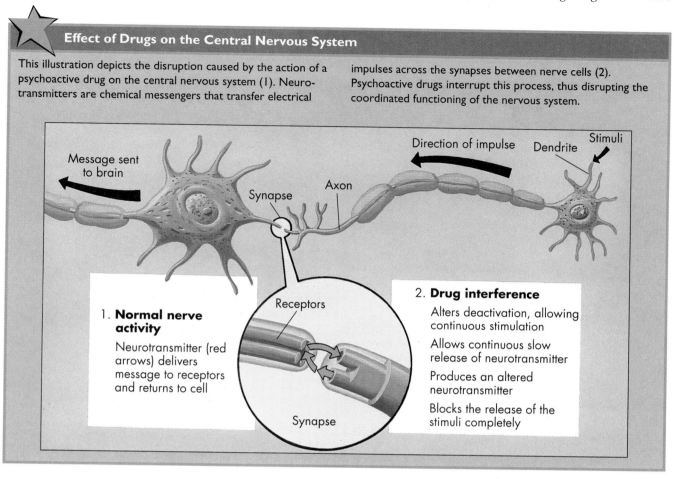

Message sent to brain

Direction of impulse   Dendrite   Stimuli

Synapse   Axon

1. **Normal nerve activity**

Neurotransmitter (red arrows) delivers message to receptors and returns to cell

Receptors

Synapse

2. **Drug interference**

Alters deactivation, allowing continuous stimulation

Allows continuous slow release of neurotransmitter

Produces an altered neurotransmitter

Blocks the release of the stimuli completely

---

to send information to the brain for interpretation and to relay appropriate response commands outward to the tissues of the body.

The role of neurotransmitters is critically important to the relay of information within the system. A substance that has the ability to alter some aspect of neurotransmitter function has the potential to seriously disrupt the otherwise normally functioning system. Psychoactive drugs are capable of exerting these disruptive influences on the neurotransmitters. Drugs "work" by changing the way neurotransmitters work, often by blocking the production of a neurotransmitter or forcing the continued release of a neurotransmitter (see the Star Box above).

Drug Classifications

Drugs can be categorized according to the nature of their physiological effects. Most psychoactive drugs fall into one of six general categories: stimulants, depressants, hallucinogens, cannabis, narcotics, and inhalants (Table 7-1).

Stimulants

In general, **stimulants** excite or increase the activity of the CNS. Also called "uppers," stimulants alert the CNS by increasing heart rate, blood pressure, and the rate of brain function. Users feel uplifted and less fatigued. Examples of stimulant drugs include caffeine, amphetamines, and cocaine. Most stimulants produce psychological dependence and tolerance relatively

gateway drug   an easily obtainable legal or illegal drug that represents a user's first experience with a mind-altering drug; this drug can serve as the "gateway" to the use of other drugs.

neuron   a nerve cell.

dendrite   the portion of a neuron that receives electrical stimuli from adjacent neurons; neurons typically have several such branches or extensions.

axon   the portion of a neuron that conducts electrical impulses to the dendrites of adjacent neurons; neurons typically have one axon.

synapse (**sinn** aps)   the location at which an electrical impulse from one neuron is transmitted to an adjacent neuron; also referred to as a *synaptic junction*.

neurotransmitters   chemical messengers that transfer electrical impulses across the synapses between nerve cells.

stimulants   psychoactive drugs that stimulate the function of the central nervous system.

Table 7-1 Psychoactive Drug Categories

Drugs	Trade or Common Names	Medical Uses	Possible Effects
Stimulants			
Cocaine*	Coke, crack, gin, girlfriend, girl, double bubble, California cornflakes, caballo, bouncing powder, flake, snow	Local anesthetic	Increased alertness, excitation, euphoria, increased pulse rate and blood pressure, insomnia, loss of appetite
Amphetamines	Biphetamine, Delcobese, Desoxyn, Dexedrine, mediatric, methamphetamine (ice), black Mollies, aimies, amps, bam, beans, benz	Hyperactivity, narcolepsy, weight control	
Phendimetrazine	Prelu-2		
Methylphenidate	Ritalin, Methidate		
Other stimulants	Adipex, Bacarate, Cylert, Didrex, Ionamin, Plegine, PreSate, Sanorex, Tenuate, Tepanil, Voranil		
Depressants			
Chloral hydrate	Noctec, Somnos	Hypnotic	Slurred speech, disorientation, drunken behavior without odor of alcohol
Barbiturates	Amobarbital, Butisol, phenobarbital, phenoxbarbital, secobarbital, Tuinal, blockbusters, black bombers, blue devils, blue dogs, blue tips, tombica	Anesthetic, anticonvulsant, sedative, hypnotic	
Glutethimide	Doriden	Sedative, hypnotic	
Methaqualone	Optimil, Parest, Quaalude, Somnafec, Sopor		
Benzodiazepines	Ativan, Azene, Clonopin, Dalmane, diazepam, Librium, Serax, Tranxene, Valium, Vestran	Antianxiety, anticonvulsant, sedative, hypnotic	
Other depressants	Equanil, Miltown, Noludar, Placidyl, Valmid	Antianxiety, sedative, hypnotic	
Hallucinogens			
LSD	Acid, brown dot, microdot, cap, California sunshine, brown bomber	None	Delusions and hallucinations, poor perception of time and distance
Mescaline and peyote	Mesc, buttons, cactus, chief	None	
Amphetamine variants (designer drugs)	2,5-DMA, DOM, DOP, MDA, MDMA, PMA, STP, TMA, clarity, chocolate chips, booty juice	None	
Phencyclidine	Angel dust, AD, hog, PCP, boat, black whack, amoeba, angel hair, angel smoke	Veterinary anesthetic	

continued

*Designated a narcotic under the Controlled Substances Act.

quickly, but they are unlikely to produce significant physical dependence when judged by life-threatening withdrawal symptoms. The important exception is cocaine, which seems to be capable of producing psychological dependence and withdrawal so powerful that continued use of the drug is inevitable in some users.

Caffeine

The methylxanthines are a family of chemicals that includes three compounds: caffeine, theophylline, and theobromine. Of these, caffeine is the most heavily consumed.

Caffeine is a tasteless drug found in coffee, tea, cocoa, many soft drinks, and several groups of over-the-counter drugs. It is a relatively harmless CNS stimulant when consumed in moderate amounts (Table 7-2). Many coffee drinkers believe that they cannot start the day successfully without the benefit of a cup or two of coffee.

The chronic effects of long-term caffeine use are less clear. Chronic users show evidence of tolerance and withdrawal, indicating that they are physically dependent. Researchers have attempted to link caffeine to coronary heart disease, pancreatic cancer, and fibrocys-

Table 7-1 Psychoactive Drug Categories—*Continued*

Drugs	Trade or Common Names	Medical Uses	Possible Effects
Hallucinogens— *continued*			
Phencyclidine analogs	PCE, PCPy, TCP	None	Euphoria, relaxed inhibitions, increased appetite, disoriented behavior
Other hallucinogens	Bufotenin, DMT, DET, ibogaine, psilocybin, psilocyn	None	
Cannabis			
Marijuana	Acapulco gold, black Bart, black mote, blue sage, bobo, butterflower, cannabis-T, cess, cheeba, grass, pot, sinsemilla, Thai sticks	Under investigation	Euphoria, drowsiness, respiratory depression, constricted pupils, nausea
Tetrahydro-cannabinol	THC	Under investigation	
Hashish	Hash	None	
Hashish oil	Hash oil	None	
Narcotics			
Opium	Dover's powder, paregoric, Parapectolin, cruz, Chinese tobacco, China	Analgesic, antidiarrheal	
Morphine	Morphine, Pectoal syrup, emsel, first line	Analgesic, antitussive	
Codeine	Codeine, Empirin compound with codeine, Robitussin A-C	Analgesic, antitussive	
Heroin	Diacetylmorphine, horse, smack, courage pills, dead on arrival (DOA)	Under investigation	
Hydromorphone	Dilaudid	Analgesic	Intoxication, excitation, disorientation, aggression, hallucination, variable effects
Meperidine (pethidine)	Demerol, Pethadol	Analgesic	
Methadone	Dolophine, Methadone, Methadose	Analgesic, heroin substitute	
Other narcotics	Darvon,† Dromoran, Fentanyl, LAAM, Leitine, Levo-Dromoran, Percodan, Tussionex, Talwin,† Lomotil	Analgesic, antidiarrheal, antitussive	
Inhalants			
Anesthetic gases	Aerosols, petroleum products, solvents	Surgical anesthesia	
Vasodilators (amyl nitrite, butyl nitrite)	Aerosols, petroleum products, solvents	None	

†Not designated a narcotic under the Controlled Substances Act.

tic breast disease. So far, the results have been inconclusive, or, in some cases, inconsistent with other studies.

One study advised pregnant women to consume caffeine sparingly.[10] In another study, babies born to women who drank more than three cups of coffee a day had a slightly increased risk of low birth weight and smaller head size.[11]

For the average healthy adult, moderate consumption of caffeine is unlikely to pose any serious health threat. However, excessive consumption (equivalent to ten or more cups of coffee daily) could lead to anxiety, diarrhea, restlessness, delayed onset of sleep or frequent awakening, headache, and heart palpitations.

Do you use caffeine to help you meet the demands of your daily life? Are you overly dependent on caffeine? For a closer look at caffeine and tips on curtailing excessive use, see the Topics for Today article on page 229.

Amphetamines

Amphetamines produce increased activity and mood elevation in almost all users. The amphetamines include several closely related compounds: amphetamine,

Table 7-2   Caffeine Content of Beverages, Food, and Drug Preparations

Coffee (5 oz cup)	Caffeine (mg)	Soft Drinks (12 oz)	Caffeine (mg)	Pain Relievers	Caffeine (mg)
Drip method	110–150	Mountain Dew	54	Anacin	32
Percolated	64–124	Mello Yello	52	Excedrin	65
Instant	40–108	TAB	46	Midol	32
Decaffeinated	2–5	Coca-Cola	46	Plain aspirin	0
		Diet Coke	46	Vanquish	33
Tea (5 oz cup)		Shasta Cola	44		
1-min brew	9–33	Mr. Pibb	40	**Diuretics**	
3-min brew	20–46	Dr. Pepper	40	Aqua Ban	100
5-min brew	20–50	Diet Dr. Pepper	40		
Instant tea	12–28	Pepsi Cola	38		
Iced tea (12 oz)	22–36	Diet Pepsi	36	**Cold Remedies**	
				Coryban-D	30
				Dristan	0
Cocoa		**Stimulants**		Triaminicin	30
Made from mix	6	NoDoz tablets	100		
Milk chocolate (1 oz)	6	Vivarin tablets	200	**Weight-Control Aids**	
Baking chocolate	35			Dexatrim	200
				Prolamine	140
				Prescription Pain Relievers	
				Cafergot	100
				Darvon compound	32
				Fiorinal	40
				Migralam	100

dextroamphetamine, and methamphetamine. These compounds do not have any natural sources and are completely manufactured in the laboratory. Medical use of amphetamines is limited primarily to the treatment of obesity, **narcolepsy**, and **attention deficit disorder (ADD)**.

Amphetamines can be ingested, injected, or snorted (inhaled). At low-to-moderate doses, amphetamines elevate mood and increase alertness and feelings of energy by stimulating receptor sites for two naturally occurring neurotransmitters. They also slow the activity of the stomach and intestine and decrease hunger. In the 1960s and 1970s, amphetamines were commonly prescribed for dieters, but when it was discovered that the appetite suppression effect of amphetamines lasted only a few weeks, most physicians stopped prescribing them. At high doses, amphetamines can increase heart rate and blood pressure to dangerous levels. As amphetamines are eliminated from the body, the user becomes tired.

When chronically abused, amphetamines produce rapid tolerance and strong psychological dependence. Other effects of chronic use include impotence and episodes of psychosis. When use is discontinued, periods of depression may develop.

Today the abuse of amphetamines is a more pressing concern than it has been in the recent past.

Underlying this sharp increase in abuse is methamphetamine. Known by a variety of names and forms, including "crank," "ice," "crystal," "meth," "speed," "crystal meth," and "Zip," methamphetamine is produced in illegal home laboratories.

Crystal Methamphetamine

Crystal methamphetamine, or ice, is among the most recent and dangerous forms of methamphetamine. Ice is a very pure form of methamphetamine that looks like rock candy. When smoked, the effects of ice are felt in about seven seconds as a wave of intense physical and psychological exhilaration. This effect lasts for several hours (much longer than the effects of crack), until the user becomes physically exhausted.

Recently, Mexican drug labs and outlaw entrepreneurs in the United States have been using the main ingredient in over-the-counter cold remedies to produce vast amounts of illegal methamphetamine. A boom in meth's popularity has led to reports of violence, psychotic behavior, and homicide. "The problem is so bad," reports Senator Diane Feinstein of California, "that in one Sacramento hospital, methamphetamine babies now outnumber crack babies as much as 7 to 1."

Chronic use leads to nutritional difficulties, weight loss, reduced resistance to infection, and damage to the liver, lungs, and kidneys. Psychological de-

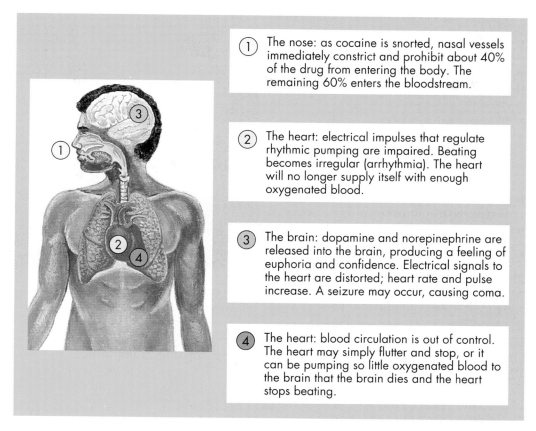

① The nose: as cocaine is snorted, nasal vessels immediately constrict and prohibit about 40% of the drug from entering the body. The remaining 60% enters the bloodstream.

② The heart: electrical impulses that regulate rhythmic pumping are impaired. Beating becomes irregular (arrhythmia). The heart will no longer supply itself with enough oxygenated blood.

③ The brain: dopamine and norepinephrine are released into the brain, producing a feeling of euphoria and confidence. Electrical signals to the heart are distorted; heart rate and pulse increase. A seizure may occur, causing coma.

④ The heart: blood circulation is out of control. The heart may simply flutter and stop, or it can be pumping so little oxygenated blood to the brain that the brain dies and the heart stops beating.

Figure 7-2 Cocaine's effects on the body.

pendence is quickly established. Withdrawal causes acute depression and fatigue but not significant physical discomfort.

Ritalin

Although Ritalin has not historically been considered a significant drug of abuse, the recent surge in the prescribing of Ritalin for children and teens has become a subject of debate. About 2.8 percent of people under age nineteen, about 1.5 million, are taking this stimulant drug.[12]

Ritalin is typically prescribed to elementary-age children to help focus attention if they are hyperactive or cannot concentrate. More girls than boys now take it, and more children continue taking the drug through adolescence. Critics argue that the drug is being prescribed to treat a variety of problems, when the better course would be to identify and treat the root cause of the problems. Supporters respond that Ritalin enables their children to pay attention in school.

Cocaine

Cocaine, perhaps the strongest of the stimulant drugs, has received much media attention. Cocaine is the primary psychoactive substance found in the leaves of the South American coca plant. The effects of cocaine last only briefly—from five to thirty minutes (Figure 7-2). Regardless of the form in which it is consumed, cocaine produces an immediate, near-orgasmic "rush," or feeling of exhilaration. This euphoria is quickly followed by a period of marked depression. Used only occasionally as a topical anesthetic, cocaine is usually inhaled (snorted), injected, or smoked (typically as crack). There is overwhelming scientific evidence that users quickly develop a strong psychological dependence on cocaine. Considerable evidence suggests that physical dependence also rapidly develops. However, physical dependence on cocaine does not lead to death on withdrawal.

The status of cocaine as a substitute for amphetamines (during the 1960s), as a recreational drug for the wealthy (during the 1970s), and as a widely abused

narcolepsy   a sleep-related disorder in which a person has a recurrent, overwhelming, and uncontrollable desire to sleep, often at inappropriate times.

attention deficit disorder (ADD)   an above-normal rate of physical movement; often accompanied by an inability to concentrate well on a specified task; also called *hyperactivity*.

crystal methamphetamine   a dangerous form of methamphetamine that quickly produces intense physical and psychological exhilaration when smoked.

drug by many segments of society (during the 1980s) is well documented. During the 1990s, overall cocaine use has decreased, although heavy use has increased. In addition, the proportion of high school seniors who have used cocaine at least once has increased from a low of 5.9 percent in 1994 to 8.7 percent in 1997, according to the annual *Monitoring the Future Study* of drug use.[3] Today, the smoking of crack has replaced the inhalation of "lines" of cocaine, which was the primary route of administration in the 1980s.

Crack Cocaine Crack is made by combining cocaine hydrochloride with common baking soda. When this pastelike mixture is allowed to dry, a small rocklike crystalline material remains. This crack is heated in the bowl of a small pipe, and the vapors are inhaled into the lungs. A single dose of crack currently sells for $20 to $30. Some crack users spend hundreds of dollars a day to maintain their habit.

The effect of crack is almost instantaneous. Within ten seconds after inhalation, cocaine reaches the CNS and influences the action of several neurotransmitters at specific sites in the brain. As with the use of other forms of cocaine, convulsions, seizures, respiratory distress, and cardiac failure have been reported with this sudden, extensive stimulation of the nervous system.

Within about six minutes, the stimulating effect of crack has been completely expended, and users frequently become depressed. Dependence develops within a few weeks, because users consume more crack in response to the short duration of stimulation and rapid onset of depression.

Intravenous administration has been the preferred route for cocaine users who are also regular users of heroin and other injectable drugs. Intravenous injection results in an almost immediate high, which lasts about ten minutes. A "smoother ride" is said to be obtained from a "speedball," the injectable mixture of heroin and cocaine (or methamphetamine).[6] However, such a mixture can be volatile and even fatal.

Freebasing Like crack, freebasing developed as a technique for maximizing the psychoactive effects of cocaine. Freebasing first requires that the common form of powdered cocaine (cocaine hydrochloride) be chemically altered (alkalized). This altered form is then dissolved in a solvent such as ether or benzene. This liquid solution is heated to evaporate the solvent. The heating process leaves the freebase cocaine in a powder form that can then be smoked, often through a water pipe. Because of the large surface area of the lungs, smoking cocaine facilitates fast absorption into the bloodstream.

One danger of freebasing cocaine is the risk related to the solvents used. Ether is a highly volatile

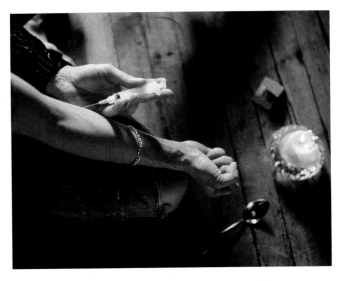

Intravenous injection of cocaine results in an almost immediate high for the user.

solvent capable of exploding and causing serious burns. Benzene is a known carcinogen associated with the development of leukemia. Clearly, neither solvent can be used without increasing the level of risk normally associated with cocaine use. This method of making smokeable cocaine led to the epidemic of smoking crack cocaine.

Cocaine and Society It is beyond the scope of this book to chronicle the ways in which cocaine use has profoundly damaged our nation. However, we encourage students to watch or read the daily media reports about this topic. A few of the central reasons why civic and government leaders have declared war on the use of illegal drugs, especially cocaine, follow.

The use of crack cocaine has tremendous costs in U.S. cities. The eventual plight of those who lose control over crack cocaine has become clear. They use up all their immediate resources, including their own financial resources and perhaps those of family or friends. They may then turn to crime, such as dealing in drugs, prostitution, or stealing, to pay for their crack cocaine. The users cease to be productive members of society and instead become a burden.

Although cocaine use hurts people from all walks of life, it most critically affects people from inner-city groups and the urban poor.[13] Cocaine use provides an instant temporary escape from an unpromising future. For many inner-city youths, selling cocaine or crack is the easiest way to escape poverty. However, drug dealing also brings with it an escalation of involvement in street gangs, crime, and violence.[14] Crack houses are also notorious for promoting the spread of HIV infection and other serious diseases. Tragically, thousands of babies are born in large city hospitals to crack-addicted mothers. These babies have both physical and neurological difficulties. Many of these babies are born with severe deformities, such as heart defects, brain damage, deformed arms and thumbs, and perforated bowels. Some are born with an HIV infection that soon leads to AIDS. Society is left to bear the burden of the treatment and care of these children. Indeed, the personal and social cost of cocaine use is enormous.

Depressants

Depressants (or sedatives) sedate the user, slowing down CNS function. Drugs included in this category are alcohol (see Chapter 8), barbiturates, and tranquilizers. Depressants produce tolerance in abusers, as well as strong psychological and physical dependence.

Barbiturates

Barbiturates are the so-called sleeping compounds that function by enhancing the effect of inhibitory neurotransmitters. They depress the CNS to the point where the user drops off to sleep or, as is the case with surgical anesthetics, the patient becomes anesthetized. Medically, barbiturates are used in widely varied dosages as anesthetics and for treatment of anxiety, insomnia, and epilepsy.[5] Regular use of a barbiturate quickly produces tolerance—eventually such a high dose is required that the user still feels the effects of the drug throughout the next morning. Some abusers then begin to alternate barbiturates with stimulants, producing a vicious circle of dependence. Other misusers combine alcohol and barbiturates or tranquilizers, inadvertently producing toxic or even lethal results. Abrupt withdrawal from barbiturate use frequently produces a withdrawal syndrome that can involve seizures, delusions, hallucinations, and even death.

Methaqualone (Quaalude, "ludes," Sopor) was developed as a sedative that would not have the dependence properties of other barbiturates.[5] Although this did not happen, Quaaludes were occasionally prescribed for anxious patients. Today, compounds resembling Quaaludes are manufactured in home laboratories and sold illegally so that they can be combined with small amounts of alcohol for an inexpensive, drunklike effect.

Tranquilizers

Tranquilizers are depressants that are intended to reduce anxiety and to relax people who are having problems managing stress. They are not specifically designed to produce sleep but rather to help people cope during their waking hours. Such tranquilizers are termed *minor tranquilizers,* of which diazepam (Valium) and chlordiazepoxide (Librium) may be the most commonly prescribed examples. Unfortunately,

some people become addicted to these and other prescription drugs.

Some tranquilizers are further designed to control hospitalized psychotic patients who may be suicidal or who are potential threats to others. These major tranquilizers subdue people physically but permit them to remain conscious. Their use is generally limited to institutional settings. All tranquilizers can produce physical and psychological dependence and tolerance.

Rohypnol

Rohypnol is a prescription drug manufactured in South America, Mexico, Europe, and Asia and illegally imported into the United States. Currently Rohypnol is being abused by a growing number of middle-class youths in the United States.

Known informally as "roofies," Rohypnol sells for $1 to $5 a tablet. It is ten times stronger than Valium and causes a drunk, sleepy feeling that lasts up to eight hours.

Some observers consider Rohypnol a serious threat and predict that Rohypnol will become as popular as crack because of its low price and intense effect. Law enforcement officials and other observers allege that young men have begun using Rohypnol to incapacitate young women before raping them. A recent federal law adds up to twenty years to the sentences of rapists who subdue their victims with Rohypnol.

High school and college students should not accept drinks from people they do not know. This recommendation extends to all parties where drinkers do not know what has been added to the punch or other drinks.

Hallucinogens

As the name suggests, hallucinogenic drugs produce hallucinations—perceived distortions of reality. Also known as *psychedelic drugs,* or *phantasticants,* **hallucinogens** reached their height of popularity during the 1960s (see the Learning from Our Diversity box on p. 218). At that time, young people were encouraged to use hallucinogenic drugs to "expand the mind," "reach an altered state," or "discover reality." Not all of the reality distortions, or "trips," were pleasant. Many users reported "bummers," or trips during which they perceived negative, frightening distortions.

Hallucinogenic drugs include laboratory-produced lysergic acid diethylamide (LSD), mescaline

---

depressants a category of drugs that sedate the user by slowing CNS function; they produce tolerance and strong psychological and physical addiction in users.

hallucinogens psychoactive drugs capable of producing hallucinations (distortions of reality).

Learning
From Our Diversity

Drugs, Religion, and the Law: Native Americans' Sacred Tradition at Risk

When we hear the word *hallucinogen*, most of us probably think of the 1960s, when millions of hippies and self-styled truth seekers looked for wisdom in substances ranging from mushrooms to mescaline. Some claimed to experience extraordinary visions, whereas years later other users were still suffering terrifying flashbacks to "bad trips" on LSD.

Unlike some other hallucinogens, mescaline—derived from the peyote cactus found in Mexico and the American Southwest—wasn't new to the sixties. Early Indian tribes in Mexico used peyote in religious ceremonies to enhance their spiritual experience. The practice later spread to Indian tribes in the United States. Today the Native American Church of North America still uses peyote in religious ceremonies.

Consumption of peyote in religious rituals is now permitted in almost thirty states, and the number of states that allow it has been growing steadily during recent years. Significantly, the Pentagon ruled in the spring of 1997 that members of the U.S. Armed Forces who belong to the Native American Church may use peyote as part of their religious ceremonies.

Practitioners of this ritual, however, still face significant legal hurdles. In a 1990 decision known as the Smith case, the Supreme Court rejected the claim of two Native Americans in Oregon who had sought unemployment compensation after losing their jobs for consuming peyote, which is a controlled substance. In 1993 President Bill Clinton signed into law the Religious Freedom Restoration Act (RFRA), which set stronger limits on government authority than the Supreme Court thought were necessary in the Smith case. The act was later declared unconstitutional, and in the summer of 1997 it was struck down by the Supreme Court.

The Religious Freedom Restoration Act was passed unanimously by the U.S. House of Representatives and by a vote of 97 to 2 in the Senate. Proponents of the law claimed it was essential to prevent the government from exercising too heavy a hand in religious activities; they contended further that, as the American population becomes increasingly diverse, government must recognize and accept the practices of religions other than the familiar mainstream denominations. Some opponents of RFRA argued that the law impermissibly reversed a Supreme Court decision based on an interpretation of the Constitution; others objected that RFRA permitted otherwise illegal practices—like the consumption of peyote in religious rituals—that may pose a threat to the common welfare.

The Supreme Court's action in affirming the unconstitutionality of the Religious Freedom Restoration Act will clearly have a far-reaching impact, both on Native Americans, to whom peyote is a sacred substance, and on everyone who is concerned with issues of religious freedom.

Do you think the consumption of otherwise illicit substances like peyote should be permitted in the practice of religion? Why or why not?

(from the peyote cactus plant), and psilocybin (from a particular genus of mushroom). Consumption of hallucinogens seems to produce not physical dependence but mild levels of psychological dependence. The development of tolerance is questionable. **Synesthesia**, a sensation in which users report hearing a color, smelling music, or touching a taste, is sometimes produced with hallucinogen use.

The long-term effects of hallucinogenic drug use are not fully understood. Questions about genetic abnormalities in offspring, fertility, sex drive and performance, and the development of personality disorders have not been fully answered. One phenomenon that has been identified and documented is the development of flashbacks—the unpredictable return to a psychedelic trip that occurred months or even years earlier. Flashbacks are thought to result from the accumulation of a drug within body cells.

LSD

The best-known, and most powerful, of all hallucinogens is lysergic acid diethylamide (LSD). LSD was first isolated in 1938 by Albert Hoffmann, who was studying a group of chemicals that were extracted from a fungus that infects rye and other cereal grains. Five years later, he accidentally discovered its hallucinogenic effects. Dr. Timothy Leary helped to spread the popularity of LSD in the 1960s by promoting the use of LSD in mind expansion and experimentation. LSD helped define the counterculture movement of the 1960s. During the 1970s and the 1980s, this drug lost considerable popularity. However, in the 1990s, LSD is making a comeback, with some studies showing that about one in ten high school students and one in twenty college students has experimented with LSD. Fear of cocaine and other powerful drugs, boredom, low cost, and an attempt to revisit the culture of the 1960s are thought to have increased LSD's attractiveness to today's young people.

LSD is manufactured in home laboratories and frequently distributed in blotter paper decorated with cartoon characters. Users place the paper on their tongue or chew the paper to ingest the drug. LSD is similar in structure to the neurotransmitter serotonin and produces psychedelic effects by interfering with the normal activity of this neurotransmitter. The effects can include altered perception of shapes, images, time, sound, and body form. Synesthesia is common to LSD users. LSD is metabolized in the liver and excreted. Its effects last an average of ten to twelve hours. Doses or "hits" range in price from $3 to $5.[15]

Users may describe LSD experiences as positive and "mind-expanding," or negative and "mind-constricting," depending on the user's mood and the social setting in which the drug is taken. Positive sensations include feelings of creativity, deep understanding of oneself and the universe, and feelings of grandeur. Although LSD users report feelings of insight and creativity, a real increase in these skills has not been demonstrated. At the same time, some reports of bad trips on LSD are thought to have been caused by other substances, such as PCP, that were sold to the user as LSD. Deaths resulting from bizarre behavior after taking LSD have been reported. Dangerous side effects include panic attacks, flashbacks, and occasional prolonged psychosis.

Although the hits today are about half as powerful as those in the 1960s, users still tend to develop high tolerance to LSD. Users do not develop physical dependence.

Designer Drugs

In recent years, chemists who produce many of the illegal drugs in home laboratories have designed versions of drugs listed on **FDA Schedule 1.** These designer drugs are similar to the controlled drugs on the FDA Schedule 1 but are sufficiently different so that they escape governmental control. The designer drugs are either newly synthesized products that are similar to already outlawed drugs but against which no law yet exists, or they are reconstituted or renamed illegal substances. Designer drugs are said to produce effects similar to their controlled drug counterparts.

People who use designer drugs do so at great risk because the manufacturing of these drugs is unregulated. The neurophysiological effect of these homemade drugs can be quite dangerous. So far, a synthetic heroin product (MPPP) and several amphetamine derivatives with hallucinogenic properties have been designed for the unwary drug consumer.

DOM (STP), MDA (the "love drug"), and MDMA ("ecstasy" or "XTC") are examples of amphetamine-derivative, hallucinogenic designer drugs. These drugs produce mild LSD-like hallucinogenic experiences, positive feelings, and enhanced alertness. They also have a number of potentially dangerous effects. Experts are particularly concerned that MDMA can produce strong psychological dependence and can deplete serotonin, an important excitatory neurotransmitter associated with a state of alertness. Permanent brain damage is possible.[5]

Phencyclidine

Phencyclidine (PCP, "angel dust") is unique because it not only produces hallucinogenic effects but also acts as an analgesic, a depressant, a stimulant, and an anesthetic. This makes the typical PCP experience impossible to predict or describe. The physical effects of PCP begin a few minutes after consumption and continue for four to six hours. PCP was studied for years during the 1950s and 1960s and was found to be an unsuitable animal and human anesthetic.

Manufactured in tablet or powder form, PCP can be injected, inhaled, taken orally, or smoked. Some users report mild euphoria, although most report bizarre perceptions, paranoid feelings, and aggressive behavior. PCP overdose may cause convulsions, cardiovascular collapse, and damage to the brain's respiratory center.

In a number of cases the aggressive behavior caused by PCP has led users to commit brutal crimes against both friends and innocent strangers. PCP accumulates in cells and may stimulate bizarre behavior months after initial use.

PCP is an extremely unpredictable drug. Although PCP has been blamed in many reports of bizarre, even homicidal, behavior, it continues to be abused. Because PCP is easily and cheaply manufactured in home laboratories, authorities have difficulty limiting its availability.

Cannabis

Cannabis (marijuana) has been labeled a mild hallucinogen for a number of years. However, most experts now consider it to be a drug category in itself. Marijuana produces mild effects like those of stimulants and depressants. The recent implication of marijuana in a large number of traffic fatalities makes this drug one whose consumption should be carefully considered. Marijuana is actually a wild plant (*Cannabis sativa*) whose fibers were once used in the manufacture of hemp rope. When the leafy material and small stems are dried and crushed, users can smoke the mixture in rolled cigarettes ("joints") or pipes. The resins collected from scraping the flowering tops of the plant yield a marijuana product called hashish, or hash, commonly smoked in a pipe.

The potency of marijuana's hallucinogenic effect is determined by the percentage of the active ingredient, tetrahydrocannabinol (THC), present in the product. Based on the analysis of samples from drug

synesthesia a sensation of combining of the senses, such as perceiving color by hearing or perceiving taste by touching.

FDA Schedule 1 a list of drugs that have a high potential for abuse but no medical use.

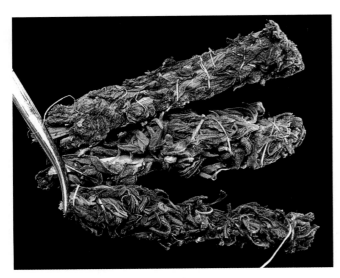

Thai sticks are a potent form of marijuana.

seizures and street buys in the United States, the concentration of THC averages about 6 percent for marijuana, 7 percent to 9 percent for higher-quality marijuana (sinsemilla), 8 percent to 14 percent for hashish, and as high as 50 percent for hash oil.[5]

Others believe the potency to be much higher, as a result of more scientific growing techniques. "Potency is 4 to 5 times higher today," says Lee Brown, former director of the White House's Office on Drug Control Policy. The increased potency can cause "paranoia and anxiety," Brown adds.

THC is a fat-soluble substance and thus is absorbed and retained in fat tissues within the body. Before being excreted, THC can remain in the body for up to a month. With the sophistication of today's drug tests, trace amounts of THC can be detected for up to three weeks after consumption.[5] It is possible that the THC that comes from passive inhalation (for example, during an indoor rock concert) can also be detected for a short time after exposure.

Once marijuana is consumed, its effects vary from person to person. Being "high" or "stoned" means different things to different people. Many people report heightened sensitivity to music, cravings for particular foods, and a relaxed mood. There is widespread consensus that marijuana's behavioral effects include four probabilities: (1) Users must learn to recognize what a marijuana high is like, (2) marijuana impairs short-term memory, (3) users overestimate the passage of time, and (4) users lose the ability to maintain attention to a task.[5]

The long-term effects of marijuana use are still being studied. Chronic abuse may lead to an amotivational syndrome in some people. Heavy marijuana users have trouble paying attention and retaining new information for at least a day after last using the drug, according to a recent study. This contradicts the notion that marijuana users are fine after the marijuana high wears off.[16]

The irritating effects of marijuana smoke on lung tissue are more pronounced than those of cigarette smoke, and some of the more than 400 chemicals in marijuana are now linked to lung cancer development. In fact, one of the most potent carcinogens, benzopyrene, is found in higher levels in marijuana smoke than in tobacco smoke. Marijuana smokers tend to inhale deeply and hold the smoke in the lungs for long periods. It is likely that at some point the lungs of chronic marijuana smokers will be damaged.

Long-term marijuana use is also associated with damage to the immune system and to the male and female reproductive systems and with an increase in birth defects in babies born to mothers who smoke marijuana. Chronic marijuana use lowers testosterone levels in men, but the effect of this change is not known. The effect of long-term marijuana use on a variety of types of sexual behavior is also not fully understood.

Because the drug can distort perceptions and thus perceptual ability (especially when combined with alcohol), its use by automobile drivers clearly jeopardizes the lives of many innocent people.

The only medical uses for marijuana are to relieve the nausea caused by chemotherapy, to improve appetite in AIDS patients, and to ease the pressure that builds up in the eyes of glaucoma patients. However, a variety of other drugs, many of which are nearly as effective, are also used for these purposes. Voters in two states recently passed propositions legalizing the medical use of marijuana when it is recommended by a physician (see the Star Box on p. 221).

From 1996 to 1997, the use of marijuana at least once (lifetime use) increased among twelfth and tenth graders, continuing the trend seen in recent years, according to the *Monitoring the Future Study.*[3] The rate of lifetime marijuana use among high school seniors was found to be higher than any year since 1987, but all rates remain well below those seen in the late 1970s and early 1980s, suggesting that the sharp increases of recent years may be slowing. Daily marijuana use in the past month increased among twelfth graders but decreased among eighth graders. This pattern of increase among older students and stability or decrease among younger students was found with several indicators in the 1997 study.

Another study[17] found that the resurgence in marijuana use continues, especially among adolescents, with rates of emergency department mentions of marijuana increasing in several cities. The researchers identified two possible causes for these dramatic consequences: higher potency and the use of marijuana mixed with or in combination with other dangerous drugs.

Our national debate over the medical uses of marijuana hit the headlines again recently, when voters in California and Arizona passed propositions legalizing the medical use of marijuana by patients when it is recommended by a physician. These new state laws conflict with federal laws against the possession of marijuana. How this conflict will be resolved remains to be seen.

The Clinton administration reacted quickly against these measures. Officials argued that these new laws could increase adolescent drug use or possibly threaten the process by which drugs now gain approval for medical use. "Marijuana use is illegal, dangerous, unhealthy, and wrong," said Donna Shalala, Health and Human Services secretary.

"There are thousands of people who are using [marijuana] now as medicine," said Dr. Lester Grinspoon of Harvard Medical School. "We're making these people criminals." Proponents argue that marijuana can act as an appetite stimulant, muscle relaxant, and pain reliever, and that it can treat the following conditions:

- Nausea resulting from cancer treatment
- Appetite loss in people with AIDS
- Pain from diseases such as multiple sclerosis
- Eye pressure and pain resulting from glaucoma

Have you known anyone who has used marijuana for medical purposes? Where do you stand on this issue?

Personal Applications

- Why do you think that today's young people believe that marijuana use is not dangerous? How widespread is marijuana use on your campus?

Narcotics

The **narcotics** are among the most dependence-producing drugs. Medically, narcotics are used to relieve pain and induce sleep. On the basis of origin, narcotics can be subgrouped into the natural, quasisynthetic, and synthetic narcotics.

Natural Narcotics

Naturally occurring substances derived from the Oriental poppy plant include opium (the primary psychoactive substance extracted from the Oriental poppy), morphine (the primary active ingredient in opium), and thebaine (a compound not used as a drug). Morphine and related compounds have medical use as analgesics in the treatment of mild to severe pain.

Quasisynthetic Narcotics

Quasisynthetic narcotics are compounds created by chemically altering morphine. These laboratory-produced drugs are intended to be used as analgesics, but their benefits are largely outweighed by a high dependence rate and a great risk of toxicity. The best known of the quasisynthetic narcotics is heroin. Although heroin is a fast-acting and very effective analgesic, it is extremely addictive. Once injected into a vein or "skin-popped" (injected beneath the skin surface), heroin produces dreamlike euphoria and, like all narcotics, strong physical and psychological dependence and tolerance.

Heroin has enjoyed an explosion in popularity in the United States recently. Some studies now put the number of heroin addicts in the United States at 1 million. Major cities reported dramatic jumps in heroin use and deaths from overdose in 1995 and 1996.[18] Particularly alarming is a trend toward heroin use by younger people, including high school students. Some observers report that heroin has overtaken cocaine in popularity.

The reasons for the burst of heroin use include the greatly increased supply now coming from Colombia and the drug's relatively low price. In some cities, heroin is used to prolong the high of crack use and to soften the shock of depression when crack wears off. Such drug combinations are particularly risky and often fatal.

As with the use of all other injectable illegal drugs, the practice of sharing needles increases the likelihood of transmission of various communicable diseases, including HIV (see Chapter 12). Abrupt withdrawal from heroin use is rarely fatal, but the discomfort during **cold turkey** withdrawal is reported to be overwhelming.

Synthetic Narcotics

Meperidine (Demerol) and propoxyphene (Darvon), common postsurgical painkillers, and methadone, the drug prescribed during the rehabilitation of heroin addicts, are synthetic narcotics. These opiatelike drugs are manufactured in medical laboratories. They are not natural narcotics or quasisynthetic narcotics because they do not originate from the Oriental poppy plant. Like true narcotics, however, these drugs can rapidly induce physical dependence. One important criticism of methadone rehabilitation

narcotics opiates; psychoactive drugs derived from the Oriental poppy plant; narcotics relieve pain and induce sleep.

cold turkey immediate, total discontinuation of use of a drug; associated withdrawal discomfort.

programs is that they merely shift the addiction from heroin to methadone.

Inhalants

Inhalants are a class of drugs that includes a variety of volatile (quickly evaporating) compounds that generally produce unpredictable, drunklike effects in users. Users of inhalants may also have some delusions and hallucinations. Some users may become quite aggressive. Drugs in this category include anesthetic gases (chloroform, nitrous oxide, and ether), vasodilators (amyl nitrite and butyl nitrite), petroleum products and commercial solvents (gasoline, kerosene, plastic cement, glue, typewriter correction fluid, paint, and paint thinner), and certain aerosols (found in some propelled spray products, fertilizers, and insecticides).

Most of the danger in using inhalants lies in the damaging, sometimes fatal effects on the respiratory system. Furthermore, users may unknowingly place themselves in dangerous situations because of the drunklike hallucinogenic effects. Aggressive behavior might also make users a threat to themselves and others.

Combination Drug Effects

Drugs taken in various combinations and dosages can alter and perhaps intensify effects.

A **synergistic effect** is a dangerous consequence of taking different drugs in the same general category at the same time. The combination exaggerates each individual drug's effects. For example, the combined use of alcohol and tranquilizers produces a synergistic effect greater than the total effect of each of the two drugs taken separately. In this instance, a much-amplified, perhaps fatal sedation will occur. In a simplistic sense, "one plus one equals four or five."

When taken at or near the same time, drug combinations produce a variety of effects. Drug combinations have additive, potentiating, or antagonistic effects. When two or more drugs are taken and the result is merely a combined total effect of each drug, the result is an **additive effect.** The sum of the effects is not exaggerated. In a sense, "one plus one plus one equals three."

When one drug intensifies the action of a second drug, the first drug is said to have a **potentiated effect** on the second drug. One popular drug-taking practice during the 1970s was the consumption of Quaaludes and beer. Quaaludes potentiated the inhibition-releasing, sedative effects of alcohol. This particular drug combination produced an inexpensive but potentially fatal drunklike euphoria in the user.

An **antagonistic effect,** on the other hand, is a drug's action in reducing another drug's effects. Knowledge of this principle has been useful in the medical treatment of certain drug overdoses, as in the use of tranquilizers to relieve the effects of LSD or other hallucinogenic drugs.

Because of these possible synergistic drug effects, patients should always inform their doctors and dentists of any illegal drugs they have taken.

Society's Response to Drug Use

During the last twenty years, society has responded to illegal drug use with growing concern. Most adults see drug abuse as a clear danger to society. This position has been supported by the development of community, school, state, and national organizations interested in the reduction of illegal drug use. These organizations have included such diverse groups as Parents Against Drugs, Parents for a Drug-Free Youth, Mothers Against Drunk Driving (MADD), Narcotics Anonymous, and the federal Drug Enforcement Administration. Certain groups have concentrated their efforts on education, others on enforcement, and still others on the development of laws and public policy.

The personal and social issues related to drug abuse are very complex. Innovative solutions continue to be devised. Some believe that only through early childhood education will people learn alternatives to drug use. Starting drug education in the preschool years may have a more positive effect than waiting until the upper elementary or junior high school years. Recently, the focus on reducing young people's exposure to gateway drugs (especially tobacco, alcohol, and marijuana) may help slow down the move to other addictive drugs. Some people advocate much harsher penalties for drug use and drug trafficking, including extreme measures such as public executions.

Others support legalizing all drugs and making governmental agencies responsible for drug regulation and control, as is the case with alcohol. Advocates of this position believe that drug-related crime and violence would virtually cease once the demand for illegal products is reduced. Sound arguments can be made on both sides of this issue. What is your opinion?

Unless significant changes in society's response to drug use take place soon, the disastrous effects of virtually uncontrolled drug abuse will continue to be felt. Families and communities will continue to be plagued by drug-related tragedies. Law enforcement officials will be pressed to the limits of their resources in their attempts to reduce drug flow. Our judicial system will be heavily burdened by thousands of court cases. Health care facilities could face overwhelming numbers of patients.

In comparison with other federally funded programs, the "war on drugs" is less expensive than farm support, food stamps, Medicare, and national defense. However, it remains to be seen whether any amount of money spent on enforcement, without adequate support for education, treatment, and poverty reduction, can reduce the illegal drug demand and supply. Currently, approximately $15 billion is spent to fight the drug war in the United States—$10 billion on law enforcement and $5 billion on education, prevention, and treatment.

Personal Applications

• What public policy measures do you support to curb the drug problem? Do you know how your elected state and federal representatives vote on drug-related issues?

Drug Testing

Drug testing is one of society's responses to drug use and is becoming an increasingly popular prevention tool. Depending on how drug testing is used, it can be considered a primary, secondary, or tertiary prevention method. When used to prevent initial drug use, drug testing can be considered a primary prevention tool. When used to detect drug use that has already begun, testing can be considered a secondary prevention method. Drug testing of long-term abusers is a tertiary method of prevention.

In 1986 the federal government instituted drug-testing policies for federal employees in safety-sensitive jobs. In 1988 the Drug Free Workplace Act extended the drug-free federal policy to include all federal grantees (including universities) and most federal contractors. Although this act did not mandate drug testing, it encouraged tougher approaches to prevent and deal with drug problems at the worksite.

Private companies have developed drug-testing procedures similar to those used with federal agencies. More than half of Fortune 500 companies use drug testing to screen applicants or monitor employee drug use.

The five largest drug-testing laboratories in the United States process more than 1 million urine specimens per month combined.[19] Most of the specimens come from corporations that screen employees for commonly abused drugs. Among these drugs are amphetamines, barbiturates, benzodiazepines (the chemical bases for prescription tranquilizers such as Valium and Librium), cannabinoids (THC, hashish, and marijuana), methaqualone, opiates (heroin, codeine, and morphine), and PCP. With the exception of marijuana, most traces of these drugs are eliminated by the body within a few days after use. Marijuana can remain detectable for weeks after use.

How accurate are the results of drug testing? At typical cutoff standards, drug tests are likely to identify 90 percent of recent drug users. This means that about 10 percent of recent users will pass undetected. (These 10% are considered false negatives.) Nonusers whose drug tests indicate drug use (false positives) are quite rare. (Follow-up tests on these false positives would nearly always show negative results.) Human errors are probably more responsible than technical errors for inaccuracies in drug tests.[19]

Recently, scientists have been refining procedures that use hair samples to detect the presence of drugs.[20] These procedures seem to hold much promise, although certain technical obstacles remain. Watch for refinements in hair-sample drug testing in the near future.

Do you think that the possibility of having to take a drug test would have any effect on college students' use of drugs? Do you think that drug testing is an acceptable method of prevention? See the Star Box on page 224 for differing viewpoints.

College and Community Support Services for Drug Dependence

Students who have drug problems and realize they need assistance might select assistance based on the services available on campus or in the surrounding community and the costs they are willing to pay for treatment services.

One recently developed approach to convince drug-dependent people to enter treatment programs is the use of *confrontation* (see the Personal Assessment on p. 206). People who live or work with chemically dependent people are being encouraged to confront them directly about their addiction. Direct confrontation helps chemically dependent people realize the effect their behavior has on others. Once chemically dependent people realize that others will no longer tolerate their behavior, the likelihood of their entering treatment programs is increased significantly. Although effective, this approach is very

---

inhalants psychoactive drugs that enter the body through inhalation.

synergistic effect a heightened, exaggerated effect produced by the concurrent use of two or more drugs.

additive effect the combined (but not exaggerated) effect produced by the concurrent use of two or more drugs.

potentiated effect a phenomenon whereby the use of one drug intensifies the effect of a second drug.

antagonistic effect the effect produced when one drug reduces or offsets the effects of a second drug.

Drug abuse in the workplace is a growing concern. In factories, stores, and offices, employee drug use is suspected to be the cause of one-third to one-half of all absenteeism, accidents, medical claims, insubordination, thefts, and loss of productivity. About 61 percent of adults say they know people who have gone to work under the influence of alcohol or drugs.[22]

In response, more than half of Fortune 500 companies have instituted mandatory preemployment drug screening. Prospective employees of these firms are required to pass one or more drug tests to be considered for employment. Preemployment screening is also becoming more popular in the public employment sector. Such drug testing is controversial in several ways.

Supporters of mandatory preemployment drug screening argue that employers have an obligation to provide a safe and healthy work environment. They also contend that drug abuse is driving the cost of health care to ever-higher levels. Worker's compensation costs are also high, perhaps in part because of an increase in drug-related accidents and the chronic nature of drug-related illnesses. Employers also say that those who have taken drugs and have failed a drug screening have already broken the law and thus have forfeited their right to be considered for employment.

Opponents of preemployment screening express two concerns. First, they argue that the validity and reliability of screening tests are too low. If 1 million tests are performed in a year, a conservative estimate, and .05 percent of those tests yield false positives, also a conservative estimate, then 50,000 people may be fired from their jobs or not offered jobs for which they are qualified, according to the American Civil Liberties Union (ACLU).

The second concern is that employers invade the privacy of applicants by assuming them guilty until proved innocent by the testing laboratory. Privacy is invaded in two ways, says the ACLU. First, the specimen-collection process itself often involves direct or indirect observation to prevent tampering by the employee. Even indirect observation can be degrading. Typically, employees must remove all outer garments and urinate in a bathroom in which the water supply has been cut off. A second search takes place in the lab. Urinalysis can reveal not only the presence of illegal drugs, but also many other physical and medical conditions, such as medication for epilepsy, hypertension, or diabetes; a genetic predisposition to heart disease or cancer; and pregnancy. Employees are usually required to fill out forms listing all the medications they currently are taking, a clear invasion of privacy, says the ACLU.

Do you feel that mandatory preemployment drug screening is justified? Do you feel that it is an invasion of privacy? Would you agree to take a preemployment drug test as a condition of employment?

stressful for family members and friends and requires the assistance of professionals in the field of chemical dependence. These professionals can be contacted at a drug treatment center in your area.

Treatment

Comprehensive drug treatment programs are available in very few college or university health centers. College settings for drug dependence programs are more commonly found in the university counseling center. At such a center the emphasis will probably be not on the medical management of dependence but on the behavioral dimensions of drug abuse. Trained counselors and psychologists who specialize in chemical dependence counseling will work with students to (1) analyze their particular concerns, (2) establish constructive ways to cope with stress, and (3) search for alternative ways to achieve new "highs" (see the Personal Assessment on p. 225).

Medical treatment for the management of drug problems may need to be obtained through the services of a community treatment facility administered by a local health department, community mental health center, private clinic, or local hospital. Treatment may be on an inpatient or outpatient basis. Medical management might include detoxification, treatment of secondary health complications and nutritional deficiencies, and therapeutic counseling related to chemical dependence.

Some communities have voluntary health agencies that deliver services and treatment programs for drug-dependent people. Check your telephone book for listings of drug treatment facilities. Some communities have drug hot lines that offer advice for people with questions about drugs (see the Star Box on p. 226 for a list of anti–drug abuse organizations and hot line numbers).

Costs of Treatment for Dependence

Drug treatment programs that are administered by colleges and universities for faculty and students usually require no fees. Local agencies may provide either free services or services based on a **sliding scale**. Private hospitals, physicians, and clinics are the most expensive forms of treatment. Inpatient treatment at a private facility may cost as much as $1,000 per day. Since the length of inpatient treatment averages three to four weeks, a patient can quickly accumulate a very large bill. However, with many types of health insurance policies now providing coverage for alcohol addiction and other types of drug dependence, even these services may not require additional out-of-pocket expenses.

> **sliding scale** a method of payment by which patient fees are scaled according to income.

Personal Assessment

Experts agree that drug use provides only short-term, ineffective, and often destructive solutions to problems. We hope that you have found (or will find) innovative, invigorating drug-free experiences that make your life more exciting. Circle the number for each activity that reflects your intention to try that activity. Use the following guide:

I   No intention of trying this activity
2   Intend to try this within two years
3   Intend to try this within six months
4   Already tried this activity
5   Regularly engage in this activity

1. Take an aerobics or dance class	I	2	3	4	5	11. Tutor a disadvantaged youngster	I	2	3	4	5
2. Go backpacking	I	2	3	4	5	12. Go rockclimbing	I	2	3	4	5
3. Complete a marathon race	I	2	3	4	5	13. Play a role in a theater production	I	2	3	4	5
4. Start a vegetable garden	I	2	3	4	5	14. Give a speech on a favorite topic	I	2	3	4	5
5. Ride in a hot air balloon	I	2	3	4	5	15. Volunteer for a worthy cause	I	2	3	4	5
6. Tell someone you love them	I	2	3	4	5	16. Learn to swim	I	2	3	4	5
7. Donate blood	I	2	3	4	5	17. Learn to speak another language	I	2	3	4	5
8. Learn a martial art	I	2	3	4	5	18. Compose a song	I	2	3	4	5
9. Learn to play a musical instrument	I	2	3	4	5	19. Travel to a foreign country	I	2	3	4	5
10. Bicycle 100 miles	I	2	3	4	5	20. Write the first chapter of a book	I	2	3	4	5

YOUR TOTAL POINTS _____

Interpretation

61–100   You participate in many challenging experiences

41–60   You are willing to try some challenging new experiences

20–40   You take few of the challenging risks described here

To Carry This Further . . .

Looking at your point total, were you surprised at the degree to which you are aware of alternative activities? What activities would you add to this list?

National Anti–Drug Abuse Groups and Hot Lines

National Groups

PRIDE (Parent's Resource Institute for Drug Education):
Atlanta (404) 577-4500; in Georgia (900) 998-7743

National Federation of State High School Associations
Target Programs: Kansas City, Mo (816) 464-5400

National Health Information Clearinghouse:
(800) 336-4797

National Clearinghouse for Alcohol and Drug
Information: Silver Spring, Md (800) 729-6686;
(301) 468-2600

Narcotics Anonymous: Van Nuys, Calif (818) 780-3951

Toughlove: Doylestown, Penn (215) 348-7090

Alcoholics Anonymous, P.O. Box 459, Grand Central
Station, New York, NY, 10163 (212) 686-1100

Hot Lines

National Institute on Alcohol and Drug Abuse Hot Line:
(800) 662-HELP

National Cocaine Hot Line: (800) COCAINE

Alcohol Hot Line: (800) ALCOHOL

Cocaine Abuse Hot Line: (800) 888-9383;
(800) 234-0420

Cocaine Anonymous (Central Offices)

National Office: Culver City, Calif (213) 839-1141

California: Los Angeles (800) 347-8998
Los Angeles area (818) 447-2887
San Francisco (415) 821-6155
Solana Beach (619) 268-9109

Connecticut: New Haven (203) 387-1664

Georgia: Atlanta (404) 255-7787

Illinois: Chicago (312) 202-8898

New Jersey: Summit (908) 273-4530

New York: Manhattan (212) 496-4266

Tennessee: Nashville (615) 747-5483

Real Life
Real choices

Your Turn

- Is marijuana addictive?
- What are the risks to Barry of continuing to smoke marijuana?
- Is Barry in a position to give his daughters good advice about drug use?

And Now, Your Choices . . .

- What would you do if you found out that one of your parents was using drugs, despite having told you repeatedly never to use drugs yourself?
- If you use drugs, what would you tell a younger brother or sister who asked you for guidance about drug use?

Summary

- Abuse of drugs takes a tremendous toll on human lives and has a devastating effect on society.
- Primary prevention of drug abuse targets individuals and groups, such as schools and workplaces, to reach people who have not used illegal drugs and reduce their desire to try drugs.
- Secondary prevention targets people who are beginning to use drugs. Detection, screening, intervention, and treatment of early drug abuse are used to help these people avoid further drug use.
- Tertiary prevention (third-level prevention) targets people who are drug dependent, such as crack or heroin addicts, and their families. Rehabilitation, maintenance, hospitalization, outpatient care, support groups, after-care programs, relapse prevention, and other methods are used to help people recover from drug use.

- The addiction process has three components: exposure, compulsion, and loss of control.
- People who are close to the drug addict, such as family members, may need to free themselves from codependence.
- A drug is any substance, other than food, that by its chemical nature alters structure or function in the living organism.
- Psychoactive drugs alter the user's feelings, behavior, perceptions, or moods.
- Physical drug dependence occurs when body cells become reliant on a drug, causing withdrawal illness if the drug is not taken.
- Tolerance to a drug has developed when continued intake of the same dose has diminishing effects.
- Psychological drug dependence occurs when a user has a strong desire to continue using a

particular drug and believes that he or she must use the drug to maintain a sense of well-being.

- Drug misuse is the inappropriate use of legal drugs intended to be medications.
- Drug abuse is any use of an illegal drug or use of a legal drug in a way that is detrimental to health and well-being.
- Individual factors that affect drug abuse include genetic predisposition, personality traits, attitudes and beliefs, interpersonal skills, and unmet developmental needs.
- Environmental factors that affect drug abuse include the home and family, school, peers, and the community.
- Societal factors that affect drug abuse include the youth subculture, modeling and advertising, and the self-care movement.

- Drugs affect the CNS by altering neurotransmitter activity on neurons.
- Psychoactive drugs are classified as stimulants, depressants, hallucinogens, cannabis, narcotics, or inhalants.
- Combination drug effects include synergistic, additive, potentiated, and antagonistic effects.
- Society has responded to drug use with educational programs, law enforcement efforts, and legislation and public policy. Some support the legalization of drugs.
- Drug testing can be used as a means of primary, secondary, or tertiary prevention.
- College and community drug treatment services are available.

Review Questions

1. Explain the terms *primary prevention, secondary prevention,* and *tertiary prevention,* and give examples of each.
2. Identify and explain the three steps in the process of addiction.
3. How is the term *drug* defined in this chapter? What are psychoactive drugs? How do medicines differ from drugs?
4. Explain what *dependence* means. Identify and explain the two types of dependence.
5. Define the word *tolerance.* What does *cross-tolerance* mean? Give an example of cross-tolerance.
6. Differentiate between drug misuse and drug abuse.
7. Identify some individual, environmental, and societal factors that affect drug abuse.

8. Describe how neurotransmitters work.
9. List the six general categories of drugs. For each category, give several examples of drugs and explain the effects they would have on the user. What are designer drugs?
10. What is the active ingredient in marijuana? What are its common effects on the user? What are the long-term effects of marijuana use?
11. Explain the terms *synergistic effect, additive effect, potentiated effect,* and *antagonistic effect.*
12. Describe some of the ways society has responded to drug abuse.
13. How accurate is drug testing?
14. Describe several drug treatment services that are available. Who administers these services and how do their approaches differ?

References

1. Levy D. Drug-caused emergency room visits drop, *USA Today,* December 31, 1997, 3–A.
2. Manning A. Teens starting substance abuse at younger ages. *USA Today* 1997 August 14:8-D.
3. *Monitoring the future study.* 1997. University of Michigan: Institute for Social Research.
4. U.S. Department of Justice, Office of Justice Programs. *Drugs, crime, and the justice system.* Washington, DC: U.S. Government Printing Office, 1992.
5. Ray O, Ksir C. *Drugs, society, & human behavior.* 7th ed. St Louis: Mosby, 1996.
6. Pinger RR, Payne WA, Hahn DB, Hahn EJ. *Drugs: issues for today.* 3rd ed. Dubuque, Iowa: WCB/McGraw-Hill, 1998.
7. *Give 'em the facts: prescription & over-the-counter drug abuse.* Rockville, Maryland: The National Clearinghouse for Alcohol and Drug Information, a service of the Substance Abuse and Mental Health Services Administration and the National Institute on Drug Abuse.
8. Jalil GD. *Street-wise drug prevention.* Reading, Penn: No More Drugs 1996.
9. U.S. Department of Health and Human Services, Substance Abuse and Mental Health Services

Administration. *National drug survey results released with new youth public education materials* [press release], pp 1–3, Sept 12, 1995.
10. Armstrong BG, McDonald AD, Sloan M. Cigarette, alcohol, and caffeine consumption and spontaneous abortion. *Am J Public Health* 1991; 82(1):85–87.
11. Mills JL et al. Moderate caffeine use and the risk of spontaneous abortion and intrauterine growth retardation. *JAMA* 1993; 269(5):593.
12. Ritalin use up among youth. *USA Today* 1996 Dec 11.
13. Cocaine: the first decade. *Rand Drug Policy Research Center Issue Paper* 1992; 1(1):1–4.
14. U.S. Department of Justice, Bureau of Justice Statistics. *Drugs and crime facts, 1994.* Washington, DC: U.S. Government Printing Office, 1994.
15. Urban J. Thirty years later, LSD again becoming the drug of choice. *The Muncie Star* 1993 March 21:6B.
16. Heavy marijuana use may impair learning. *USA Today* 1996 Feb 21.
17. Community Epidemiology Work Group. *Epidemiologic trends in drug abuse.* Volumes I and II. December 1996.
18. Flores I. Heroin has its deadly hooks in teens across the nation. *USA Today* 1996 Oct 9.
19. Ackerman S. Drug testing: the state of the art. *Am Sci* 1989; 77:19–23.
20. Mieczkowski T. New approaches in drug testing: a review of hair analysis. *Ann Am Acad Pol Soc Sci* 1992; 521:132–50.
21. Just Say Life Skills. *Time* 1996 November 11, 70.
22. Drug abuse on the job. *USA Today* 1997 Feb 25.
23. Swan N. *Response to escalating methamphetamine abuse builds on NIDA-funded research.* National Institute on Drug Abuse (NIDA), NIDA Notes, November/December 1996.

Suggested Readings

West, JD. *The Betty Ford Center book of answers: help for those struggling with substance abuse and the people who love them.* New York: Pocket Books, 1997. The author of this book is a physician who is a former director of the Betty Ford Center. He draws on his expertise in the field of substance abuse to answer many commonly asked questions about drugs and addiction. The book provides comprehensive coverage of drug abuse issues for addicts and their families.

James WH, Johnson SL. *Doin' drugs: patterns of African-American addiction.* Austin, TX: University of Texas Press, 1997. This is a scholarly work for those who want to learn about historical and current patterns of drug use in the African-American community. The book begins with a solid historical overview, followed by chapters that focus on specific drugs, such as alcohol and cocaine. Separate chapters discuss gangs and the role of the church in dealing with drug-related problems.

Twerski AJ. *Addictive thinking: understanding self-deception.* Central City, MN: Hazelden, 1997. This book focuses on overcoming the denial that usually accompanies addiction. This newly revised edition features expanded coverage of depression and affective disorders. The author, a physician, writes in an authoritative yet accessible style.

As We Go To PRESS

Abuse of methamphetamine is spreading to large areas of the West, Midwest, and elsewhere.[23] The growing abuse is blamed on increased availability. Until recently, methamphetamine was manufactured in small, rural operations, but now organized groups operating out of Mexico and southern California are producing larger quantities.

Methamphetamine is a synthetic, highly addictive CNS stimulant. Scientists are currently studying its effects on nerve cells, particularly in the brain, and warn that meth use over time may reduce brain levels of dopamine, which can cause symptoms of Parkinson's disease, a severe motor disorder. Animal studies over the past 20 years have shown that high doses of meth damage nerve cells, and in some cases, one high dose has been enough to cause damage. Prolonged use makes the damage worse.

Drug treatment professionals report that meth users have more difficulty "staying clean" than do cocaine abusers. The meth users are more likely to need medical treatment, are more damaged, and show paranoia and hallucinations.

topics for Today

Caffeine: America's Most Popular Drug

Coffee is definitely hip again. On two popular television sitcoms, "Friends" hang out at Central Perk and Drs. Frasier and Niles Crane solve many of life's problems over cups of gourmet brew. Starbucks, a coffeehouse chain based in Seattle, has swept the West Coast and is becoming a national phenomenon.[1] They're not the only ones jumping at the chance to serve you your favorite cup of espresso, cappuccino, or latte. Bookstores, fast-food restaurants, and even gas stations are beginning to offer these specialty brews. This is just the latest twist on a very old habit.

Tea, so the story goes, was discovered in 2737 B.C. by Chinese emperor Shen Nung when leaves from a local plant fell into water he was boiling.[2] Thousands of years later, around A.D. 600, coffee berries were being used as food and currency in parts of Africa. Coffee emerged as a beverage in these same regions a little later. From there, coffee consumption spread to the Middle East and then to Europe.[3] Soft drinks and over-the-counter (OTC) medications are part of caffeine's more recent history, and the very latest caffeinated product is caffeinated water, marketed under the brand names Water Joe and Crank. David Marcheschi, a twenty-nine-year-old Chicago mortgage banker, invented Water Joe while trying to stay awake in college. A 16.9-ounce bottle has the caffeine equivalent of an eight-ounce cup of coffee and retails for 99 cents.[4] It's coffee without the bitterness and a soft drink without the sweetness.

Economics

Coffee is one of the most widely consumed beverages in the world. An estimated 1.5 billion cups of coffee are drunk worldwide every day.[5] The coffee trade competes with wheat in global importance, and these commodities are second only to oil in international trade.[5] Five million tons are produced annually in fifty countries. South American countries lead production, with 42 percent of the market. Next is Africa, with 20.4 percent; Asia, with 18.5 percent; and North and Central America, with 17.9 percent. Oceania completes the picture, contributing 1.2 percent of the

world's coffee.[5] The larger producers ship most of their crop abroad to countries like the United States. Although coffee consumption in the United States has dropped since the 1960s, 50 percent of American adults still drink one or more cups a day.[6] Many people are banking on the renewed interest in coffee and this loyal customer base to keep the more than 10,000 specialty coffeehouses (total projected for the year 2000) in business.[1]

Social Issues

Coffee breaks are a time to socialize. Midmorning or midafternoon caffeine, conversation, and company improves the rest of the workday for many people. Whether it's at work or in a high-style downtown brasserie, a homey neighborhood cafe, or a philosophical college hangout, coffee consumption is a social activity.[1]

Historically, leaders in many countries have tried to ban coffeehouses for this very reason: Being the meeting places that they are, coffeehouses tended to breed revolutionary political ideas.[3] There may be a few revolutionaries who frequent today's coffeehouses in the United States, but by and large the clientele is more mainstream. A typical day at a Washington, D.C. coffeehouse sees mothers and their babies gathering after dropping older children at school. Later in the morning, retirees come in. In the afternoon, people who work at home stop in. After school, the same coffeehouse becomes a high school hangout. After dark, young professionals and couples on dates arrive. This is evidence that coffeehouses are nongenerational meeting places that everyone can enjoy. The coffeehouse is so popular in some towns that it's even threatening to replace the local pub.[6]

The draw of the coffeehouse is manyfold. It provides a relaxing atmosphere, a refuge from unpaid bills and unmade beds, a place to work where you're not entirely alone, a place to engage in conversation and life, a place to watch the world go by, and a familiar place where you'll probably run into someone you know in the next fifteen minutes.

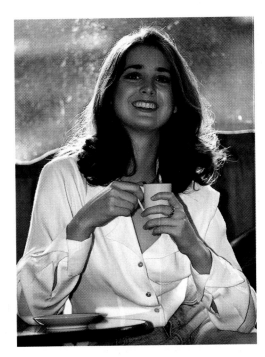

Coffeehouses have become popular places to relax, work, or spend time with friends.

Health Effects

Although caffeine does have pharmacological effects on the function of cardiovascular, respiratory, renal, and nervous systems, at the low fixed pattern of consumption that most people enjoy, caffeine is merely a mild stimulant.[5] But withdrawal from even a mild caffeine habit may cause headaches, fatigue, and difficulty concentrating. These symptoms peak in 24 to 48 hours, causing many weekday coffee drinkers to experience weekend withdrawal headaches.[7] In high doses, acute effects such as restlessness, agitation, tremors, cardiac dysrhythmias (irregular heartbeat), gastric disturbance, and diarrhea have been reported. Chronic problems such as heart and vascular disease, breast and ovarian fibrocystic conditions, breast and ovarian cancer, and infertility have largely been dismissed by the scientific community as not being linked to caffeine.[5,8]

Caffeine is just one of the more than 100 active substances present in coffee.[5] Even if caffeine does have certain effects on the body, they may not be apparent because other chemicals in the coffee counteract them or because the effects themselves may be short lived. Results of studies of caffeine's effect on the cardiovascular system have not been consistent. It seems, though, that caffeine does trigger a rise in blood pressure and a lowering of heart rate. These effects last only for a matter of hours initially, and after a few days of consumption, caffeine tolerance sets in and these conditions no longer occur. It seems that the only permanent toll that coffee takes on the cardiovascular system is not even related to caffeine. If the coffee is unfiltered, fats from the coffee beans can raise cholesterol levels.[5]

Suspicion that caffeine causes cancer is undeserved as well. A recent literature review of coffee and cancer epidemiology reported no meaningful association of coffee with most common cancers, including those of the digestive tract, breast, and genital tract.[5] Neither has any dose-response relationship between coffee/caffeine consumption and delayed conception or persistent infertility been demonstrated.[5]

In children, caffeine causes inattentiveness, distraction, and impulsivity. Parents are wise to monitor the caffeine intake of their children. One soda to a four-year-old is like two cups of coffee to an adult.[9] Pregnant women should avoid caffeine use. Three or more cups of coffee or tea a day during the first 4 months of pregnancy seems to increase the risk of miscarriage.[10] This finding may not be entirely attributable to caffeine, though, because coffee consumption increases with age, and aging itself is a risk factor in pregnancy.[5]

Breaking the Habit

You may want to break the caffeine habit because it generates dependence and you don't like the headache you get when you can't find a vending machine or when nobody at the office made coffee. You may want to set a good example for your children to avoid caffeine, or you may simply want to live as drug-free as possible. Whatever your reasons, the following list offers suggestions that will help you to attain your goal.[11]

1. Keep a log of where, when, how much, and with whom you consume coffee, tea, caffeinated soda, or caffeinated pills.
2. To avoid withdrawal symptoms such as headaches, don't quit cold turkey. Instead, reduce your consumption slowly, by one cup, can, or pill per day.
3. If you are a coffee drinker, gradually switch from regular to decaffeinated coffee by mixing them before brewing, or substitute decaffeinated instant coffee for some of the caffeinated instant you drink. Increase the decaffeinated proportion each day. Choose a premium decaf to reward yourself and to keep your coffee routine enjoyable.
4. Substitute decaffeinated tea for your regular caffeinated tea, and replace caffeinated soda with a caffeine-free drink.
5. Drink from smaller cups instead of large mugs or glasses. Avoid the huge mugs made popular by the television show "Friends." If your favorite mug is a comfort to you, don't discard it, but fill it with a caffeine-free beverage. If, on the other hand, you find your coffee paraphernalia to be a temptation, get rid of those mugs, pots, filters,

and grinders. Change your daily routine by taking a walk instead of your usual coffee break.

6. Use more low-fat milk in your coffee or tea to reduce the amount of caffeinated beverage you consume while increasing your calcium consumption.

7. Consider an alternative to a caffeinated beverage, such as bouillon, cider, herbal tea, or a grain-based beverage such as Postum.

8. Do not restructure your home and work routines to avoid caffeine so much that you lose the healthful aspects of a coffee break or an evening at your favorite hangout. Remember that noncaffeinated beverages are available; simply plan ahead.

9. When you find yourself getting sleepy while studying, driving, or working and feel tempted to drink a caffeinated beverage, take a break, open a window, breathe deeply and stretch, jog in place, go for a walk, get a cold drink, or take a short nap!

If you get enough sleep, exercise regularly, and follow a healthy diet, you'll be less reliant on the artificial "pep" that caffeine provides.

For Discussion . . .

Of the caffeinated beverages—coffee, tea, and soda—which do you prefer? Do you consume more than three cups or glasses a day? If so, have you thought about why you rely so heavily on caffeine? Would you like to reduce your consumption?

Are you part of the coffeehouse craze? What's special about your hangout?

References

1. Schultz K. Coffee, conversation and company. *Theta* 1996; 111(1):3–4.
2. Anonymous. Tea, a story of serendipity. *FDA Consumer* 1996; 30(2):22–26.
3. Morse M. Across the country, it's all happening at the coffeehouse. *Smithsonian* 1996; 27(6):104–13.
4. Anonymous. Jolting Joe. *Time* 1996; 148(12):51.
5. Garattini S, ed. Caffeine, coffee and health. New York: Raven Press, 1993.
6. DePriest T. Java goes mocha: African Americans are getting in on the coffeehouse craze. *Black Enterprise* 1995; 25(11):316.
7. *Caffeine withdrawal.* OnHealth, May 28, 1997. (www.onhealth.com)
8. *Caffeine.* Johns Hopkins InteliHealth online newsletter, November 10, 1998. (www.intelihealth.com)
9. Anonymous. Caffeine dependency "brewing". *Tufts University Diet and Nutrition Letter* 1995; 13(9):2.
10. Anonymous. Health report. *Time* 1996; 147(18):34.
11. Anonymous. 1996 *Tips for breaking the caffeine habit.*

InfoLinks
www.gardfoods.com/coffee/
    index.htm
www.roble.com/marquis/caffeine

Using Alcohol Responsibly

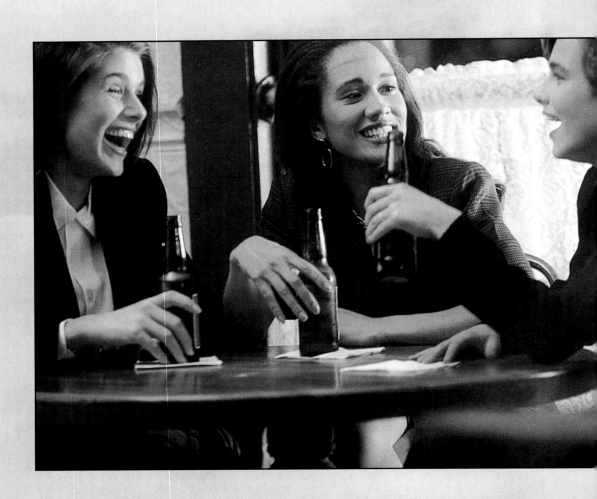

The push for zero tolerance laws, the tightening of standards for determining legal intoxication, and the growing influence of national groups concerned with alcohol misuse show that our society is more sensitive than ever to the misuse of alcohol.

People are concerned about the consequences of drunk driving, alcohol-related crime, and lowered job productivity.[1] Alcohol use remains quite high among young people in the United States and has not changed much in the last few years. Alcohol use remains the preferred form of drug use for most adults (including college students), but as a society, we are increasingly uncomfortable with the ease with which alcohol can be misused.

HEALTHY PEOPLE: LOOKING AHEAD TO 2010

The *Health People 2000 Midcourse Review* highlighted significant progress toward achieving several important alcohol-related objectives. The most notable and encouraging change was the reduction in the number of alcohol-related traffic fatalities. The original 1990 goal was easily surpassed in this area. This success was largely attributable to the passage of state laws that revoked drunk drivers' licenses and lowered the legal limit for blood alcohol concentration (BAC) from .10% to .08%.

At mid-decade, the number of deaths caused by cirrhosis (alcohol-related liver disease) had declined, and per capital alcohol consumption had dropped. When the *Midcourse Review* was issued, the nation was about halfway toward reaching the specific targets for these two objectives.

The *Healthy People 2010* document will probably contain objectives aimed at reducing binge drinking (measured by the number of people who report heavy drinking during the past two weeks) among youth and college-age students. These objectives will be critical ones, especially in light of the 1997 *Monitoring the Future Study,* which indicated that binge drinking was still on the rise among America's youth.[2]

Real Life
Real choices

• Name: Ricardo Diaz
• Age: 38
• Occupation: Vice squad detective

"I'll never be like that."

Those words—whispered, shouted, sobbed—were the anthem of Ricardo (Rick) Diaz's youth. The years that should have been carefree and adventuresome for Rick and his three younger brothers were instead an endlessly running horror movie. Rick tried to be a substitute dad to his siblings as their father, Geraldo, drank his way from life of the party to menacing bully, from successful machine-shop foreman to unemployed loafer, from proud family man to shameful secret. Geraldo died of **cirrhosis** of the liver in Rick's senior year in high school, and although he grieved his father's loss, he also secretly felt relief.

Now 38, Rick was recently promoted to detective lieutenant in a big-city police department. His wife, Maria, is a successful accountant, and their two daughters and son are excellent students and all-around good kids. Rick and Maria don't

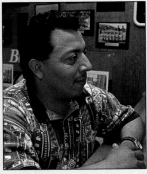

drink, and he's proud that his life reflects his vow: "I'll never be like that."

Rick's not like that—but the same can't be said for his youngest brother, Rodrigo. Now 28, he seems to be headed into the same dark tunnel as his father, taking with him his frightened wife and 4-year-old twin daughters. Rick, ever the protective big brother, has tried everything to help Rodrigo, from "lending" him money and bringing him home from bars to "taking care of" his citations for drunk driving and making excuses for his behavior at family get-togethers.

As you study this chapter, think about Rick and Rod's situation and prepare yourself to answer the questions in **Your Turn** at the end of the chapter.

Choosing to Drink

Clearly, people drink for many different reasons (see the Star Box on the right). We believe that most people drink because alcohol is an effective, affordable, and legal substance for altering the brain's chemistry. As **inhibitions** are removed by the influence of alcohol, behavior that is generally held in check is expressed. At least temporarily, drinkers become a different version of themselves—more outgoing, relaxed, and adventuresome. If alcohol did not make these changes in people, it would not be consumed as much. Do you agree or disagree?

Alcohol Use Patterns

From magazines to billboards to television, alcohol is one of the most heavily advertised consumer products in the country.[3] You cannot watch television, listen to the radio, or read a newspaper without being encouraged to buy a particular brand of beer, wine, or liquor. The advertisements create a warm aura about the nature of alcohol use. The implications are clear: Alcohol use will bring you good times, handsome men or seductive women, exotic settings, and a chance to forget the hassles of hard work and study.

Perhaps as a consequence of the many pressures to drink, it is not surprising that most adults drink alcoholic beverages. Two-thirds of all American adults are classified as drinkers. Yet one in three adults does not

Why Do I Choose an Alcoholic Beverage?

• I think alcoholic beverages are more thirst quenching than nonalcoholic alternatives.

• Alcoholic beverages taste better—their flavor is unique and satisfying.

• My friends always choose alcoholic beverages—I've learned to do the same.

• Alcoholic drinks are an important part of the larger statement I am making about myself. They reflect that I am an adult.

• Drinking alcoholic beverages makes me feel different—I like the changes that come about when I drink.

drink. In the college environment, where surveys indicate that 85 percent to 90 percent of all students drink, it is difficult for many students to imagine that every third adult is an abstainer. Complete the Personal Assessment on page 236 to rate your own alcohol use.

Alcohol consumption figures are reported in many different ways, depending on the researchers' criteria. Figures from various sources support the contention that about one-third of adults eighteen years of age and older are abstainers, about one-third are light drinkers, and one-third are moderate-to-heavy drinkers (see the Star Box on p. 235). As a single category, heavy drinkers make up about 10 percent of the adult drinking population.

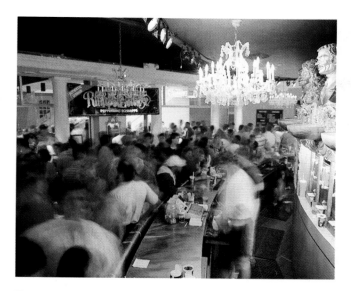

Two-thirds of American adults, including most of those in this Atlanta nightclub, are classified as drinkers. Only one-third choose to abstain from using alcohol.

Moderate Drinking Redefined

Alcohol Alert, a publication of the National Institute on Alcohol Abuse and Alcoholism (NIAAA), defines moderate drinking as no more than two drinks each day for most men and one drink each day for women. These cutoff levels are based on the amount of alcohol that can be consumed without causing problems, either for the drinker or society. (The gender difference is due primarily to the higher percentage of body fat in women and to the lower amount of an essential stomach enzyme in women.) Elderly people are limited to no more than one drink each day, again due to a higher percentage of body fat.

These consumption levels are applicable to most people. Indeed, people who plan to drive, women who are pregnant, people recovering from alcohol addiction, people under age twenty-one, people taking medications, and those with existing medical concerns should not consume alcohol. In addition, although some studies have shown that low levels of alcohol consumption may have minor psychological and cardiovascular benefits, the NIAAA does not advise nondrinkers to start drinking.

Drinking on Campus

Students who drink in college tend to classify themselves as light-to-moderate drinkers. It comes as a shock to students, though, when they read the criteria for each drinking classification. Many students will find that they fall into the category of heavy drinkers. The criteria are based on a combination of quantity of alcohol consumed per occasion and the frequency of drinking, as shown in Table 8-1.

Recent studies[4,5] have reported that 44 percent to 48 percent of college males are heavy drinkers, with women close behind at 39 percent. High percentages of college fraternity residents are presumed to be heavy drinkers. Many students, faculty members, and administrators now believe that alcohol abuse is a serious problem on their campuses.

Personal Applications

• Do you think that about one-third of the students on your campus seem to be heavy drinkers? If you think more or fewer students drink heavily, how might you explain these figures?

Binge Drinking

Alcohol abuse by college students usually takes the form of a drinking pattern called **binge drinking**. Binge drinking refers to the consumption of five drinks in a row, at least once during the previous two-week period.[6] One large study of more than 17,000 students on 140 campuses found that 44 percent of students (50% of men and 39% of women) binged.[7] The strongest predictors for bingeing were living in a fraternity or sorority, adopting a party-centered lifestyle, and engaging in other risky behavior. The study also suggested that many college students began binge drinking in high school.

By its very nature, binge drinking can be dangerous. Drunk driving, physical violence, property destruction, date rape, police arrest, and lowered academic performance are all highly associated with binge drinking. Besides the role that heavy drinking may play in the aggressor in date rape, a recent study found that more than half the victims in sexual assaults also were at least somewhat drunk (see the Star Box on p. 237).

Reducing binge drinking is one of the *Healthy People 2000* objectives. The direct correlation between the amount of alcohol consumed and lowered academic performance is crystal clear. Frequently, the

cirrhosis (sir oh sis)   pathological changes to the liver resulting from chronic, heavy alcohol consumption; a frequent cause of death among heavy alcohol users (see Figure 8-1).

inhibitions   inner controls that prevent a person from engaging in certain types of behavior.

binge drinking   the consumption of five drinks or more on one drinking occasion.

Personal Assessment

Answer the following questions about your own alcohol use. Record your number of "yes" and "no" responses at the end of the questionnaire.

Do you:

	Yes	No
1. Drink more often than you did a year ago?	___	___
2. Drink more heavily than you did a year ago?	___	___
3. Plan to drink, sometimes days in advance?	___	___
4. Gulp or "chug" your drinks, perhaps in a contest?	___	___
5. Set personal limits on the amount you plan to drink but then consistently disregard these limits?	___	___
6. Drink at a rate greater than two drinks per hour?	___	___
7. Encourage or even pressure others to drink with you?	___	___
8. Frequently want a nonalcoholic beverage but then end up drinking an alcoholic drink?	___	___
9. Drive your car while under the influence of alcohol or ride with another person who has been drinking?	___	___
10. Use alcoholic beverages while taking prescription or OTC medications?	___	___
11. Forget what happened while you were drinking?	___	___
12. Have a tendency to disregard information about the effects of drinking?	___	___
13. Find your reputation fading because of alcohol use?	___	___
TOTAL	___	___

Interpretation

If you answered yes to any of these questions, you may be using alcohol irresponsibly. Two or more yes responses indicate an unacceptable pattern of alcohol use and may reflect problem drinking behavior.

To Carry This Further . . .

Ask your friends or roommates to take this assessment. Are they willing to take this assessment and then talk about their results with you? Be prepared to discuss any follow-up questions they might have about their (or your) alcohol consumption patterns. Your willingness to talk about drinking behavior might help someone realize that this topic can and should be discussed openly. Finally, be aware of how people in your area can get professional help with drinking or other drug concerns.

Table 8-1 Criteria for Drinking Classifications

Classification	Alcohol-Related Behavior
Abstainers	Do not drink or drink less often than once a year
Infrequent drinkers	Drink once a month at most and drink small amounts per typical drinking occasion
Light drinkers	Drink once a month at most and drink medium amounts per typical drinking occasion, or drink no more than three to four times a month and drink small amounts per typical drinking occasion
Moderate drinkers	Drink at least once a week and small amounts per typical drinking occasion or three to four times a month and medium amounts per typical drinking occasion or no more than once a month and large amounts per typical drinking occasion
Moderate/heavy drinkers	Drink at least once a week and medium amounts per typical drinking occasion or three to four times a month and large amounts per typical drinking occasion
Heavy drinkers	Drink at least once a week and large amounts per typical drinking occasion

Note:
Small amounts = One drink or less per drinking occasion
Medium amounts = Two to four drinks per drinking occasion
Large amounts = Five or more drinks per drinking occasion (binge drinking)
Drink = 12 fluid oz of beer, 4 fluid oz of wine, or 1 fluid oz of distilled spirits

Alcohol Plays a Dual Role in Sexual Assaults

We know that binge drinkers cause a variety of problems on college campuses, such as attacking and sexually assaulting other students. The victims in many cases are nondrinkers.

A recent study, however, reports that most victims of sexual assault on college campuses, 55 percent of the total victims, also were at least somewhat drunk at the time of the attack.[8] The victims who felt they were at least somewhat drunk reported engaging in higher levels of consensual sexual activity with the aggressor immediately before the attack and reported they had lower levels of resistance to the attack than those who were not drunk.

This *does not* mean that we should blame the victim in sexual assaults! It stresses the importance, however, of exercising common sense and control in the consumption of alcohol, and avoiding potentially dangerous situations.

social costs of binge drinking can be very high, especially when intoxicated people demonstrate their level of immaturity. How common is binge drinking on your campus?

For large numbers of students who drink, the college years are a time when they will drink more heavily than at any other period during their lifetime. Some will suffer serious consequences as a result. These years will also mark the entry into a lifetime of problem drinking for some.

Personal Applications

• Do you think your drinking pattern will change after you finish college?

Drinking Games

Drinking games are one form of binge drinking that seeks to make binge drinking socially acceptable. A recent study found that drinking games especially present a risk to light and moderate drinkers.[9]

Heavy drinkers experience many drinking-related problems regardless of whether they play drinking games, according to the study. Among the light and moderate drinkers, however, those who played drinking games experienced more drinking-related problems than those who did not. The authors of the study conclude that light and moderate drinkers need to know that drinking games can increase their risk of drinking-related problems, such as injuries, property destruction, legal problems, and sexual assaults.

Personal Applications

• Have you ever had more to drink than you wanted to because you were participating in a drinking game? If so, what negative consequences did you experience?

Declining Alcohol Use

As you learned in Chapter 7, "Living Drug-Free," being able to decline drugs and alcohol when others around are using these substances is a challenge that you can learn to meet. For example, if you are fit, participating in a long bicycle ride or run can leave you with an excellent sense of well-being produced by endorphins, natural painkillers produced by the brain. Such a "high" is enhanced by the knowledge that you have earned the good feeling through your efforts. Consider some additional techniques for avoiding alcohol:

- Avoid parties where you can logically expect heavy drinking.
- Avoid people who are drinking heavily or becoming erratic or threatening.
- Request a nonalcoholic beer, soft drink, or glass of water instead of alcohol.
- Participate in activities that can provide a nonchemical high. See the Personal Assessment on page 225 of Chapter 7 for a variety of suggestions.
- Cultivate friends who find their highs through natural, positive activities in which you share an interest.

Alcohol and the Family

The alcohol abuser hurts more than just himself or herself. Everyone around the addicted person suffers.[10] Alcoholism is a family disease, and a family can be a person, a family, a fraternity, a sorority, a dormitory floor, even a therapy group or a 12-step group. Eventually everyone around the alcoholic suffers, including the spouse, parents, children, siblings, friends, boyfriend/girlfriend, and even roommates.

Following are some of the behaviors that the dysfunctional family teaches:[11]

- Lives in fear, teaching you to fear others different from yourself in race, religion, color, nationality, appearance, and so forth.
- Teaches that the family members should depend on each other to the exclusion of the outside world. An exception can be made for outsiders who are identical to the family members.
- Teaches that, to be successful, you must make, marry, or have money.
- Teaches that the authority figures in the family are right.
- Teaches every member of the family to adapt to the emotional sickness of the family and feels threatened when a member attempts to recover.
- Teaches conditional love.
- Teaches that, to have a worthwhile identity, you must gain the approval of the outside world, and especially the group itself.
- Feels threatened and abandoned at the death or departure of a loved member of the group.
- Tries to maintain the group through guilt and pity, which it calls "love."
- Expects all members to like the same things and people.
- Thrives on excitement, and teaches that if you are not excited, you are not alive.

As a result of these constant lessons, the person living with alcoholism can develop many of the following problems. The person living with alcoholism can tend to:

- Become isolated and afraid of people and authority figures.
- Become an approval-seeker and lose his or her identity in the process.
- Become frightened by angry people and any criticism.
- Become an alcoholic, marry one, or find another compulsive personality such as a workaholic to continue the sickness.
- Develop a victim mentality and can be attracted by weakness in potential friends or loved ones.
- Have an extreme sense of responsibility and focus on others to the detriment of himself or herself.
- Feel guilty when being assertive or saying no.
- Become addicted to excitement.
- Confuse pity with love.
- Lose the ability to feel or express feelings.
- Be terrified of abandonment and may tolerate abuse to hold on to a relationship.
- Develop all the symptoms of an alcoholic without actually drinking.

The good news is that many resources, such as recovery and support groups, have become available in the last few years for both the alcoholic and those who live with the alcoholic. See the sections on alcohol self-assessment, codependence, rehabilitation and recovery, and adult children of alcoholic parents beginning on page 250.

Those who have lived with an alcoholic will face their own issues as they work through their own recovery. They may find that they learned compulsions from the alcoholic, or they may transfer the compulsions to other behaviors, such as food, gambling, house cleaning, or taking up lost causes or people. Those who know, or are still living with, an active alcoholic also can consider intervention to urge the alcoholic to seek help. For advice on planning an intervention, see the Health Action Guide on page 201.

The Nature of Alcoholic Beverages

Alcohol (also known as *ethyl alcohol* or *ethanol*) is the principal product of **fermentation**. In this process, yeast cells act on the sugar content of fruits and grains to produce alcohol and carbon dioxide.

The alcohol concentration in distilled beverages (such as whiskey, gin, rum, and vodka) is expressed by the term *proof*, a number that is twice the percentage of alcohol by volume in a beverage. Thus 70 percent of the fluid in a bottle of 140 proof gin is pure alcohol. Most proofs in distilled beverages range from

No Fear? Not Smart

Are you a fearless, easily bored thrill-seeker? If so, you might have a recently identified "thrill-seeking gene." Unfortunately, this gene may put you at risk for alcoholism and other problems.

Several researchers recently identified the genetic difference,[12] a slightly longer form of the D4–dopamine receptor (D4DR) gene, in subjects who had higher levels of novelty-seeking behavior than deliberate, reflective people did. Dopamine is a neurotransmitter that studies have linked to pleasure-seeking behavior. Some researchers suggest that abnormal dopamine regulation may contribute to drug abuse, alcoholism, criminality, and other mental and behavioral problems.

A study in Sweden[13] found that children who are curious, fearless, assertive, and easily bored are three times more likely than other children to become alcoholics as adults. The reasons are unclear. These children might be simply imitating thrill-seeking alcoholic adults, or they might be showing the effects of the "thrill-seeking gene." In any case, parents of such children, and those who exhibit such behavior, should beware of this risk and ask their physician for help.

Considering that the thrill-seeking gene is linked to criminality and a higher risk of death, we might wonder how such a gene could have survived evolution. One observer has suggested[14] that the thrill-seeking gene might have been genetically advantageous in human history. For example, these individuals could have taken risks that would have benefitted the entire group, such as determining which foods were safe and which were poisonous, or exploring new territories. In a safer modern society, however, such tendencies may more often lead to self-destructive or other-destructive behavior.

---

80 to 160. The pure grain alcohol that is often added to fruit punches and similar beverages has a proof of almost 200.

The nutritional value of alcohol is extremely limited. Alcoholic beverages produced today through modern processing methods contain nothing but empty calories—about 100 calories per fluid ounce of 100-proof distilled spirits and about 150 calories per each twelve-ounce bottle or can of beer. Clearly, alcohol consumption is a significant contributor to the additional pounds of fat that many college students accumulate. Pure alcohol contains only simple carbohydrates; it has no vitamins and minerals, and no fats or protein.

Recently, some researchers have suggested that moderate consumption of alcoholic beverages, particularly wine, can reduce the risk of coronary heart disease, but the evidence so far is inconclusive.[16] Such announcements are controversial because of the risk that they could encourage problem drinking in some people. For a detailed look at this issue, see the Star Box on page 311 in Chapter 10.

"Light" beer and low-calorie wines have been introduced in response to concerns about the number of calories in alcoholic beverages. These light beverages are not low-alcohol beverages but merely low-calorie beverages. Only beverages marked "low alcohol" contain a lower concentration of alcohol than the usual beverages of that type.

The popular new ice beers actually contain a higher percentage of alcohol than other types of beer. The term *ice* refers to the way in which this beer is processed. After brewing and fermentation, it is deep-chilled at 24 to 28 degrees Fahrenheit, which causes ice crystals to form in the mixture. When these ice crystals are removed, the remaining liquid contains a higher percentage of alcohol. Most regular and light beers contain less than 5 percent alcohol, whereas ice beer generally contains 5 percent to 6 percent alcohol. Do you think beer drinkers are choosing this beer for its reportedly rich flavor or simply because it contains more alcohol?

The Physiological Effects of Alcohol

First and foremost, alcohol is classified as a drug—a very strong CNS depressant. The primary depressant effect of alcohol occurs in the brain and spinal cord. Many people think of alcohol as a stimulant because of the way most users feel after consuming a serving or two of their favorite drink. Any temporary sensations of jubilation, boldness, or relief are attributable to alcohol's ability as a depressant drug to release personal inhibitions and provide temporary relief from tension.

Factors That Influence the Absorption of Alcohol

The **absorption** of alcohol is influenced by several factors, most of which can be controlled by the individual. These factors include the following:

Strength of the Beverage

The stronger the beverage, the greater the amount of alcohol that will accumulate within the digestive tract.

---

fermentation a chemical process whereby plant products are converted into alcohol by the action of yeast cells on carbohydrate materials.

absorption the passage of nutrients or alcohol through the walls of the stomach or intestinal tract into the bloodstream.

Number of Drinks Consumed

As more drinks are consumed, more alcohol is absorbed.

Speed of Consumption

If consumed rapidly, even relatively few drinks will result in a large concentration gradient that will lead to high blood alcohol concentration.

Presence of Food

Food can compete with alcohol for absorption into the bloodstream, thus slowing the absorption of alcohol. When you slow your alcohol absorption, your body can remove alcohol already in the bloodstream. Serving food at a party is a healthy idea.

Body Chemistry

Each person has an individual pattern of physiological functioning that may affect the ability to process alcohol. For example, in some conditions, such as that marked by "dumping syndrome," the stomach empties more rapidly than is normal, and alcohol seems to be absorbed more quickly. The emptying time may be either slowed or quickened by anger, fear, stress, nausea, and the condition of the stomach tissues.

Gender

A significant study published in the *New England Journal of Medicine* reported that women produce much less alcohol dehydrogenase than do men.[17] This enzyme is responsible for breaking down alcohol in the stomach. With less alcohol dehydrogenase action, women absorb about 30 percent more alcohol into the bloodstream than men, even with an identical number of drinks and equal body weight.

Three other factors help explain why women tend to absorb alcohol more quickly than men of the same body weight: (1) Women have proportionately more body fat than men. Because alcohol is not very fat soluble, it enters the bloodstream relatively quickly. (2) Women's bodies have proportionately less water than men's bodies of equal weight. Thus consumed alcohol does not become as diluted as in men. (3) Alcohol absorption is influenced by a woman's menstrual cycle. Alcohol is more quickly absorbed during the premenstrual phase of a woman's cycle. Also, there is evidence that women using birth control pills absorb alcohol more quickly than usual.[15]

With the exception of a person's body chemistry and gender, all factors that influence absorption can be moderated by the alcohol user.

Blood Alcohol Concentration

A person's **blood alcohol concentration (BAC)** rises when alcohol is consumed faster than it can be removed (oxidized) by the liver. A fairly predictable

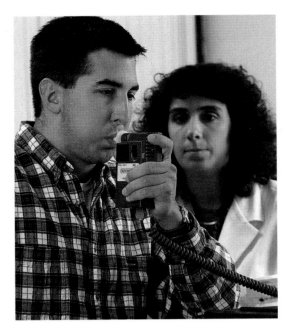

A breathanalysis test can measure a person's blood alcohol concentration indirectly, through analysis of exhaled air.

sequence of events takes place when a person drinks alcohol at a rate faster than one drink every hour. When the BAC reaches 0.05 percent, initial measurable changes in mood and behavior take place. Inhibitions and everyday tensions appear to be released, while judgment and critical thinking are somewhat impaired. This BAC would be achieved by a 160-pound person taking about two drinks in an hour (see Table 8-2).

At a level of 0.10 percent (one part alcohol to 1,000 parts blood), the drinker typically loses significant motor coordination. Voluntary motor function becomes quite clumsy. At this BAC, most states consider a drinker legally intoxicated and thus incapable of safely operating a vehicle. Although physiological changes associated with this BAC do occur, certain users do not feel drunk or appear impaired.

As a person continues to elevate the BAC from 0.20 percent to 0.50 percent, the health risk of **acute alcohol intoxication** increases rapidly. A BAC of 0.20 percent is characterized by the loud, boisterous, obnoxious drunk person who staggers. A 0.30 percent BAC produces further depression and stuporous behavior, during which time the drinker becomes so confused that he or she may not be capable of understanding anything. The 0.40 percent or 0.50 percent BAC produces unconsciousness. At this BAC a person can die, because brain centers that control body temperature, heartbeat, and respiration may virtually shut down.

An important factor influencing the BAC is the individual's blood volume. The larger the person, the greater the amount of blood into which alcohol can be distributed. Conversely, the smaller person has less

Table 8-2   Blood Alcohol Concentration and Symptoms

Blood Alcohol Concentration	Sporadic Drinker	Chronic Drinker	Hours for Alcohol to be Metabolized
.05%	Congenial euphoria; decreased tension	No observable effect	2–3
.75%	Talkative	Often no effect	
.10%	Uncoordinated; legally drunk (as in drunk driving) in most states; a level of 0.08% is legal drunkenness in 12 states	Minimal signs	4–6
.125%–.150%	Unrestrained behavior; episodic uncontrolled behavior; legally drunk at 0.15% in all states.	Pleasurable euphoria or beginning of uncoordination	6–10
.200%–.250%	Alertness lost; sluggish	Effort required to maintain emotional and motor control	10–24
.300%–.350%	Stupor to coma	Drowsy and slow	
7.50%	Some will die	Coma	>24

blood into which alcohol can be distributed, and as a result, a higher BAC will develop.

Sobering Up

Alcohol is removed from the bloodstream principally through the process of **oxidation.** Oxidation occurs at a constant rate (about one-fourth to one-third ounce of pure alcohol per hour) that cannot be appreciably altered. Because each typical drink of beer, wine, or distilled spirits contains about one-half ounce of pure alcohol, it takes about two hours for the body to fully oxidize one typical alcoholic drink.[18]

Although people have attempted to sober up by drinking hot coffee, taking cold showers, or exercising, the oxidation rate of alcohol is unaffected. Thus far the FDA has not approved any commercial product that can help people achieve sobriety. Passage of time remains the only effective way to sober up.

Personal Applications

• Has anyone told you about a "foolproof" way to sober up quickly? How would you explain why it is ineffective?

First Aid for Acute Alcohol Intoxication

Not everyone who goes to sleep, passes out, or even becomes unconscious after drinking has a high BAC. People who are already sleepy, have not eaten well, are sick, or are bored may drink a little alcohol and quickly fall asleep. However, people who drink heavily in a rather short time may be setting themselves

up for an extremely unpleasant, toxic, potentially life-threatening experience because of their high BAC.

Although responsible drinking would prevent acute alcohol intoxication (poisoning), such responsible drinking will never be a reality for everyone. As caring adults, what should we know about this health emergency that may help us save a life?

The first real danger sign we need to recognize is **shock** and its typical signs. By the time these signs are evident, a drinker will already have become unconscious. He or she cannot be aroused from a deep stupor. The person will probably have a weak, rapid pulse (over 100 beats per minute). The skin will be cool and damp, and breathing will be increased to once every three or four seconds. These breaths may be shallow or deep but will certainly occur in an irregular pattern. The skin will be pale or bluish. (In a person with dark skin, these color changes will be more evident in the fingernail beds or in the mucous

blood alcohol concentration (BAC)   the percentage of alcohol in a measured quantity of blood; BAC can be determined directly, through the analysis of a blood sample, or indirectly, through the analysis of exhaled air.

acute alcohol intoxication   a potentially fatal elevation of BAC, often resulting from heavy, rapid consumption of alcohol.

oxidation   the process that removes alcohol from the bloodstream.

shock   profound collapse of many vital body functions; evident during acute alcohol intoxication and other serious health emergencies.

membranes inside the mouth or under the eyelids.) Whenever any of these signs are present, seek emergency medical help immediately (see the Health Action Guide below for a summary of these signs).

Involuntary regurgitation (vomiting) can be another potentially life-threatening emergency for a person who has drunk too much alcohol. When a drinker has consumed more alcohol than the liver can oxidize, the pyloric valve at the base of the stomach tends to close. Additional alcohol remains in the stomach. This alcohol irritates the lining of the stomach so much that involuntary muscle contractions force the stomach contents to flow back through the esophagus. By removing alcohol from the stomach, vomiting may be a life-saving mechanism for conscious drinkers.

An unconscious drinker who vomits, however, may be lying in such a position that the airway becomes obstructed with the vomitus from the stomach. This person is in great risk of dying from **asphyxiation.** As a first-aid measure, unconscious drinkers should always be rolled onto their sides to minimize the chance of airway obstruction. If you are with a person who is vomiting, make certain that his or her head is positioned lower than the rest of the body. This position minimizes the chance that vomitus will obstruct the air passages.

It is also important to keep a close watch on anyone who passes out from heavy drinking. Unfortunately, partygoers sometimes make the mistake of carrying these people to bed and then forgetting about them. You should do your best to monitor the physical condition of anyone who becomes unconscious from heavy drinking because of the risk of death. If you really care about these people, you will observe them at regular intervals until they appear to be clearly out of danger. Although this may mean an evening of interrupted sleep for you, you might save a friend's life.

HEALTH ACTION GUIDE

Acute Alcohol Intoxication

You should seek emergency help for acute alcohol intoxication when you find that a person drinking heavily:

- Cannot be aroused
- Has a weak, rapid pulse
- Has an unusual or irregular breathing pattern
- Has cool (possibly damp), pale, or bluish skin

InfoLinks
www.ncadd.org

Alcohol-Related Health Problems

The relationship of chronic alcohol use to the structure and function of the body is reasonably well understood. Heavy alcohol use causes a variety of changes in the body that lead to an increase in morbidity and mortality. Figure 8-1 describes these changes. Some of these health problems are specifically addressed in the *Healthy People 2000* objectives.

Research clearly shows that chronic alcohol use also damages the immune system and the nervous system. Thus chronic users are at high risk for a variety of infections and neurological complications.

Fetal Alcohol Syndrome and Fetal Alcohol Effects

A growing body of scientific evidence shows that alcohol use by pregnant women can cause birth defects in unborn children. When alcohol crosses the **placenta,** it enters the fetal bloodstream in a concentration equal to that in the mother's bloodstream. Because the fetal liver is underdeveloped, it oxidizes this alcohol much more slowly than the alcohol in the mother. During this time of slow detoxification, the developing fetus is certain to be overexposed to the toxic effects of alcohol. Mental retardation frequently develops.

This exposure has additional disastrous consequences for the developing fetus. Low birth weight, facial abnormalities, such as a small head and widely spaced eyes, and heart problems are often seen in such infants (Figure 8-2). This combination of effects is called **fetal alcohol syndrome (FAS).** Recent studies estimate that the full expression of this syndrome occurs at a rate of 1 to 3 per 1,000 births. Partial expression (*fetal alcohol effects, [FAE]*) can be seen in 3 to 9 per 1,000 live births. In addition, it is likely that many cases of FAE go undetected.

Is there a safe limit to the number of drinks a woman can consume during pregnancy? Because no one can accurately predict the effect of drinking even small amounts of alcohol during pregnancy, the wisest plan is to avoid alcohol altogether.

asphyxiation   death resulting from lack of oxygen to the brain.

placenta   the structure through which nutrients, metabolic wastes, and drugs (including alcohol) pass from the bloodstream of the mother into the bloodstream of the developing fetus.

fetal alcohol syndrome (FAS)   characteristic birth defects noted in the children of some women who consume alcohol during their pregnancies.

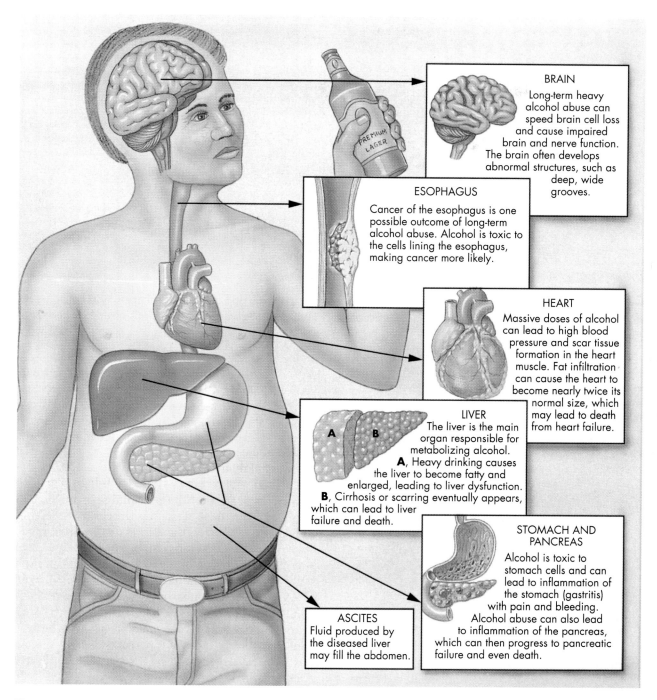

Figure 8-1 Effects of alcohol use on the body. The mind-altering effects of alcohol begin soon after it enters the bloodstream. Within minutes, alcohol numbs nerve cells in the brain. The heart muscle strains to cope with alcohol's depressive action. If drinking continues, the rising BAC causes impaired speech, vision, balance, and judgment. With an extremely high BAC, respiratory failure is possible. Over time, alcohol abuse increases the risk for certain forms of heart disease and cancer and makes liver and pancreas failure more likely.

Because of the critical growth and development that occur during the first months of fetal life, women who have any reason to suspect they are pregnant should stop all alcohol consumption. Furthermore, women who are planning to become pregnant and women who are not practicing effective contraception should also keep their alcohol use to a minimum.

Personal Applications

• What role should men play in the prevention of fetal alcohol syndrome?

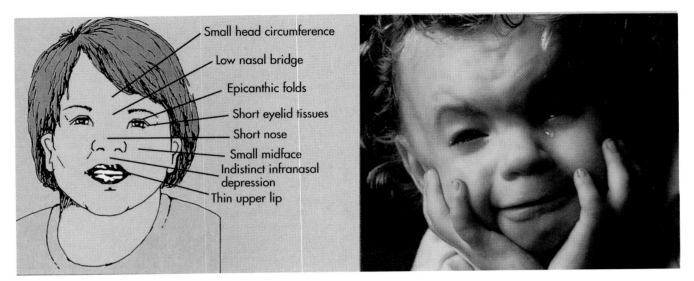

Figure 8-2 Fetal alcohol syndrome. The facial features shown are characteristic of affected children. Additional abnormalities in the brain and other internal organs accompany fetal alcohol syndrome but are not obvious in the child's appearance.

Alcohol-Related Social Problems

Beyond personal health problems, alcohol abuse is related to a variety of social problems. These problems affect the quality of interpersonal relationships, employment stability, and the financial security of both the individual and family. Clearly, alcohol's negative social consequences damage our quality of life. For example, we spend $5 billion a year for treatment of alcohol abuse in this country.[19] An increasing share of these expenses are paid by the public.

Accidents

The four leading causes of accidental death in the United States (motor vehicle collisions, falls, drownings, and fires and burns) have significant statistical connections to alcohol use. Approximately 40 percent of all fatal traffic crashes are alcohol related. Further, the likelihood of being involved in a fatal collision is about eight times higher for a drunk driver (0.10% BAC) than for a sober one.

Many people are surprised to learn that falls are the second leading cause of accidental death in the United States, with about 13,000 deaths per year. Alcohol use increases the risk for falls. Various studies suggest that alcohol is involved in 17 percent to 53 percent of deadly falls and 21 percent to 77 percent of nonfatal falls.

Drownings are the third leading cause of accidental death in the United States. Studies have shown that alcohol use is implicated in approximately 38 percent of these deaths. Over one-third of boaters have been found to drink alcohol while boating.

Fires and burns are responsible for an estimated 6,000 deaths each year in the United States, the fourth leading cause of accidental death. This cause is also connected to alcohol use: Studies indicate that nearly half of burn victims have BACs above the legal limit.

Alcohol and Driving

Reports indicate that the percentage of traffic deaths resulting from alcohol use has dropped to well below 50 percent. However, the 20,000 deaths attributed annually to drunk driving remain unacceptable, and the additional number of serious injuries is great. All states have raised the legal drinking age to twenty-one years. Most states have set 0.10 percent as the BAC at which drivers are considered to be legally drunk (Figure 8-3). However, sixteen states have lowered this standard to 0.08 percent (see As We Go to Press on p. 256). Much of the credit for this trend goes to public-interest groups such as Mothers Against Drunk Driving (MADD). In addition, all fifty states have enacted **zero tolerance laws** to help prevent underage drinking and driving. These laws set BAC limits for drivers under 21 years of age to 0.02 percent or lower. Already, studies show that the first 12 states that enacted these zero tolerance laws for young drivers have cut fatal crashes among young people by 20 percent compared with states that do not have such laws.[20] These laws may help the United States achieve some of its major health objectives for the year 2000.

Other programs and policies are being implemented that are designed to prevent intoxicated people from driving. Included are efforts to educate bartenders to recognize intoxicated customers, to

Number of drinks
in 2-hour period
(1 1/2-oz 86-proof liquor
or 12-oz beer)

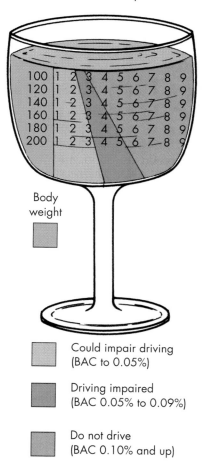

100	1	2	3	4	5	6	7	8	9
120	1	2	3	4	5	6	7	8	9
140	1	2	3	4	5	6	7	8	9
160	1	2	3	4	5	6	7	8	9
180	1	2	3	4	5	6	7	8	9
200	1	2	3	4	5	6	7	8	9

Body
weight

Could impair driving
(BAC to 0.05%)

Driving impaired
(BAC 0.05% to 0.09%)

Do not drive
(BAC 0.10% and up)

Figure 8-3 For most states, a BAC of 0.10% constitutes legal intoxication. However, a BAC as low as 0.05% can impair functioning enough to cause a serious accident.

encourage people to establish designated drivers, to use off-duty police officers as observers in bars, to use police roadblocks, and to develop mechanical devices that prevent intoxicated drivers from starting their cars.

Personal Applications

• Do you believe it is your responsibility to make sure friends do not drink and drive?

Crime and Violence

You may have noticed at your college that most of the violent behavior and vandalism on campus is related to alcohol use. Indeed, the connection of alcohol to

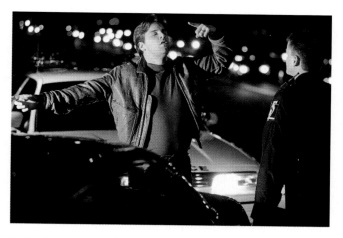

Police have stepped up their efforts to keep drunk drivers off the road by using sobriety checkpoints and roadside sobriety tests for people suspected of being intoxicated.

crime has a long history. Prison populations have large percentages of alcohol abusers and alcoholics; people who commit crimes are more likely to have alcohol problems than people in the general population. This is especially true for young criminals. Furthermore, alcohol use has been reported in 67 percent of all homicides, with the victim, the perpetrator, or both found to have been drinking. In more than half of rape cases, both the rapist and the victim are intoxicated when the crime is committed. Drinking may also increase the risk of becoming a robbery victim.[21]

Because of research methodological problems, pinpointing alcohol's connection to family violence is difficult. However, it seems clear that among a large number of families, alcohol is associated with violence and other harmful behavior, including physical abuse, child abuse, psychological abuse, and abandonment.[15] Alcohol use is present in over half of all domestic violence cases, and frequent drunkenness for husbands appears to be associated with partner abuse.[21] One study estimated that the incidence of spousal abuse was almost 15 times higher for households where husbands were described as often drunk compared with never drunk.

The first question that arises when discussing the relationship between alcohol use and violence is whether a link can be proved. Obviously, not everyone who drinks becomes violent, but in many violent crimes at least one person involved has been drinking. The answer is perhaps that alcohol by itself is not

zero tolerance laws laws that severely restrict the right to operate motor vehicles for underage drinkers who have been convicted of driving under the influence of alcohol or any other drug.

enough to cause violence, but use of alcohol may be one of several factors that act in combination to cause violent behavior in some instances.

Who is most likely to be involved in an alcohol-related violent crime? A nine-year study of more than 4,000 Los Angeles homicide victims suggests that men are much more likely to be involved than women. In the study, 51.3 percent of the male victims had detectable blood alcohol concentrations, compared with 25.8 percent of the female victims.[21] Other studies have shown that people under age thirty are more likely than older people to be involved in both sexual and nonsexual assault when alcohol is a factor. Data on race and ethnicity are inconclusive; some studies show that whites are more likely to be involved in alcohol-related homicides, whereas others show that African-Americans are. In the Los Angeles study, 38.2 percent of Hispanic homicide victims had detectable blood alcohol concentrations; this places them between the percentage figures for male victims and female victims and thus shows no tendency for or against involvement in alcohol-related violence. Alcohol-related homicides and assaults are more likely to occur on weekends than weekdays, in part because more people tend to drink on weekends.[21]

Alcohol and Types of Violent Crime

The risk of a person committing a violent crime is higher among heavy drinkers than light drinkers. Heavy drinkers are also at higher risk of being victims of violent crime and are more likely to inflict and to receive violent injuries.[22] A Johns Hopkins University study shows that being a victim of sexual abuse or assault is also linked to high rates of alcohol use.[23] An environment in which alcohol use is prevalent is a risk factor associated with gun injuries, particularly deaths among youths.[24] Alcohol-related violence tends to be more prevalent in urban environments. It is estimated that eliminating the glut of inner-city alcohol outlets could cut the U.S. homicide rate by 10 percent and could save 2,000 lives annually.[25]

Suicide

The *Seventh Special Report to the U.S. Congress on Alcohol and Health* points out alcohol's relationship to suicide. Between 20 percent and 36 percent of suicide victims have a history of alcohol abuse or were drinking shortly before their suicides. In addition, alcohol use is associated with impulsive suicides rather than with premeditated ones. Drinking is also connected with more violent and lethal means of suicide, such as the use of firearms.

For many of these social problems, alcohol use impairs critical judgment and allows a person's behavior to quickly become reckless, antisocial, and deadly. Acting responsibly when we host a party can help prevent a deadly situation.

Personal Applications

• What alcohol-related social problems have touched your life? How could you contribute to finding solutions to these problems?

Hosting a Party Responsibly

Some people might say that no party is totally safe when alcohol is served. These people are probably right, considering the possibility of unexpected **drug synergism,** overconsumption, and the consequences of released inhibitions. Fortunately, an increasing awareness of the value of responsible party hosting seems to be spreading among college communities. The impetus for this awareness has come from various sources, including respect for an individual's right to choose not to drink alcohol, the growing recognition that many automobile crashes are alcohol related, and the legal threats posed by **host negligence.**

For whatever reasons, responsibly hosting parties at which alcohol is served is becoming a trend, especially among college-educated young adults. The Education Commission of the States' Task Force on Responsible Decisions about Alcohol has generated a list of guidelines for hosting a social event at which alcoholic beverages are served. The list includes the recommendations shown in the Health Action Guide on page 247.

In addition to these suggestions, the use of a **designated driver** is an important component of responsible alcohol use. By planning to abstain from alcohol or to carefully limit their own alcohol consumption, designated drivers are able to safely transport friends who have been drinking.

Designated drivers have indisputably saved many lives. However, there may be a down side. Some health professionals are concerned that the use of designated drivers allows the nondrivers to drink more heavily than they might otherwise. In effect, designated drivers "enable" drinkers to be less responsible for their own behavior. This freedom from responsibility might eventually lead to further problems for the drinkers. What do you think?

Organizations That Support Responsible Drinking

The serious consequences of the irresponsible use of alcohol have led to the formation of a number of concerned-citizen groups. Although each organization has a unique approach, all attempt to deal objectively with two indisputable facts: alcohol use is part of our society, and irresponsible alcohol use can be deadly. You can find the telephone numbers of the following organizations in the Health Reference Guide at the end of this book.

Mothers Against Drunk Driving

Mothers Against Drunk Driving (MADD) is a national network of more than 500 local chapters in the United States and Canada. MADD attempts to educate people about alcohol's effects on driving and to influence legislation and enforcement of laws related to drunk drivers. MADD clearly had a strong influence on the passage of a federal law requiring states to raise the legal drinking age to twenty-one or risk losing federal highway funds.

Students Against Destructive Decisions

Students Against Destructive Decisions (SADD), formerly called Students Against Driving Drunk, recently changed its name to reflect not only its opposition to drinking and driving, but also to underage and other irresponsible drinking and to illegal drug use. The group also educates students about seat belt use and takes a stand on other issues, such as suicide and teen pregnancy. The organization is well known for its "Contract for Life," a pact that encourages both students and their parents to seek safe transportation

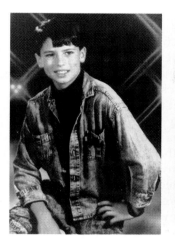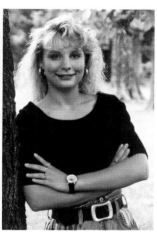

Paul William Chambers, age twelve, was killed on Christmas Eve 1992 by a drunk driver who was traveling the wrong way and struck the family van and three other vehicles. The driver was sentenced to fifteen years in prison. Kimberly Ann Mosley, age nineteen, was a passenger in a car in which the drunk driver lost control, resulting in a fatal crash. She had been a student at Poplar Bluff Senior High School in Missouri when she died in August 1994.

if they or a person offering them a ride has been drinking or using drugs. The agreement stipulates that the consequences of the teen's behavior will not be addressed until a later, perhaps calmer, time.

Boost Alcohol Consciousness Concerning the Health of University Students

BACCHUS is an acronym for Boost Alcohol Consciousness Concerning the Health of University Students. Run by student volunteers, this college-based organization promotes responsible drinking among university students who choose to drink. BACCHUS supports responsible party hosting, including providing quantities of food and nonalcoholic beverages. The individual chapters of BACCHUS (which now total more than 500) are encouraged to use a number of innovative educational approaches to promote alcohol awareness.

HEALTH ACTION GUIDE

Guidelines for Hosting a Party Responsibly[26]

- Provide other social activities as a primary focus when alcohol is served.
- Respect an individual's decision about alcohol if that decision is either to abstain or to drink responsibly.
- Recognize the decision not to drink and the respect it warrants by providing equally attractive and accessible nonalcohol drinks when alcohol is served.
- Recognize that drunkenness is neither healthy nor safe. One should not excuse otherwise unacceptable behavior solely because the individual had "too much to drink."
- Provide food when alcohol is served.
- Serve diluted drinks, and do not keep filling glasses.
- Keep the cocktail hour before dinner to a reasonable time and consumption limit.
- Recognize your responsibility for the health, safety, and pleasure of both the drinker and the nondrinker by avoiding intoxication and helping others do the same.
- Make contingency plans for intoxication. If it occurs in spite of your efforts to prevent it, assume responsibility for the health and safety of guests—for example, by providing transportation home or overnight accommodations.
- Serve or use alcohol only in environments conducive to pleasant and relaxing behavior.

InfoLinks
www.madd.org

---

drug synergism (sin er jism)   enhancement of a drug's effect as a result of the presence of additional drugs within the system.

host negligence   a legal term that reflects the failure of a host to provide reasonable care and safety for people visiting the host's residence or business.

designated driver   a person who abstains from or carefully limits alcohol consumption to be able to safely transport other people who have been drinking.

Other Approaches

Other responsible approaches to alcohol use are surfacing nearly every day. Even among college fraternity organizations, attitudes toward the indiscriminate use of alcohol are changing. Most fraternity rush functions are now conducted without the use of alcohol.

Another encouraging sign seen on college campuses is the increasing number of alcohol use task forces. Although each of these study committees has its own focus and title, many of these groups are meeting to discuss alcohol-related concerns on their particular campus. These task forces often attempt to formulate detailed, comprehensive policies for alcohol use across the entire campus community. Members of these committees often include students (on-campus and off-campus, graduate and undergraduate), faculty and staff members, academic administrators, residence hall advisers, university police, health center personnel, alumni, and local citizens. Does your college have such a committee?

Problem Drinking and Alcoholism

Problem Drinking

At times the line separating problem drinking from alcoholism is difficult to distinguish (see the Star Box in the next column). There may be no true line, with the exception that an alcoholic is unable to stop drinking. **Problem drinking** is a pattern of alcohol use in which a drinker's behavior creates personal difficulties or difficulties for other people. What are some of these behaviors? Examples might be drinking to avoid life stressors, going to work intoxicated, drinking and driving, becoming injured or injuring others while drinking, solitary drinking, morning drinking, an occasional **blackout,** and being told by others that you drink too much. For college students, two clear indications of problem drinking are missing classes and lowered academic performance caused by alcohol involvement. The Health Action Guide on this page offers suggestions that can help you keep drinking under control.

Problem drinkers are not always heavy drinkers; they might not be daily or even weekly drinkers. Unlike alcoholics, problem drinkers do not need to drink to maintain "normal" body functions. However, when they do drink, they (and others around them) experience problems . . . sometimes with tragic consequences. It is not surprising that problem drinkers are more likely than other drinkers to eventually develop alcoholism. Do you know people who show signs of problem drinking?

Alcoholism

In 1992 a revised definition of **alcoholism** was established by a joint committee of experts on alcohol dependence.[27] This committee defined alcoholism as follows: *Alcoholism is a primary, chronic disease with genetic, psychosocial, and environmental factors influencing its development and manifestations. The disease is often*

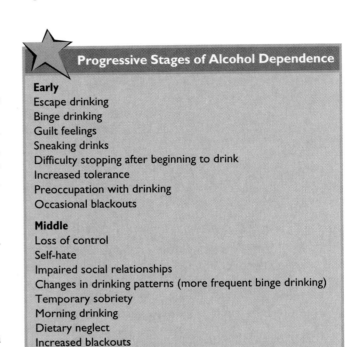

Progressive Stages of Alcohol Dependence

Early
Escape drinking
Binge drinking
Guilt feelings
Sneaking drinks
Difficulty stopping after beginning to drink
Increased tolerance
Preoccupation with drinking
Occasional blackouts

Middle
Loss of control
Self-hate
Impaired social relationships
Changes in drinking patterns (more frequent binge drinking)
Temporary sobriety
Morning drinking
Dietary neglect
Increased blackouts

Late
Prolonged binges
Alcohol used to control withdrawal symptoms
Alcohol psychosis
Nutritional disease
Frequent blackouts

HEALTH ACTION GUIDE

Tips to Help You Keep Drinking Under Control

- Do not drink before a party.
- Avoid drinking when you are anxious, angry, or depressed.
- Measure the liquor you put in mixed drinks (use only 1.5 oz).
- Eat ample amounts of food and drink lots of water before and during the time you are drinking.
- Avoid salty foods that may make you drink more than you had planned.
- Drink slowly.
- Do not participate in drinking games.
- Do not drive after drinking; use a designated nondrinking driver or use public transportation.
- Consume only a predetermined number of drinks.
- Stop alcohol consumption at a predetermined hour.

InfoLinks
www.bacchusgamma.org

progressive and fatal. It is characterized by impaired control over drinking, preoccupation with the drug alcohol, use of alcohol despite adverse consequences, and distortions in thinking, most notably denial. Each of these symptoms may be continuous or periodic.

This definition incorporates much of the knowledge gained from addiction research during the last two decades. It is well recognized that alcoholics do not drink for the pleasurable effects of alcohol but to escape being sober. For alcoholics, being sober is stressful.

Unlike problem drinking, alcoholism involves a physical addiction to alcohol. For the true alcoholic, when the body is deprived of alcohol, physical and mental withdrawal symptoms become evident. These withdrawal symptoms can be life threatening. Uncontrollable shaking can progress to nausea, vomiting, hallucinations, shock, and cardiac and pulmonary arrest. Uncontrollable shaking combined with irrational hallucinations is called *delirium tremens (DT)*, an occasional manifestation of alcohol withdrawal.

The complex reasons for the physical and emotional dependence of alcoholism have not been fully explained. Why, when more than 100 million adults use alcohol without becoming dependent on it, do 10 million or more others become unable to control its use?

Could alcoholism be an inherited disease? Studies in humans and animals have provided strong evidence that genetics plays a role in some cases of alcoholism. Two forms of alcoholism are thought to be inherited: type I and type II. Type I is thought to take years to develop and may not surface until midlife. Type II is a more severe form and appears to be passed primarily from fathers to sons. This form of alcoholism frequently begins earlier in a person's life and may even start in adolescence.

Genetics may also help protect some Asians from developing alcoholism. About half of all Far East Asians produce low levels of an important enzyme that helps metabolize alcohol. These people cannot tolerate even small amounts of alcohol. In addition, genetic factors influencing the absorption rates of alcohol in the intestinal tract have been hypothesized to predispose some Native Americans to alcoholism. More research is needed about the role of genetic factors in all forms of chemical dependence.

The role of personality traits as conditioning factors in the development of alcoholism has received considerable attention. Factors ranging from unusually low self-esteem to an antisocial personality have been implicated. Additional factors making people susceptible to alcoholism may include excessive reliance on denial, hypervigilance, compulsiveness, and chronic levels of anxiety. Always complicating the study of personality traits is the uncertainty of whether the personality profile is a predisposing fac-

tor (perhaps from inheritance) or is caused by the alcoholism itself.

Denial and Enabling

Problem drinkers and alcoholics frequently use the psychological defense mechanism of *denial* to maintain their drinking behavior. By convincing themselves that their lives are not affected by their drinking, problem drinkers and alcoholics are able to maintain their drinking patterns. A person's denial is an unconscious process that is apparent only to rational observers.

Formerly, alcoholics were required to admit that their denial was no longer effective before they could be admitted to a treatment program. This is not the case today. Currently, family members, friends, and coworkers of alcohol-dependent people are encouraged to intervene (with the help and supervision of a professional) and force an alcohol-dependent person into treatment.

During treatment, chemically dependent people must break through the security of denial and admit that alcohol controls their lives. This process is demanding and often time consuming, but there is no alternative path to recovery.

For family and friends of chemically dependent people, denial is part of a process known as *enabling*. In this process, people close to the problem drinker or alcoholic inadvertently support drinking behavior by denying that a problem really exists. Enablers unconsciously make excuses for the drinker, try to keep the drinker's work and family life intact, and in effect make the continued abuse of alcohol possible. For example, college students enable problem drinkers when they clean up a drinker's messy room, lie to professors about a student's class absences, and provide class notes or other assistance to a drinker who cannot perform academically. Even the use of designated drivers has been criticized as enabling behavior.

Alcohol counselors contend that enablers can significantly delay the onset of effective therapy. Do you know of a situation in which you or others have enabled a person with alcohol problems?

problem drinking   an alcohol use pattern in which a drinker's behavior creates personal difficulties or difficulties for other people.

blackout   a temporary state of amnesia experienced by an alcoholic; an inability to remember events that occurred during a period of alcohol use.

alcoholism   a primary, chronic disease with genetic, psychosocial, and environmental factors influencing its development and manifestations.

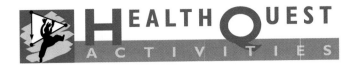

- The alcohol self-assessment activity in Module 8 will help you understand your current drinking behavior and determine how that behavior may affect your health. You can assess your beliefs about alcohol and take a critical look at your ideas about whether alcohol use harms various aspects of your life, such as your friendships, family relationships, and appearance. *HealthQuest* will help you estimate your risk of becoming a problem drinker or alcoholic. After completing the assessment activity, briefly record your answers to the following questions: Do your beliefs about alcohol reflect your own drinking behavior? What factors might cause a person's beliefs and behaviors to be incompatible? What life experiences or influences, such as family, religion, and advertising, have helped form your own beliefs about alcohol? Do you think your beliefs and behavior patterns are fixed, or will they change over time?

- The *Alcohol Decision Maze*, found in Module 8, simulates an evening out with a friend. The activity prompts you to make a variety of choices throughout the evening that may influence whether or how much you drink. First you will choose among several companions for the evening. Then you must decide where to go. At each location, such as a restaurant or sporting event, you can choose from a list of activities in which to participate. The choice to buy or drink alcohol surfaces often. *HealthQuest* will then provide feedback on the outcome of the evening and estimate your blood alcohol content. Complete this activity several times, making different decisions each time. Does the outcome of the evening reflect the drinking behavior you entered? Why or why not?

Codependence

A new term has been coined in the last decade to describe the relationship between drug-dependent people and those around them—codependence. This term implies a kind of dual addiction. The alcoholic and the person close to the alcoholic are both addicted, one to alcohol and the other to the alcoholic. People who are codependent often find themselves denying the addiction and enabling the alcohol-dependent person.

Unfortunately, this kind of behavior damages both the alcoholic and the codependent. The alcoholic's intervention and treatment may be delayed for a considerable time. Codependent people often pay a heavy price as well. They often become drug or alcohol dependent themselves, or they may suffer a variety of psychological consequences related to guilt, loss of self-esteem, depression, and anxiety. Codependents may be at increased risk for physical and sexual abuse.

Fortunately, researchers continue to explore this dimension of alcoholism. Many students have found some of the sources listed at the end of this chapter to

be especially helpful. To determine whether you could benefit from a support program such as Al-Anon or Alateen, answer the questions in the Personal Assessment on page 251.

Helping the Alcoholic: Rehabilitation and Recovery

When an alcoholic realizes that alcoholism is not a form of moral weakness but rather a clearly defined illness, the chances for recovery are remarkably good. It is estimated that as many as two-thirds of alcoholics can recover. Recovery is especially improved when the addicted person has a good emotional support system, including concerned family members, friends, and employer. When this support system is not well established, the alcoholic's chances for recovery are considerably lower.

AA is a voluntary support group of recovering alcoholics who meet regularly to help each other get and stay sober. There are more than 19,000 AA groups in the United States. AA encourages alcoholics to admit their lack of power over alcohol and to turn their lives over to a higher power (although the organization is nonsectarian).[28] Members of AA are encouraged not to be judgmental about the behavior of other members. They support anyone with a problem caused by alcohol.

Al-Anon and Alateen are parallel organizations that give support to people who live with alcoholics. Al-Anon is geared toward spouses and other relatives, whereas Alateen focuses on children of alcoholics. Both organizations help members realize that they are not alone and that successful adjustments can be made to nearly every situation. AA, Al-Anon, and Alateen chapter organizations are usually listed in the telephone book or in the classified sections of local newspapers.

For people who feel uncomfortable with the concept that their lives are controlled by a higher power, secular recovery programs are becoming popular. These programs maintain that sobriety comes from within the alcoholic. Secular programs strongly emphasize self-reliance, self-determination, and rational thinking about one's drinking. Secular Organizations for Sobriety (SOS) and Rational Recovery are examples of secular recovery programs.

SOS can be reached at (310) 821-8430, and Rational Recovery can be reached at (530) 621-2667. Because these programs are relatively new, they might not yet be listed in your local telephone book.

Personal Applications

- What could you do to support a friend or family member who is recovering from alcoholism? What could you do to help yourself through this process?

Personal Assessment

The following questions are designed to help you decide whether you are affected by someone's drinking and could benefit from a program such as Al-Anon. Record your number of yes and no responses in the boxes at the end of the questionnaire.

	Yes	No
1. Do you worry about how much someone else drinks?	___	___
2. Do you have money problems because of someone else's drinking?	___	___
3. Do you tell lies to cover up for someone else's drinking?	___	___
4. Do you feel that if the drinker loved you, he or she would stop drinking to please you?	___	___
5. Do you blame the drinker's behavior on his or her companions?	___	___
6. Are plans frequently upset or meals delayed because of the drinker?	___	___
7. Do you make threats, such as, "If you don't stop drinking, I'll leave you?"	___	___
8. Do you secretly try to smell the drinker's breath?	___	___
9. Are you afraid to upset someone for fear it will set off a drinking bout?	___	___
10. Have you been hurt or embarrassed by a drinker's behavior?	___	___
11. Are holidays and gatherings spoiled because of the drinking?	___	___
12. Have you considered calling the police for help in fear of abuse?	___	___
13. Do you search for hidden alcohol?	___	___
14. Do you often ride in a car with a driver who has been drinking?	___	___
15. Have you refused social invitations out of fear or anxiety that the drinker will cause a scene?	___	___
16. Do you sometimes feel like a failure when you think of the lengths to which you have gone to control the drinker?	___	___

	Yes	No
17. Do you think that if the drinker stopped drinking, your other problems would be solved?	___	___
18. Do you ever threaten to hurt yourself to scare the drinker?	___	___
19. Do you feel angry, confused, or depressed most of the time?	___	___
20. Do you feel there is no one who understands your problems?	___	___
TOTAL	___	___

Interpretation

If you answered yes to three or more of these questions, Al-Anon or Alateen may be able to help. You can contact Al-Anon or Alateen by looking in your local telephone directory or by writing to Al-Anon Family Group Headquarters, Inc., 1600 Corporate Landing Parkway, Virginia Beach, VA 23454-5617, or you may call (800) 356-9996.

To Carry This Further . . .

Sometimes the decision to seek help from a support group is a difficult one. If you answered yes to any of the questions above, spend a few moments reflecting on your responses. How long have you been experiencing problems because of someone else's drinking? How would sharing your feelings with others—people who have dealt with very similar problems—help you cope with your own situation? Knowing you're not alone can often be a great relief; it's up to you to take the first step.

Alcohol and the Elderly: A Hidden Problem

We know that children, adolescents, and adults all can succumb to the risks of alcohol abuse. Unfortunately, we should not assume that the risk goes away as we age.

About 1.8 million women over the age of 59 in the United States need treatment for alcohol abuse, according to one recent study.[29] Other studies report that the problem is even worse among older men[30] and that up to 10 percent of all elderly people are heavy drinkers.[31]

As the number of elderly is expected to grow over the next few decades while baby boomers begin retiring, we will see an increase in the number of older problem drinkers. Likewise, we can expect alcohol to continue to contribute to motor vehicle accidents involving the elderly, as alcohol already appears at a relatively high frequency in crashes involving the elderly, especially men.[32]

Health-care professionals need to be aware of this growing problem and offer help to elderly people facing the risks of alcohol abuse. In particular, we need to realize that the elderly have special needs:

- The elderly may experience problems even at lower levels of alcohol consumption.[33]
- Signs and symptoms of alcohol problems in the elderly may differ from those of younger problem drinkers.
- Those most at risk are men, especially the younger elderly in transition from work to retirement.
- Older alcoholics tend to do well in alcohol treatment.

Common Traits of Adult Children of Alcoholics

Adult children of alcoholics may:

- Have difficulty identifying normal behavior
- Have difficulty following a project from beginning to end
- Lie when it would be just as easy to tell the truth
- Judge themselves without mercy
- Have difficulty having fun
- Take themselves very seriously
- Have difficulty with intimate relationships
- Overreact to changes over which they have no control
- Constantly seek approval and affirmation
- Feel that they are different from other people
- Be super-responsible or super-irresponsible
- Be extremely loyal, even in the face of evidence that the loyalty is undeserved
- Tend to lock themselves into a course of action without considering the consequences

Medical Treatment for Alcoholism

Could there be a medical cure for alcoholism? For nearly fifty years, the only prescription drug physicians could use to help drinkers stop drinking was antabuse. Antabuse would cause drinkers to become extremely nauseated whenever they used alcohol.

In 1995 the Food and Drug Administration approved a drug called naltrexone that works by reducing the craving for alcohol and the pleasurable sensations felt when drinking. Combining naltrexone with conventional behavior modification has been shown to reduce alcohol relapse significantly.

Current Alcohol Concerns

Adult Children of Alcoholic Parents

In recent years a new dimension of alcoholism has been identified—the unusually high prevalence of alcoholism among adult children of alcoholics (ACAs). It is estimated that these children are about four times more likely to develop alcoholism than children whose parents are not alcoholics. Even the ACAs who do not become alcoholics may have a difficult time adjusting to everyday living. Janet Geringer Woititz,

author of the best-selling book *Adult Children of Alcoholics*,[34] describes thirteen traits that, to some degree, most ACAs exhibit (see the Star Box on this page).

In response to this concern, support groups have been formed to prevent the adult sons and daughters of alcoholics from developing the condition that afflicted their parents. If a stronger link for an inherited genetic predisposition to alcoholism is found, these groups may play an even greater role in the prevention of alcoholism.

Women and Alcohol

For decades, women have consumed less alcohol and had fewer alcohol-related problems than men. Evidence is mounting that a greater percentage of women are choosing to drink and that some subgroups of women, especially young women, are drinking more heavily. A greater number of admissions of women to treatment centers may also reflect that alcohol consumption among women is on the rise.

Studies show that there are now almost as many female as male alcoholics. However, differences appear to exist between men and women when it comes to alcohol abuse:[35] (1) More women than men can point to a specific triggering event, such as a divorce, death of a spouse, a career change, or children leaving home, that started them drinking heavily. (2) Alcoholism among women often starts later and progresses more quickly than alcoholism among men. (3) Women tend to be prescribed more mood-altering

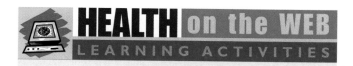

Rating Your Risk for Alcoholism

For traditional-age students, the college years can mark the beginning of a lifetime of problem drinking. A self-assessment can help you determine your risk. Go to www.glness.com/ndhs/risk.html and use the educational tool "Are You at Risk?" This site will help you evaluate your drinking patterns and review the role alcohol plays in your life. The simple yes/no questions incorporate many common symptoms of alcoholism and should raise a "red flag" if your drinking is problematic. However, this is not a diagnostic test.

Understanding Denial and Enabling

In the process of denying and enabling, family members and friends of problem drinkers or alcoholics support their drinking by refusing to acknowledge that a problem really exists. If you are a friend of someone whose drinking concerns you, go to the Mayo Clinic Health Oasis website, at www.mayohealth.org/mayo/9707/htm/quiz3.htm, and answer nine simple yes and no questions about that person's drinking pattern. Consult a substance abuse professional if you suspect the friend's problem may require intervention and treatment.

Estimating Your BAC

The world's leading manufacturer of alcohol breath-testing instruments, Intoximeters, Inc., has a website at which you can instantly estimate your BAC. The site's primary purpose is to provide useful information about the responsible use of alcohol. Go to www.intox.com, select *Drink Wheel*, and complete the form listed. Your BAC will be instantly estimated based on the information you have provided. Try entering different amounts of alcohol consumed over various time periods. Were you surprised that so few drinks could raise your BAC above the legal limit? What strategies might you use to keep your BAC lower the next time you drink alcohol?

drugs than men. Thus women face a greater risk of drug interaction or cross-tolerance. (4) Nonalcoholic men tend to divorce their alcoholic spouses nine times more often than nonalcoholic women divorce their alcoholic spouses. Thus alcoholic women are not as likely to have a family support system to aid them in their recovery attempts. (5) Female alcoholics do not tend to receive as much social support as men in their treatment and recovery. (6) Unmarried, divorced, or single-parent women tend to have significant economic problems that may make entry into a treatment program especially difficult. In light of the generally recognized educational, occupational, and social gains made by women during the last two decades, it will be interesting to see whether these male-female differences continue. What's your best guess?

Alcohol Advertising

Every few years, careful observers can see subtle changes in the ways the alcoholic beverage industry markets its products. Recently, the marketing push appears to be directed toward minorities (through advertisements for malt liquor and fortified wines), women (through wine and wine cooler ads), and youth (through trendy, young adult-oriented commercials).

On the college campus, aggressive alcohol campaigns have used rock stars, beach party scenes, athletic event sponsorships, and colorful newspaper supplements to encourage the purchase of alcohol. Critics claim that most of the collegiate advertising is directed at minors and that the prevention messages are not strong enough to offset the potential health damage to this population. As a college student, how do you feel about alcohol advertising on your campus? If you are a nontraditional-age student, do you find the advertising campaigns amusing or potentially dangerous?

Some beer and liquor companies have begun using websites on the Internet to promote their products. Critics contend that the colorful graphics, hip language, games, chat rooms, and "virtual bars" are designed to recruit underage drinkers.

The Center for Media Education, a group that wants television and other media to become more educational, charges that the sites are particularly appealing to high school and college-age youth. The Distilled Spirits Council denies the charge.

In another medium, distiller Seagram recently began advertising its liquor products on television stations, breaking the industry's forty-seven-year voluntary ban on advertising hard liquor on television (see the Topics for Today article on p. 257). Other distillers plan to follow suit.

President Clinton charges that the television advertising of hard liquor will increase the number of underage drinkers and thus threaten the health and safety of young people. He has asked the FCC to study the possibility of curbing television ads for distilled spirits. In addition, some members of Congress have proposed banning liquor commercials on television altogether.

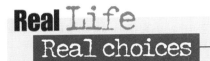

Your Turn

• What role did Rick Diaz play as the oldest child in an alcoholic family?
• What is the term for the way Rick is behaving toward his alcoholic brother now?
• How could Rick be most helpful to his brother?

And Now, Your Choices . . .

• How do you think you would feel and behave if one of your parents were an alcoholic? If you have an alcoholic parent, how do you deal with the situation?
• How would you deal with a younger brother or sister you believed was drinking alcohol excessively?

Summary

• Alcohol is the drug of choice among college students and the rest of American society.
• Most people drink because alcohol is an effective, affordable, legal substance for altering the brain's chemistry.
• People are categorized as abstainers, light drinkers, moderate drinkers, or heavy drinkers, according to their alcohol use patterns.
• Binge drinking is dangerous and can lead to drunk driving, violence, lowered academic performance, and social problems.
• People who do not want to drink can use a variety of techniques to decline alcohol use.
• Alcohol is a product of fermentation, and its nutritional value is extremely limited.
• Alcohol is a drug that is a strong CNS depressant.
• Many factors affect the rate of absorption of alcohol into the bloodstream.
• As BAC rises, predictable depressant effects take place and the risk of acute alcohol intoxication increases; people with this condition are in danger and must receive first aid immediately.
• Alcohol is removed from the bloodstream through the process of oxidation.
• Chronic alcohol use causes a variety of serious health problems for the drinker and can cause fetal alcohol syndrome in infants when a woman drinks during pregnancy.
• Alcohol-related social problems include accidents (motor vehicle crashes, falls, drownings, and fires and burns), crime and violence, and suicide.
• People who host events at which alcohol is served should follow certain guidelines, such as providing

nonalcoholic alternative beverages, to help ensure the safety of their guests.
• Several groups of concerned citizens, such as MADD, SADD, and BACCHUS, promote responsible alcohol use.
• Problem drinking is an alcohol use pattern in which a drinker's behavior creates personal difficulties or problems for others.
• Alcoholism is a primary, chronic disease characterized by addiction to alcohol; it has a variety of possible causes and manifestations.
• Problem drinkers and alcoholics often use the psychological defense mechanism of denial to maintain their drinking behavior.
• Enabling is a behavior pattern in which people close to the problem drinker or alcoholic make the continued use of alcohol possible by keeping the drinker's work and family life intact.
• An alcoholic's family members may unintentionally delay the alcoholic's intervention and treatment by becoming codependent.
• Alcoholics Anonymous and other support groups may help an alcoholic recover from the disease.
• The drugs antabuse and naltrexone are sometimes prescribed to discourage alcohol use.
• Children of alcoholic parents often have characteristic adjustment problems in adulthood.
• Women who abuse alcohol have unique problems and concerns.
• Alcohol advertising is often targeted at minorities, women, and youth.

Review Questions

1. What percentage of American adults consume alcohol? Approximately what percentage of adults are classified as abstainers? What percentage of college students drink?
2. What is binge drinking?
3. What is meant by the term *proof*?
4. What is the nutritional value of alcohol? How do "light" and low-alcohol beverages compare?
5. Identify and explain the various factors that influence the absorption of alcohol. Why is it important to be aware of these factors?
6. What is BAC? Describe the general sequence of physiological events that takes place when a person drinks alcohol at a rate faster than the liver can oxidize it.
7. What are the signs and symptoms of acute alcohol intoxication? What are the first-aid steps you should take to help a person with this problem?
8. Describe the characteristics of fetal alcohol syndrome and fetal alcohol effects.
9. Explain the differences between problem drinking and alcoholism.
10. What roles do denial and enabling play in alcoholism? What is codependence?
11. What are some common traits of ACAs?
12. What unique alcohol-related problems do women face?

References

1. U.S. Department of Health and Human Services. *Alcohol and health: seventh special report to the U.S. Congress.* DHHS Pub No (ADM) 90-1656. Washington, DC: U.S. Government Printing Office, 1990.
2. *Monitoring the future study* (press release). University of Michigan: Institute for Social Research, December 20, 1997.
3. U.S. Bureau of the Census. *Statistical abstract of the United States, 1998, annual.* 118th ed., Washington, DC: U.S. Government Printing Office, 1998.
4. Binge drinking: a big killer. *Reader's Digest* 1998 Nov.
5. Numbers. *Time* 1997 October 13:27.
6. Presley CA, Meilman PW. *Alcohol and drugs on American college campuses: a report to college presidents.* U.S. Department of Education, Drug Prevention in Higher Education Program (FIPSE Grant), Southern Illinois University Student Health Program Wellness Center, June 1992.
7. Wechsler H et al. Correlates of college student binge drinking. *Am J Public Health* 1995 July; 85(7):921–26.
8. Harrington NT, Leitenberg H. Relationship between alcohol consumption and victim behaviors immediately preceding sexual aggression by an acquaintance. *Violence and Victims* 1994 Winter; 9(4):315–24.
9. Engs RC, Hanson DJ. Drinking games and problems related to drinking among moderate and heavy drinkers. *Psychological Reports* 1993 Aug; 73(1):115–20.
10. Sekorska M. Co-dependence—diagnosis and therapy. *Przegl Lek* 1997; 54(6):441–45.
11. Adult Children Educational Foundation Computer Bulletin Board. *Sick families.* 1998. http://www.recovery.org/acoa/families.html
12. *Crime Times* 1996; 2(1):6.
13. Physicians of the Geisinger Health System. *Thrill-seeking children may become alcoholics.* 1997. http://www.geisinger.edu/ghs/pubtips/T/Thrill-SeekingChildrenMayBecomeAlcoholics.htm
14. Roberts P. Risk. *Psychology Today* 1994 NovDec:27.
15. Pinger et al. *Drugs: issues for today.* 3rd ed. Dubuque, IA: WCB/McGraw-Hill, 1998.
16. Klatsky AL. Alcohol, coronary disease, and hypertension. *Ann Rev Med* 1996; 47:149–60.
17. Frezza M et al. High blood alcohol levels in women: the role of decreased gastric alcohol dehydrogenase activity and first-pass metabolism. *N Engl J Med* 1990; 322(4):95–99.
18. Ray O, Ksir C. *Drugs, society, and human behavior.* 8th ed. Dubuque, IA: WCB/McGraw-Hill, 1999.
19. The National Clearinghouse for Alcohol and Drug Information, a service of the Substance Abuse and mental Health Services Administration. *National expenditures for mental health, alcohol, and other drug abuse treatment, 1996,* September 15, 1998.
20. U.S. Department of Health and Human Services. National Institute on Alcohol Abuse and Alcoholism. *Alcohol alert.* No 34 (PH 370) October 1996.
21. Messerschmidt PM: Epidemiology of alcohol related violence, *Alcohol Health and Research World* 1993; 17(2).
22. Cherpitel CJ: What emergency room studies reveal about alcohol involvement in violence-related injuries, *Alcohol Health and Research World* 1993; 17(2).
23. Violence, drugs, alcohol spur decline of youth health across U.S., study says, *Jet* June 1995; 88(7).
24. Voelker R: Taking aim at handgun violence, *JAMA* 1995; 273(22).
25. Abramson H: Quick fix for violence: cut back on liquor stores, *Nation's Cities Weekly* 1995; 18(3).
26. Task Force on Responsible Decisions about Alcohol. Interim report No 2. Denver: Education Commission of the States.
27. Morse RM et al. The definition of alcoholism. *JAMA* 1992; 268(8):1012–14.

28. Alcoholics Anonymous. *This is AA: an introduction to the AA recovery program.* Alcoholics Anonymous World Services, Inc., March 1992, pp 1–21.

29. Glassman M. Doctors slow to spot alcohol abuse in older women. *USA Today* 1998 June 8:1D.

30. Adlaf EM, Smart RG. Alcohol use, drug use, and well-being in older adults in Toronto. *Int J Addict* 1995; 30(13-14):1985–2016.

31. Adams WL, Cox NS. Epidemiology of problem drinking among elderly people. *Int J Addict* 1995; 30(13-14):1693–1716.

32. Higgins JP, Wright SW, Wrenn KD. Alcohol, the elderly, and motor vehicle crashes. *Am J Emerg Med* 1996; 14(3):265–67.

33. Dufour M, Fuller RK. Alcohol in the elderly. *Ann Rev Med* 1995; 46:123–32.

34. Woititz JG. *Adult children of alcoholics.* Pompano Beach, FL: Health Communications Inc, 1990.

35. Kinney J, Leaton G: *Loosening the grip: a handbook of alcohol information,* ed 6. St. Louis, WCB/McGraw-Hill, 1998.

Suggested Readings

Makela K. (editor) *Alcoholics Anonymous as a mutual-help movement: a study in eight societies,* Madison, WI, 1996, University of Wisconsin Press. This book is one of the first comprehensive studies of Alcoholics Anonymous as a social movement and a model for small-group interaction. Experts collaborated to examine the history of an organization that was founded in the 1930s and now has nearly 2 million members worldwide. The book describes what happens at AA meetings, how AA is organized, and how it serves as a professional health care provider across many cultures.

Schaefer D. *Choices and consequences: what to do when a teenager uses alcohol or drugs.* Minneapolis, MN, 1996, The Johnson Institute. This paperback book, published by the highly regarded Johnson Institute, is a useful guide that can help parents, teachers, youth leaders, and other adults recognize and better understand all types of drinking behavior or drug use by teenagers. Schaefer helps adults receognize the role that intervention can play in working against a teenager's denial and resistance.

West JW et al. *The Betty Ford Center book of answers: help for those struggling with substance abuse and for the people who love them.* Pocket Books, 1997. A guide for sufferers and their supporters; answers vital questions about substance abuse, from understanding addictions, to obtaining help, to evaluating recovery options.

As We Go To PRESS

By late March 1999, sixteen states had lowered the BAC at which drivers are considered legally drunk. These states were: Alabama, California, Florida, Hawaii, Illinois, Idaho, Kansas, Maine, New Hampshire, New Mexico, North Carolina, Oregon, Utah, Vermont, Virginia, and Washington. Is your state included in this list? If not, what is the status of this type of proposal in your state?

Success in a Bottle? A Look at Alcohol Advertising

Did the Budweiser frogs, Bud Ice penguin or Schlitz malt liquor bull have anything to do with your recent beverage purchases? Did the scantily clad, frolicking female models get you to belly up to the bar? Despite the brewing industry's claim that marketing does not influence attitudes, behaviors, or beliefs,[1] it spends $600 million per year on radio and TV ads and another $90 million per year on print ads. The hard liquor industry spends $230 million per year on print ads, until recently its only medium of advertising.[2] Controversy over just what alcohol ads accomplish and who they are aimed at was renewed and intensified last year, when Seagrams defied the voluntary ban on TV hard liquor advertising and began marketing its Crown Royal Canadian Whiskey in Texan TV markets. Seagrams's action was followed by the repeal by the Distilled Spirits Council of the United States of the voluntary ban its members had honored against radio and television advertising since 1936 and 1948, respectively.[2]

A growing body of research suggests that alcohol advertising influences the consumption of alcoholic beverages by younger people.[3] Children and adolescents are frequently exposed to beer and liquor advertising because these ads run during shows and at times when most of the audience is under twenty-one. A Schlitz malt liquor commercial appeared on MTV during "My So-Called Life," a show about teenage girls. Molson beer ads appeared during "Beavis and Butt-Head," and a number of Coors and Anheuser-Busch–sponsored shows had viewing audiences of 52 percent to 70 percent minors.[4] Some of these incidents were said to be programming mistakes, but in light of the public outcry, Anheuser-Busch shifted its ads from MTV to VH-1 in order to reach a more adult audience.[5]

Most youth exposure to alcohol advertising, however, occurs through sports programming. These ads are especially troublesome because they often depict the mixture of alcohol and fast driving, water sports, or other dangerous activity. The retention of beer ads by fifth and sixth graders revealed that those most familiar with the ads had more positive beliefs about alcohol and expressed an intention to drink more heavily as adults.[1]

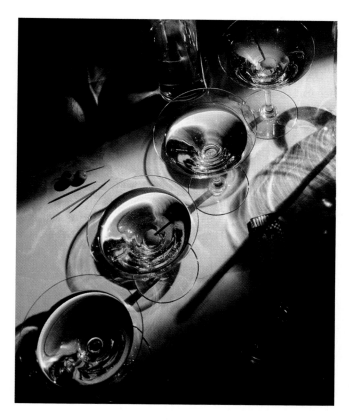

Will television advertisements for hard liquor encourage minors to drink alcohol?

Even before the voluntary ban was lifted, consumer groups had taken up the cause of sheltering young people from the alcohol advertising that *was* allowed; this action just intensifies their efforts. A coalition of minority, religious, and antialcoholism groups, led by the Center on Alcohol Advertising, recently finished a successful campaign to keep Santa Claus out of beer ads. They are now targeting Halloween-themed beer advertising, pointing out that Halloween is generally regarded as a children's holiday.[6] Halloween ads are just one of MADD's (Mothers Against Drunk Driving) targets. They have released a new policy statement denouncing all ads with "special appeal to youth," including those displayed at rock concerts and sporting events.[7] The marketing of so-called "designer drinks" to young people also has become a concern.[8]

Major broadcasting networks still will not air the hard liquor ads, but Continental Cablevision and Black Entertainment Television have been airing them.[2] Targeting of African-Americans also occurs in print ads. One study compared alcohol ads in *Ladies Home Journal*, which has a primarily white readership, and *Ebony* and *Essence*, women's magazines for a black audience. *Ladies Home Journal* had virtually no alcohol ads, whereas 47 percent of the advertising in *Ebony* and *Essence* was alcohol related.[9] Billboards in primarily African-American neighborhoods further push alcohol to this market.[10]

Consumption of Alcohol Among Youth

Although the legal drinking age in all states is twenty-one, fake IDs are readily obtainable and commercially accepted. Many times fake IDs are not even needed. Adults often provide alcohol to underage drinkers. One survey reported that 46 percent of ninth graders, 60 percent of twelfth graders, and 68 percent of eighteen- to twenty-year-old drinkers received their alcohol from a source over twenty-one.[11] According to the U.S. Inspector General, junior high and high school students consume 1.1 billion cans of beer per year, netting $200 million in revenues for the brewing industry.[1] Not to be outdone, college students, most of them still underage, spend $5.5 billion on alcohol annually. This figure is more than they spend on nonalcoholic drinks and books combined.[12]

Of course, some students don't drink (16% of college students, no figure available for high school students), and 40 percent of college students surveyed would be considered moderate drinkers,[13] but 30 percent of high school seniors[1] and 44 percent of college students can be classified as binge drinkers, defined in this survey as those who drink five or more drinks consecutively on one or more occasions per month, drink three or more times per month, or drink to get drunk.[1,14,15]

Availability and price of alcohol, the attitudes and behavior of parents and peers, a need for belonging, and pressure to perform academically, athletically, and socially all influence adolescent drinking behavior. Binge behavior can be roughly predicted by residence in a fraternity or sorority house, marijuana use, history of binge drinking in high school, and involvement in sports.[13,16] That is not to say that all students involved in these activities become binge drinkers—it's just more likely that binge drinkers fall into one or more of these categories. As a general rule, students over twenty-three years old drink significantly less than their younger counterparts.[14] In a national study, another set of trends was revealed. Regionally, students in the Northeast drank more heavily than students in other regions of the country. Racially, white male students drank far more than white females and more than African-Americans and Hispanic-Americans of both sexes. Overall, students at historically black colleges and commuter colleges drank less than any other group.[12,14]

Control of Alcohol Abuse and Regulation of Advertising

What are colleges, the alcohol and advertising industries, and the federal government doing to regulate the abuse of alcohol and its advertising? Some college campuses are dry, not allowing anyone to have alcohol on campus property. Other campuses attempt to segregate heavy drinkers from the rest of the resident population. Alcohol awareness programs are common on all types of college campuses. Still, administrators find themselves having to punish rule-breakers, from individuals to entire athletic teams. For example, a starting linebacker at the University of Nebraska–Lincoln was suspended following a DUI citation, and the entire University of North Carolina–Chapel Hill men's soccer team was put on probation and prohibited from playing in two tournament games because a freshman on the team was hospitalized for acute alcohol intoxication after attending a team party.[13] Alcohol doesn't just cause problems for students—a University of Michigan–Ann Arbor football coach resigned after a drunken outburst in a restaurant, and a football coach at the Citadel was suspended after a DUI incident.[13] Numerous colleges have banned the sale of alcohol at football games and restricted tailgate parties.

The alcohol industry does not view itself as part of the problem. In its defense, industry executives point to voluntary codes that prohibit marketing to underage consumers, emphasize their public service announcements discouraging underage drinking,[1] and maintain that only current or would-be consumers of a product pay any attention to its advertising.[16] Thus, they do not believe that they persuade anyone to drink who was not already going to do so. The advertising industry simply writes off regulation of alcohol advertising as impossible, calling attempts to regulate "age restricted" product advertising "not feasible in the current circumstances."[5]

The government, on the other hand, finding the voluntary rules of the alcohol industry to be vague, too narrow, and unenforceable,[1] is confident of its own regulatory abilities. The Federal Trade Commission is currently investigating alcohol advertising on television. If the content of the commercials or the times and shows during which they air suggest a pattern of targeting youth, fines could be imposed, orders to pull the ads issued, and screening of future advertising mandated.[4] A bipartisan group in Congress has called for a separate Federal Communications Commission investigation, and Representative Joseph Kennedy has introduced the Comprehensive Alcohol Abuse Prevention Act of 1996. If this legislation passes, it would require publications with under-twenty-one readership of 15 percent or 2 million, whichever is less, to run black and white, text-only ads.[17] It would also ban radio and television advertising of alcohol from 7 A.M. to 10 P.M. and require health warnings on all forms of alcohol advertising.[4] Alcohol, media, and advertising lobbies are very powerful and may tie up or kill this legislation. The bill may also be ruled an unconstitutional prohibition of commercial speech. Protection of commercial speech was strengthened by the May 1996 Supreme Court ruling in *44 Liquormart v. Rhode Island.* Rhode Island wanted to restrict alcohol advertising on public transit, but the justices ruled that any restriction must have a chance of solving the problem and must be narrowly tailored,[17] both of which are extremely hard to accomplish.

Money is also a concern. A recent ban on alcohol and tobacco advertising in Russia could cost that country $500 million to $1 billion in Western investment in the next five years and could also cost 20 percent of Russian television station employees their jobs.[18] There, advertising is in its infancy, since the economy opened up only after the fall of the Soviet Union. The effects in lost advertising dollars and jobs in the United States would be much more serious.

Taking Action—What You Can Do

Many people are concerned about the effect alcohol advertising is having on our nation's children and adolescents. The following list suggests steps that each of us can take to address this serious problem:

- Write to alcohol producers, such as Seagrams, to voice your concern.
- Boycott the products of companies that continue inappropriate advertising.
- Write to television and cable stations.
- Boycott programming that is supported by alcohol advertising that targets youth.
- Write to your representatives in Washington.
- Talk to youth about alcohol awareness issues.
- Be conscious of the example you set for others.
- Do not force, prod, or cajole anyone to drink.
- Do not provide alcohol to minors.

Alcohol abuse among minors is a complicated problem for which there is no simple solution, but can we afford to leave American youth to drown in images of success in a bottle?[2]

For Discussion . . .

Do you consider beer and wine ads to be different from hard liquor ads? Do you think advertising encourages young people to drink? If so, how? If not, what does? What alcohol policies does your college have? In your view, are they sufficient, overly stringent, or insufficient?

References

1. Mosher JF. Alcohol advertising and public health: an urgent call for action. *Am J Public Health* 1994; 84(2):180–81.
2. Ingersoll B. FTC opens investigation of TV alcohol advertising; Seagram, Stroh targeted; placement and content of ads to be examined. *The Wall Street Journal* 1996 Nov 26:A3.
3. Wyllie A, Zhang JF, Casswell S. Positive responses to televised beer advertisements associated with drinking and problems reportedly by 18- to 29-year-olds. *Addiction* 1998; 93(5):749–60.
4. Beatty SG. Are beer ads on "Beavis and Butt-Head" aimed at kids? *The Wall Street Journal* 1997 Jan. 6:B1.
5. Staff. Ad industry group rejects alcohol, tobacco system. *The Wall Street Journal* 1996 Dec. 23:B6.
6. Baldauf S. Family groups fight Halloween beer ads. *Christian Science Monitor* 1995; 87(232):4
7. Colford SW. MADD's mood turns tougher on liquor ads. *Advertising Age* 1994; 65(47):18.
8. Hughes K et al. Young people, alcohol, and designer drinks: quantitative and qualitative study. *Br Med J* 1997; 314(7078):414–18.
9. Pratt CA, Pratt CB. Nutrition advertisements in consumer magazines: health implications for African Americans. *Black Studies* 1996; 26(4):504–23.
10. Hackbarth DP, Silvestri B, Cosper W. Tobacco and alcohol billboards in 50 Chicago neighborhoods: market segmentation to sell dangerous products to the poor. *J Pub Health Policy* 1995; 16(2):213–30.
11. Wagenaar AC, Toomey TL, Murray DM, Short BJ, Wolfson M, Jones-Webb R. Sources of alcohol for underage drinkers. *Studies on Alcohol* 1996; 57(3):325–33.
12. Alder J. The endless binge. *Newsweek* 1994; 124(25):72–73.
13. Naughton J. Alcohol abuse by athletes poses big problems for colleges: some educators say that sports programs are "a center of binge drinking." *Chron High Ed* 1996; 43(4):A47–48.
14. Shea C. New look at college drinking. *Chron High Ed* 1994; 41(16):A39.
15. Wechsler H, Moeykens B, Davenport A, Castillo S, Hansen J. The adverse impact of heavy episodic drinkers on other college students. *J Studies on Alcohol* 1995; 56(6):628–34.
16. Calfee JE, Scheraga C. The influence of advertising on alcohol consumption: a literature review and an econometric analysis of four European nations. *Int J Advertising* 1994; 13(4):287–310.
17. Schnuer J. Liquor bill could hurt publishers. *Folio: The Magazine for Magazine Management* 1996; 25(10):18.
18. Specter M. Yelstin move has delighted the doctors. *The New York Times* 1995; 144:A8.

InfoLinks
www.arf.org/isd/bib/advert.html
www2.postdam.edu/alcohol-info/

chapter
nine

Rejecting
Tobacco Use

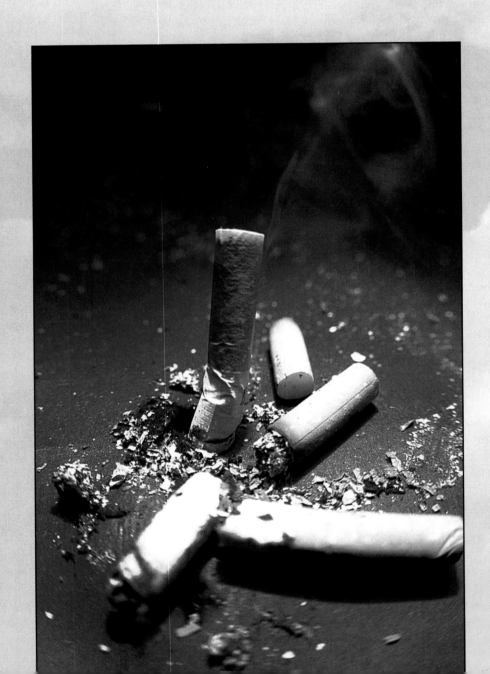

The extent of the tobacco industry's knowledge of the addictive and life-shortening nature of its products, particularly cigarettes, is being revealed daily in the news media. The protective wall of denial built by the tobacco industry over the past forty years to protect its products and profits crumbled in November 1998 when 46 states joined four others that had settled earlier in reaching a final settlement with the tobacco industry regarding current and future class action lawsuits. In that settlement the tobacco industry agreed to pay $206 billion (over 25 years) to reimburse the states for Medicaid expenditures accrued in treating smoking-related illnesses; to stop advertisements intended to influence tobacco use by children; and to find antismoking education program development and implementation. In turn, the states agreed not to initiate further class action lawsuits against the tobacco industry.

Today the evidence linking tobacco use to impaired health is beyond any serious challenge and has, in fact, been "admitted" by the tobacco industry via internal documents released by the Liggett Group in conjunction with the litigation just mentioned. These documents detail activities on the part of the tobacco industry to disprove, mask, and deny their own knowledge that nicotine was addictive and that cigarette smoking caused cancer and chronic obstructive lung disease and increased the risk of developing cardiovascular diseases. It was also revealed that concerted marketing efforts were directed to children and young adolescents in an attempt to move them in the direction of entry-level use (see the Star Box on p. 262). Of course, prior to this "unmasking" of the tobacco industry, health experts knew that regular users of tobacco products, and those who are exposed to tobacco smoke, were more likely to experience serious health problems and even die prematurely. It is estimated that tobacco use, and cigarette smoking in particular, will result in 2 million deaths between 1986 and the year 2000, with nearly 419,000 deaths occurring annually.[1]

HEALTHY PEOPLE: LOOKING AHEAD TO 2010

Several of the original *Healthy People 2000* objectives were aimed at reducing the use of tobacco products, especially cigarettes, to prevent heart disease, stroke, and lung cancer and to promote physical activity, fitness, and oral health.

Although the 1995 *Midcourse Review* did not assess progress in these areas, other sources of information indicated that neither lung cancer nor chronic obstructive lung disease rates had declined at mid-decade. Smoking rates had leveled off for men and nearly leveled off for women but had increased among adolescents. Accordingly, no progress was expected toward preventing the other tobacco-related diseases.

Healthy People 2010 will focus on several areas related to tobacco use, such as reducing the incidence of chronic disease, increasing levels of physical activity, improving environmental health, reducing the incidence of oral disease, and improving maternal and child health. A principal goal of *Healthy People 2010* is to increase years of healthy life among Americans; therefore, decreasing tobacco use and reducing exposure to secondhand smoke are absolute necessities.

Reducing the prevalence of smoking are the initiatives set into place by the legal settlement just described above. Depending on the effectiveness of widespread primary prevention through antismoking education and the efforts to eliminate youth-oriented advertising, and due to the consumer response to the increased price of cigarettes (necessary to fund the $206 billion settlement), a reduction in the number of smokers of all ages could occur. However, increases in the size of the smoking population that began in the early 1990s may negate these factors entirely, resulting in no significant reduction in the overall percentage of the population who smoke.

Real Life
Real choices

Smoking Can Be Hazardous to Your Health—and Relationships

- Names: Karen Heilmann and Steven Chu
- Ages: 24 and 23
- Occupation: Graduate students in molecular biology

Little more than a generation ago, smoking was considered sophisticated, sociable, and safe. Today there's ever-decreasing tolerance for smoking, and those who still cling to the habit may find it causes them heart problems—not only cardiovascular but also romantic.

That's the unhappy reality confronting Karen Heilmann and Steven Chu, who are both top students in their university's graduate program in molecular biology. They met as undergraduates and have been involved in a serious relationship for nearly three years. Although they don't plan to marry until they receive their doctorates, they intend to announce their engagement in the spring.

Karen and Steven seem to have everything going for them. But there's one big hang-up, at least in Steven's mind: Karen smokes. As a former smoker, Steven understands how easy it is to get hooked on nicotine and how difficult it can be to quit, but he's been putting increasing pressure on Karen to give it up. She smokes less than a pack a day, doesn't light up in Steven's apartment or car, and says she'll quit when she finishes her demanding graduate program. In the meantime, Steven and Karen have begun to spend more time arguing about smoking than enjoying each other's company, and last night Steven told Karen he wouldn't consider becoming engaged unless Karen agrees to quit smoking completely before they make the announcement.

As you study this chapter, think about steps Karen and Steven might take to resolve their conflict, and prepare yourself to answer the questions in **Your Turn** at the end of the chapter.

Key Facts about Children and Tobacco

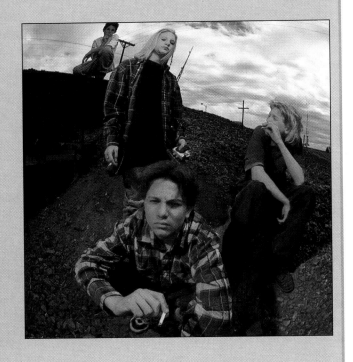

Adults Don't Start Smoking; Kids Do
Almost 9 out of 10 adult smokers began using tobacco products as kids. The average teen smoker begins at age 13 and becomes a daily smoker by 14½. Two-thirds of teen smokers say they want to quit smoking, and 70 percent say that if they could choose again, they would never have started.

Every Day 3,000 Kids Become Regular Smokers
And 1,000 of them will eventually die from their use of cigarettes. Tobacco kills more people than AIDS, alcohol, drugs, fires, homicide, motor vehicles, and suicide combined.

Five Million Deaths
More than 5 million children under age 18 alive today will die prematurely from smoking-related diseases, unless current rates are reversed.

Buying Influence
Tobacco companies gave more than $10 million over the past 10 years to candidates running for Congress in order to buy influence and stop efforts to protect people from tobacco.

Tobacco Advertisements Attract Kids
Eighty-six percent of underage smokers, compared with less than one-third of adults, buy the three most heavily advertised brands: Marlboro, Newport, and Camel. Without suggesting that one specific factor can fully explain why young people experiment with and subsequently adopt smoking, it is interesting to note that during the "Joe Camel era" (1988–1997), the incidence of smoking among American youth increased by 73 percent.[2]

Tobacco Use in American Society

If you were to visit certain businesses, entertainment spots, or sporting events in your community, you might leave convinced that virtually every adult is a tobacco user. Certainly, for some segments of society, tobacco use is the rule rather than the exception. You may be quite surprised to find out that the great majority of adults do not use tobacco products.

Following the Surgeon General's 1964 report (the first official statement of concern by the federal government regarding the dangers of smoking), the prevalence of smoking began a decline that lasted until 1991, when a leveling off was noted that lasted for the next three years. Since 1994 the percentage of the population who smoke has risen slowly but progressively due to the increasing number of adolescents who are smoking. On the basis of our most current statistics reported in the 1995 National Health Interview Survey (NHIS), a recent broadly based study of smoking behavior, 24.7 percent of adults reported that they were current smokers (daily or nearly daily). Men were more likely to smoke (27%) than were women (22.6%).[3]

Cigarette Smoking Among College Students and Young Adults

Smoking among college students and young adults dropped significantly between 1977 and 1981 and then remained relatively constant until 1991. In 1991 the rates of daily smoking actually increased in both groups. Young adults aged nineteen to twenty-eight who were not students had higher smoking rates (21.7%) than college students (13.8%).[4] Most of these smokers began smoking as teenagers.

Over the last few years a dramatic increase in cigarette smoking by people in late adolescence has been widely reported. Most recently (1997) it was reported that 39.6 percent of high school seniors had smoked at least once during the month before data were collected, with 19.4 percent doing so on a near daily basis.[5] Equally recent figures show that the very low incidence of smoking among college students tra-

---

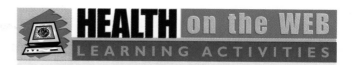

Evaluating Your Smokeless Tobacco Use

If you use smokeless tobacco, you may think you don't have to worry about illness and premature death. However, chewing tobacco can cause cancer of the mouth, digestive system, and urinary system. To find out more, go to www.quitnet.org and select *Beat the Smokeless Habit.* Take the short quiz on smokeless tobacco, and then score yourself on-line.

Exploring the Benefits of Quitting Smoking

If you or someone you know has been smoking for a long time, you may think it's too late for quitting to be beneficial. No so! Even in long-term smokers, quitting greatly improves both short-term and long-term health. For more encouraging news about quitting, go to the Wellness Web page, www.wellweb.com/smoking/SMOKIQ.HTM, and take the I.Q. quiz for older smokers, which was developed by the National Heart, Lung, and Blood Institute. Just answer true or false to the 10 statements listed. The answers that follow include excellent information about the effects of smoking and the benefits of quitting.

Learning the Tobacco Marketers' Tricks

Tobacco companies spend $700,000 an hour to convince people, especially adolescents, that smoking is fun and exciting. Read about some of the ways tobacco companies try appealing to and influencing impressionable young people. Go to www.quitsmoking.miningco.com, select *Teenage Smoking,* and then select *Ways Tobacco Companies Try to Trick You.* What can you do to help young people resist the lure of these tobacco ads?

For more activities, log on to our Online Learning Center at www.mhhe.com/hper/health/payne

---

ditionally anticipated, relative to the general population, has undergone a dramatic change, increasing 28 percent since mid-decade.[5] Whereas the college population once was comprised of only about 14 percent smokers, today the figure exceeds 20 percent.

The most disturbing aspect of the increase in reported smoking among college students, beyond the eventual influence it will have on health and life expectancy, is its negation of the traditional belief that the college and university experience "protected" this segment of the society from making some ill-informed choices. As recently as the mid-1990s it was still possible to believe that the college population was "too well informed" and "too future oriented" to engage widely in an addictive behavior that fosters dependence, compromises health, and eventually shortens life. Today that proposition seems to lack some of its former validity.

A particularly distressing aspect of the increase in tobacco use by college students involves a group that previously was the least likely to smoke cigarettes—African-Americans. The most recent data reporting smoking behavior among high school seniors

---

Personal Applications

• During a traditional commencement ceremony, graduates are welcomed into the "community of educated men and women." To what extent would you support the contention that those who began (or continue) cigarette use during this period have not earned the privilege of membership in this community?

Personal Assessment

Assumption

1. There are now safe cigarettes on the market.
2. A small number of cigarettes can be smoked without risk.
3. Most early changes in the body resulting from cigarette smoking are temporary.
4. Filters provide a measure of safety to cigarette smokers.
5. Low-tar, low-nicotine cigarettes are safer than high-tar, high-nicotine brands.
6. Mentholated cigarettes are better for the smoker than are nonmentholated brands.
7. It has been scientifically proven that cigarette smoking causes cancer.
8. No specific agent capable of causing cancer has ever been identified in the tobacco used in smokeless tobacco.
9. The cure rate for lung cancer is so good that no one should fear developing this form of cancer.
10. Smoking is not harmful as long as the smoke is not inhaled.
11. The "smoker's cough" reflects underlying damage to the tissue of the airways.
12. Cigarette smoking does not appear to be associated with damage to the heart and blood vessels.
13. Because of the design of the placenta, smoking does not present a major risk to the developing fetus.
14. Women who smoke cigarettes and use an oral contraceptive should decide which they wish to continue because there is a risk in using both.
15. Air pollution is a greater risk to our respiratory health than is cigarette smoking.
16. Addiction, in the sense of physical addiction, is found in conjunction with cigarette smoking.
17. Among the best "teachers" a young smoker has are his or her parents.
18. Nonsmoking and higher levels of education are directly related.
19. About as many women smoke cigarettes as do men.
20. Fortunately, for those who now smoke, stopping is relatively easy.

Discussion

F Depending on the brand, some cigarettes contain less tar and nicotine; none is safe, however.

F Even a low level of smoking exposes the body to harmful substances in tobacco smoke.

T Some changes, however, cannot be reversed—particularly changes associated with emphysema.

T However, the protection is far from adequate.

T Many people, however, smoke low-tar, low-nicotine cigarettes in a manner that makes them just as dangerous as stronger cigarettes.

F Menthol simply makes cigarette smoke feel cooler. The smoke contains all of the harmful agents found in the smoke from regular cigarettes.

T Particularly lung cancer and cancers of the larynx, esophagus, oral cavity, and urinary bladder.

F Unfortunately, smokeless tobacco is no safer than the tobacco that is burned. The user of smokeless tobacco swallows much of what the smoker inhales.

F Approximately 10% of people who have lung cancer will live the 5 years required to meet the medical definition of "cured."

F Because of the toxic material in smoke, even its contact with the tissue of the oral cavity introduces a measure of risk in this form of cigarette use.

T The cough occurs in response to an inability to clear the airway of mucus as a result of changes in the cells that normally keep the air passages clear.

F Cigarette smoking is in fact the single most important risk factor in the development of cardiovascular disease.

F Children born to women who smoked during pregnancy show a variety of health impairments, including smaller birth size, premature birth, and more illnesses during the first year of life. Smoking women also have more stillbirths than nonsmokers.

T Women over 35 years of age, in particular, are at risk of experiencing serious heart disease should they continue using both cigarettes and an oral contraceptive.

F Although air pollution does expose the body to potentially serious problems, the risk is considerably less than that associated with smoking.

T Dependence, including true physical addiction, is widely recognized in cigarette smokers.

T There is a strong correlation between cigarette smoking of parents and the subsequent smoking of their children. Parents who do not want their children to smoke should not smoke.

T The higher one's level of education, the less likely one is to smoke.

T Although in the past, more men smoked than did women, the gap is narrowing.

F Unfortunately, relatively few smokers can quit. The best advice is never to begin smoking.

To Carry This Further . . .

Were you surprised at the number of items that you answered correctly? In what areas did you hold misconceptions regarding cigarette smoking? Do you think that most university students are as knowledgeable as you?

Where do you see the general public in terms of its understanding of cigarette smoking? How can the health care community do a better job in educating the public about tobacco use?

indicates that cigarette use has risen most dramatically among African-American students, increasing 80 percent during 1991–1997.[6] Those of this group who attend college could reverse the most health-enhancing pattern of tobacco use seen among any group of American students.

The Influence of Education

Despite the trend seen among today's students, a higher level of formal education completed is associated with a lower rate of smoking. Among those with less than twelve years of formal education, 37.5 percent smoked during 1995, whereas only 14 percent of those with sixteen or more years of education were cigarette smokers.[3] Clearly, education appears to assist people in understanding the risks of cigarette smoking. In contrast to the general population, where higher percentages of men than women smoke, college women are more likely to smoke than college men, perhaps because they wish to control their weight. Approximately 13.7 percent of college-educated women smoke, and 14.3 percent of college-educated men smoke.[3]

How much do you know about smoking? Find out by completing the Personal Assessment on page 264.

Cigarette Consumption and Preferences

The production of cigarettes in this country has fluctuated in the last two decades. In 1981 the annual production of cigarettes in the United States reached a peak of 744 billion. From that point, production declined each year through 1986, when only 658 billion were produced. Today production is again higher, with 747 billion cigarettes produced in 1995.[7] In terms of consumption patterns, however, the per capita consumption of cigarettes has declined from 4,287 cigarettes per person in 1966 to 3,000 per person in 1995.[7] Regardless of decreasing domestic use, the tobacco industry continues to enjoy strong sales, as noted in 1995, when $45.1 billion was spent for cigarettes.[7]

In recent years the type of cigarettes preferred by smokers has changed. Today only a small percentage of all smokers prefer the small unfiltered cigarettes that were popular before and just after World War II. Even the king-sized filtered cigarettes popular during the 1960s are losing popularity. Today low-tar and low-nicotine brands (15 mg of tar or less) and ultralow-tar and ultralow-nicotine brands (less than 4 mg of tar) have the major share of the total cigarette market. In regard to these cigarettes, however, it should be noted that documents from inside the tobacco industry indicate that tar levels may be understated because of the method of testing used by the Federal Trade Commission.[8]

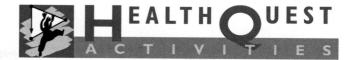

- Module 7 of HealthQuest allows you to assess your risk of disease caused by exposure to tobacco smoke. If you're a smoker, you can evaluate the reasons you may be ready to quit or cut back. If you have loved ones or friends who smoke, you will also benefit from this exercise. The feedback you'll receive in the personal risk section takes into account both direct and indirect exposure to tobacco smoke. Feedback about reasons for quitting is based on the relative importance of each reason to the smoker. For example, you might want to quit for health reasons, while a friend of yours might want to quit because smoking is inconvenient at work.

- The *Tobacco Ads and You* activity in Module 7 introduces you to the messages that tobacco advertisements send to consumers and the ways in which young people are manipulated to become smokers. This exploration activity helps you examine your beliefs and feelings about cigarette advertising by rating how each ad appeals to you. You can also participate in a survey about the messages the ads are trying to convey and your own use of tobacco products and promotional items.

Marketing of Tobacco Products

Shredded plant material, wrapped in paper or leaf, ignited with a flame, and then placed on or near the delicate tissues of the mouth . . . what other human behavior does this resemble? If you answered *None!* to this question, then you appreciate that smoking is unique, and, therefore, that it must be learned. How it is learned is currently a less than fully understood process that most likely requires a variety of stimuli ranging from modeling to actual experimentation. The role of advertising as a source of models has long been suspected and intensely debated. Today, as in the past, controversy surrounds the intent of the tobacco industry's advertising. Are the hedonistic commercials and familiar logos seen in a variety of media intended to challenge the brand loyalty of those who have already decided to smoke, as the industry claims? For example, the new emphasis on the "natural" menthol of Kool cigarettes is seen by some as racially targeted advertising. Mentholated cigarettes are popular among African-American consumers and, as mentioned above, young people in this group seem particularly interested in smoking. Or are they intended to entice new smokers, older children and young adolescents, in sufficient numbers to replace the 3,000 smokers who die each day from the consequences of tobacco use? This latter objective is now known, by admission of the tobacco industry, to have been pursued for decades. Its effectiveness has also been documented through

---

⭐ **Thanks, But No Cigar**

Ten million Americans smoke cigars, which is an increase of about two million since 1993. If cigar smoking appeals to you, as it does to many college students, consider the following facts from the American Lung Association:

- *Secondhand (sidestream) cigar smoke is more poisonous than secondhand cigarette smoke. The smoke from one cigar equals that of three cigarettes. Carbon monoxide emissions from one cigar are 30 times higher than for one cigarette.*

- *Cigar smoking can cause cancer of the larynx (voice box), mouth, esophagus, and lungs. Cancer death rates for cigar smokers are 34 percent higher than for nonsmokers.*

- *Ninety-nine percent of cigar smokers have atypical cells found in the larynx. These cells are the first step toward malignancy (cancer).*

- *Cigar smokers are three to five times more likely to die of lung cancer than nonsmokers.*

- *Cigar smokers have five times the risk of emphysema as nonsmokers.*

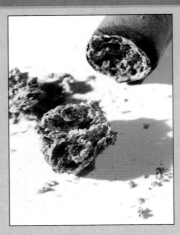

- *Nicotine does not have to be inhaled to damage the heart and blood vessels. It is absorbed into the bloodstream through the mucous membranes of the mouth. Nicotine increases the heart rate and constricts the blood vessels, which reduces blood flow to the heart.*

---

recent research.[9] The cartoon character Joe Camel has been an especially successful tool for enticing children and teens to begin smoking.

Over the years the tobacco industry has used all aspects of mass media advertising, including radio, television, print, billboards, and sponsorship of televised athletic events and concerts, to sell its products. In addition, it has often distributed free samples and sold merchandise bearing the company or product logo.

Today the tobacco industry has been denied access to television and radio, and it can no longer distribute free samples, but the industry continues to be active and innovative in other aspects of the media to which it has access. For example, Philip Morris has introduced an upscale lifestyle magazine called *Unlimited: Action, Adventure, Good Times,* to be provided free to over 1 million smokers. Interestingly, the magazine features articles about healthful activities that many longtime smokers would be unable to engage in because of the effects of smoking.

In addition to the magazine just described, the development of nonmarket brands of cigarettes for free distribution to patrons of bars and restaurants who are attempting to "bum" cigarettes represents a second form of "advertising." This "premarketing" introduction of a prototype brand technically does not violate the law regarding the distribution of samples. To date, several hundred establishments in several major cities have participated.

A final current example of the tobacco industry's subtle but effective presence in the mind of the public is that of tobacco use in motion pictures. In spite of a 1990 tobacco industry policy prohibiting

"brand placement" of tobacco products in films, cigarette and cigar smoking continue to be disproportionately represented in current films. Unfortunately, children and adolescents can easily identify with these characters (and their smoking), since they are generally depicted in a positive light.

Personal Applications

- The tobacco industry continues to contend that its advertising is intended only to challenge the brand loyalty of current smokers, not to attract new smokers. Which goal do you believe motivates the tobacco industry to spend hundreds of millions annually on advertising and promotion?

Pipe and Cigar Smoking

Many people believe that pipe or cigar smoking is a safe alternative to cigarette smoking. Unfortunately, this is not the case. All forms of tobacco present users with a series of health threats (see the Star Box above).

When compared with cigarette smokers, pipe and cigar smokers have cancer of the mouth, throat, larynx (voice box), and esophagus at the same frequency. Cigarette smokers are more likely than pipe and cigar smokers to have lung cancer, chronic obstructive lung disease (COLD), also called chronic obstructive pulmonary disease (COPD), and heart disease. However, the incidence of respiratory disease and heart disease in pipe and cigar smokers is greater than that among nonusers of tobacco.

In comparison to cigarette smokers, pipe and cigar smokers are considerably fewer in number. Interestingly, however, cigar smoking is enjoying a resurgence. In 1995 cigars generated sales of $1 billion, mainly to younger adults, including a very small but growing percentage of women, and the magazine *Cigar Aficionado,* an upscale publication devoted to cigar smoking, is enjoying rapid growth in readership.

Perhaps because of the increase in cigar smoking noted above, the National Cancer Institute commissioned the first extensive study of regular cigar smoking. That report confirmed and expanded upon the health risks identified in earlier smaller studies.[10] In addition, the FTC announced that cigar manufacturers must now disclose, in addition to expenditures, the tobacco content and additives in their products.[11] The use of smokeless tobacco, a third alternative to cigarette smoking, is discussed later in the chapter.

Tobacco Use and the Development of Dependence

Although not true for every tobacco user (see discussion of "chippers" later in this section), the vast majority of users, particularly cigarette smokers, will develop a dependency relationship with the nicotine contained in tobacco. This state of **dependence** causes users to consume greater quantities of nicotine over extended periods of time, further endangering their health.

Dependence can imply both a physical and psychological relationship. Particularly with cigarettes, *physical dependence* or *addiction*, with its associated *tolerance*, *withdrawal*, and **titration,** is strongly developed by 40 percent of all smokers. Most of the remaining population of smokers will experience lesser degrees of physical dependence. Psychological *dependence* or *habituation*, with its accompanying psychological components of *compulsion* and *indulgence*, is almost universally seen.

Compulsion is a strong emotional desire to continue tobacco use despite restrictions on smoking and the awareness of health risks. Very likely, users are "compelled" to engage in continual tobacco use in fear of the unpleasant physical, emotional, and social effects that result from discontinuing use. In comparison to compulsion, indulgence is seen as "rewarding" oneself for aligning with a particular behavior pattern—in this case, smoking. Indulgence is made possible by the existence of various reward systems built around the use of tobacco, including a perceived image, group affiliation, and even appetite suppression intended to foster weight control.

Much to the benefit of the tobacco industry, dependence on tobacco is easily established. Many experts believe that physical dependence on tobacco is far more easily established than is physical dependence on alcohol, cocaine (other than crack), or heroin. Of all people who experiment with cigarettes, 85 percent develop various aspects of a dependence relationship.

A small percentage of smokers, known as "chippers," can smoke on occasion without becoming dependent. Experts now believe that a defective gene increases the toxic effect of nicotine in these occasional smokers.[12] Because they "enjoy" the effects of smoking less, they smoke fewer cigarettes and smoke less frequently, thus reducing the likelihood of dependency. They may be truly "social smokers" in that they smoke with only a few selected friends or in a very limited number of places. Unfortunately, many inexperienced smokers feel that they too are only social smokers; however, a few additional months of this type of occasional smoking could be a transitional period into a dependence pattern of tobacco use.

Theories of Nicotine Addiction

The establishment and maintenance of physical dependence or addiction is less than fully understood. Most experts, however, believe that for a specific individual, addiction has a personal and multifaceted etiology, or cause. Accordingly, several theories have been proposed to explain the development of dependence. We will present a brief account of some of the more familiar theories. The more emotional aspects of dependence formation will be discussed later in the chapter.

Bolus Theory

In the **bolus theory** of nicotine addiction, each inhalation of smoke releases into the blood a concentrated quantity of nicotine (a ball or bolus) that reaches the brain and results in a period of neurohormonal excitement.[13] The smoker perceives this period of stimulation as pleasurable but, unfortunately, short lived. Accordingly, the smoker attempts to reestablish this pleasurable feeling by again inhaling and sending another bolus of nicotine on its way to the brain. The 70,000 or more inhalations during the first year of smoking serve to condition the novice smoker, resulting in a lifelong pattern of cigarette dependence. The level needed for arousal is different for each individual

---

dependence   a physical and/or psychological need to continue the use of a drug.

titration (tie **tray** shun)   the particular level of a drug within the body; adjusting the level of nicotine by adjusting the rate of smoking.

bolus theory   a theory of nicotine addiction based on the body's response to the bolus (ball) of nicotine delivered to the brain with each inhalation of cigarette smoke.

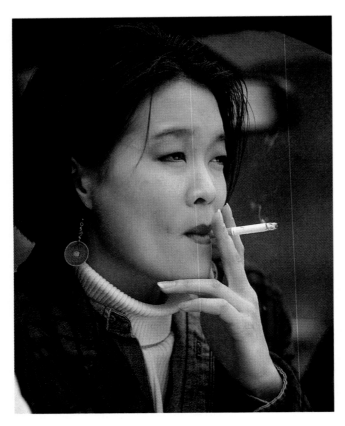

A smoker inhales about 70,000 times during the first year of smoking, resulting in a nicotine addiction that often lasts a lifetime.

smoker, depending on the length of addiction, the level of tolerance, inherited characteristics, and other factors.

Adrenocorticotropic Hormone (ACTH) Theory

A second theory of dependence suggests that nicotine stimulates the release of adrenocorticotropic hormone (ACTH) from the anterior pituitary, or "master gland" of the endocrine system (see Chapter 3). It has been shown that ACTH causes the release of **beta endorphins** (naturally occurring opiate-like chemicals) that produce mild feelings of euphoria. Perhaps this stresslike response mechanism involving ACTH may also account for the increased energy expenditure seen in smokers and thus their tendency to maintain a lower body weight than nonsmokers.

When these physiological responses are viewed collectively, nicotine may be seen as biochemically influencing brain activity by enhancing the extent and strength of various forms of "communication" between different brain areas[14] and even glands of the endocrine system. If this is the case, it is apparent why, once addicted, the functioning of the smoker's control systems is much altered in comparison with that of nonsmokers.

Self-Medication Theory

Yet another explanation, called self-medication, suggests that nicotine, through the effects of mood-enhancing dopamine, may allow smokers to "treat" feelings of tiredness and lack of motivation. In other words, a smoke lifts the spirits, if only briefly. Eventually, however, smokers become dependent on tobacco as a "medication" to make themselves feel better. Thus, because tobacco is a legal drug that is readily available, it becomes preferred to prescription medications and illegal drugs, such as cocaine and the stimulants, that elevate mood.

Regardless of the mechanism involved, as tolerance to nicotine develops, smoking behavior is adjusted to maintain titration and prevent the occurrence of withdrawal symptoms. At some point the desire for constant arousal is probably superseded by the smoker's desire not to experience withdrawal. Thus people smoke to protect themselves from the withdrawal effects rather than for the pleasure of being aroused.

The importance of nicotine as the primary factor in establishing dependence on tobacco is supported by research that demonstrates that smokers will not select a nontobacco cigarette if a tobacco cigarette is available. Even tobacco cigarettes with a very low level of nicotine seem to be unacceptable to most smokers, as do cigarettes with very low nicotine but with high tar content. Interestingly, users of low-nicotine cigarettes tend to inhale more frequently and deeply to obtain as much nicotine as possible.

Evidence that nicotine is addictive is so substantial that Liggett and Meyer (L & M) has placed the statement "Smoking is addictive" on packages of its cigarette brands. Chesterfield, Lark, Eve, and L & M generic brands now carry this additional warning.

Personal Applications

• What do your experience and observations tell you about the addictive potential of nicotine?

• To what extent would you support the control of tobacco by the FDA on the grounds that cigarettes are drug delivery systems?

Snuff and Chewing Tobacco as a Source of Nicotine

Although not burned, snuff and chewing tobacco deliver nicotine effectively through the mucous membranes of the mouth and nose. Cigar and pipe smoke, when not inhaled, manage to transmit some nicotine to the smoker, but in amounts considerably below those associated with cigarettes.

Acute Effects of Nicotine on Nervous System Function

In comparison with the more chronic effects of nicotine on the central nervous system (CNS) that eventually result in physical dependence or addiction, nicotine also produces changes of short duration. In the CNS, nicotine activates receptors within the brain. Stimulation of the brain is seen by changes in electroencephalogram (EEG) patterns, reflecting an increase in the frequency of electrical activity. This is part of a general arousal pattern signaled by the release of the neurotransmitters **norepinephrine**, dopamine, acetylcholine, and serotonin. Heavy use of tobacco products, resulting in high levels of nicotine in the bloodstream, eventually produces a blocking effect as more and more receptor sites are filled. The result is a generalized depression of the CNS. When blood levels of nicotine reach a critical point, the brain's vomiting center may be activated. This response is a built-in mechanism of protection against poisoning.

The level of plasma nicotine associated with normal levels of heavy smoking (one to two packs per day) would not likely produce the depressive effect just described. However, in chain smokers (four to eight packs per day), plasma nicotine levels would be sufficient to have a depressive influence on nervous system function. In fact, it has been suggested that chain smoking is driven by the fruitless effort to counter the depressive influence of chronically high levels of nicotine.

In carefully controlled studies involving both animals and humans, nicotine increased the ability of subjects to concentrate on a task. It must be noted, however, that the duration of this improvement was limited. Most would agree that this brief benefit is not enough to justify the health risks associated with chronic tobacco use.

Non-Nervous System Acute Effects of Nicotine

Outside the CNS, nicotine affects the transmission of nerve signals at the point where nerves innervate muscle tissue (called the *neuromuscular junction*) by mimicking the action of the neurotransmitter acetylcholine. Nicotine occupies receptor sites at the junction and prevents the transmission of nerve impulses from nerve cell to muscle cell. Because of its ability to act in this manner, nicotine has been used successfully as an insecticide in greenhouses.

Nicotine also causes the release of epinephrine from the adrenal medulla (see Chapter 3), which results in an increase in respiration rate, heart rate, blood pressure, and coronary blood flow. These changes are accompanied by the constriction of the blood vessels beneath the skin, a reduction in the motility in the bowel, loss of appetite, and changes in sleep patterns.

Although a lethal dose of nicotine could be obtained through the ingestion of a nicotine-containing insecticide, to "smoke oneself to death" in a single intense period of cigarette use would be highly improbable. In humans, 40 to 60 mg (.06–.09 mg/kg) is a lethal dose.[15] A typical cigarette supplies .05 to 2.5 mg of nicotine, and that nicotine is relatively quickly broken down for removal from the body.

Psychosocial Factors Related to Dependence

You will recall that a psychological aspect of dependence (habituation) exists and is important in maintaining the smoker's need for nicotine. Both research and general observation support many of the powerful influences this aspect of dependence possesses, especially for beginning smokers, prior to the onset of physical addiction. Consequently, in the remainder of this section, we will explore factors that may contribute to the development of this aspect of dependence.

Modeling

Because tobacco use is a learned behavior, it is reasonable to accept that modeling acts as a stimulus to experimental smoking. Modeling suggests that susceptible people smoke to emulate, or model their behavior after, smokers whom they admire or with whom they share other types of social or emotional bonds. Particularly for young adolescents (ages fourteen to seventeen), smoking behavior correlates with the smoking behavior of slightly older peers and very young adults (ages eighteen to twenty-two), older siblings, and to some degree, parents. Is it possible that the very young and attractive models used in tobacco (and beer) advertisements may be seen by young adolescents as being closer to their own age than they really are?

beta endorphins mood-enhancing, pain-reducing, opiatelike chemicals produced within the smoker's body in response to the presence of nicotine.

norepinephrine (nor epp in **eff** rin) an adrenaline-like chemical produced within the nervous system.

Modeling is particularly evident when smoking is a central factor in peer group formation and peer group association and can lead to a shared behavioral pattern that differentiates the group from others and from adults. Further, when risk-taking behavior and disregard for authority are common to the group, smoking becomes the behavioral pattern that most consistently identifies and bonds the group. Particularly for those young people who lack self-directedness or the ability to resist peer pressure, initial membership in a tobacco-using peer group may become inescapable.

In addition, when adolescents have lower levels of self-esteem and are searching for an avenue to improve self-image, a role model who smokes is often seen as tough, sociable, and sexually attractive. These three traits have been played up by the tobacco industry in their carefully crafted advertisements.

Manipulation

In addition to modeling as a psychosocial link with tobacco use, cigarette use may meet the beginning smoker's need to manipulate something and at the same time provide the manipulative "tool" necessary to offset boredom, feelings of depression, or social immaturity. Clearly the availability of affordable smoking paraphernalia provides smokers with ways to reward themselves. A new cigarette lighter, a status brand of tobacco, or a beach towel with a cigarette's logo are all reinforcements to some smokers. For others, the ability to take out a cigarette or fill a pipe adds a measure of structure and control to situations in which they might otherwise feel somewhat ill at ease. The cigarette becomes a readily available and dependable "friend" to turn to during stressful moments.

Personal Applications

• If you saw a person who appeared to be a minor being sold cigarettes, would you feel comfortable expressing your concerns to the merchant? Would you report the incident to the police or to the prosecutor's office?

Susceptibility to Advertising

The images of the smoker's world portrayed by the media can be particularly attractive. For adolescents, women, minorities, and other carefully targeted groups of adults, the tobacco industry has paired suggestions of a better life with the use of its products (see the Topics for Today article on p. 290). To these users and potential users, the self-reward of power, liberation, affluence, sophistication, or adult status is achieved by using the products that they are told are associated with these desired states. Thus the self-rewarding use of tobacco products becomes a means of achievement.

With this multiplicity of forces at work, it is possible to understand why so many who experiment with tobacco use find that they quickly become dependent on tobacco. Human needs, both physiological and psychosocial, are many and complex. Tobacco use meets the needs on a short-term basis, whereas dependence, once established, replaces these needs with a different, more immediate set of needs.

As part of the proposed agreement between the Liggett Group and the over forty states that brought suit for reimbursement of Medicaid funds, and as a point of discussion among other tobacco companies and the federal government, the use of humans in tobacco advertisements would be discontinued. These "humanless" advertisements are already being used. For example, in one ad a cigarette is shown assuming a human role—resting in a hammock, as if to suggest that the "good life" is still associated with tobacco products.[16]

In spite of the needs that are met by continuing to use tobacco, in a recent study approximately 68.2 percent of adult smokers have, on at least one occasion, expressed a desire to quit, but only 45.8 percent were actually able to quit, some for only a day.[3] It therefore seems apparent that tobacco use is a source of **dissonance**. This dissonance stems from the need to deal emotionally with a behavior that is enjoyable, dangerous, but known to be difficult to stop. The degree to which this dissonance exists and the extent to which it negates the effectiveness of tobacco use as a coping technique probably varies from user to user.

Preventing Teen Smoking

Even before the 1997 release of tobacco industry documents confirming the targeting of young adolescents, the federal government stated its intention to curb these cigarette advertisements. In August 1995 the FDA described the specific actions that it hoped it would be given authority to implement. Collectively, the restrictions described in the following list were intended to discourage cigarette smoking among America's teens, resulting in 50 percent fewer adolescents beginning smoking in the year 2002 than in 1995.[17]

1. Limit tobacco advertising in publications that appeal to teens and restrict billboards with tobacco-related content to no closer than 1,000 feet of schools and playgrounds. (An August 1995 study in California found that stores near schools displayed significantly more tobacco-related advertisements than those farther from schools.)
2. Restrict the use of logo and other tobacco-related images on nontobacco-related products, such as towels, T-shirts, and caps.

Learning
From Our Diversity

World No-Tobacco Day Seeks Support from Athletes and Artists

Sports and smoking seem to make strange bedfellows—but not in the world of advertising. For decades, cigarette manufacturers have worked hand-in-glove with professional athletes and teams, exchanging huge sums of money for endorsements of tobacco products or for the promotion and sponsorship of major sporting events. Although cigarette advertising has been banned from American television for nearly 30 years, the cozy connections continue, with perhaps the most notable example being the women's tennis tournament sponsored by Virginia Slims cigarettes (whose slogan, "You've come a long way, baby," resonated with women of a generation ago but is increasingly quoted in tones ranging from irony to contempt).

A step in the opposite direction is World No-Tobacco Day, promoted annually since 1988 by the World Health Organization (WHO), an autonomous unit of the United Nations whose headquarters are in Switzerland. On a designated day each year, WHO urges tobacco users to abstain for at least that day—and, ideally, for good. WHO says the annual observance of World No-Tobacco Day "is a unique opportunity to mobilize athletes, artists, and the media, as well as the public in general,

in support of the objective of promoting a society and a way of life where tobacco use is no longer an accepted norm."

In sponsoring World No-Tobacco Day, WHO has focused on smoking in public places, on public transportation, in the workplace, and in medical facilities. A recent campaign escalated the stop-smoking effort with a theme of "United Nations and Specialized Agencies Against Tobacco," with the aim of sharply reducing tobacco use worldwide by the end of the twentieth century.

As noted earlier, tobacco interests continue to promote many sporting events, as well as some cultural events. As far as sports are concerned, however, WHO officials see reason for encouragement in the recent smoke-free history of the Olympic Games. Beginning with the 1988 Winter Games in Calgary, all Olympic Games—both summer and winter—have been smoke-free.

While a major cigarette manufacturer congratulates its (female) customers on having "come a long way, baby," the World Health Organization is strongly conveying the message that you'll go a lot farther if you don't smoke.

Which tactic do you think is most likely to reduce the rate of tobacco use worldwide: legal bans and restrictions, campaigns of persuasion like World No-Tobacco Day, or a combination of these two approaches?

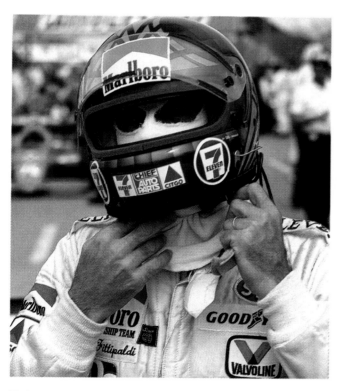

Tobacco company logos are seen by millions of viewers of televised sporting events.

3. Bar certain sources of access to tobacco products, such as mail order sales, the distribution of free samples, and vending machines.

4. Halt sponsorship of high-visibility events, such as auto racing and athletic contests in which brand names appear on highly televised surfaces, including hoods, fenders, uniforms, and arena sign boards. (It is estimated that the Marlboro logo is seen 5,933 times during the course of a 90-minute televised Winston Cup auto race.)

5. Require merchants to obtain proof of age when selling tobacco products to adolescents. (This particular component of the initial plan became law in 1997. Merchants are required to validate the age of people whom they suspect to be younger than twenty-seven years of age before selling cigarettes to those eighteen years of age and older. If found in violation, both the salesperson and the store owner will be fined $500.)

dissonance (dis´ son ince) a feeling of uncertainty that occurs when a person believes two equally attractive but opposite ideas.

By mid-1998 the federal government's desire to reduce youth smoking through implementation of the steps just described was mired in a larger package of tobacco-related policies being debated in Congress. This undertaking was related to the class action suit filed by all 50 states against the tobacco industry in an attempt to recoup Medicaid expenditures for treating tobacco-related illnesses. As Congress attempted to construct a settlement that would be acceptable to all parties, the impasse fragmented attempts to reduce youth smoking. Nonetheless, four states (Mississippi, Florida, Texas, and Minnesota) have settled with the tobacco industry. In each case the settlements were more favorable to these states than the collective settlement being debated in Washington; unfortunately, this outcome diluted some restrictions on tobacco advertisements, as well as the FDA's ability to reduce smoking by defining cigarettes as drug delivery systems.

As noted earlier in the chapter, the November 1998 settlement by 46 states in which the tobacco industry is to pay the states $206 billion restricts some forms of youth-oriented advertising and funds antismoking education, both of which may accomplish some of the changes initially proposed.

Early Childhood Intervention

Although significant concern centers on the onset of smoking behavior by adolescents in the eleven- to fourteen-year-old age group and later teen years, the decision to smoke (or use other forms of tobacco) may be made at a much earlier age. Accordingly, parents (and other adults) who do not want their children to smoke or use tobacco in other forms should begin educating their children as preschoolers and certainly by school age. The following recommendations, and many additional ones as well, can be found in *A Parent's Guide to Prevention*, available from the National Clearinghouse for Drug and Alcohol Information.[18]

When dealing with preschool children, it should be remembered that facts are unlikely to be comprehended. Accordingly, the following activities are suggested:

- Set aside regular time when you can give your child your full attention. Playing and reading together builds a strong parent-child bond.
- Point out poisonous and harmful substances that can be found in the home.
- Explain how medicines can be harmful if used incorrectly.
- Provide guidelines that teach the child what kind of behavior is expected.
- Encourage the child to follow instructions.
- Help the child learn decision-making skills; give positive feedback when appropriate decisions have been made.

For children in kindergarten through third grade, new skills and insights need to be developed to deal with drugs, including tobacco products. Adults should attempt to:

- Help the child recognize and understand family rules.
- Discuss how television advertisements try to persuade people to buy their products.
- Practice ways in which the child can say no to other people.
- Develop a "helper" file made up of the names and phone numbers of people the child can turn to when confronted by others who want them to try smoking or smokeless tobacco.

As children approach the preteen years, more focused presentations can be made regarding the dangers associated with smoking and the use of other substances. Adults working with children in grades four through six should focus on the following activities:

- Create special times when an adult is available to talk with the child about whatever he or she wants to talk about.
- Encourage participation in a variety of activities that are both fun and allow the child to meet new friends.
- Teach the child how drugs, including tobacco products, are promoted and how their messages can be "defused."
- Continue to assist the child in learning how to say no.
- Become acquainted with the parents of the child's friends so that you will be able to work with them in support of antismoking activities in the community.
- Participate in providing support for supervised activities for children of this age.

Although nothing is certain regarding the decision that older preadolescents or teens make about beginning to smoke, the activities just listed may be effective in countering the influences of the peer group and the mass media.

Tobacco: The Source of Physiologically Active Compounds

When burned, the tobacco in cigarettes, cigars, and pipe mixtures is the source of an array of physiologically active chemicals, many of which are closely linked to significant changes in normal body structure and function. At the burning tip of the cigarette, the

900° C (1,652° F) heat oxidizes tobacco (as well as paper, wrapper, filter, and additives). With each puff of smoke, the body is exposed to more than 4,000 chemical compounds, hundreds of which are known to be physiologically active, toxic, and carcinogenic (cancer causing). An annual 70,000 puffs taken in by the one-pack-a-day cigarette smoker results in an environment that makes the most polluted urban environment seem clean by comparison.

Particulate Phase

Cigarette, cigar, and pipe smoke can be described on the basis of two phases. These phases include a particulate phase and a gaseous phase. The **particulate phase** includes **nicotine**, water, and a variety of powerful chemicals known collectively as tar. **Tar** includes phenol, cresol, pyrene, DDT, and a benzene-ring group of compounds that includes benzo[a]pyrene. Most of the carcinogenic compounds are found within the tar. A person who smokes one pack of cigarettes per day will collect four ounces of tar in his or her lungs in a year. Only the gases and the smallest particles reach the small sacs of the lungs, called the *alveoli*, where oxygen exchange occurs. The carcinogen-rich particles from the particulate phase are deposited somewhere along the air passage leading to the lungs.

Gaseous Phase

The **gaseous phase** of tobacco smoke, like the particulate phase, is composed of a variety of physiologically active compounds, including carbon monoxide, carbon dioxide, ammonia, hydrogen cyanide, isopyrene, acetaldehyde, and acetone. At least forty-three of these compounds have been determined to be **carcinogens**, thus capable of stimulating the development of cancer. Carbon monoxide is, however, the most damaging compound found in this component of tobacco smoke. Its impact is discussed next.

Carbon Monoxide

Like every inefficient engine, a cigarette, cigar, or pipe burns (oxidizes) its fuel with less than complete conversion into carbon dioxide, water, and heat. As a result of this incomplete oxidation, burning tobacco forms **carbon monoxide** (CO) gas. Carbon monoxide is one of the most harmful components of tobacco smoke.

Carbon monoxide is a colorless, odorless, tasteless gas that possesses a very strong physiological attraction for hemoglobin, the oxygen-carrying pigment on each red blood cell. When CO is inhaled, it quickly bonds with hemoglobin and forms a new compound, carboxyhemoglobin. In this form, hemoglobin is unable to transport oxygen to the tissues and cells where it is needed.

Although it is true that normal body metabolism always keeps an irreducible minimum of CO in our blood (0.5% to 1%), the blood of smokers may have levels of 5 percent to 10 percent CO saturation.[19] We are exposed to additional CO from environmental sources such as automobiles and buses and other combustion of fossil fuels. By combining a smoker's CO with environmental CO, it is little wonder that smokers more easily become out of breath than nonsmokers. The half-life of CO combined with hemoglobin is approximately four to six hours.[20] Most smokers replenish their level of CO saturation at far shorter intervals than this.

As mentioned, the presence of excessive levels of carboxyhemoglobin in the blood of smokers leads to shortness of breath and lowered endurance. Because an adequate oxygen supply to all body tissues is critical for normal functioning, any oxygen reduction can have a serious impact on health. Brain function may be reduced, reactions and judgment are dulled, and of course, cardiovascular function is impaired. Fetuses are especially at risk for this oxygen deprivation (hypoxia) because fetal development is so critically dependent on a sufficient oxygen supply from the mother.

Illness, Premature Death, and Tobacco Use

For people who begin tobacco use as adolescents or young adults, smoke heavily, and continue to smoke, the likelihood of premature death is virtually ensured. Two-pack-a-day cigarette smokers can expect to die seven to eight years earlier than their nonsmoking counterparts. (Only nonsmoking-related deaths that can afflict smokers and nonsmokers alike keep the difference at this level rather than much higher.) Not

---

particulate phase portion of the tobacco smoke composed of small suspended particles.

nicotine physiologically active, dependence-producing drug found in tobacco.

tar a chemically rich, syrupy, blackish-brown material obtained from the particulate matter within cigarette smoke when nicotine and water are removed.

gaseous phase portion of the tobacco smoke containing carbon monoxide and many other physiologically active gaseous compounds.

carcinogens environmental agents, including chemical compounds within cigarette smoke, that stimulate the development of cancerous changes within cells.

carbon monoxide (CO) chemical compound that can "inactivate" red blood cells.

Table 9-1 Selected Established and Suspected Health Effects of Cigarette Smoking

Category of Condition	Established and Suspected Effects	Category of Condition	Established and Suspected Effects
1 Lung Disease	lung cancer, chronic obstructive lung disease; increased severity of asthma; increased risk of developing various respiratory infections	10 Complications in Obstetrics and Gynecology	infertility; miscarriage; fetal growth retardation; prematurity; stillbirth; transmission of HIV to the fetus from the infected biological mother; birth defects; intellectual impairment of offspring; sudden infant death syndrome; earlier menopause
2 Cancer Risk	esophageal, laryngeal, oral, bladder, kidney, stomach, pancreatic, vulvar, cervical, and colorectal cancers	11 Male Infertility and Sexuality Dysfunctions	decreased sperm motility; decreased sperm density; impotence
3 Heart Disease	coronary heart disease; angina pectoris; heart attack; repeat heart attack; arrhythmia; aortic aneurysm; cardiomyopathy	12 Neurological Disorders	transient ischemic attack; stroke; worsened multiple sclerosis
4 Peripheral Vascular Disease	pain and discomfort in the legs and feet resulting from restricted blood flow into the extremities	13 Brain and Behavior	depression
		14 Abnormialities of the Ears, Nose, and Throat	snoring and hearing loss
5 Skin Changes	wrinkling; fingernail discoloration; psoriasis; palmoplantar pustulosis	15 Eyes	cataracts; complications from Graves' disease; macular degeneration; optic neuropathy
6 Surgical Risk	need for more anesthesia; increased risk of postsurgical respiratory infection; increased need for supplemental oxygen following surgery; delayed wound healing	16 Oral Health	periodontal disease
		17 Endocrine System	increased metabolic rate; blood-sugar abnormalities; increased waist-to-hip ratio; redistribution of body fat
7 Orthopedic Problems	disc degeneration; less successful back surgery; musculoskeletal injury; delayed fracture healing	18 Gastrointestinal Diseases	stomach and duodenal ulcers; Crohn's disease
		19 Immune System	impaired humoral and cell-mediated immunity
8 Rheumatologic Conditions	osteoporosis and osteoarthritis	20 Emergency Medicine	injuries from fires; occupational injuries
9 Environmental Tobacco Smoke and Pediatric Illnesses	infections of the lower respiratory tract; more severe asthma; middle ear infections; Crohn's disease and ulcerative colitis; sudden infant death syndrome; impaired delivery of oxygen to body tissues		

only will these people die sooner, but they will also probably be plagued with painful, debilitating illnesses for an extended time. Smoking is responsible for nearly 420,000 premature deaths each year.[4] An overview of illnesses known to be caused or worsened by tobacco use is presented above in Table 9-1.[21]

Personal Applications

• Table 9-1 lists twenty categories of health conditions closely associated with tobacco use, several of which are very serious and can even cause premature death. In light of this evidence, why do you believe that smokers somehow see themselves as being safe from developing one or more of these conditions?

Cardiovascular Disease

Cardiovascular disease is the leading cause of death among all adults, accounting for 960,000 deaths in the United States in 1996.[22] Tobacco use, and cigarette smoking in particular, is clearly one of the major factors contributing to this cause of death. Although overall progress is being made in reducing the incidence of cardiovascular-related deaths, tobacco use impedes these efforts. So important is tobacco use as a contributing factor in deaths from cardiovascular disease that the cigarette smoker more than doubles the risk of experiencing a **myocardial infarction,** the leading cause of death from cardiovascular disease. Smokers also increase their risk of **sudden cardiac death** by two to four times.[22] Fully one-third of all cardiovascular disease can be traced to cigarette smoking.

The relationship between tobacco use and cardiovascular disease is centered on two major components of tobacco smoke: nicotine and carbon monoxide.

Nicotine and Cardiovascular Disease

The influence of nicotine on the cardiovascular system occurs when it stimulates the nervous system to release norepinephrine. This powerful stimulant increases the heart rate. In turn, an elevated heart rate increases cardiac output, thus increasing blood pressure. The extent to which this is dangerous depends in part on the coronary circulation's ability to supply blood to the rapidly contracting heart muscle. The development of **angina pectoris** and the possibility of sudden heart attack are heightened by this sustained elevation of heart rate, particularly in those individuals with existing coronary artery disease (see Chapter 10).

Nicotine is also a powerful vasoconstrictor of the peripheral blood vessels. As these vessels are constricted by the influence of nicotine, the pressure against their walls increases. Recent research shows that irreversible atherosclerotic damage to major arteries also occurs with smoking.

Nicotine also increases blood **platelet adhesiveness.**[23] As the platelets become more and more likely to "clump," a person will be more likely to develop a blood clot. In people already prone to cardiovascular disease, more rapidly clotting blood is an unwelcome liability. Heart attacks occur when clots form within the coronary arteries or are transported to the heart from other areas of the body.

In addition to other influences on the cardiovascular system, nicotine possesses the ability to decrease the proportion of high-density lipoproteins (HDLs) and to increase the proportion of low-density lipoproteins (LDLs) and very-low-density lipoproteins that constitute the body's serum cholesterol. Low-density lipoproteins appear to support the development of atherosclerosis and are clearly increased in the bloodstreams of smokers. (See Chapter 10 for further information about cholesterol's role in cardiovascular disease.)

Carbon Monoxide and Cardiovascular Disease

A second substance contributed by tobacco influences the type and extent of cardiovascular disease found among tobacco users. Carbon monoxide interferes with oxygen transport within the circulatory system.

As described earlier in the chapter, carbon monoxide is a component of the gaseous phase of tobacco smoke and readily joins with the hemoglobin of the red blood cells. Carbon monoxide has an affinity for hemoglobin 206 times that of oxygen. Once the hemoglobin of a red cell has accepted carbon monoxide molecules, the hemoglobin is transformed into carboxyhemoglobin. Thereafter, the carboxyhemoglobin permanently weakens the red blood cell's ability to transport oxygen. These red blood cells remain relatively useless during the remainder of their 120-day lives. Levels of carboxyhemoglobin in heavy smokers are associated with significant increases in the incidence of myocardial infarction.

When a person has impaired oxygen-transporting abilities, physical exertion becomes increasingly demanding on both the heart and the lungs. The cardiovascular system will attempt to respond to the body's demand for oxygen, but these responses are themselves impaired as a result of the influence of nicotine on the cardiovascular system. If tobacco does create the good life, as advertisers claim, it also unfortunately lessens the ability to participate actively in that life.

Cancer

Over the past forty-five years, research from the most reputable institutions in this country and abroad has consistently concluded that tobacco use is a significant factor in the development of virtually all forms of cancer and the most significant factor in cancers involving the respiratory system.

In describing cancer development, the currently used reference is twenty pack-years, or an amount of smoking equal to smoking one pack of cigarettes a

---

myocardial infarction heart attack; the death of heart muscle as a result of a blockage in one of the coronary arteries.

sudden cardiac death immediate death resulting from a sudden change in the rhythm of the heart.

angina pectoris (an jie nuh **peck** tor is) chest pain that results from impaired blood supply to the heart muscle.

platelet adhesiveness tendency of platelets to clump together, thus enhancing the speed at which the blood clots.

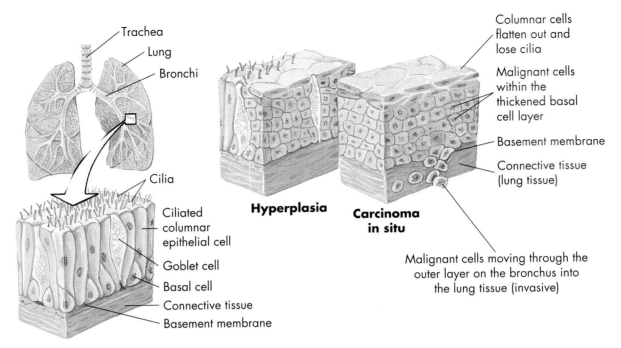

Figure 9-1   Histologic changes associated with bronchogenic carcinoma (lung cancer).

day for twenty years. Thus the two-pack-a-day smoker can anticipate cancer development in as few as ten years, while the half-pack-a-day smoker may have forty years to wait. Regardless, the opportunity is there for all smokers to confirm these data by developing cancer as predicted. It is hoped that most people will think twice before disregarding this evidence.

Data supplied by the American Cancer Society (ACS) indicate that during 1998 an estimated 1,228,600 Americans developed cancer.* These cases were nearly equally divided between the sexes and resulted in approximately 534,310 deaths.[24] In the opinion of the ACS, 30 percent of all cancer cases are heavily influenced by tobacco use.[1] Lung cancer alone accounted for about 171,500 of the new cancer cases and 160,100 deaths in 1998.[24] Fully 87 percent of men with lung cancer were cigarette smokers.[1] Recently a genetic "missing link" between smoking and lung cancer was established, when mutations to an important tumor suppressor gene were identified. If it was necessary to have a final "proof" that smoking causes lung cancer, that proof now appears to be in hand.[25]

Cancer of the entire respiratory system, including lung cancer and cancers of the mouth and throat, accounted for about 218,200 new cases of cancer and 173,600 deaths.[24] Despite these high figures, not all smokers develop cancer.

*Excluding cases of nonmelanoma skin cancer.

Respiratory Tract Cancer

Recall that tobacco smoke produces both a gaseous and a particulate phase. As noted, the particulate phase contains the tar fragment of tobacco smoke. This rich chemical environment contains more than 4,000 known chemical compounds, hundreds of which are known to be carcinogens.

In the normally functioning respiratory system, particulate matter suspended in the inhaled air settles on the tissues lining the airways and is trapped in **mucus** produced by specialized *goblet cells*. This mucus, with its trapped impurities, is continuously swept upward by the beating action of hairlike **cilia** of the ciliated columnar epithelial cells lining the air passages (Figure 9-1). On reaching the throat, this mucus is swallowed and eventually removed through the digestive system.

When tobacco smoke is drawn into the respiratory system, however, its rapidly dropping temperature allows the particulate matter to accumulate. This brown, sticky tar contains compounds known to harm the ciliated cells, goblet cells, and the basal cells of the respiratory lining. As the damage from smoking increases, the cilia become less effective in sweeping mucus upward to the throat. When cilia can no longer clean the airway, tar accumulates on the surfaces and brings carcinogenic compounds into direct contact with the tissues of the airway.

At the same time that the sweeping action of the lining cells is being slowed, substances in the tar are stimulating the goblet cells to increase the amount of

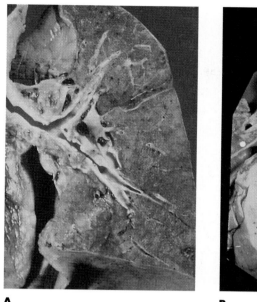 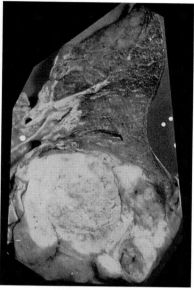

A　　　　**B**

Figure 9-2 **A,** Normal lung. **B,** Cancerous lung.

mucus they normally produce. The "smoker's cough" is the body's attempt to remove this excess mucus.

With prolonged exposure to the carcinogenic materials in tar, predictable changes will begin to occur within the respiratory system's basal cell layer (Figure 9-1). The basal cells begin to display changes characteristic of all cancer cells. In addition, an abnormal accumulation of cells occurs. When a person stops smoking, these cells do not repair themselves as quickly as once thought.[26]

By the time lung cancer is usually diagnosed, its development is so advanced that the chance for recovery is very poor. Still today, only 14 percent of all lung cancer victims survive for five years or more after diagnosis.[1] Most die in a very uncomfortable, painful way (Figure 9-2).

Cancerous activity in other areas of the respiratory system, including the larynx, and within the oral cavity (mouth) follows a similar course. In the case of oral cavity cancer, carcinogens found within the smoke and within the saliva are involved in the cancerous changes. Tobacco users, such as pipe smokers, cigar smokers, and users of smokeless tobacco, have a very high rate of cancer of the mouth, tongue, and voice box.

In addition to drawing smoke into the lungs, tobacco users swallow saliva that contains an array of chemical compounds from tobacco. As this saliva is swallowed, carcinogens are absorbed into the circulatory system and transported to all areas of the body. The filtering of the blood by the liver, kidneys, and bladder may account for the higher-than-normal levels of cancer in these organs among smokers.

As reported earlier in the chapter, newly released documents from within the tobacco industry clearly show that the major tobacco companies were aware of tobacco's role in the development of cancer and had made a concerted effort to deprive the American public access to such knowledge.

Chronic Obstructive Lung Disease

Chronic obstructive lung disease (COLD), also known as chronic obstructive pulmonary disease (COPD), is a chronic disorder in which the amount of air that flows in and out of the lungs becomes progressively limited. COLD is a disease state that is made up of two separate but related diseases: **chronic bronchitis** and **pulmonary emphysema.**

With chronic bronchitis, excess mucus is produced in response to the effects of smoking on airway tissue, and the walls of the bronchi become inflamed and infected. This produces a characteristic narrowing of the air passages. Breathing becomes difficult,

mucus　clear, sticky material produced by specialized cells within the mucous membranes of the body; mucus traps much of the suspended particulate matter within tobacco smoke.

cilia (sill ee uh)　small, hairlike structures that extend from cells that line the air passages.

chronic bronchitis　persistent inflammation and infection of the smaller airways within the lungs.

pulmonary emphysema　an irreversible disease process in which the alveoli are destroyed.

and activity can be severely restricted. With cessation of smoking, chronic bronchitis is reversible.[27]

Emphysema causes irreversible damage to the tiny air sacs of the lungs, the **alveoli**. Chest pressure builds when air becomes trapped by narrowed air passages (chronic bronchitis) and the thin-walled sacs rupture. Emphysema patients lose the ability to ventilate fully. They feel as though they are suffocating. You may have seen people with this condition in malls and other locations as they walk slowly by, carrying or pulling their portable oxygen tanks.

More than 10 million Americans suffer from COLD. It is responsible for a greater limitation of physical activity than any other disease, including heart disease.[27] COLD patients tend to die a very unpleasant, prolonged death, often from a general collapse of normal cardiorespiratory function that results in congestive heart failure (see Chapter 10).

Additional Health Concerns

In addition to the serious health problems stemming from tobacco use already described, other health-related changes are routinely seen. These include a generally poor state of nutrition, the gradual loss of the sense of smell, and premature wrinkling of the skin. Tobacco users are also more likely to experience strokes (a potentially fatal condition), lose bone mass leading to osteoporosis, experience more back pain and muscle injury, and find that fractures heal more slowly. Further, smokers who have surgery spend more time in the recovery room. Although not perceived as a health problem by people who continue smoking in order to control weight, smoking does appear to minimize weight gain. In studies using identical twins, twins who smoked were six to eight pounds lighter than their nonsmoking siblings.[28] Current thought about why smoking results in lower body weight is centered on two areas: an increase in BMR brought about by the influence of nicotine on sympathetic nervous system function (see Chapter 3) and a "reprogramming" of the set point (see Chapter 6) in the direction of lower body weight.[21]

Smoking and Reproduction

In all of its dimensions, the reproductive process is impaired by the use of tobacco, particularly cigarette smoking. Problems can be found in association with infertility, problem pregnancy, breastfeeding, and the health of the newborn. So broadly based are reproductive problems and smoking that the term *fetal tobacco syndrome* or *fetal smoking syndrome* is regularly used in clinical medicine. Some physicians even de-

fine a fetus being carried by a smoker as a "smoker" and, upon birth, as a "former smoker."

Infertility

Recent research indicates that cigarette smoking by both men and women can reduce levels of fertility. Among men, smoking adversely affects blood flow to erectile tissue, sperm motility and sperm shape, and causes an overall decrease in the number of viable sperm. Among women, the effects of smoking are seen in terms of abnormal ovum formation, including a lessened ability on the part of the egg to prevent polyspermia, or the fertilization by multiple sperm.[21] Smoking also negatively influences estrogen levels, resulting in underdevelopment of the uterine wall and ineffective implantation of the fertilized ovum. Lower levels of estrogen may also influence the rate of transit of the fertilized egg through the fallopian tube, making it arrive in the uterus too early for successful implantation or, in some cases, restricting movement to the point that an *ectopic*, or *tubal*, pregnancy may develop. Also, the early onset of menopause is associated with smoking.[21]

Problem Pregnancy

The harmful effects of tobacco smoke on the course of pregnancy are principally the result of the carbon monoxide and nicotine to which the mother and her fetus are exposed. Carbon monoxide from the incomplete oxidation of tobacco is carried in the maternal blood to the placenta, where it diffuses across the placental barrier and enters the fetal circulation. Once in the fetal blood, the carbon monoxide bonds with the fetal hemoglobin to form fetal carboxyhemoglobin. As a result of this exposure to carbon monoxide, the fetus is progressively deprived of normal oxygen transport and eventually becomes compromised by chronic **hypoxia.**

Nicotine also exerts its influence on the developing fetus. Thermographs of the placenta and fetus show signs of marked vasoconstriction within a few seconds after inhalation by the mother. This constriction further reduces the oxygen supply, resulting in hypoxia, an abnormally low level of oxygen in the blood. In addition, nicotine stimulates the mother's stress response, placing the mother and fetus under the potentially harmful influence of elevated epinephrine and corticoid levels (see Chapter 3). Any fetus exposed to all of these agents is more likely to be miscarried, stillborn, or born prematurely.[21] Even when carried to term, children born to mothers who smoked during pregnancy have lower birth weights and may show other signs of a stressful intrauterine life.

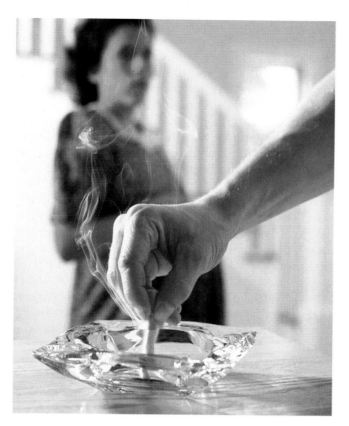

Pregnant women and those around them should refrain from smoking to protect the health of the developing fetus.

Personal Applications

• To what extent do you believe that a woman who is attempting to become pregnant or is pregnant is responsible for neglect of her child if she is a smoker at the time? Should this responsibility be applied to a smoking spouse or other person with whom the pregnant woman has regular contact?

Breastfeeding

For women who decide to breastfeed their infants, smoking during this period will continue to expose their children to the harmful effects of tobacco smoke. It is well recognized that nicotine appears in breast milk and thus is capable of exerting its vasoconstricting and stress-response influences on nursing infants. Mothers who stop smoking during pregnancy should be encouraged to continue to refrain from smoking while they are breastfeeding.

Neonatal Health Problems

Babies born to women who smoked during pregnancy will, on average, be shorter and have a lower birth weight than children born to nonsmoking mothers. During the earliest months of life, babies born to mothers who smoke experience an elevated rate of death caused by sudden infant death syndrome.[29] Statistics also show that infants are more likely to develop chronic respiratory problems, be hospitalized, and have poorer overall health during their early years of life. These problems are compounded when the children are exposed to involuntary smoking (see p. 281) in the household environment. Recent studies, in fact, suggest that the harmful effect of passive smoke exposure may approach that seen when the biological mother smoked during pregnancy.[30]

Parenting, in the sense of assuming responsibility for the well-being of children, does not begin at birth, but during the prenatal period. In the case of smoking, this is especially true. Pregnant women who continue smoking are disregarding the well-being of the children they are carrying. Other family members, friends, and coworkers who subject pregnant women to cigarette, pipe, or cigar smoke are, in a sense, exhibiting their own disregard for the health of the next generation.

Oral Contraceptives and Tobacco Use

Women who smoke and use oral contraceptives, particularly after age 35, are placing themselves at a much greater risk of experiencing a fatal cardiovascular accident (heart attack, stroke, or **embolism**) than oral contraceptive users who do not smoke. This risk of cardiovascular complications increases further for oral contraceptive users twenty-five years of age or older. Women who both smoke and use oral contraceptives are four times more likely to die from myocardial infarction (heart attack) than women who only smoke.[31] Because of this adverse relationship, *it is strongly recommended that women who smoke should not use oral contraceptives.*

---

alveoli (al vee oh lie) thin, saclike terminal ends of the airways; the site at which gases are exchanged between the blood and inhaled air.

hypoxia oxygenation deprivation at the cellular level.

embolism a potentially fatal condition in which a circulating blood clot lodges in a smaller vessel.

Combining Tobacco and Alcohol Use

Although there are exceptions to every generalization, it is very common to see tobacco and alcohol being used by the same people, often at the same time. Younger people who use both tobacco and alcohol are also more likely to use additional drugs. Accordingly, both tobacco and alcohol are considered *gateway drugs* because they are often introductory drugs that "open the door" for a more broadly based polydrug use pattern (see Chapter 7).

Beyond the potential for polydrug use initiated by the use of tobacco and alcohol is the simple reality that the use of both tobacco products and alcoholic beverages is associated with a wide array of illnesses and with premature death. As you have seen in this chapter and in Chapter 8 regarding alcohol use, the negative health impact of using both is significant. When use is combined, of course, the risks of living less healthfully and dying prematurely are accentuated.

Smokeless Tobacco Use

What do Red Man, Skoal, and Copenhagen have in common? They have all served to introduce nearly 16 percent of male high school seniors (1997) to a bit of the past—the use of smokeless tobacco.

Thanks to the resurgence of smokeless tobacco use, no longer are professional baseball players the only Americans to know the value of an empty coffee can or soft drink cup. These discarded containers are becoming standard equipment for people who dip and chew smokeless tobacco.

As the term implies, smokeless tobacco is not burned; rather, it is placed into the mouth. Once in place, the physiologically active nicotine and other soluble compounds are absorbed through the mucous membranes and into the blood. Within a few minutes, chewing tobacco and snuff generate blood levels of nicotine in amounts equivalent to those seen in cigarette smokers.

Chewing tobacco is taken from its foil pouch, formed into a small ball (called a "wad," "chaw," or "chew"), and placed into the mouth. Once in place, the bolus of tobacco is sucked and occasionally chewed, but not swallowed.

Snuff, a more finely shredded smokeless tobacco product, is marketed in small round cans. Snuff is formed into a small mass (or "quid") for dipping. The quid is placed between the jaw and the cheek; the user sucks the quid, then spits out the brown liquid. Snuff, as once used, was actually a powdered form of tobacco that was inhaled through the nose.

Although smokeless tobacco would seem to free the tobacco user from many of the risks associated with smoking, chewing and dipping are not without their own substantial risks. The presence of *leukoplakia* (white spots) and *erythroplakia* (red spots) on the tissues of the mouth indicate precancerous changes. In addition, an increase in **periodontal disease** (with the pulling away of the gums from the teeth, resulting in later tooth loss), the abrasive damage to the enamel of the teeth, and the high concentration of sugar in processed tobacco all contribute to health problems among users of smokeless tobacco. In those who develop oral cancer, the risk is dramatically heightened if the cancer metastasizes from the site of origin in the mouth to the brain. Clearly, it is important that users be aware of any signs of damage being done by their use of smokeless tobacco (see the Health Action Guide below). The validity of this warning was made clear in 1998 when 59 percent of smokeless tobacco-using major league players were found to have tobacco-related lesions when oral examinations were performed by team physicians on the first day of spring training.[32]

In addition to the damage done to the tissues of the mouth, the need to process the inadvertently swallowed saliva that contains dissolved carcinogens places both the digestive and urinary systems at risk of cancer.

In the opinion of health experts, the use of smokeless tobacco and its potential for life-threatening disease is presently at the place cigarette smoking was forty years ago. Consequently, television advertisements have been banned, and the following warnings have been placed in rotation on all smokeless tobacco products:

WARNING: THIS PRODUCT MAY CAUSE MOUTH CANCER
WARNING: THIS PRODUCT MAY CAUSE GUM DISEASE AND TOOTH LOSS
WARNING: THIS PRODUCT IS NOT A SAFE ALTERNATIVE TO CIGARETTE SMOKING

HEALTH ACTION GUIDE

Smokeless Tobacco Use

If you use smokeless tobacco, you are at risk for serious health problems. If you have any of the following signs, see your dentist or physician immediately:

- Lumps in the jaw or neck area
- Color changes or lumps inside the lips
- A red spot or sore on the lips or gums or inside the mouth that does not heal in two weeks
- Repeated bleeding in the mouth
- Difficulty or abnormality in speaking or swallowing

InfoLinks
www.kidsource.com/index.html

Clearly, smokeless tobacco is a dangerous product, and little doubt exists that continued use of tobacco in this form is a serious problem to health in all of its dimensions.

The Risks of Involuntary (Passive) Smoking

The smoke generated by the burning of tobacco can be classified as either **mainstream smoke** (the smoke inhaled and then exhaled by the smoker) or **sidestream smoke** (the smoke that comes from the burning end of the cigarette, pipe, or cigar that simply disperses into the air without being inhaled by the smoker). When either form of tobacco smoke is diluted and stays within a common source of air, it can eventually be referred to as **environmental tobacco smoke.** All three forms of tobacco smoke lead to involuntary or passive smoking and can present health problems for both nonsmokers and smokers.

Surprisingly, mainstream smoke makes up only 15 percent of our exposure to the harmful substances associated with involuntary smoking. Sidestream smoke is responsible for 85 percent of the harmful substances associated with secondhand smoke exposure. Because it is not filtered by the tobacco, the filter, or the smoker's body, sidestream smoke contains more free nicotine and produces higher yields of carbon dioxide and carbon monoxide. Much to the detriment of nonsmokers, sidestream smoke has a much higher quantity of highly carcinogenic compounds, called *N-nitrosamines*, than mainstream smoke has.

Current scientific opinion suggests that smokers and nonsmokers are exposed to very much the same smoke when tobacco is used within a common airspace. The important difference is the quantity of smoke inhaled by smokers and nonsmokers. It is likely that for each pack of cigarettes smoked by a smoker, nonsmokers who must share a common air supply with the smokers will involuntarily smoke the equivalent of three to five cigarettes per day. Even today, because of the small size of the particles produced by burning tobacco, environmental tobacco smoke cannot be completely removed from a workplace, restaurant, or shopping mall by the most effective ventilation system.

Recently reported research indicates that involuntary smoke exposure may be responsible for 10,000 to 20,000 premature deaths per year among nonsmokers in the United States (other estimates range upward to 53,000 premature deaths).[33] In addition, large numbers of people exposed to involuntary smoke develop eye irritation, nasal symptoms, headaches, and a cough. Furthermore, most nonsmokers dislike the odor of tobacco smoke.

For these reasons, state, local, and private-sector initiatives to restrict smoking have been introduced. Most buildings in which people work, study, play, reside, eat, or shop now have some smoking restrictions. Some have complete smoking bans. Nowhere is smoking more noticeably prohibited than in the U.S. airline industry. Currently, smoking is banned on all domestic plane flights of less than six hours, and on most American Airlines has extended the ban on smoking to selected international flights as well.

Involuntary smoking poses major threats to nonsmokers within residential settings. Spouses and children of smokers are at greatest risk for involuntary smoking. Scientific studies suggest that nonsmokers married to smokers are three times more likely to experience heart attacks than nonsmoking spouses of nonsmokers, and they have a 30 percent greater risk of lung cancer than nonsmoking spouses of nonsmokers.

The children of parents who smoke are twice as likely as children of nonsmoking parents to experience bronchitis or pneumonia during the first year of life. In addition, throughout childhood these children will experience more wheezing, coughing, and sputum production than children whose parents do not smoke. Otitis media (middle ear infection), one of the most frequently seen conditions in pediatric medicine, is also significantly more common in children under age three who reside with one or more adults who smoke.[34]

In July 1998, the tobacco industry challenged in court the salient 1993 EPA report that was the basis for restricting smoking in a wide array of public places and work sites. The federal judge who heard the case concluded that the principal study used in the report was flawed in its methodology and that its conclusions therefore were of questionable validity.[35] In response to this finding, the scientific community rallied to the EPA's defense by reporting on more recent and more carefully controlled studies demonstrating the damaging effects of secondhand smoke. Many of these studies used members of the Seventh-Day Adventist church as controls, because they represent nonsmokers who are also unlikely to have been exposed to secondhand smoke.

---

periodontal disease destruction of soft tissue and bone that surround the teeth.

mainstream smoke smoke inhaled and then exhaled by a smoker.

sidestream smoke smoke that comes from the burning end of a cigarette, pipe, or cigar.

environmental tobacco smoke tobacco smoke, regardless of source, that stays within a common source of air.

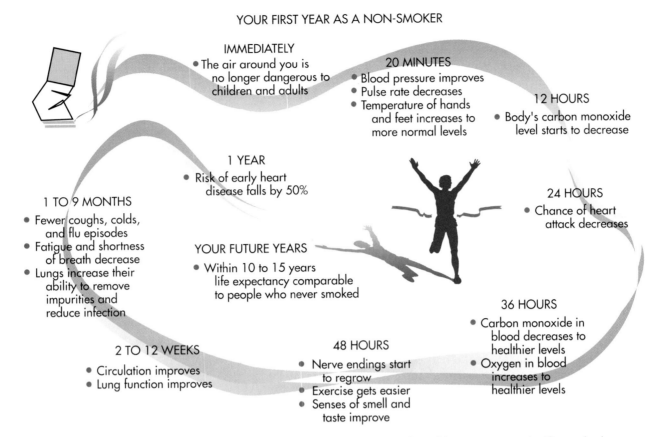

YOUR FIRST YEAR AS A NON-SMOKER

IMMEDIATELY
- The air around you is no longer dangerous to children and adults

20 MINUTES
- Blood pressure improves
- Pulse rate decreases
- Temperature of hands and feet increases to more normal levels

12 HOURS
- Body's carbon monoxide level starts to decrease

1 YEAR
- Risk of early heart disease falls by 50%

24 HOURS
- Chance of heart attack decreases

1 TO 9 MONTHS
- Fewer coughs, colds, and flu episodes
- Fatigue and shortness of breath decrease
- Lungs increase their ability to remove impurities and reduce infection

YOUR FUTURE YEARS
- Within 10 to 15 years life expectancy comparable to people who never smoked

36 HOURS
- Carbon monoxide in blood decreases to healthier levels
- Oxygen in blood increases to healthier levels

2 TO 12 WEEKS
- Circulation improves
- Lung function improves

48 HOURS
- Nerve endings start to regrow
- Exercise gets easier
- Senses of smell and taste improve

Figure 9-3   The health benefits of quitting smoking begin immediately and become more significant the longer you stay smoke-free.

A newly developed "smoking system" named Accord represents the latest attempt to develop a low-smoke cigarette. This system uses a battery-powered, device into which a special small cigarette is inserted. The user inhales through the device and the cigarette is electrically ignited only when inhaling, thus reducing sidestream smoke.

Stopping What You Started

Experts in health behavior contend that before people will discontinue harmful health behaviors, such as tobacco use, they must appreciate fully what they are expecting of themselves. This understanding grows in relationship to the following:

1. *Knowledge* about the health risks associated with tobacco use
2. *Recognition* that these health risks are applicable to all tobacco users
3. *Familiarity* with steps that can be taken to eliminate or reduce these risks
4. *Belief* that the benefits to be gained by no longer using tobacco will outweigh the pleasures gained through the use of tobacco

5. *Certainty* that one can start and maintain the behaviors required to stop or reduce the use of tobacco

On closer examination it is evident that these steps combine both knowledge and desire (or motivation). Being knowledgeable about risks, however, will not always stop behaviors that involve varying degrees of psychological and physical dependence. The 75 percent failure rate thought to be common among tobacco cessation programs suggests that the motivation is not easy to achieve or maintain. In fact, on the basis of information reported by the Hazelden Foundation, for persons who are successful in quitting, approximately 18.6 years elapses between the first attempt to stop and the actual time of quitting. The many health benefits of quitting smoking are shown in Figure 9-3.

A variety of smoking cessation programs exist, including those using highly organized formats, with or without the use of prescription or OTC nicotine replacement systems. In past years, most of the 1.3 million people who managed to quit smoking each year did so by throwing away their cigarettes (going cold turkey) and paying the physical and emotional price of waiting for their bodies to adjust to life without nicotine. Today, however, the use of nicotine replacement products in combination with external programs (such as those listed in the next paragraph), or programs accompanying the nicotine replacement product itself are more frequently turned to. The Health Action Guide on page 284 provides a plan for smoking cessation that incorporates nicotine replacement products. For those who are concerned about weight gain following smoking cessation, the Health Action Guide on page 284 offers some helpful weight management tips.

Programs to help people stop their tobacco use are available in a variety of formats, including educational programs, behavior modification, aversive conditioning, hypnosis, acupuncture, and various combinations of these approaches. Programs are offered in both individual and group settings and are operated by hospitals, universities, health departments, voluntary health agencies, churches, and private practitioners. The better programs will have limited success rates—20 percent to 50 percent as measured over one year (with self-reporting), whereas the remainder will have even poorer results.

Two methods for weaning smokers from cigarettes to a nontobacco source of nicotine are nicotine-containing chewing gum (Nicorette), in either prescription or OTC versions, and transdermal patches, in either prescription or OTC versions (Nicoderm, Nicotrol, Habitrol, Prostep), using either single-strength or step-down formulas. A brief description of both gum and the transdermal patch is provided next, although subtle variations exist between prescription and OTC formulations and between brands.[36,37]

Nicotine-containing chewing gum. Correct use of nicotine-containing chewing gum requires an immediate cessation of smoking, an initial determination of dosage (4 mg or 2 mg of nicotine per piece), knowledge of the appropriate manner of chewing each piece of gum, the appropriate time to chew each piece, the maximum number of pieces to be chewed each day, and time to begin withdrawal from the therapy. When used in combination with physician guidance or program support provided by the manufacturer, cessation using nicotine-containing gum may have a success rate of 40 percent or more. Nicotine-containing chewing gum therapy ranges in cost from an initial $50 kit to weekly refills of approximately $30.

Transdermal nicotine patches. The more recently developed transdermal (through the skin) nicotine patches appear to be less effective (25%) than the gum just described, but in many ways are more easily used. If a step-down version (21 mg, 14 mg, 7 mg) is employed, determinations must be made as to the appropriate initial dosage (based on number of cigarettes smoked per day and body weight), the length of time at the initial dosage before stepping down, and the manner of withdrawal after a usual eight- to

twelve-week treatment period. The single dose (15 mg) version, of course, eliminates the step-down component. Costs associated with transdermal nicotine replacement therapy are similar to those for the gum-based program.

In all delivery forms and formulations, nicotine replacement therapy can be associated with contraindications and adverse reactions, including skin irritation, redness, and irregular heart rates.

A recently developed prescription medication, mecamylamine, used in combination with the transdermal nicotine patch improves the latter's effectiveness rate to the 40 percent level reported for nicotine-containing chewing gum. The drug affects receptors in the CNS, reducing the pleasurable effects of nicotine and thus decreasing dependency.

In addition to the drugs just described, Nicotrol Inhaler, a nicotine-replacement therapy, has been approved (in prescription form) by the FDA. This new delivery technique uses a nicotine cartridge inserted into a cigarette holder-like device through which the user inhales. Because of the large surface area of the lungs and rapid absorption into the blood, inhalation-based delivery of nicotine should become a very attractive alternative to transdermal and oral routes of replacement.

Several nicotine-free prescription medications to aid smoking cessation have now been approved or are nearing approval. These agents can be used alone or with nicotine replacement therapy. Zyban and Wellbutrin are antidepressant drugs that increase the production of dopamine, a neurotransmitter. Production of dopamine declines when a smoker quits, creating the craving to smoke. Prozac, the serotonin-reuptake inhibitor antidepressant approved for the treatment of depression, bulimia nervosa, and obsessive-compulsive disorder, has also shown promise as an adjunct to smoking cessation.

Those who are concerned that nicotine-replacement therapies are simply a "trade-off" of addictions (from cigarettes to gum or patches) should remember that while using the therapy the former smoker is no longer being exposed to carbon monoxide and carcinogens, while the step-down feature allows for a gradual return to a totally nicotine-free lifestyle. Therefore a short period of cross-addiction should be seen as simply a "cost" of recovery for the 40 percent who will be successful.

Personal Applications

• In the absence of a clear indication that a smoker has tried to stop but was unable to do so, should tax-paying citizens restrict access to the health care services the smoker will eventually need but most likely be unable to pay for?

Countdown to Quit Day: A Plan for Smoking Cessation

Make a decision to quit smoking on a particular day during the next week. Then use the following steps to begin preparing yourself for that day.

Five Days before Quit Day

- Keep a daylong record of each cigarette you smoke. List the time you smoked, whom you were with, and why you decided to light up (for example, for stimulation, tension reduction, or social pleasure, or because you had a craving or wanted something to do with your hands). Once you know why you smoke, you can plan intervention strategies for use during the two-minute periods of craving you will feel during the first weeks of your smoke-free life.
- Contact your physician to help you decide whether to use prescription or OTC nicotine replacement therapy. Make sure you understand all directions for its safe and effective use.
- Draw up a contract in which you formally state your intention to quit smoking. Sign and date the contract and clearly display it in your home or workplace.

Four Days before Quit Day

- Solicit support from family, friends, and coworkers by sharing your intention with them and asking for their help and encouragement.
- Organize your intervention strategies and assemble needed supplies, such as gum, bottled water, diet soda, handwork (for example, needlepoint or wood carving), and walking shoes.

Three Days before Quit Day

- Review your quitting contract and touch bases with several people in your support group to bolster your resolve.
- Study all nicotine-replacement therapy product information and any material supplied by your physician.
- Continue preparing your intervention supplies.
- Reschedule your personal calendar and work schedule to minimize situations that could tempt you to smoke during the first several days of your smoke-free life.

Two Days before Quit Day

- Continue or revisit any earlier tasks that you have not yet finished.
- Practice your intervention strategies as appropriate. For example, map out a safe walking route and practice your deep breathing exercises.
- Obtain a large glass or other container, such as an empty milk jug, that will serve as a bank into which you will deposit daily the money that you would have otherwise spent on cigarettes.
- If you feel comfortable doing so, construct a yard sign to inform outsiders that your home is a smoke-free environment and to report your daily success toward a smoke-free life.
- Smoke-proof your home and workplace by removing and destroying all materials and supplies associated with tobacco use, saving only enough tobacco products needed for today and tomorrow.

One Day before Quit Day

- Complete all preparations described above, including the almost total removal and destruction of smoking-related materials.
- As the end of the day approaches, review your contract and call a few people in your support network for last-minute words of encouragement.
- Smoke your last cigarette and flush any remaining cigarettes down the toilet.
- Begin your nicotine replacement therapy as directed by your physician or by product insert information.
- Publicly display your yard sign, if you decided to make one.
- Retire for the night and await your rebirth in the morning as a former smoker.

InfoLinks
http://kickbutt.org

Avoiding Weight Gain When You Stop Smoking

For many smokers, particularly women, an important "plus" for smoking is weight management. In their minds the risks associated with tobacco use are more than offset by the cigarette's ability to curb appetite and thus serve as an aid in restricting caloric intake. Accordingly, the fear of weight gain frequently prevents any serious attempts at stopping smoking or permits easy relapse back into cigarette use.

The fear described above is in fact true. Most people who quit smoking do gain weight during the ten years after cessation and in amounts greater than that seen in people who continue smoking or who have never smoked. It is also true, however, that this weight gain is relatively small (2.4 pounds for women and 3.8 pounds for men) and only slightly greater than that experienced by agemates who smoke or have never smoked. Certainly, the weight gained is a minimal health risk compared with the risks associated with continued smoking.

The keys to minimizing weight gain after smoking cessation are centered in two areas: (1) the ability to manage the "smoking urges" associated with the first several months of being a former smoker without resorting to eating and (2) the willingness to adopt healthy eating and exercise behaviors.

In regard to the management of smoking urges, people who are attempting to quit smoking should recognize that these powerful urges are very temporary, usually lasting only about two minutes. During these periods of intense desire for a cigarette, coping activities such as taking a short walk, drinking water or a diet beverage, or talking with a coworker or family member will distract the mind from a cigarette until the urge has passed. If one "must" eat during these times, then healthy low-calorie snacks, such as apple slices, should be selected.

To minimize weight gain (or actually achieve a lower weight than when smoking) in the years after stopping smoking, a serious wellness-oriented lifestyle change involving both exercise and diet should be implemented. Specific information regarding adult fitness and sound nutrition can be found in Chapters 4 and 5, respectively.

InfoLinks
www.ash.org/papers/h3.htm

Tobacco Use: A Question of Rights

For those readers who have found themselves involved (or nearly so) in confrontation situations involving smokers' versus nonsmokers' rights, we hope the section that follows will be helpful in allowing you to see more clearly the positions that you have taken. For those who have somehow remained removed from this discussion, consideration of these issues now may be good preparation for the future. Regardless, consider these two important questions:

1. To what extent should smokers be allowed to pollute the air and endanger the health of nonsmokers?
2. To what extent should nonsmokers be allowed to restrict the personal freedom of smokers, particularly since tobacco products are sold legally?

At this time, answers to these questions are only partially available, but one trend is developing: The tobacco user is being forced to give ground to the nonsmoker. Today, in fact, it is becoming more a matter of where the smoker will be allowed to smoke, rather than a matter of where smoking will be restricted. Smoking is becoming less and less tolerated. The health concerns of the majority are prevailing over the dependence needs of the minority.

Personal Applications

- If you are a smoker, have you ever been asked to extinguish your cigarette? How did you react?
- If you are the nonsmoker doing the asking, what response do you most often receive? How do you feel about your right to breathe the most smoke-free air possible?

Enhancing Communication Between Smokers and Nonsmokers

Exchanges between smokers and nonsmokers are sometimes strained and, in many cases, friendships are damaged beyond the point of repair. As you have probably observed, roommates are changed, dates are refused, and memberships in groups are withheld or rejected because of the opposing rights of these two groups.

Recognizing that social skills development is an important task for young adults, the following simple considerations or approaches for *smokers* can reduce some conflict presently associated with smoking:

- Before lighting up, ask whether smoking would bother others in close proximity to you.
- When in a neutral setting, seek physical space in which you will be able to smoke and in a reasonable way not interfere with nonsmokers' comfort.
- Accept the validity of the nonsmoker's statement that your smoke causes everything and everyone to smell.
- Respect stated prohibitions against smoking. If a nonsmoker requests that you refrain from smoking, respond with courtesy, regardless of whether you intend to comply.
- Practice "civil smoking" by applying a measure of restraint when you recognize that smoking is offensive to others. Particularly, respect the aesthetics that should accompany any act of smoking—ashes on dinner plates, cigarette butts in flower pots, and emptying car ashtrays on shopping center parking lots are hardly popular with others.

The preceding suggestions can become skills for the social dimension of your health that can be applied to other social conflicts. Remember that as a smoker you are part of a statistical minority living in a society that often makes decisions and resolves conflict based on majority rule.

For *nonsmokers*, we suggest several approaches we believe will make you more sensitive and skilled in dealing with smoking behavior:

- Attempt to develop a sensitivity to the power of the dependence that smokers have on their cigarettes.
- Accept the reality of the smoker's sensory insensitivity—an insensitivity so profound that the odors you complain about are not even recognized by the smoker.
- When in a neutral setting, allow smokers their fair share of physical space in which to smoke. So long as the host does not object to smoking, you, as a guest, do not have the right to infringe on a person's right to smoke.
- When asking a person not to smoke, use a manner that reflects social consideration and skill. State your request clearly, and accept a refusal gracefully.
- Respond with honesty to inquiries from the smoker as to whether the smoke is bothering you.

If you are contemplating smoking, examine closely whether the social isolation that appears to be more and more common for smokers will be offset by the benefits you might receive from cigarettes. The ability to find satisfaction through social contact may be one of the most important avenues to a sense of well-being.

Real Life
Real choices

- Do you identify more strongly with Karen or with Steven in this situation? Give reasons for your answer.
- If you smoke, how do friends, classmates, and others treat you, and how do you feel about their behavior?
- If you don't smoke, what is your attitude toward smoking and smokers? Why do you think and feel the way you do?

And Now, Your Choices . . .
- If you were a smoker and your partner didn't smoke, would you be willing to quit to save the relationship?
- If you didn't smoke and were involved with someone who did, would you consider ending the relationship if your partner refused to quit?

Final Thoughts About Tobacco and Health

Recalling the alternative definition of the role and composition of health presented in Chapter 1, we raise this question for readers who currently use tobacco in some form: "Are you healthy (resourceful) enough to continue your use of tobacco?" We ask you to think about the degree to which tobacco use functions as a resource in each of the multiple dimensions of your health. For example, to what degree does tobacco use enhance the structure and function of the physical body? To what degree does it increase the positive feelings that comprise the emotional dimension of health versus increase those more negative or uncomfortable feelings that all people feel to various degrees? How does smoking or smokeless tobacco use serve as a social lubricant, making its users more desirable people with whom to spend time? To what extent does tobacco use reflect the intellect's role in

shaping important behavioral choices? How is tobacco use a contributing factor in workplace relationships and the effective use of time for which employees are financially compensated? Certainly, in our opinion, tobacco use decreases resourcefulness in each of health's seven dimensions.

When the mastery of developmental tasks that compose each life cycle segment is assessed in terms of the contribution (or lack thereof) made by tobacco use, the picture seems no more positive. Simply stated, what are the positive contributions of tobacco use to a growing sense of responsibility for self and others, desired independence, intimacy with others, success in developing social skills, parenting, and making a statement about your adult identity? Again, we see little contribution to adult growth and development from the use of tobacco products. We believe the compromising of your resourcefulness caused by tobacco use and its detrimental effect on adult growth and development will quickly become evident.

Summary

- The percentage of American adults who smoke is continuing to decline.
- The incidence of adolescent and young-adult smoking is increasing.
- Cigarette smoking is inversely related to level of formal education.
- The tobacco industry continues to aggressively market its products to potential smokers.
- In spite of denial by the tobacco industry, tobacco-related advertisements appear to be directed to older children and younger adolescents.
- Pipe and cigar smoking present their own unique contributions to the development of tobacco-related health problems.
- Dependence, including addiction and habituation, is established quickly through tobacco use.
- Multiple theories regarding nicotine's role in dependence have been advanced.

- Nicotine exerts acute effects both within the central nervous system and on a variety of other tissues and organs.
- Modeling, self-reward, and self-medication play important psychological roles in the development of tobacco dependence.
- The tobacco industry is continually targeting new markets, such as women, minorities, and adolescents, although the huge fines and restrictions associated with lawsuits may severely curtail these efforts.
- The federal government has proposed a broadly based program intended to reduce the use of cigarettes by adolescents.
- Early childhood intervention may be effective in stemming the current rise in adolescent tobacco use.

- Tobacco smoke can be divided into gaseous and particulate phases. Each phase has its unique chemical composition.
- Nicotine, carbon monoxide, and phenol have damaging effects on various body tissues.
- Thousands of chemical components and hundreds of carcinogenic agents are found in tobacco smoke.
- Nicotine and carbon monoxide have predictable effects on the function of the cardiovascular system.
- The development of nearly one-third of all cancers can be attributed to tobacco use, and virtually every form of cancer is found more frequently in smokers than in nonsmokers.
- Components in tobacco smoke, principally phenol, alter the structure and function of airway tissue in the direction of eventual lung cancer.
- Chronic obstructive lung disease (COLD), also called chronic obstructive pulmonary disease, (COPD) is a likely consequence of long-term cigarette smoking, with early symptoms appearing shortly after beginning regular smoking.
- Smoking alters normal structure and function of the body, as seen in a wide variety of noncardiovascular and noncancerous conditions, such as infertility, problem pregnancy, and

neonatal health concerns. Additional health concerns include the diminished ability to smell and bone loss leading to osteoporosis.
- Cigarette smoking and long-term use of oral contraceptives are not compatible.
- The combined use of tobacco and alcohol is associated with an above-normal tendency to use additional types of drugs; thus both are referred to as gateway drugs.
- Smokeless tobacco carries its own health risks, including oral cancer.
- The presence of secondhand smoke results in involuntary (or passive) smoking by those who must share a common air source with smokers. This secondhand smoke threatens the health of the spouse, children, and coworkers of the smoker.
- Stopping smoking can be undertaken in any one of several ways, including going cold turkey.
- Nicotine gum and transdermal nicotine patches, in both prescription and OTC formulations, can be effective in a smoking cessation program.
- Both smokers and nonsmokers have certain rights regarding the use of tobacco. Effective communication can be established between smokers and nonsmokers.

Review Questions

1. What percentage of the American adult population smokes? In what direction has change been occurring? What is the current direction that adolescent smoking is taking? What position has the tobacco industry traditionally taken regarding the focus of its advertising?
2. In comparison to cigarettes, what health risks are associated with pipe and cigar smoking?
3. What are the two principal components of nicotine dependence? What specific components compose each of these? What percentage of smokers appear to be strongly physically dependent? To which aspect of dependence does compulsion belong? What is a "chipper" and how does this smoking pattern differ from that seen in most tobacco users?
4. Identify each of the three theories of nicotine addiction discussed in the chapter. In amounts consumed by the typical regular smoker, what is the effect of nicotine on central nervous system function? How does this differ in chain smokers?
5. What effects does nicotine have on the body outside of the central nervous system? How does the influence of nicotine resemble that associated with the stress response?
6. How do modeling and manipulation explain the development of emotional dependence on

tobacco? How do self-esteem, self-image, and self-directedness relate to tobacco use? How does the tobacco industry "address" these needs through their advertisements?
7. How is the federal government attempting to limit the exposure that children and adolescents currently have to tobacco products and tobacco advertisements? What techniques have been developed by the tobacco industry to market its products to children and adolescents? What is the status of lawsuits against the tobacco industry now pending?
8. How might concerned parents begin to "tobacco-proof" their children to keep them from becoming smokers in the future?
9. What are the principal components of the gaseous and particulate phases of tobacco smoke? What is tar?
10. What detrimental effect does carbon monoxide have on oxygen transport capabilities? What relationship exists between maternal smoking and oxygen transport capabilities in the fetus?
11. In what ways do nicotine and carbon monoxide contribute to cardiovascular disease? How does smoking compromise the normal function of blood platelets? How are cholesterol profiles influenced by smoking?

12. To what extent is tobacco use a factor in cancer? What percentage of all cancers are thought to be causally related to smoking? How does smoking alter airway tissue to promote eventual lung cancer?

13. What is the traditional progression of chronic obstructive lung disease (COLD) or chronic obstructive pulmonary disease (COPD)? What is fetal tobacco syndrome? In what ways does tobacco use impair reproductive health, in terms of infertility, breastfeeding, and neonatal health?

14. How does smoking relate to the long-term use of oral contraceptives?

15. Why are both tobacco and alcohol referred to as gateway drugs?

16. In what ways is smokeless tobacco equal to smoking in the development of serious health concerns?

17. What is involuntary or passive smoking? What are the forms of secondhand tobacco smoke? Which is the most highly concentrated form of smoke? Which form has been "filtered" by the smoker prior to its release into the common air supply? What is the effect of secondhand smoke on the spouses and children of smokers?

18. What are the several basic realities that smokers must be aware of before they are likely to change their behavior? In what way does a "cold turkey" approach to smoking cessation differ from the prevailing approaches built around nicotine replacement therapy? What, in a general sense, is the level of effectiveness seen in the better smoking abatement programs?

19. What rights do smokers and nonsmokers have in public places? How can communication be enhanced between smokers and nonsmokers?

References

1. *Cancer facts & figures—1998.* Atlanta: American Cancer Society, 1998.

2. Since Joe Camel's debut, new teen smoking up 73%. *USA Today* 1998 Oct 9:10A.

3. Cigarette smoking among adults—United States, 1995. *MMWR* 1997 Dec; 46(51):1217–20.

4. Johnson LS, O'Malley PM, Bachman JG. *Smoking, drinking, and illicit drug use among American secondary school students, college students and young adults, 1975–1991,* vol. 2. *College students and young adults,* NIH Pub No. 93–3481. Rockville, MD: National Institute on Drug Abuse, USDHHS, USPHS, 1992.

5. Wechsler H et al. Increased levels of cigarette use among college students: a cause for national concern. *JAMA* 1998 Nov 18; 280(19):1673–78.

6. Tobacco use among high school students—United States, 1997. *MMWR* 1998 Apr; 45(12):229–33.

7. U.S. Department of Commerce, Bureau of the Census. *Statistical abstract of the United States 1998.* 118th ed. Washington, DC: U.S. Government Printing Office, 1998.

8. Levy D. Firm knew cigarette tar tested low. *USA Today* 1995 Aug 2: ID.

9. Pollay RW, Siddarth S, Siegel M. The last straw? Cigarette advertising and realized market shares among youths and adults, 1979–1993. *J Marketing* 1996 Apr; 60:1–16.

10. Burns DM, ed. *Cigars: health effects and trends.* Cancer Monograph Series (No. 9). National Cancer Institute, April 1998.

11. *FTC requires cigar companies to supply data on cigar sales and advertising expenditures.* Washington: DCFTC's Consumer Response Center, Feb, 1998. http://www.ftc.gov

12. Pianezza ML, Sellers EM, Tyndale RF. Nicotine metabolism defect reduces smoking (letter). *Nature* 1998 June 25; 393(6687):750.

13. Russell M. Cigarette smoking: natural history of a dependency disorder. *Br J Med Psych* 1971; 44:1.

14. McGehee D. Nicotine enhancement of fast excitatory synaptic transmission in CNS by presynaptic receptors. *Science* 1995 Sept 22; 269: 1692–96.

15. Clancy C. Poison pearls and perils. *A bulletin from the National Capital Poison Center* 1996 Oct; 2(4):1–3. http://www.poison.org/nicotine.htm

16. Cigarettes strike pose. *USA Today* 1997 Apr 23:IB.

17. Page S, Woodyard C. In new climate, tobacco industry fights to breathe. *USA Today* 1998 Apr 9:12A.

18. National Clearinghouse for Alcohol and Drug Information. *Growing up drug free: a parent's guide to prevention.* Washington DC: U.S. Department of Education, 1992.

19. Saladin KS. *Anatomy & physiology: the unit of form and function.* Dubuque, IA: WCB/McGraw Hill, 1998.

20. Hecht ML. *Smoking cessation: pre-operative.* University of Wisconsin Anesthesia Topics, Nov 1998. http://www.anesthesia.wisc.edu/Topics/Coexisting_Disease/smo

21. Kapier KN et al. *Cigarettes: what the warning label doesn't tell you.* New York: American Council on Science and Health, 1997.

22. American Heart Association. *1998 heart and stroke facts: 1998 statistical update.* Dallas: The Association, 1997.

23. Howard G et al. Cigarette smoking and progression of atherosclerosis. *JAMA 1998; 279(2):119–24.*

24. Landis H et al. *Cancer statistics 1998: epidemiology and surveillance publication.* Atlanta: American Cancer Society, 1998.

25. Denissenko MF, Pao A, Pfeifer GP. Preferential formation of benzol[a]pyrene adducts at lung cancer

mutational hotspot in p53. *Science* 1996;274(5288):430–32.

26. Wistuba I et al. Molecular damage in the bronchial epithelium of smokers. *J. Natl Cancer Inst* 1997; 89(18):1366–73.

27. Crowley LV. *Introduction to human disease.* 4th ed. Boston: Jones & Bartlett, 1996.

28. Eisen S et al. The impact of cigarette and alcohol consumption on weight and obesity: an analysis of 1911 monozygotic male twin pairs. *Arch Intern Med* 1993; 153(21):2457–63.

29. Kahn A et al. Parental exposure to cigarettes in infants with obstructive sleep apneas. *Pediatrics* 1994; 93(5):778–83.

30. Eliopoulos C et al. Hair concentrations of nicotine in women and their newborn infants. *JAMA* 1994; 271(8):621–23.

31. Hatcher RA et al. *Contraceptive technology* 17th ed. New York: Ardent Media, 1998.

32. Bad news for players who chew tobacco. *USA Today* 1998 Apr 1:3C.

33. Glantz SA, Parmely WW. Passive smoking and heart disease: epidemiology, physiology, and biochemistry. *Circulation* 1991; 83(1):1–12.

34. Adair-Bischoff CE, Sauve RS. Environmental tobacco smoke and middle ear disease in preschool-age children. *Arch Pediatr Adolesc Med* 1998 Feb; 152(2):127–33.

35. *Order and judgment.* In the United States District Court for the Middle District of North Carolina, Winston-Salem Division, District Judge Osteen, July 17, 1998. http://www.rjrt.com/immediate/ruling.htm

36. *Physicians desk reference.* 52nd ed. Montvale, NJ: Medical Economics, 1998.

37. *Physicians desk reference for nonprescription drugs.* 19th ed. Montvale NJ: Medical Economics, 1998.

Suggested Readings

Glantz S. (ed.). *The cigarette papers.* Berkeley, CA: University of California Press, 1996. Staton Glantz, a professor of medicine at the University of California–San Francisco, is a true thorn in the side of the tobacco industry. His book gives readers an array of information obtained from 4,000 recently released tobacco industry documents. He and a panel of experts tell the inside story of how the industry manipulated the product, the government, and the public in order to retain smokers and disclaim the dangers of tobacco.

Kapier KN. *Cigarettes: what the warning label doesn't tell you.* New York: American Council on Science and Health, 1997. Drawing on the expertise of clinicians and researchers in many areas, this 20-chapter book investigates virtually every area of human structures and function harmed by smoking. The information in the book would be of interest to both health-care providers and laypeople.

Gebhardt J. *The enlightened smoker's guide to quitting.* Boston: Element Books, 1998. To some degree a smoking cessation program must be tailored to the smoking history of the people attempting to quit. Using a seven-step approach, the author discusses tailoring these components for participants in order to enhance their success. The approach described is frequently employed by programs approved by the American Cancer Society.

Hirschfelder AB. *Kick butts: a kid's guide to a tobacco-free America.* Parsippany, NJ: Silver Burdett Press, 1998. The decision to smoke is made at a surprisingly early age, often well before the actual behavior is seen. Accordingly, the author skillfully focuses the information and activities of her book to the children she wants to reach. Her account of the last 100 years of tobacco use is informative to all readers, but the activities described in the latter portion of the book are well suited for and will be well received by young children. Recommended for both parents and teachers.

As We Go To PRESS

A recent study suggests that marriages in which one partner is a smoker are among the most difficult of all marriages to sustain. Researchers at the University of Chicago found that these couples were 53 percent more likely to divorce than married couples who were both nonsmokers. How can this higher divorce rate be explained? Some observers have suggested that people who begin smoking in their teens have some adjustment problems, which eventually affect their marital relationships. Others point out that the educational attainment of smokers is generally lower than average, thus causing stress in their marriages. What do you think?

Smoking among Women: Troubling Trends

Cigarette smoking among women was virtually nonexistent 100 years ago. But by 1934, when First Lady Eleanor Roosevelt smoked a cigarette in public, 17 percent of American women had taken up the habit. Thirty years later that proportion had doubled[1]. In the last 30 years the percentage of women smokers has declined, but there remains cause for grave concern. More female adolescents are lighting up. The proportion of heavy smokers among women is on the rise. And health problems associated with tobacco use that were once virtually unknown in women, such as lung cancer, are now taking a significant toll on the health and lives of American women.

In 1993, 73 percent of the 22 million women smokers in the United States wanted to quit.[2] An increasing number of women are breaking the habit, but this does not hold true for teenage smokers.[3] Some research suggests that it may be more difficult for women to quit than for men. Women report perceptions of greater physical and emotional dependence on cigarettes, use more nicotine gum while trying to quit, and are more likely to relapse than men.[1] To find out why it's hard to stop, let's examine some of the predictors in women's lives that may lead them to start smoking and reasons that they continue to smoke.

Predictors and Reasons for Smoking

Ninety percent of smokers take up the habit before age 20, so it is instructive to look at this age group for predictors of smoking onset. Low academic achievement, low socioeconomic status, exhibition of problem behavior, such as truancy and suspensions, and infrequent church attendance, although not absolute predictors of youth smoking, are certainly seen in young females known to be smokers. Whereas male teens smoke to cope with insecurity and demonstrate male assertiveness, female teens tend to smoke to symbolize autonomy and rebelliousness. Ironically, modeling the smoking behaviors of the peers that she is autonomous from and the parents she is rebelling against seems to heavily influence a female teen's decision to smoke. She may be indoctrinated with the benefits of smoking by the advertisers, but she learns of its acceptability from her friends and family. Young women are four times more likely to smoke if an older sibling or parent smokes, and the odds further increase if her smoking parent is her mother. Having a close friend who is a smoker makes a girl nine times more likely to become a smoker herself.[4]

Many teens begin using nicotine as an appetite suppressant. The possibility of weight gain keeps many women from quitting and encourages relapse among those who have quit. Smokers who quit do tend to gain weight in the first year,[5] but weight gain slows after the first 6 months cigarette-free. Efforts to diet right after quitting increase the chance of relapse.[5] It is best for a woman to become comfortable with being a nonsmoker before tackling the weight issue. A woman who wants to quit smoking should also remember that weight gain associated with smoking cessation is much less detrimental to health than continuing to smoke. In addition to preoccupation with ideal weight, women are more likely than men to smoke to cope with the anxiety, tension, anger, aggression, and stressors produced by family and career demands.[1]

Smoking and Pregnancy

A woman may value nicotine over her own health, but she has an obligation to consider her children. Maternal smoking has been associated with spontaneous abortion, low birth weight, sudden infant death syndrome (SIDS), asthma, and major birth defects, including mental retardation.

Most recently, urine samples from newborns collected in Germany and analyzed at the University of Minnesota demonstrated the presence of a family of strong carcinogens in the infants whose mothers smoked during pregnancy. These carcinogens, the NNKs, are among the strongest known carcinogens in tobacco smoke. These substances were not found in the urine from babies of nonsmoking mothers.[6]

Smoking is detrimental to the fetus, newborn, and infant, and its effects can follow children into adulthood. Effects of children's exposure to sidestream smoke can lead to severe respiratory disease and hinder growth of the lungs.[3] Yet smoking by pregnant women continues to be a problem, especially among teenage mothers. Between 28 percent and 42 percent of pregnant teens continue to smoke.[4] They do so to cope with increased weight gain, to deliver smaller infants and thus decrease the pain of delivery, and to counteract feelings of anxiety from the loneliness of their situation. It is common for the father of the baby to be uninvolved with the woman during her pregnancy, and her own parents are more than likely disapproving. Even friends may stop calling.

Health Concerns Unique to Women

In addition to risks associated with pregnancy, nicotine and other chemicals in cigarettes pose a variety of unique and increased health risks to women. In general, the veins, arteries, and airways are smaller in women than in men, which makes blockage and damage more severe. Smoking destroys the unique hormonal protection that women of reproductive age have against heart disease by reducing estrogen and high-density lipoprotein (HDL) levels. Consequently, smoking increases women's risk of heart attack by six times, compared with a threefold increase for men. Female smokers also have four times the risk of developing cervical cancer than do nonsmoking women.[1] Women who smoke go through menopause earlier, and after menopause have five times the risk of dying from smoking-related cancer than premenopausal smokers.[1,7] The odds are bad for women smokers no matter what group is used in comparison.

Lung cancer from smoking recently surpassed breast cancer as the leading cause of cancer deaths in women, with 24.7 percent and 16 percent of cancer deaths, respectively.[8] Although the connection between smoking and lung cancer is widely recognized, tobacco use also contributes to breast cancer and is associated with cervical cancer, osteoporosis, and complications with the use of oral contraceptives.[1,7]

Advertising That Targets Women

Advertisers don't mention the disease and death or even the bad breath, cough, shortness of breath, smelly clothes, stained teeth, and deep wrinkles smoking is known to cause. Instead, the ads present smoking as the key to financial success, sports participation, and female independence and social acceptance.[4,7] In fact, the opposite holds true. Cigarettes take a big bite out of the smoker's budget and leave her out of breath and on the sidelines at sporting events. Smokers are forced into designated areas as social acceptance continues to plummet, and the idea of independence through addiction is ridiculous. Many brands also have thin spokeswomen pushing "slim" and "light" cigarettes in order to cash in on women's fear of weight gain.

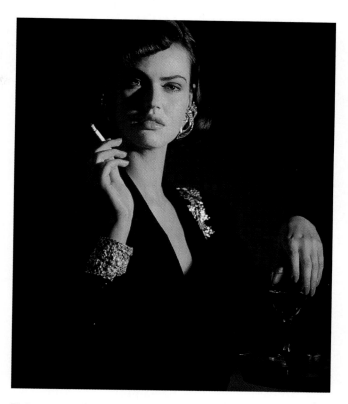

Tobacco advertisers want women to think smoking will make them appear glamorous, sophisticated, and financially successful. Do you think women smokers convey this image?

This chapter discussed a number of specific ways in which tobacco companies target women. In addition, tobacco companies are heavy sponsors of women's sports, fashion, and artistic and political activities. High concentrations of tobacco ads are found in women's magazines, and the more ads are found, the less likely the magazine is to cover smoking and health issues.[7]

Quitting Smoking

The effects of nicotine withdrawal include craving, irritability, anxiety, headache, difficulty concentrating, restlessness, and increased appetite. These symptoms peak within twenty-four to forty-eight hours and usually diminish after two weeks, but they may persist for months. Nicotine replacement therapy with transdermal patches or nicotine-containing gum reduces physical withdrawal symptoms while the ex-smoker learns to deal with the behavioral and psychological issues of her past addiction. These methods are the most effective that can be offered, yet unfortunately only about 40 percent of the people who use these methods in an attempt to quit smoking are successful.

Nicotine gum, unlike the patch, provides nicotine on demand and involves a habitual behavior substitute. The patch, however, is easier to use because it is simply applied once a day. For maximum benefit, the gum must be chewed on a specific schedule, and soda, juice, and other acidic substances that reduce nicotine absorption in the mouth must be consciously regulated.[1] Hypnosis, nasal spray with nicotine blockers, and other drugs are also being used to kick the habit.

These therapies are not long-term alternatives to smoking. Instead, support and motivation determine long-term success. If you are a smoker who is trying to quit, tell family and friends of your decision. They'll support you, and the fact that they know you're trying to quit will bolster your resolve. Join a smoking cessation group through your doctor or at work. Remove cigarettes from your environment, identify the situations that tempt you to smoke, and take control. If you do relapse, it is important to view the relapse as a learning experience, rather than a failure, and try again.[1]

Of course, it's much easier never to start than to quit. School-based programs with community intervention have been shown to work. Other methods to prevent smoking initiation include enforcement of laws that prohibit the sale of tobacco products to minors, ad campaigns that deglamorize smoking, and increased pricing of cigarettes.[2] Maybe then we can all breathe a little easier.

For Discussion . . .

Are you, or were you once, a smoker? Have you ever tried to quit? What did you find the most difficult? Before reading this chapter, did you realize how harmful even sidestream smoke is to children before and after birth? Have you ever tried to help someone else quit smoking?

References

1. Bjornson WM, Fiore MC, Oogan-Morrison BA. The growing problem of smoking in women. *Patient Care* 1996; 30(13):142–54.
2. CDC. *Indicators of nicotine addiction among women 1991–1992.* 1995; 44(6):102–5.
3. Dreker N. The facts about women and smoking. *Current Health 2* 1995; 21(8):16–19.
4. Lawson EJ. The role of smoking in the lives of low-income pregnant adolescents: a field study. *Adolescence* 1994; 29(11):61–79.
5. Caan B et al. Women gain weight 1 year after smoking cessation while dietary intake temporarily increases. *J Am Diet Assoc* 1996; 96(11):1150–55.
6. Hecht SS. *Metabolites of the tobacco-specific lung carcinogen 4-(methylnitrosamino)-1-(3pyridly)-Ibitampme (NNK) in the urine of newborns.* Boston: Meeting of the American Chemical Society, August 24, 1998.
7. Ernster VL. Women and smoking. *Am J Public Health* 1993; 83(9):1202–1203.
8. *Cancer facts & figures—1998.* Atlanta: American Cancer Society, 1998.

InfoLinks

www.arhp.org/clinical/index.html

www.amhrt.org/heart/
   womensheart.html

MASTERING TASKS

Addictive Substances

Your decisions about substance use affect all five of the developmental tasks. Look within the chapters of this unit for specific information to support our beliefs about drugs, alcohol, and tobacco use and their effects on developmental task mastery.

Forming an Initial Adult Identity

For most of you, this period of life is a time when you will discover more about yourself—about who you really are. All of life's experiences will help you find out who you are. With these experiences, you begin to take on an identity that probably differs somewhat from the one you had a few years ago, when you were less independent. The relative freedom you now have allows you to develop a unique identity that might carry you through all of your adult life. Decisions to use or avoid drugs, alcohol, and tobacco will reflect your uniqueness and how you view yourself. Some people will judge you either positively or negatively solely on your use or misuse of these substances. Will your current drug use patterns support or hinder your self-identity as you wish it to be fifteen years from now?

Establishing Independence

Living where you want, pursuing a career for which you have prepared, and marrying the person of your choice are among the more obvious dimensions of the independence enjoyed by many adults. However, less obvious dimensions of independence can also be important. Substance use, such as smoking, can influence independence in these less obvious dimensions. You may have seen a substance abuser experience a partial loss of independence—not the absence of independence to reside, work, or marry as you choose—but rather the independence to make decisions free from substance addiction. Although none of us is totally independent, the user of dependence-producing substances is relatively less independent.

Developing Social Skills

Not only is the use or misuse of substances such as alcohol, psychoactive drugs, and tobacco damaging to the user, but it also injures the health and well-being of others with whom the user has contact. Alcohol and drug abusers frequently find themselves unable (physically and psychologically) to interact socially with a wide range of people. As a result, the user may cease social communication. With tobacco use in particular, we see substance abuse having a negative effect on others' health. For those who are contemplating using dependence-producing substances, explore thoroughly whether the social isolation that appears to be more and more common for users will be offset by the benefits you might receive from the substance. The importance of social acceptance cannot be taken lightly.

Assuming Responsibility

College requires students to accept increasing levels of academic responsibility. Adult life in general demands additional responsibilities—everything from paying taxes to managing a growing family. Job requirements force us to assign priorities to schedules and personal activities. Clearly, adulthood is marked by our assumption of additional responsibility. Will you be able to accept these complex responsibilities if you find yourself incapable of functioning because of substance abuse? If you recognize now that your preferred method of coping with stress is to rely on alcohol or drugs, then you need to explore alternatives in light of the responsibilities that lie ahead of you.

Developing Intimacy

As suggested, the misuse or abuse of drugs, alcohol, and tobacco can easily diminish social resourcefulness. Consider the role that social interaction skills play in all forms of intimacy; reducing the effectiveness of these skills through substance misuse and abuse eventually limits intimacy. The search for illegal drugs and the loss of control resulting from chronic heavy alcohol use can diminish the quality of an intimate relationship very quickly. In addition, smoking can have a powerful influence in reducing the opportunity to be a friend, mentor, and even a dating partner.

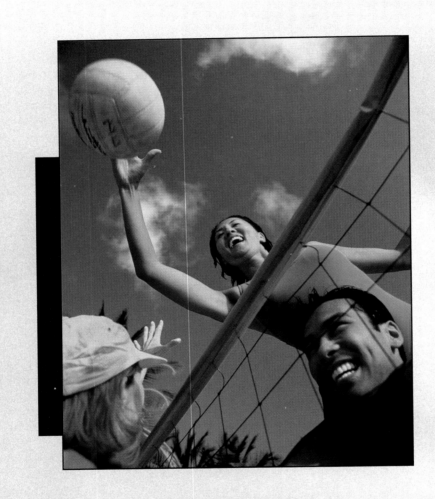

Preventing Diseases

Unit Four consists of four chapters that focus on disease prevention. Each illness you contract or develop can harm your health in each of its dimensions; therefore, prevention should be a high priority.

① Physical Dimension

We usually associate illness with pain, fear, discomfort, and limitations. But paradoxically, health problems can also improve the physical dimension of health. For example, exposure to certain infectious diseases may allow your body to develop immunity. Illness can also force you to rest, reduce your workload, and reconsider your health behavior. Weight loss, smoking cessation, improved dietary practices, genetic counseling, or a renewed commitment to fitness may follow your recovery from an illness.

② Emotional Dimension

Emotionally healthy people feel good about themselves and others and are able to cope with most of life's demands. Being diagnosed with an illness or disease can jeopardize your emotional resources. You may feel anxious, isolated, and vulnerable. Fortunately, many diseases can be prevented or at least managed or treated successfully.

③ Social Dimension

People rarely face an illness or manage a chronic health condition alone. People who have heart disease, cancer, diabetes, or AIDS often join support groups or establish friendships with others who have the same condition. In addition, you probably interact with people during activities aimed at preventing diseases. For example, you might exercise with a partner or meet people at a weight loss group.

④ Intellectual Dimension

We can best use our intellect when we are free from health problems. In some cases, diseases or medications can impair our intellectual functioning. However, managing a condition or recovering from an illness can allow you to learn about your body, your personality, and the health care system. Learning how to reduce your risk of certain diseases will also require you to draw on your intellectual resources.

⑤ Spiritual Dimension

Your ability to serve others can be hindered by an illness or chronic condition. In addition, your faith can be shaken when a family member falls ill or when you are diagnosed with a serious disease. For most people, however, this initial questioning leads to an even stronger faith or spirituality than they had before the experience.

⑥ Occupational Dimension

Diseases and your efforts to prevent them can have a significant effect on your job performance. If you have an acute illness, you probably will not be able to work temporarily. If you have a chronic condition or disease, you must try to manage it well enough that you are still able to work. Some conditions are so severe that employment becomes impossible. On the other hand, your efforts to prevent illness, such as fitness activities, will enhance your job performance.

⑦ Environmental Dimension

Diseases such as cancer and cardiovascular disease and conditions such as asthma and certain congenital abnormalities are caused or worsened by various environmental pollutants and toxins. Avoiding or minimizing these hazards is an important part of disease prevention.

chapter
ten

Reducing Your Risk of Cardiovascular Disease

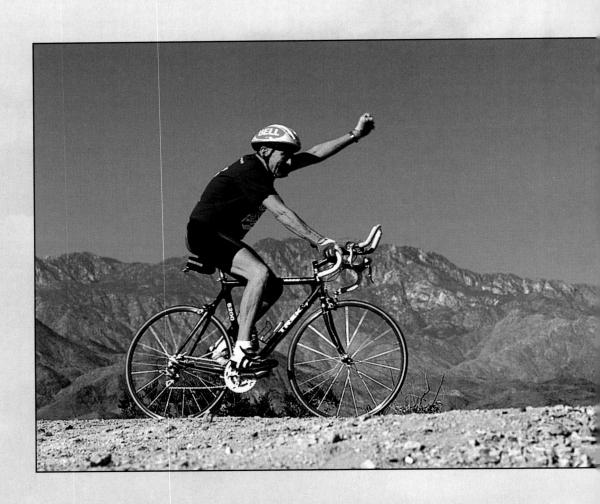

This section of the book contains four chapters that deal with diseases. Although uninformed people claim that "there is nothing you can do to avoid disease," ample evidence indicates that positive personal health choices can help reduce your risk of developing many diseases, from cardiovascular disease to cancer to sexually transmitted diseases, including HIV and AIDS.

In this chapter we will explain what you can do to reduce your risk of developing cardiovascular disease. Prevention efforts are most effective when started in childhood, but it is never too late to adopt a wellness lifestyle. Quitting smoking, becoming physically active, following a nutritious, low-fat diet, and controlling your blood pressure are important ways of reducing your risk of heart disease and improving your overall health.

HEALTHY PEOPLE: LOOKING AHEAD TO 2010

The *Midcourse Review* reported that we have successfully moved toward achieving 15 of the 17 *Healthy People 2000* objectives in the priority area of cardiovascular disease. This was not surprising, since widespread public education programs have been developed and implemented during the last 25 years. Measures to identify high-risk groups have been initiated and refined. The ability to control high blood pressure and blood cholesterol levels has improved markedly. A great deal of evidence now indicates that heart disease can indeed be prevented through lifestyle changes.

Nevertheless, cardiovascular disease remains the nation's number one cause of death and disability, considerably outdistancing the number two cause. The *Midcourse Review* reminded us that premature morbidity (sickness) is devastating for many heart disease patients. Affected people often cannot participate fully in daily activities, and many become unable to function independently. The annual economic impact of heart disease is estimated to be $259 billion, which includes health care expenses, medications, and lost work productivity resulting from disability and death.[1] Heart disease will certainly be among the most important chronic conditions addressed in the *Healthy People 2010* objectives now being drafted.

Real Life
Real choices

- Name: Greg Chulick
- Age: 10
- Occupation: Student, Boy Scout, Little Leaguer

"Enjoy being a kid—you'll be a grown up soon enough!"

If Greg Chulick had a nickel for every time he's heard those words from an older relative, he'd be a lot closer to affording that Duke Snider card at the Baseball Bonanza store downtown. He knows there are a lot of great things about being his age: like lazy afternoons fishing for carp in the Criders' pond, playing first base on the Little League team, and going on overnights with his scout troop.

As much as he has going for him, though, right now Greg is terrified. Why? Because for the last 3 days he's had a sore throat, and this morning it isn't any better. Like most kids, Greg ordinarily tells one of his parents when he isn't feeling well. But not this time.

If Greg were somebody else, a sore throat would be no bigger deal than a scrape, a bruise, or a belly-flop in the Y pool. But Greg isn't somebody else: he's the former big brother of Joey, a chunky, spunky 5-year-old who 3 years ago woke up

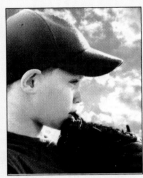

one morning with a sore throat and a month later was buried in All Saints Cemetery. Joey's sore throat turned out to have been caused by an infection that wasn't treated in time to prevent him from developing the disease that killed him—rheumatic fever.

Greg never talks about his little brother, because who would understand the hole in his life Joey left when he died? Who but Greg shared a room with him, traded secrets and jokes and kid crimes, helped him climb out on the roof one August night so they could watch a meteor shower while the rest of the family slept?

And now it's Greg's turn. He's got the sore throat that won't go away, the sore throat that isn't just *any* sore throat, except that's what everyone thought Joey had . . .

As you study this chapter, think about what Greg is experiencing and prepare yourself to answer the questions in **Your Turn** at the end of the chapter.

Great progress has been made with respect to **cardiovascular** disease (CVD), the focus of this chapter. Although heart disease continues to be the number one killer of Americans, between 1984 and 1994 the death rates from CVD declined 22.4 percent.[1] Still, CVD claimed nearly a million lives in 1995.[2] By comparison, cancer caused about 538,000 deaths, accidents caused about 93,000, and HIV/AIDS caused about 43,000. This means CVD caused 41.5 percent of all deaths, or one out of every 2.4 deaths in 1995. Today, more than 2,600 Americans die each day of CVD, an average of one death every 33 seconds. Interestingly, if all forms of cardiovascular disease were eliminated, life expectancy in the United States would increase by almost ten years.[3]

This chapter provides material to help you understand how the heart works. Beyond this, it will help you identify your CVD risk factors and suggest ways you can alter certain lifestyle behaviors to reduce your risk of developing heart disease.

Prevalence of Cardiovascular Disease

Cardiovascular diseases are directly related to more than 40 percent of deaths in the United States and indirectly related to a large percentage of additional deaths.[1] Fortunately, the rate of deaths from coronary heart disease has been falling. The decrease averaged 3 percent during the 1980s, but the decrease has slowed to 2.6 percent in the 1990s (Figure 10-1 and Table 10-1).[4]

Normal Cardiovascular Function

The cardiovascular system, also called the circulatory system, uses a muscular pump to send a complex fluid on a continuous trip through a closed system of tubes. The pump is the heart, the fluid is blood, and the closed system of tubes is the network of blood vessels.

The Vascular System

The term *vascular system* refers to the body's blood vessels. Although we might be familiar with the arteries (vessels that carry blood away from the heart) and the veins (vessels that carry blood to the heart), arterioles, capillaries, and venules are also part of the vascular system. Arterioles are the farther, smaller-diameter extensions of arteries. These arterioles lead eventually to capillaries, the smallest extensions of the vascular system. At the capillary level, oxygen, food, and waste are exchanged between cells and the blood.

After the blood leaves the capillaries and begins its return to the heart, it drains into small veins, or venules. The blood in the venules flows into in-

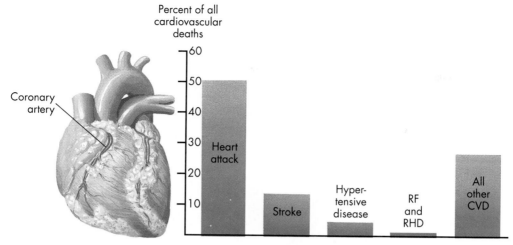

Figure 10-1 Of the 960,592 deaths in the United States in 1995 caused by cardiovascular diseases, half were attributable to heart attack.

Table 10-1	Estimated Prevalence of Major Cardiovascular Diseases*
Coronary heart disease	13,900,000
Hypertension	50,000,000
Stroke	4,000,000
Rheumatic heart disease	1,800,000
Total	69,700,000

*58,200,000 people total. The sum of the individual estimates exceeds 58,200,000 because so many people have more than one cardiovascular disorder.

creasingly larger vessels called *veins*. Blood pressure is highest in arteries and lowest in veins, especially the largest veins, which empty into the right atrium of the heart.

The Heart

The heart is a four-chambered pump designed to create the pressure required to circulate blood throughout the body. Usually considered to be about the size of a person's clenched fist, this organ lies slightly tilted between the lungs in the central portion of the **thorax**. The heart does not lie completely in the center of the chest. Rather, approximately two-thirds of the heart is to the left of the body midline and one third is to the right.[5]

Two upper chambers, called *atria*, and two lower chambers, called *ventricles*, form the heart. The thin-walled atrial chambers are considered collecting chambers, whereas the thick-walled muscular ventricles are considered the pumping chambers. The right and left sides of the heart are divided by a partition called the *septum*. Study Figure 10-2 and follow the flow of blood through the heart's four chambers.

To function well, the heart muscle must receive adequate amounts of oxygen. The two main **coronary arteries** (and their many branches) accomplish this. These arteries are located outside of the heart. If the coronary arteries are diseased and not functioning well, a heart attack is possible.

Heart Stimulation

The heart contracts and relaxes through the delicate interplay of **cardiac muscle** tissue and cardiac electrical centers, called *nodes*. Nodal tissue generates the electrical impulses necessary to contract heart muscle.[6] The heart's electrical activity is measured by an instrument called an *electrocardiograph (ECG or EKG)*, which provides a printout called an *electrocardiogram* that can be evaluated to determine cardiac electrical functioning.

Blood

The average-sized adult has approximately six quarts of blood in his or her circulatory system. Blood's functions, which are performed continuously, are quite

cardiovascular pertaining to the heart (cardio) and blood vessels (vascular).

thorax the chest; portion of the torso above the diaphragm and within the rib cage.

coronary arteries vessels that supply oxygenated blood to heart muscle tissues.

cardiac muscle specialized smooth muscle tissue that forms the middle (muscular) layer of the heart wall.

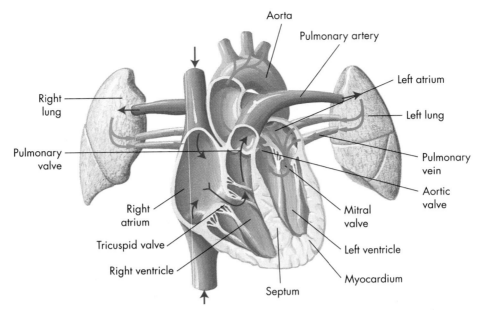

Figure 10-2 The heart functions like a complex double pump. The right side of the heart pumps deoxygenated blood to the lungs. The left side of the heart pumps oxygenated blood through the aorta to all parts of the body. Note the thickness of the walls of the ventricles. These are the primary pumping chambers.

similar to the overall functions of the circulatory system and include the following:

- Transportation of nutrients, oxygen, wastes, hormones, and enzymes
- Regulation of water content of body cells and fluids
- Buffering to help maintain appropriate pH balance of body fluids
- Regulation of body temperature; the water component in the blood absorbs heat and transfers it
- Prevention of blood loss; by coagulating or clotting, the blood can alter its form to prevent blood loss through injured vessels
- Protection against toxins and microorganisms, accomplished by chemical substances called *antibodies* and specialized cellular elements circulating in the bloodstream.

Cardiovascular Disease Risk Factors

As you have just read, the heart and blood vessels are among the most important structures in the human body. By protecting your cardiovascular system, you lay the groundwork for a more exciting, productive, and energetic life. The best time to start protecting and improving your cardiovascular system is early in life, when lifestyle patterns are developed and reinforced (see the Star Box on p. 301). Of course, it is difficult to move

backward through time, so the second best time to start protecting your heart is today. Improvements in certain lifestyle activities can pay significant dividends as your life unfolds. Complete the Personal Assessment on page 302 to estimate your risk for heart disease.

The American Heart Association encourages people to protect and enhance their heart health by examining the ten cardiovascular risk factors that are related to various forms of heart disease. A *cardiovascular risk factor* is an attribute that a person has or is exposed to that increases the likelihood that he or she will develop some form of heart disease. Three risk factors are those you will be unable to change. An additional six risk factors are those you can clearly change. One final risk factor is thought to be a contributing factor to heart disease. The American Heart Association recently moved obesity and diabetes from the category of contributing risk factors to the category of risk factors that you can clearly change.[7] These risk factors are summarized in the Star Box on page 303. Let's look at these three groups of risk factors separately.

Risk Factors That Cannot Be Changed

The three risk factors that you cannot change are increasing age, male gender, and heredity. Despite the fact that these risk factors cannot be changed, your knowledge that they might be an influence in your life should encourage you to make a more serious commitment to the risk factors you *can* change.

Prevention of Heart Disease Begins in Childhood

For many aspects of wellness, preventive behaviors are often best learned in childhood, where they can be repeated and reinforced by family members and caregivers. This is especially true for behaviors to prevent heart disease. Although many problems related to heart disease are seen most frequently at midlife and beyond, the roots of heart disease start early in life.

For example, researchers studying children and using autopsies have found that hypertension, or high blood pressure, begins in early childhood. Intervention programs that target children have been shown to be effective in preventing hypertensive cardiovascular disease.[8]

Likewise, atherosclerotic cardiovascular disease, the type of disease that can result in heart attacks, reaches substantial levels in men beginning at age 45 and in women at age 55, but the disease has its onset in childhood. The disease progresses according to each individual's level of risk factors. That is, the unhealthier the person's lifestyle, with behaviors such as smoking, lack of exercise, or poor diet, the more quickly the disease develops. Even in people who are genetically predisposed for cardiovascular disease, the disease usually requires an unhealthy lifestyle for it actually to take effect.[9]

So, we now know that efforts to promote cardiovascular health in childhood can have a dramatic effect after the child grows up. In response, experts have identified five major areas as targets for cardiovascular health promotion in childhood: obesity, cardiovascular fitness, hypertension, hypercholesterolemia (high blood levels of cholesterol), and smoking prevention.[10]

Sadly, the present state of health of America's youth shows severe deficiencies in these areas. Children's diets lack nutrient density and remain alarmingly high in overall fat. Teenage children are becoming increasingly overweight and obese. Studies consistently show a deterioration in the amount of physical activity by today's youth, as television and video games have become the after-school companions for large numbers of children. Sadly, cigarette smoking continues to rise among schoolchildren, especially teenagers.

These unhealthy behaviors are laying the foundation for coronary artery disease, hypertension, and stroke in the future. Rather than trying to repair sick people in their older years, increased efforts on childhood prevention should be a focus for today's adults.

Programs that seek to instill healthy behaviors in children can have a real benefit. One study found that, of all children, those most at risk of cardiovascular disease also showed the greatest benefit from lifestyle intervention programs. The study found the greatest benefit in two types of programs: improving home nutrition and improving fitness.[11]

Those of us who are parents must make better efforts to encourage our children to eat more nutritiously and be physically active. We can discourage cigarette use. Perhaps the best thing all adults can do for our youth is to set a good example by adopting our own heart-healthy behaviors. Following the Food Guide Pyramid and exercising regularly are excellent strategies that can be started early in life.

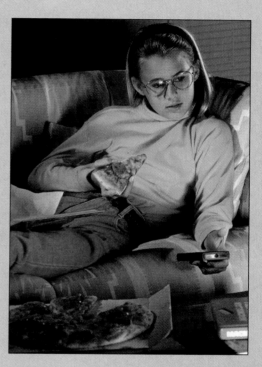

Physical inactivity and a poor diet can set the stage for heart disease later in life.

Increasing Age

Heart disease tends to develop gradually over the course of one's life. Although we may know of a person or two who experienced a heart attack in their thirties or forties, most of the serious consequences of heart disease become evident as we age. For example, nearly 85 percent of people who die from heart attack are aged sixty-five and older.

Being Male

Young men have a greater risk of heart disease than young women. Yet when women move through menopause (typically in their fifties), their rates of heart disease become similar to men's rates (see the Star Box on p. 304). It is thought that women are somewhat more protected from heart disease than men because of their natural production of the hormone estrogen during their fertile years.

Heredity

Obviously, you have no input in determining whom your biological parents are. Like increasing age and male gender, this risk factor cannot be changed. By the luck of the draw, some people are born into families where heart disease has never been a serious problem, whereas others are born into families where

Personal Assessment

Cholesterol

Your serum cholesterol level is:

0	190 or below
+ 2	191 to 230
+ 6	231 to 289
+12	290 to 319
+16	Over 320

Your HDL cholesterol is:

− 2	Over 60
0	45 to 60
+ 2	35 to 44
+ 6	29 to 34
+12	23 to 28
+16	Below 23

Smoking

You smoke now or have in the past:

0	Never smoked, or quit more than 5 years ago
+1	Quit 2 to 4 years ago
+3	Quit about 1 year ago
+6	Quit during the past year

You now smoke:

+ 9	½ to 1 pack a day
+12	1 to 2 packs a day
+15	More than 2 packs a day

The quality of the air you breathe is:

0	Unpolluted by smoke, exhaust, or industry at home **and** at work
+2	Live **or** work with smokers in unpolluted area
+4	Live **and** work with smokers in unpolluted area
+6	Live **or** work with smokers **and** live or work in air-polluted area
+8	Live **and** work with smokers **and** live and work in air-polluted area

Blood Pressure

Your blood pressure is:

0	120/75 or below
+ 2	120/75 to 140/85
+ 6	140/85 to 150/90
+ 8	150/90 to 175/100
+10	175/100 to 190/110
+12	190/110 or above

Exercise

Your exercise habits are:

0	Exercise vigorously 4 or 5 times a week
+2	Exercise moderately 4 or 5 times a week
+4	Exercise only on weekends
+6	Exercise occasionally
+8	Little or no exercise

Weight

Your weight is:

0	Always at or near ideal weight
+1	Now 10% overweight
+2	Now 20% overweight
+3	Now 30% or more overweight
+4	Now 20% or more overweight and have been since before age 30

Stress

You feel overstressed:

0	Rarely at work or at home
+ 3	Somewhat at home but not at work
+ 5	Somewhat at work but not at home
+ 7	Somewhat at work **and** at home
+ 9	Usually at work **or** at home
+12	Usually at work **and** at home

Diabetes

Your diabetic history is:

0	Blood sugar always normal
+2	Blood glucose slightly high (prediabetic) or slightly low (hypoglycemic)
+4	Diabetic beginning after age 40 requiring strict dietary or insulin control
+5	Diabetic beginning before age 30 requiring strict dietary or insulin control

Alcohol

You drink alcoholic beverages:

0	Never or only socially, about once or twice a month, or only one 5-ounce glass of wine or 12-ounce glass of beer or 1½ ounces of hard liquor about 5 times a week
+2	Two to three 5-ounce glasses of wine or 12-ounce glasses of beer or 1½-ounce cocktails about 5 times a week
+4	More than three 1½-ounce cocktails or more than three 5-ounce glasses of wine or 12-ounce glasses of beer almost every day

Interpretation

Add all sources and check below

0 to 20: Low risk. Excellent family history and lifestyle habits.

21 to 50: Moderate risk. Family history or lifestyle habits put you at some risk. You might lower your risks and minimize your genetic predisposition if you change any poor habits.

51 to 74: High risk. Habits and family history indicate high risk of heart disease. Change your habits now.

Above 75: Very high risk. Family history and a lifetime of poor habits put you at very high risk of heart disease. Eliminate as many of the risk factors as you can.

To Carry This Further . . .

Were you surprised with your score on this assessment? What were your most significant risk factors? Do you plan to make any changes in your lifestyle to reduce your cardiovascular risks? Why or why not?

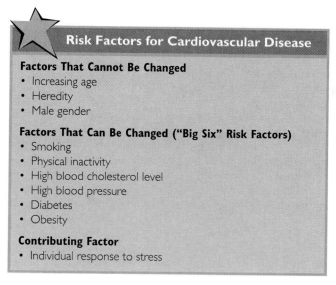

Risk Factors for Cardiovascular Disease

Factors That Cannot Be Changed
- Increasing age
- Heredity
- Male gender

Factors That Can Be Changed ("Big Six" Risk Factors)
- Smoking
- Physical inactivity
- High blood cholesterol level
- High blood pressure
- Diabetes
- Obesity

Contributing Factor
- Individual response to stress

heart disease is quite prevalent. In this latter case, children are said to have a genetic predisposition (tendency) to develop heart disease as they grow and develop throughout their lives. These people have every reason to be highly motivated to reduce the risk factors they can control.

Race is also a consideration related to heart disease. African-Americans have moderately high blood pressure at rates twice that of whites and severe hypertension at rates three times higher than whites[1] (for a detailed discussion of this topic, see the Topics for Today article on p. 321). Hypertension significantly increases the risk of both heart disease and stroke. Fortunately, as you will soon read, hypertension can be controlled through a variety of methods. It is especially important for African-Americans to take advantage of every opportunity to have their blood pressure measured so that preventive actions can be started immediately if necessary.

Risk Factors That Can Be Changed

Six cardiovascular risk factors are influenced, in large part, by our lifestyle choices. These risk factors are smoking, physical inactivity, high blood cholesterol level, high blood pressure, diabetes, and obesity. Healthful behavior changes you make concerning these "big six" risk factors can help you protect and strengthen your cardiovascular system.

Smoking

Although the other three controllable risk factors are important, this one may be the most critical risk factor. Smokers have a heart attack risk that is more than twice that of nonsmokers. Smoking cigarettes is the major risk factor associated with sudden cardiac death. In fact, smokers have two to four times the risk of dying from sudden cardiac arrest than nonsmokers. Smokers who experience a heart attack are more

likely to die suddenly (within an hour) than those who don't smoke.

Smoking also adversely affects nonsmokers who are exposed to environmental tobacco smoke. Studies suggest that the risk of death caused by heart disease is increased about 30 percent in people exposed to secondhand smoke in the home. The risk of death caused by heart disease may even be higher in people exposed to environmental tobacco smoke in work settings (for example, bars, casinos, enclosed offices, some bowling alleys and restaurants), since higher levels of smoke may be present at work than at home. Because of the health threat to nonsmokers, restrictions on indoor smoking in public areas and business settings are increasing tremendously in every part of the country.

For years it was commonly believed that if you had smoked for many years, it was pointless to try to quit; the damage to one's health could never be reversed. However, the American Heart Association now indicates that by quitting smoking, regardless of how long or how much you have smoked, your risk of heart disease declines rapidly (see Figure 9-3, on p. 282). For people who have smoked a pack or less of cigarettes per day, within three years after quitting smoking, their heart disease risk is virtually the same as those who never smoked.[3]

This news is exciting and should encourage people to quit smoking, regardless of how long they have smoked. Of course, if you have started to smoke, the healthy approach would be to quit now . . . before the nicotine controls your life and damages your heart. (For additional information about the health effects of tobacco, see Chapter 9.)

Physical Inactivity

Lack of exercise is a significant risk factor for heart disease. Regular aerobic exercise (discussed in Chapter 4) helps strengthen the heart muscle, maintain healthy blood vessels, and improve the ability of the vascular system to transfer blood and oxygen to all parts of the body. In addition, physical activity helps lower overall blood cholesterol levels for most people, encourages weight loss and retention of lean muscle mass, and allows people to moderate the stress in their lives.

With all the benefits that come with physical activity, it amazes health professionals that so many Americans refuse to participate in regular exercise. Perhaps people feel that they do not have enough time or that they must work out strenuously. However, you will recall from Chapter 4 that only twenty to sixty minutes of moderate aerobic activity three to five times each week is recommended. This is not a large price to pay for a lifetime of cardiovascular health. Find a partner and get started!

Women and Heart Disease

Do you think heart disease is a problem just for men? You might be surprised to discover that data from the American Heart Association indicate that 52 percent of all cardiovascular disease deaths are in women. There are 20,800 women under age 65 who die from heart attack each year, and 29 percent of women who die from coronary artery disease are under age 55. In addition, 44 percent of women who have a heart attack will die within 1 year, compared with 27 percent of men. A total of 60 percent of the deaths from stroke and high blood pressure are in women, compared with 40 percent in men. Women who smoke and also take oral contraceptives are 39 times more likely to have a heart attack and 22 times more likely to have a stroke than women who neither smoke nor use oral contraceptives.[12]

For many years, it was thought that men were at much greater risk than women for the development of cardiovascular problems. It is now known that younger men are more prone to heart disease than young women, yet once women reach menopause (usually in their early to middle 50s), their rates of heart-related problems quickly equal those of men.

Among people having heart attacks, one study found the drug TPA to save 17 lives per 1,000 women and 7 per 1,000 men.[13] TPA benefits women more than men because women are at greater risk of dying from their heart attacks. The study also found that women delayed seeking treatment for their heart attack 18 minutes longer than men, and once they were in the hospital, doctors took longer to treat women. In both cases, the study suggested, the reason may be that women may not recognize the symptoms of a heart attack. Women often experience abdominal pain and fatigue with chest pain. On the other hand, those who do experience chest pain in response to stress are more likely to be women, according to a recent study.[14] In this study of people with heart disease, those who experienced chest pain during stress were more likely to be women, have a history of high blood pressure, and have greater increases in heart rate than those without chest pain. Such symptoms can have a silver lining, in that they may motivate people to seek medical help. For a look at the differences in the way women and men are diagnosed and treated in cases of cardiovascular disease, see the Star Box below.

The protective mechanism for young women seems to be the female hormone estrogen. Estrogen appears to help women maintain a beneficial profile of blood fats. When the production of estrogen is severely reduced at menopause, this protective factor no longer exists. This is one of the reasons that increasing numbers of physicians are prescribing estrogen replacement therapy (ERT) for many postmenopausal women. For women who already have coronary disease, however, hormone therapy appears to have no benefit and may in fact be harmful.[15]

Of course, young women should not rely solely on naturally produced estrogen to prevent heart disease. The general recommendations for maintaining heart health through a good diet, adequate physical activity, monitoring blood pressure and cholesterol levels, controlling weight, avoiding smoking, and managing stress will benefit women at every stage of life.

Do Women Receive Equal Treatment in Cardiovascular Disease?

The short answer is no; women do not receive the same level of diagnosis or treatment for cardiovascular disorders as do men. In addition, the procedures and therapies we currently use were developed predominantly or completely for men.[16]

Researchers report that the history of medicine shows a disregard for women's health problems that may prevail even today. Women are older and sicker when they have cardiovascular treatments such as angioplasty or bypass grafting, and they receive far fewer heart transplants.

These differences may be a result of the difference in the way women experience cardiac symptoms. For example, women often experience abdominal pain and fatigue with chest pain. Other possibilities are problems in the referrals women receive, or in the way women perceive themselves and their illness.

In response, medical professionals are now attempting to provide equitable health care for women and to conduct research that will describe women's cardiac symptoms and their responses to cardiovascular treatments.

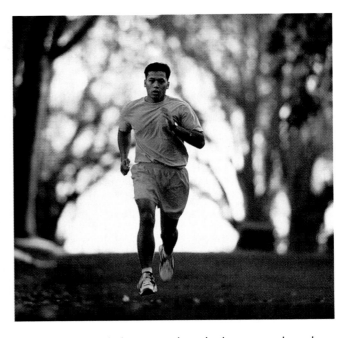

Regular exercise helps strengthen the heart muscle and lower overall blood cholesterol.

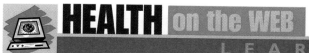

HEALTH on the WEB

LEARNING ACTIVITIES

Determining Your Risk of Heart Disease

The American Heart Association encourages people to protect and enhance their heart health by examining the ten cardiovascular risk factors that are related to various forms of heart disease. Visit the American Heart Association's website, at www.amhrt.org. Click on *What's Your Risk of Heart Disease?* How can you change your behavior to reduce your risk?

Avoiding High-Fat Diets

A controllable risk factor for heart disease is having a high blood cholesterol level. People with high blood cholesterol are encouraged to follow a heart-healthy diet. Most people can lower their serum cholesterol level by adopting three dietary changes: lowering their intake of saturated fats, reducing dietary cholesterol, and controlling caloric intake. Go to

www.olen.com/food, and use the interactive *Fast-Food Facts* list to determine the amount of fat in your favorite fast foods. How can you use this information to make sound decisions about your food selections?

Raising Your Awareness of High Blood Pressure

A controllable risk factor for heart disease is high blood pressure, or hypertension. To find out more about this "silent killer," visit the Hypertension Network's home page, www.bloodpressure.com. Select *Q & A*, and then select *Lifestyles*. Choose a topic that you would like to learn more about. How can you make better lifestyle choices to reduce your risk of high blood pressure?

For more activities, log on to our Online Learning Center at www.mhhe.com/hper/health/payne

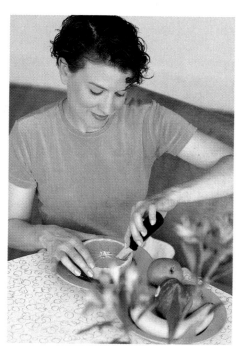

People who have high cholesterol should follow a heart-healthy diet based on the Food Guide Pyramid.

If you are middle-aged or older and have been inactive, you should consult with a physician before starting an exercise program. Also, if you have any known health condition that could be aggravated by physical activity, check with a physician first.

High Blood Cholesterol Level

The third controllable risk factor for heart disease is high blood cholesterol level. Generally speaking, the higher the blood cholesterol level, the greater the risk for heart disease. When high blood cholesterol levels

are combined with other important risk factors, the risks become much greater.

Fortunately, blood cholesterol levels are relatively easy to measure. Many campus health and wellness centers provide cholesterol screenings for employees and students. These screenings help identify people whose cholesterol levels (or profiles) may be dangerous. Medical professionals have linked people's diets with their cholesterol levels. People with high blood cholesterol levels are encouraged to consume a heart-healthy diet (see Chapter 5) and to become physically active. In recent years, researchers have developed a variety of drugs that are very effective at lowering cholesterol levels. In a later section in this chapter, you will read more about cholesterol.

High Blood Pressure

The fourth of the six cardiovascular risk factors that can be changed is high blood pressure, or hypertension. High blood pressure can seriously damage a person's heart and blood vessels. High blood pressure causes the heart to work much harder, eventually causing the heart to enlarge and weaken. High blood pressure increases the risk of stroke, heart attack, congestive heart failure, and kidney disease.

When high blood pressure is seen with other risk factors, the risk for stroke or heart attack is increased tremendously. As you will soon see, this "silent killer" is easy to monitor and can be effectively controlled through a variety of approaches.

Personal Applications

• In the last week, what have you done to improve your cardiovascular system?

Diabetes

Diabetes mellitus (discussed in detail in Chapter 12) is a debilitating chronic disease that has a significant effect on the human body. In addition to increasing the risk of developing kidney disease, blindness, and nerve damage, diabetes increases the likelihood of developing heart and blood vessel diseases. More than 80 percent of people with diabetes die of some type of heart or blood vessel disease. The cardiovascular damage is thought to occur when diabetes begins to alter normal cholesterol and blood fat levels. With weight management, exercise, dietary changes, and drug therapy, diabetes can be relatively well controlled in most people. Despite careful management of this disease, diabetic patients remain quite susceptible to eventual heart and blood vessel damage.

Obesity

Even if they have no other risk factors, obese people are more likely than nonobese people to develop heart disease and stroke. Obesity places considerable strain on the heart, and it tends to worsen both blood pressure and blood cholesterol levels. Obese men and women can expect a greater risk of heart disease, and as a result, a greater cost of medical care for the treatment of their heart disease throughout their lives.[17] Also, obesity tends to trigger diabetes in predisposed people.[3] Maintaining body weight within a desirable range minimizes the chances of obesity ever happening. To accomplish this, you can elect to make a commitment to a reasonably sound diet and an active lifestyle.

Other Risk Factor That Contributes to Heart Disease

The American Heart Association identifies one other risk factor that is associated with an increased risk of heart disease. This risk factor is individual response to stress.

Individual Response to Stress

Unresolved stress over a long period may be a contributing factor to the development of heart disease. Certainly, people who are unable to cope with stressful life experiences are more likely to develop negative dependence behaviors (for example, smoking, underactivity, poor dietary practices), which can then lead to cardiovascular problems through changes in blood fat profiles, blood pressure, and heart workload. To discover ways of coping with stress, you might wish to return to the discussion in Chapter 3.

Personal Applications

• Are you comfortable talking with your relatives about their possible risk factors for heart disease?

Forms of Cardiovascular Disease

The American Heart Association describes the three major forms of CVD as coronary heart disease, hypertension, and stroke. These three diseases account for 70 percent of the deaths due to CVD.[2] Additionally, many other diseases can affect the heart and blood vessels, such as congenital heart disease, rheumatic heart disease, peripheral artery disease, congestive heart failure, and arrhythmias. (These other CVDs will be discussed later in the chapter.)

A person may have just one of these three diseases or a combination of forms at the same time. Each form exists in varying degrees of severity. All forms are capable of causing secondary damage to other body organs and systems.

Coronary Heart Disease

This form of CVD, also known as *coronary artery disease*, involves damage to the vessels that supply blood to the heart muscle. The bulk of this blood is supplied by the coronary arteries. Any damage to these important vessels can cause a reduction of blood flow (with its vital oxygen and nutrients) to specific areas of heart muscle. The ultimate result of an inadequate blood supply is a heart attack.

Atherosclerosis

The principal cause of coronary heart disease is **atherosclerosis** (Figure 10-3). Atherosclerosis produces a narrowing of the coronary arteries. This narrowing stems from the long-term buildup of fatty deposits, called *plaque*, on the inner walls of the arteries. This buildup reduces the blood supply to specific portions of the heart. Some arteries of the heart can become so blocked (occluded) that all blood supply is stopped. Heart muscle tissue begins to die when it is deprived of oxygen and nutrients. This damage is known as **myocardial infarction**. In lay terms, this event is called a heart attack. The Health Action Guide on page 307 explains how to recognize the signs of a heart attack and what to do next.

Cholesterol and Lipoproteins For many years, scientists have known that atherosclerosis is a complicated disease that has many causes. Some of these

atherosclerosis the buildup of plaque on the inner walls of arteries.

myocardial infarction heart attack; the death of part of the heart muscle as a result of a blockage in one of the coronary arteries.

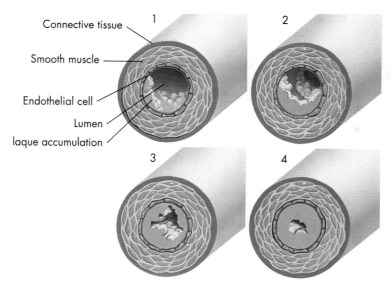

Figure 10-3 Progression of atherosclerosis. This diagram shows how plaque deposits gradually accumulate to narrow the lumen (interior space) of an artery. Although enlarged here, coronary arteries are only as wide as a pencil lead.

Labels on figure: Connective tissue, Smooth muscle, Endothelial cell, Lumen, Plaque accumulation

HEALTH ACTION GUIDE

Recognizing Signs of a Heart Attack and Taking Action

Warning Signs of a Heart Attack

- Uncomfortable pressure, fullness, squeezing, or pain in the center of your chest, and for women, in the abdomen, lasting 2 minutes or longer
- Pain spreading to your shoulders, neck, or arms
- Severe pain, dizziness, fainting, sweating, nausea, or shortness of breath

   Not all of these warning signs occur with every heart attack. If some start to occur, don't wait. Get help immediately!

What to Do in an Emergency

- Find out which hospitals in your area have 24-hour emergency cardiac care.
- Determine (in advance) the hospital or medical facility that is nearest your home and office, and tell your family and friends to call this facility in an emergency.
- Keep a list of emergency rescue service numbers next to your telephone and in your pocket, wallet, or purse.

- If you have chest discomfort that lasts for 2 minutes or more, call the emergency rescue service.
- If you can get to a hospital faster by going yourself and not waiting for an ambulance, have someone drive you there.

Be a Heart Saver

- If you are with someone experiencing the signs of a heart attack and the warning signs last for 2 minutes or longer, act immediately.
- Expect a denial. It is normal for someone with chest discomfort to deny the possibility of something as serious as a heart attack. Don't take no for an answer. Insist on taking prompt action.
- Call the rescue service (911), or get to the nearest hospital emergency room that offers 24-hour emergency cardiac care.
- Give CPR (mouth-to-mouth breathing and chest compression) if it is necessary and if you are properly trained.
- If you do not know CPR, enroll in a CPR class as soon as possible! The American Red Cross and the American Heart Association are two organizations that offer CPR training.

InfoLinks

www.columbia-utah.com/heartattack.html

causes are not well understood, but others are clearly understood. Cholesterol, a soft, fatlike material, is manufactured in the liver and small intestine and is necessary in the formation of sex hormones, cell membranes, bile salts, and nerve fibers. Elevated levels of serum cholesterol (200 mg/dl or more for adults aged twenty and older, and 170 mg/dl or more for young people under age 20) are associated with an increased risk of developing atherosclerosis.[3]

Some 52 percent of American adults aged twenty and older exceed the "borderline high" 200 mg/dl cholesterol level. Experts estimate that nearly 40 percent of American youth aged nineteen and under have "borderline high" cholesterol levels of 170 mg/dl or above. Twenty percent of American adults have "high" blood cholesterol levels, that is, 240 mg/dl or greater.[1]

Initially, most people can help lower their serum cholesterol level by adopting three dietary changes: lowering the intake of saturated fats, lowering the intake of dietary cholesterol, and lowering caloric intake to a level that does not exceed body requirements. The aim is to reduce excess fat, cholesterol, and calories in our diet while promoting sound nutrition. By carefully following such a diet, people with elevated serum cholesterol levels are typically able to reduce their cholesterol levels by 30 to 55 mg/dl.[18] However, dietary changes do not affect people equally; some will experience greater reductions than others. Some will not respond at all to dietary changes and may need to take cholesterol-lowering medications and increase physical activity.

Cholesterol is attached to structures called *lipoproteins*. Lipoproteins are particles that circulate in the blood and transport lipids (including cholesterol).[3] The two major classes of lipoproteins are **low-density lipoproteins (LDLs)** and **high-density lipoproteins (HDLs)**. A person's total cholesterol level is essentially determined by the amount of the LDLs and HDLs in a measured sample of blood. (For example, a person's total cholesterol level of 200 mg/dl could be represented by an LDL level of 160 and an HDL level of 40, or an LDL level of 140 and an HDL level of 60.)

After much study, researchers have determined that high levels of LDL are a significant cause of atherosclerosis. This makes sense because LDLs carry the greatest percentage of cholesterol in the bloodstream. LDLs are more likely to deposit excess cholesterol into the artery walls. This contributes to plaque formation. For this reason, LDLs are often called the "bad cholesterol."[1] High LDL levels are determined partly by inheritance, but they are also clearly associated with smoking, poor dietary patterns, obesity, and lack of exercise.

On the other hand, high levels of HDLs are related to a decrease in the development of atherosclerosis. HDLs are thought to transport cholesterol out of the bloodstream. Thus HDLs have been called the "good cholesterol." Certain lifestyle alterations, such as quitting smoking, reducing obesity, increasing physical activity, and decreasing dietary fats, help many people increase their level of HDLs.

Reducing total serum cholesterol levels is a significant step in reducing the risk of death from coronary heart disease. For people with elevated cholesterol levels, a 1 percent reduction in serum cholesterol level yields about a 2 percent reduction in the risk of death from heart disease. Thus a 10 percent to 15 percent cholesterol reduction can reduce risk by 20 percent to 30 percent.[22] For high-risk patients, especially those with heart disease or very high cholesterol levels, a group of cholesterol-reducing drugs known as the "statin" drugs have dramatically reduced the risk of death from heart disease.[23] For most people, however, the decision to take such drugs to reduce cholesterol depends on each individual's risk.

Ritalin Heart Risk Concern

Along with the explosive popularity of Ritalin (methylphenidate) as a treatment for children with attention deficit disorder (ADD) has some concern that the drug might pose a risk of sudden cardiac death. The concern is "overblown," however, says the American Heart Association, and can be eliminated during the examination before Ritalin is prescribed.[19] The use of Ritalin as a treatment for conditions such as ADD has increased twofold from 1990 to 1995. Nearly 3 percent of all U.S. young people ages 5 to 18 were receiving this medication in 1995.[20]

The fear of possible heart damage was sparked by seven reports since the late 1980s of sudden death in children taking psychotropic medications. Psychotropic medications can interfere with the conduction system of the heart and should not be given to children with conduction abnormalities. One study using rats and mice found that Ritalin damaged the myocardium of the heart.[21] The American Heart Association stresses the need for the physician to take a careful history of the patient before prescribing Ritalin.[19] Electrocardiograms can help identify the rare cases involving children who are at risk of sudden cardiac death.

Personal Applications

- Do you know your total cholesterol reading? Do you know your levels of LDLs and HDLs?

Angina Pectoris When coronary arteries become narrowed, chest pain, or angina pectoris, is often felt. This pain is caused by a reduced supply of oxygen to heart muscle tissue. Usually, a patient feels angina when he or she becomes stressed or exercises too strenuously. Angina reportedly can range from a feeling of mild indigestion to a severe viselike pressure in the chest. The pain may extend from the center of the chest to the arms and even up to the jaw. Generally, the more severe the blockage, the more pain is felt.

Some cardiac patients relieve angina with the drug nitroglycerin, a powerful blood vessel dilator.

HEALTHQUEST ACTIVITIES

- The *Heart Attack Risk* and *Cardiovascular Exploration* activities in Module 5 allow you to assess your risk for cardiovascular disease. In the first of these activities, *Heart Attack Risk*, answer the questions about your health history, behavioral practices, and knowledge about heart disease. HealthQuest will then provide the correct answers and point out any health risks indicated by your responses. In the *Cardiovascular Exploration* section, fill out all of the items, and then click on the "Show Me!" button to find out your overall risk. You can get more specific feedback on each risk factor by clicking on the underlined words.

- Many traditional-age college students have difficulty understanding how cardiovascular disease affects quality of life. Heart disease seems only a distant possibility, but for many, it can become all too real. To learn more, read about heart disease among women and minority groups in the *Social Perspectives* section. List several health choices that can increase the likelihood of developing cardiovascular disease, and explain how one's family history can affect the risk. Finally, describe what you would do if you observed someone having a heart attack.

This prescription drug, available in slow-release transdermal patches or small pills that are placed under the patient's tongue, causes the coronary arteries to dilate and allow a greater flow of blood into heart muscle tissue. Other cardiac patients may be prescribed drugs such as **calcium channel blockers** or **beta blockers**.

Emergency Response to Heart Crises

Heart attacks are not always fatal. The consequences of any heart attack depend on the location of the damage to the heart, the extent to which heart muscle is damaged, and the speed with which adequate circulation is restored. Injury to the ventricles may very well prove fatal unless medical countermeasures are immediately undertaken. Recognizing a heart attack is critically important (see the Health Action Guide on p. 307).

Cardiopulmonary resuscitation (CPR) is one of the most important immediate countermeasures that trained people can use when confronted with a person having a heart attack. Public education programs sponsored by the American Red Cross and the American Heart Association teach people how to recognize, evaluate, and manage heart attack emergencies. CPR trainees are taught how to restore breathing (through mouth-to-mouth resuscitation) and circulation (through external chest compression) in people who require such emergency countermeasures. Frequently, colleges offer CPR classes through health science or physical education departments. We encourage each student to enroll in a CPR course.

Diagnosis

After a person's vital signs have stabilized, further diagnostic examinations can reveal the type and extent of damage to heart muscle. Initially an ECG might be taken. This test analyzes the electrical activity of the heart. Heart catheterization, also called *coronary arteriography*, is a minor surgical procedure that starts by placing a thin plastic tube into an arm or leg artery.

This tube, called a *catheter*, is guided through the artery until it reaches the coronary circulation, where a radiopaque dye is then released. X-ray pictures called *angiograms* then record the progress of the dye through the coronary arteries. Areas of blockage are relatively easily identified.

Recently, researchers have greatly expanded the use of magnetic resonance imaging (MRI) in cardiovascular diagnosis. In the past, MRI has been used to illustrate the cardiac anatomy, congenital malformations, thrombi, and masses. Now MRI is also used to illustrate the anatomy of coronary arteries and the function of the heart, enabling physicians to evaluate such problems as valvular disease and cardiac shunts.[24] MRI is combined with electrocardiogram (ECG) studies to illustrate the function of the left ventricle.

Nuclear medicine is another important tool in the diagnosis of cardiac disease. Nuclear medicine uses radiopharmaceuticals such as Thallium-201 to map blood flow and perfusion of tissues. Physicians use such tools to study the function of the heart and diagnose cardiac problems. Other radiopharmaceuticals are used to reveal metabolic disorders, hypoxia, and disturbances in the function of the myocardium of the heart.[25]

---

low-density lipoprotein (LDL)   the type of lipoprotein that transports the largest amount of cholesterol in the bloodstream; high levels of LDL are related to heart disease.

high-density lipoprotein (HDL)   the type of lipoprotein that transports cholesterol from the bloodstream to the liver, where it is eventually removed from the body; high levels of HDL are related to a reduction in heart disease.

calcium channel blockers   drugs that prevent arterial spasms; used in the long-term management of angina pectoris.

beta blockers   drugs that prevent overactivity of the heart, which results in angina pectoris.

Treatment

After the extent of damage has been determined, a physician or team of physicians can decide on a medical course of action. Treatments can be divided into two broad categories: surgical and nonsurgical.

Surgical Treatments   Currently popular is an extensive form of surgery called **coronary artery bypass surgery.** About 400,000 bypass surgeries are performed each year. The purpose of such surgery is to detour (bypass) areas of coronary artery obstruction by using a section of a vein from the patient's leg (often the saphenous vein) or an artery from the patient's chest (the internal mammary artery) and grafting it from the aorta to a location just beyond the area of obstruction. Multiple areas of obstruction result in double, triple, or quadruple bypasses. The average cost of coronary bypass surgery exceeds $50,000.[1]

Surgeons have recently begun performing heart bypass surgery through a three-inch incision in the rib cage, along with two to four small incisions in the patient's chest, rather than the traditional large, twelve- to fifteen-inch incision. Physicians manipulate the coronary arteries through the small ports, and they view their work through a fiber-optic camera called a *thoracoscope.* This new technique results in much less pain and blood loss, a shorter hospital stay, and a quicker recovery for the patient. This method has been nicknamed "keyhole" surgery and is still considered to be somewhat experimental.

Angioplasty. Angioplasty, an alternative to bypass surgery, involves the surgical insertion of a doughnut-shaped "balloon" directly into the narrowed coronary artery (Figure 10-4). When this balloon is inflated, plaque and fatty deposits are compressed against the artery walls, widening the space through which blood flows. These balloons usually remain within the artery for less than an hour. Renarrowing of the artery will occur in about one-quarter of angioplasty patients.[3] Each year, about 400,000 people with heart disease undergo angioplasty.

Balloon angioplasty can be used for blockages in the heart, kidneys, arms, and legs. The decision whether to have angioplasty or bypass surgery can be a difficult one to make.[26]

The FDA has approved a new device for clearing heart and leg arteries. This device is called a *motorized scraper.* Inserted through a leg artery and held in place by a tiny inflated balloon, this motor-driven cutter shaves off plaque deposits from inside the artery. A nose cone in the scraper unit stores the plaque until the device is removed.

The use of laser beams to dissolve plaque that blocks arteries has been slowly evolving. The FDA has approved three laser devices for use in clogged leg arteries. In February 1992 the FDA approved the

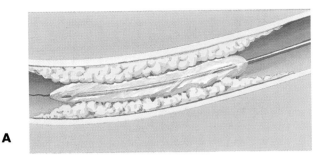

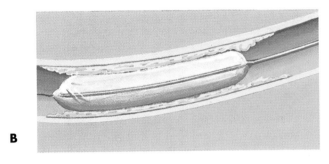

Figure 10-4   Angioplasty. **A,** A "balloon" is surgically inserted into the narrowed coronary artery. **B,** The balloon is inflated, compressing plaque and fatty deposits against the artery walls.

use of an excimer laser for use in coronary arteries.[27] Recently, refinements in the use of the excimer laser for coronary angioplasty have improved the success rate to 90 percent.[28]

Heart transplants and artificial hearts. For approximately thirty years, surgeons have been able to surgically replace a person's damaged heart with that of another human being. Although very risky, these transplant operations have added years to the lives of a number of patients who otherwise would have lived only a short time.

Artificial hearts have also been developed and implanted in humans. These mechanical devices have extended the lives of patients and have also served as temporary hearts while patients wait for a suitable donor heart. One of the important difficulties with artificial heart implantation has been the control of blood clots that may form, especially around the artificial valves.

Nonsurgical Treatments

IIa/IIIb Inhibitors. This new class of drugs has been shown to prevent the formation of blood clots, a major cause of heart attacks, chest pain, and artery tightening after angioplasty. One study found that the IIa/IIIb inhibitors reduce heart attacks in patients with unstable angina, or severe chest pain, by about half.[29] Observers say this new class of drugs will have a tremendous effect on the treatment of heart problems.

Can Alcohol Be Good for Your Heart?

You have probably seen the controversial headlines over the past couple of years, stating that moderate consumption of alcohol may actually reduce your risk of coronary heart disease. Such research is controversial because experts fear they may encourage problem drinkers or turn abstainers into problem drinkers.

Nevertheless, the evidence is strong that drinking alcohol in moderate amounts indeed reduces the risk of heart attack and death from coronary heart disease, according to a recent report. Cardiologist Arthur Klatsky reports that the best evidence comes from population studies that show a 30 percent reduction in coronary risk among moderate drinkers when compared with abstainers. The results are similar in both men and women, and among various ethnic groups. Moderate drinking is typically defined as one or two daily small drinks.

Klatsky identifies two possible explanations for the cardiovascular benefits: (1) that alcohol raises the level of protective high-density lipoprotein (HDL) cholesterol in the blood, making atherosclerosis less likely, and (2) that alcohol inhibits blood clotting by helping to dissolve clots in blood vessels.

Researchers are looking at specific types of alcohol, such as red wine, but the results are not yet strong enough to justify

recommending that people switch to wine from beer or liquor. It appears that the benefits come from any type of alcohol product.

Grape juice, the dark purple kind, may convey the same cardiovascular benefit as alcohol. Studies have demonstrated that compounds called "flavonoids" in purple grape juice reduce the activity of platelets, the blood cells that stick together to form clots.[30,31]

These are the same compounds that are at least partly responsible for the apparent health effects of red wine. Purple grape juice, of course, would be a safer alternative, since it does not carry the risks of alcohol abuse that must be considered when drinking alcohol.

Because of the consistent evidence for the beneficial effects (and potentially negative effects) of alcohol consumption, the American Heart Association makes the following recommendations:[32]

- The beneficial effects of alcohol are limited to one or two drinks a day.
- Heavier consumption is related to many health problems.
- People with medical or social conditions that are worsened by alcohol should not consume any alcohol.

Aspirin and Clopidogrel. Studies released in the late 1980s highlighted the role of aspirin in reducing the risk of heart attack in men who had no history of previous attacks. Specifically, the studies concluded that for men with hypertension, elevated cholesterol levels, or both, taking one aspirin per day was a significant factor in reducing their risk of heart attack. Aspirin works by making the blood less able to clot, which reduces the likelihood of blood vessel blockages. Experts currently disagree about the age at which this preventive action should begin. The safest advice is to check with your physician before starting aspirin therapy. Fortunately, recent evidence presented in the *American Journal of Cardiology* indicates that women who are at highest risk for heart disease also benefit significantly from aspirin therapy.[33]

More recently, one study has found that the experimental drug Clopidogrel reduces the risk of heart attack, stroke, and death by about 35 percent, versus 27 percent for aspirin.[34] Others say the new drug is much more expensive than aspirin and has not been proved to save more lives overall than aspirin.

Alcohol. For years, scientists have been uncertain about the extent to which alcohol consumption is related to a reduced risk of heart disease. The current thinking is that moderate drinking (defined as no more than two drinks per day for men and one drink per day for women) is related to a lower heart disease risk (see the Star Box above). However, the benefit is much smaller than proven risk reduction behavior,

such as stopping smoking, reducing cholesterol level, lowering blood pressure, and increasing physical activity. Experts caution that heavy drinking increases cardiovascular risks and that nondrinkers should not start to drink just to reduce heart disease risk.

Hypertension

Just as your car's water pump recirculates water and maintains water pressure, your heart recirculates blood and maintains blood pressure. When the heart contracts, blood is forced through your arteries and veins. Your blood pressure is a measure of the force that your circulating blood exerts against the interior walls of your arteries and veins.

Blood pressure is measured with a *sphygmomanometer.* A sphygmomanometer is attached to an arm-cuff device that can be inflated to stop the flow of blood temporarily in the brachial artery. This artery is a major supplier of blood to the lower arm. It is located on the inside of the upper arm, between the biceps and triceps muscles.

A physician, nurse, or technician using a stethoscope listens for blood flow while the pressure in the cuff is released. Two pressure measurements are

---

coronary artery bypass surgery   a surgical procedure designed to improve blood flow to the heart by providing alternative routes for blood to take around points of blockage.

recorded: The **systolic pressure** is the blood pressure against the vessel walls when the heart contracts, and the **diastolic pressure** is the blood pressure against the vessel walls when the heart relaxes (between heartbeats). Expressed in millimeters of mercury displaced on the sphygmomanometer, blood pressure is recorded in the form of a fraction, for example, 115/82. Because blood pressure drops when the heart relaxes, the diastolic pressure is always lower than the systolic pressure.

Although many people still consider 120/80 as a "normal" or safe blood pressure for a young adult, variations from this figure do not necessarily indicate a medical problem. In fact, many young college women of average weight display blood pressures that seem to be relatively low (100/60, for example), yet these lowered blood pressures are quite "normal" for them. Any wide deviation from 120/80 in your blood pressure should be discussed with a physician.

Hypertension refers to a consistently elevated blood pressure. Generally, concern about a young adult's high blood pressure begins when he or she has a systolic reading of 140 or above or a diastolic reading of 90 or above.[3] Approximately 50 million American adults and children have hypertension. The American Heart Association reports that African-American adults have significantly higher rates (28.4%) of high blood pressure than white Americans (24.7%). Nearly 19 percent of Cuban-Americans, 15 percent of Mexican-Americans, and about 14 percent of Puerto Ricans have high blood pressure. Asian/Pacific Islanders (9%) and American Indian/Alaska Natives (12%), however, have significantly lower rates of hypertension.[1]

The causes of 90 to 95 percent of the cases of hypertension are unknown. However, the health risks are real. Throughout the body, hypertension makes arteries and arterioles become less elastic and thus incapable of dilating under a heavy workload. Brittle, calcified blood vessels can burst unexpectedly and produce serious strokes (brain accidents), kidney failure (renal accidents), or eye damage (**retinal hemorrhage**). Furthermore, it appears that blood and fat clots are more easily formed and dislodged in a vascular system affected by hypertension. Thus hypertension can be a cause of heart attacks. Clearly, hypertension is a potential killer.

Hypertension is referred to as "the silent killer" because people with hypertension often are not aware that they have the condition. People with this disorder cannot feel the sensation of high blood pressure. The condition does not produce dizziness, headaches, or memory loss unless one is experiencing a medical crisis. Because it is a silent killer, it is estimated that nearly 35 percent of the people who have hypertension do not realize they have it.[12] Many who are aware of their hypertension do little to control it. Only a small percentage (21%) of people who have hypertension control it adequately, generally through dietary control, supervised fitness, relaxation training, and drug therapy.

Hypertension is not thought of as a curable disease; rather, it is a controllable disease. When therapy is stopped, the condition returns. As a responsible adult, you should use every opportunity you can to measure your blood pressure regularly.

Prevention and Treatment

Weight reduction, physical activity, moderation in alcohol use, and sodium restriction are often used to reduce hypertension. For overweight or obese people, a reduction in body weight may produce a significant drop in blood pressure. Physical activity helps lower blood pressure by expending calories (which leads to weight loss) and improving overall circulation. Reducing alcohol intake helps reduce blood pressure in some people.

The restriction of sodium (salt) in the diet also helps some people reduce hypertension. Interestingly, this strategy is effective only for those who are **salt sensitive**—estimated to be about 25 percent of the population. Reducing salt intake would have little effect on the blood pressure of the rest of the population. Nevertheless, because our daily intake of salt vastly exceeds our need for salt, the general recommendation to curb salt intake still makes good sense.

Many of the stress reduction activities we discuss in Chapter 3 are receiving increased attention in the struggle to reduce hypertension. In recent years, behavioral scientists have reported the success of meditation, biofeedback, controlled breathing, and muscle relaxation exercises in reducing hypertension. Look for further research findings in these areas in the years to come.

Drugs used to lower high blood pressure are called *antihypertensives. Diuretic drugs* work by forcing fluid from the bloodstream, thereby reducing blood volume. *Vasodilators* relax the muscles in the walls of blood vessels (especially the arterioles), allowing the vessels to dilate (widen). Also used are calcium channel blockers, beta blockers, and other drugs that work in various ways to relax blood vessels. The most disturbing aspect of drug therapy for hypertension is that many patients refuse to take their medication on a consistent basis, probably because of the mistaken notion that "you must feel sick to be sick."

Some people taking these medications report uncomfortable side effects, including depression, reduced libido (sex drive), muscle weakness, impotence, dizziness, and fainting. Thus the treatment's side effects may seem worse than the disease. Because of the poor record of patient compliance with hypertension drug therapy, many television and radio public service announcements are geared to the hypertensive patient. Nutritional supplements, such as

Learning
From Our Diversity

Dancing Their Hearts Out: African-American and Hispanic-American Adolescents Improve Cardiovascular Fitness

Try telling a teenager that he or she is at risk for cardiovascular disease, and you'll probably get a reaction ranging from polite skepticism to a burst of laughter. Kids have always seen themselves as immortal: immune to the ailments that plague their elders, and magically shielded from the consequences of unhealthful behaviors like smoking, drinking, eating junk food, and being a couch spud instead of an exercise buff.

The bad news is that cardiovascular disease (CVD) doesn't suddenly appear when we get old. It starts early in life, when habits of eating and exercise are learned. Particularly at risk are African-American and Hispanic-American adolescents, in whom low levels of fitness and increased body mass index are common.[35] Not surprisingly, cardiovascular disease is the major cause of death among Hispanic-Americans and African-Americans in the United States.

A key to preventing or delaying the onset of CVD is regular physical activity, and school physical education programs can encourage students to participate by making activities appealing and enjoyable. That was the rationale behind Dance for Health,

an intervention program designed to provide an enjoyable aerobic routine for low-income African-American and Hispanic-American adolescents. In the first year of the intervention, some 110 boys and girls ages ten to thirteen took part in the aerobic dance pilot program for twelve weeks. The next year, a culturally sensitive health education curriculum was added. Participants attended the health education class twice a week and went to a dance-oriented physical education class three times a week. Meanwhile, another group of students took part in the school's usual playground-based activity.

The results? The students who participated in the intervention program experienced a significantly greater decrease in body mass index and resting heart rate than did the students who engaged only in playground activities. Program participants also learned culturally appropriate information about nutrition, exercise, obesity and unhealthy weight regulation practices, smoking prevention, substance abuse, stress management, and peer pressure.[35]

The bottom line? Efforts aimed at preventing cardiovascular disease can't begin too early, especially among high-risk populations—and a great way to get started is to offer kids the chance to have fun while getting healthy.

Do you have a favorite aerobic activity? Why do you like it, and how often do you do it?

---

calcium, magnesium, potassium, and fish oil, are not effective in lowering blood pressure.

Personal Applications

- When was the last time you had your blood pressure checked? What were the readings?

Stroke

The third major CVD is stroke. *Stroke* is a general term for a wide variety of crises (sometimes called cerebrovascular accidents [CVAs] or brain attacks) that result from blood vessel damage in the brain. African-Americans have a 60 percent greater risk of stroke than white Americans do, probably because African-Americans have a greater likelihood of having hypertension than white Americans. About a half million people suffer a stroke in the United States each year, and of these, about a third die. A total of 154,350 Americans died of stroke in 1994.[1] Just as the heart muscle needs an adequate blood supply, so does the brain. Any disturbance in the proper supply of oxygen and nutrients to the brain can pose a threat.

Cerebrovascular Occlusions

Perhaps the most common form of stroke results from the blockage of a cerebral (brain) artery. Similar to coronary occlusions, **cerebrovascular occlusions** can be started by a clot that forms within an artery, called a *thrombus,* or by a clot that travels from another part of the body to the brain, called an *embolus* (Figure 10-5 A and B). The resultant accidents (cerebral thrombosis or cerebral embolism) cause 70 percent to 80 percent

---

systolic pressure (sis **tol** ick)   blood pressure against blood vessel walls when the heart contracts.

diastolic pressure (**dye** uh stol ick)   blood pressure against blood vessel walls when the heart relaxes.

retinal hemorrhage   uncontrolled bleeding from arteries within the eye's retina.

salt sensitive   term used to describe people whose bodies overreact to the presence of sodium by retaining fluid, thus increasing blood pressure.

cerebrovascular occlusions (ser ee bro **vas** kyou lar) blockages to arteries supplying blood to the cerebral cortex of the brain; strokes.

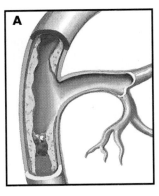

Thrombus
A clot that forms within
a narrowed section of a
blood vessel and remains
at its place of origin.

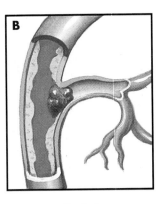

Embolus
A clot that moves through
the circulatory system
and becomes lodged at
a narrowed point within
a vessel.

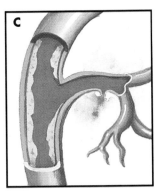

Hemorrhage
The sudden bursting
of a blood vessel.

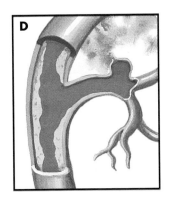

Aneurysm
A sac formed when a
section of a blood vessel
thins and balloons; the
weakened wall of the sac
can burst, or rupture, as
shown here.

Figure 10-5 Causes of stroke.

of all strokes. The portion of the brain deprived of oxygen and nutrients can literally die.

Cerebral Hemorrhage

A third type of stroke can result from an artery that bursts to produce a crisis called *cerebral hemorrhage* (Figure 10-5 C). Damaged, brittle arteries can be especially susceptible to bursting when a person has hypertension.

Cerebral Aneurysm

A fourth form of stroke is a *cerebral aneurysm.* An aneurysm is a ballooning or outpouching on a weakened area of an artery (Figure 10-5 D). Aneurysms may occur in various locations of the body and are not always life threatening. The development of aneurysms is not fully understood, although there seems to be a relationship between aneurysms and hypertension. It is quite possible that many aneurysms are congenital defects. In any case, when a cerebral aneurysm bursts, a stroke results. See the Health Action Guide on this page to learn the warning signs of stroke.

Diagnosis

A person who reports any warning signs of stroke or any small stroke, called a **transient ischemic attack (TIA)**, is given a battery of diagnostic tests, which could include a physical examination, a search for possible brain tumors, tests to identify areas of the brain affected, electroencephalogram, cerebral arteriography, and **CAT** (computerized axial tomography) **scan** or **MRI** (magnetic resonance imaging) **scan**. Many other tests can also be used.

Treatment

Researchers recently made a breakthrough in the treatment of stroke, with the discovery that the clot-dissolving drug TPA and the cell-rebuilding drug citicoline could reduce the severity of strokes.

In the past, physicians essentially waited for a stroke to end before assessing damage and beginning rehabilitation. Now, experts find that TPA can actually reduce the severity of a stroke as it is occurring. TPA was previously used to dissolve clots in the treatment of heart attacks. This same effect, applied during a stroke, can help prevent brain cells from "starving" to death because of a lack of blood supply.[36]

HEALTH ACTION GUIDE

Recognizing Warning Signs of Stroke

Although many stroke victims have little warning of an impending crisis, there are some warning signals of stroke that you should recognize. The American Heart Association encourages everyone to be aware of the following signs:

- Sudden, temporary weakness or numbness of the face, arm, and leg on one side of the body
- Temporary loss of speech or trouble in speaking or understanding speech
- Temporary dimness or loss of vision, particularly in one eye
- Unexplained dizziness, unsteadiness, or sudden falls

Many severe strokes are preceded by "little strokes," warning signals like the above, experienced days, weeks, or months before the more severe event. Prompt medical or surgical attention to these symptoms may prevent a fatal or disabling stroke.

InfoLinks
www.amhrt.org

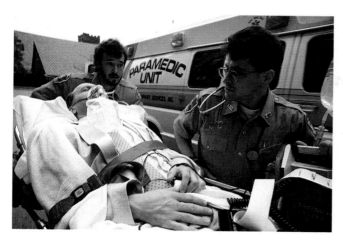

A stroke is a medical emergency that must be treated quickly to minimize damage to brain cells.

As a result, experts are reclassifying stroke as a medical emergency that must be treated as quickly as possible. To be effective, TPA must be administered in the first 3 hours of the stroke. After that time, brain cells have been damaged and TPA can worsen the damage. In addition, TPA is useful only for ischemic stroke, which occurs when arteries clog (embolism or thrombosis), the most common type. Because 500,000 people suffer strokes and about one-third of these die each year, TPA has the potential to save thousands of lives a year.

More recently, researchers have found that the drug citicoline, administered within twenty-four hours of a stroke, appears to help injured brain cell membranes repair themselves.[37] This limits the number of brain cell deaths and enables the brain to repair damaged circuits or create new ones. In addition, citicoline can be given with both ischemic strokes and other types of strokes.

Other treatment after a stroke depends on the nature and extent of the damage the patient has suffered. Some patients require surgery (to repair vessels and relieve pressure) and acute care in the hospital.

The advances made in the rehabilitation of stroke patients are amazing. Although some severely affected patients have little hope of improvement, our continuing advances in the application of computer technology to such disciplines as speech and physical therapy offer encouraging signs for stroke patients and their families.

Other Heart Diseases

Congenital Heart Disease

A congenital defect is one that is present at birth. The incidence of congenital heart disease is about 1 percent in newborn babies.[38] In infants who die before reaching term, however, the incidence is much higher.

A variety of abnormalities may be produced by congenital heart disease, including valve damage, holes in the walls of the septum, blood vessel transposition, and an underdevelopment of the left side of the heart. All of these problems ultimately prevent a newborn baby from receiving adequate oxygenation of tissues throughout the body. A bluish skin color (cyanosis) is seen in some infants with such congenital heart defects.

The cause of congenital heart defects is not clearly understood, although one cause, rubella, has been identified. The fetuses of mothers who contract the rubella virus during the first three months of pregnancy are at great risk of developing congenital rubella syndrome (CRS), a catch-all term for a wide variety of congenital defects, including heart defects, deafness, cataracts, and mental retardation. Other hypotheses about the development of congenital heart disease implicate environmental pollutants, maternal use of drugs, including alcohol, during pregnancy, and unknown genetic factors (see the Star Box above).

Treatment of congenital defects usually requires surgery, although some conditions may respond well

transient ischemic attack (TIA) (tran see ent iss **key** mick) strokelike symptoms caused by temporary spasm of cerebral blood vessels.

CAT scan computerized axial tomography scan; an x-ray procedure designed to illustrate structures within the body that would not normally be seen through conventional x-ray procedures.

MRI scan magnetic resonance imaging scan; an imaging procedure that uses a giant magnet to generate an image of body tissue.

to drug therapy. Defective blood vessels and certain malformations of the heart can be surgically repaired. This surgery is so successful that many children respond quickly to the increased circulation and oxygenation. Many are able to lead normal, active lives.

Rheumatic Heart Disease

Rheumatic heart disease is the final stage in a series of complications started by a streptococcal infection of the throat (strep throat). The Star Box on page 315 lists common symptoms of strep throat. This bacterial infection, if untreated, can result in an inflammatory disease called rheumatic fever (and a related condition, scarlet fever). Rheumatic fever is a whole-body (systemic) reaction that can produce fever, joint pain, skin rashes, and possible brain and heart damage. A person who has had rheumatic fever is more susceptible to subsequent attacks. Rheumatic fever tends to run in families. About 1.8 million people suffer from various stages of rheumatic heart disease.[2]

Damage from rheumatic fever centers on the heart's valves. For some reason the bacteria tend to proliferate in the heart valves. Defective heart valves may fail either to open fully (stenosis) or to close fully (insufficiency). A physician initially might diagnose valve damage when she hears a backwashing or backflow of blood (a **murmur**). Further tests, including chest X rays, cardiac catheterization, and echocardiography, can reveal the extent of valve damage. After it is identified, a faulty valve can be replaced surgically with a metal or plastic artificial valve or a valve taken from an animal's heart.

Peripheral Artery Disease

Peripheral artery disease (PAD), also called peripheral vascular disease (PVD), is a blood vessel disease characterized by pathological changes to the arteries and arterioles in the extremities (primarily the legs and feet but sometimes the hands). These changes result from years of damage to the peripheral blood vessels. Important causes of PAD are cigarette smoking, a high-fat diet, obesity, and sedentary occupations. In some cases, PAD is aggravated by blood vessel changes resulting from diabetes.

PAD severely restricts blood flow to the extremities. The reduction in blood flow is responsible for leg pain or cramping during exercise, numbness, tingling, coldness, and loss of hair on the affected limb. The most serious consequence of PAD is the increased

likelihood of developing ulcerations and tissue death. These conditions can lead to gangrene and may eventually necessitate amputation.

PAD is treated in multiple ways, including efforts to improve blood lipid levels (through diet, exercise, or drug therapy), to reduce hypertension, to reduce body weight, and to eliminate smoking. Blood vessel surgery may be a possibility.

Congestive Heart Failure

Congestive heart failure is a condition in which the heart lacks the strength to continue to circulate blood normally throughout the body. During congestive heart failure, the heart continues to work, but it cannot function well enough to maintain appropriate circulation. Venous blood flow starts to "back up." Swelling occurs, especially in the legs and ankles. Fluid can collect in the lungs and cause breathing difficulties and shortness of breath, and kidney function may be damaged.[6]

Congestive heart failure can result from heart damage caused by congenital heart defects, lung disease, rheumatic fever, heart attack, atherosclerosis, or high blood pressure. Generally, congestive heart failure is treatable through a combined program of rest, proper diet, modified daily activities, and the use of appropriate drugs. Without medical care, congestive heart failure can be fatal.[39]

Arrhythmias

Arrhythmias are disorders of the heart's normal sequence of electrical activity. They result in an irregular beating pattern of the heart. Arrhythmias can be so brief that they do not affect the overall heart rate. Some arrhythmias, however, can last for long periods of time and cause the heart to beat either too slowly or too fast. A slow beating pattern is called a **bradycardia** (fewer than 60 beats per minute) and a fast beating pattern is called a **tachycardia** (more than 100 beats per minute).

Hearts that beat too slowly are unable to pump a sufficient amount of blood throughout the body. The body becomes starved of oxygen, and loss of consciousness and even death can occur. Hearts that beat too rapidly do not allow the ventricles to fill sufficiently. When this happens, the heart cannot pump enough blood throughout the body. The heart becomes, in effect, a very inefficient machine. It beats rapidly but cannot pump much blood from its ventricles. This pattern may lead to fibrillation, which is the life-threatening, rapid uncoordinated contractions of the heart. Interestingly, whether the heart pumps too slowly or too rapidly, the result is the same: inadequate blood flow throughout the body.

The person most prone to arrhythmia is a person with some form of heart disease, including atherosclerosis, hypertension, or inflammatory or degenerative conditions.[3] The prevalence of arrhythmia tends to increase with age. Certain congenital defects may make a person more likely to have an arrhythmia. Some chemical agents, including high or low levels of minerals (potassium, magnesium, and calcium) in the blood, addictive substances (alcohol, tobacco, other drugs), and various cardiac medications, can all provoke arrhythmias.

Arrhythmias are most frequently diagnosed through an ECG (electrocardiogram), which records electrical activity of the heart. After diagnosis, a range of therapeutic approaches can be used, including simple monitoring (if the problem is relatively minor), drug therapy, use of a pacemaker, or the use of implantable defibrillators.

Related Cardiovascular Conditions

Besides the cardiovascular diseases already discussed, the heart and blood vessels are also subject to other pathological conditions. Tumors of the heart, although rare, occur. Infectious conditions involving the pericardial sac that surrounds the heart (*pericarditis*) and the innermost layer of the heart (*endocarditis*) are more commonly seen. Some people develop serious diseases of the heart valves. In addition, inflammation of the veins (*phlebitis*) is troublesome to some people.

---

rheumatic heart disease   chronic damage to the heart (especially the heart valves) resulting from a streptococcal infection within the heart; a complication of rheumatic fever.

murmur   an atypical heart sound that suggests a backwashing of blood into a chamber of the heart from which it has just left.

peripheral artery disease (PAD)   damage resulting from restricted blood flow to the extremities, especially the legs and feet.

congestive heart failure   inability of the heart to pump out all the blood that returns to it; can lead to dangerous fluid accumulations in veins, lungs, and kidneys.

bradycardia   slowness of the heartbeat, as evidenced by a resting pulse rate of less than 60.

tachycardia   excessively rapid heartbeat, as evidenced by a resting pulse rate of greater than 100.

Real Life
Real choices

Your Turn

- What specific kind of throat infection might Greg Chulick be dealing with?
- What can happen to someone who has this kind of throat infection and doesn't get medical treatment?
- What is your reaction to Greg's fear of telling his parents about his sore throat?

And Now, Your Choices . . .
- If you were one of Greg's parents, how could you encourage Greg to tell you when he got a sore throat without adding to his fears arising from his brother's death?
- If you were Greg's older brother or sister and he told you about his sore throat, how would you try to help him?

Summary

- Cardiovascular diseases are responsible for more disabilities and deaths than any other disease.
- The cardiovascular system consists of the heart, blood, and blood vessels.
- The vascular system comprises the body's blood vessels, including arteries, veins, arterioles, capillaries, and venules.
- The heart is a four-chambered pump designed to create the pressure required to circulate blood throughout the body.
- The blood continuously performs many functions, including transportation of nutrients and oxygen.
- A cardiovascular risk factor is an attribute that a person has or is exposed to that increases the likelihood of heart disease.

- Increasing age, being male, and heredity are risk factors that cannot be changed.
- The "big six" risk factors are smoking, physical inactivity, high blood cholesterol level, high blood pressure, diabetes and obesity. These are risk factors that can be changed.
- A contributing risk factor for heart disease is individual response to stress.
- Smokers have a heart attack risk that is more than twice that of nonsmokers. However, the risk of heart disease declines rapidly if the smoker quits.
- Regular aerobic exercise helps strengthen the heart muscle, maintain healthy blood vessels, and improve the vascular system's ability to transport blood and oxygen to the body. Physical activity can

also help lower blood cholesterol, encourage weight loss and retention of lean muscle mass, and allow people to moderate stress.

- People with high blood cholesterol should eat a heart-healthy diet and become physically active.
- Risk factors that can be changed are smoking, physical inactivity, high blood cholesterol, high blood pressure, diabetes, and obesity.
- The three most significant and common forms of heart disease are coronary artery disease, high blood pressure, and stroke.
- Each form of heart disease develops in a unique way and requires specialized treatment that may be surgical, such as coronary artery bypass surgery, or nonsurgical, such as the use of aspirin or other drugs.
- Moderate alcohol consumption may be related to a lower risk of heart disease. However, heavy drinking increases cardiovascular disease risk.

- Hypertension is consistently elevated blood pressure; the condition can produce strokes, kidney failure, eye damage, and other serious problems.
- Weight reduction, physical activity, lowering alcohol use, sodium restriction, and antihypertensive drugs are often used to control hypertension.
- There are four types of strokes: cerebral thrombosis, cerebral embolism, cerebral hemorrhage, and cerebral aneurysm.
- The new clot-dissolving drug TPA can reduce the severity of a stroke as it occurs.
- Other heart diseases include congenital heart disease, rheumatic heart disease, peripheral artery disease, congestive heart failure, and heart arrhythmias.

Review Questions

1. Identify the principal components of the cardiovascular system. Trace the path of blood through the heart and cardiovascular system.
2. How much blood does the average adult have? What are some of the important functions of blood?
3. Define *cardiovascular risk factor*. What relationship do risk factors have to cardiovascular disease?
4. Identify the risk factors for cardiovascular disease that cannot be changed. Identify the risk factors that can be changed. Identify the risk factor that is a contributing factor.
5. Describe the relationship between smoking and heart disease, including the role of environmental tobacco smoke. Explain the cardiovascular benefits of quitting smoking.
6. Describe the cardiovascular benefits of aerobic exercise.

7. What are the three major forms of cardiovascular disease? For each of these diseases, describe the disease, its cause (if known), and its treatment. Describe some additional CVDs.
8. Describe how high-density lipoproteins differ from low-density lipoproteins.
9. What problems does atherosclerosis produce?
10. Why is hypertension called the "silent killer"? What serious health problems can hypertension cause?
11. What are the warning signals of stroke? Identify and describe each of the four types of stroke.
12. What is a heart arrhythmia and what are its consequences? Identify the two main heart arrhythmia patterns.

References

1. The American Heart Association. *1997 heart and stroke statistical update.* Dallas: The Association, 1997.
2. The American Heart Association. *1998 heart and stroke statistical update.* Dallas: The Association, 1998.
3. The American Heart Association. *Heart and stroke facts.* Dallas: The Association, 1996.
4. Heart disease deaths declining. *USA Today* 1997 Feb 21.
5. Thibodeau GA. *Structure and function of the body.* 9th ed. St Louis: Mosby, 1992.
6. Thibodeau GA, Patton KT. *The human body in health and disease.* St Louis: Mosby, 1992.
7. American Heart Association. Risk factors and coronary heart disease. *Heart and stroke A to Z guide.* Dallas: The Association, 1998.
8. Berenson GS et al. Epidemiology of early primary hypertension and implications for prevention: the

Bogalusa Heart Study. *J Hum Hypertension* 1994 May; 8(5):303–11.

9. Kannel WB, D'Agostino RB, Belanger AJ. Concept of bridging the gap from youth to adulthood (review). *Am J Med Sci* 1995 Dec; 310 (suppl) 1:S15–S21.

10. Bronfin DR, Urbina EM. The role of the pediatrician in the promotion of cardiovascular health (review). *Am J Med Sci* 1995 Dec; 310 (suppl) 1:S42–S47.

11. Beilin L, Burke V, Milligan R. Strategies for prevention of adult hypertension and cardiovascular risk behavior in childhood. An Australian perspective. *J Hum Hypertension* 1996 Feb; 10 (suppl) 1:S51–S54.

12. The American Heart Association. *Heart and stroke facts: 1995 statistical supplement.* Dallas: The Association, 1995.

13. Friend T. Pros, cons of clot drugs for women's hearts. *USA Today* 1996 Mar 13:9D.

14. American Heart Association Meeting Report. *"Silent" heart damage not so quiet for some women with heart disease* (press release). Dallas, November 11, 1998.

15. Estrogen and the heart: does estrogen protect the heart? New findings, troubling questions. *Women's Health Advocate Newsletter* 1998; 5(8)1–6.

16. Beery TA: Gender bias in the diagnosis and treatment of coronary artery disease (review), *Heart Lung,* 1995 Nov-Dec.; 24(6):427–35.

17. American Heart Association Meeting Report. *Lifetime risks and costs of heart disease much higher for obese.* (press release). Dallas, November 10, 1998.

18. U.S. Department of Health and Human Services. *Report of the expert panel on detection, evaluation, and treatment of high blood cholesterol in adults.* U.S. Department of Health and Human Services, Public Health Service, NIH Pub. No. 89-2925, Washington, DC: U.S. Government Printing Office, 1989.

19. Reuters Health. *Psychotropic drugs safe for children.* Dallas, November 9, 1998.

20. Safer DJ, Zito JM, Fine EM. Increased methylphenidate usage for attention deficit disorder in the 1990s. *Pediatrics* 1996; 98(6 Pt 1): 1084–88.

21. Henderson TA, Fischer VW. Effects of methylphenidate (Ritalin) on mammalian myocardial ultrastructure. *Am J Cardiovasc Pathol* 1995; 5(1):68–78.

22. Cholesterol: up with the good. *Harvard Heart Letter* 1995; 5(11):3–4.

23. Lowering cholesterol: drugs for everyone? *Women's Health Advocate* 1998 August; 4–6.

24. Colletti PM, Terk MR. Magnetic resonance imaging applications to cardiac diagnosis (review). *Biomed Instrument Tech* 1996 July–Aug; 30(4):354–58.

25. Pauwels E, DeRoos A. Nuclear medicine techniques and magnetic resonance imaging in coronary artery disease (review). *Q J Nuclear Med* 1996 Mar; 40(1):132–41.

26. Best choice: bypass or angioplasty? *Johns Hopkins Medical Letter: Health After 50* 1995; 7(5):1–2.

27. Friend T. Laser OK'd to unclog heart arteries. *USA Today* 1992 Feb 7:1D.

28. Bittl JA. Clinical results with excimer laser coronary angioplasty. *Semin Interv Cardiol* 1996; 1(2):129–34.

29. Levy D. New heart drugs to have big impact. *USA Today* 1997 Mar 24:8D.

30. American Heart Association Meeting Report. *The heart-healthy cup runneth over—with grape juice* (press release). Dallas, November 10, 1998.

31. Levy D. A glass of grape juice may help your heart. *USA Today* 1997 Mar 19:1D.

32. Pearson TA. *Alcohol and heart disease.* American Heart Association Medical/Scientific Statement, Nutrition Committee of the American Heart Association. *Circulation* 1996; 94:3023–25.

33. Harpaz D, Benderly M, et al. Effect of aspirin on mortality in women with symptomatic or silent myocardial ischemia. *Am J Cardiology* 1996 Dec; 78(11):1215–19.

34. Friend T. A new drug beats aspirin in preventing clots. *USA Today* 1996 Nov 14:1D.

35. Flores R. Dance for health: improving fitness in African American and Hispanic adolescents. *Public Health Reports,* 1995 Mar-Apr; 110(2):189.

36. Levy D. Experts urge swift treatment of strokes. *USA Today* 1996 Dec 16:5D.

37. Friend T. Drug reduces stroke effects. *USA Today* 1996 Mar 29:1D.

38. Hoffman JI. Incidence of congenital heart disease: II. Prenatal incidence. *Pediatr Cardiol* 1995; 16(4):155–65.

39. Klieman C, Osborne K. *If it runs in your family: heart disease: reducing your risk.* New York: Bantam Books 1991.

40. American Heart Association Meeting Report. *Risk factors for cardiovascular disease tied to mental decline* (press release). Dallas, November 9, 1998.

Suggested Readings

Kowalski RE, Kattus AA. *The 8-week cholesterol cure: how to lower your blood cholesterol by up to 40 percent without drugs or deprivation.* New York: HarperCollins, 1990. Kowalski's program offers a general diet modification that includes niacin supplements and oat bran. This book includes recipes for reducing cholesterol and methods of testing cholesterol.

Goldberg B, the editors of *Alternative Medicine Digest. Alternative medicine guide to heart disease.* Tiburon, CA: Future Medicine Publishing, 1997. With a goal of helping you to prevent heart disease, stroke, and high blood pressure, and avoid the risks of angioplasty, bypass, and other invasive surgeries, this book offers the heart-saving strategies of 12 physicians.

Epps RP, ed., American Medical Women's Association, ed. *The American Medical Women's Association guide to cardiovascular health.* New York: Bantam Books, 1997. Because women have different symptoms from men, receive less care from medical professionals, die more often in the hospital, and are misdiagnosed more often than men, this book was published to help women understand the risk factors for cardiovascular disease, their signs and symptoms, and their treatment options.

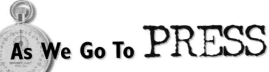

As We Go To PRESS

Risk Factors for Cardiovascular Disease Can Also Damage Mental Ability

Those who ignore the risk factors for heart disease and stroke—cigarette smoking, obesity, high blood pressure, and diabetes—may be hurting themselves in more ways than simply raising their risk of heart disease. They also may be damaging their ability to think and remember, according to a new study.[40]

The risk of mental decline worsens with each risk factor that the person carries. People with one risk factor have a 32 percent greater chance of decline in memory and learning than people with no risk factors. The chance of decline increased by another 32 percent with each additional risk factor. The study tracked the thinking and memory abilities of about 1,800 people for about 50 years.

The findings tell us that, among the many payoffs for stopping smoking, losing weight, and controlling blood pressure and diabetes, we can add the benefit of preventing or slowing mental decline.

Hypertension in African-Americans: Targeting Prevention

Development of disease is an area in which each societal group is disadvantaged in one way or another. Practically every group has a tendency to develop one or more afflictions at a higher rate than the general population. For the African-American community, one particular problem is hypertension.

The existing data show that hypertension is more common in African-Americans.[1,2] Whereas one in four adults in the general population has hypertension, the proportion rises to one in three among African-Americans. This disease is also more aggressive and less well managed in African-Americans than in whites. African-Americans also have higher rates of morbidity and mortality from diseases related to high blood pressure, such as stroke and renal (kidney) failure. The natural nocturnal fall in blood pressure is less pronounced in African-Americans, and their systolic blood pressure while awake is higher than in people of other races.[1] In addition, black women face four times greater risk of dying before age 60 from heart disease or stroke than white women.[3] This gap has not improved in 30 years.

The exact causes of these differences have not been pinpointed, but research seems to be focused in two general areas. Some research suggests that certain physical and genetic factors contribute to increased incidence of hypertension in African-Americans, whereas other studies have shown that hypertension in African-Americans is related to environmental stress. This debate involves not just medical data but socioeconomic factors as well. In short, it is a nature versus nurture debate, and supporting data exist for both arguments.

Nature versus Nurture

Studies have shown that environmental stress may contribute to increased hypertension in African-Americans. A study conducted by Dr. Norman Anderson of Duke University[4] shows that chronic stress may lead to an increase in the release of the hormone norepinephrine to the bloodstream. Norepinephrine reduces the amount of salt eliminated from the kidneys, and the resulting increase in blood salt content can lead to increased blood pressure. This chain reaction has been shown to occur in animal studies. The high rate of chronic exposure to stress in many African-American communities has been well documented.[4] If these studies hold true for humans, it would lend credence to the idea that certain stressful factors found in some African-American communities could cause hypertension. Stressors such as poverty, unemployment, the threat of violence, and racial discrimination could be shown to cause kidneys to reduce elimination of salt and thus may also increase the risk of hypertension.[4]

One recent study[5] found that factors such as unemployment, poverty, alcohol and drug abuse, and lack of health insurance among African-American males ages 18 to 54 increased their environmental stress and raised their blood pressure. In addition, these men had low rates of hypertension awareness, treatment, and control. Fortunately, the study also found that new approaches to managing and treating their hypertension could significantly help control their hypertension.

Such conclusions seem to suggest that socioeconomic factors are the main cause of hypertension among African-Americans. A study performed on twenty-six African-American women on strict low-fat diets seems to support this. The data showed that women of higher socioeconomic status had more excretion of salt than those of lower status.[4] Since proportionately more African-Americans are in lower socioeconomic classes than whites, increased stress from lower status could be the main factor behind the inflated rate of hypertension among the African-American population.

Another link between socioeconomic status and hypertension has recently been discovered. Babies born to mothers of low socioeconomic status are typically small for their age because of intrauterine growth retardation. Because their kidneys do not develop adequately, they retain excess sodium. Sodium draws fluid into the bloodstream and increases the pressure in blood vessels. Many groups of these small babies, the majority of whom are African-American, were followed by researchers over a period of years and confirmed to be more likely to have hypertension in adulthood than their more developed counterparts of any race.[6]

But is it all due to environment? Perhaps not. Other groups of traditionally lower socioeconomic status, such as Hispanics, Asians, and Native Americans, have been found to have the same incidence of hypertension as whites.[1] African-American children have been found to have higher blood pressure in general than white children;[1] it is not known whether stress plays a significant role in affecting the blood pressure of these children so early in life.

Some evidence also shows that African-Americans may be predisposed to hypertension at the cellular level. Microscopic studies of blood vessels in African-Americans with severe hypertension revealed that renal arterioles were thickened and had reduced flow. This thickening, not found in the renal arterioles of hypertensive whites, was caused by hypertrophy (excess growth) of smooth muscle cells in the muscle walls of the arterioles. This thickening reduced the size of the lumen (inside opening) of the vessels, and the resulting reduced blood flow may have caused increased blood pressure. The smooth muscle cells were thought to be responding abnormally to growth factors, which caused the hypertrophy to occur.[2] The reason behind this abnormal reaction was not determined, however.

The best explanation of why African-Americans are more prone to develop hypertension may not involve environment or genetics alone, but a combination of the two. Stress factors unique to the African-American community may serve to aggravate or intensify an existing physical predisposition toward hypertension. It has already been shown that the tendency toward developing hypertension can be passed from parents to their children. Add several unique stress factors to a population already predisposed to high blood pressure, and the potential exists for high numbers of people to develop hypertension.

Treatment of Hypertension in African-Americans

The good news is that African-Americans respond to medical treatment in a manner similar to whites. The treatment regimen for African-Americans may be somewhat different, however, since they do not respond as well to some hypertension medications as people of other races. For unknown reasons, drugs such as beta blockers and ACE (angiotensin converting enzyme) inhibitors do not work as well in African-Americans and may need to be supplemented by other medications, such as diuretics.[1]

Lifestyle changes may also be needed and may be a more effective tool in lowering blood pressure in African-Americans than in people of other races (see the table on p. 323).[1] An effort should be made to ex-

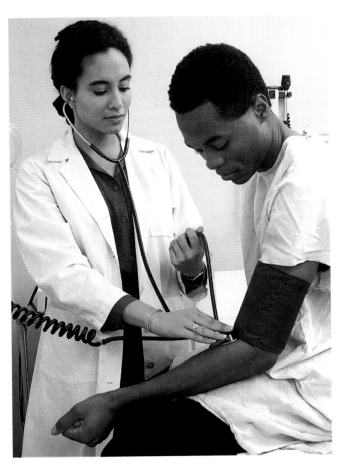

A combination of genetic factors and stress may be responsible for the high incidence of hypertension among African-Americans.

ercise and lose weight if needed, since excess weight can be a contributing factor in hypertension. African-American women may need to make a strong effort to control their weight, since data suggest that African-American women have a greater tendency to become overweight.[7,8] Thirty-five percent of all adult women are overweight, but the proportion of overweight African-American women is between 38 percent and 48.6 percent.[9,10] This may be due in part to the higher percentage of African-American women (68%) than white women (56%) with sedentary lifestyles.

Hypertensive African-Americans tend to have lower intakes of potassium and calcium, so diet changes should be made to ensure that these minerals are in adequate supply. A reduction in sodium may also be desirable, since research suggests that African-Americans may be more sensitive to the effects of sodium on the cardiovascular system.[1]

Although African-Americans are more likely to develop high blood pressure, prevention and treatment can help keep hypertension from becoming a deadly affliction. Proper diagnosis is essential, so people at risk should see their doctors to determine

Suggested Lifestyle Modifications to Control or Reduce the Risk of Hypertension[6,10]

Stop smoking	A first heart attack convinces many people to quit smoking, but don't wait—you may not get a second chance.
Lose weight if you are overweight or obese	Losing 5% to 10% of your body weight drastically reduces your disease risk factors
Reduce sodium intake	Consume < 2,400 mg of sodium per day. Excess sodium raises blood pressure in salt-sensitive people.
Moderate alcohol intake	Intake of alcohol above moderate levels increases blood pressure. Men should have no more than two drinks a day, and women should have no more than one drink a day.
Exercise regularly	Sedentary people have a 50% greater chance of developing hypertension. One simple plan for increasing your physical activity is to walk briskly 30 to 45 minutes three to five times per week.
Increase potassium intake	Potassium works to control blood volume and therefore blood pressure. Eat at least five servings of fruits and vegetables a day. Good sources of potassium are potatoes, tomatoes, and orange juice.
Maintain an adequate intake of calcium and magnesium	These minerals are important to blood pressure regulation. Eat two to three portions of low-fat milk or cheese per day.
Seek appropriate prenatal care during pregnancy	Prenatal visits help to ensure delivery of healthy babies whose kidneys are adequately developed.
Take prescribed medication as directed	Hypertension is called the "silent killer" because people who have it don't feel sick. It is critical to take your medication no matter how good you feel.
Consult your physician regularly	He or she can help you comply with and personalize your hypertension control program.

whether they have hypertension or are at risk for developing it. By recommending lifestyle modifications, prescribing medications, or both, a physician can help manage this condition or help prevent its onset. The keys to living with hypertension are awareness, treatment, and control.

For Discussion . . .

Were you aware of how serious hypertension can be? Even if you're not in a particularly high-risk group, would you consider adopting some of the suggested lifestyle modifications to improve your general health? Which ones would be the easiest to follow? The most difficult?

References

1. Kaplan NM. Ethnic aspects of hypertension. *Lancet* 1994; 344:8920.
2. Dustan HP. Growth factors and racial differences in severity of hypertension and renal diseases. *Lancet* 1992; 339:8805.
3. American Heart Association Meeting Report. *Premature death due to heart disease and stroke takes much larger toll on black women* (press release). Dallas, November 9, 1998.
4. Burt VL. Prevalence of hypertension in the U.S. adult population: results from the Third National Health and Nutrition Examination Survey, 1988–1991. *JAMA* 1995; 274(16):1254H.
5. InteliHealth, Johns Hopkins Health Information. *Hopkins: environmental factors contribute to high blood pressure in African-American males.* Baltimore, November 9, 1998.
6. Kaplan NM. High blood pressure—why do we have it? And what are we doing about it? *Saturday Evening Post* 1997; 269(1):48–52.
7. Morrison JA et al. Mother-daughter correlations of obesity and cardiovascular disease risk factors in black and white households: the NHLBI growth and health study. *Am J Public Health* 1994; 84(11):176.
8. Garn SM. Obesity in black and white mothers and daughters. *Am J Public Health* 1994; 84(11):1727–28.
9. CDC. Prevalence of selected risk factors for chronic disease by educational level in racial/ethnic populations—United States 1991–1992. *JAMA* 1995; 273(2):102.
10. Alkinson RL Jr., Calloway CW, St. Jeor S, Wolf-Novak L. A sane approach to weight loss. *Patient Care* 1995; 29(18):152–55.

InfoLinks
www.libov.com
www.womensheartinstitute.com

Living with Cancer

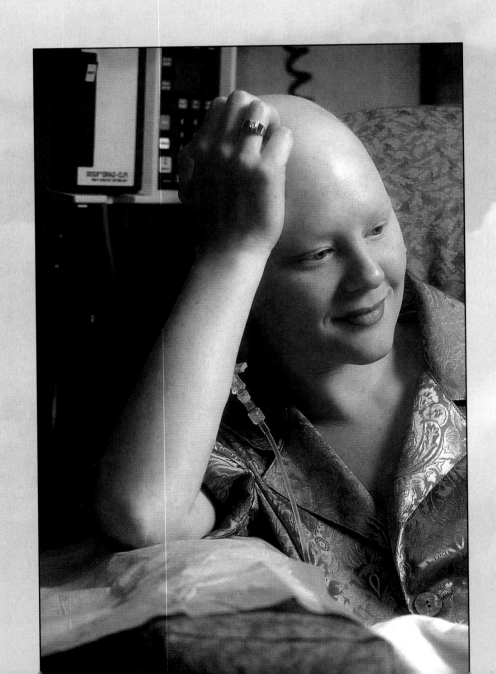

Most people can attest to the disruptive influence an illness can have on their ability to participate in day-to-day activities. When we are ill, school, employment, and leisure activities are replaced by periods of lessened activity and even periods of bed rest or hospitalization. When an illness is chronic, the effect of being ill may extend over long periods, perhaps even an entire lifetime. People with chronic illness must eventually find a balance between day-to-day function and the continuous presence of their condition. Cancer is usually a chronic illness.

HEALTHY PEOPLE: LOOKING AHEAD TO 2010

Reversing the rise in the incidence of cancer-related deaths was a key objective of *Healthy People 2000*. The *Midcourse Review* reported encouraging success in reducing the death rate of some cancers, but overall mortality remained near the same level.

Since the *Midcourse Review* was issued, other sources have indicated encouraging progress. In men, the incidence of deaths from lung cancer, colorectal cancer, and prostate cancer has declined, particularly among African-American men. In women, the death rate from breast cancer, colorectal cancer, and some types of gynecologic cancer has also declined. This modest progress is encouraging.

Healthy People 2010 will set goals for the nation of increasing years of healthy life and eliminating disparities in health care. To accomplish these goals, a broad-based approach to cancer reduction is likely to be continued. It will focus on reducing particular types of cancer, risk reduction initiatives for selected segments of the population, and broad-based lifestyle modifications for the general population. We also can anticipate continued basic and applied research leading to specialized therapies designed to affect cancer cells at the molecular level.

Real Life
Real choices

Sunny Side Up: Dying for a Tan

- Name: Tina Mavrakos
- Age: 19
- Occupation: College student/camp counselor

"Let's hit the beach!"

If Tina Mavrakos has a signature phrase, it's those four words. She's lived all her life in a small seaside town in southern New Jersey where her father and older brothers operate a small fishing boat, and she's loved the ocean and the shore ever since she picked up her first shell. When it came time to choose a college, Tina went straight for the "Sunshine State"; she's now a marketing major at a large university in southeastern Florida, where the palm-lined beach is her second home. During the summer she returns to New Jersey and works as a counselor at—what else?—a sailing camp for kids.

Tina loves the whole ocean experience, and she's got the tan to prove it. Her naturally olive-toned skin, a gift of her Greek heritage, is always the deep bronze of people in high-fashion magazines. Unlike her fair-haired friends, who apply the maximum-SPF sunscreen before even walking to the beach,

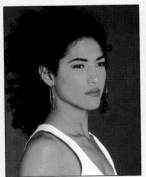

Tina never uses sun protection and laughs when someone advises her to be careful. Whatever she'd put on would just wash off, she says breezily, because she's always getting wet while swimming, sailing, or helping her father and brothers unload a day's catch from their boat.

Anyway, she's never gotten sunburned—well, *almost* never. A few times—or maybe it's more than that—Tina has felt her unprotected skin begin to tighten and tingle after a couple of hours in the sun. She never wears more than a swimsuit or cutoffs and a tank top, and she can't understand why her father and brothers always go out in their boat clad in long pants, T-shirts or jerseys, and long-billed caps.

As you study this chapter, think about the risks of Tina's sun-worshiping life, and prepare yourself to answer the questions in **Your Turn** at the end of the chapter.

In spite of our understanding of its relationship to human health and our ceaseless attempts to prevent and cure it, progress in "the war on cancer" has been at best limited. In this regard, cancer is clearly an "expensive" condition, both in terms of its human consequences and its monetary costs. Current estimates indicate that about 1,228,600 people develop invasive cancer each year. Since 1990, it is estimated that nearly 11 million new cases of cancer have developed in this country. Once diagnosed, approximately 58 percent (adjusted for other causes of death) of this group will be alive five years later.[1] Regardless of survivability, for those who develop cancer, the physical, emotional, and social costs will be substantial.

The financial cost of cancer to society is also troublesome. For example, since 1971, $107 billion has been spent on cancer in the form of direct medical care, lost productivity, and death benefits.[1] This figure does not include the sizable amount of money spent on primary cancer prevention, such as school-based programs, public education efforts, and lobbying efforts intended to remove harmful products and pollutants from the environment.

No single explanation can be given for why progress in eliminating cancer has been so limited. It is a combination of factors, including the aging of the population, continued use of tobacco, the high fat American diet, the continuing urbanization and pollution of our environment, the lack of health insurance for nearly 20 percent of the population to pay for

early diagnosis and proper treatment,[1] or simply our recognition of cancer's true role in deaths once ascribed to other causes. Regardless, we continue to be challenged to control this array of abnormal conditions that we collectively call cancer.

Personal Applications

- Do you know anyone who has or has had cancer? How did cancer affect that person's life?

Cancer: A Problem of Cell Regulation

Just as a corporation depends on individuals to staff its various departments, the body depends on its basic units of function, the cells. Cells band together as tissues, such as muscle tissue, to perform a prescribed function. Tissues in turn join to form organs, such as the heart, and organs are assembled into the body's several organ systems, such as the cardiovascular system. Such is the "corporate structure" of the body.

If individuals and cells are the basic units of function for their respective organizations, the failure of either to perform in a prescribed, dependable manner can erode the overall organization to the extent that it might not be able to continue. Cancer, the second leading cause of death among adults,[2] is a condition reflecting cell dysfunction in its most extreme form.[2] In cancer, the normal behavior of cells ceases.

Cell Regulation

Most of the body's tissues lose cells over time. This continual loss requires that replacement cells come from areas of young and less specialized cells. The process of specialization required to turn the less specialized cells into mature cells is controlled by genes within the cells. On becoming specialized, these newest cells copy, or replicate, themselves. These two processes are carefully monitored by the cells' **regulatory genes.** Failure to regulate specialization and replication results in abnormal, or cancerous, cells.[3]

In addition to genes that regulate specialization and replication, cells also have genes designed to repair mistakes in the copying of genetic material (the basis of replication) and genes to suppress the growth of abnormal cells should it occur. Thus, repair genes and tumor suppressor genes, such as the *p53* gene (altered or missing in half of all cancers), can also be considered regulatory genes in place to prevent the development of abnormal cells.[3] Should these genes fail to function properly, resulting in the development of malignant (cancerous) cells, the immune system (see Chapter 13) will ideally recognize their presence and remove them before a clinical (diagnosable) case of cancer can develop.

Because specialization, replication, repair, and suppressor genes can become cancer-causing genes, or **oncogenes,** when not working properly, these four types of genes could also be referred to as **proto-oncogenes,** or potential oncogenes.[3] How proto-oncogenes become oncogenes is a question that cannot be completely answered at this time. Regardless, abnormal cells produce abnormal proteins, and the absence of normal proteins alters the body's ability to function appropriately, from the molecular to the organ system level.

Oncogene Formation

Recognizing that all cells have proto-oncogenes, what events alter otherwise normal regulatory genes so that they become cancer-causing genes? Three mechanisms, genetic mutations, viral infections, and carcinogens, have received much attention.

Genetic mutations develop when dividing cells miscopy genetic information. If the gene that is miscopied is a gene that controls specialization, replication, repair, or tumor suppression (a proto-oncogene), the oncogene that results will allow the formation of cancerous cells. A variety of factors, including aging, free radical formation, and radiation, are associated with the miscopying of the complex genetic information that comprises the genes found within the cell, including those intended to prevent cancer.

In both animals and humans, cancer-producing viruses, such as the feline leukemia virus in cats and the HIV virus in humans (see Chapter 13), have been identified. These viruses seek out cells of a particular type, such as cells of the immune system, and alter their genetic material to convert them into virus-producing cells. In so doing, however, they change the makeup of the specialization, replication, repair, or suppressor genes, converting the proto-oncogenes into oncogenes. Once converted into oncogenes, the altered genes are passed on through cell division.

A third possible explanation for the conversion of proto-oncogenes into oncogenes involves the presence of environmental agents known as *carcinogens.* Over an extended period, carcinogens, such as chemicals found in tobacco smoke, polluted air and water, toxic wastes, and even high fat foods, may convert proto-oncogenes into oncogenes. These carcinogens may work alone or in combination (co-carcinogens). Thus people might develop lung cancer only if they are exposed to the right combination of carcinogens over an extended period.

You may already see that some of the specific risk factors in each area—such as radiation in the development of mutations, sexually transmitted viruses in cancers of the reproductive tract, and smoking-induced carcinogens in the development of lung cancer—can be moderated by adopting health-promoting behaviors. Look for information on cancer prevention throughout this chapter.

Our understanding of the role of genes in the development of cancer is expanding rapidly. Through the Human Genome Project, the scientific community has now identified over 36 genes that function as oncogenes in a variety of cancers. On occasion the public learns the identity of selected oncogenes. Very likely many readers have heard of the *BRCA1* and *BRAC2* genes associated with breast and ovarian cancer, the *RAS* oncogene thought to influence 30 percent of all cancers, and the *p53* suppressor oncogene involved in virtually half of all forms of cancer.[3] As geneticists continue to map the **human genome** and discover additional genetic links to cancer, the possibility of some form of oncogene suppressor technology becomes a more realistic possibility in the war against cancer.

regulatory genes   genes that control cell specialization replication, DNA repair, and tumor suppression.

oncogenes   faulty regulatory genes that are believed to activate the development of cancer.

proto-oncogenes (pro toe **on** co genes)   normal regulatory genes that may become oncogenes.

human genome   the sum total of all genes within a single human gamete (sperm or ovum).

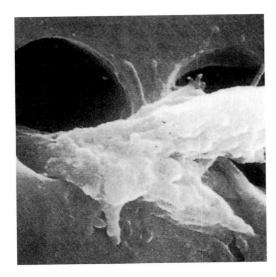

Figure 11-1 How cancer spreads. Locomotion is integral to the process of metastasis. Scientists have identified a protein that causes cancer cells to grow arms, or pseudopodia, enabling them to move to other parts of the body.

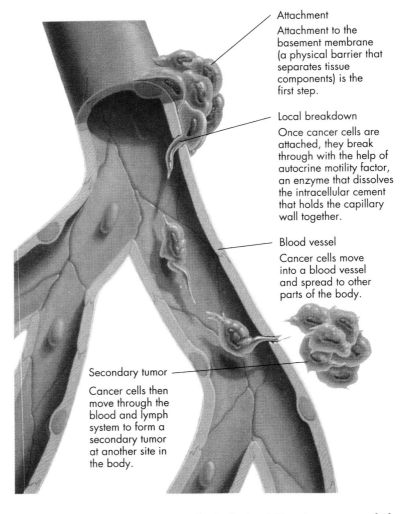

Attachment
Attachment to the basement membrane (a physical barrier that separates tissue components) is the first step.

Local breakdown
Once cancer cells are attached, they break through with the help of autocrine motility factor, an enzyme that dissolves the intracellular cement that holds the capillary wall together.

Blood vessel
Cancer cells move into a blood vessel and spread to other parts of the body.

Secondary tumor
Cancer cells then move through the blood and lymph system to form a secondary tumor at another site in the body.

The Cancerous Cell

Compared with noncancerous cells, cancer cells function in similar and dissimilar ways. It is the dissimilar aspects that often make them unpredictable and difficult to manage.

Perhaps the most unusual aspect of cancerous cells is their infinite life expectancy. Specifically, it appears that cancerous cells can produce an enzyme, *telomerase*, that blocks the cellular biological clock that informs normal cells that it is time to die. In spite of this ability to live forever, cancer cells do not necessarily divide more quickly than normal cells. In fact, they can divide at the same rate or even at a slower rate.[4]

In addition, cancerous cells do not possess the *contact inhibition* (a mechanism that influences the number of cells that can occupy a particular space at a particular time) of normal cells. In the absence of this property, cancer cells accumulate, altering the functional capacity of the tissue or organ they occupy.[5] Further, the absence of *cellular cohesiveness* (a property seen in normal cells that "keeps them at home") allows cancer cells to spread through the circulatory or lymphatic system to distant points via **metastasis** (Figure 11-1).[5] A final unique characteris-

tic of cancerous cells is their ability to command the circulatory system to send them additional blood supply to meet their metabolic needs and to provide additional routes for metastasis. This *angiogenesis* capability of cancer cells makes them extremely hardy compared with noncancerous cells.[5]

Benign Tumors

Noncancerous, or **benign**, tumors can also form in the body. These **tumors** are usually enclosed by a membrane and do not spread from their point of origin. Benign tumors can be dangerous when they crowd out normal tissue within a confined space.

Types of Cancer

Cancers are named according to the types of tissues from which they originate. Physicians use the following classifications to describe malignancies to the layperson:[1]

carcinoma—Found most frequently in the skin, nose, mouth, throat, stomach, intestinal tract, glands, nerves, breasts, urinary and genital structures, lungs, kidneys, and liver;

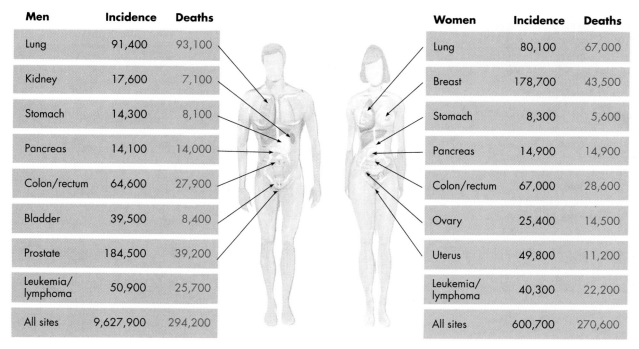

Men	Incidence	Deaths
Lung	91,400	93,100
Kidney	17,600	7,100
Stomach	14,300	8,100
Pancreas	14,100	14,000
Colon/rectum	64,600	27,900
Bladder	39,500	8,400
Prostate	184,500	39,200
Leukemia/lymphoma	50,900	25,700
All sites	9,627,900	294,200

Women	Incidence	Deaths
Lung	80,100	67,000
Breast	178,700	43,500
Stomach	8,300	5,600
Pancreas	14,900	14,900
Colon/rectum	67,000	28,600
Ovary	25,400	14,500
Uterus	49,800	11,200
Leukemia/lymphoma	40,300	22,200
All sites	600,700	270,600

Figure 11-2 These 1998 estimates of cancer incidence and deaths reveal some significant similarities between men and women. Note that lung cancer is the leading cause of cancer deaths for both genders.

approximately 85 percent of all malignant tumors are classified as carcinomas

sarcoma—Formed in the connective tissues of the body; bone, cartilage, and tendons are the sites of sarcoma development; only 2 percent of all malignancies are of this type

melanoma—Arises from the melanin-containing cells of skin; found most often in people who have had extensive sun exposure, particularly a deep, penetrating sunburn; although once rare, the amount of this cancer has increased markedly in recent years; remains among the most deadly forms of cancer

neuroblastoma—Originates in the immature cells found within the central nervous system; neuroblastomas are rare; usually found in children

adenocarcinoma—Derived from cells of the endocrine glands

hepatoma—Originates in cells of the liver; although not thought to be directly caused by alcohol use, seen more frequently in people who have experienced **sclerotic changes** in the liver

leukemia—Found in cells of the blood and blood-forming tissues; characterized by abnormal, immature white blood cell formation; several forms are found in children and adults

lymphoma—Arises in cells of the lymphatic tissues or other immune system tissues; includes lymphosarcomas and Hodgkin's disease; characterized by abnormal white cell production and decreased resistance

Figure 11-2 presents information about the incidence of cancer and the deaths from cancer at various sites in both men and women.[1]

Cancer at Selected Sites in the Body

A second and more familiar way to describe cancer is on the basis of the organ (or tissue) site at which it occurs. The following discussion relates to some of these more familiar sites. Regular screening procedures can lead to early identification of cancer at these sites (see the Health Action Guide on p. 331).

---

metastasis (muh **tas** ta sis)   the spread of cancerous cells from their site of origin to other areas of the body.

benign   noncancerous; tumors that do not spread.

tumor   mass of cells; may be cancerous (malignant) or noncancerous (benign).

sclerotic changes (skluh **rot** ick)   thickening or hardening of tissues.

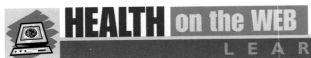

Learning About Cancer

The American Cancer Society is a nationwide, community-based, voluntary health organization dedicated to preventing cancer, saving lives, and diminishing suffering from cancer through research, education, advocacy, and service. Visit the American Cancer Society's website at www.cancer.org/frames. Scroll down and click on *Cancer Info,* and then choose *Specific Cancers.* Select a cancer that interests you, and read about its causes, prevention, diagnosis, and treatment. What did you learn?

Becoming Informed About Breast Cancer

Surpassed only by lung cancer, breast cancer is the second leading cause of cancer deaths among women. Nearly one in eight women will develop breast cancer in her lifetime. As women age, their risk of developing breast cancer increases. Are you informed about breast health and breast cancer detection? Go to the Electra Health site, www.electra.com/electraquiz/admin/Breast_Health_Qu.html, and complete the quiz on breast cancer. How did you do? If you are a woman, are you taking appropriate steps for breast cancer prevention and detection?

Preventing Skin Cancer

A golden tan may look great now, but are you willing to pay for it later? Make sure you are informed about skin health and skin cancer detection. Go to www.naturalland.com/quizzes/sun.htm to take the *Sun Savvy* quiz. How did you score? What steps can you take right now to reduce your risk of skin cancer?

For more activities, log on to our Online Learning Center at www.mhhe.com/hper/health/payne

Lung Cancer

Lung cancer is one of the most lethal and frequently diagnosed forms of cancer. Primarily because of the advanced stage of the disease at the time symptoms first appear, only 14 percent of all people with lung cancer (all stages) survive five years beyond diagnosis.[1] By the time a person is sufficiently concerned about having a persistent cough, blood-streaked sputum, and chest pain, it is often too late for treatment to be effective.

Risk Factors

Today it is known that a genetic predisposition is important in the development of lung cancer. Perhaps as many as 70 percent of the people who develop this form of cancer have an inherited "head start."[6] When people who are genetically at risk also smoke, their level of risk for developing lung cancer is hundreds of times greater than it is for nonsmokers. About 30 percent of lung cancer cases appear in people who smoke but are not genetically predisposed.

Cigarette smoking is unquestionably the single most important factor in the development of lung cancer. For men who smoke, the rate of lung cancer is twenty-three times higher than for men who do not smoke. For women who smoke, the rate is eleven times higher than for women who do not smoke. Smokers account for 87 percent of all reported cases of lung cancer, and lung cancer itself produces nearly 29 percent of all cancer-caused deaths.[1] A recent study also links smoking marijuana and crack cocaine with the same precancerous cellular changes to airway tissues seen in cigarette smoking. It is assumed that, like tobacco smoke, the smoke generated by marijuana and crack contains compounds capable of damaging the important *p53* tumor suppressor gene.[7]

Since 1987, lung cancer has exceeded breast cancer as the leading cause of cancer deaths in women.[1] The incidence of lung cancer has shown an encouraging decline in men that parallels their declining use of tobacco products. Environmental agents, such as radon, asbestos, and air pollutants, make a smaller contribution to the development of lung cancer. Radon alone may have accounted for 21,800 of the estimated 160,100 lung cancer deaths in 1998.[8]

Prevention

The preceding information clearly suggests that not smoking or quitting smoking (see p. 281) and avoidance of environmental tobacco smoke (see p. 281) are the most important factors in the prevention of lung cancer. In addition, choices of occupation and place of residence might reduce the risk of lung cancer. Nonsmokers who are considering living with a smoker or working in a confined area where environmental tobacco smoke is prevalent should carefully consider the risk of developing lung cancer.

Personal Applications

• Given the causal relationship between smoking and lung cancer, would you feel differently about a smoker who developed this form of cancer than you would about a person whose lung cancer was caused by occupational exposure?

Treatment

The prognosis for surviving lung cancer remains extremely guarded. Depending on the type of lung cancer, its extent, and factors related to the patient's overall health, various combinations of surgery, radiation,

HEALTH ACTION GUIDE

Cancer-Related Checkups

Following are guidelines for the early detection of cancer in people without symptoms. Talk with your doctor—ask how these guidelines relate to you. Remember, these guidelines are not rules and apply only to people without symptoms. If you have any of the seven warning signs of cancer, see your doctor or go to your clinic without delay.

Ages 20 to 40
Cancer-Related Checkup Every 3 Years

Should include the procedures listed below plus health counseling (such as tips on quitting smoking) and examinations for cancers of the thyroid, testes, prostate, mouth, ovaries, skin, and lymph nodes. *Some people are at higher risk for certain cancers and may need to have tests more frequently.*

Breast
• Examination by doctor every 3 years
• Self-examination every month
• One baseline mammogram between ages 35 and 40

Higher risk for breast cancer: personal or family history of breast cancer, never had children, first child after 30

Uterus
• Pelvic examination every 3 years

Cervix
• Pap test—after three initial negative tests 1 year apart—*at least* every 3 years; includes women under 20 if sexually active

Higher risk for cervical cancer: early age at first intercourse, multiple sex partners

Testes
• Self-examination every month
• Consult doctor when an abnormality is present

Higher risk for testicular cancer: personal or family history of testicular cancer, undescended testicles not corrected during early childhood, more prevalent in whites and in men under 35 years of age

Age 40 and Over
Cancer-Related Checkup Every Year

Should include the procedures listed plus health counseling (such as tips on quitting smoking) and examinations for cancers of the thyroid, testicles, prostate, mouth, ovaries, skin, and lymph nodes. *Some people are at higher risk for certain cancers and may need to have tests more frequently.*

Breasts
• Examination by doctor every year
• Self-examination every month
• Mammogram every year after age 50 (between ages 40 and 50, ask your doctor)

Higher risk for breast cancer: personal or family history of breast cancer, never had children, first child after 30

Uterus
• Pelvic examination every year

Cervix
• Pap test—after three initial negative tests 1 year apart—*at least* every 3 years

Higher risk for cervical cancer: early age at first intercourse, multiple sex partners

Endometrium
• Endometrial tissue sample at menopause if at risk

Higher risk for endometrial cancer: infertility, obesity, failure of ovulation, abnormal uterine bleeding, estrogen therapy

Testes
• Self-examination every month
• Consult doctor when an abnormality is present

Higher risk for testicular cancer: personal or family history of testicular cancer, undescended testicles not corrected during early childhood, more prevalent in whites, risk declines with increasing age

Colon and Rectum
• Digital (manual) rectal examination every year
• Guaiac slide test every year after age 50
• Proctoscopic exam—after two initial negative tests 1 year apart—every 3 to 5 years after age 50

Higher risk for colorectal cancer: personal or family history of colon or rectal cancer, personal or family history of polyps in the colon or rectum, ulcerative colitis

Prostate
• Digital rectal examination and PSA test every year

Higher risk for prostate cancer: a history of previous urinary tract infections and over 50 years of age

InfoLinks
www.cancer.org

---

and chemotherapy remain the physicians' primary approach to treatment. New drugs, such as Navelbine, have recently become available for use in combination with older therapies. Even so, recovery remains unlikely in all but a small percentage of cases.

Breast Cancer

Surpassed only by lung cancer, breast cancer is the second leading cause of death from cancer in women. It is the third leading cause of cancer deaths overall.[1]

Nearly one in eight women will develop breast cancer in her lifetime, resulting in an estimated 178,700 new invasive cases and 43,500 deaths in 1998.[1] In men, an estimated 1,600 new cases and 400 deaths will occur in 1997.[2] As they age, women's risk of developing breast cancer increases. Regardless of age, however, waiting to learn whether a suspicious lump is benign or is a relatively harmless fluid-filled cyst will be stressful. Early detection is the key to complete recovery. Ninety-four percent of women who discover their

Learning
From Our Diversity

A Story of Strength: A Breast Cancer Survivor Gives Back

At the age of 29, Dani Grady was on top of the world. Her business was booming, she had found the man of her dreams, and she was planning a year-long trip around the world.[9]

Then she was diagnosed with cancer. A biopsy of a breast lump showed an advanced cancer, and she underwent a lumpectomy. She began chemotherapy, but her therapy failed, and, in the middle of it, she had a recurrence. She had such an aggressive cancer that she went through two treatment cycles. After this high-dose protocol, Dani was finally able to have a mastectomy.

During the next 7 months, she endured several hospital stays and an infection that almost killed her. Then her fiancé left. "I learned that people who aren't good for you fall by the wayside," Grady says. "Cancer acts as a sieve or funnel in that way. My family, friends, and other cancer survivors helped me get through the difficult times."

Grady's cancer treatment lasted 18 months. She experienced such temporary side effects as blindness in one eye and early menopause. But the 6-foot avid body surfer and basketball player hasn't let cancer and its treatment get her down. "I had

to learn to see this as a new start, a second chance. This is who I am now. I don't compare myself to who I was before," she says. "I have a different life. Living with cancer taught me self-reliance. It gave me the skills I have now to live my life to the fullest—and to go beyond."

In 1993 Grady launched the Thriver's Network in San Diego, a clearinghouse for information on cancer, treatment, and support services. She also has the proud distinction of launching the CHEMOCare program on the west coast through the University of California, San Diego. "I tell cancer patients to search out the available resources," she says. "Follow survivors around, because they are role models. Learn from them."

After her long struggle with cancer, Grady says she's on top of the world once again. "Fear is not a word for me. I am a realist. I know that the cancer can reoccur, but I've chosen not to let it detract from what's happening now. I'd regret wasting time being worried about cancer. There are different seasons of survivorship. They get better and better as you practice over time."

Think about someone you know who is a cancer survivor, or imagine what it would be like to be a survivor yourself. How do you think you would feel and behave if you had a life-threatening disease like cancer?

---

breast cancer before it has spread (metastasized) will survive more than five years.[1]

Risk Factors

Although all women and men are at some risk of developing breast cancer, the following groups of women have a higher risk:[10,11]

- Women whose menstrual periods began at an especially early age and women in whom menopause occurred late (both of whom have had longer exposure to higher estrogen levels)
- Women who had no children (high risk seen later in life)
- Women who had their first child later in life (nursing helps lower risk, however)
- Women with a family history of breast cancer
- Women whose diets are high in saturated fats, those who are sedentary, and those who have excessive fat in the waist-hip area (the exact role of dietary fats remains contested)

In addition to the risks just identified, alcohol consumption, use of oral contraceptives, and use of estrogen replacement therapy (ERT) still foster controversy regarding their contribution to breast cancer. Alcohol consumption appears to be related to higher levels of estrogen.[12] Concern about the use of ERT,

even in women who have had breast cancer, may soon abate, however, since a major study released in 1997 indicates that ERT poses less risk than initially thought.[13]

The effects of environmental pollutants and regional influences have recently been introduced as causative factors in the development of breast cancer.[14,15] Environmental pollutants vary from region to region and are influenced by a number of factors, including the type of industrial and agricultural activity in a particular area. A wide array of regional factors may be involved, including genetic background of people in a given area and lifestyle differences involving diet, alcohol consumption, and exercise patterns.

Perhaps 5 percent of women with breast cancer have inherited or developed mutations in one or both of two tumor suppressor genes (proto-oncogenes), *BRCA1* and *BRCA2*. Discovered in 1994 and 1995, respectively, and currently the focus of extensive research, more than 200 mutations in these genes have been identified. In a recent study involving 5,000 Ashkenazi Jews (Jews of Central and Eastern European descent) living in the Washington, D.C., area, mutation in the *BRCA1* gene resulted in a 56 percent greater chance of developing breast cancer by age seventy (versus a 13% greater risk for people without a mutated version of the gene).[16] A similar course of events was seen on a much smaller scale in men who carry a mutated *BRCA1* gene. A mutation in the *BRCA2* gene has been found to be less likely to foster the development of breast cancer than the *BRCA1* mutation.[16]

Both of these genes are also associated with increased risk of developing ovarian cancer (see p. 339) and, perhaps, prostate cancer in men. Of course, breast cancer and ovarian cancer have been observed in the same woman, most likely as the result of carrying one or both of the mutated suppressor genes.

Uncertainty exists regarding the use of screening tests to determine the status of the *BRCA1* and *BRCA2* oncogenes. Central to this concern is that a complex set of circumstances must accompany the genetic mutation for breast or ovarian cancer to actually develop. Therefore, it cannot be definitively determined whether a given carrier of a mutated gene will actually develop cancer.[17] For a detailed discussion of the issues surrounding screening tests for cancer and other genetic diseases, see the Topics for Today article on page 353.

Other genetic links to breast cancer have been identified. One of these is a mutation of the gene that codes for a protein called *MAP kinase*. This protein functions as a "chemical switch" that controls cell replication. Another genetic link to breast cancer is a gene (*CYP17*) that codes for an enzyme that helps synthesize estrogen from cholesterol. This gene has three variations, two of which are associated with higher levels of estrogen production and probably a higher incidence of breast cancer, particularly in older women. Most recently a mutation in the APC tumor suppressor gene, thought to be associated with an increased risk of several cancers, including breast cancer, was identified in a population of Ashkenazi Jews.[18] The Personal Assessment on page 334 may be helpful in determining your relative level of risk for developing breast cancer.

Prevention

As already discussed, a variety of risk factors are thought to be important in the development of most cases of breast cancer. Accordingly, some degree of prevention is possible when factors such as diet; alcohol use; physical activity level; decisions about contraception, pregnancy, and breastfeeding; occupational exposure to toxins; and even place of residence are considered.

For women who have a primary family history of breast cancer (sisters, mother, or grandmothers with the disease) and who have been found to carry one or both of the mutated suppressor genes discussed, an extreme form of prevention is also possible—**prophylactic mastectomy**.[18] In this surgical procedure, both noncancerous breasts are removed, in an attempt to eliminate the possibility of future cancer

development. When carefully planned, breast reconstruction surgery can be undertaken immediately, with satisfactory results. Initial research indicates that, for women who have inherited a mutated *BRCA1* gene, the probability of developing breast cancer after a prophylactic mastectomy is reduced to a very low level.

One important consideration related to this procedure is that not every person who carries a mutated tumor suppressor gene will develop cancer, making the surgery unnecessary. Accordingly, some physicians recommend against the surgery, preferring to monitor susceptible women very carefully and frequently.

Pharmacological prevention of breast cancer may become routine in the near future. A recent study of tamoxifen, an estrogen-receptor blocker, showed that tamoxifen reduced the risk of developing breast cancer by 45 percent in a group of high-risk women.[19] Additionally, a seven-year study of raloxifene, an osteoporosis medication, is underway to confirm earlier studies that indicated it was nearly twice as effective as tamoxifen, and without the risk of inducing uterine cancer.[20]

Personal Applications

• If a young woman in your family had a *BRCA1* and/or *BRCA2* mutation (confirmed by genetic testing) and a family history of breast cancer, would you support her decision to undergo prophylactic mastectomy?

Early Detection: Breast Self-Examination

For several decades a fundamental component of early detection of breast cancer has been breast self-examination (BSE). Generally recommended for women twenty years of age and older, the procedure should be performed during the menstrual period or during the day immediately following the end of the menstrual period, when estrogen levels are at their lowest and cystic activity in breast tissue is minimal (or on the same day of each month by postmenopausal women). The proper technique is illustrated in the Health Action Guide on page 336. Although breast self-examination is an easily learned technique and should be undertaken on a regular basis, it is important to know that BSE as the sole form of cancer screening is of limited value in reducing the number of deaths resulting from breast cancer.

---

prophylactic mastectomy surgical removal of the breasts to prevent breast cancer in women who are at high risk of developing the disease.

Personal Assessment

Some people may have more than an average risk of developing particular types of cancer. These people can be identified by certain risk factors.

This simple self-testing method is designed by the American Cancer Society to help you assess your risk factors for three common types of cancer. These are the major risk factors but by no means represent the only ones that might be involved.

Check your response to each risk factor. Add the numbers in the parentheses to arrive at a total score for each cancer type. Find out what your score means by reading the information in the "Interpretation" section. You are advised to discuss the information with your physician if you are at a higher risk.

Skin Cancer

1. Frequent work or play in the sun
   a. Yes (10)   b. No (1)
2. Work in mines, around coal tars, or around radio-activity
   a. Yes (10)   b. No (1)
3. Complexion—fair skin or light skin
   a. Yes (10)   b. No (1)

Your total points _____

Explanation

Excessive ultraviolet light causes skin cancer. Protect yourself with a sunscreen.
These materials can cause skin cancer.

Light complexions need more protection than others.

Interpretation

Numerical risks for skin cancer are difficult to state. For instance, a person with a dark complexion can work longer in the sun and be less likely to develop cancer than a light-complected person. Furthermore, a person wearing a long-sleeved shirt and a wide-brimmed hat may work in the sun and be less at risk than a person who wears a bathing suit and stays in the sun for only a short period. The risk increases greatly with age.

The key here is if you answered "yes" to any question, you need to realize that you have above-average risk.

Breast Cancer

1. Age group
   a. 20–34 (10)   b. 35–49 (40)   c. 50 and over (90)
2. Race/nationality
   a. Asian (5)   c. White (25)
   b. Black (20)   d. Mexican American (10)
3. Family history of breast cancer
   a. Mother, sister, or grandmother (30)
   b. None (10)

4. Your history
   a. No breast disease (10)
   b. Previous noncancerous lumps or cysts (25)
   c. Previous breast cancer (100)
5. Maternity
   a. First pregnancy before age 25 (10)
   b. First pregnancy after age 25 (15)
   c. No pregnancies (20)

Your total points _____

Interpretation

Under 100   Low-risk women should practice monthly breast self-examination (BSE) and have their breasts examined by a doctor as part of a cancer-related checkup.

100–199   Moderate-risk women should practice monthly BSE and have their breasts examined by a doctor as part of a cancer-related checkup. Periodic mammograms should be included as your doctor may advise.

200 or more High-risk women should practice monthly BSE and have the examinations and mammograms described earlier.

Cervical Cancer*

1. Age group
   a. Less than 25 (10)   c. 40–54 (30)
   b. 25–39 (20)   d. 55 and over (30)

2. Race/nationality
   a. Asian (10)   d. White (10)
   b. Puerto Rican (20)   e. Mexican American (20)
   c. Black (20)

3. Number of pregnancies
   a. 0 (10)   c. 4 and over (30)
   b. 1 to 3 (20)

4. Viral infections
   a. Herpes and other viral infections or ulcer
      formations on the vagina (10)
   b. Never (1)

5. Age at first intercourse
   a. Before 15 (40)   c. 20–24 (20)
   b. 15–19 (30)   d. 25 and over (10)

6. Bleeding between periods or after intercourse
   a. Yes (40)   b. No (1)

Your total points _____

Explanation

The highest occurrence is in the 40-and-over age group.
The numbers represent the relative rates of cancer for different age groups. A 45-year-old woman has a risk three times higher than a 20-year-old.

Puerto Ricans, blacks, and Mexican Americans have higher rates of cervical cancer.

Women who have delivered more children have a higher occurrence.

Viral infections of the cervix and vagina are associated with cervical cancer.

Women with earlier intercourse and with more sexual partners are at a higher risk.

Irregular bleeding may be a sign of uterine cancer.

Interpretations/To Carry This Further . . .

40–69   This is a low-risk group. Ask your doctor for a Pap test. You will be advised how often you should be tested after your first test.

70–99   In this moderate-risk group, more frequent Pap tests may be required.

100 or higher You are in a high-risk group and should have a Pap test (and pelvic examination) as advised by your doctor.

---

*Lower portion of uterus. These questions would not apply to a woman who has had a complete hysterectomy.

HEALTH ACTION GUIDE

Breast Self-Examination

The following explains how to do a breast self-examination:

1. *In the shower:* Examine your breasts during a bath or shower; hands glide more easily over wet skin. With your fingers flat, move gently over every part of each breast. Use your right hand to examine the left breast, your left hand to examine the right breast. Check for any lump, hard knot, or thickening. This self-examination should be done monthly, preferably a day or two after the end of your menstrual period.

2. *Before a mirror:* Inspect your breasts, with arms at your sides. Next, raise your arms high overhead. Look for any changes in contour of each breast, swelling, dimpling of skin, and changes in the nipple. Then rest your palms on your hips and press down firmly to flex your chest muscles. The left and right breasts will not match exactly—few women's breasts do.

3. *Lying down:* To examine your right breast, put a pillow or folded towel under your right shoulder. Place your right hand behind your head—this distributes breast tissue more evenly on the chest. With your left hand, fingers flat, press gently in small circular motions around an imaginary clock face. Begin at the outermost top of your right breast for 12 o'clock, then move to 1 o'clock, and so on around the circle back to 12 o'clock. A ridge of firm tissue in the lower curve of each breast is normal. Then move in an inch toward the nipple; keep circling to examine every part of your breast, including the nipple. This requires at least three more circles. Now slowly repeat the procedure on your left breast, with a pillow under your left shoulder and your left hand behind your head. Notice how your breast structure feels. Finally, squeeze the nipple of each breast gently between your thumb and index finger. Any discharge, clear or bloody, should be reported to your doctor immediately.

Breast cancer can occur in men too. Therefore, this examination should be performed monthly by men. Regular inspection shows what is normal for you and will give you confidence in your examination.

InfoLinks

www.mskcc.org/pd.htm

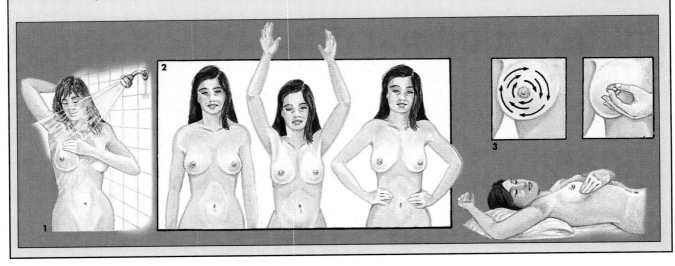

Monthly BSE is an important adjunct to regularly scheduled breast examination conducted by a physician and to the routine use of mammography. Beyond the possibility of finding a malignant lesion at an early stage, BSE is also recommended because it regularly reinforces the importance of breast health, and thus the importance of regularly scheduled comprehensive breast cancer screening.[21,22]

Early Detection: Mammography

Although researchers currently disagree about the age at which women should begin routine mammography and the extent to which mammography is effective in finding masses in dense breast tissue, mammograms are physicians' best tool for the early detection of breast cancer. In January 1997 the National Cancer Institute (NCI), after considering current research, softened its previous position, in which it had recommended routine mammography for women beginning at age forty and now recommended fifty as a starting point for mammography. This raising of the age, however, was widely criticized by health professionals and women's health groups. The NCI's current position states that the value of mammography varies depending on age, and therefore the decision as to when to begin the procedure should be made by each individual woman and her physician.[23] In 1997 an American Cancer Society advisory board recommended that the ACS change its position and begin recommending regular mammography beginning at age 40.[23] This re-

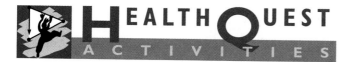

placed a long-standing policy of not beginning routine mammography for most women until age 50. In spite of this difference in recommendation, however, the ultimate decision rests in the hands of women and their physicians.

Whether women begin routine mammography at forty, forty-five, or fifty years of age, it is critical that they do begin to use this highly effective approach to the early identification of breast cancer. Many physicians recommend beginning mammograms as early as thirty-five years of age, particularly for women with earlier symptoms or a family history of breast cancer.

Because of the important role routine mammography plays in the early identification of breast lesions, the Mammography Quality Standards Act (MQSA), formulated by the FDA (April 1998), is a valuable step toward ensuring that mammography is performed by experienced technicians, using correctly calibrated equipment, and interpreted by skilled radiologists. Every woman should be certain that her mammography is being performed in a MQSA-certified facility.

To secure the highest quality images for interpretation, the soft-tissue X-ray-based mammography of the past is rapidly being supplemented by newer technologies, including MRI, contrast media-based MRI, ultrasound, and the Image-Checker, in which MRI images are quickly checked against a computerized library of normal breast images and any suspicious areas are "tagged" for further evaluation,

including biopsy. Ideally these newer approaches will reduce the percentage of false-positive results associated with traditional mammography procedures.

Treatment

Regardless of the method of detection, if a lump is found, a breast biopsy can determine whether the lump is cancerous. If the lump is cancerous but localized, treatment is highly effective, with cure rates at nearly 100 percent. The most frequently used treatments are **lumpectomy** combined with radiation, lumpectomy without radiation, and mastectomy. Today the injection of a radioactive "tag" prior to surgery allows identification of the most distant lymph node (the *sentinel node*), to which breast cancer cells may have spread, thus allowing the surgeon to spare noncancerous nodes. When the cancer is invasive or has metastasized, more radical surgery (mastectomy with lymph node removal) combined with chemotherapy and/or various forms of radiation may be the most effective course of treatment.[24,25]

When drug therapy is deemed desirable in treating breast cancer, oncologists may consider two drugs that have recently become available or whose earlier protocols have been redefined. The first, tamoxifen, discussed earlier in terms of breast cancer prevention, is a hormonelike drug that prevents estrogen from stimulating cancer cell growth. The use of tamoxifen reportedly has reduced breast cancer recurrence by approximately one-third.[26] Used for many years for more localized tumors, today its use has been extended to highly metastasized breast cancers. Tamoxifen's ability to stimulate uterine cancer development, however, is a potentially serious side effect of the drug's use and must be closely monitored.

The second drug, herceptin, is an antibody-like agent used in combination with other chemotherapeutic drugs in highly advanced breast cancer. This newly approved drug interferes with the activity of a protein produced by the HER-2 oncogene that normally fosters tumor cell division. In initial studies, the use of herceptin extended life by approximately three months.[27] Both of these drugs gained FDA approval in 1998.

Cervical Cancer

In 1998 an estimated 13,700 new cases of cancer of the cervix (the anatomical neck of the uterus) will occur in the United States.[2] Fortunately, the death rate from cervical cancer has dropped greatly since 1950, largely

---

lumpectomy a surgical treatment for breast cancer in which a minimal amount of breast tissue is removed; when appropriate, this procedure is an alternative to mastectomy, in which the entire breast and underlying tissue is removed.

because of the **Pap test.** This test screens for precancerous cellular changes (called *cervical intraepithelial neoplasia,* or *CIN*) and malignant cells. If malignant cells are found, it is hoped that they represent only cancer in situ, rather than a more advanced invasive stage of the disease. Unfortunately, this simple and relatively inexpensive screening test is still underused, particularly in women over age sixty, the group in which cervical cancer is most frequently found.

Risk Factors

Because of the clear association between sexually transmitted infections and cervical cancer, risk factors for this form of cancer include early age of first intercourse, large number of sexual partners, history of infertility (which may indicate chronic pelvic inflammatory disease), and clinical evidence of human papillomavirus infections (see p. 407 in Chapter 13). Cigarette smoking and socioeconomic factors are also risk factors for cervical cancer. The latter most likely relates to less frequent medical assessment, including infrequent Pap tests. The Personal Assessment on page 334 will help women evaluate their risk of developing cervical cancer.

Prevention

Sexual abstinence would be the most effective way of reducing the risk of developing cervical cancer (for example, Catholic nuns have extremely low rates of cervical cancer). However, since this is unlikely to be the choice for most women, other alternatives include fewer sexual partners, more careful selection of partners to minimize those at high risk, the use of condoms, and the use of spermicides. In addition, of course, regular medical assessment, including annual Pap tests, represents prevention through early detection.

Early Detection

The importance of women having Pap tests for cervical cancer performed on a regular basis cannot be overemphasized. Without screening, a twenty-year-old woman of average risk has a 250 in 10,000 chance of developing cervical cancer and a 118 in 10,000 chance of dying from it. With screening, a twenty-year-old woman of average risk has a 35 in 10,000 chance of developing this form of cancer and only an 11 in 10,000 chance of dying from it.[28] The American Cancer Society estimates that cervical cancer will claim the lives of 4,800 women in 1998.[1]

The Pap test is not perfect, however. When tests are read in laboratories highly experienced in interpreting Pap slides, about 7 percent will be false negatives, resulting in a 93 percent accuracy rate.[30] In less-experienced laboratories, false negatives may be as high as 20 percent. In addition, not all women whose test results are accurately assessed as abnormal receive adequate follow-up care, nor do they have subsequent Pap tests regularly enough.[29] On a more positive note, potentially more effective tests have been developed and are gaining acceptance. AutoPap and PAPNET are automated tests, while ThinPrep represents a new technology that enhances the clarity of the cell samples to be evaluated by the cytotechnologist. Some, however, fear that ThinPrep and the automated Pap tests are too expensive and lack data from large-scale studies of effectiveness.[30]

In addition to changes discovered by a Pap test, symptoms that suggest potential cervical cancer include abnormal vaginal bleeding between periods and frequent spotting.

Because cervical cancer is closely related to sexually transmitted *human papillomavirus (HPV)* infections, the development of a screening test capable of identifying the early presence of viral infections was greatly anticipated. However, preliminary studies of the "viralpap" test indicate a false negative rate approaching 40 percent. The ideal result, of course, would be an effective vaccine against the viral infections that are so frequently the cause of cervical cancer. At this time of writing, human trials (Stage I) are underway on a vaccine designed to protect against human papillomavirus (HPV) infections.[31]

Treatment

Should precancerous cellular changes (CIN) be identified, treatment can include one of several alternatives. Physicians can destroy areas of abnormal cellular change using cryotherapy (freezing), electrocoagulation, laser destruction, or surgical removal of abnormal tissue.[1] More advanced (invasive) cancer of the cervix can be treated with a hysterectomy combined with other established cancer therapies.

Uterine (Endometrial) Cancer

The American Cancer Society estimates that in 1998, 36,100 cases of uterine cancer (cancer within the inner wall of the body of the uterus, rather than within the cervix or neck of the uterus) will be diagnosed in American women. In addition, 6,300 women will die of the disease.[1]

Risk Factors

Unlike cervical cancer, in which a strong viral link has been identified, the principal risk factor related to the development of endometrial cancer is a high estrogen level.[32] Accordingly, the following factors are related to higher levels of estrogen and, thus, to the development of endometrial cancer:

* Early menarche (early onset of menstruation)
* Late menopause
* Lack of ovulation
* Never having given birth

- Estrogen replacement therapy (ERT not moderated with progesterone)
- Use of tamoxifen (a drug used in breast cancer therapy).

To some degree, endometrial cancer is seen more frequently in people who are diabetic, obese, or hypertensive or who have gallbladder disease.[1]

Prevention

The risk factors associated with high levels of estrogen are areas in which prevention might be targeted. In addition, the need for regular gynecological care that includes pelvic examination is a principal factor in minimizing the risk of uterine cancer. Pregnancy and the use of oral contraceptives both provide some protection from endometrial cancer.[1]

Early Detection

Compared with cervical cancer, which is routinely identified through Pap tests, endometrial cancer is much more likely to be suspected on the basis of symptoms (irregular or postmenopausal bleeding) and confirmed by biopsy. Although more invasive, biopsy is a more effective method than ultrasound to diagnose uterine cancer.[33]

Treatment

The treatment for early or localized endometrial cancer is generally surgical removal of the uterus (hysterectomy). Other therapies, such as radiation, chemotherapy, and hormonal therapy, may then be added to the treatment regimen. Because estrogen is important to cardiovascular and bone health after menopause, hormone replacement therapy (HRT), in which estrogen is combined with progesterone, is often prescribed in older women even though they have had endometrial cancer.

Vaginal Cancer

Although rare, cancer of the vagina (the passage leading to the uterus) is of concern to a particular group of women: the daughters of more than 3 million mothers who were given the drug DES (diethylstilbestrol) to prevent miscarriages. Because of the effects of DES on the development of the fetal reproductive system, these daughters now face the risk of developing a form of vaginal (and cervical) cancer called *clear cell cancer*. Since the risk was identified over forty years ago, the medical community has been following large groups of daughters to better assess their level of risk. To date, 1 in every 1,000 exposed daughters has developed this form of cancer, some as early as fifteen years of age.

Outside of this unique group of women, vaginal cancer is a relatively rare form of cancer. The Ameri-can Cancer Society estimates that in 1998, 2,000 new cases will be diagnosed and 600 women will die as the result of vaginal cancer.[2] Early detection can be accomplished using a Pap test when vaginal wall cell samples are taken. Treatment centers on surgical removal of the vagina and associated lymph nodes. Other supportive therapies may also be included in the treatment regimen.

Ovarian Cancer

Since the death in 1989 of actress Gilda Radner, a star in the early years of *Saturday Night Live*, public awareness of ovarian cancer has increased in the United States. The American Cancer Society estimates that in 1998, 25,400 new cases will be diagnosed and 14,500 women will die of the disease.[2] Most cases develop in women over age forty who have not had children or began menstruation at an early age. The highest rate is in women over age sixty. Today ovarian cancer causes more deaths than any other form of female reproductive system cancer.

For a relatively small percentage of all women (10%), the inheritance of either the *BRCA1* or *BRCA2* suppressor gene mutation (see p. 332) significantly increases the risk of developing both breast and ovarian cancer. When the *BRCA2* mutation is present, the risk of developing ovarian cancer is greater than with *BRCA1*. Today it is estimated that about 20 percent of all cases of ovarian cancer stem from these genetic mutations. For women with a *BRCA* mutation, the risk of developing ovarian cancer may be as high as 85 percent.[16]

Prevention

Methods of preventing or lowering the risk of developing ovarian cancer are very similar to those recommended for breast cancer. These include using oral contraceptives, giving birth and breastfeeding (for at least three months), reducing dietary fat intake, abstaining from alcohol use, and performing regular physical activity.

For the small group of women with a strong family history of ovarian cancer, a **prophylactic oophorectomy** should be seriously considered. In this surgical procedure, both ovaries are removed. Carefully monitored hormone replacement therapy is then used to provide the protective advantages of estrogen in maintaining cardiovascular health and bone density.

Pap test   a cancer screening procedure in which cells are removed from the cervix and examined for precancerous changes.

prophylactic oophorectomy   surgical removal of the ovaries to prevent ovarian cancer in women at high risk of developing the disease.

Although not nearly as effective as oophorectomy, use of the oral contraceptive may provide some protection for women in this high-risk group.[34]

Early Detection

Because of its vague symptoms, ovarian cancer has been referred to as a *silent cancer*. Women in whom ovarian cancer has been diagnosed often report that the only symptoms of their cancer's presence were digestive disturbances, gas, and stomach distention. For this reason, annual pelvic examinations are important.

For women with a strong family history of ovarian cancer (four primary family members who have had breast or ovarian cancer, with two or more cases occurring before age fifty) or women of Ashkenazi Jewish descent (see p. 332), genetic screening and transvaginal ultrasound screening are likely to be recommended. These women may also be referred for participation in one of several prevention trials now under way.

Treatment

At this time, treatment of ovarian cancer requires surgical removal of the ovary, followed by aggressive use of chemotherapy. Use of the chemotherapeutic drug Taxol, obtained from the bark and needles of the Pacific yew tree, results in a 50 percent survival rate nineteen months after the completion of therapy. Most recently, use of an experimental three-drug combination—cyclophosphamide, paclitaxel, and cisplatin—has resulted in a 70 percent survival rate twenty-two months after chemotherapy.

Prostate Cancer

If the names Bob Dole, General Norman Schwarzkopf, Jerry Lewis, and Jesse Helms are familiar, then you know four older men who have been diagnosed with and treated for prostate cancer. In fact, prostate cancer is so common that in 1998 an estimated 184,500 new cases will be diagnosed and 39,200 men will die of the disease.[1] Prostate cancer is the second leading cause of cancer deaths in American men, exceeded only by lung cancer deaths.[1] Cancer of the prostate is the third most common form of cancer in men and a leading cause of death from cancer in older men.

The prostate gland is a walnut-size gland located near the base of the penis. It surrounds the neck of the bladder and the urethra. The prostate secretes a number of components of semen, such as nutrients used to fuel sperm motility.

Risk Factors

Compared with other cancers, the risk factors for prostate cancer are less clearly defined. The most pre-

Symptoms of Prostate Disease

- Difficulty urinating
- Frequent urination, particularly at night
- Continued wetness for a short time after urination
- Blood in the urine
- Low back pain
- Ache in the upper thighs

dictable risk factor is age. Nearly 80 percent of all prostate cancer cases are diagnosed in men over sixty-five years of age, while cases in men under age fifty are infrequent. African-American men and men with a family history of prostate cancer are at greater risk of developing this form of cancer. A link between prostate cancer and dietary fat intake, including excessive red meat and dairy product consumption, has also been suggested.[35] With the discovery of the *BRCA1* and *BRCA2* genes related to breast and ovarian cancer, a genetic link with prostate cancer was also established. Men with one of these genetic mutations have an increased risk of developing prostate cancer.

Prevention

Although the American Cancer Society does not specifically address prevention of prostate cancer, prevention is not an unrealistic goal.[1] Clearly, moderation of dietary fat intake is a preventive step. Recently, increased dietary intake levels of vitamin E and the micronutrient selenium have been shown to play a preventive role in prostate cancer.[36,37] In addition, effective treatment of benign prostatic hyperplasia (BPH) (prostate enlargement) may reduce the risk of developing prostate cancer in the future.

Early Detection

The symptoms of prostate disease, including prostate cancer, are listed in the Star Box above. A physician should be consulted if any of these symptoms appear, particularly in men aged fifty or older. Screening for prostate cancer should begin by age forty. This screening consists of an annual rectal examination performed by a physician and a blood test, the **prostate-specific antigen (PSA) test,** administered every two years. Although the initial version of the PSA test was very successful in diagnosing prostate cancer, new, age-specific test values are now employed. These new interpretive standards allow increased specificity in determining risk. Another version of the PSA test has also been developed. This test can identify the "free" antigen most closely associated with the more aggressive forms of prostate cancer, thus cutting down on the false positives and extensive use of biopsies. In addition, an ultrasound rectal examination is used in men whose PSA scores are abnormally high. In men who have been diagnosed with prostate cancer, a new test, Prostascint, is now available to determine how extensively the cancer has spread.

Treatment

Today prostate cancer is treated surgically, or through the use of external radiation or the implantation of radioactive seeds (brachytherapy) into the gland. The latter form of radiation therapy is highly effective for early-stage disease.[38] One form of prostate cancer grows so slowly that men whose cancer is of this type, whose tumors are very localized, and whose life expectancy is less than ten years at the time of diagnosis will not receive treatment but rather will be closely monitored for any progression of the cancer. For men who have the more aggressive form of the cancer, or whose tumor is no longer localized, physicians can employ a range of therapies, including surgery, radiation, chemotherapy, and hormonal therapy. In addition, an experimental vaccine has recently been tested on humans. The five-year survival rate for men with localized prostate cancer is very high.

Testicular Cancer

Cancer of the testicle is among the least common forms of cancer; however, it is the most common solid tumor in men ages fifteen to thirty-four. Awareness of this type of cancer was raised in 1996 and 1997, when world-class bicyclist Lance Armstrong and champion figure skater Scott Hamilton were diagnosed with testicular cancer. In both men, chronic fatigue and abdominal discomfort were the first symptoms of the disease. The American Cancer Society estimates that in 1998 testicular cancer will be diagnosed in 7,600 men and cause the deaths of 400.[2]

Four forms of testicular cancer have been described: seminoma, teratoma, carcinoma, and choriocarcinoma. The most prevalent, seminoma, forms in the seminiferous tubules (where sperm originate) and is generally first observed during testicular self-examination as a small, hard mass on the side (or near the front) of the testicle. Fortunately, this form of testicular cancer is now highly curable.

Risk Factors

Risk factors for testicular cancer are variable, ranging from family history to environmental factors. The disease is more frequently seen in African-Americans and in men whose testicles were undescended during childhood. Additional risk factors, such as difficulty during the mother's pregnancy, elevated temperature in the groin, and mumps during childhood, have been

reported. The incidence of this cancer has been increasing in recent decades, while a corresponding drop in sperm levels has also been observed. Although no single explanation can be given for these changes, environmental factors such as agricultural pesticide toxicity may be involved. Once pesticides are concentrated in the tissues of the human body, during pregnancy they mimic estrogen and exert a **teratogenic** effect on male fetal development.

Testicular cancer is more frequently seen among white-collar workers than among people in blue-collar occupations. The suspicion that testicular cancer is linked to vasectomies appears to be unfounded.

Prevention

Because risk factors for testicular cancer are so variable, prevention is limited to regular self-examination of the testicles. Symptoms such as fatigue, abdominal discomfort, and enlargement of the testicle should be reported to a physician, since these can be associated with other disease processes. A male infant with one or both testicles in the undescended position (resulting in an empty scrotum) should be seen promptly by a physician so that corrective procedures can be undertaken.

Early Detection

In addition to the fatigue and abdominal distress reported by both Armstrong and Hamilton, other symptoms of testicular cancer include a small, painless lump on the side or near the front of the testicle, a swollen or enlarged testicle, and a heaviness or dragging sensation in the groin or scrotum. The importance of testicular self-examination, as well as early diagnosis and prompt treatment, cannot be overemphasized for men in the at-risk age group of fifteen to thirty-four years. The Health Action Guide on page 342 explains how to perform a testicular self-examination.

Treatment

Depending on the type, stage, and degree of localization of the tumor, surgical intervention generally includes removal of the testicle, spermatic cord, and regional lymph nodes. Chemotherapy and radiation might also be used. Today, treatment is very effective, with 95 percent of all testicular cancer patients surviving five years and 99 percent surviving five years when the cancer was localized at the time of diagnosis.

prostate-specific antigen (PSA) test a blood test used to identify prostate-specific antigen, an early indicator that the immune system has recognized and mounted a defense against prostate cancer.

teratogenic capable of causing birth defects (congenital abnormalities) in a fetus.

It should be noted, however, that suspicion is growing regarding effective treatment for a second cancer later in life.[39]

Colorectal Cancer

Cancer of the colon and rectum (colorectal cancer) has a death rate second only to that of lung cancer. Two types of tumors, carcinoma and lymphoma, can be found in both the colon and rectum. Fortunately, when diagnosed in a localized state, colorectal cancer has a relatively high survival rate (92% when localized and 64% for all stages).[1]

Risk Factors

Underlying the development of colorectal cancer are at least two potentially important areas of risk: genetic susceptibility and dietary patterns. Genes have recently been discovered that lead to familial colon cancer and familial polyposis (abnormal tissue growth that occurs before formation of cancer) and are believed to be responsible for the tendency of colorectal cancer to run in families. Dietary risk factors include diets that are high in saturated fat from red meat and low in fruits and vegetables, which contain antioxidant vitamins and fiber. In addition, an association between colorectal cancer and smoking has been identified.

Prevention

Small outpouchings in the lower intestinal tract wall, called *polyps*, are frequently important in the eventual development of colorectal cancer. Prompt removal of polyps has been shown to lower the risk of colorectal cancer. Further, some evidence indicates that the development of colorectal cancer may be prevented or slowed through regular exercise, the regular use of aspirin, an increase in dietary calcium intake, and long-term folic acid supplementation.[40,41,42] Additionally, oral contraceptive use may be protective for women.

Again, routine screening for colorectal cancer should be considered a form of prevention, much as PSA testing is for prostate cancer and mammography is for breast cancer.

Early Detection

Symptoms of colorectal cancer include bleeding from the rectum, blood in the stool, and a change in bowel habits. In addition, a family history of inflammatory bowel disease, polyp formation, or colorectal cancer should make one more alert to symptoms. In people over age fifty, any sudden change in bowel habits that lasts ten days or longer should be evaluated by a physician. The American Cancer Society recommends preventive health care that includes digital (manual) rectal examination after age forty, a stool blood test after age fifty, and proctoscopic examination every three to five years and **colonoscopy** every ten years after age fifty.

Treatment

When one or more of these screening procedures suggests the possibility of disease within the lower intestinal tract, a careful visual evaluation of the entire length of the colon will be undertaken. During colonoscopy, areas of concern can be biopsied and the presence of a malignancy confirmed. Upon diagnosis, a localized and noninvasive malignancy will be removed surgically. When an invasive tumor is identified, supportive treatment with radiation or chemotherapy is necessary. Metastatic cancer requires chemotherapy. The creation of a **colostomy** is necessary in only 15 percent of colorectal cancer cases.

Pancreatic Cancer

Pancreatic cancer is one of the most lethal forms of cancer, with a survival rate of only 4 percent five years

---

HEALTH ACTION GUIDE

Testicular Self-Examination

The best method of early detection of testicular cancer is a simple three-minute monthly self-examination. The following steps explain how to do a testicular self-examination. The ideal time to perform the examination is after a warm bath or shower, when the scrotal skin is most relaxed.

1. Roll each testicle gently between the thumb and fingers of both hands.
2. If you find any hard lumps or nodules, see your doctor promptly. They may not be malignant, but only your doctor can make the diagnosis.

After a thorough physical examination, your doctor may perform certain x-ray studies to make the most accurate diagnosis possible.

InfoLinks
www.mskcc.org/document/WICTEST.htm

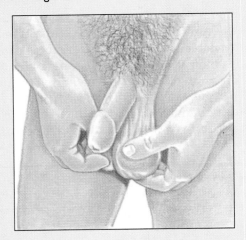

Testicular self-examinations are as important for men as breast self-examinations are for women.

after diagnosis.[1] Because of this gland's important functions in both digestion and metabolic processes related to glucose utilization (see the discussion of diabetes mellitus on p. 367), its destruction by a malignancy leaves the body in a state incompatible with living.

In 1998 an estimated 29,000 new cases of pancreatic cancer will be diagnosed and 28,900 deaths will occur.[2]

Risk Factors

Pancreatic cancer is more common in men than women, occurs more frequently with age, and develops most often in African-American men. Smoking is clearly a risk factor for this form of cancer, with smokers more than twice as likely to develop the disease. Other risk factors have been tentatively suggested, such as chronic inflammation of the pancreas (pancreatitis), diabetes mellitus, alcohol-induced liver deterioration (cirrhosis), and high-fat diets.[1] Relatively little else is known about risk factors and, thus, prevention.

Prevention

Not smoking and abstaining from alcohol use are the most effective steps toward preventing this form of cancer. Further, reducing the risk of type II diabetes mellitus (see p. 367) would also make an important contribution to prevention. Annual medical examinations are, of course, associated with overall cancer prevention.

Early Detection

Early detection of this cancer is difficult because of the absence of symptoms until late in its course. Perhaps for people with a history of chronic pancreatitis, physicians might consider routine ultrasound assessment or computerized axial tomography scans (CAT scans). Once symptoms appear, a biopsy will be performed.

Treatment

At this time there is no effective treatment for pancreatic cancer. Surgical removal of malignant sites within the gland, in addition to radiation and chemotherapy, is usually tried. Certainly, if a particular patient with pancreatic cancer qualifies, enrollment in a clinical trial would be worth consideration.

Lymphatic Cancer

In 1996 sports fans were saddened by the news that National Hockey League great Mario LeMeux had been diagnosed with cancer of the lymphatic system, the basis of the body's immune capabilities. LeMeux's cancer was Hodgkin's disease, a form of lymphoma. Following treatment in 1996, he appears to be in complete remission.

An estimated 62,500 new cases of lymphoma (7,100 cases of Hodgkin's disease and 55,400 cases of non-Hodgkin's lymphoma) will be diagnosed in 1998. The number of deaths from both forms of lymphoma is expected to be near 26,300.[2] The incidence of Hodgkin's disease has declined over the last twenty-five years, while the incidence of non-Hodgkin's disease has increased by more than 80 percent.[1]

Risk Factors

Risk factors for lymphoma are difficult to determine. Some possible factors are a general reduction in immune protection, exposure to toxic environmental chemicals such as pesticides and herbicides, and viral infections.[1] As you will learn in Chapter 13, the virus that causes AIDS (HIV) is a leukemia/lymphoma virus that was initially called HTLV-III (human T-cell leukemia/lymphoma virus-type III). A related leukemia/lymphoma virus, HTLV-I, is also suspected in the development of lymphatic cancer.

Prevention

Beyond limiting exposure to toxic chemicals and sexually transmitted viruses, few recommendations can be made about prevention. Again, early detection and diagnosis can serve as a form of prevention, since early-stage cancer is more survivable than advanced disease.

Early Detection

Unlike other cancers, the early symptoms of lymphoma are diverse and similar to symptoms of other illnesses, most of which are not serious. These symptoms include enlarged lymph nodes (frequently a sign of any infection that the immune system is fighting), fever, itching, weight loss, and anemia.

Treatment

Although surgery (beyond a biopsy) is usually not associated with the treatment of lymphoma, a variety of other therapies are employed. Depending on the stage and type of lymphoma, therapy may involve only radiation treatment of localized lymph nodes, as is seen in non-Hodgkin's lymphoma. Radiation combined with chemotherapy is generally used in the treatment of late-stage non-Hodgkin's lymphoma. More recently,

---

colonoscopy (co lun **os** ko py) examination of the entire length of the colon, using a flexible fiberoptic scope to inspect the structure's inner lining.

colostomy (co **los** to my) a surgically created opening through which body wastes can exit; created by attaching the terminal end of the colon to an incision in the abdominal wall.

other therapies, including more aggressive chemotherapy, monoclonal antibody therapy, and bone marrow transplantation, have been employed.[1]

Among the most recent innovations in treatment are the use of low-dose arsenic trioxide to treat acute promyelocytic leukemia, the use of umbilical cord blood as an alternative to bone marrow transplants in childhood leukemia, and a new technology that "washes" bone marrow cells to reduce tissue rejection.[43,44,45]

After completion of therapy, one-year survival rates for Hodgkin's disease are near 92 percent and near 71 percent for non-Hodgkin's lymphoma. By the end of five years, these rates have dropped to 81 percent and 51 percent, respectively.[1] Lower rates of survival are seen at ten years and beyond.

Skin Cancer

Thanks largely to our desire for a fashionable tan, many teens and adults have spent more time in the sun (and in tanning booths) than their skin can tolerate. As a result, skin cancer, once common only among people who had to work in the sun, is occurring with alarming frequency. In 1998, nearly 1 million Americans will develop basal or squamous cell skin cancer and 41,600 cases of highly dangerous malignant melanoma will be diagnosed.[1]

Deaths from skin cancer do occur, with 9,200 anticipated in 1998. More than 80 percent of these deaths will be the result of malignant melanoma.

Risk Factors

Severe sunburning during childhood and chronic sun exposure during adolescence and younger adulthood are largely responsible for the "epidemic" of skin cancer being reported. The current emphasis on screening for skin cancer may also be increasing the incidence of early-stage cancer being reported. Progress is being made in deterring people from pursuing the perfect tan. The American Academy of Dermatology reports that the incidence of deliberate tanning is down, and the use of sunscreens has increased. Occupational exposure to some hydrocarbon compounds can also cause skin cancer.

Prevention

Prevention of skin cancer should be a high priority for people who enjoy the sun or must work outdoors. The use of sunscreen with an SPF of 15 or greater is very important. In addition, parents can help their children prevent skin cancer later in life by restricting their outdoor play from 11:00 A.M. to 2:00 P.M., requiring them to wear hats that shade their faces, and applying a sunscreen with an SPF of 15 on them regardless of skin tone. A recent evaluation of sunscreen effectiveness studies by Sloan-Kettering Cancer Center, however, suggests that sunscreens provide lit-

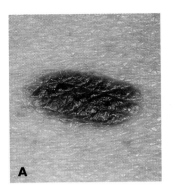 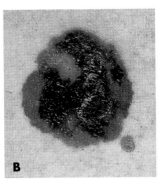

Figure 11-3 **A,** Normal mole. This type of lesion is often seen in large numbers on the skin of young adults and may affect any body site. Note its symmetrical shape, regular borders, uniform color, and relatively small size (about 6 millimeters). **B,** Malignant melanoma. Note its asymmetrical shape, irregular borders, uneven color, and relatively large size (about 2 centimeters).

tle protection against the deeply penetrating UV-A rays associated with the development of melanoma in susceptible people, and less protection than once thought against the UV-B rays associated with burning and wrinkling of the skin. Practicing dermatologists nonetheless continue to recommend their use.

A further rationale for preventing the development of skin cancer is the recently described relationship between skin cancer and the heightened probability of developing other forms of cancer later in life. Research now suggests that people who have had skin cancer carry a 20 percent to 30 percent greater risk of developing other types of cancer than do people who have never developed skin cancer.[46] The Personal Assessment on page 334 will help you determine your own risk of developing this kind of cancer.

Early Detection

Although many doctors do not emphasize this point enough, the key to the successful treatment of skin cancer is early detection. For basal cell or squamous cell cancer, a pale, waxlike, pearly nodule or red, scaly patch may be the first symptom. Other types of skin cancer may be indicated by a gradual change in the appearance of an existing mole. A physician should be consulted if such a change is noted. Melanoma usually begins as a small, molelike growth that increases progressively in size, changes color, ulcerates, and bleeds easily. To help detect melanoma, the American Cancer Society recommends using the guidelines below:

A is for asymmetry.

B is for border irregularity.

C is for color (change).

D is for a diameter greater than 6 mm.

HEALTH ACTION GUIDE

How to look for melanoma

1. Examine your body front and back in the mirror, then right and left sides with arms raised.

2. Bend your elbows and carefully look at your palms, forearms, and under your upper arms.

3. Look at the backs of your legs and feet, the spaces between your toes, and the soles of your feet.

4. Examine the back of your neck and scalp with a hand mirror. Part your hair for a closer look.

5. Finally, check your back and buttocks with a hand mirror.

What to look for
Potential signs of malignancy in moles or pigmented spots:

Asymmetry
One half unlike the other half

Irregularity
Border irregular or poorly circumscribed

Color
Color varies from one area to another; shades of tan, brown, or black

Size
Diameter larger than 6 mm as a rule (diameter of a pencil eraser)

InfoLinks
www.asds-net.org/scfactsheet.html

Figure 11-3 shows a mole that would be considered harmless and one that clearly demonstrates the ABCD characteristics just described. The Health Action Guide above shows how to make a regular inspection of the skin.

Most recently, a relationship between the presence of abnormal moles, called *dysplastic nevi* (flat, irregularly shaped, mottled in color, with irregular edges), and the risk of developing malignant melanoma has been established. By counting these "indicator moles," physicians can judge the relative risk of developing this serious form of skin cancer before it first appears.[47]

Treatment

When nonmelanoma skin cancer is found, an almost 100 percent cure rate can be expected. Treatment of these skin cancers can involve surgical removal by traditional excising or laser vaporization, destruction by burning or freezing, or destruction using x-ray therapy. When the more serious melanomas are found at an early stage, a high cure rate (95%) is accomplished using the same techniques. However, when malignant melanomas are more advanced, extensive surgery and chemotherapy will be necessary. The five-year survival rate for regionalized forms of the disease drops to 61 percent, and, unfortunately, long-term disease recovery is uncommon (16%).[1]

However, a new treatment for malignant melanoma offers a ray of hope to people with the disease. A vaccine has been developed that stimulates the immune system to attack the melanoma cells more aggressively. This treatment-centered (rather than prevention-centered) vaccine uses components of the patient's own cancer cells to mobilize more white blood cells and produce more antibodies to fight the cancer.

The Future of Cancer Prevention, Diagnosis, and Treatment

Is the "war on cancer" being won? For the first time, according to National Cancer Institute data, the answer is a guarded "Yes!" Between 1992 and the end of 1995 (the last year for which data were available), the reported rate of new cancer cases fell 0.07 percent per year, while the cancer death rate fell 0.05 percent per year. In the opinion of some experts, these changes are too small to support a claim that much progress has been made.[48] Nonetheless, the likelihood of an individual's survival (defined as living at least five years after diagnosis) depends greatly on the promptness of identification, diagnosis, and treatment.

Thus the chances for recovery from cancer are best when cancer is detected early. The list of "cancer's seven warning signals" can serve as a basis for early detection (see the Star Box). In addition, unexplained weight loss can signal the presence of a malignancy. Weight loss, however, is not usually an early indicator of cancer. Persistent headaches and vision changes should be evaluated by a physician. In fact, almost any clearly evident change in the structure or function of the body should be called to the attention of a health care provider.

In addition to the recognition of danger signals, undergoing regularly scheduled screening for malignancy-related changes is important. Breast self-examination for all women over age twenty is recommended (see the discussion of BSE effectiveness on p. 333). Testicular self-examination is strongly recommended for men. Step-by-step procedures for both of these self-examinations are provided in the Health Action Guides on pages 336 and 342. The remaining screening procedures require the services of medical practitioners or laboratories.

Personal Applications

• How regularly do you perform either breast or testicular self-examination?

Treatment

In today's approach to cancer treatment, proven therapies and promising new experimental approaches are often combined. The traditional therapies are surgery,

---
⭐ **Cancer's Seven Warning Signals**

Listed below are the seven warning signs of cancer, which the acronym CAUTION will help you remember:

1. **C**hange in bowel or bladder habits
2. **A** sore that does not heal
3. **U**nusual bleeding or discharge
4. **T**hickening or lump in the breast or elsewhere
5. **I**ndigestion or difficulty in swallowing
6. **O**bvious change in a wart or mole
7. **N**agging cough or hoarseness

If you have a warning signal that persists for more than 5 days, see your doctor!

---

radiation, and chemotherapy. Used independently or in combination, they form the backbone of our increasingly successful efforts in treating cancer. Newer, more experimental therapies are also being used on a limited basis. For example, a mutated cold virus is being used to genetically invade and then inactivate the *p53* oncogene. And a genetically altered lymphocyte is being developed that secretes a toxin in response to the presence of a specific protein produced by malignant breast cells. In the future, however, the strategy of killing cancer cells (and other healthy cells) will be replaced by methods to return cancer cells to normal functioning.

Personal Applications

• If you were diagnosed as having a terminal illness, would you be willing to serve as a subject in a research project to test a potentially toxic experimental drug?

Surgery

Surgical removal of tissue suspected of containing cancerous cells is the oldest approach to cancer therapy. When undertaken early in the course of the disease, surgery is particularly suited for cancers of the skin, gastrointestinal tract, breast, uterus, cervix, prostate gland, and testicle. Minimal procedures are undertaken whenever possible, and radiation or chemotherapy is often used with surgery to ensure maximum effectiveness.

Radiation

Radiation is capable of killing cancer cells by altering their genetic material while it is in an exposed state during cell division. Of course, since neighboring cells also divide, they are exposed to the damaging effects of radiation as well. However, by carefully planning the length of exposure and time of treatment, and by focusing the radiation precisely, damage to noncancerous cells can be held to a minimum.

Chemotherapy

The important advances in successful cancer treatment can be attributed to advances in chemotherapy, both in terms of new drugs and the more effective combination of new drugs and familiar chemotherapeutic agents. Most often, these drugs work by destroying cancer cells' ability to use important substrates in various metabolic processes or carry out cell division in a normal manner. Because chemotherapy influences cell division, it will affect noncancerous cells that divide frequently. Among the cells most susceptible to this influence are those that make up bone marrow, the lining of the intestinal tract, and the hair follicles. People who are undergoing chemotherapy often have side effects directly related to these changes, such as immune system suppression, diarrhea, and hair loss. Controversy exists regarding the effectiveness of marijuana versus conventional (and newly introduced) drugs designed to suppress the nausea or control the pain associated with cancer.

Immunotherapy

Immunotherapy refers to the use of a variety of substances to trigger a person's own immune system to attack cancer cells or prevent cancer cells from becoming activated. Among these new forms of immunotherapy are the use of interferon, monoclonal antibodies (often with radioactive isotopes attached), interleukin-2, tumor necrosis factor (TNF), and certain bone marrow growth regulators. These products are being manufactured using genetic engineering technology.

Alternative (Complementary) Cancer Therapies

In spite of the advances made in the diagnosis and treatment of cancer during this century, cancer rates are climbing as we move toward the next century. In response to spiraling rates and to requests made by cancer patients and many clinicians to expand the range of treatments, the National Institutes of Health has begun an in-depth study of alternative or nonconventional cancer treatments. Through the use of new and carefully controlled studies and the reassessment of research and records already available, the NIH will attempt to better understand the benefits of alternative or complementary therapies.

Among the treatments to be given closer consideration are chiropractic (the manipulation of the spine), acupressure (finger and thumb pressure to relieve pain), and acupuncture (needles inserted to relieve pain and promote the flow of energy within the body). Additional areas of investigation will include ayurveda (a traditional Indian lifestyle that involves the use of herbs and a specific diet), biofeedback (monitoring of body functions to control body processes), homeopathy (use of minuscule doses of toxic substances), and naturopathy (use of natural remedies, including sunshine and vitamins). Further focus will be on antioxidants (substances believed to prevent free-radical formation), reflexology (the massaging of points on the feet), therapeutic touch (redirecting of "life forces" through touching areas of the body), and visualization (learning to "see" a cure occurring).

Time and study will answer many questions about the effectiveness of these methods of treating cancer. Should these areas prove to be more effective than traditional medical science now believes, their incorporation will probably be very gradual.

Prevention Through Risk Reduction

Because cancer will probably continue to be the second most common cause of death among adults, it is important that you explore ways to reduce your risk of developing cancer. The following factors, which could make you vulnerable to cancer, can be controlled or at least recognized.

• *Know your family history.* You are the recipient of the genetic strengths and weaknesses of your biological parents and your more distant relatives. If cancer is prevalent in your family medical history, you cannot afford to disregard this fact. It may be appropriate for you to be screened for certain types of cancer more often or at a young age. The importance of family history was clearly seen in our discussion of the *BRCA1/BRCA2* inheritance pattern and related decisions about prophylactic mastectomy and prophylactic oophorectomy.

• *Select and monitor your occupation carefully.* Because of recently discovered relationships between cancer and occupations that bring employees into contact with carcinogenic agents, you must be aware of the risks posed by certain job selections and assignments. Worksites where you will come into frequent contact with pesticides, strong solvents, volatile hydrocarbons, and airborne fibers could pay well but also shorten your life. The importance of this point is evident in reviewing the current list of environmental carcinogens studies funded by the National Cancer Institute. Included are studies that focus on indoor air pollution (tobacco smoke and cooking oils), dust (cotton, grain, plastic, and wood), organic solvents (benzene, carbon tetrachloride, toluene, xylene, and chlordane), organophosphates (diazinon, dichlorvos, malathion, triazines, and cyaniazine), polybrominated biphenyls, polychlorinated biphenyls, fumigants (ethylene), water pollution (chloride, phosphene, and fluoride), petroleum products (diesel fuel, gasoline, jet fuel), radiation (radon, neutron therapy, and reactor accidents), biological agents (chlamydia, helicobacter, hepatitis B and C) and radioisotopes (iodine and radium).[49]

• *Do not use tobacco products.* You may want to review Chapter 9 on the overwhelming evidence link-

Resources from the Home Front

Although we typically envision the treatment and management of cancer as being conducted in or near the confines of a medical center, certain aspects of our personal "war on cancer" can be conducted from home. In fact, these aspects of our overall fight against cancer are often minimal in cost and based on readily available technology.

One particularly useful component in managing the pain and discomfort often associated with cancer is social involvement and the support of family, friends, and coworkers. Studies now suggest that many cancer victims who maintain active involvement in the community and who maintain contact with other people demonstrate less pain and discomfort than those who cannot or choose not to be so involved. Unknown at this time, however, is whether less than average amounts of pain and discomfort have allowed these people to remain involved, or whether their decision to remain connected has helped lessen their level of discomfort. Unfortunately, the carefully controlled study needed to determine which is cause and which is effect would be difficult to conduct on a double-blind basis.

Another potential home front aid in dealing with cancer is music therapy. Using the professional expertise of a certified music therapist, cancer victims have been helped in reducing their level of discomfort by listening to carefully selected music recorded for their use. The exact neurological mechanism through which auditory stimuli (the music) reduces discomfort is not fully understood. Nonetheless, music therapy has moved into the mainstream of clinical practice in the management of cancer, as well as in gait restoration (physical therapy) and the labor phase of childbirth. Fortunately, it is now easier for patients to receive Medicare/Medicaid and third-party reimbursement for music therapy services than once was the case.

A final area of low-tech assistance for improving the long-term management of cancer is the use of stress management to enhance the function of the immune system. Experts in the field of psychoneuroimmunology (PNI) have contended, on the basis of both animal and human subject research and anecdotal reports, that reduction of stress enhances immune system function. Accordingly, oncological treatment plans increasingly involve the inpatient and outpatient services of a medical psychologist or other stress management experts in helping patients maintain a stress-reducing lifestyle. As discussed in Chapter 3, family, friends, coworkers, and the community in general can be active participants in helping others (including cancer victims) develop and use effective coping strategies intended to reduce distress and/or foster eustress.

ing all forms of tobacco use (including smokeless tobacco) to the development of cancer. Smoking is so detrimental to health that it is considered the number one preventable cause of death.

• *Follow a sound diet.* As mentioned in conjunction with folic acid and colorectal cancer and high-fat diets and prostate cancer, dietary patterns are known to play both a causative and a preventive role in cancer. Review Chapter 5 for information about dietary practices and the incidence of various diseases, including cancer. In that chapter, the role of fruits and vegetables known to be sources of cancer-preventing phytochemicals is introduced. Good sources include a wide variety of fruits and vegetables, particularly the cruciferous vegetables, including cauliflower, broccoli, and brussels sprouts, and fruits high in beta-carotene, vitamin C, and fiber. Should research demonstrate an even clearer role for nutrients,

Resources for People Living with Cancer

For people with cancer and their families, many telephone hot lines have been set up offering information and referrals:

• American Cancer Society National Hotline: (800) ACS-2345. Also, the ACS recommends calling local ACS chapters for support group information.

• National Cancer Institute Cancer Information Service: (800) 4-CANCER.

• National Coalition for Cancer Survivorship (an umbrella group for cancer survivor units nationwide): (301) 650-8868.

• Candlelighters Childhood Cancer Foundation: Information on support groups for children with cancer and their families: (301) 657-8401 and (800) 366-2223.

• Surviving: Support group. Publishes a newsletter for Hodgkin's disease survivors. Stanford University Medical Center, Radiology Dept, Room C050, 300 Pasteur Dr, Stanford, CA 94305.

• Vital Options: Support group for people 17 to 40 who are cancer survivors: (818) 508-5657.

• The Resource Center: American College of Obstetricians and Gynecologists, 409 12th St. S.W., Washington, DC 20224-2188. Send a self-addressed, business-size envelope for Detecting and Treating Breast Problems.

• American College of Radiology, for accredited mammography centers, (800) ACR-LINE (members only) or (703) 648-8900, ask for mammography.

chemoprevention cancer prevention using food, food supplements, or medications thought to bolster the immune system or reduce the damage caused by carcinogens.

chemoprevention may become an even more widely practiced component of cancer prevention. Chemoprevention is not limited to food items and dietary supplements but can also involve pharmaceutical agents, such as aspirin, estrogen replacement therapy, and hormone replacement therapy.

• *Control your body weight.* For women, obesity is related to a higher incidence of cancer of the uterus, ovary, and breast because obesity correlates with high estrogen levels. Maintaining a desirable body weight could improve overall health and lead to more successful management of cancer should it develop.

• *Exercise regularly.* Chapter 4 discusses in detail the importance of regular moderate exercise to all aspects of health, including reducing the risk of chronic illnesses. Moderate exercise increases the body's ability to deliver oxygen to its tissues and thus to reduce the formation of cancer-enhancing free radicals formed during incomplete oxidation of nutrients. Moderate exercise also stimulates the production of enzymes that remove free radicals. Some researchers are concerned, however, that extensive exercise might actually reduce the body's ability to produce the enzymes mentioned above and thus contribute to the development of free-radical-based cellular changes, including cancer.[50]

• *Limit your exposure to the sun.* It is important to heed this message even if you enjoy many outdoor activities. Particularly for people with light complexions, the radiation received through chronic exposure to the sun may foster the development of skin cancer.

• *Consume alcohol in moderation if at all.* Heavier users of alcohol have an increased prevalence of several types of cancer, including cancer of the oral cavity, larynx, and esophagus. Whether this results directly from the presence of carcinogens in alcohol or is more closely related to the alcohol user's tendency to smoke has not yet been established.

Cancer and Wellness

When you carefully consider the preceding suggestions, it should be obvious that you can do a great deal to prevent or at least minimize the development of cancer. A wellness-oriented lifestyle is the best weapon in your "personal war against cancer." However, all risk factor reduction is relative. Observation and experience tell us that life cannot be totally structured around the desire to achieve maximum longevity or reduce morbidity at all costs. Most people need to strike a balance between life that is emotionally, socially, and spiritually satisfying and life that is structured solely for the purpose of living a long time and minimizing exposure to illness. Regardless of our personal lifestyle, however, we can educate others, provide comfort and support to those who are living with cancer, and support the funding of continuing and innovative new cancer research. Resources available for people with cancer and their families are listed in the Star Boxes on page 348.

Real Life
Real choices

Your Turn

• What health risks does Tina Mavrakos face as a consequence of her prolonged exposure to the sun?
• Is it safe for darker-skinned people like Tina to swim and sunbathe without using a sunscreen? Why or why not?
• What are the ABCD guidelines for detecting melanomas?

And Now, Your Choices . . .
• Have you ever gotten a severe sunburn? If so, did you change your attitude and behavior related to sunbathing?
• If you were a friend of Tina's, what do you think would be the most helpful advice you could give her?

Summary

• More than one half million people in the United States develop cancer each year.
• Cancer is a condition in which the body is unable to control the specialization, replication, repair of cells, or suppression of abnormal cell formation.
• Genes that control replication, specialization, repair of cells, and suppression of abnormal cellular activity have the potential to become oncogenes and thus can be considered proto-oncogenes.

• A variety of agents, including genetic mutations, viruses, and carcinogens, stimulate the conversion of regulatory genes (proto-oncogenes) into oncogenes.
• Cancer can be described on the basis of the type of tissue from which it originates, such as carcinoma, sarcoma, and melanoma.
• Cancer can be described on the basis of its location within the body, such as lung, breast, and prostate cancer.

- Cigarette smoking and genetic predisposition are both related to the development of lung cancer.
- Most cases of breast cancer do not demonstrate a clear familial pattern that suggests a genetic predisposition.
- Long-term exposure to high levels of estrogen is an important risk factor for breast cancer.
- Mammograms are an important component of breast cancer identification.
- Regular use of Pap tests is related to the early detection of cervical cancer. Sexually transmitted viral infections are strongly suspected of causing cervical cancer.
- Uterine (endometrial) cancer is more common than cervical cancer. High levels of estrogen are strongly associated with this form of cancer.
- A group of middle-aged women who are the daughters of mothers given the drug DES during pregnancy have a high incidence of vaginal cancer.
- Ovarian cancer is often "silent" in its presentation of symptoms.
- Prostate cancer is the second leading cause of cancer deaths in men.
- The PSA test improves the ability to diagnose prostate cancer. Age, high-fat diets, and inheritance of a mutated suppressor gene are known risk factors.

- Regular self-examination of the testicles leads to early detection of testicular cancer. Environmental factors may be associated with an increasing rate of testicular cancer.
- Colorectal cancer has a strong familial link and is seen in populations that consume diets high in fat and low in fruits and vegetables. Polyp formation is associated with an increased risk of this form of cancer.
- Pancreatic cancer is very difficult to survive, in part because of the absence of symptoms early in the disease's course.
- Lymphatic cancers display a wide array of initial symptoms that reflect failure of the immune system to function fully. Viral infections and environmental toxins are suspected causative agents.
- Basal cell and squamous cell carcinomas are highly curable forms of skin cancer when detected early. Malignant melanoma is life threatening if not detected early.
- Skin cancer prevention requires protection from excessive sun exposure.
- Early detection based on self-examination and screening is the basis for the identification and successful treatment of many cancers.
- Conventional treatments, including surgery, radiation, chemotherapy, and immunotherapy, as well as alternative treatments, can be used.

Review Questions

1. What is the relationship between regulatory genes and tumor suppressor genes in the development of cancer? Why are regulatory genes called both proto-oncogenes and oncogenes?
2. What are some of the major types of cancer, based on the tissue from which they originate?
3. What are the principal factors that contribute to the development of lung cancer? Of breast cancer?
4. When should regular use of mammography begin, and which women should begin using it earliest?
5. How does the PSA test contribute to the early detection of prostate cancer?
6. What signs indicate the possibility that a skin lesion has become cancerous?
7. What important information can be obtained with the use of Pap tests? What innovations are associated with the newest Pap tests?
8. What are the steps for effective self-examination of the breasts and testicles?
9. Why is ovarian cancer described as a "silent" cancer?
10. What are the conventional and alternative cancer methods most often used in the treatment of cancer?
11. What are the risk reduction activities identified in this chapter?

References

1. American Cancer Society. *Cancer facts & figures—1998.* Atlanta: The Society, 1998.
2. Landis SH et al. *Cancer statistics 1998: epidemiology and surveillance publication.* Atlanta: American Cancer Society, 1998.
3. Songer J (oncologist). Personal interviews, Nov 1998.
4. Otto SE. *Oncology nursing.* St. Louis: Mosby, 1997.
5. Cooper GM. *Elements of human cancer.* Boston: Jones & Bartlett, 1992.
6. Sellers TA et al. Evidence of Mendelian inheritance in the pathogenesis of lung cancer. *J Nat Cancer Inst* 1990; 82(15):1272–79.
7. Barsky SH et al. Histopathologic and molecular alterations in bronchial epithelium in habitual smokers

of marijuana, cocaine, and/or tobacco. *J Natl Cancer Inst* 1998; 90(16):1198–1205.

8. Radon increases lung cancer risk. *National research council's radon study committee report,* as reported by Cancer Research Foundation of America, Feb 1998. http://www.crfa.org/radon.html

9. Equal Opportunity Publications. *Independent Living* 1994; 9(7):67.

10. Sellers TA et al. Effect of family history, body fat distribution, and reproductive factors on the risk of postmenopausal breast cancer. *N Engl J Med* 1992; 326(20):1323–29.

11. Ballard-Barbash R et al. Body fat distribution and breast cancer in the Framingham study. *J Natl Cancer Inst* 1990; 82(24):1943–44.

12. Alcohol, estrogen, and breast cancer. *Harvard Women's Health Watch* 1997; 4(6):6.

13. Col NF et al. Patient-specific decisions about hormone replacement therapy in postmenopausal women. *JAMA* 1997; 227(14):1140–47.

14. Kliewer EV, Smith KB. Breast cancer mortality among immigrants in Australia and Canada (reports). *J Natl Cancer Inst* 1995; 87(15):1161.

15. Blot WJ, McLaughlin JK. Geographic patterns of breast cancer among American women. *J Natl Cancer Inst* 1995; 87(24):1819–20.

16. Krainer M et al. Differential contributions of BRCA1 and BRCA2 to early-onset breast cancer. *N Engl J Med* 1997; 336(20):1416–21.

17. Healy B. BRCA genes—bookmarking, fortunetelling, and medical care (editorials). *N Engl J Med* 1997; 336(20):1148–49.

18. Woodage T et al. The APCI1307K allele and cancer risk in a community-based study of Ashkenaza Jews. *Nat Genet* 1998; 20(1):62–65.

19. Fisher B et al. Tamoxifen for prevention of breast cancer: report of the National Surgical Adjuvant Breast and Bowel Project P-1 Study. *J Natl Cancer Inst* 1998; 90(16):1371–88.

20. Cummings Sr et al. Raloxifene reduces the risk of breast cancer and may decrease the risk of endometrial cancer in postmenopausal women. Two-year findings from the multiple outcomes of Raloxifene evaluation (MORE) trial. *Publication Year: 1998.* http://www.asco.org/prof/me/html/98abstracts/p/m3.htm

21. Screening for breast cancer in the Breast Cancer Demonstration Project. PDQ screening/prevention summary for health professionals. *J Natl Cancer Inst* 1998 Nov 11; 80(19):1540–47.

22. Screening for breast cancer. *PDQ—screening & prevention—patients.* National Cancer Institute, Aug 1998. http://www.cancernet.nic.clinpdq/screening/Screening_1

23. Neus B. Mammograms yearly urged for women in 40s. *USA Today* 1997 March 10:ID.

24. Jacobson JA et al. Ten-year results of a comparison of conservation with mastectomy in the treatment of stage I and II breast cancer. *N Engl J Med* 1995; 332(14):907–11.

25. Fisher BF et al. Reanalysis and results after 12 years follow-up in a randomized clinical trial comparing total mastectomy with lumpectomy with or without irradiation in the treatment of breast cancer. *N Engl J Med* 1995; 333(22):1456–61.

26. Tamoxifen: its history and future. *InteliHealth.* Johns Hopkins Health Information. http://www.intelihealth.com (search: tamoxifen)

27. Herceptin—a new breast cancer drug. *InteliHealth.* Johns Hopkins Health Information. http://www.intelihealth.com (search: herceptin)

28. Eddy DM. Screening for cervical cancer. *Ann Intern Med* 1990; 113(7):560–61.

29. Janerich DT et al. The screening histories of women with invasive cervical cancer, Connecticut. *Am J Public Health* 1995; 85(6):791–94.

30. *Some doctors say traditional is better.* http://www.cancer.org/bottomsearch.html

31. Company testing vaccine against cervical cancer (The Associated Press). *USA Today* 1998 June 18:6D.

32. Crowley LV. *Introduction to human disease.* 4th ed. Boston: Jones & Bartlett, 1996.

33. Langer RD et al. Transvaginal ultrasonography compared with endometrial biopsy for the detection of endometrial disease (for The Postmenopausal Estrogen/Progestin Trial). *N Engl J Med* 1997 Dec 18; 337(25):1792–98.

34. Narod SA et al. Oral contraceptives and the risk of hereditary ovarian cancer. Hereditary Ovarian Cancer Clinical Study Group. *N Engl J Med* 1998; 339(7):424–28.

35. Hebert JR et al. Nutritional and socioeconomic factors in relation to prostate cancer mortality: a cross-national study. *J Natl Cancer Inst* 1998; 90(21):1631–47.

36. Heinonen OP et al. Prostate cancer and supplementation with alpha-tocopherol and beta-carotene: incidence and mortality in a controlled trial. *J Natl Cancer Inst* 1998; 90(6):440–46.

37. Yoshizawa K et al. Study of prediagnostic selenium level in toenails and the risk of advanced prostate cancer. *J Natl Cancer Inst* 1998; 90(16):1219–24.

38. Ragde H et al. Ten-year disease free survival after transperineal sonography-guided iodine-125 brachytherapy with or without 45-gray external beam irradiation in the treatment of patients with clinically localized, low to high Gleason grade prostate carcinoma. *Cancer* 1998; 83(45):989–1001.

39. Travis LB et al. Risk of second malignant neoplasms among long-term survivors of testicular cancer. *J Natl Cancer Inst* 1997; 89(19):1429–39.

40. Giovannucci E et al. Aspirin and the risk of colorectal cancer in women. *N Engl J Med* 1995; 333(10):609–14.

41. Holt PR et al. Modulation of abnormal colonic epithelial cell proliferation and differentiation by low-fat dairy foods: a randomized controlled trial. *JAMA* 1998; 280(12):1074–79.

42. Giovannucci E et al. Multivitamin use, folate, and colon cancer in women in the Nurses' Health Study. *Ann Intern Med* 1998; 129(7):517–24.

43. Soignet SL et al. Complete remission after treatment of acute promyelocytic leukemia with arsenic trioxide. *N Engl J Med* 1998; 339(19):1341–48.

44. Kline RM et al. Umbilical cord blood transplantation: providing a donor for everyone needing a bone marrow transplant? *South Med J* 1998; 91(9):821–28.

45. Aversa F et al. Treatment of high-risk acute leukemia with T cell-depleted stem cells from related donors with one fully mismatched HLA haplotype. *N Engl J Med* 1998; 339(17):1186–93.

46. Kahn HS et al. Increased cancer mortality following a history of nonmelanoma skin cancer. *JAMA* 1998; 280(10):910–12.

47. Tucker MA et al. Clinically recognized dysplastic nevi: a central risk factor for cutaneous melanoma. *JAMA* 1997; 277(18):1439–44.

48. Wilcken N. Winning the war on cancer (comment). *N Engl J Med* 1997; 337(13):937–38. (seven additional comments on topic included)

49. Highlights of NCI's carcinogenesis studies. *Cancer facts,* May 23, 1997. http://www.icic.nci.nih.gov

50. Fink W (exercise physiologist). Personal interview, December, 1995.

Suggested Readings

Piver MS, Wilder G, Bull J. *Gilda's disease: sharing personal experiences and a medical perspective on ovarian cancer.* New York: Bantam Doubleday Dell Publishing, 1998. For those who remember the more public aspects of comedienne Gilda Radner's death from ovarian cancer in 1989, a moving new dimension, her husband's profoundly personal relationship with his wife and her disease, is added to the story. The addition of medical perspectives by Steven Piver, MD, regarding ovarian cancer and the array of available treatment options makes this book an important resource for persons interested in the "silent cancer."

Walsh PC, Worthington JF. *The prostate: a guide for men and the women who love them.* New York: Warner Books, 1997. The prostate, a small but important gland in the male's urogenital system, plays a central role in reproductive health, yet it also can be the basis of life-threatening cancer. This book details the pathological changes that occur within the prostate and describes the available medical treatment options. A unique family perspective makes this book important not only to men, but also to the women and other family members who love them.

Arnot RB. *The breast cancer prevention diet: the powerful foods, supplements, and drugs that can save your life.* New York:

Little Brown, 1998. The author, a physician and NBC's chief medical correspondent, advances a diet-based approach to the prevention of breast cancer that has failed to impress many of his peers. Respected nutritionists applaud the book's emphasis on better nutrition, but at the same time remind readers that many of the author's contentions regarding the role of specific nutrients and supplements in preventing cancer are simply not supported by research. Nevertheless, the book will appeal to many people who wish to be proactive in their attempt to prevent cancer and other chronic conditions of adulthood.

Kenet B, Lawler P. *Saving your skin: prevention, early detection, and treatment of melanoma and other skin cancers.* New York: Four Walls Eight Windows, 1998. Malignant melanoma is not the garden-variety skin cancer so frequently experienced by adults. Rather, it is a potentially lethal form of cancer that is very difficult to treat in its more advanced stages. This book proves valuable insights into the prevention as well as the medical terminology and treatment options associated with this serious form of skin cancer.

As We Go To PRESS

An article published recently in the *New England Journal of Medicine* indicates that prophylactic mastectomy is indeed effective in preventing breast cancer among women at high risk. Researchers at the Mayo Clinic studied sisters with strong family histories of breast cancer. One sister in each pair had undergone prophylactic breast removal, and one had not. The results showed that the risk of developing the disease was cut by 90 percent in the sister who had elected to have the surgery. The study's authors concluded that prophylactic mastectomy may be the best course of action for women with the BRCA-1 or BRCA-2 mutation.

topics for Today

Cancer and Genetic Testing: Answers Raise New Questions

Cancer is essentially cell resolution that is out of control. The resulting mass of overactive cells is a tumor. But what causes our systems to go awry? Genetic mutations can be inherited or caused by exposure to chemicals, radiation, or viruses. Normal functioning of our cells also produces cancer-causing chemicals.[1] These carcinogens act on two types of genes that function in opposite ways. Proto-oncogenes code for proteins that stimulate cell division; mutations in these genes cause overstimulation, which results in excessive cell division. Tumor-suppressor genes, on the other hand, normally code for proteins that inhibit cell division; mutations of these genes inactivate them, which also results in excessive cell division.[1]

Carcinogenesis is a multistep process. It normally takes many decades to accumulate all the mutations necessary to produce cancer. This process is accelerated, however, when mutated genes are inherited. Not only are the mutations already in place, but certain inherited defects impair the normally efficient repair of DNA, which allows the mutations to accumulate.[1] Consequently, these inherited cancers develop earlier in life.

The structure of DNA itself wasn't understood until the 1950s, but genetic advances since then have been amazingly rapid and numerous. In the 1980s, a gene linked to retinoblastoma, a rare eye cancer, was identified. However, it was the recent discovery of *BRCA1* and *BRCA2*, two breast cancer genes, that brought genetic testing to the public's attention.[2] These genes are also linked to ovarian cancer and possibly prostate cancer, which increases scientists' and the public's interest in them.

Most women with breast cancer do not have a genetic predisposition for the disease.[3] In fact, of the 108,300 new cases of breast cancer estimated in the United States in 1998, an inherited gene is a factor in only a small percentage of cases.[3] Still, possession of the mutated gene is of critical concern because inherited cancers develop earlier in life and the risk in this subpopulation is so much higher than in the population as a whole. For example, an average woman's lifetime risk for breast cancer is 11 percent, but a woman with the *BRCA1* mutation has a risk of 85%.[2] Even male members of families with strong histories of breast cancer are at risk for developing the disease.

Genetic Testing

Until recently, genetic testing focused on rare single-gene disorders, such as Tay-Sachs disease, cystic fibrosis, Huntington's disease,[4] and sickle cell anemia. Such tests, conducted before marriage or childbearing, identified carriers of the mutated gene and allowed them to consider their reproductive options. The emphasis in genetic testing is now shifting to common chronic diseases, which pose the major health threat in Western countries. Genetic testing is called upon to identify multiple genes associated with such conditions as cancer, atherosclerosis, and hypertension.[4] However, unlike in testing for single-gene disorders, cases will be missed if the test does not detect all mutations.[5] Another difference is that the tests reveal a predisposition in the patient herself or himself for acquiring the disease, rather than only the chance for passing it on to future offspring.

With frequent public announcements of the discovery of "new" genes linked to normal and pathological functions, tests for common diseases are expected to shift from being research screening devices for high-risk patients to being the standard of good medical practice. Medical schools are introducing DNA diagnostics into their curricula in anticipation of this trend.

Isolating genes is a scientifically valid method of investigating biological processes and environmental influences. However, understanding of the genetic basis for diseases such as cancer has thus far outpaced advances in medical treatment.[6] This creates a gap between what technology can tell us and what's best for patients and their families. This gap can lead even the most likely candidates for such testing to decline.

Would You Want to Know?

A positive test indicates only a probability for developing a given disease; it is not a diagnosis of disease.

However, having knowledge of one's high risk could lead to serious depression. In addition, a positive finding in one patient implies that other family members are also at risk. This situation forces doctors to weigh the patient's right to confidentiality against the family members' right to make informed decisions concerning their own health.[7]

Problems are created even if the test results are not positive. A negative test result may foster a false sense of security that causes the patient to ignore symptoms and delay doctor's visits. A negative result can also cause feelings of guilt if other family members test positive. There are only 1,000 trained genetic counseling specialists in the United States qualified to help a patient deal with the psychological issues surrounding disease predisposition. Although not a substitute for professional counseling, family genetic disease support groups fund research and provide assistance and guidance in an effort to lessen the heartache of inherited disease factors. Those at risk should consider contacting the National Cancer Institute's National Cancer Genetics Network. Working with physicians and educational institutions, they can enroll people in research studies, inform them of their genetic status, and provide necessary counseling.

What If You Knew?

How would you feel if you knew that you possessed a mutated gene that could later result in disease? The answer to this question hinges on cultural norms, concepts of disease, religious beliefs, possibly a history of the same disease claiming those close to you, and in the case of breast cancer, a woman's own view of the importance of her breasts.[8] Some women who believe themselves to be at high risk for breast cancer are undergoing bilateral prophylactic mastectomies. This radical procedure involves removal of both breasts before any cancer is detected. Although this procedure is done with some frequency within high-risk groups, its long-term effectiveness is not yet fully known. In addition, the desirability of reconstructive surgery is difficult to address at this time. Sites of future disease in vital organs, of course, cannot be removed.

A positive genetic test would ideally allow you to be eligible for clinical trials of chemoprevention drugs. In the future, as the new field of pharmacogenetics (the prevention and treatment of genetic diseases with drugs) grows, genetic information will help to match diagnosis and treatment more effectively than is now possible.[9] Beyond that, genetic knowledge gives you an increased awareness of your body's signals so that disease may be detected early.

What If Someone Else Found Out?

Without adequate regulation, one's genetic makeup could become the basis for discrimination by insurance companies, employers, and society at large. Insurance companies already use family history, an estimate of your genetic makeup, to make insurability decisions.[5] Their power grows as information becomes more definite, as in the form of genetic test results. Employers are also concerned with insurance risk, and they may discriminate against employees because of the projected absenteeism and productivity lost to illness. And society discriminates against people with certain illnesses, especially when a particular disease is not fully understood.

Legislatures have begun to pass laws to prevent discrimination by insurance companies against carriers of genetic mutations.[5] The California state legislature, for example, voted to ban all discrimination on the basis of genetic status, but the bill was vetoed by the governor.[9] Many fear that the widespread use of genetic testing will occur before adequate standards are in place, thus doing the patient and his or her family more harm than good.

The Boundary Between Health and Disease

Testing for genetic predispositions is an area in which the boundary between health and disease is blurred. To clarify this boundary as much as possible and to guard against the psychosocial risks of anxiety, loss of privacy, stigmatization, and discrimination, the use of any available test should conform to the following guidelines:

- The test should have well-defined goals, specifically those concerning associated disease reduction measures.
- The overall testing procedure should have a patient education and counseling program in place and rely solely on informed consent.
- The test itself must be accurate and reliable, with appropriate quality control, acceptable costs, and adequate follow-up. (Currently the costs run from several hundred to several thousand dollars per test.)

Genetic makeup is a powerful tool for individual and familial health risk assessment. No one is completely healthy; thus, ultimately, responsible decision making concerning genetic testing is of benefit to everyone.

For Discussion . . .

If a mutated gene for cancer ran in your family, would you want to know if you had it or not? What would you do with the information? What kinds of regulations do you think should be placed on genetic testing and the privacy of results? Are the current costs of genetic testing acceptable? Why or why not?

References

1. Weinberg R. How cancer arises. *Scientific American* 1996; 275(3):62–70.

2. Mutation detection of the breast/ovarian cancer genes BRCA1 and BRCA2 in Ashkenazi Jewish population, Dec 1998. http://www.harc.edu/dna/brcaz.html

3. The American Cancer Society. *Cancer facts & figures—1998.* Atlanta: The Society, 1998.

4. Dewanjee MK. Detecting cancer in the body. *Chemtech* 1994; 24(11):21–24.

5. Sidransky D, Stix G. Advances in cancer detection. *Scientific American* 1996; 275(3):104–6.

6. Harper PS. Genetic testing, common diseases, and health service provision. *The Lancet* 1995; 346(8991-2): 1645–46.

7. Dickens BM. Legal and ethical issues in genetic testing and counseling for susceptibility to breast, ovarian, and colon cancer. *JAMA* 1996; 276(20):1621.

8. Parker LS. Breast cancer, genetic screening and critical bioethics gaze. *JAMA* 1996; 276(20):1622.

9. Pap MZ et al. Breast cancer prevention in high risk individuals—the surgical aspect. *Women's Health Weekly* (research from conferences) 1998 April 6; 18–19.

InfoLinks
www.ornl.gov/TechResources/
 Human_Genome/home.html
www.ncifcrf.gov/

chapter
twelve

Managing Chronic Conditions

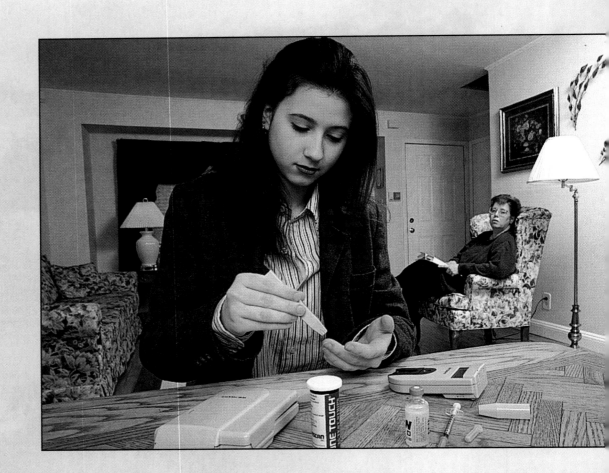

To successfully manage their condition, people with insulin-dependent (type I) diabetes mellitus must periodically test their blood glucose level.

I n clinical medicine, thousands of diseases, illnesses, and conditions can be diagnosed and treated. For ease of communication among health-care professionals and between professionals and laypeople, these diseases and illnesses have been individually named and categorized. We have chosen a set of categories—*genetic/inherited*, *congenital*, *metabolic*, *degenerative*, and *infectious*—with which to organize a sample of conditions that we believe you will be interested in learning about.[1] Knowledge of these conditions will increase your understanding of chronic disease processes and how they differ from infectious diseases. Where appropriate, you will also find useful information about risk factors and lifestyle changes you can make to reduce your risk of developing a chronic condition.*†

HEALTHY PEOPLE: LOOKING AHEAD TO 2010

The *Healthy People 2000* document gave little attention to chronic conditions. In fact, it addressed only diabetes mellitus type II (non-insulin-dependent diabetes) and asthma. Because of this narrow focus on chronic conditions, we elected to discuss the four factors we believed would influence the nature and extent of progress made in this important area. One factor was the need to better understand the genetic underpinnings of many of the most important chronic conditions. We speculated that such enhanced understanding would spur the development of new medications, screening procedures, and counseling services. The remaining three factors, however, were presented in a less optimistic light. These were: the aging of the population, which raises the probability that people will have more time to develop chronic illnesses; the lack of comprehensive health care, which is due partly to the lack of health insurance coverage among a large group of people; and the unhealthful lifestyle choices that maturing adults continue to make.

If the *Healthy People 2010* project continues to emphasize diabetes mellitus, we must consider two recent recommendations regarding the medical management of that condition. The first recommendation is to lower the standard at which a blood sugar level is considered normal; the second is that all persons age 25 and above should be screened regularly for early indicators of glucose intolerance. The task of creating a delivery model to implement the latter recommendation would be both comprehensive and expensive, making it unlikely that significant progress could be achieved by 2010.

Further, if *Healthy People 2010* continues to emphasize asthma, implementation may be achieved by using a delivery model based on disparities (for example, children forced to live in major urban areas with high levels of pollution) and/or leading contributors (such as children residing in a family with one or more adult smokers). Today, people affected by asthma come into the health-care community on their own, generally after an initial serious attack. By 2010 the health-care system may be seeking them out so they can receive regular preventive services.

---

*Only a clinician can diagnose and treat these conditions. The information contained in this chapter is intended only to inform.

†We have placed each condition into its most appropriate category. However, the characteristics of a given condition may overlap with those in a second group. We will point this out when it occurs.

Real Life
Real choices

- Names: Penny Christenson
- Age: 31
- Occupation: Urban planner

- Jay Christenson
- Age: 30
- Occupation: Sales representative

"I can't believe this . . . Please tell me this isn't happening . . ." The last words trail off into a whisper as Penny Christenson turns tear-filled eyes to her husband. Jay, known to family and friends for being brave to the point of stoicism, grips Penny's hand so tightly that his knuckles whiten. With tears standing unshed in his own eyes, he shakes his head despondently. "I wish it weren't . . . I never thought . . ." Like Penny's, his voice fades to silence. Sitting on the hospital lounge bench padded in garish orange vinyl, Jay and Penny stare helplessly at each other. Outside, a cloudless blue-and-gold September day seems to mock their anguish as they contemplate a future far from what they'd planned and dreamed.

The Christensons have just met with a genetic counselor at the most prestigious medical center in their region. Eagerly planning their first pregnancy, they'd consulted the specialist on the advice of their family practitioner, who was concerned because Penny's younger sister, Jill, has a 7-year-old son, Tad, who suffers from cystic fibrosis. Fearing Penny might also be a CF carrier, her physician recommended she and Jay seek genetic counseling before becoming pregnant.

By means of sophisticated tests, the genetics lab at the medical center has been able to identify the specific genetic mutation that caused young Tad to be born with CF. Further testing re-

vealed that Penny is positive for the same mutation, meaning she definitely is a carrier of the chronic, debilitating lung disease.

Ever since Tad was born, Penny had known she had a chance of passing CF to a child of her own. Reassured by one doctor that the risk probably wasn't significant, she and Jay happily made plans for the family they wanted. Like any other prospective parents, they talked excitedly about the sound, healthy kids they'd have and the fun they'd have teaching them to swim, ski, and canoe.

But Penny knows from watching her nephew Tad that a child with cystic fibrosis often has barely enough energy to walk, let alone run, swim laps, or paddle a canoe. Fighting to breathe through thick mucous secretions in their lungs, CF kids usually are frail, thin, and unable to tolerate anything more than mild activity.

Penny and Jay both love Tad dearly and admire his brave effort to enjoy life in spite of his condition. They also credit Jill and her husband, Randy, with doing everything in their power to help Tad live as normal a life as possible and to make the most of his considerable talent and intelligence. But they also see the endless struggle as Jill and Randy try to give Tad every opportunity and at the same time meet the needs of their older son, Jerry, and carve out some time for themselves.

Can we do this? Penny wonders. *Should* we do this? How, Jay asks himself, is our child going to feel when he or she realizes we knew Penny was a CF carrier and went ahead anyway? Do we have the love and courage to deal with this every day—and to deal with the possible death of our child from this wretched disease?

As you study this chapter, think about Jay and Penny's situation and prepare to answer the questions in **Your Turn** at the end of the chapter.

The first four categories of conditions—genetic/inherited, congenital, metabolic, and degenerative—are discussed in the sections that follow. They have in common a slow, gradual course of development and remain a part of people's lives for long periods of time; thus they are said to be **chronic** conditions. Conversely, the infectious diseases are often quickly contracted and, once treatment has begun, stay active for a limited amount of time. These are referred to as the **acute** conditions (although HIV/AIDS is now defined as a chronic condition because of its extended duration). This fifth category, the infectious conditions, comprises illnesses caused by pathogenic organisms transmitted from person to person.[1] These conditions are discussed separately, in Chapter 13. The worldwide HIV/AIDS epidemic, the increasing threat of infectious diseases from the tropical rain forests, such as Ebola, and the comeback of familiar infections that are now resistant to antibiotics makes this separate coverage necessary.

Two types of chronic diseases, cardiovascular disease and cancer, are also addressed separately (in

Chapters 10 and 11, respectively) because of their importance to so many families and to the health of the nation. Many other chronic conditions are addressed in appropriate chapters throughout the book. For example, low back pain is discussed in Chapter 4, osteoporosis in Chapter 5, and chronic obstructive lung disease in Chapter 9, as well as many others. Even though these conditions are not discussed in this chapter, they too fit into one or more of the categories described and are either chronic or acute in nature.

Genetic/Inherited Conditions

The first category, genetic or inherited conditions, can occur in any of three ways: (1) abnormal genetic material (genes) are transmitted from one or both biological parents at conception; (2) abnormal genetic material is formed by mutation of normal genetic material at a very early stage of cellular replication and, subsequently, passed on with each cell doubling; or (3) an abnormal number of chromosomes—more or fewer than the normal number of forty-six—is inherited or formed.[1] We will present several conditions from this broad category, including Klinefelter's syndrome, Turner's syndrome, supermasculinity, Down syndrome, cystic fibrosis, Tay-Sachs disease, and Duchenne muscular dystrophy.

Abnormal Number of Sex Chromosomes

At the time of conception (fertilization) an ovum (egg) from the biological mother containing twenty-three chromosomes is penetrated by a sperm from the biological father that also contains twenty-three chromosomes. This fusion of genetic material results in an initial human cell that contains forty-six chromosomes, the number found in virtually every human cell. Of these chromosomes, forty-four (twenty-two from each biological patent) are **autosomes** (body chromosomes or nonsex chromosomes), and the remaining two are **sex chromosomes** (an X from the biological mother and an X or Y from the biological father). A normal male would thus possess a 44XY chromosomal profile, and a normal female would be depicted as 44XX.[2] Occasionally people are born who possess more or fewer than the normal forty-six chromosomes because they have more than or fewer than the normal two sex chromosomes.

Klinefelter's Syndrome

Klinefelter's syndrome is one condition in which an abnormal number of sex chromosomes is present. It occurs in males and is a relatively rare (1 in 1,000 male births)[3] condition in which a Y sex chromosome from the biological father is combined with two X sex chromosomes from the biological mother. Klinefelter's syndrome would be graphically depicted as 44XXY, for a total of forty-seven chromosomes.[4] Advanced maternal age is thought to be related to the development of this syndrome.

Although they look normal at birth, male children with Klinefelter's syndrome gradually show signs of the condition by the time they reach puberty. Men with Klinefelter's syndrome are often tall, very thin, and have gynecomastia (breast enlargement).[4] In addition, a small penis, small testicles, and underdeveloped secondary sexual characteristics are typical. Men with Klinefelter's syndrome are infertile and have some impairment in learning ability and personality adjustment. The unique components of Klinefelter's syndrome are thought to reflect the feminizing influence of the additional X chromosome.

Prevention, Diagnosis, and Management Klinefelter's syndrome cannot, of course, be cured. Hormonal treatment is often used to minimize feminization, although fertility is not restored by testosterone therapy.

Turner's Syndrome

Another genetic condition caused by an altered sex chromosome number is Turner's syndrome. It occurs in females (1 in 5,000 female births)[3] when one of the two X chromosomes is missing, resulting in a chromosomal number of forty-five. This pattern is graphically depicted as 44X0, with 0 reflecting the absence of the second X chromosome.[4] Women with Turner's syndrome have equivalent versions of many of the problems seen in men with Klinefelter's syndrome: infertility, a characteristic body type, and diminished secondary sex characteristics.[5]

Supermasculinity

A final sex chromosome abnormality is referred to as supermasculinity (1 in 1,000 male births),[3] a syndrome in which males possess more than a single Y chromosome, such as a 44XYY pattern. Once thought to be associated with higher-than-normal levels of aggression, the behavioral consequences of this condition are now unclear. Because their distinguishing physical characteristics are subtle, men with this syndrome are not easily identifiable. They may be slightly taller than normal and more inclined to outbursts of anger, although this may be largely environmentally determined.

Abnormal Number of Autosomes

Down Syndrome

In about 1 of every 600 live births, a child with Down syndrome is born. Bearing a chromosomal number of forty-seven, the infant with Down syndrome has an additional chromosome number 21.[4] In almost all cases, this extra twenty-first chromosome is obtained through the biological mother's ovum. Pregnancy late in a woman's reproductive years appears to be the single most important risk factor for this condition.[4]

Children with Down syndrome have several characteristic physical features. Among these are a short but broad neck, folds of tissue over the eyelids, a thick, protruding tongue, short hands with curving of the little finger, and a body build characterized by shortness and obesity. A variety of internal problems may also be seen in infants and children with Down

chronic develops slowly and persists for an extended period of time.

acute has a sudden onset and a prompt resolution.

autosomes body chromosomes; chromosomes other than the X and Y sex chromosomes.

sex chromosomes the X and Y chromosomes that determine sex; chromosomes other than the autosomes.

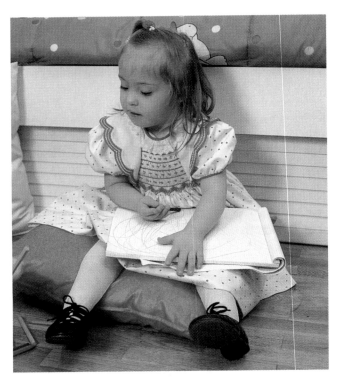

Early intervention programs have improved the functional abilities of people with Down syndrome.

syndrome. These include heart defects, atherosclerotic vessel damage, chronic respiratory problems, intestinal obstructions, and a variety of vision-related abnormalities. With advancing age, dementia resembling that in Alzheimer's disease can develop.

Prevention, Diagnosis, and Management In recent years, the functional abilities and average life span of people with Down syndrome have increased. Early intervention programs, including home visits, speech therapy, and educational enrichment, combined with a regular school experience and comprehensive parental involvement, have made it possible for children with Down syndrome to become more independent.[6] In addition, improved medical treatment of physical problems has extended life expectancy into middle adulthood.

Screening tests for Down syndrome can be performed when a pregnancy meets any of the following criteria: (1) there is a family history of Down syndrome; (2) the biological mother has undergone in vitro fertilization; or (3) the mother is over age thirty-five at the time of conception. A new blood test, which eliminates the need for amniocentesis and/or chorionic villus sampling, can identify the existence of Down syndrome by the ninth week of pregnancy.[7] The woman or couple can then make an informed decision about whether to terminate the pregnancy.

Inherited Genetic Mutations

Cystic Fibrosis

No inherited condition claims more children's and young adults' lives than cystic fibrosis (CF). In the United States, in about 1 of every 2,000 live births an infant is born with this inherited condition. In past decades, life expectancy for children with cystic fibrosis was only about eight years. Today, however, with a fuller understanding of the disease and with more effective forms of treatment, life expectancy has increased significantly, to about thirty years. Unfortunately, the disease is very demanding, and effective management requires daily intervention.[25]

Cystic fibrosis causes a profound disruption in the function of the **exocrine glands** in several areas of the body. This impaired function is due to the body's inability to produce a protein that helps regulate chloride content within the secretory cells of various exocrine glands. In the absence of this protein, the glands cannot produce certain enzymes needed to carry out important bodily functions.

For example, cystic fibrosis impairs the ability of the pancreas, an exocrine gland, to produce digestive enzymes. Thus the disease was once called *cystic fibrosis of the pancreas*. But today CF is known to affect other exocrine glands as well. It reduces the ability of sweat glands to conserve electrolytes, the ability of mucous glands lining the airway to control mucus production, and the ability of secretory glands within the digestive tract to produce digestive enzymes. These impairments of normal function underlie significant problems in respiration and digestion.[8] For example, a person with CF may have compromised growth and development from malnutrition, liver disease, and pancreatic deterioration. In addition, the long strands of mucus that accumulate in inflamed airways can cause life-threatening episodes of respiratory distress.[25]

Prevention, Diagnosis, and Management Although CF is sometimes not identified until later in life, the diagnosis is usually made during childhood. Infants and young children with CF present a combination of the following symptoms:

- Poor growth
- Frequent, foul-smelling stools
- Chronic coughing and wheezing
- Recurrent pneumonia
- Nasal polyps
- Enlarged fingertips
- Skin that has a salty taste

When CF is suspected on the basis of these symptoms, a diagnosis is made using a blood test with which the presence of an abnormal gene on chromosome number 7 is identified.[4]

The management of CF has improved dramatically in recent years. Diets designed to maintain weight and support growth, respiratory therapy to maintain the health of the airways, a newly approved inhaled antibiotic, and drugs to break up mucus plugs have improved the quality of life and increased the life expectancy of people with CF.[9] Recently, **gene replacement therapy** through viral inhalation and virus-containing microscopic beads (liposomes) has been attempted, but the effectiveness of this treatment has not yet been established. Accordingly, CF remains an incurable, life-shortening disease process.

Like sickle-cell disease and Tay-Sachs disease, which are described later, CF shows a **recessive inheritance pattern.** Genetic testing can determine whether a person who is apparently free from CF might, in fact, carry a copy of the recessive gene. If one biological parent does not carry the defective gene and one does, 25 percent of their children will be carriers of the defective gene. When both biological parents are carriers, 25 percent of their children will have CF, 50 percent will be carriers (but not have CF), and 25 percent will neither have CF nor be carriers.[4] A panel of scientists assembled by the National Institutes of Health in 1997 recommended that all couples anticipating a pregnancy be offered genetic screening for CF. In addition, chorionic villus sampling or amniocentesis can be performed. When the embryo is positive for CF, parents can seek counseling regarding their options, including whether to continue the pregnancy.

Personal Applications

• How do you feel about pregnancy termination when conditions such as cystic fibrosis or Down syndrome are discovered early in the course of a pregnancy?

Tay-Sachs Disease

Tay-Sachs disease is among the rarest of the genetic diseases within the general population, yet it is frequently seen among people of Eastern European Jewish heritage. Tay-Sachs disease is a fatal disorder that develops in one-quarter of the children conceived by two biological parents who carry the abnormal gene. Approximately 30 percent of American Jews carry this recessive gene.

In the most common type of Tay-Sachs disease, called juvenile Tay-Sachs, affected children appear normal at birth but begin to display clear and increasing signs of neurological abnormality by the age of six months. Blindness, deafness, profound muscle atrophy, paralysis, and the total inability to swallow then develop before the child dies at about five years of age. In rare cases of the disease, called intermediate-

onset Tay-Sachs, symptoms first appear during adolescence. The neurological abnormalities are similar to those listed earlier, but also include slurred speech, cramps, tremors, and sometimes mental illness. Death occurs by age fifteen. In the even rarer cases when Tay-Sachs develops during young adulthood, called late-onset Tay-Sachs disease, symptoms progress slowly, with debilitating physical and mental disorders eventually noted.

Tay-Sachs disease is caused by a genetic inability to manufacture an enzyme that is necessary in the breakdown of a lipid (fat) produced in the nervous system. In the absence of the enzyme, this lipid accumulates within the tissues of the brain, resulting in irreversible damage and eventual death.

Prevention, Diagnosis, and Management As with cystic fibrosis, people with a family history of Tay-Sachs and people of Eastern European Jewish heritage are encouraged to have their carrier status determined. If the carrier status of the biological parents is not known at the time of pregnancy or if the biological parents are both carriers, chorionic villus sampling or amniocentesis can be used to determine whether the fetus is affected.[9]

Sickle-Cell Trait and Sickle-Cell Disease

Of all the chemical compounds found within the body, few occur in as many forms as hemoglobin, which helps bind oxygen to red blood cells. Two forms of hemoglobin are associated with sickle-cell trait and sickle-cell disease. African-Americans can possess either form of this abnormal hemoglobin. Those who inherit the trait form do not develop the disease but are capable of transmitting the gene for abnormal hemoglobin to their offspring. Those who inherit the disease form face a shortened life characterized by periods of pain and impairment called *crises.*

Approximately 8 percent of African-Americans carry the recessive gene for sickle-cell trait; they experience little impairment, and they can transmit the gene to their children. For approximately 1.5 percent of African-Americans, however, sickle-cell disease is a painful, incapacitating, and life-shortening condition.[4]

---

exocrine glands glands whose secretions are released through tubes or ducts, such as sweat glands.

gene replacement therapy an experimental therapy in which a healthy human gene is incorporated into a harmless virus to be delivered to cells that lack the gene.

recessive inheritance pattern the inheritance of traits whose expression requires that they be carried by both biological parents.

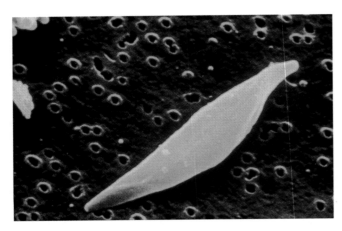

Figure 12-1 A sickled (crescent-shaped) red blood cell in a person with sickle-cell disease. The red blood cells are elongated and thus cannot pass through the body's minute capillaries, causing periods of pain and impairment called *crises*.

Red blood cells are elongated, crescent-shaped (or sickled), and unable to pass through the body's minute capillaries (Figure 12-1). The body responds to the presence of these abnormal red blood cells by removing them very quickly. This sets the stage for anemia—thus the condition is often called *sickle-cell anemia*. In addition to anemia, this form of the condition is associated with many serious medical problems, including impaired lung function, congestive heart failure, gallbladder infections, bone changes, and abnormalities of the eyes and skin. Living beyond early adulthood was until recently not possible. Today, however, with effective screening and new medications, people with sickle-cell disease may live to reach fifty years of age.[8]

Prevention, Diagnosis, and Management In about 1 percent of people with sickle-cell disease, a bone marrow transplant may be able to give the body the ability to produce a normal form of hemoglobin. Early results are promising and raise hope of a "cure" of sorts, although the number of patients who might be helped by this therapy is small. In addition, a newly introduced drug, hydroxyurea, has provided some relief from the pain caused by the clogging of vessels and the discomfort of acute chest congestion. The drug also reduces the number of blood transfusions normally needed to relieve pain.

Screening to determine whether a woman or her partner carries the recessive gene may be the only key for preventing sickle-cell trait and disease. Genetic counseling can then help couples weigh the risk of passing on the gene to their children, allowing them to make informed reproductive decisions based on this knowledge.[4] The Star Box at right provides useful information about genetic counseling.

Genetic Counseling

Consider genetic counseling if you find yourself in any of the following situations:

- You know that certain disorders with a definite or possible genetic component run in your family and you want to find out more about the risks.

- You are pregnant or planning a pregnancy and you are in your mid-thirties or older.

- You have previously given birth to a child with a genetic (inherited) or congenital abnormality.

- You are planning a pregnancy and belong to an ethnic group with a high incidence of genetic disorders. For example, African-Americans have a high incidence of sickle-cell disease and trait, and Jews of Eastern European descent have a high incidence of Tay-Sachs disease.

How to Find a Genetic Counselor
You should not regard any form of genetic testing as "just another blood test." You should understand the benefits and costs. Your primary care physician or obstetrician/gynecologist should refer you for counseling. Counselors usually work in hospitals or clinics as part of a multidisciplinary medical team; they are certified by the American Board of Genetic Counseling and may be either Board Certified or in Active Candidate Status (authorized to take the next certification examination). An accredited counselor will be trained in both prenatal and general genetic counseling. You should ask the counselor about his or her experience and qualifications. For a free brochure and a list of counselors in your area, contact the National Society of Genetic Counselors at 233 Canterbury Drive, Dept. WL, Wallingford, PA 19086-6617 (telephone 610-872-7608, mailbox 7). The society is not a source of medical information about specific genetic diseases.

What a Counselor Can Tell You
A genetic counselor should be able to help you decide, first, whether you need testing. Some tests are widely available. Others must be performed by a specialized laboratory. It is important to discuss issues of confidentiality. For example, who will know you have been tested and who will know the results of the tests? You should also find out what will happen if the test shows you have a genetic risk for or are a carrier of the disease for which you are being tested. What are your options if you are already pregnant? Will your health insurance be threatened? How accurate are the tests? With thorough answers to these and other questions, you can make an informed decision about whether to undergo or decline genetic testing.

Sex Chromosome–Linked Inherited Genetic Mutations

Duchenne Muscular Dystrophy
Genetic mutations located on a maternal sex chromosome (which is always an X chromosome) present a unique problem for male offspring. The crux of the

problem lies in the male's inability to "offset" or "override" the mutated gene's influence because he lacks a second X chromosome containing a normal version of the mutated gene. Females can carry the mutated gene but cannot be affected by the abnormal trait because they have a normal second X chromosome.

Duchenne muscular dystrophy (DMD) is an inherited condition in which muscle fibers lack the ability to produce a protein called *dystrophin,* which is necessary for normal muscular function. In the absence of this protein, skeletal muscles deteriorate, impairing the ability to stand, walk, and, eventually, even breathe. Death occurs prematurely, generally due to respiratory collapse. Some people with DMD die during the their teen years and some live to reach their thirties, but most die in their twenties.

Prevention, Diagnosis, and Management Muscular dystrophy can be relatively easily diagnosed by an experienced physician, but the symptoms are usually not apparent until after the age of two. Before this age the signs of the disease are unlikely to be recognized, unless parents' concern about delayed walking prompts them to have the child seen by a physician. After age two, however, falls, changes in gait, the development of distinct scoliosis (spinal curvature), and the appearance of muscle wasting become obvious, and the disease is identified. The diagnosis is generally made using a blood test that assesses the level of creatine kinase, an enzyme that leaks out of the muscle in response to the inadequate presence of dystrophin. Abnormally high levels of creatine kinase confirm the diagnosis. Electrical activity within the muscle may also be measured in diagnosing DMD.[10]

The medical management of DMD centers on the prompt and effective use of physical therapy and occupational therapy to maintain the highest level of function possible. By the teen years, people with DMD usually can no longer walk and have begun to use a wheelchair. Scoliosis can be surgically corrected to provide relief from chest compression caused by the increasing rotation of the spine. Some people choose to use mechanical ventilation when breathing is no longer possible.[10] Even with the best care, however, the course of the disease is irreversible.

A study of a controversial therapy for MD is now being funded by the FDA. This therapy involves the injection of myoblasts (muscle cells) that have been grown outside the body of the MD patient from donor cells provided by people who do not have MD. Researchers hope that these cells will bond with themselves and with the patient's own muscle cells to form new muscle tissue. To date, no scientific evidence supports the effectiveness of this therapy.

Several other forms of MD exist, including Becker, limb girdle, and a rare adult-onset form

(Miyoshi myopathy). These, too, result from the mutation of genes on the X chromosome, but are present at different ages and in different areas of the body than in Duchenne muscular dystrophy.

In very rare cases, muscular dystrophy is seen in females. The occurrence of the disease in females is almost certainly caused by a mutation in the person's genetic makeup that takes place during an early stage of development, rather than by inheritance.

Personal Applications

• If you knew you carried a gene for a disease such as MD that would be passed on to any male biological children, what reproductive decisions would you make? Which reproductive options would be acceptable to you?

Congenital Abnormalities

The second group of conditions, congenital abnormalities, refers to abnormalities that are present at birth. These conditions are caused by inappropriate changes in tissues (and thus in organs and organ systems) during embryonic development.[1] Although both inherited (genetic) and congenital conditions are present at birth, congenital abnormalities differ in that they do not involve abnormal genetic material or an atypical number of chromosomes.

During the first three months of pregnancy (the first trimester), the embryo is "constructed" within the protective confines of the uterus. Tissues, organs, and organ systems are formed and take their proper positions according to the complex genetic blueprint established at conception. The embryo will be fully formed by the end of this three-month period. Subsequent enlargement (growth) and refinement (maturation) will occur during the fetal period, which comprises the second and third trimesters.[2]

A congenital abnormality is a condition caused by the inappropriate or incomplete development of a particular embryonic structure or the failure of a structure to function properly at birth. In the section that follows, we will describe selected types of congenital abnormalities. Some congenital abnormalities are so severe that they are incompatible with life, even within the uterus. Thus the embryo is spontaneously aborted by the body (this event is commonly known as a *miscarriage*). Some other congenital abnormalities are life threatening, but the pregnancy can be carried to full term. And in many other cases the abnormality is recognized early in the child's life and can be corrected, or may even be so minor that it is not problematic.

No single factor is responsible for causing congenital abnormalities. They generally form early in pregnancy, during the critical weeks when the

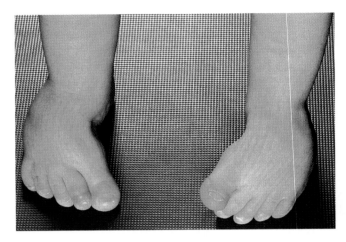

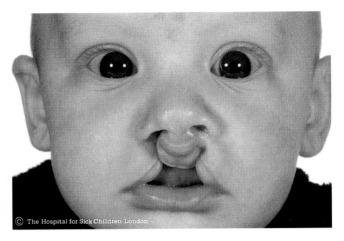

© The Hospital for Sick Children·London

Figure 12-2 An infant with talipes (clubfoot). Treatment for this common congenital abnormality usually begins soon after birth, using plaster casts and manipulation of the foot. Surgery can be performed to give the foot a more normal appearance.

Figure 12-3 An infant with cleft lip and cleft palate. This common congenital abnormality is repaired before the child is two years old. Surgical correction is usually quite successful, both cosmetically and functionally.

embryo's organs are being formed. They may be the result of genetic abnormalities or environmental factors, such as infections and drugs. Most congenital abnormalities, however, are caused by a complex interplay of factors, some genetic and some environmental. Thus their cause is considered to be **multifactorial.**

Talipes (Clubfoot)

Talipes (clubfoot) is among the most common congenital abnormalities, affecting 1 of every 1,000 infants (Figure 12-2).[5] A clubfoot is turned so that the heel points inward while the rest of the foot points inward and downward. The arch of the foot is prominent, and the muscles of the lower leg appear atrophied. This form of talipes is the most common form of the abnormality.[5] Although there appears to be a genetic predisposition for talipes, the specific cause or causes are unknown. Early amniocentesis (11 to 12 weeks) also may foster the formation of talipes.[11]

Prevention, Diagnosis, and Management

Treatment of talipes begins soon after birth, with a combination of manipulation of the foot followed by a series of plaster casts.[12] You may have seen infants in lower leg casts that contain a spacer board between one leg and the other. When the foot is profoundly deformed, tendon reassignment surgery can be performed to give the foot a more normal appearance. Some forms of talipes have responded well to stretching exercises performed regularly, combined with splinting or casting if necessary.

Cleft Palate and Cleft Lip

In the early weeks of embryonic life, the structures of the face, including the lips and roof of the mouth, form as separate halves on each side of the midline. During the fourth through twelfth weeks of development, these halves must move toward each other so that fusion may occur. Failure of the upper lip to fuse results in a split or cleft lip. Failure of the roof of the mouth to fuse causes cleft palate.[13] One of these conditions (or both) occurs in about 1 of every 800 live births.

Although a genetic predisposition may be a factor is some cases of cleft lip and palate, the cause of these conditions is unknown. Environmental factors, such as the use of certain medications during pregnancy, alcohol use, and smoking, may contribute to varying degrees.[14]

If a child's cleft lip or cleft palate is not corrected, he or she may have trouble eating or speaking clearly. In addition, cosmetic concerns may be at issue, an adequate bone foundation for tooth stability may not be established, and significant hearing loss may occur.[15] For these reasons, surgery is recommended to correct both conditions and prevent these difficulties. Figure 12-3 shows a child with cleft lip and cleft palate before surgery.

Prevention, Diagnosis, and Management

Cleft lip and cleft palate are diagnosed at delivery, when the newborn is screened for the presence of these and other abnormalities. A diverse team of health-care specialists then assists parents in understanding the condition(s) and in planning the infant's presurgical and postsurgical care. This medical team would include a plastic surgeon, pediatrician, otolaryngologist (nose/throat specialist), speech pathologist, audiologist (hearing specialist), dentist, dietitian, and nurse. These health-care professionals will collectively determine the child's treatment plan.

Surgery to repair a cleft lip is usually performed when the infant is three to four months old, while

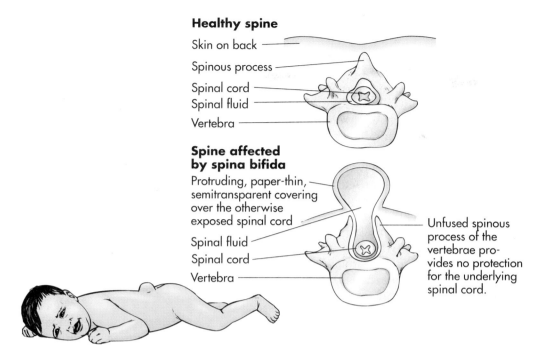

Healthy spine

Skin on back
Spinous process
Spinal cord
Spinal fluid
Vertebra

Spine affected by spina bifida

Protruding, paper-thin, semitransparent covering over the otherwise exposed spinal cord
Spinal fluid
Spinal cord
Vertebra

Unfused spinous process of the vertebrae provides no protection for the underlying spinal cord.

Figure 12-4   Spina bifida is a congenital abnormality in which the fetal neural tube (the forerunner of the brain and spinal cord) fails to close completely.

surgery to repair a cleft palate is usually completed before the child reaches his or her second birthday. If the nasal passages and throat structures are involved, additional surgeries may be required to achieve the high level of success that characterizes today's medical care of these facial abnormalities.[13]

Spina Bifida

In the earliest weeks of intrauterine life, the developing embryo's central nervous system initially forms as an open, trough-shaped **neural tube.** Soon after its formation, the neural tube begins to close, giving rise to the brain and spinal cord. In 1 to 2 per 1,000 live births, a child is born with spina bifida, a condition caused by incomplete closure of the neural tube. In the most common form of the disorder, the spinal cord and its covering lie exposed in an opening in the skin (Figure 12-4). Additionally for some babies with spina bifida, a resulting accumulation of cerebrospinal fluid in the head causes a condition known as **hydrocephalus,** which can lead to mental retardation. Neurological impairment caused by spina bifida may range from minimal to total paralysis.[16]

Prevention, Diagnosis, and Management

Spina bifida can now be detected at sixteen to twenty weeks of pregnancy, using a new blood test that measures the level of a specific protein associated with spinal cord development.[17] Ultrasonography can also be used to visualize abnormalities in the fetus. When the condition is identified at this stage, the woman or couple can decide whether to continue the pregnancy.

Screening for this condition is strongly recommended when any of the following risk factors is present: a family history of the condition; nutritional or environmental deprivation; use of drugs known to affect skull and spinal cord development.

When a child is born with spina bifida, consultation between the parents and several medical specialists will be required to plan a course of action. Surgical repair and closure of the neural tube will be undertaken within two days of birth.

In recent years, significant progress has been made in the prevention of spina bifida. Researchers discovered that as little as .4 mg of folic acid (folacin) consumed daily before pregnancy and during the first trimester greatly reduces the risk of spina bifida and other neural tube defects.[18] If you are a sexually active woman of childbearing age, follow a diet that includes foods high in folic acid, such as orange juice, broccoli, dark leafy greens, whole grains, beans, and peanut butter.

multifactorial   requiring the interplay of many factors; refers to the cause of a disease or condition.

neural tube   the embryonic structure that is the forerunner of the brain and spinal cord.

hydrocephalus   a condition caused by the accumulation of cerebrospinal fluid in the brain, leading to enlargement of the head and structural damage of brain tissue.

Patent Foramen Ovale (PFO)

During intrauterine life, blood flow in the fetal heart bypasses the right ventricle, the chamber that normally pumps unoxygenated blood to the lungs for oxygenation (see Chapter 10). The lungs are bypassed because the fetus is in effect "under water" and, thus, cannot use its lungs. A hole (the foramen ovale) in the interatrial septum, the wall that divides the upper right chamber of the heart from the upper left chamber, provides the necessary passageway around the lungs. At the time of birth, however, when the fetus begins to breathe air, this hole is normally closed by a small flap of tissue. The blood is then redirected into the right ventricle to be sent to the lungs.[2]

In about one in five live births, the foramen ovale fails to close completely, without any apparent leakage of blood. In the absence of other cardiac abnormalities, this patent foramen ovale does not cause any problems, is rarely identified, and, thus, prompts no medical attention. In some infants or children, however, a patent foramen ovale may leak, allowing unoxygenated blood to flow into the left atrium of the heart and out into the general circulation. This leakage may result in some **cyanosis** and cause a heart murmur to develop.[19]

Prevention, Diagnosis, and Management

Patent foramen ovale is usually diagnosed by the child's primary care physician. No treatment is needed unless other heart abnormalities exist or the volume of unoxygenated blood reaching the left side of the heart is too great.

The possible worsening of the leakage of PFO (both diagnosed and undiagnosed) in adults who regularly scuba dive has recently caused concern. Researchers speculate that pressure changes on the chest wall during descents may not only increase the right-to-left movement of blood but also reduce to a dangerous level the amount of oxygenated blood reaching the brain. Experts disagree about whether scuba divers should undergo an echocardiogram to test for the presence of a patent foramen ovale.[20] If you are concerned, discuss the issue with your physician.

Scoliosis

Most cases of scoliosis (abnormal lateral spinal curvatures) have no known cause and are thus classified as *idiopathic*. For a small percentage, particularly when present at birth, a genetic basis is thought to exist. In general, curvatures that are less than 10 degrees (or 20 degrees and nonprogressive) are considered postural malalignments and do not require treatment.[12]

Most spinal curvatures begin as a lateral deviation of the spine (curvature to the side) in either the thoracic (upper back) or lumbar (lower back) region.

The normally aligned spine above or below the initial curvature then begins to curve in the opposite direction to offset the original curvature. This eventually gives the spine an "S" shape. If it is not corrected, the increasing curvature of the spine causes the vertebrae that form the spinal column to rotate. As the vertebrae rotate forward, the ribs follow accordingly, eventually altering the entire architecture of the chest cavity. This causes noticeable postural problems, including uneven positioning of the shoulder blades and a "rib hump" deformity. In addition, the changing shape of the chest compresses the heart, lungs, and related structures that pass through the middle of the chest. Increasing disfiguration and discomfort accompany each degree of additional curvature and rotation.

Prevention, Diagnosis, and Management

For most people with scoliosis, the curvature that initially develops during the preteen years progressively worsens until the spine stops growing after puberty. Since treatment is the key to preventing these problems, most American elementary schools screen students between the fourth and sixth grades to identify children who need additional evaluation. Children should be screened every six to nine months until growth of the spine slows and then stops. Curvatures of 20 degrees but less than 30 degrees when initially found may require treatment but will generally not

---

HEALTH ACTION GUIDE

Recognizing Signs of Scoliosis

If you are the parent of a daughter or son in late childhood or early adolescence, use the following checklist to evaluate your child's posture. If you answer yes to any of the questions, your child should be promptly evaluated by a physician for possible scoliosis.

1. The shoulders appear to be uneven in height when viewed from the front or back.
2. The shoulder blades are excessively prominent when viewed from the back or the side.
3. There is an unequal amount of space between the arms and the sides of the body.
4. The waistline appears to be uneven when viewed from the front or back.
5. The hips appear to be uneven when viewed from the front or back.
6. The body appears to lean sideways when viewed from the front.
7. When the child sits in a chair and bends toward you with his or her head down, a hump or bump is formed by the rib cage on one side of the spine and not on the other.

InfoLinks

http://www.ami-med.com/mhc/top/001241.htm

progress after skeletal growth stops. Curvatures greater than 30 degrees will, however, usually continue to increase well after skeletal growth has stopped and into adulthood unless effective treatment is undertaken. The Health Action Guide on page 366 lists several signs of scoliosis.

In this country, scoliosis is treated by orthopedic surgeons. Once the spine has been radiographically evaluated and the precise nature of the condition determined, one of the following three treatment options is chosen:[21]

- *Do nothing.* Depending on the patient's age and the degree of curvature, it may be appropriate to do nothing and simply monitor the condition to see whether further change occurs.
- *Use a brace.* In children and adolescents, a curve in the mild range (between 25 and 35 degrees) is most effectively treated by bracing the back with a specially fitted metal brace for twenty-three hours per day. This treatment continues until the spine has moved into acceptable alignment. Needless to say, the adolescent who must wear the brace generally sees bracing as uncomfortable, unattractive, and a challenge to self-esteem.
- *Undergo surgery.* When a curvature in a preteen or adolescent is near or beyond 45 degrees, the treatment of choice may well be surgical realignment of several vertebrae within and beyond the curvature.

At this time, no other treatment options appear to be effective in correcting scoliosis, including exercise, chiropractic, or dietary modification. Electrical stimulation of muscles in the back is used by some physicians as an adjunct to bracing of the back.

Only about 2 percent of females and 1 percent of males have scoliosis. For those who do, prompt and effective treatment is important to ensure both physical and emotional well-being.

Personal Applications

- If you had a child with scoliosis, would you subject your child to surgery or to extended periods of bracing, or would you prefer to do nothing and have the child periodically reassessed? Would you be willing to try an alternative therapy?

Metabolic Disorders

The third category of conditions is metabolic. Metabolic disorders are caused by the body's inability to control chemical processes that regulate the building

up (anabolism) and tearing down (catabolism) of tissue.[1] Diabetes mellitus type II and diabetes mellitus type I are, perhaps, the most familiar of the metabolic disorders.

Congenital abnormalities, which you learned about in the last section, are caused by abnormal structure that leads to abnormal function. The metabolic disorders, on the other hand, are caused directly by abnormal function. The body is unable to normally utilize various nutrients in the growth and repair of tissues and in the regulation of body processes. The conditions described in this section have clear metabolic components. They may also have some characteristics that overlap with other categories of conditions. For example, a genetic predisposition is associated with non-insulin-dependent diabetes mellitus (type II).

Non-Insulin-Dependent Diabetes Mellitus (Type II)

In people who do not have diabetes mellitus, the body's need for energy is met through the "burning" of glucose (blood sugar) within the cells. Glucose is absorbed from the digestive tract and carried to the cells by the blood. Glucose passes into the cell through a transport system that moves the glucose molecule across the cell's membrane. Activation of this glucose transport mechanism requires the hormone **insulin** (Figure 12-5). Specific receptor sites for insulin can be found on the cell membrane. Insulin is also required for the conversion of glucose into glycogen in the liver and for the formation of fatty acids in adipose cells. Insulin is produced in the islet cells of the pancreas. The release of insulin from the pancreas corresponds to the changing levels of glucose within the blood.[2]

In adults with a genetic predisposition for developing non-insulin-dependent diabetes mellitus (type II), trigger mechanisms (most likely obesity and inactivity) begin a process through which the body cells become increasingly less sensitive to the presence of insulin, although a normal (or slightly greater than normal) amount of insulin is produced by the pancreas. The growing ineffectiveness of insulin in moving glucose into cells causes the buildup of glucose in the blood. Elevated levels of glucose give rise to **hyperglycemia,** a hallmark symptom of non-insulin-dependent diabetes mellitus.

---

cyanosis   blue coloration of the lips, skin, and nail beds caused by inadequate oxygenation of the blood.

insulin   a hormone produced by the islet cells of the pancreas that is necessary for the normal utilization of glucose.

hyperglycemia   the condition of having an abnormally high blood glucose level.

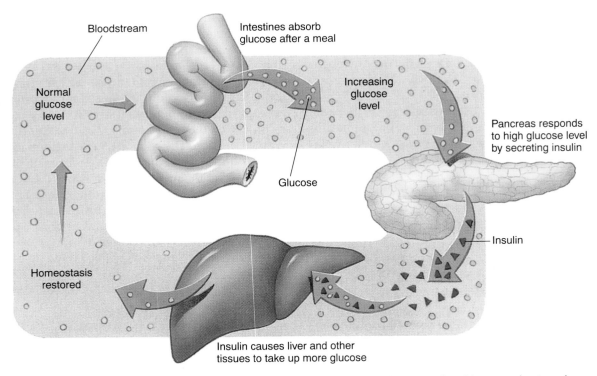

Figure 12-5 Normal blood glucose regulation. The secretion of insulin is regulated by a mechanism that tends to reverse any deviation from normal. Thus an increase in blood glucose level triggers secretion of insulin. Since insulin promotes glucose uptake by cells, blood glucose level is restored to its lower, normal level.

In response to this buildup, the kidneys begin the process of filtering glucose from the blood. Excess glucose then spills over into the urine. This removal of glucose in the urine demands large amounts of water, a condition called **diuresis,** a second important symptom of adult-onset diabetes. Increased thirst, a third symptom of developing diabetes, occurs in response to the movement of fluid from extracellular spaces into the circulatory system to maintain homeostasis.[22]

Prevention, Diagnosis, and Management

For many adults with diabetes, dietary modification (with an emphasis on monitoring total carbohydrate intake, not just sugar) and regular exercise is the only treatment required to maintain an acceptable level of glucose.[1] Weight loss improves the condition by "releasing" more insulin receptors, and exercise increases the actual number of receptor sites. With better insulin recognition, the person can return to a more normal state of functioning.

For people whose condition is more advanced, dietary modification and weight loss alone will not be effective in managing the condition, and oral drugs that stimulate insulin output, called hypoglycemic agents, will be required. Troglitazone, a drug that enhances insulin recognition, and metformin, a drug that influences glucose production in the liver, may

also be used.[23] Increasingly, very aggressive management, including these drugs and insulin, is successfully reducing risks associated with the disease. Many persons, however, have difficulty controlling blood sugar levels even with the use of insulin.

In addition to genetic predisposition and obesity as important factors in non-insulin-dependent diabetes mellitus, unresolved stress appears to play a role in the development of hyperglycemic states. Although stress alone probably cannot produce a diabetic condition, it is likely that stress can induce a series of endocrine changes that can lead to a state of hyperglycemia.

Diabetes can cause serious damage to several important body structures. The extent to which people with diabetes develop these pathological changes can be markedly influenced by the nature of their particular condition and the type of management with which they comply. Today, in addition to the 16 million persons known to have type II diabetes, there may be another 15 million persons who are affected but not yet diagnosed. Accordingly, the medical community is now recommending routine blood glucose screening for persons age 25 and older and is urging the establishment of a more rigorous standard for defining normal blood glucose levels. Of course, prevention is always the best solution. The Star Box on page 369 presents a wellness plan for preventing this type of diabetes.

A Wellness Plan for Preventing Non-Insulin-Dependent Diabetes Mellitus (Type II)

The rate at which Americans develop non-insulin-dependent diabetes mellitus (type II) is on the rise, partly because the population is aging. The disease typically affects older people and thus is sometimes called *adult-onset diabetes*. African-Americans, Hispanic-Americans, and Native Americans are at greater risk than other ethnic groups, but anyone can develop the disease. There is no foolproof way to prevent diabetes, but you can take steps to lower your risk.

Obesity and Overweight
Not all obese people become diabetic, but 90 percent of people with diabetes are overweight. In addition, body fat distribution is important—those who are heavy around the middle ("apple shaped") are more susceptible to the disease than those whose fat is stored in the buttocks and thighs ("pear shaped"). Evidence indicates that both men and women who gain weight in adulthood increase their risk of diabetes. A recent study conducted at Harvard University showed that women who had gained 11 to 17 pounds since age 18 doubled their risk of diabetes; those who had gained between 18 and 24 pounds tripled their risk.

If diabetes runs in your family and you are overweight, you are four times as likely to become diabetic as a person with neither risk factor and twice as likely as a person with only one of these risk factors. Whatever your family history, staying within a healthy weight range and losing weight if you are overweight (see Chapter 6) will lower your risk of diabetes. If you tend to weight-cycle (repeatedly lose weight and then gain it back), keep trying. It is not true, as was once believed, that weight-cycling (yo-yo dieting) is in itself harmful to health.

Genetics
Some progress has been made in identifying the genes that predispose a person to become obese or develop diabetes, but many more years of research will undoubtedly be required before this knowledge is of any practical use. As already mentioned, a family history of diabetes puts you at increased risk. This does not mean that people with a family history are certain to develop diabetes. But if the disease runs in your family, you should try to reduce other risk factors.

Diet
Following a sound diet is a worthwhile step toward preventing diabetes. A semivegetarian diet (see Chapter 5) is known to lower the risk of heart disease and cancer and may also lower the risk of diabetes. It is low in fat, especially animal fat, and rich in fruits, grains, vegetables, and low-fat or nonfat dairy products. Such a diet is unlikely to promote weight gain and often promotes weight loss. It also provides the vitamins, minerals, and other nutrients you need to help prevent chronic diseases.

Exercise
Direct evidence shows that regular physical activity helps prevent diabetes. In one study, researchers from the University of California at Berkeley and Stanford University found that men who were very active—expending 3,500 calories in exercise per week—were only half as likely to develop diabetes as men who were sedentary, expending less than 500 calories per week in leisure-time activity. In fact, those who benefited most from exercise were those at highest risk for diabetes.

Other strong evidence indicates that vigorous exercise, even if done only once a week, has a protective effect against diabetes in both women and men. This is not just because exercise can promote weight loss—physical activity lowers blood sugar whether or not you lose weight.

Vitamin and Mineral Supplements
There is no evidence that any supplement can prevent diabetes, despite manufacturers' claims for chromium and other supplements. People with diabetes are often deficient in some vitamins and minerals, such as vitamin E, zinc, magnesium, and occasionally chromium. But these deficiencies may be caused in part by a reduced ability to absorb and utilize these nutrients. Thus they may be a result of the disease, not the cause.

Smoking
Smoking boosts your risk of diabetes and exacerbates the disease if you already have it. If you are a smoker, do whatever it takes to quit (see Chapter 9). Diabetes is just one of the many serious threats to your health that will be greatly reduced if you stop smoking now.

Insulin-Dependent Diabetes Mellitus (Type I)

A second type of diabetes mellitus is insulin-dependent diabetes mellitus (type I). The onset of this type of diabetes usually occurs before age thirty-five, most often during childhood. In contrast to type II diabetes, in which insulin is produced but is ineffective because of insensitivity, in type I diabetes the body produces no insulin at all. Destruction of the insulin-producing cells of the pancreas by the immune system (possibly in search of a viral infection within the islet cells of the pancreas) accounts for this sudden and irreversible loss of insulin production.[24]

Prevention, Diagnosis, and Management

In most ways the two forms of diabetes are similar, with the important exception that insulin-dependent diabetes mellitus always requires the use of insulin from an outside source (see the Star Box on p. 370, left). Today this insulin is obtained from either animals or genetically engineered bacteria. It is taken by injection (one to four times per day) or through the use of an insulin pump, which provides a constant

diuresis (die yoo **ree** sis)   a physiological condition in which an excessive amount of water leaves body cells and is excreted in the urine.

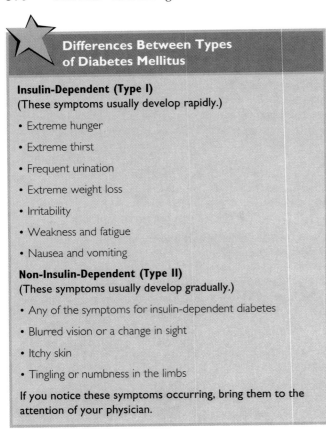

- Cataract formation
- Glaucoma
- Blindness
- Dental caries
- Stillbirths/miscarriages
- Neonatal deaths
- Congenital defects
- Cardiovascular disease
- Kidney disease
- Gangrene
- Impotence

supply of insulin. Delivery of insulin by inhalation in aerosol or powdered form is also being tested. Transdermal delivery of insulin (by a patch) may someday be used as well. Development of the glucometer, a highly accurate device for measuring the amount of glucose in the blood, allows better management of this condition. Progress toward development of an immunization for type I diabetes mellitus and inpancreas cell transplantation also have occurred.

With both forms of diabetes mellitus, sound dietary practices, planned activity, and control of stress are important for keeping blood glucose levels within a normal range. When diabetes mellitus is not properly managed, several serious problems can result, including blindness, gangrene of the extremities, kidney disease, and heart attack. These and other common complications of diabetes are listed in the Star Box at the top of the right column on this page. People who cannot establish good control of the disease are likely to die prematurely.

Personal Applications

- What would you do if you had a friend with diabetes who was purposely disregarding the dietary restrictions necessary to manage the disease?

Hypoglycemia

When people with insulin-dependent diabetes mellitus do not eat enough, exercise too much, or take too much insulin, they may develop excessively low levels of blood sugar (blood glucose), resulting in a state of **hypoglycemia.** In nondiabetic people, difficulty maintaining high enough blood glucose levels may also be associated with drug use, liver damage, partial removal of the stomach, fasting, pancreatic tumors, and rare forms of adrenal and breast tumors, or as a prediabetic symptom.[25] People who have hypoglycemia experience headaches, mild confusion, low energy levels, anxiety, sweating, and tremors. They may look pale and behave somewhat abnormally.[26]

A rare form of hypoglycemia called *reactive hypoglycemia* is seen in people who are hypersensitive to the presence of sugar in the blood. In these people, a meal that is high in simple carbohydrates (sugars) stimulates excessive insulin production. This insulin removes blood sugar too quickly, leading to a state of hypoglycemia. People with reactive hypoglycemia have the same symptoms seen in hypoglycemia caused by other factors.

Prevention, Diagnosis, and Management

Before reactive hypoglycemia can be definitively diagnosed, the many other causes of low blood sugar (including diabetes mellitus) must first be ruled out. Confirmation of the diagnosis is made on the basis of "Whipple's triad": symptoms of hypoglycemia, a blood glucose level less than 45mg/dl of blood, and complete resolution of symptoms following administration of glucose.[27]

Treatment of reactive hypoglycemia involves dietary modification centered on the consumption of

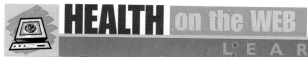

frequent, small meals that contain high levels of complex carbohydrates and few simple carbohydrates.[25] These dietary modifications make the movement of glucose into the bloodstream more gradual, thus eliminating high glucose loads. This "spacing out" of glucose delivery to the blood reduces the body's tendency to over-produce insulin.

In the 1970s the diagnosis of hypoglycemia was made by some physicians to placate patients who complained of vague symptoms of anxiety, moodiness, fatigue, and a loss of interest in normal activities. Once serious clinical conditions such as depression were ruled out, patients were told that they "must be experiencing hypoglycemia." Patients were then put on a special diet and assured that they would begin to feel better "now that the problem was known." In many cases, patients reported dramatic improvement. Thus hypoglycemia gained a reputation for being over-diagnosed. A decade later, some physicians initially approached the treatment of premenstrual syndrome (PMS) as if it were the "hypoglycemia of the 1990s."

PKU (Phenylketonuria)

PKU (phenylketonuria) is a well-understood recessive genetic disorder with strong metabolic consequences. Accordingly, both biological parents must be carriers of the gene for PKU. One-fourth of their children will have the condition, and one-half of their children will themselves be carriers.

PKU is an inherited inability to produce (or produce enough of) an enzyme needed to convert the amino acid phenylalanine into the amino acid tyrosine. In the absence of this enzyme, phenylalanine accumulates in the body. The toxic effects of phenylalanine on the nervous system are profound, including extreme brain deterioration and severe mental retardation. However, not all infants with PKU have a total inability to convert phenylalanine into tyrosine; thus they are at less risk of serious damage. PKU affects only about 1 in 10,000 live-born infants.

Prevention, Diagnosis, and Management

Because of PKU's potential to cause profound harm, all hospitals in the United States screen for the disorder by testing a blood sample drawn at birth. Infants with PKU are then placed on an extremely restrictive diet that contains no concentrated (animal) sources of protein or products made with regular flour. A person with PKU would thus not be able to consume meat, fish, poultry, milk, eggs, cheese, other dairy products, legumes (beans, peas), nuts, and bakery products, such as bread, that contain regular flour—unquestionably an extremely limited diet.[5]

In the management of PKU during infancy, the baby is fed a synthetic formula that is expensive but well tolerated. With increasing age, the child's diet is shifted to a selection of specially formulated low-protein foods, combined with carefully evaluated

> **hypoglycemia**   the condition of having an abnormally low blood glucose level.

types and amounts of fruits, vegetables, and some grain products. The extent to which a particular child can tolerate "normal" foods containing phenylalanine must be determined, since people with PKU are not affected equally. Over time, some phenylalanine can usually be included in the diet.

These dietary restrictions were once thought to be unnecessary beyond childhood (ages six through ten). However, serious problems, such as personality disorders, and subsequent brain tissue changes were seen in people who had gone off the diet. Thus the diet is now deemed to be lifelong.[28] Adult women with PKU must follow an appropriate diet for this condition before becoming pregnant and throughout the course of the pregnancy. Babies born to mothers with PKU are generally healthy.

Degenerative Diseases

A fourth category of chronic conditions is degenerative diseases. These conditions, many of which are diagnosed late in life, reflect the increasing vulnerability to disease that occurs with age.[1] The term **degenerative** refers not just to structural degeneration over time, but also to functional degeneration. In some degenerative conditions, the structure of the body is clearly changed by the disease process. In others, however, the degeneration changes the way an organ or organ system works but does not affect its structure. The first two conditions we will learn about, fibromyalgia and asthma, are caused by functional degeneration.

Fibromyalgia

Fibromyalgia syndrome (FMS) is a chronic condition with symptoms that are so complex an affected person might never be diagnosed and treated despite years of discomfort. For the 2 percent of the adult population believed to have FMS, intermittent periods of morning stiffness, muscle pain, fatigue, numbness and tingling, poor sleep, chronic headaches, jaw discomfort, and many other problems are often seen simply as signs of aging or stress. To trained physicians (often rheumatologists), however, these symptoms may indicate FMS. Accordingly, this syndrome can be diagnosed and effectively treated.[29] Of course, other chronic conditions can coexist with FMS.

The cause of fibromyalgia is unclear at this time. Theories focus on altered neurotransmitter regulation, immune system dysfunction, hormonal abnormalities (cortisol and HGH), and subtle brain dysfunction. Additionally, certain trigger events—infections, emotional stress, physical trauma such as a fall—thyroid dysfunction, and connective tissue disorders, such as lupus (see page 376), may cause or exacerbate FMS.[29]

Prevention, Diagnosis, and Management

Preventive measures for fibromyalgia syndrome and this condition's irregular and sometimes subtle symptoms might be to reduce stress, avoid infections, and maintain a high level of overall health. Another preventive strategy is the appropriate diagnosis and treatment of associated conditions, such as lupus, rheumatoid arthritis, and thyroid disease.

The diagnosis of FMS is based on medical history and the assessment of discomfort in 18 so-called *tender-point locations*. For research purposes, people who experience pain in at least 11 of the 18 tender points are diagnosed with FMS.[30] A lower number of "hits" is considered to be diagnostic in a nonresearch setting. Most people with chronic discomfort will be found to have several tender points during the examination. People who lack tender points and morning stiffness, but have other symptoms of FMS, may have chronic fatigue syndrome (CFS).[30]

The treatment of fibromyalgia centers on improving sleep and reducing pain. Physicians can prescribe medications to enhance the effectiveness of sleep-inducing neurotransmitters (such as serotonin and norepinephrine). Nonsteroidal anti-inflammatory drugs (NSAIDs), such as ibuprofen, are used for pain relief. Other therapies include injection of synthetic narcotics into tender points, acupuncture, and therapeutic massage.[30]

The prognosis for people with FMS is unclear, since few long-term studies have been carried out. For most patients, the condition will remain chronic, with periods of remission and active discomfort occurring intermittently. Whether daily functioning will be significantly impaired later in life remains to be seen.[29]

Asthma

Bronchial asthma is a chronic respiratory disease characterized by acute attacks of breathlessness and wheezing caused by chronic airway inflammation with episodes of narrowing of the bronchioles. Although the mechanisms associated with asthmatic attacks are understood, the reason that some people develop asthma is not fully known. The recent discovery of a gene (which may be one of several) related to asthma suggests a genetic predisposition that is expressed during exposure to one or more triggering agents.[31] If other genes are identified, perhaps someday asthma will be viewed primarily as an inherited condition.

Two main types of asthma have been identified: extrinsic and intrinsic.[5] In extrinsic asthma, allergens such as pollen, dust mites, mold spores, animal fur or dander, and feathers produce sudden and severe bronchoconstriction that narrows the airways. Increased sputum production further narrows the bronchioles and restricts the passage of air. This narrowing fosters the development of chronic inflammation of the airways, which is the most damaging aspect of

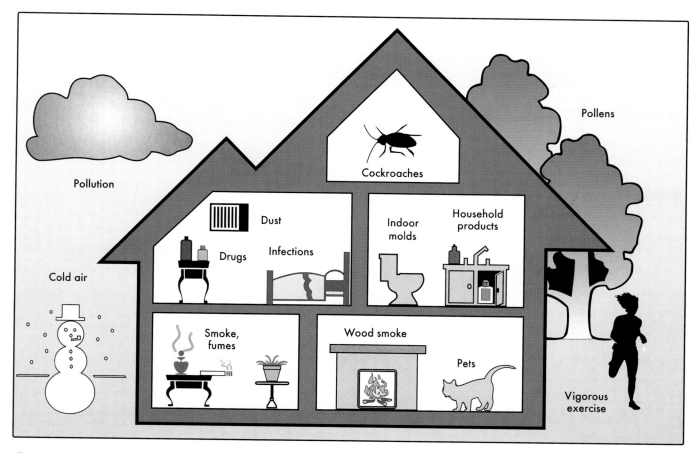

Figure 12-6 Common asthma triggers. If you have asthma, do you know which triggers are troublesome for you?

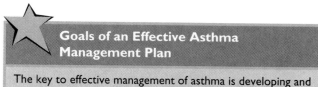

Goals of an Effective Asthma Management Plan

The key to effective management of asthma is developing and following a management plan that is appropriate for your condition and fits your lifestyle. According to the *Guidelines for Diagnosis and Management of Asthma*, published by the National Heart, Lung, and Blood Institute of the National Institutes of Health, the goals of a successful asthma management plan are the following:

• To maintain normal activity levels (including exercise)

• To maintain near-normal pulmonary function rates

• To prevent chronic and troublesome symptoms, such as coughing or breathlessness at night, in the morning, or after exertion

• To prevent recurrent asthma attacks

• To avoid adverse effects from asthma medications

• To avoid emergency room visits and hospitalizations

asthma. Wheezing is most pronounced when the person attempts to exhale air through the narrowed air passages. For many people with asthma, exercise, cigarette smoke, and certain foods or drugs can cause an asthma attack (Figure 12-6).

The incidence of extrinsic asthma is increasing within the general population. This increase probably reflects the growing urban population, who must breathe more polluted air, and the tendency for people to spend more time indoors, often in structures that are well insulated and relatively airtight, where air containing allergens is recirculated. The increase may also relate to our success in immunizing children against infectious diseases. In immunized children, the absence of pathogens for the immune system to fight may allow the system to respond overly aggressively to allergens through the release of *leukotrienes* and other immune system elements.

Intrinsic asthma, the less common form, has similar symptoms but is caused by stress or by frequent respiratory tract infections. Allergens play a lesser role in this form of asthma, which may be more strongly influenced by genetic predisposition.[5]

Prevention, Diagnosis, and Management

Prevention or effective management of asthma is often possible using a combination of approaches. Most

degenerative a slow but progressive deterioration of the body's structure or function.

Personal Assessment

Place a check mark next to each statement that applies to you.

Reducing or Avoiding Asthma Triggers

_____ I have identified my asthma triggers.

_____ I do not smoke, and I avoid environmental tobacco smoke as much as possible.

_____ I use and properly maintain an air filter and an air conditioner to keep my home cleaner and more comfortable.

_____ I avoid vacuuming or I use a dust mask.

_____ I avoid mowing the lawn or I use a dust mask.

_____ I avoid wood stoves and fireplaces.

_____ I use dustproof encasings on my pillows, mattress, and box spring.

_____ I use a dehumidifier as necessary in my home to reduce indoor mold.

_____ I use window shades or curtains made of plastic or other washable material for easy cleaning.

_____ My closets contain only needed clothing; clothing I do not currently wear is stored in plastic garment bags.

_____ I do not sleep or lie down on upholstered furniture.

_____ If I have a pet, it does not sleep in or go into the bedroom.

_____ I avoid perfume and cologne, cleaning chemicals, paint, and talcum powder as much as possible.

Preventing and Managing Asthma Attacks

_____ I have learned everything I can about asthma.

_____ I take medications as prescribed by my physician whether or not I am having an attack.

_____ I carry my inhaler with me at all times.

_____ I have asked my physician to help me develop a crisis plan for managing a severe asthma attack.

_____ I keep emergency numbers by the phone.

_____ I have learned about my asthma medications and know how quickly they should work.

_____ I use a peak flow meter to anticipate and respond quickly to asthma attacks.

Interpretation

17 or more items checked: You are doing a great job avoiding asthma triggers and preventing and managing asthma attacks.

14 to 16 items checked: In many ways you are doing a good job of managing your asthma. However, you may be unnecessarily exposing yourself to common asthma triggers, or your plan for preventing and managing asthma attacks may need some work.

13 or fewer items checked: You could be managing your asthma much more effectively. Modify your home and activities as necessary to avoid common asthma triggers. Talk to your physician right away about establishing an asthma management plan and an emergency plan. Remember, asthma can be fatal, and poor preventive asthma management is an important contributing factor. Don't let it happen to you!

To Carry This Further . . .

Discuss this assessment with other members of your family or your roommates. Secure their cooperation in helping you maintain a clean home free of dust, pet hair, smoke, and other asthma triggers. Make sure they know what to do to help you in case of a severe asthma attack.

HEALTH ACTION GUIDE

Tips for Controlling Exercise-Induced Asthma

- Obtain a treatment and prevention plan from your physician.
- Alert instructors and coaches about the existence of any treatment plan.
- Medicate before exercising according to your physician's instruction.
- Warm up slowly to increase heart rate gradually and cool down slowly after exercise.
- Carry your bronchodilator with you at all times if one was prescribed.
- Wear a scarf or mask over your mouth and nose during cold weather to warm and moisten the air you breathe.
- Wear an allergy mask over the mouth and nose when exercising during pollen season.

InfoLinks

http://www.mdnet.de/asthma/

HEALTH ACTION GUIDE

Managing Inflammatory Bowel Disease

In addition to the management strategy recommended by your doctor, the following steps may help ease the symptoms of Crohn's disease and other inflammatory bowel disorders:

- Eat a low-fat diet. Avoid cream, butter, whole milk, and high-fat salad dressings, cheeses, and meats.
- Eat more high-fiber foods, such as fruits, grains, and vegetables. This should help if you are constipated. But take a gradual approach. Sudden increases in fiber may cause gas and diarrhea.
- Avoid sorbitol, a sugar substitute used in many products; it can cause diarrhea. Fructose, found in fruits and often in processed foods, may also be a problem.
- Try switching to lactose-free milk in case you have trouble digesting milk sugar.
- Cut down on or eliminate alcohol and caffeine.
- If you are taking medications, particularly antibiotics, ask your doctor if they could exacerbate the disease.
- Try eating several small meals a day rather than two or three large ones.
- If emotional stress is involved, try dealing with it directly by talking with a counselor.
- Regular exercise and other lifestyle alterations may help.

InfoLinks

http://members.aol.com/bospol/homepage/crohns.htm

important, of course, is the maintenance of high-level wellness through a healthful lifestyle that includes a sound diet, regular exercise, and effective stress management. Each person who has asthma should work with his or her physician to develop a sound, individually tailored management plan. The goals of such a plan are listed in the Star Box on page 373. If you have asthma, complete the Personal Assessment on page 374 to determine whether you are doing all you can to manage your condition effectively.

A number of components can be included in an asthma management plan. Exercises that are well tolerated, such as swimming, can help maintain a more normal level of respiratory function. Immunotherapy, in which the patient with extrinsic asthma is desensitized through injections of weakened allergens, is often attempted. In addition, the careful use of corticosteroid drugs several times per day reduces inflammation. Four additional drugs have recently been introduced. Two of these, zafirlukast (Accolate) and zileuton (Zyflo), both *antileukotrienes,* reduce the immune system's ability to foster inflammation.[32] The remaining two, montelukast (Singulair) and salmeterol (Serevent), are used to reduce the effects of exercise and cold air to trigger asthma attacks.[33,34]

Despite the use of older drugs, such as the bronchodilators that open constricted airways and the newer drugs that counter specific allergens or immune system inflammation, asthma remains a serious and potentially fatal condition. Each year in this country, several thousand people die as the result of asthma attacks. Some experts believe that this number could be reduced if physicians were more aggressive in their treatment of the bronchial inflammation component of the condition.

People with exercise-induced asthma (EIA), a common type of extrinsic asthma, should take several important steps when attempting to exercise (see the Health Action Guide above).

Many children who have asthma manage well with the proper use of exercise and medication. They may experience less asthma, or none at all, when they reach adulthood.

Crohn's Disease

A wide array of chronic conditions that involve the gastrointestinal system are collectively referred to as *inflammatory bowel disease (IBD).* One type of IBD is Crohn's disease, an erosive deterioration of the inner surface and muscular layer of the intestinal wall that affects nearly 500,000 Americans, many of whom are of traditional college age. The disease most often affects the terminal end of the small intestine and the beginning of the large intestine, or colon. When the disease is active (it frequently has long periods of remission), symptoms include abdominal pain in the lower right quadrant, fever, diarrhea, weight loss, and rectal bleeding that leads to anemia.

Although the cause of Crohn's disease is not fully understood, a genetic predisposition and an autoimmune response may be the principal factors. Multiple forms of Crohn's disease are thought to exist, with each reflecting different genetic components. Genes located on chromosomes 3, 7, 12, and 16 are under investigation.[35]

Prevention, Diagnosis, and Management

When a patient reports the symptoms just described, the physician quickly suspects some form of IBD, such as Crohn's disease. Accordingly, blood tests are ordered and a complete series of gastrointestinal (GI) X-rays is taken. Additional diagnostic procedures could include a CT scan of the GI tract, endoscopic examination of the colon, and a biopsy of the intestinal wall.[5] Positive results of these tests confirm the diagnosis of Crohn's disease.

Today an array of pharmacological agents are available or in development for use in the management of Crohn's disease. Sulfasalazine, a widely used medication, is now available in new forms. In addition, a variety of monoclonal antibodies and proteins will soon be available to reduce the impact of tumor necrosis factor in some forms of the disease, as will other immunosuppressive drugs and a variety of newer steroids with fewer side effects.[36]

Although Crohn's disease can often be well managed, intestinal obstructions can occur due to the progressive thickening of the intestinal wall in the area of inflammation. Surgery may be necessary to remove the obstruction. However, obstructions may form in neighboring areas of the intestinal tract, requiring additional surgery. **Fistulas** can develop between the intestinal tract wall and adjacent structures, such as the vagina or urinary bladder. These, too, will be corrected surgically. People with Crohn's disease may encounter further complications, including gallstones, arthritis, and chronic irritation of the skin. The Health Action Guide on page 375 offers suggestions for managing Crohn's disease and other inflammatory bowel diseases.

Systemic Lupus Erythematosus (SLE)

Systemic lupus erythematosus, or simply *lupus*, is perhaps the most familiar of a class of chronic degenerative conditions known as **autoimmune disorders**, or connective tissue disorders. These conditions are caused by an extensive and inappropriate attack by the body's immune system on its own tissues, which then serve as **self-antigens** (see Chapter 13 for a discussion of the immune response).

The word **systemic** refers to the widespread destruction of fibrous connective tissue and other tissues. *Erythematosus* (*erythema*- means "red") refers to the reddish rash that imparts a characteristic "mask" to the face of a person with SLE. The disease is seen in women twenty-five times more often than in men and first appears during young adulthood. The course of

the condition is gradual, with intermittent periods of inflammation, stiffness, fatigue, pleurisy (chest pain), and discomfort over wide areas of the body, including muscles, joints, and skin. Similar changes may take place in the tissues of the nervous system, kidneys, and heart.[37]

Researchers do not know why the immune system attacks the body in such an extensive and aggressive way. It is likely, however, that a combination of genetic predisposition and an earlier viral infection may be involved in its development.

Prevention, Diagnosis, and Management

A physician may suspect lupus based on the patient's description of her symptoms and make a diagnosis using a number of laboratory tests, including the identification of an SLE factor in the blood.[5] A skin biopsy may be taken to confirm structural changes in the connective tissue layer below the skin.

Management of lupus generally involves the occasional or long-term use of nonsteroidal anti-inflammatory drugs (NSAIDs), malarial drugs for the skin rash, and a low dose of prednisone (a corticosteroid) to reduce fever, treat episodes of pleurisy, and minimize certain neurological symptoms. The immune system itself may be medically suppressed as well. These treatments must be carefully monitored because they have serious side effects.[37]

Management of lupus centers on the prevention of episodes of the disease called *flares*. These periods of active lupus are often triggered by exposure to the sun, periods of fatigue, or an infectious disease, all of which should be avoided as much as possible.

Multiple Sclerosis (MS)

For proper nerve conduction to occur within portions of the brain and spinal cord, an insulating sheath of myelin must surround the neurons (nerve cells). In the progressive disease multiple sclerosis (MS), the cells that produce myelin are destroyed, myelin production ceases, and the underlying nerves are badly damaged.[38] Neurological functioning eventually becomes so disrupted that vital functions are significantly impaired. The cause of MS is not known. Research continues to focus on multiple virus-induced autoimmune mechanisms in which T cells attack viral-infected myelin-producing cells.

Prevention, Diagnosis, and Management

Multiple sclerosis usually appears for the first time during the young adult years. It may take one of three forms, depending on the interplay of periods of stabilization (remitting), renewed deterioration (relapsing), and continuous deterioration (progressive). The initial symptoms of the condition are often visual impairment, prickling and burning in the extremities,

Learning
From Our Diversity

Fighting Multiple Sclerosis: Women's Winning Strategies

What do Letitia McQuay, a recent Miss Delaware; Susan Unger, a freelance art buyer; and Elin Silveous, an entrepreneur, have in common?

If you think the answer is brains, talent, poise, and success, you're absolutely right. But these three women—and thousands of others—also share something that's far from glamour and accolades: They all have multiple sclerosis.

Multiple sclerosis (MS) is a disease that attacks the central nervous system, typically appearing during early adulthood. Women are two to three times as likely to develop the disease as men. Through courage and determination, however, many women with MS are able to lead productive and rewarding lives.

MS is characterized by a loss of myelin, the fatty tissue that surrounds and protects nerve fibers and helps conduct electrical impulses to and from the brain. How MS manifests itself depends on which areas—brain, spinal cord, or optic nerve—have been damaged. In addition to problems with fatigue, poor balance, tingling, numbness, and impaired vision, patients may have muscle stiffness, slurred speech, bowel or bladder problems, difficulties with sexual function, sensitivity to heat, and trouble with short-term memory or reasoning. Although no cure has yet been found for MS, recent research has yielded exciting advances in drug therapies that lessen the frequency and severity of attacks in some forms of the disease.

How are women coping with MS while living balanced and fulfilling lives? Letitia McQuay's disease was diagnosed in 1992, but she was not deterred from pursuing her goals. Competing for and winning the Miss Delaware title in 1994 is an example of how she copes with her chronic illness. She's now married and has undertaken graduate studies in public administration. "Multiple sclerosis is simply something I have to deal with," she says. "The disease affects my body but doesn't change who I am."

Susan Unger of New York City, who has produced a documentary about living with MS, says that life between flare-ups can be perfectly normal. "You'd never know I had MS," she says, noting, however, that her healthy appearance sometimes prevents others from realizing when she's not feeling well. Although no longer able to run, Unger keeps fit by swimming and bicycling.

For Elin Silveous, who runs her own multimedia health communications company, one challenge of being diagnosed with MS at age 33 was finding a way to continue a favorite activity: driving. Because of weakness in her leg, she had to give up driving a stick shift and change to an automatic transmission, which she describes as a traumatic decision. "But I learned that there is life after an MS diagnosis," she says. "We're not broken or damaged goods. We can still be sexy and romantic, date and have relationships, and certainly enjoy life."

These women, and thousands of others like them, are living full, active lives because they refuse to let a chronic condition define who they are and where they're going.

Think about someone you know who lives with a chronic condition. How does this person's life reflect his or her attitude toward the condition and the limitations it imposes?

---

and an altered gait. In its most advanced stages, movement is greatly impaired and mental deterioration may be present.

Treatment of MS is aimed at reducing the severity of symptoms and extending the periods of remission. Today a variety of therapies are used, including immune system–targeted drugs, steroid drugs, drugs to relieve muscle spasms, injections of nerve blockers, and physical therapy.

The development of immune system–related medications is at the center of the fight against MS. Interferon beta-1b (Betaseron), a genetically engineered form of interferon, effectively reduces the symptoms of MS but may not slow the progression of the disease. More recently, interferon beta-1a (Avonex) and Glatiramer acetate (Copaxone), drugs that slow the development of the disease and delay periods of relapse, have been approved by the FDA.[39] Newly designed monoclonal antibodies are being tested to determine their ability to shorten periods of relapse by preventing the movement of immune cells from the blood into nerve tissue.[40] A new drug called Zanaflex, intended to reduce the muscle spasticity that accompanies MS, has also won approval from the FDA.

Psychotherapy is an important adjunct to the treatment of MS. Profound periods of depression often accompany the initial diagnosis of this condition. Emotional support is helpful in dealing with the progressive impairment associated with the condition.

---

fistula   a fissure, break, or hole in the wall of an organ.

autoimmune disorders   disorders caused by the immune system's failure to recognize the body as "self"; thus the body mounts an attack against its own cells and tissues.

self-antigens   the cells and tissues that stimulate the immune system's autoimmune response.

systemic (sis **tem** ic)   distributed or occurring throughout the entire body system.

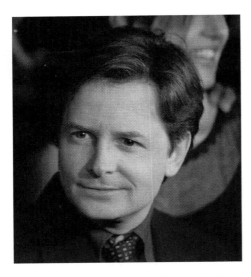

Actor Michael J. Fox recently revealed that he has Parkinson's disease.

Parkinson's Disease

Once called "shaking palsy," Parkinson's disease is now recognized as a specific neurological disorder belonging to a family of conditions called *motor system disorders*. Parkinson's disease involves the chronic progressive loss of dopamine production within specific areas of the brain. These areas, called the substantia nigra and striatum, transmits signals required to produce purposeful muscle activity that leads to more highly coordinated movement. The four primary signs of the disease reflect this loss of muscular coordination: (1) tremor or trembling in the hands, arms, legs, jaw, and face; (2) rigidity or stiffness of the limbs or trunk; (3) slowness of movement; and (4) postural instability and impaired balance. As these symptoms worsen, people with Parkinson's disease become progressively less able to talk, walk, and perform simple tasks associated with daily living.[37]

Parkinson's-like symptoms are associated with other conditions, such as head injury, tumors, prolonged use of tranquilizers, and manganese and carbon monoxide poisoning. The labels *Parkinson's syndrome* and *atypical Parkinson's* are used to describe these conditions. A recent study indicates that as many as one in five elderly Americans shows some Parkinsonian signs.[41]

About 500,000 Americans have been diagnosed with primary Parkinson's disease, and about 50,000 new cases are diagnosed annually. The exact number of people with this condition has always been difficult to establish with certainty, since some people assume that these changes are the result of aging and thus do not seek medical evaluation. The incidence of Parkinson's disease is the same in men and women. The condition is usually first seen in people over age fifty, with sixty being the average age at first diagnosis. Compared with African-Americans and Asian-Americans, whites are more likely to be diagnosed with Parkinson's disease. A relatively small percentage of people develop the disease as early as age forty. Slightly fewer cases of Parkinson's disease are seen among smokers than among nonsmokers (the risks of smoking, however, greatly outweigh the slightly lower risk of Parkinson's disease among smokers).

Three explanations of the cause of Parkinson's disease have been proposed. The first involves the formation of highly excited unstable chemical compounds known as *free radicals*.[42] These compounds are formed in greater and greater quantities with age, as the body gradually loses its ability to completely oxidize substrates. These free radicals seek stability by physically altering the chemical structure of tissues with which they have contact, including the cells of the substantia nigra. Once damaged, the cells of the substantia nigra die; thus their dopamine production is lost and the symptoms of Parkinson's appear.

The second possible explanation relates to environmental toxins that are known to produce Parkinson's-like symptoms in humans. However, no widely occurring environmental toxins of this nature have been discovered that could account for the large number of cases of Parkinson's disease in this country and around the world.[42]

The third and most credible theory about the cause of Parkinson's disease suggests an inherited predisposition associated with genetic material found within the mitochondria of cells. Mitochondria are cell structures in which energy is produced to fuel specific cellular tasks, such as the production of dopamine.[42] In November 1996 a genetic marker was identified within the mitochondrial DNA of members of a family with a long history of Parkinson's disease.[43] The specific gene was identified in June 1997.[44] This discovery provides some evidence that a genetic predisposition may, in addition to other factors, be necessary for Parkinson's disease to develop.

Prevention, Diagnosis, and Management

Parkinson's disease is usually diagnosed by a neurologist after the patient is referred by a primary care physician. Although there is no single test for diagnosing Parkinson's disease, medical imaging, such as CT scans and MRI scans, may be helpful in ruling out conditions that mimic the disease.

Several medications are used to delay the progression of the disease. Most of these drugs affect dopamine production. Two drugs, carbidopa/levodopa, an older medication, and tolcapone (Tasmar), a newer drug, enhance the conversion of levodopa into dopamine. As helpful as these medications are, however, their influence is temporary and at best they only slow the progress of the disease.

In addition to drug therapy, electrodes have been surgically implanted into the brain. This procedure appears to reduce tremors to the extent that affected people can achieve and maintain a more functional level of activity for as long as two years.[45]

Alzheimer's Disease (AD)

Although it affects only 1 percent to 2 percent of elderly people, organic brain syndrome, in either its acute or chronic form, is a collection of incapacitating, heart-rending, and costly afflictions. Alzheimer's disease is the best known of these conditions, affecting between 2 and 4 million adults. Today, more than ever before, it is the disease associated with longevity.

The initial signs of Alzheimer's disease are often subtle and may be confused with mild depression. At this stage of the disease process, however, the person might have some difficulty answering questions like these:

- Where are we now?
- What month is it?
- What is today's date?
- When is your birthday?
- Who is the president?

During the ensuing months, people with this condition experience greater memory loss, confusion, and **dementia.** In the most advanced stage, people with Alzheimer's disease are incontinent (unable to control bladder and bowel function), display infantile behavior, and finally become totally incapacitated as a result of the destruction of brain tissue. Patients with advanced Alzheimer's disease must be institutionalized.

Several theories have been advanced about the cause of Alzheimer's disease. Increasing evidence indicates that genetic mutations in chromosomes 14, 19, or 21 may encourage the development of the disease. Other theories suggest links between Alzheimer's disease and abnormal protein development, deficiencies in acetylcholine (a neurotransmitter) production, abnormal blood flow, or exposure to infectious agents or toxins. Most recently, researchers have been investigating the role of nerve cell mitochondria, where energy needed to synthesize important enzymes is produced. Current thought holds that, because of faulty genes within the mitochondrial DNA, inadequate energy is produced, resulting in faulty enzymes. Because of errors in the design of these enzymes, damaging free radicals (see p. 378) are produced and nerve cells are irreversibly damaged.[46]

Prevention, Diagnosis, and Management

The precise diagnosis of Alzheimer's disease and similar disorders is difficult to make before the patient dies. Only during an autopsy can the characteristic signs of the disease, such as loss of neurons, be identi-

Estrogen Replacement Therapy and Alzheimer's Disease

Many women going through menopause have chosen to take estrogen replacement therapy. Estrogen, which women's bodies produce bountifully during the reproductive years but in lesser amounts with age, can quell the unpleasant symptoms of menopause, such as hot flashes and mood swings, and help lower the risk of heart disease and osteoporosis. Now it appears that estrogen may be beneficial in another way: It might help prevent Alzheimer's disease.

Richard Mayeux and his colleagues at Columbia University interviewed 1,124 women over age 70 about their use of estrogen over the years. Only 156 of them had ever used estrogen replacement therapy. None of the women showed any signs of Alzheimer's disease at the start of the study. But when the researchers repeated their examinations between one and five years later, 16 percent of the women who had never taken estrogen had developed Alzheimer's, compared with about 6 percent of the women who had taken estrogen supplements.

However, it is too early to draw firm conclusions: Women who take estrogen tend to get better overall medical care, and that or another factor may be responsible for the lower incidence of the disease. But other researchers have found similar results in smaller studies, and scientists have some theories about how estrogen might help. It is thought to improve blood flow in the brain and stimulate nerve cell growth in regions affected by Alzheimer's.

In Mayeux's study, women who used estrogen for the longest period of time had the lowest rate of Alzheimer's disease, but even those who took it for as little as a year saw a benefit. Estrogen replacement therapy does carry some risks, of course, including an increased chance of uterine and ovarian cancers. But for women with a family history of Alzheimer's, the chance that estrogen could help fend off the disease may make it worth the risk.

fied to confirm the diagnosis. Before death, all other conditions capable of causing dementia must be individually ruled out. Thus, tentative or probable diagnosis of Alzheimer's disease is made by a process of elimination.[5] Newer medical imaging technologies, such as MRI scans and PET scans, have become so refined that it is now *nearly* possible to confirm the diagnosis of Alzheimer's disease before death.

Effective drugs to treat Alzheimer's disease have not yet been developed. Although more than ten experimental drugs are currently being tested, none has been shown to reverse the disease. One drug, tacrine (Cognex), brings about minor temporary improvement in Alzheimer's patients when used early in the

dementia the loss of cognitive abilities, including memory and reason.

disease process. A newer drug, donepezil (Aricept), was approved in 1997 and appears to work as well as tacrine, with a similar mechanism of action. Both slow the course of the disease only slightly.

Researchers have recently announced two possible means of preventing Alzheimer's disease. The first is the use of ibuprofen (a nonsteroidal anti-inflammatory agent) to reduce the inflammation associated with cells damaged by the disease. In a study involving long-term ibuprofen use, the risk of developing Alzheimer's disease was reduced by 50 percent, compared with people who took aspirin and acetaminophen. However, some risks are associated with long-term high-dosage ibuprofen use. The second possible way of preventing Alzheimer's disease is the use of estrogen replacement

Personal Applications

• How do you feel about institutionalizing people with Alzheimer's disease? Do you believe you could institutionalize one of your own parents if his or her condition warranted this step?

therapy in postmenopausal women (see the Star Box on page 379). Both potential preventive therapies will require much additional evaluation.

Chronic Disease Prevention

With the well-deserved emphasis placed on the prevention of heart disease and cancer, you might expect that virtually all diseases are preventable if you follow a healthy lifestyle. While it is true that many diseases are strongly linked to the lifestyle choices you make, we know little about how to prevent most of the chronic diseases described in this chapter. Learning about these conditions reminds us that even the most carefully tended human body is vulnerable to the effects of aging and the array of diseases that, in many cases, we do not yet understand. Accordingly, we are challenged to move beyond our perception of health as the absence of disease and illness. Only then can we see that the value of health is not what it prevents, but rather what it makes possible—a life characterized by growth and development through each stage of the life cycle.

Real Life
Real choices

Your Turn

• Have you, or has someone you know, been in a situation similar to that of Penny and Jay Christenson?
• If so, what did you/they do on learning you/they were the carrier of a serious chronic condition that would be passed on to children?

And Now, Your Choices . . .
• If you haven't been in a situation like Jay and Penny's, what do you think you'd do if you were? Would you choose to go ahead and have a child, knowing it might (or definitely would) be born with a serious chronic condition? What alternatives might you consider (adoption, artificial insemination, remaining childless)?

Summary

• Diseases, illnesses, and conditions can be classified into five categories: genetic/inherited, congenital, metabolic, degenerative, and infectious.
• Chronic conditions are those that develop slowly and last a long time, while acute conditions are those that develop quickly and are generally resolved in a short period of time.
• Klinefelter's syndrome is a genetic condition caused by the presence of one or more additional X chromosomes; it results in feminization of the male body.
• Turner's syndrome occurs in females who lack one of the normal two X chromosomes, resulting in a total of forty-five chromosomes.

• Supermasculinity occurs in males who possess one or more additional Y chromosomes.
• Down syndrome results from an extra twenty-first chromosome obtained through the mother's ovum.
• Cystic fibrosis is caused by the inheritance of a recessive gene that prevents the body from producing a protein required for the normal function of exocrine glands.
• Sickle-cell disease results from inheriting a gene for an abnormal form of hemoglobin associated with crescent-shaped red blood cells that have limited oxygen transport capabilities. People with

sickle-cell trait are carriers of the abnormal hemoglobin gene.

- Duchenne muscular dystrophy is an X-linked recessive trait, thus seen almost exclusively in males, in which the body lacks the ability to produce dystrophin. The disease causes a progressive loss of muscular control and premature death.
- Talipes (clubfoot) is a common congenital abnormality in which, during embryonic formation of the lower extremity, the foot is turned inward and tipped into a clearly abnormal position.
- Cleft palate and cleft lip are caused by lack of fusion in the bones of the face during embryonic formation of the mouth and nasal cavity.
- Spina bifida results when the embryonic neural tube, the forerunner of the brain and spinal cord, fails to close, leaving the spinal cord and its coverings exposed rather than covered by skin.
- Patent foramen ovale is a congenital heart abnormality in which a hole linking the right atrium to the left atrium fails to close completely at birth, allowing unoxygenated blood to enter the systemic circulation.
- Scoliosis, an abnormal lateral curvature of the spine, can begin to develop before birth; thus it is classified as a congenital abnormality, although most cases develop during later childhood and adolescence.
- Diabetes mellitus type II, or non-insulin-dependent diabetes mellitus, occurs when the body's cells lose the ability to recognize insulin and thus are unable to utilize blood glucose normally.
- Diabetes mellitus type I, or insulin-dependent diabetes mellitus, occurs when the cells of the pancreas are destroyed, thus depriving the body of insulin, the hormone needed for the normal utilization of blood glucose.
- Reactive hypoglycemia is a relatively rare condition in which a high level of glucose in the blood after a meal stimulates the overproduction of insulin; thus glucose is removed from the blood too quickly, and the amount of glucose in the blood falls to an abnormally low level.
- Fibromyalgia is characterized by stiffness, poor sleep, chronic headaches, and other symptoms. Diagnosis is based on soreness in specific tender-point locations. Treatment is primarily aimed at reducing discomfort and enhancing sleep.
- PKU or phenylketonuria is an autosomal recessive inherited defect in the body's ability to convert the amino acid phenylalanine into the amino acid tyrosine. This results in a toxicity that destroys brain tissue, leading to mental retardation.
- Asthma is a chronic respiratory disease characterized by acute attacks of respiratory distress caused by abnormal narrowing of the airways.
- Crohn's disease, a type of inflammatory bowel disease, results from the erosion of the inner and middle layers of the intestinal tract wall, leading to pain, fever, weight loss, and rectal bleeding that causes anemia.
- Systemic lupus erythematosus is an autoimmune disorder in which the body's own immune system attacks connective tissue in the skin, muscles, nervous system, kidneys, and other areas.
- Multiple sclerosis is thought to be an autoimmune disorder in which the body loses the ability to produce myelin, an insulation material needed for proper conduction of nerve impulses.
- Parkinson's disease is characterized by loss of fine muscular control caused by the gradual cessation of dopamine production within the brain cells.
- Alzheimer's disease is a form of dementia (or loss of cognitive ability) caused by the gradual loss of the brain's ability to produce acetylcholine, a neurotransmitter essential for normal mental functioning.

Review Questions

1. Identify and describe the four categories of chronic conditions presented in this chapter. What is a fifth category of illnesses that was not covered in this chapter?
2. Compare and contrast the terms *chronic* and *acute* in terms of the onset and duration of each type of illness. Which term most appropriately describes a condition such as Down syndrome? Which describes a cold or the flu?
3. What is the genetic basis of Klinefelter's syndrome? What physical characteristics would a person with Klinefelter's syndrome have?
4. What is the genetic basis of Turner's syndrome? What physical features characterize the person with Turner's syndrome?
5. What is the genetic basis of supermasculinity? What behavioral characteristics were once ascribed to people with this genetic pattern?
6. What is the genetic basis of Down syndrome? What physical features do people with Down syndrome usually have?
7. Cystic fibrosis is a *recessive genetic disorder*; explain this term. What functional difficulties are experienced by people with cystic fibrosis? What is the condition's long-term prognosis? Why are

genetic screening and counseling important for this condition?

8. What complex protein structure is present in an abnormal form in people with sickle-cell disease? What shape are the red blood cells in people with this condition? Why are genetic screening and counseling considered important for sickle-cell disease and trait?

9. Duchenne muscular dystrophy is an *X-linked recessive disorder;* explain this term. Which gender carries this trait and which is affected by it?

10. Describe the appearance of talipes. What is this condition's more common name? How and when is this condition generally treated?

11. What medical complications could arise if cleft palate and cleft lip are not corrected?

12. What structures are exposed when the neural tube fails to close completely? What is the most serious consequence of spina bifida? Why is nutrition education an important component of prenatal care in the prevention of spina bifida?

13. What is the function of the foramen ovale in the fetal heart? What recreational pursuit may be compromised by the presence of a patent foramen ovale?

14. What structures in the upper body are at risk if scoliosis is not corrected? What are the two principal methods of treating scoliosis?

15. What are the differences between non-insulin-dependent diabetes mellitus (type II) and insulin-dependent diabetes mellitus (type I)? How does treatment for each condition differ? How important is genetic predisposition in each form of diabetes?

16. How does a person with reactive hypoglycemia respond physiologically to a large blood glucose load? How is dietary management used to treat this condition?

17. Identify three symptoms that characterize fibromyalgia. What role do tender points play in the diagnosis and treatment of fibromyalgia?

18. Although it is an inherited condition, why is PKU appropriately classified as a metabolic disorder? What is the consequence of untreated phenylketonuria? Why is long-term dietary management now being stressed?

19. How are intrinsic asthma and extrinsic asthma similar? In what important way are they different? How is exercise-induced asthma treated differently today than in the past? Why is the incidence of asthma apparently increasing?

20. How is Crohn's disease different from other forms of inflammatory bowel disease? What is currently believed to be the cause of Crohn's disease? What are some of the potentially serious consequences of this condition? How is the condition managed?

21. Systemic lupus erythematosus is an *autoimmune disorder;* explain this term. What environmental factors seem to trigger outbreaks or "flares" of SLE?

22. In multiple sclerosis, what important material associated with nervous system function cannot be produced? Why does the body lose its ability to produce this important material? To what important immune system material are several of the more effective MS drugs related?

23. What neurotransmitter is inadequately produced in people with Parkinson's disease? In which specific area of the brain is the production of this neurotransmitter lost? How do drugs used to manage the condition work?

24. Alzheimer's disease is classified as a form of *dementia;* explain this term. Which neurotransmitter is involved in Alzheimer's disease? How effective is drug treatment? What are the long-term consequences of Alzheimer's disease?

References

1. Crowley LV. *Introduction to human disease.* 4th ed. Boston: Jones & Bartlett, 1996.
2. Mader SS. *Understanding human anatomy & physiology.* 3rd ed. Dubuque, IA: WC Brown, 1997.
3. Griffiths AJF et al. *An introduction to genetic analysis.* 6th ed. New York: Freeman & Co., 1996.
4. Mange EJ, Mange AP. *Basic human genetics.* 2nd ed. Sunderland, MA: Sinauer Assoc., 1998.
5. McMahon E et al., eds. *Diseases.* Springhouse, PA: Springhouse, 1993.
6. *Our early prevention programme.* Kiwanis Down's Syndrome Foundation. The Network Connections, 1995. http://ngo.asiapac.net/down/early.html
7. Haddow JE et al. Screening of maternal serum for fetal Down's syndrome in the first trimester. *N Engl J Med* 1998; 338(14):955–61.
8. Fauci AS et al., eds. *Harrison's principles of internal medicine: companion handbook.* New York: McGraw-Hill, 1998.
9. *A family guide to cystic fibrosis genetic testing.* MSU Human Genetics, 1997. http://www.phd.msu.edu/cf/fam.html
10. *Duchenne muscular dystrophy.* Muscular Dystrophy Association of Australia, 1996. http://mda.org.au/descript.html
11. The Canadian Early and Mid-trimester Amniocentesis Trial (CEMAT) Group. Randomized trial to assess safety and fetal outcome of early and mid-trimester amniocentesis. *Lancet* 1998; 351(9098):242–47.

12. Wong DL. *Essentials of pediatric nursing.* 5th ed. St. Louis: Mosby, 1997.

13. *Cleft lip and palate surgery.* The Cleft Palate Foundation, Pittsburgh, 1997. http://plasticsurgery.org./surgery/cleft.htm

14. Means M. *Questions and answers about cleft lip and palate.* University of Iowa Hospitals & Clinics, Iowa City, IA: The Cleft Lip/Palate Service, 1997.

15. *Cleft palate.* Jacksonville, FL: Nemours Children's Clinic, 1997. http://kidshealth.org.ncc/service/cleft.html

16. *Understanding spina bifida.* Chicago: National Easter Seal Society, 1996.

17. Epstein F. *Spina bifida: prenatal detection.* New York: Institute for Neurology and Neurosurgery, Beth Israel Medical Center, 1997.

18. Whitney EN, Cataldo CB, Rolfes SR. *Understanding normal and clinical nutrition.* 5th ed. Belmont, CA: West/Wadsworth, 1997.

19. *Patent foramen ovale.* Applied Medical Information, 1996. http://www.familyinternet.com/peds/scr/001113sc.htm

20. Cohort study of multiple brain lesions in sports divers: role of a patent foramen ovale. *Br Med J* 1997 Mar 8. http://www.aceology.com/med/mpneu/ovale.htm

21. Blackman R et al. *Scoliosis treatment.* Oakland, CA: Kaiser Permanente Hospital, 1996. http://www.scoliosis.com/option1

22. Thibodeau G, Patton K. *The human body in health and disease.* 2nd ed. St. Louis: Mosby, 1996.

23. Inzucchi SE et al. Efficacy and metabolic effects of metformin and troglitazone in type II diabetes mellitus. *N Engl J Med* 1998; 338(13):867–72.

24. Conrad B et al. Evidence of superantigen involvement in insulin-dependent diabetes mellitus aetiology. *Nature* 1994; 371(6495):351–53.

25. Clayman CB, ed. *The American Medical Association home medical encyclopedia.* New York: Random House, 1989.

26. *Hypoglycemia.* National Diabetes Information Clearinghouse (NIDDK), Feb 1997. http://www.niddk.nih.gov/health/diabetes/pubs/hypo/hypo

27. *Hypoglycemia.* Information Network, 1995–1997. http://www.medicinenet.com/mainmenu/encyclop/art_h/hypoglyc.htm

28. Battistini S et al. Unexpected white matter changes in an early treatment. *Functional Neurol* 1991; 6(2):177–80.

29. *Fibromyalgia basics: symptoms, treatments and research.* 1998. http://www.fmnetnews.com/pages/basics.html

30. *Diagnostic criteria for fibromyalgia and CFS.* 1998. http://www.fmnetnews.com/pages/criteria.html

31. Asthma (medical essay). *Mayo Clinical Health Letter* (suppl) 1996; 14(2):1–8.

32. New asthma drugs add another dimension to treatment. *Mayo Clinic Health Letter* 1997; 15(3):4.

33. Nelson JA et al. Effect of long-term salmeterol treatment on exercise-induced asthma. *N Engl J Med* 1998; 339(3):141–46.

34. Leff JA et al. Montelukast, a leukotriene-receptor antagonist, for the treatment of mild asthma and exercise-induced bronchoconstriction. *N Engl J Med* 1998; 339(3)147–52.

35. Sartor RB. IBD researchers are breaking new ground. *Under the Microscope* (research news bulletin from the Crohn's & Colitis Foundation of America) 1998; 5:2.

36. Sandborn WJ. Progress in IBD: update from the scientific community. *Under the Microscope* (research news bulletin from the Crohn's & Colitis Foundation of America) 1998; 5:4.

37. Price SA, Wilson L, eds. *Pathophysiology: clinical concepts of disease processes.* 5th ed. St. Louis: Mosby, 1996.

38. Waxman SG. Demyelinating diseases—new pathological insights, new therapeutic targets. *N Engl J Med* 1998; 338(5):323–25.

39. King M. Treatment options—now there are three. *Inside MS* 1997 Spring; 15(1):3.

40. Can monoclonal antibodies shorten MS attacks? *Inside MS* 1997 Fall; 15(3):15.

41. Bennett D et al. Prevalence of Parkinsonian signs and associated mortality in a community population of older people. *N Engl J Med* 1996; 3334(2):71–76.

42. *Parkinson's disease: hope through research.* NIH Pub. No. 94-139, Sept. 1994.

43. Polymeropoulos M et al. Mapping of a gene for Parkinson's disease to chromosome 4q21–q23. *Science* 1996; 274(5290):1197–99.

44. Friend T. Gene defect is linked to Parkinson's. *USA Today* 1997 June 27:1D.

45. Limousin P et al. Electrical stimulation of the subthalamic nucleus in advanced Parkinson's disease. *N Engl J Med* 1998; 339(16):1105–11.

46. Sano M. A controlled trial of selegiline, alphatocopherol, or both as treatment for Alzheimer's disease. *N Engl J Med* 1997; 336(17)1216–22.

Suggested Readings

Berkow R, Beers MH, Fletcher AJ, eds. *The Merck manual of medical information: home edition.* Rahway, NJ: Merck & Co., 1997. Few medical reference books are as valuable as the "Merck Manual." Now a useful, home version is available. Topics range from basic science-related information such as anatomy and physiology to informative descriptions of hundreds of medical conditions. In addition, a section on medication provides information similar to that found in a *Physicians Desk Reference (PDR).*

Iams BA. *From MS to wellness.* San Diego, CA: Iams House, 1998. For persons diagnosed with a serious lifelong illness, it is often as important to have encouragement from others as it is to have technical information about the condition. Betty Iams' book provides that encouragement as she shares with readers her journey along the course of progressive MS and her decision to look inward for new resources. This book does not provide technical information about the disease or information regarding alternative forms of treatment.

topics for Today

Managing Chronic Pain: New Treatments Offer Solutions for Sufferers

Carlotta loved to spend her spare time puttering around in her flower garden. Every weekend she worked outside for hours, tilling soil, putting in new plants, pruning, and landscaping. One Saturday afternoon, as she was lifting some railroad ties to install a new border for her plant paradise, she heard a loud popping noise and felt a sharp pain in her lower back. She tried aspirin, bed rest, massage, and heat, but the pain was still excruciating even after two weeks. She went to see her doctor, who prescribed pain medication and a brief course of physical therapy, but the pain persisted. Finally, after nearly a year passed with little relief, her doctor recommended back surgery. Carlotta spent almost 3 months recovering from the surgery, after which she hoped to be able to lead a normal, pain-free life.

Unfortunately, Carlotta's pain persists even today, almost 2 years after her initial injury. Carlotta suffers from chronic pain, a type of pain that persists beyond the expected healing time of an injury or illness. Chronic pain differs from most ordinary encounters with pain, such as pain resulting from a headache, a fall, or surgery. According to the American Pain Society, chronic pain is difficult to treat because it does not respond to normal pain treatments. Also, many of the signs that usually accompany acute pain, such as sweating, increased heart rate, and dilated pupils, are absent in people with chronic pain.[1] Despite these obstacles, impressive progress has been made in the management of chronic pain. Today physicians who are board certified in pain management, most often anesthesiologists, are routinely found in the anesthesiology services of larger hospitals.[2] Of the 60 million Americans who suffer from chronic pain, an increasing number are receiving the most technologically advanced care available.

Causes of Chronic Pain

In some patients, chronic pain may be linked to injury of the central or peripheral nervous systems, according to John D. Loeser, M.D., director of the Multidisci-plinary Pain Center at the University of Washington School of Medicine.[1] In these patients, no tissue damage ever occurred in the part of their body that hurts. When the nervous system heals itself, the functions of the nerve cells lost in the injury are not restored. As a result, the patient's neurological function is impaired. This type of pain can be caused by limb amputation, shingles, diabetes, or surgery.[1]

A second cause of chronic pain is linked to degenerative changes in joints. In these cases, tissue damage that has occurred may not heal properly. Patients have both inflammation of the joints and chronic degenerative problems.[1] This cause of pain usually accompanies diseases such as arthritis and lupus.

Another "cause" of pain is the catchall category "no known pathological mechanism."[1] Doctors are unsure why these patients are having pain. The one criterion used to place a patient in this category is whether the patient's pain complaints exceed the physician's expectations based on the illness or injury the patient has suffered.

An increasingly common source of pain is repetitive strain injuries (RSIs). Three times as many cases of RSIs were reported in 1993 as in 1986.[3] These injuries are caused mainly by awkward postures or repetitive motion. This type of injury is a product of the computer age and is therefore often encountered by college students.

Conditions Associated with Chronic Pain

Several types of conditions, such as headaches, are commonly associated with chronic pain. Up to 57 percent of men and 76 percent of women in the adolescent and young adult age-groups have recurrent headaches. The National Headache Foundation estimates that 45 million Americans suffer from chronic headaches. Of these sufferers, 86 percent are women. Although doctors have identified 55 types of headaches, the four most commonly associated with chronic pain are tension headaches, migraines, cluster headaches, and sinus headaches.[4]

Like Carlotta in our previous example, four out of five Americans experience back pain at some point in their lives. The problem usually resolves itself for most people; however, researchers estimate that more than 11 million Americans have enough back pain to cause impairment. This cause of chronic pain is particularly troublesome because of its economic effect on society. Attorney's costs for pursuing back injuries as a result of worker's compensation and other accidents approach $5 billion per year. The indirect costs of lost wages and homemakers' potential lost earnings are near $3.6 billion. Based on all analyses of possible cost factors, back pain costs society anywhere from $75 billion to $100 billion annually.[1]

Another debilitating condition commonly associated with chronic pain is arthritis. More than 35 million Americans have a form of this disease. Two types of arthritis exist. Osteoarthritis is the breaking down of the cartilage found at the ends of the long bones. Weight-bearing and frequently used joints are the areas most commonly affected. Rheumatoid arthritis is an autoimmune disorder in which the patient's own immune system produces antibodies that attack the tissues in the joints of the body.[5] Symptoms of both types include stiffness and swelling of the joints.

Cancer and Chronic Pain

Although cancer is one of the conditions often associated with chronic pain, pain experts put it into a class by itself because of its special circumstances. Chronic cancer pain is complex because the pain can occur as a result of bone invasion, tumors compressing nerves, tumors affecting internal organs, obstruction of blood vessels, surgery, chemotherapy, or radiation treatment.[1]

Effects of Chronic Pain

Because chronic pain is such a disruptive, continuing phenomenon, it can affect almost every aspect of a person's life. Richard Linchitz, M.D., a pain specialist and chronic pain sufferer, describes what his life was like after a disk in his lower back became herniated: "As bad as the pain was, the worst aspect for me was the growing and quite depressing sense that my days of vigorous exercise were over. My doctor began ruling out, one by one, the very activities—running, bicycling, weightlifting—that had become a part of my identity."[6] Veronica, one of Dr. Norman J. Marcus's patients, found it difficult not only to pursue hobbies but even to complete simple everyday tasks, such as washing the dishes.[4]

The devastation of losing a job is another potential effect of suffering with chronic pain. Because the pain is so disruptive and persistent, it affects a person's ability to concentrate, perform essential job duties, or even go to work. Toni, another of Dr. Marcus's patients, had been the manager of a high-pressure department of a busy store. She had always been conscientious and hardworking until she began having pain in her hip. Because of the pain, she had difficulty performing her job, and she also had to take time off from work frequently either because of doctor's appointments or because her pain was so severe. As a result, Toni was fired.[4]

Sleep disorders are a third potential effect of chronic pain. Sleep disorders can come about in two ways. Either a patient is unable to sleep because of the pain, or the individual becomes dependent on a pain or sleep medication that disrupts the sleep cycle. Toni, who was described in the previous paragraph, was on many medications, including both painkillers and sleeping pills, yet she continually had trouble falling and staying asleep. On being admitted to a pain management center, Toni was taken off all her medications and given a mild antidepressant instead. She slept for 10 hours that night, "the first good night's sleep I'd had in four years."[4]

Pain sufferers often lose their friends as well as their jobs. Society tends to judge chronic pain sufferers harshly. Other people may doubt the severity of the sufferer's symptoms, especially if no medical cause can be identified or the pain does not respond to traditional treatments. Acquaintances may distance themselves from the person, considering him or her to be lazy, or faking, or somehow responsible for the injury.

Serious psychological problems can also result from chronic pain. Depression is one of the most common ailments. Henry, another patient at Dr. Marcus's pain clinic and a former construction worker, had always been a calm, easygoing person who got along well with others and was the chief provider for his family. One day at work, Henry was struck in the back of the neck by a steel beam. He suffered pain not just in his neck but also throughout his body. As time went on and the pain did not go away, Henry's entire personality began to change. He went from being easygoing to being a chronic worrier because he was concerned about the family's financial security. He isolated himself from his family and friends, and he began to snap at anyone who asked him questions about his condition. The more Henry hurt, the more he worried about hurting; the more he worried about hurting, the more he hurt. Henry was caught in a downward spiral of depression that set him apart from his family and friends.[4]

The final significant side effect of chronic pain is the potential damage it can do to the immune system. This effect can be particularly troublesome in patients whose chronic pain is the result of cancer. Studies have shown that pain can suppress the immune system, thus causing cancer patients to have difficulty recovering.[7] Because of this potentially fatal problem, it is especially important for cancer patients to have their pain treated promptly and effectively.

Methods of Managing Chronic Pain

Although chronic pain has several negative side effects, many of these effects can be controlled using proper pain management methods. Most pain specialists recommend that sufferers be treated with a multidisciplinary approach that uses a combination of methods to achieve maximal relief.

One of the most common and effective methods of relieving chronic pain is the use of opioid drugs, also known as Schedule II drugs. These drugs provide quick relief of pain, particularly among cancer patients and headache sufferers.[7] However, physicians are often reluctant to prescribe these drugs for several reasons. First, doctors are afraid that if they are perceived as prescribing too many opioids, they could be reported to the medical board and ultimately lose their licenses. Second, American society in general disapproves of prescribing narcotics because of the fear of addiction and the idea that all narcotics are bad, despite their potential for providing pain relief. Finally, medical personnel tend to underestimate the amount of pain that patients suffer. Most people who suffer severe pain and request narcotics will not become addicts, but some medical personnel who work with pain sufferers believe that people with chronic pain do not hurt as badly as they claim to.[7]

The mention of the term *narcotics* commonly brings images of drug addicts to mind. Although the potential for abuse exists, the overwhelming majority of patients do not become addicted and can gradually eliminate their intakes as their condition improves. As Dr. Richard Patt, of the Anderson Cancer Center of Houston, points out, a major difference is seen between addicts and pain patients. "When addicts use drugs, they become less functional, more isolated and they move away from the mainstream," he explains, "When pain patients use drugs, they become more functional, much less isolated, and they move toward the mainstream."[8]

Today effective pain-reducing drugs can be delivered in a variety of ways. Depending on the nature of the pain and the patient's experience with more conservative treatments, medication can be delivered through tender-point injections, epidural injections, injections in specific sympathetic nerves and ganglia, or injections into joints such as tiny facet joints of the vertebral column.[9]

For chronic headache sufferers, several other types of drugs offer hope as well. Small doses of tricyclic antidepressants taken at bedtime seem to help headache sufferers sleep better and have some preventive effect during the day. Other drugs that provide relief include beta-blockers, calcium channel blockers, and anticonvulsants. Doctors may try several combinations of these drugs to see which will most effectively relieve headache symptoms, with the eventual goal of removing as many medications as possible from the patient's daily regimen.[6]

For patients with arthritis, two classes of drugs appear to offer the most relief. The first type is known as *nonsteroidal anti-inflammatory drugs (NSAIDs)*. The most well-known types of these drugs are Advil, Nuprin, Naprosyn, and Anaprox. They provide relief within two hours. A second type of antiarthritic medicine is known as *slow-acting antirheumatic drugs (SAARDs)*. These drugs provide time-released, long-lasting relief. Other treatments that may be used in combination with these two types of drugs include injectable gold and corticosteroids.[10]

Surgery is another option for managing chronic pain. This choice is most effective in helping patients with cancer. Removing diseased cells or tumors often removes the source that is causing pain for the patient. Surgery may also become necessary for the arthritis pain sufferer. Replacement of cartilage or an affected joint will often help a sufferer lead a more normal, less painful life.

Because the mind is such a powerful instrument of healing, pain specialists often recommend that patients undertake psychological methods of pain relief along with traditional methods. For example, many headache specialists recommend biofeedback techniques so that patients can learn to control their responses to pain. Pain specialists teach their patients to do deep-breathing exercises and then advance them to meditation techniques to promote relaxation. In addition, positive thinking about one's situation and prospects for recovery can help patients need fewer medications, according to a recent British study.[10]

Physical methods are another dimension of chronic pain management. One time-tested method of relief is massage. Other helpful treatments include nerve blocks to the affected area, physical therapy, exercises prescribed by a physical therapist or physician, hydrotherapy, and acupuncture.[11] Finally, a patient can make some lifestyle changes to lessen the pain. Eating regularly, getting plenty of rest, and reducing caffeine intake have all been found to be particularly helpful to headache sufferers but may also help others who have chronic pain.

The Future of Chronic Pain Management

Although they were virtually unheard of just a few years ago, pain clinics, or pain centers, are becoming more prevalent in the medical community. These centers feature physicians and other health-care professionals who use the multidisciplinary approach to pain management. Personnel on-site might include physicians, physical therapists, exercise physiologists, psychologists, and psychiatrists.[4] Pain centers are also at the forefront of pain research. A pain center in Dallas is currently studying the possibility of using gene therapy to conquer chronic pain. The new genes would enable patients to grow new, undamaged nerves, which would also enhance endorphin production.[2] Whether through medication, therapy, or research, the goal of all pain centers is the same: to improve the patient's condition so that on leaving the center, the person will be able to resume normal activities, need a minimal amount of medication, and maintain a positive attitude.[4]

An additional hope for better chronic pain management is the training of tomorrow's doctors. The American Medical Association (AMA) has called for better education about pain and pain management in both undergraduate and postgraduate medical training. In particular, the AMA hopes to make the use of opioid drugs more acceptable to health-care personnel as an option for relieving pain. Hospitals are also instituting quality assurance programs so that patients can be more empowered to demand and receive the pain relief they need. There is even a new field of medicine developing to train physicians in the initial diagnosis of chronic pain so that only appropriate referrals are made to specialists in pain management. Known as *manual* or *musculoskeletal medicine,* this new medical field emphasizes detailed physical examination techniques.[12]

An option for terminally ill cancer patients who are in need of relief from chronic pain is the hospice movement. Hospices put into practice a philosophy that allows medical personnel to focus on the patients rather than their diseases (see Chapter 21). The main goals of hospices are to provide pain relief and to give psychological support to both the patient and his or her family. Hospices also use a multidisciplinary approach that includes physicians, nurses, social workers, physical therapists, and members of the clergy.[1] The hospice can provide the care and support that cancer sufferers and their families need as the patient nears the end of life.

Although a cure has not yet been found for chronic pain, it can be managed successfully with the help of trained personnel from a variety of fields. Unfortunately, chronic pain sufferers must be vocal and persistent to get the help they desperately need.

For Discussion . . .

Have you ever known someone who suffered (or still suffers) from chronic pain? What were your feelings about this person and his or her pain? If you suffered from chronic pain, what treatments do you think would be the best for you? Would you be willing to try alternative therapies like the ones described in this article, or would you be more comfortable with traditional methods of therapy? Why? Have you thought about your level of risk for an RSI? What could you do to lessen that risk?

References

1. Cowles J. *Pain relief.* New York: Mastermedia, 1993.
2. *Pain management.* West Jersey, PA: West Jersey Anesthesia Association, 1999. http://www.westjerseyanesthesia.com/pain.htm
3. Yassi A. Repetitive strain injuries. *Lancet* 1997; (349): 9056.
4. Marcus NJ. *Freedom from chronic pain.* New York: Simon & Schuster, 1994.
5. Crowley LV. *Introduction to human disease.* 4th ed. Boston: Jones & Bartlett, 1996.
6. Linchitz RM. *Life without pain.* New York: Addison-Wesley, 1987.
7. Buterbaugh L. Breaking through cancer pain barriers. *Medical World* 1993 Oct 15:10.
8. Gorman C. The case for morphine: if nothing is better for pain than narcotics, why don't more doctors prescribe them? *Time* 1997; (149):17.
9. *Treatment procedures.* St. Louis University, SLUCare Anesthesiology, 1997. http://www.slucare.edu/clinical/anesthesia/treatment/
10. Meinson M. Brain against pain. *Prevention* 1996 Jan 1:48.
11. *Chronic pain: questions and answers* (What are common treatments for chronic pain?). Allegheny General Hospital, Neurosurgical Pain Management. http://www.arsi.edu/neuro/brochure/pain.htm
12. Hill CS Jr. When will adequate pain treatment be the norm? *JAMA* 1995; (274):23.

InfoLinks
http://neurosurgery.mgh.harvard.edu/ncpainoa.htm
www.ampainsoc.org

thirteen

Preventing Infectious Disease Transmission

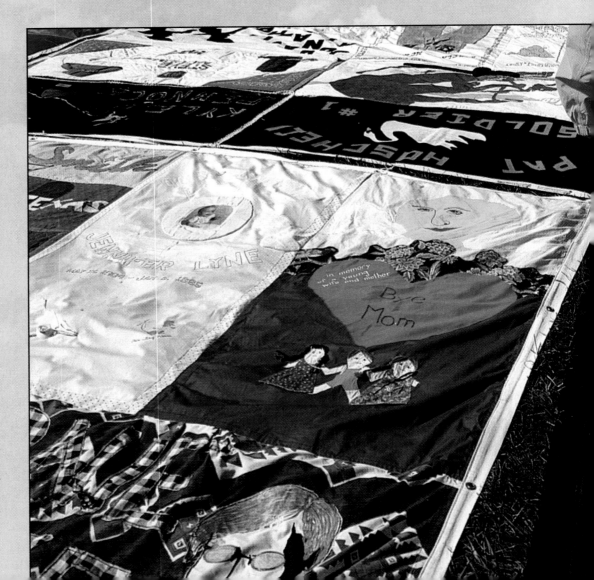

Each panel of the AIDS quilt is crafted by loved ones in memory of a family member or friend who has died. People with HIV/AIDS are living longer, and researchers are working hard to find a cure.

In the nineteenth century, infectious diseases were the leading cause of death. These deaths came after exposure to the organisms that produced such diseases as smallpox, tuberculosis (TB), influenza, whooping cough (pertussis), typhoid, diphtheria, and tetanus. However, since the early 1900s, improvements in public sanitation, the widespread use of antibiotic drugs, and vaccinations have considerably reduced the number of people who die from infectious diseases. People now die more often from chronic disease processes.

Today, however, we have a new respect for infectious diseases. We have learned that AIDS threatens millions of people in many areas of the world. We are witnessing the resurgence of TB. We recognize the role of pelvic infections in infertility. We also know that failure to fully immunize children has laid the groundwork for a return of whooping cough, polio, and other serious childhood diseases. In fact, some experts suggest that because of HIV/AIDS and the emergence and re-emergence of infectious diseases, today's young adults may have a lower life expectancy than the generation immediately ahead of them.

HEALTHY PEOPLE: LOOKING AHEAD TO 2010

Progress was uneven in achieving the *Healthy People 2000* objectives in the area of infectious disease prevention. On the positive side, the nation moved steadily toward reducing the incidence of vaccine-preventable infectious diseases in people under 25. In addition, the *Midcourse Review* reported an increase in condom use, an important aspect of controlling transmission of HIV/AIDS. At the same time, the use of new drug combinations has significantly reduced the HIV/AIDS death rate in just a few years.

Healthy People 2010 will, of course, continue to recommend federally supported efforts to control infectious diseases. The objectives related to infectious conditions will focus on several important areas,

including substance abuse, sexual health, food safety, maternal-child health, delivery of health services, and improvement of public health care. Education and community health promotion will probably be emphasized. The new initiative will also continue to support basic research in infectious diseases.

Because of the broad scope of infectious disease transmission, it is likely that almost every health-care model described in Chapter 1 will be employed to direct resources appropriately. Virtually everyone is affected by infectious diseases, either directly or indirectly; and many diseases, such as HIV/AIDS and pandemic flu outbreaks, have national and international implications.

Real Life
Real choices

• Name: Chris Karasawa
• Age: 53
• Occupation: Electrical engineer

"What if he uses my coffee mug?" "He shouldn't be allowed in our restroom." "I don't want him working anywhere near me."

Those are just a few of the comments Chris Karasawa has heard from some of his employees since the beginning of this week, when he interviewed a young engineer for a newly created position in his department. Of all the candidates Chris has met with, John Travers is by far the best qualified for the position Chris has been seeking to fill for the past 2 months. He graduated summa cum laude from one of the top engineering programs in the country, has impeccable references, is enthusiastic, energetic—and openly gay. His partner recently died of AIDS, and John (who has consistently tested negative for the HIV virus) wants to relocate from the West Coast to this New England city.

Those of Chris's employees who object to his hiring John know intellectually that he won't inevitably contract AIDS. They also know that HIV isn't spread by casual contact, so even if a coworker did have AIDS, the risk to fellow employees is extremely low.

Overall, the people on Chris's staff are a diverse and tolerant group who attach little importance to differences in race, sex, religion, and lifestyle. Chris knows, however, that when it comes to AIDS, reasonable and accepting people with otherwise open minds often slam the door shut. AIDS is often a fatal disease, and it's most prevalent among gay men. John Travers is gay, his partner died of AIDS, and therefore some of Chris's staffers perceive his presence as a threat to their physical and emotional well-being.

As you study this chapter, think about Chris Karasawa's challenges and choices in hiring John Travers, and prepare yourself to answer the questions in **Your Turn** at the end of the chapter.

Several new types of infectious disease have appeared, and new concerns have been raised about the spread of familiar infectious diseases. These include the following:

• The extremely virulent viruses, such as the Ebola virus in Zaire, which is fatal to 75 percent of those who contract it, for which we do not have an immunization, and whose transmission we do not understand (see the Topics for Today article on p. 418); and the Sabia virus, released in a Yale laboratory accident
• The increasing resistance of bacteria such as *Staphylococcus aureus*, *Enterococcus*, and *Mycobacterium* (which causes tuberculosis) to antibiotics as the result of overuse, improper use, and biological "redesign" of the organisms themselves
• The role of a bacterium (*Helicobacter pylori*) in the development of gastric ulcers
• The growing concern over transmission of infectious organisms through contaminated food, improper preparation of food, and contamination of water

Infectious Disease Transmission

Infectious diseases can generally be transmitted from person to person, although the transfer is not always direct. Infectious diseases can be especially dangerous because they can spread to large numbers of people, producing epidemics or pandemics. The following

sections explain the process of disease transmission and the stages of infection.

Pathogens

For a disease to be transferred, a person must come into contact with the disease-producing agent, or **pathogen,** such as a virus, bacterium, or fungus. When pathogens enter our bodies, the pathogens can sometimes resist body defense systems, flourish, and produce an illness. We commonly call this an *infection.* Because of their small size, pathogens are sometimes called *microorganisms, microbes,* or *germs.* Table 13-1 describes familiar infectious disease agents and some of the illnesses they produce.

Chain of Infection

The movement of a pathogenic agent through the various links in the chain of infection (Figure 13-1) explains how diseases spread.[1] Not every pathogenic agent moves all the way through the chain of infection, because various links in the chain can be broken. Therefore, the presence of a pathogen creates only the potential for causing disease.

Agent

The first link in the chain of infection is the disease-causing **agent.** Whereas some agents are very **virulent** and lead to serious infectious illnesses such as HIV, which causes AIDS, others produce far less serious infections, such as the common cold. Through mutation, some pathogenic agents, particularly viruses, can become more virulent.

Table 13-1   Pathogens and Common Infectious Diseases

Pathogen	Description	Representative Disease Processes
Viruses	Smallest common pathogens; nonliving particles of genetic material (DNA) surrounded by a protein coat	Rubeola, mumps, chickenpox, rubella, influenza, warts, colds, oral and genital herpes, shingles, AIDS, genital warts
Bacteria	One-celled microorganisms with sturdy, well-defined cell walls; three distinctive forms: spherical (cocci), rod shaped (bacilli), and spiral shaped (spirilla)	Tetanus, strep throat, scarlet fever, gonorrhea, syphilis, chlamydia, toxic shock syndrome, Legionnaires' disease, bacterial pneumonia, meningitis, diphtheria, food poisoning, Lyme disease
Fungi	Plantlike microorganisms; molds and yeasts	Athlete's foot, ringworm, histoplasmosis, San Joaquin Valley fever, candidiasis
Protozoa	Simplest animal form, generally one-celled organisms	Malaria, amebic dysentery, trichomoniasis, vaginitis
Rickettsia	Viruslike organisms that require a host's living cells for growth and replication	Typhus, Rocky Mountain spotted fever, rickettsialpox
Parasitic worms	Many-celled organisms; represented by tapeworms, leeches, and roundworms	Dirofilariasis (dog heartworm), elephantiasis, onchocerciasis

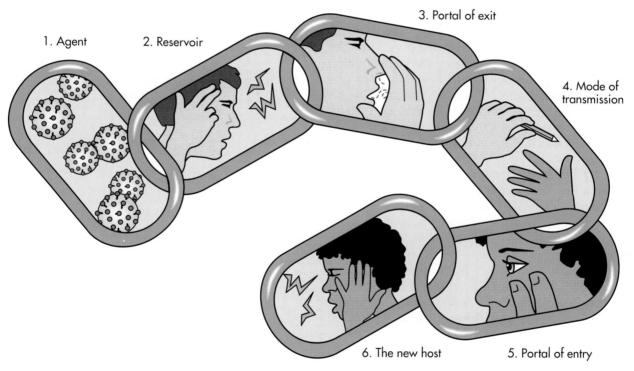

Figure 13-1   The six links in the chain of infection. The example above shows a rhinovirus, which causes the common cold, being passed from one person to another. 1, The *agent* (pathogen) is a rhinovirus; 2, The *reservoir* is the infected person; 3, The *portal of exit* is the respiratory system (coughing); 4, The *mode of transmission* is indirect hand contact; 5, The *portal of entry* is the mucous membranes of the uninfected person's eye; 6, The virus now has a *new host.*

Reservoir

Infectious agents require the support and protection of a favorable environment to survive. This environment forms the second link in the chain of infection and is called the *reservoir,* in which the agent resides.

---

pathogen   a disease-causing agent.

agent   the causal pathogen of a particular disease.

virulent (**veer** yuh lent)   capable of causing disease.

For many of the most common infectious diseases, the reservoirs are the bodies of people who are already infected. Here the agents thrive before being spread to others. These infected people are, accordingly, the hosts for particular disease agents. In some infectious illnesses a person's reservoir status may be restored after treatment and apparent recovery from the original infection. This is because some pathogens, particularly viruses, can remain sequestered (hidden), emerging later to give rise to another infection.

For other infectious diseases, however, the reservoirs are the bodies of animals. Rabies is a well-known animal-reservoir disease. The infected animals are not always sick and do not always show symptoms similar to those seen in infected people.

The third type of reservoir in which disease-causing agents can live is in a nonliving environment, such as the soil. The spores of the tetanus bacterium, for example, can survive in soil for up to fifty years, entering the human body in a puncture wound.

Portal of Exit

For pathogenic agents to cause diseases and illnesses in others, they must leave their reservoirs. Thus the third link in the chain of infection is the portal of exit, or the point at which agents leave their reservoirs.

The principal portals of exit are familiar—the digestive system, urinary system, respiratory system, reproductive system, and the blood, especially with infectious diseases that infect humans.

Mode of Transmission

The fourth link in the chain of infection is the mode of transmission, or the way in which pathogens move from reservoirs to susceptible hosts. Two principal methods are direct transmission and indirect transmission.

We see three types of direct transmission in human-to-human transmission. These include contact between body surfaces (such as kissing, touching, and sexual intercourse), droplet spread (inhalation of contaminated air droplets), and fecal-oral spread (feces on the host's hands are brought into contact with the new host's mouth).

Indirect transmission between infected and uninfected people occurs when infectious agents travel by means of nonhuman materials. Vehicles of transmission include inanimate objects, such as water, food, soil, towels, clothing, and eating utensils.

Infectious agents can also be indirectly transmitted through vectors. The term *vector* describes living things, such as insects, birds, and other animals, that carry diseases from human to human. An example of a vector is the deer tick, which transmits Lyme disease.

Airborne indirect transmission includes the inhalation of infected particles that have been sus-pended in an air source for an extended time. Unlike droplet transmission, in which both infected and uninfected people must be in close physical proximity, noninfected people can become infected through airborne transmission by sharing air with infected people who were in the same room hours earlier. Viral infections such as German measles can be spread this way.

Portal of Entry

The fifth link in the chain of infection is the portal of entry. As with the portals of exit, portals of entry have three primary methods that allow pathogenic agents to enter the bodies of uninfected people. These are through the digestive system, respiratory system, and reproductive system. In addition, a break in the skin provides another portal of entry. In most infectious conditions, the portals of entry are the same systems that served as the portals of exit for the infected people. In HIV, however, we see cross-system transmission. Oral and anal sex allow infectious agents to pass between the warm, moist tissues of the reproductive and digestive systems.

Personal Applications

• How do you feel when a classmate or coworker comes to class or work ill? Is it fair for this person to expose others to his or her illness?

The New Host

All people are, in theory, at risk for contracting infectious diseases and thus could be called susceptible hosts. In practice, however, factors such as overall health, acquired immunity, health-care services, and health-related behavior can affect susceptibility to infectious diseases.

Stages of Infection

When a pathogenic agent assaults a new host, a reasonably predictable sequence of events begins. That is, the disease moves through five distinctive stages.[2] You may be able to recognize these stages of infection each time you catch a cold.

1. *The incubation stage.* This stage lasts from the time a pathogen enters the body until it multiplies enough to produce signs and symptoms of the disease. The duration of this stage can vary from a few hours to many months, depending on the virulence of the organisms, the concentration of organisms, the host's level of immune responsiveness, and other health problems. This stage has been

called a *silent stage.* The pathogen can be transmitted to a new host during this stage, but this is not likely. A host may be infected during this stage but not infectious. HIV infection is an exception to this rule.

2. *The prodromal stage.* After the incubation stage, the host may experience a variety of general signs and symptoms, including watery eyes, runny nose, slight fever, and overall tiredness for a brief time. These symptoms are nonspecific and may not be severe enough to force the host to rest. During this stage the pathogenic agent continues to multiply. Now the host is capable of transferring pathogens to a new host. One should practice self-imposed isolation during this stage to protect others. Again, HIV infection is different in this stage.

3. *The clinical stage.* This stage, also called the *acme* or *acute stage,* is often the most unpleasant stage for the host. At this time the disease reaches its highest point of development. Laboratory tests can identify or analyze all of the clinical (observable) signs and symptoms of the particular disease. The likelihood of transmitting the disease to others is highest during this peak stage; all of our available defense mechanisms are in the process of resisting further damage from the pathogen.

4. *The decline stage.* The first signs of recovery appear during this stage. The infection is ending or, in some cases, falling to a subclinical level. People may suffer a relapse if they overextend themselves. In HIV and AIDS, this is almost always the last stage before death.

5. *The recovery stage.* Also called the *convalescence stage,* this stage is characterized by apparent recovery from the invading agent. The disease can be transmitted during this stage, but this is not probable. Until the host's overall health has been strengthened, he or she may be especially susceptible to another (perhaps different) disease pathogen. Fortunately, after the recovery stage, further susceptibility to the pathogenic agent is typically lower because the body has built up immunity. This buildup of immunity is not always permanent; for example, many sexually transmitted diseases can be contracted repeatedly.

Body Defenses: Mechanical and Cellular Immune Systems

Much as a series of defensive alignments protect a military installation, so too is the body protected by sets of defenses. These defenses can be classified as either mechanical or cellular (Figure 13-2). Mechanical defenses are first-line defenses, because they physically separate the internal body from the external environment. Examples include the skin, the mucous membranes that line the respiratory and gastrointestinal tracts, earwax, the tiny hairs and cilia that filter incoming air, and even tears. These defenses serve primarily as a shield against foreign materials that may contain pathogenic agents. These defenses can, however, be disarmed, such as when tobacco smoke kills the cilia that protect the airway, resulting in chronic bronchitis, or when contact lenses reduce tearing, leading to irritation and eye infection.

The second component of the body's protective defenses is the cellular system or, more commonly, the **immune system.** The cellular component is far more specific than the mechanical defenses. Its primary mission is to eliminate microorganisms, foreign proteins, and foreign cells from the body. A wellness-oriented lifestyle, including sound nutrition, effective stress management, and regular exercise, supports this important division of the immune system. The microorganisms, foreign proteins, or abnormal cells that activate this cellular component are collectively called *antigens.*[3]

Divisions of the Immune System

Closer examination of the immune system, or cellular defenses, reveals two separate but highly cooperative groups of cells. One group of cells originates in the fetal thymus gland and thus has become known as *T cell-mediated immunity,* or simply *cell-mediated immunity.* The second group of cells that make up cellular immunity are the B cells (bursa of Fabricius), which are the working units of *humoral immunity.*[3] Cellular elements of both cell-mediated and humoral immunity can be found within the bloodstream, the lymphatic tissues of the body, and the fluid that surrounds body cells.

Although we are born with the structural elements of both cell-mediated and humoral immunity, developing an immune response requires that

---

Personal Applications

• Which infectious disease have you had in the recent past? What effect did this infection have on your day-to-day activities?

---

immune system the system of cellular elements that protects the body from invading pathogens and foreign materials.

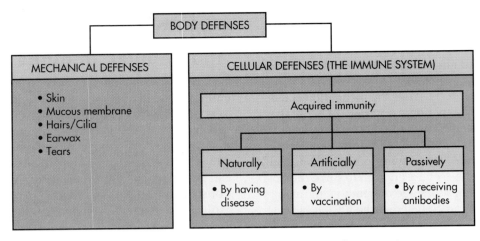

Figure 13-2   The body has a variety of defenses against invading organisms. Mechanical defenses are the first means of protection, because they separate the internal body from the external environment. Cellular defenses include chemicals and specialized cells that produce immunity to subsequent infections.

Table 13-2   Recommended Immunization Schedule*†

			Months					Years
	Birth	**1–2**	**2**	**4**	**6**	**6–18**	**12–15**	**4–6**
Diphtheria/pertussis^v/ tetanus (DPT)			X	X	X		X‡	X
Polio (OPV) (IPV)^∝			X	X	X			X
Measles/mumps/ rubella (MMR)							X	X
Haemophilus influenza (Hib)			X	X	X§		X	
Hepatitis B‖ (Hep B)	X	X				X		
or:		X		X		X		

*Foreign travelers: renew immunizations for diseases prevalent in the countries of travel.

†Influenza: yearly for elderly adults, workers in occupations (such as health-care workers and teachers) exposed to infected persons, and for all adults with chronic respiratory and heart disease.

‡As early as 12 months, as long as at least 6 months since last DPT dose.

§May not be required, depending on which Hib vaccine is used.

‖Anyone exposed to infected individuals or contaminated food and water, and foreign travelers and health-care workers.

For referral to an immunization clinic or for other information, contact the Centers for Disease Control and Prevention National Immunization Program: (800) 232-2522 in English or TDD; (800) 232-0233 in Spanish.

^vA new pertussis vaccine has far fewer serious side effects than older pertussis components of the DPT series.

^∝The first two inoculations use injected polio vaccine (IPV), a killed-virus vaccine, with the third and fourth using oral polio vaccine, a live polio vaccine. (Recommended by the American Academy of Pediatrics.)

components of these cellular systems encounter and successfully defend against specific antigens. When the immune system has done this once, it is primed to respond quickly and effectively if the same antigens appear again. This confrontation produces a state of **acquired immunity (AI).** Acquired immunity develops in different ways, as seen in Figure 13-2.

- **Naturally acquired immunity (NAI)** develops when the body is exposed to infectious agents. Thus when we catch an infectious disease, we fight the infection and in the process become immune (protected) from developing that illness again if we encounter the agent again.

- **Artificially acquired immunity (AAI)** occurs when the body is exposed to weakened or killed infectious agents introduced through vaccination or immunization. As in NAI, the body fights the infectious agents and records the method of fighting the agents. Young children, older adults, and adults in high-risk occupations should consult their physicians about immunizations. See Table 13-2 for an immunization schedule.

- **Passively acquired immunity (PAI),** a third form of immunity, results when antibodies are introduced into the body. These antibodies are for a variety of specific infections, and they are produced outside the body (either in animals or by the genetic manipulation of microorganisms). When introduced into the human body, they provide immediate protection until the body can develop a more natural form of immunity.

Collectively, these forms of immunity can provide important protection against infectious disease.

Immunizations

Although the incidence of several childhood communicable diseases is at or near the lowest level ever, we are risking a resurgence of diseases such as measles, polio, diphtheria, and rubella. This possible increase in childhood infectious illnesses is based on the disturbing finding that fewer than half of American preschoolers are adequately immunized, which is principally due to the failure of many parents to complete their children's immunization programs. Today health professionals are attempting to raise the level of immunization to 90 percent of all children under the age of two years.

Vaccinations against several potentially serious infectious conditions are available and should be given. These include the following:

- *Diphtheria:* A potentially fatal illness that leads to inflammation of the membranes that line the throat, to swollen lymph nodes, and to heart and kidney failure
- *Whooping cough:* A bacterial infection of the airways and lungs that results in deep, noisy breathing and coughing
- *Hepatitis B:* A viral infection that can be transmitted sexually or through the exchange of blood or bodily fluids; seriously damages the liver
- *Haemophilus influenzae type B:* A bacterial infection that can damage the heart and brain, resulting in meningitis, and can produce profound hearing loss
- *Tetanus:* A fatal infection that damages the central nervous system; caused by bacteria found in the soil
- *Rubella (German measles):* A viral infection of the upper respiratory tract that can cause damage to a developing fetus when the mother contracts the infection during the first trimester of pregnancy
- *Measles (red measles):* A highly contagious viral infection leading to a rash, high fever, and upper respiratory tract symptoms

- *Polio:* A viral infection capable of causing paralysis of the large muscles of the extremities
- *Mumps:* A viral infection of the salivary glands
- *Chicken pox:* A varicella zoster virus spread by airborne droplets, leading to a sore throat, rash, and fluid-filled blisters

Parents of newborns should take their infants to their family-care physicians, pediatricians, or well-baby clinics operated by county health departments to begin the immunization process. The schedule shown in Table 13-2 is recommended by the Centers for Disease Control and Prevention (CDC). The new chicken pox vaccine, VariVax, is now available. In addition, a vaccine against infant diarrhea caused by rotaviruses has been approved.[4] Researchers are also attempting to develop a single immunization that would combine many individual vaccines now used. In addition, research is being conducted on new delivery systems, including a skin patch, nasal spray, and vaccine-enriched foods, such as potatoes.[5,6]

Personal Applications
- How do you feel about parents who do not have their children immunized?

The Immune Response

Fully understanding the function of the immune system requires a substantial understanding of human biology and is beyond the scope of this text. Figure 13-3 presents a simplified view of the immune response.

When antigens (whether microorganisms, foreign substances, or abnormal cells) are discovered within the body, various types of white blood cells confront and destroy some of these antigens. At the same time, macrophages (very large white blood cells) encounter other antigens and signal agents of

acquired immunity (AI) the major component of the immune system; forms antibodies and specialized blood cells capable of destroying pathogens.

naturally acquired immunity (NAI) a type of acquired immunity resulting from the body's response to naturally occurring pathogens.

artificially acquired immunity (AAI) a type of acquired immunity resulting from the body's response to pathogens introduced into the body through immunizations.

passively acquired immunity (PAI) a temporary immunity achieved by providing antibodies to a person exposed to a particular pathogen.

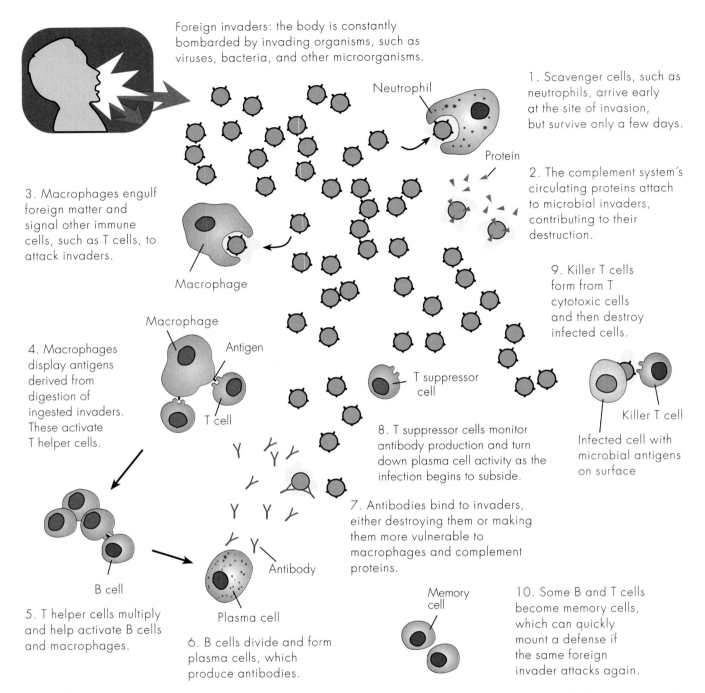

Foreign invaders: the body is constantly bombarded by invading organisms, such as viruses, bacteria, and other microorganisms.

Neutrophil

1. Scavenger cells, such as neutrophils, arrive early at the site of invasion, but survive only a few days.

Protein

2. The complement system's circulating proteins attach to microbial invaders, contributing to their destruction.

3. Macrophages engulf foreign matter and signal other immune cells, such as T cells, to attack invaders.

Macrophage

9. Killer T cells form from T cytotoxic cells and then destroy infected cells.

Macrophage

Antigen

4. Macrophages display antigens derived from digestion of ingested invaders. These activate T helper cells.

T cell

T suppressor cell

Killer T cell

Infected cell with microbial antigens on surface

8. T suppressor cells monitor antibody production and turn down plasma cell activity as the infection begins to subside.

7. Antibodies bind to invaders, either destroying them or making them more vulnerable to macrophages and complement proteins.

B cell

5. T helper cells multiply and help activate B cells and macrophages.

Plasma cell

Antibody

6. B cells divide and form plasma cells, which produce antibodies.

Memory cell

10. Some B and T cells become memory cells, which can quickly mount a defense if the same foreign invader attacks again.

Figure 13-3 Biological warfare. The body commands an army of defenders to reduce the danger of infection and guard against repeat infections. Antigens are the ultimate targets of all immune responses.

cell-mediated immunity called helper T cells to assist in the immune response.

Once helper T cells are activated by the presence of the macrophage/antigens complex, they notify a second component of cellular immunity, the killer T cells, and a component of humoral immunity, B cells. Killer T cells produce powerful chemical messengers that activate specific white blood cells that destroy antigens. At the same time, B cells are transformed into specialized cells (plasma cells) capable of producing

antibodies and into memory cells that record information about the antigen and the appropriate immune-system response.

While helper T cells and killer T cells are destroying invading antigens, two more components of cellular immunity are formed: memory T cells and suppressor T cells. As the name suggests, the memory T cells remember additional aspects of the immune system's responses so that reinfections can be repelled even more quickly and decisively. Suppressor T cells are specialized T cells that moderate B cell activity by offsetting the action of helper T cells. Their action allows the production of antibodies to be reduced when the immune system has won its battle.

Clearly, without a normal immune system employing both cellular and humoral elements, we would quickly fall victim to serious and life-shortening infections and malignancies. As you will see later, this is exactly what occurs in many people infected with HIV.

Emerging medical technology holds promise for repairing damaged immune systems. Umbilical cord blood (*cord blood*) harvested at the time of birth is already being used to supply new cells to stimulate the immune response.[7] Further, it soon may be possible to cultivate unspecialized *stem cells* from embryonic cell masses that also can be used to repair the damaged immune system.[8]

Causes and Management of Selected Infectious Diseases

This section focuses on some of the common infectious diseases and some diseases that are less common but serious. You can use this information as a basis for judging your own disease susceptibility.

The Common Cold

The common cold, an acute upper-respiratory-tract infection, must reign as humankind's supreme infectious disease. Also known as **acute rhinitis,** this highly contagious viral infection can be caused by any of the nearly 200 known rhinoviruses. Colds are particularly common when people spend time in crowded indoor environments, such as classrooms.

The signs and symptoms of a cold are fairly predictable. Runny nose, watery eyes, general aches and pains, a listless feeling, and a slight fever all may accompany a cold in its early stages. Eventually the nasal passages swell, and the inflammation may spread to the throat. Stuffy nose, sore throat, and coughing may follow (Table 13–1). The senses of taste and smell are blocked, and appetite declines.

When you notice the onset of symptoms, you should begin managing the cold promptly. After a few days, most of the cold's symptoms subside. In the meantime, you should isolate yourself from others, drink plenty of fluids, eat moderately, and rest.

Some of the many OTC cold remedies can help you manage a cold. These remedies will not cure your cold but may lessen the discomfort associated with it. Nasal decongestants, expectorants, cough syrups, and aspirin or acetaminophen can give some temporary relief. Follow label directions carefully.

If a cold persists, as evidenced by prolonged chills, fever above 103 degrees Fahrenheit, chest heav-

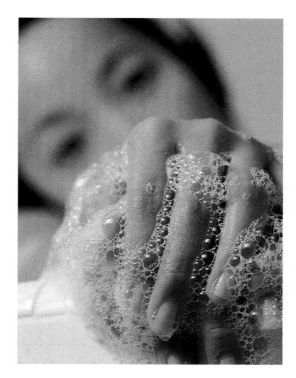

Washing your hands often is the best way to prevent the common cold.

iness or aches, shortness of breath, coughing up rust-colored mucus, or persistent sore throat or hoarseness, you should contact a physician. Because we now consider colds to be transmitted most readily by hand contact, you should wash your hands frequently.

Personal Applications

• How often do you wash your hands during the day? Do you think you would get fewer colds if you washed your hands more frequently?

Influenza

Influenza is also an acute contagious disease caused by viruses. Some influenza outbreaks have killed many people, such as the influenza pandemics of 1889 to 1890, 1918 to 1919, and 1957. The viral strains that produce this infectious disease have the potential for more severe complications than the viral strains that produce the common cold. The viral strain for a

antibodies   chemical compounds produced by the body's immune system to destroy antigens and their toxins.

acute rhinitis   the common cold; the sudden onset of nasal inflammation.

Table 13-3 Is It a Cold or the Flu?

	Cold	Flu
Symptoms		
Fever	Rare	Characteristic, high (102°–104°+ F); lasts 3–4 days
Headache	Rare	Prominent
General aches, pains	Slight	Usual; often severe
Fatigue, weakness	Quite mild	Can last up to 2–3 weeks
Extreme exhaustion	Never	Early and prominent
Stuffy nose	Common	Sometimes
Sneezing	Usual	Sometimes
Sore throat	Common	Sometimes
Chest discomfort, cough	Mild to moderate; hacking cough	Common; can become severe
Complications	Sinus congestion, earache	Pneumonia, bronchitis; can be life threatening
Prevention	Avoidance of infected people	Annual vaccination; amantadine or rimantadine (antiviral drugs)
Treatment	Temporary relief	Amantadine or rimantadine within 24–48 hours after onset of symptoms

particular form of influenza enters the body through the respiratory tract. After brief incubation and prodromal stages, the host develops signs and symptoms not just in the upper respiratory tract but throughout the entire body. These symptoms include fever, chills, cough, sore throat, headache, gastrointestinal disturbances, and muscular pain (Table 13–3).

Antibiotics are generally not prescribed for people with influenza, except when the patient has a possible secondary bacterial infection. Physicians may recommend only aspirin, fluids, and rest. Parents are reminded not to give aspirin to children because of the danger of Reye's syndrome. In addition to amantadine, the medication most frequently used to treat influenza, two new medications are under development and will soon be on the market—GS4101, in pill form, and Relenza, an inhaler. Both are intended to minimize the complications associated with the flu.[9]

Most young adults can cope with the milder strains of influenza that appear each winter or spring. However, pregnant women and older people—especially older people with additional health complications, such as heart disease, kidney disease, emphysema, and chronic bronchitis—are not as capable of handling this viral attack. People who regularly come into contact with the general public, such as teachers, should also consider annual flu shots. Some experts even recommend flu shots for children because of their role in infecting adults with whom they have contact.[10]

Tuberculosis

Experts considered TB, a bacterial infection of the lungs resulting in chronic coughing, weight loss, and even death, to be under control in this country until the mid-1980s. The number of cases surged then, however, with a peak of 26,283 cases in 1992. The number has declined since then, with 21,327 cases reported in 1996.[11] However, we must continually watch this infectious disease, as people immigrate to the United States from areas of the world in which TB is considerably more common and drug-resistant strains of the bacterium emerge.

Tuberculosis thrives in crowded places where infected people are in constant contact with others, since TB is spread by coughing. This includes prisons, hospitals, public housing units, and even college residence halls. In such settings, a single infected person can spread the TB agents to many others.

When healthy people are exposed to TB agents, their immune systems can usually suppress the bacteria enough to prevent symptoms from developing and to reduce the likelihood of infecting others. When the immune system is damaged, however, such as in some elderly people, malnourished people, and those who are infected with HIV, the disease can become established and eventually be transmitted to other people at risk.

As previously mentioned, multiple drug-resistant (MDR) TB has appeared. Increasingly prevalent in this country, MDR tuberculosis is the result of patients' inability to follow their physicians' instructions when initially treated (for whatever reason), inadequate treatment by physicians, and increased exposure of HIV-infected people to TB. Only 50 percent of people with this form of TB can be cured. Some believe that MDR tuberculosis will be the next epidemic in this country.

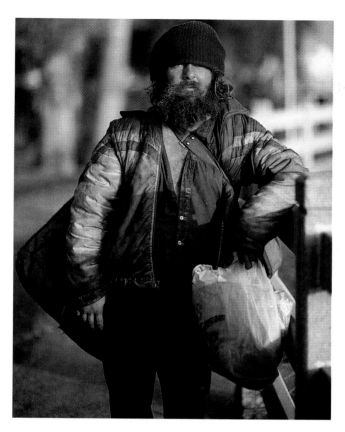

Homeless people, who are at high risk for contracting infectious diseases such as tuberculosis, often lack access to health-care services.

Health officials are again requesting that TB testing programs be implemented and that infected people be identified, isolated, and brought into treatment. The recent identification of the tuberculosis bacterium's genetic code offers promise for the development of new medications and effective immunizations.[12]

Pneumonia

Pneumonia is a general term that describes a variety of infectious respiratory conditions. There are bacterial, viral, fungal, rickettsial, mycoplasmal, and parasitic forms of pneumonia. However, bacterial pneumonia is the most common form and is often seen with other illnesses that weaken the body's immune system. In fact, pneumonia is so common in the frail elderly that it is often the specific condition causing death. *Pneumocystis carinii* pneumonia, a parasitic form, is important today because it is a principal opportunistic infection associated with the diagnosis of AIDS in HIV-infected people.

Older adults with a history of chronic obstructive lung disease, cardiovascular disease, diabetes, or alcoholism often encounter a potentially serious midwinter form of pneumonia known as *acute community-acquired pneumonia*. Characteristics of this condition are the sudden onset of chills, chest pain, and a cough producing sputum. In addition, a symptom-free form of pneumonia known as *walking pneumonia* is also commonly seen in adults and can become serious without warning.

The first known drug-resistant strain of pneumonia has been identified. As a result, some experts are calling for more comprehensive vaccination of older adults.[13]

Mononucleosis

College students who contract **mononucleosis** ("**mono**") can be forced into a long period of bed rest during a semester when they can least afford it. Other common diseases can be managed with minimal disruption. The overall weakness and fatigue seen in many people with mono, however, sometimes require a month or two of rest and recuperation.

Mono is a viral infection in which the body produces an excess of mononuclear leukocytes (a type of white blood cell). After uncertain, perhaps long, incubation and prodromal stages, the acute symptoms of mono can appear, including weakness, headache, low-grade fever, swollen lymph glands (especially in the neck), and sore throat. Mental fatigue and depression are sometimes reported as side effects of mononucleosis. After the acute symptoms disappear, the weakness and fatigue usually persist—perhaps for a few months.

Mono is diagnosed by its characteristic symptoms. The Monospot blood smear can also be used to identify the prevalence of abnormal white blood cells. In addition, an antibody test can detect activity of the immune system that is characteristic of the illness.

This disease is caused by a virus (Epstein-Barr virus), so antibiotic therapy is not recommended. Treatment usually includes bed rest and the use of OTC remedies for fever (aspirin or acetaminophen) and sore throat (lozenges). Corticosteroid drugs can be used in extreme cases. Adequate fluid intake and a well-balanced diet are also important in the recovery stages of mono. Fortunately, the body tends to develop NAI (naturally acquired immunity) to the mono virus, so repeat infections of mono are unusual.

For years, mono has been labeled the "kissing disease"; however, mono is not highly contagious and is known to be spread by direct transmission in ways other than kissing. No vaccine has been developed to confer AAI for mononucleosis. The best preventive measures are the steps that you can take to increase

mononucleosis ("mono") a viral infection characterized by weakness, fatigue, swollen glands, sore throat, and low-grade fever.

your resistance to most infectious diseases: (1) eat a well-balanced diet, (2) exercise regularly, (3) sleep sufficiently, (4) use health-care services appropriately, (5) live in a reasonably healthful environment, and (6) avoid direct contact with infected people.

Chronic Fatigue Syndrome

Chronic fatigue syndrome (CFS) may be the most perplexing "infectious" condition physicians see. First identified in 1985, this mononucleosis-like condition is most often seen in women in their thirties and forties. People with CFS, often busy professional people, report flulike symptoms, including severe exhaustion, fatigue, headaches, muscle aches, fever, inability to concentrate, allergies, intolerance to exercise, and depression. Examinations of the first people with CFS revealed antibodies to the Epstein-Barr virus. Thus observers assumed CFS to be an infectious viral disease (and initially called it *chronic Epstein-Barr syndrome*).

In the years since its first appearance, the condition has received great attention that has produced considerable confusion over its exact nature. In fact, several theories have been advanced to identify the cause (or causes) of CFS. As suggested above, some experts believe an infectious agent may be responsible, possibly a virus such as EBV, cytomegalovirus, herpes simplex 1 and 2, or human herpes virus 6. To date no specific virus has been isolated. A second explanation involves an extended challenge to the immune system, possibly activated by an initial viral infection and resulting in the overproduction of immune system chemicals that produce flulike symptoms. A final CFS model suggests the involvement of one or more factors, including emotional, environmental, genetic, and infectious factors. In this model, a stresslike response is believed to disrupt the appropriate interplay among the pituitary, hypothalamus, and adrenal glands (see Chapter 3), thus reducing cortisol production.[14] On the basis of this explanation, other conditions, such as fibromyalgia (see Chapter 12), are related to CFS.

Regardless of its cause or causes, CFS is extremely unpleasant for people who have it. Those experiencing the symptoms over an extended time need to see a physician experienced in dealing with CFS.

Measles

Red measles (also called **rubeola** or common measles) was previously considered only a childhood disease, but it has recently been seen in large numbers on some American college campuses. Red measles is the highly contagious type of measles characterized by a short-lived, relatively high fever (103° to 104° F) and a whole-body red spotty rash that lasts about a week. The other type of measles, German measles (**rubella**, or three-day measles), is a much milder form of measles that has serious implications for newborn babies of mothers who contracted this disease during pregnancy. Highly effective vaccines are now available for both varieties of measles and are usually given in the same injection. Women should get these vaccinations before they become pregnant.

The recent annual outbreaks of red measles among college students show that it is a mistake to think that most infectious diseases have been eliminated. Public health experts now realize that those who contracted the disease either had never been vaccinated or had been vaccinated with a killed-variety vaccine used before 1969. Only students who had already had red measles as children or who had been vaccinated with a live virus were guaranteed full immunity against the red measles virus. Nontraditional-age college students in particular should attempt to determine whether their immunization status is based on use of the older, less effective vaccine.

Most public school systems now require documented proof of immunization from a physician or clinic before children can attend classes. As educated parents, you should conscientiously adhere to immunization schedules for your children. In fact, measles-immunization efforts of schools and public health departments helped reduce the number of measles cases from 55,000 between 1989 and 1991 to 734 in 1996.[15]

Mumps

Mumps is one of the more familiar childhood infectious diseases. Mumps is a viral illness, characterized by inflammation and swelling in one or both salivary glands at the angle of the jaw. Common symptoms include fever, pain, and difficulty swallowing. The treatment is fluids, bed rest, painkillers, and, in children, a few days' absence from school.

When older male children, adolescents, and adults contract mumps, the risk of infection to the testicles increases. A less common condition is inflammation of the pancreas, with abdominal pain and vomiting.

Protection against mumps is produced by the standard childhood immunization series, measles-mumps-rubella (MMR). Those who contract mumps develop NAI to the disease.

Lyme Disease

Lyme disease is an infectious disease that is becoming increasingly common in eastern, southeastern, upper midwestern, and West Coast states, with 16,461 cases in 1996. This bacterial disease results when infected deer ticks, usually in the nymph (immature) state, attach to the skin and inject the infectious agent as they feed on a host's blood. Deer ticks become infected by feeding on infected white-tailed deer or white-footed mice.[16]

The symptoms of Lyme disease vary but typically appear within thirty days as small red bumps surrounded by a circular red rash at the site of bites. Flulike symptoms may accompany this phase I stage, including chills, headaches, muscle and joint aches, and low-grade fever. A phase II stage develops in about 20 percent of infected people. This phase may produce disorders of the nervous system or heart. Those who remain untreated even to this stage can develop a phase III stage, which can include chronic arthritis, lasting up to two years. Fortunately, Lyme disease can be treated with antibiotics. Unfortunately, however, no immunity develops, so infection can recur.[16] Because some physicians order tests and begin antibiotic therapy too quickly, however, the basis of concern should be the appearance of phase I symptoms, not simply having been bitten by a tick.[17] Lyme disease may be more difficult to diagnose in children than in adults.

People who live in susceptible areas and participate in outdoor activities can encounter the nearly invisible tick nymphs that have fallen from deer into the grass. Thus these people should check themselves frequently to be sure that they are tick-free. They should tuck shirts into pants, tuck pants into socks, and wear gloves and hats when possible. They should also shower after coming inside from outdoors and check clothing for evidence of ticks. Pets can carry infected ticks into the house. If you find ticks, they should be carefully removed from the skin with tweezers and the affected area washed. For adults who are at high risk of tick bites, a newly approved three-step immunization (LYMErix) should be considered. Its effectiveness is reported to be 76 percent after the third shot.[18]

The tick that carries Lyme disease has also been found to be responsible for a potentially fatal bacterial infection called *human granulocytic ehrlichiosis (HGE)*. This disease is associated with high fever, headache, muscle aches, and chills. Fortunately, HGE is successfully treated with doxycycline, an antibiotic that can also be used in the treatment of Lyme disease. People with these symptoms who live in areas of the country where Lyme disease is reported should make certain that their physician considers HGE in the diagnosis and treatment of their symptoms.

Hantavirus Pulmonary Syndrome

Since 1993 a small but rapidly growing number of people have been dying of extreme pulmonary distress caused by the leakage of plasma into the lungs. In the initial cases, the people lived in the Southwest, had been well until they began developing flulike symptoms over one or two days, then quickly experienced difficulty breathing, and died only hours later. Epidemiologists quickly suspected a viral agent such as the hantavirus, known to exist in Asia and, to a lesser degree, in Europe. Exhaustive laboratory work led to the culturing of the virus and confirmed that

all of these patients had been infected with an American version of the hantavirus. Researchers identified this latest infectious condition as *hantavirus pulmonary syndrome*.

Today this hantavirus disease has been reported in areas beyond the Southwest, including most of the western states and some of the eastern states. The common denominator in all these areas is the presence of deer mice. We now know that this common rodent serves as the reservoir for the virus.

The virus moves from deer mice to humans when people inhale dust contaminated with dried virus-rich rodent urine or saliva-contaminated materials, such as nests. Health experts now warn people who live in areas with deer mouse populations (most of the United States) to be extremely careful when cleaning houses and barns in which deer mouse droppings are likely to be found. If you must remove rodent nests, wear rubber gloves, pour Lysol or bleach on the nests and soak them thoroughly, and finally, pick up the nests with shovels and burn them or bury them in holes that are several feet deep. These procedures should greatly reduce the airborne spread of the viral particles.[19]

In addition, the first cases of human-to-human transmission of hantavirus have been reported in Argentina, with nine reported deaths. Further, the El Niño–induced wet weather in several southwestern states has created ideal conditions for a large rodent population and a heightened risk of hantavirus outbreaks in that area.[20]

Because there is no vaccine for hantavirus pulmonary syndrome, people who are likely to be exposed to the infected excrement of deer mice should seek early evaluation of flulike symptoms.

Toxic Shock Syndrome

Toxic shock syndrome (TSS) made front-page headlines in 1980, when the CDC reported a connection between TSS and the presence of a specific bacterial agent (*Staphylococcus aureus*) in the vagina associated with the use of tampons.

---

chronic fatigue syndrome (CFS)   an illness that causes severe exhaustion, fatigue, aches, and depression; mostly affects women in their thirties and forties.

rubeola (roo **bee** oh luh)   red or common measles.

rubella   German or 3-day measles.

Lyme disease   a bacterial infection transmitted by deer ticks.

toxic shock syndrome (TSS)   a potentially fatal condition caused by the proliferation of certain bacteria in the vagina that enter the general blood circulation.

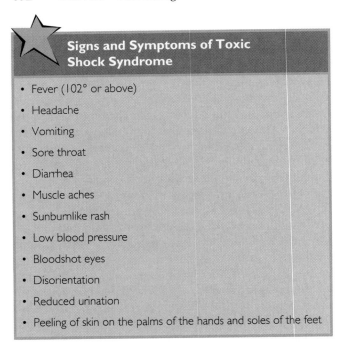

Signs and Symptoms of Toxic Shock Syndrome

- Fever (102° or above)
- Headache
- Vomiting
- Sore throat
- Diarrhea
- Muscle aches
- Sunburnlike rash
- Low blood pressure
- Bloodshot eyes
- Disorientation
- Reduced urination
- Peeling of skin on the palms of the hands and soles of the feet

Who Is Affected by AIDS?

The Centers for Disease Control and Prevention report that the people most likely to develop AIDS are homosexual or bisexual men and intravenous drug users. As of December 1996, the breakdown of AIDS cases was as follows:

Men who have sex with men	48%
Injection drug use	26%
Heterosexual contact	10%
Risk not identified	8%
Men who have sex with men and inject drugs	6%
Recipients of blood products or tissue	1%
Hemophilia or other coagulation disorders	1%
Total	100%

TSS causes the signs and symptoms listed in the Star Box above. Superabsorbent tampons can irritate the vaginal lining three times more quickly than regular tampons. This vaginal irritation is aggravated when the tampon remains in the vagina for a long time (more than five hours). When this irritation begins, the staphylococcal bacteria (which are usually present in the vagina) have relatively easy access to the bloodstream. When these bacteria proliferate in the circulatory system, their resultant toxins produce toxic shock syndrome. A woman with TSS can die, usually as a result of cardiovascular failure, if left untreated. Fortunately, less than 10 percent of women diagnosed as having TSS die.

Although the extent of this disease is still limited (only about 3 to 6 cases per 100,000 women per year) and the mortality figures are low (similar to those in women who use oral contraceptives), every woman should exercise reasonable caution in the use of tampons. Consider these recommendations: (1) tampons should not be the sole form of sanitary protection used, and (2) tampons should not remain in place for too long. Women should change tampons every few hours and intermittently use sanitary napkins. Tampons should not be used during sleep. Some physicians recommend that tampons not be used at all if a woman wants to be extraordinarily safe from TSS.

The incidence of TSS has dropped significantly since the early 1980s. Possible reasons for this decrease are the removal of some superabsorbent tampons from the market and the standardized labeling of junior, super, and super-plus tampons that began in 1990. Unfortunately, few women today read the instructions on tampon boxes about minimizing the risk of toxic shock syndrome.

Today it is estimated that about half of the 1,300 annual cases of TSS arise from tampon use and thus affect only women. The same condition, however, can be caused by infected skin sores, burns, and nasal packing. Accordingly, people at risk for these reasons should be aware of the symptoms described in the Star Box in left-hand column.

Hepatitis

Hepatitis is an inflammatory process in the liver that can be caused by several viruses. Types A, B, C (once called non-A and non-B), D, and E have been recognized. Hepatitis can also be caused indirectly from abuse of alcohol and other drugs. General symptoms of hepatitis include fever, nausea, loss of appetite, abdominal pain, and jaundice (yellowing of the skin and eyes).[16]

Type A hepatitis is often associated with consuming fecal-contaminated food, such as raw shellfish, or water. Poor sanitation, particularly in the handling of food and diaper-changing activities has produced outbreaks in child-care centers. Experts estimate that up to 200,000 people per year experience this infection. In 1995 the FDA approved a vaccine, Harvix.

Type B hepatitis (HBV) is spread in various ways, including sexual contact, intravenous drug use, tattooing, and medical and dental procedures. Chronic HBV infection has been associated with liver cirrhosis and liver cancer. An effective immunization for hepatitis B is now available. Although it is given during childhood, it should be seriously considered for older unvaccinated people and college students. An AIDS drug, 3TC (lamivudine), was recently approved for the treatment of hepatitis B.[21]

Hepatitis C is contracted in ways similar to hepatitis B (sexual contact, tainted blood, and shared needles). In the absence of immunization, the pool of infected people is in excess of four million and the death rate is expected to climb. In 1998 the FDA approved a dual-drug therapy for HCV involving multiple forms of interferon in combination with the drug ribavirin.[22]

Learning
From Our Diversity

From Terminal Illness to Chronic Condition: People with HIV Accept the Changing Face of AIDS

For almost a generation, a diagnosis of AIDS (acquired immuno-deficiency syndrome) has been a virtual death sentence. World-wide, hundreds of thousands have died from the ravages of the human immunodeficiency virus (HIV), and the search for a cure or a means of prevention is a leading focus of research scientists around the globe.

Although no cure or preventive agent has yet been found, the AIDS epidemic in America has taken a dramatic turn, holding out hope that the disease is changing from a terminal illness to a chronic condition. A "cocktail" of costly experimental drugs is forcing HIV to retreat, with much of the credit going to the protease inhibitors introduced in recent years.

The protease inhibitors attack AIDS by zeroing in on reproduction of HIV and crippling a critical enzyme it needs. Once the virus's rate of reproduction has been halted, the body's immune system can fight back. Patients' overall health also improves because they can eat and sleep better.

In the first half of 1996, U.S. deaths from AIDS fell 13 percent from 24,900 a year earlier to 22,000, according to federal health officials. This reversal of a long trend is giving patients new hope. At the same time, it's confronting them with new, unexpected dilemmas.

Until the recent success of protease inhibitors, an AIDS physician and researcher says, "People were focused on just living for the next two or three years. Now someone says to them, 'I have news for you. You're going to live.' That's not as easy to adjust to as you might think. They have to reset their minds."

A 38-year-old man was diagnosed with HIV in 1988. Over the years, he says, those with AIDS have often heard that a big breakthrough was coming. "After a while you get to the point where you don't want to set yourself up to say, I'm all better now and I can go out and do the things I did before," he says. "Because I'm not all better. The virus is not eradicated. Who's to say that next month I won't die?"

One 34-year-old patient who has had AIDS for 14 years lost her daughter to the disease, and the heartbreak only worsened her condition. Then the woman began taking protease inhibitors. "I consider it very much a miracle," says the woman, whose immune system is rapidly recovering. "I am a longtime survivor of AIDS, but this has really given me hope that I'm not going to die."

The good news about protease inhibitors is not universal. Some people can't afford the drugs. Some can't tolerate the side effects. Some wait too long. Still, the drugs have changed the lives of many patients with HIV/AIDS. Perhaps the greatest adjustment is realizing how a normal or near-normal life expectancy changes their priorities.

"They're now well enough to go back to work, but many of them say they don't want to return to their previous jobs," one AIDS physician and researcher says. "They've had time to do some thinking, and some are going back to school; others are looking at totally different careers."

Think about how you'd feel and what you'd want to do if you'd been told you were going to die in a few years. How would your attitude and desires change if you later learned you could expect to live an almost normal life span?

The newly identified type D (delta) hepatitis is very difficult to treat and is found almost exclusively in people already suffering from type B hepatitis. This virus, like type B hepatitis and HIV, makes unprotected sexual contact, including anal and oral sex, very risky.[16] Hepatitis E, associated with water contamination, is rarely seen in this country other than in people returning from HEV-endemic areas of the world.

AIDS

AIDS has become the most devastating infectious disease of modern times. Through June 1998, 665,357 Americans have been diagnosed with AIDS and 401,028 people (60.2% of all cases) have died from the disease since it was first reported in 1981.[23] The Star Box on p. 402 shows the extent to which various groups of people have been affected by the disease.

As recently as 1993, experts estimated that by the year 2000, $13.1 billion in third-party and public funds would be spent for HIV/AIDS-related illnesses.

Although the final figure is not yet available, it will likely be somewhat less because the annual cost of treating one person with AIDS has fallen to $20,000 from nearly three times that amount.[23] This reduction reflects the effectiveness of new medications, which has reduced the need for hospitalization. Nonetheless, the toll in human lives and the financial burden AIDS places on our health-care system make AIDS a demanding disease.

Cause of AIDS

AIDS is the disease caused by HIV, a virus that attacks the helper T cells of the immune system (see pp. 395–396). When HIV attacks helper T cells, people lose the ability to fight off a variety of infections that would normally be easily controlled. Because these infections develop while people are vulnerable, they are collectively called *opportunistic infections*. HIV-infected patients become vulnerable to infection by bacteria, protozoa, fungi, and several viruses. A variety of

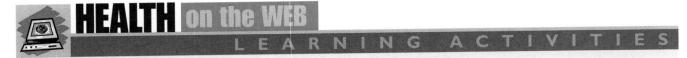

malignancies (see Chapter 11) also develop during this period of immune-system vulnerability.

HIV+ with AIDS was originally diagnosed based on the presence of specific conditions. Among these were *Pneumocystis carinii* pneumonia and Kaposi's sarcoma, a rare but deadly form of skin cancer. Gradually, experts recognized that additional conditions were associated with advancing deterioration of the immune system and thus added them to the list of AIDS conditions. This list now includes almost thirty definitive conditions, with more conditions being added as they become apparent. Among the conditions found on the current version of the list are toxoplasmosis within the brain, cytomegalovirus retinitis with loss of vision, lymphoma involving the brain, recurrent salmonella blood infections, and a wasting syndrome that includes invasive cervical cancer in women, recurrent pneumonia, and recurrent tuberculosis. Today, however, experts tend to assign the label of HIV+ with AIDS to HIV-infected people when their level of helper T cells drops below 200 cells per cubic millimeter, regardless of whether specific conditions are present.

Spread of HIV

HIV cannot be contracted easily. The chances of contracting HIV through casual contact with HIV-infected people at work, school, or home are extremely low or nonexistent. HIV is known to be spread only by direct sexual contact involving the exchange of bodily fluids (including blood, semen, and vaginal secretions), the sharing of hypodermic needles, transfusion of infected blood or blood products, and perinatal transmission (from an infected mother to a fetus or newborn baby). For HIV to be transmitted, it must enter the bloodstream of the noninfected person, such as through needles or tears in body tissues lining the

rectum, mouth, or reproductive system. Current research also indicates that HIV is not transmitted by sweat, saliva, or tears, although the virus may be found in very low concentrations in these fluids. The HIV virus cannot enter the body through the gastrointestinal system because digestive enzymes destroy the virus. However, because gingivitis and bleeding gums are so common, unprotected oral sex is now considered a route for transmission, particularly for the person whose mouth is involved.[24]

Women are at much greater risk (twelve times the risk) than men of contracting HIV through heterosexual activity because of the higher concentration of HIV in semen than in vaginal secretions. This susceptibility is seen in part by the increasing percentage of women with AIDS who were infected through heterosexual contact—from 8 percent in 1981, to 19 percent in 1993, and 39 percent in 1998.[23] Women under age 25 contract the virus principally through heterosexual contact.

Signs and Symptoms of HIV Infection

Most people infected with HIV initially feel well and have no symptoms (that is, they are asymptomatic). Experts generally consider the incubation period for HIV infection to be six months to ten or more years, with the average approximately six years. Despite the long period between infection and the first clinical observation of damage to the immune system, antibodies to HIV may appear within several weeks to three months of contracting the virus. Of course, relatively few people are tested for HIV infection at any time during the incubation period. Thus infected people could remain asymptomatic (currently described as HIV+ without symptoms) and be carriers of HIV for years before they experience signs of illness sufficient to warrant a physical examination.

Table 13-4   The Spectrum of HIV Infection

	HIV+ without Symptoms (Asymptomatic)	HIV+ with Symptoms	HIV+ with AIDS
External signs	No symptoms Looks well	Fever Night sweats Swollen lymph glands Weight loss Diarrhea Minor infections Fatigue	Kaposi's sarcoma *Pneumocystis carinii* pneumonia and/or other predetermined illnesses Neurological disorders One or more of an additional 25+ diagnosable conditions or a helper T cell count falls below 200 per cubic milliliter
Incubation	Invasion of virus to 10 years	Several months to 10 or more years	Several months to 10–12 or more years
Internal level of infection	Antibodies are produced Immune system remains intact Positive antibody test	Antibodies are produced Immune system weakened Positive antibody test	Immune system deficient Positive antibody test
Infectious?	Yes	Yes	Yes

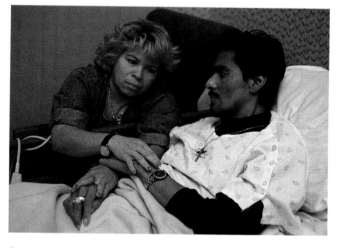

People with AIDS need strong support from their families.

Without symptoms of immune-system deterioration or AIDS-testing results, sexually active people need to redefine the meaning of monogamy. Couples must now account for the sexual partners they have both had over the past ten years. Unfortunately, people do this so infrequently that some observers are labeling today's late adolescents and young adults "a generation in jeopardy."

Most people infected with HIV eventually develop signs and symptoms of a more advanced stage of the disease. These signs and symptoms include tiredness, fever, loss of appetite and weight, diarrhea, night sweats, and swollen glands (usually in the neck, armpits, and groin). At this point, they are said to be HIV+ with symptoms. (See Table 13-4.)

Experts estimate that, given sufficient time, perhaps as long as fifteen years, most infected people will move beyond HIV with symptoms. At this point, the label HIV+ with AIDS is applied, either on the basis of clinically defined conditions or more likely on the basis of a helper T cell count below 200 per cubic millimeter of blood. A normal helper T cell range is 800 to 1,000. The efficacy of treatment is based in part on improvements in the T cell count over time.

A small percentage of infected people can suppress the infection and have survived for two decades without developing AIDS, but experts do not fully understand this ability (possibly attributing it to a suppressor compound formed by specific immune system cells).

Diagnosis of HIV Infection

HIV infection is diagnosed through a clinical examination, laboratory tests for accompanying infections, and an initial screening test. After an initial positive screening test, more sensitive tests can be administered, including the enzyme-linked immunosorbent assay (ELISA) and the Western Blot. Home tests are also available. A recently developed test can determine not only a person's infectious status but also the relative duration of infection. This information helps physicians structure treatment protocols. For people at risk for infection, an initially negative screening test should be repeated three to six months later.

Treatment of HIV and AIDS

There is no cure for HIV infection and the resultant AIDS. It is critically important, however, that treatment begin upon diagnosis. Current treatment uses a combination of drugs drawn from two distinct groups: the *reverse-transcriptase inhibitors* and the *protease inhibitors.*

The reverse-transcriptase inhibitors block (or inhibit) the action of reverse transcriptase, an enzyme the virus requires to replicate itself within the host's infected T helper cells. Currently a combination of two of the ten available reverse-transcriptase inhibitors is used to formulate the drug "cocktail" employed in treating HIV infection. The ten inhibitors are AZT, ddI, ddC, 3TC, ZVD, d4T, EFV, ABC, ADV, and APV.[25]

The introduction of the protease inhibitors, in combination with the reverse-transcriptase inhibitors, has revolutionized the treatment of HIV infection. These drugs inhibit the ability of the virus to uncouple polypeptides needed in the replication process. Four of these agents are available: Indinavir, Nelfinavir, Ritonavir, and Saquinavir.[25] In most treatment protocols, one protease inhibitor is combined with two reverse-transcriptase inhibitors to complete the drug cocktail.

A final pharmacological approach to slow the progression of HIV is interleukin-2, a naturally occurring immune system protein, to help protect helper T cells.

Protease inhibitors have revolutionized AIDS care, reducing HIV to undetectable levels in thousands of people. The number of deaths from AIDS has decreased dramatically, from 49,985 in 1995 to 21,909 in 1997.[23] However, people should not consider this improvement to mean that the emergency is over. In fact, when the drug cocktail therapy described above is discontinued, viral loads frequently moved toward pretreatment levels. This suggests the existence of well-protected sequestered (hidden) viruses within other tissues of the body.

Personal Applications

• New medications have made it possible for people who are HIV+ to live for many years without developing AIDS. Do you know anyone who is being treated for HIV? If so, how long has he or she lived with the disease?

Physicians also have a variety of medications to treat the symptoms associated with various infections and malignancies that make up AIDS. These drugs cannot reverse HIV status or cure AIDS.

Researchers continue to search for vaccines to prevent HIV infection. To date only one large-scale clinical trial involving a vaccine is under way. The vaccine, AIDSVAX, employs two genetically altered AIDS virus types.[26] In its current form the vaccine is designed for viral strains found in North America and Europe. Even if it proves successful, therefore, it can-

not influence HIV strains found in Africa and Asia. Developing a safe, effective, and affordable vaccine (as was done for other infectious diseases) has been difficult because of the unique ability of HIV to alter its outer coat and quickly incorporate its genetic material into the host's helper T cells' genetic material, thus preventing the immune system from developing immune recognition.

This ability of the virus to change its appearance is so strong that dozens of strains of HIV can be found at all times in the United States. More than one version of HIV may even be found within a single individual.

Prevention of HIV Infection

Can HIV infection be prevented? The answer is a definite yes. HIV infection rates on college campuses are considered low (approximately 0.2%), but students can be at risk. Every person can take several steps to reduce the risk of contracting and transmitting HIV. All of these steps require understanding one's behavior and the methods by which HIV can be transmitted. Some appropriate steps for college-aged people are abstinence, safer sex, sobriety, and communication with potential sexual partners. To ensure the greatest protection from HIV, one should abstain from sexual activity. Other than this, the Health Action Guide below lists recommendations for safer sex, sobriety, and the exchange of honest, accurate information about sexual histories.

HEALTH ACTION GUIDE

Reducing Your Risk of Contracting HIV

One must remember that sexual partners may not reveal their true sexual history or drug habits. If you are sexually active, you can reduce your risk of infection with HIV, as well as other STDs, by adopting the following safer sex practices.

• Learn the sexual history and HIV status of your sex partner.
• Limit your number of sex partners.
• Always use condoms correctly and consistently.
• Avoid contact with bodily fluids, feces, and semen.
• Curtail use of drugs that impair good judgment.
• Never share hypodermic needles.
• Refrain from sex with known injectable drug abusers.*
• Avoid sex with HIV-infected patients, those with signs and symptoms of AIDS, and the partners of high-risk people.*
• Get regular tests for STD infections.
• Do not insert any foreign objects into the rectum.

How easy will it be to adopt these behaviors? How real is your risk of becoming HIV positive?

*Current studies report that eliminating high-risk people as sexual partners is the single most effective safer sex practice that one can implement.

InfoLinks
www.caps.ucsf.edu/FSindex.html

The U.S. Public Health Service offers recommendations for the following groups: (1) the general public, (2) people at increased risk of infection (including health-care workers), and (3) people with a positive HIV antibody test. The Public Health Service has a toll-free AIDS telephone hot line (800-342-AIDS), and you may find local or state hot lines in your area. Stay informed about HIV infection and AIDS!

Sexually Transmitted Diseases

Sexually transmitted diseases (STDs) were once called venereal diseases (for Venus, the Roman goddess of love). Today the term *venereal disease* has been superseded by the broader term *sexually transmitted disease*. Experts currently emphasize the successful prevention and treatment of STDs rather than the ethics of sexuality. Thus one should consider the following points: (1) A person can have more than one STD at a time; (2) the symptoms of STDs can vary over time and from person to person; (3) the body develops little immunity for STDs; and (4) STDs can predispose people to additional health problems, including infertility, birth defects in their children, cancer, and long-term disability. In addition, the risk of HIV infection is higher when sexual partners are also infected with STDs. Several of the most common STDs are summarized in Table 13-5, on page 408.

This section focuses on the STDs most frequently diagnosed among college students (chlamydia, gonorrhea, human papillomavirus infection, herpes simplex, syphilis, and pubic lice). Complete the Personal Assessment on page 410 to determine your risk of contracting an STD. See the Health Action Guide on page 406 for safer sex practices.

Chlamydia (Nonspecific Urethritis)

Chlamydia is thought to be the most prevalent STD in the United States today. Chlamydia infections occur an estimated five times more frequently than gonorrhea and up to ten times more frequently than syphilis. Because of its high prevalence in sexually active adolescents, they should be screened for chlamydia twice a year, even in the absence of symptoms.[27] Because chlamydia frequently accompanies gonorrheal infections, a dual therapy is often appropriate when gonorrhea is found. Sexually active people in the 20 to 24 age range should also be considered for routine screening, particularly if they have a history of multiple sex partners and have not practiced a form of barrier contraception.[28]

Chlamydia trachomatis is the bacterial agent that causes the chlamydia infection. Chlamydia is the most common cause of nonspecific urethritis (NSU). NSU describes infections of the **urethra** and surrounding

tissues that are not caused by the bacterium responsible for gonorrhea. About 80 percent of men with chlamydia display gonorrhea-like signs and symptoms, including painful urination and a whitish pus discharge from the penis. As in gonorrheal infections and many other STDs, most women report no overt signs or symptoms. A few women might exhibit a mild urethral discharge, painful urination, and swelling of vulval tissues. The recommended treatment for chlamydia is either a single dose of azithromycin (1 g) or doxycycline (100 mg) given orally twice a day for 7 days. The infected person should carefully comply with instructions to abstain from sexual intercourse.[28]

Both sexual partners should receive treatment to avoid the ping-pong effect—the back-and-forth reinfection that occurs among couples when only one partner receives treatment. Furthermore, as with other STDs, having chlamydia once does not effectively confer immunity.

Unresolved chlamydia can lead to the same negative health consequences that result from untreated gonorrheal infections. In men the pathogens can invade and damage the deeper reproductive structures (the prostate gland, seminal vesicles, and Cowper's glands). Sterility can result. The pathogens can spread further and produce joint problems (arthritis) and heart complications (damaged heart valves, blood vessels, and heart muscle tissue).

In women the pathogens enter the body through the urethra or the cervical area. If the invasion is not properly treated, it can reach the deeper pelvic structures, producing a syndrome called **pelvic inflammatory disease (PID)**. The infection may attack the inner uterine wall (endometrium), the fallopian tubes, and any surrounding structures to produce this painful syndrome. A variety of further complications can result, including sterility, ectopic pregnancies, and **peritonitis**. Infected women can transmit a chlamydia

---

sexually transmitted diseases (STDs)
infectious diseases that are spread primarily through intimate sexual contact.

chlamydia the most prevalent sexually transmitted disease; caused by a nongonococcal bacterium.

urethra (yoo **ree** thra) the passageway through which urine leaves the urinary bladder.

pelvic inflammatory disease (PID) an acute or chronic infection of the peritoneum or lining of the abdominopelvic cavity; associated with a variety of symptoms and is a potential cause of sterility.

peritonitis (pare it ton **eye** tis) inflammation of the peritoneum, or lining of the abdominopelvic cavity.

Table 13-5   Summary of Common Sexually Transmitted Diseases

STD	Pathogen Name/Type	Symptoms
Chlamydia	*Chlamydia trachomatis* bacterium	Most women report no overt signs or symptoms. In men, gonorrhea-like signs and symptoms, including painful urination and a whitish pus discharge from the penis.
Human papillomavirus (HPV, genital warts)	Human papillomavirus	Genital warts (condylomata acuminata), pinkish-white lesions in raised clusters on the penis, scrotum, labia, cervix, or around the anus.
Gonorrhea	*Neisseria gonorrhoea* bacterium	In men, a milky-white discharge from the penis, painful urination; women tend to be asymptomatic but can report frequent, painful urination, with a slimy yellow-green discharge from the vagina or urethra.
Herpes	Herpes simplex 1 virus (HSV-1) produces labial herpes; herpes simplex 2 virus (HSV-2) produces genital herpes	HSV-1 produces common fever blisters or cold sores around the lips and oral cavity; HSV-2 produces similar blisterlike lesions in the genital area, swollen lymph glands, muscular aches and pains, and fever.
Syphilis	*Treponema pallidum* bacterium	Primary stage marked by appearance of small, painless red pustule on skin or mucous membrane anywhere on body 10 to 90 days after exposure; forms a painless but highly infectious ulcer called a *chancre*; heals spontaneously in 4 to 8 weeks. If not treated, progresses to secondary, latent, and late stages.
Pubic lice	Pubic louse (insect)	Intense itching in the genital region.

Modes of Transmission	Treatment	Consequences If Not Treated
Sexual intercourse; can be transmitted to newborn during vaginal birth	Azithromycin: 1 g orally in a single dose Doxycycline: 100 mg orally twice a day for 7 days Erythromycin and ofloxacin are alternative medications.	In men, damage to prostate gland, seminal vesicles, and Cowper's glands; sterility; joint problems; heart complications. In women, PID; infection of uterine wall (endometrium), fallopian tubes, and surrounding structures; sterility and peritonitis.
Sexual activity	*Patient-Applied:* Pondofilor solution or gel: applied by swab or finger twice a day for 3 days Imiquimod 5% cream: applied by finger 3 times a week for 16 weeks *Provider-Administered:* Cryotherapy: with liquid nitrogen Podophyllin resin: small amount applied directly to each wart within a relatively small area TCA or BCA: applied in liquid form, repeated weekly if necessary Surgical removal: scissors, shave excision, curettage, or electrosurgery	In women, precancerous changes in the cervix; can become large enough to block the birth canal. In both sexes can become large enough to block the anus.
Sexual activity; oral sex can produce a gonorrheal infection of the throat; can be transmitted to the rectal areas of both sexes; can be transmitted to a newborn during birth	Cefixine: 400 mg orally (single dose) or Ceftriaxone: 125 mg IM (single dose) or Ciprofloxacin: 500 mg orally (single dose) or Ofloxacin: 400 mg orally (single dose) + azithromycin or doxycycline	Nausea, vomiting, fever, tachycardia (rapid heart beat), infection of upper or lower genital tract; can spread to tissues surrounding liver, peritoneum, heart, joints, or other structures.
Direct contact with a person who has an active infection; shared drinking glasses or utensils; intimate sexual contact; condoms may provide insufficient protection	*Initial Infection* (episodic and suppressive therapy protols required later): Acyclovir: 400 mg orally 3/day (7–10 days) Acyclovir: 200 mg orally 5/day (7–10 days) Famciclovir: 250 mg orally 3/day (7–10 days) Valacyclovir: 1 g orally 2/day (7–10 days)	Recurrent infections are shorter and less severe than the initial episode.
Sexual intercourse	*Primary and Secondary:* Benzathine penicillin G: 2.4 million units IM (single dose) *Latent (early):* Benzathine penicillin G: 2.4 million units IM (single dose) *Latent (late):* Benzathine penicillin G: 7.2 million units (3 doses of 7.2 million once/week)	Secondary stage: general malaise, loss of appetite, fever, headache, hair loss, bone and joint pain, rash, sores in mouth and throat. Late (tertiary) stage: soft, rubbery tumors anywhere on the body that ulcerate and heal with scarring; damage to CNS and heart; disability; premature death.
Sexual contact; contact with contaminated bedsheets and clothes	Permethrin: 1% cream (applied for 10 minutes/washed off) Lindane: 1% shampoo (applied for 4 minutes/washed off) or Pyrethrins with piperonyl butoxide: (applied for 10 minutes/washed off) Bedding/clothing: wash (machine)/dry (hot cycle); no body contact for 72 hours	Lice rarely carry disease, but the itching they cause can be embarrassing and uncomfortable.

Personal Assessment

A variety of factors interact to determine your risk of contracting a sexually transmitted disease (STD). This inventory is intended to provide you with an estimate of your level of risk.

Circle the number in each row that best characterizes you. Enter that number on the line at the end of the row (points). After assigning yourself a number in each row, total the number appearing in the points column. Your total points will allow you to interpret your risk for contracting an STD.

Age

						Points
1	3	4	5	3	2	
0–9	10–14	15–19	20–29	30–34	35+	_____

Sexual Practices

0	1	2	4	6	8	
Never engage in sex	One sex partner	More than one sex partner but never more than one at a time	Two to five sex partners	Five to ten sex partners	Ten or more sex partners	_____

Sexual Attitudes

0	1	8	1	7	8	
Will not engage in nonmarital sex	Premarital sex is okay if it is with future spouse	Any kind of premarital sex is okay	Extramarital sex is not for me	Extramarital sex is okay	Believe in complete sexual freedom	_____

Attitudes toward Contraception

1	1	6	5	4	8	
Would use condom to prevent pregnancy	Would use condom to prevent STDs	Would never use a condom	Would use the birth control pill	Would use other contraceptive measure	Would not use anything	_____

Attitudes toward STD

3	3	4	6	6	6	
Am not sexually active so I do not worry	Would be able to talk about STD with my partner	Would check an infection to be sure	Would be afraid to check out an infection	Can't even talk about an infection	STDs are no problem— easily cured	_____

YOUR TOTAL POINTS _____

Interpretation

5–8	Your risk is well below average
9–13	Your risk is below average
14–17	Your risk is at or near average
18–21	Your risk is moderately high
22+	Your risk is high

To Carry This Further . . .

Having taken this Personal Assessment, were you surprised at your level of risk? What is the primary reason for this level? How concerned are you and your classmates and friends about contracting an STD?

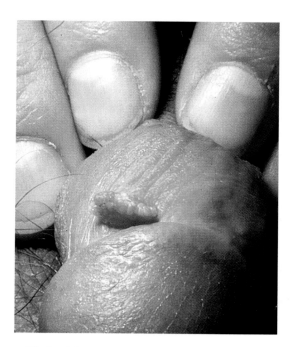

Figure 13-4 A human papillomavirus infection (genital warts).

infection to the eyes and lungs of newborns during a vaginal birth. Detecting chlamydia and other NSUs early is of paramount concern for both men and women.

Human Papillomavirus

The appearance of another STD, **human papillomavirus (HPV)**, is unwanted news. Because HPV infections are generally asymptomatic, the exact extent of the disease is unknown. A study of a group of sexually active college women found HPV infection in approximately 20 percent of the women. HPV-related changes to the cells of the cervix are found in nearly 5 percent of the Pap smears taken from women under age thirty. Researchers currently believe that risk factors for HPV infection in women include: (1) sexual activity before age twenty, (2) intercourse with three or more partners before age thirty-five, and (3) intercourse with a partner who has three or more partners.[29] The extent of HPV infection in men is even less clearly known, but it is probably widespread.

HPV infection is alarming because some of the more than fifty forms of the virus are strongly associated with sexual activity patterns. Visible genital warts (cauliflower-like, raised, pinkish-white lesions) are associated with viral forms 6 or 11, while viral forms 16, 18, 31, 33, and 35 foster changes in other areas.[28] Found most commonly on the penis, scrotum, labia, cervix, and around the anus, these lesions represent the most common symptomatic viral STD in this country. Although most genital wart colonies are small, they may become very large and block the anus or birth canal during pregnancy.

Treatment for HPV, including genital warts, may include patient-applied gels or creams or physician-administered cryotherapy, topical medication, or surgery (see Table 13-5). Regardless of treatment, however, the viral colonies will probably return. One should use condoms to attempt to prevent transmission of HPV.

Gonorrhea

Another extremely common (600,000 cases/year) STD, gonorrhea is caused by a bacterium (*N. gonorrhoea*). In men this bacterial agent can produce a milky-white discharge from the penis, accompanied by painful urination. About 80 precent of men who contract gonorrhea report varying degrees of these symptoms. This figure is approximately reversed for women: Only about 20 percent of women are symptomatic and thus report varying degrees of frequent, painful urination, with a slimy yellow-green discharge from the vagina or urethra. Oral sex with an infected partner can produce a gonorrheal infection of the throat (pharyngeal gonorrhea). Gonorrhea can also be transmitted to the rectal areas of both men and women.

Physicians diagnose gonorrhea by culturing the bacteria. Because of the paired occurrence of chlamydia and gonorrhea, dual therapy with doxycycline or azithromycin in combination with ofloxacin (see Table 13-5) is used in susceptible populations, particularly adolescent women. Outside of these groups, recommended treatment for uncomplicated cases involves the use of one of several antimicrobial drugs, including cefixine, ceftriaxone, and ciprofloxacin. Although prevalent in other areas of the world, drug-resistant strains are not extensive in the United States.[28]

Testing for gonorrhea is included as a part of prenatal care so that infections in mothers can be treated before birth. If the birth canal is infected, newborns can easily contract the infection in the mucous membranes of the eye.

Herpes Simplex

Public health officials think that the sexually transmitted genital herpes virus infection rivals chlamydia as the most prevalent STD. To date about 45 million Americans have been diagnosed, although the asymptomatic (thus undiagnosed) population could increase this figure substantially. Herpes is really a family of more than fifty viruses, some of which produce recognized diseases in humans (chicken pox,

human papillomavirus (HPV) a sexually transmitted virus some of which are capable of causing precancerous changes in the cervix; causative agent for genital warts.

shingles, mononucleosis, and others). One subgroup called herpes simplex 1 virus (HSV-1) produces an infection called labial herpes (oral or lip herpes). Labial herpes produces common fever blisters or cold sores around the lips and oral cavity. Herpes simplex 2 virus (HSV-2) is a different strain that produces similar clumps of blisterlike lesions in the genital region (Figure 13-5). Laypeople call this second type of herpes the STD type, but both types produce identical clinical pictures. About five to 30 percent of cases are caused by HSV-1.[28] Oral-genital sexual practices most likely account for this crossover infection.

Herpes appears as a single sore or as a small cluster of blisterlike sores. These sores burn, itch, and (for some) become very painful. The infected person might also report swollen lymph glands, muscular aches and pains, and fever. Some patients feel weak and sleepy when they have blisters. The lesions may last from a few days to a few weeks. Viral shedding lasts a week on average; then the blisters begin scabbing, and new skin is formed. Even when the patient has become asymptomatic, viral transmission is still possible.

Herpes is an interesting virus for several reasons. It can lie dormant for long periods. For reasons not well understood but perhaps related to stress, diet, or overall health, the viral particles can be stimulated to travel along the nerve pathways to the skin and then create an active infection. Thus herpes can be consid-

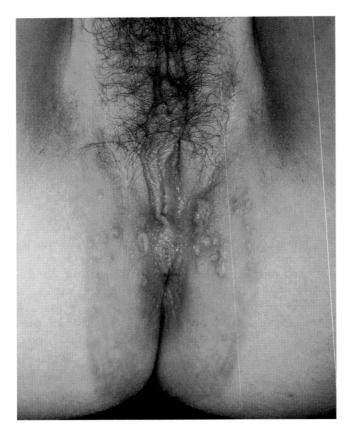

Figure 13-5 A severe herpes infection.

ered a recurrent infection. Fortunately for most people, recurrent infections are less severe than the initial episode and do not last as long. Recommended treatment for an initial outbreak of herpes calls for the use of one of three medications: acyclovir, famciclovir, or valacyclovir. These medications are taken orally, multiple times each day, for seven to ten days (see Table 13-5). Because herpes may occur at intervals following initial treatment, two choices exist. One is to treat each recurrence as it arises (episodic recurrent treatment), and the second is to attempt to suppress recurrence through continuous use of medication (daily suppressive therapy) (see Table 13-5). The treatment choices described above appear to be equally effective for HSV-1 and HSV-2.[28] Additionally, physicians may recommend other medications for relief of various symptoms. Genital herpes is almost always diagnosed through a clinical examination.

The best method of preventing herpes infection is to avoid all direct contact with a person who has an active infection. Do not kiss someone with a fever blister—or let them kiss you (or your children) if they have an active lesion. Do not share drinking glasses or eating utensils. Check your partner's genitals. Do not have intimate sexual contact with someone who displays the blisterlike clusters or rash. (Condoms are only marginally helpful and cannot protect against lesions on the female vulva or the lower abdominal area of men). Be careful not to infect yourself by touching a blister and then touching any other part of your body. The Health Action Guide on p. 413 gives helpful advice about talking with your partner if you have genital herpes.

Newborn babies are especially susceptible to the virus if they come into contact with an active lesion during birth. Newborns have not developed the defense capabilities to resist the invasion. They can quickly develop a systemic (general) infection (neonatal herpes) that is often fatal or local infections that produce permanent brain damage or blindness. Fortunately, most of these problems can be prevented through proper prenatal care. A cesarean delivery can be performed if viral particles might be present at birth, although this is done less often today than in the past.

Syphilis

Like gonorrhea, syphilis is caused by a bacterium (*Treponema pallidum*) and is transmitted almost exclusively by sexual intercourse. The incidence of syphilis, a CDC-reportable disease, is far lower than that of gonorrhea. In 1950 a record 217,558 cases of syphilis were reported in this country. The number of cases then fell steadily to less than 80,000 cases in 1980. From 1980 through 1990 the incidence climbed, reaching nearly 140,000 cases in 1990. Another decline then began, and in 1993 the number of cases dropped to 101,259. In 1997 the CDC reported that syphilis had fallen to the lowest level (8,551) in forty years, and that it may now be possible to wipe out this STD entirely.[30]

In spite of this downward trend, an alarming number of today's cases have been associated with HIV infections. See the Star Box below for more information on this disease. Observers have noted an alarming increase in infant syphilis in children born to mothers who use drugs and support their habit through sexual activity.

Pubic Lice

Three types of lice infect humans: The head louse, the body louse, and the pubic louse all feed on the blood of the host. Except for the relatively uncommon body louse, these tiny insects do not carry diseases. They are, however, very annoying.

Pubic lice, also called crabs, attach themselves to the base of the pubic hairs, where they live and lay their eggs (nits). These eggs move into a larval stage after one week; after two more weeks, they develop into mature adult crab lice.

shingles a viral infection affecting the nerve endings of the skin.

Syphilis

Syphilis is a serious disease that, left untreated, can cause death. The chance of contracting syphilis during a single sexual encounter with an infected partner is now about 30 percent. Syphilis takes a well-established course after it is contracted.

Infection
The syphilis bacterium, *Treponema pallidum,* is a spirochete. It is transmitted from an infected person to a new host through intimate contact. Moist, warm tissue, such as that lining the reproductive, urinary, and digestive tracts, offers an ideal environment for the agent.

Incubation
Syphilis incubates without symptoms for 10 to 90 days, followed by the characteristic primary stage of the disease.

Primary Stage
The primary stage of syphilis lasts 1 to 5 weeks. A small, raised, painless sore called a *chancre* forms at this time. This highly infectious lesion is not easily identified in 90 percent of women and 50 percent of men; thus these people generally do not seek treatment. The chancre heals in 4 to 8 weeks.

Secondary Stage
The extremely contagious secondary stage of the disease occurs 6 to 12 weeks after initial infection. The infectious agents are now systemic, so symptoms may include a generalized body rash, a sore throat, or a patchy loss of hair. A blood test (VDRL) will be positive, and treatment can be effectively administered. If untreated, the second stage subsides within 2 to 6 weeks. A pregnant woman can easily transmit syphilis to her fetus during this stage. Congenital syphilis often results in stillbirth or an infant born with a variety of life-threatening complications. Early treatment of infected pregnant women can prevent congenital syphilis.

Latent Stage
After the secondary stage subsides, an extended period of noninfectiousness occurs. The infectious agents remain dormant within the body cells, and the infected person displays few clinical signs during this stage.

Late Stage
Syphilis can recur for a third time 15 to 25 years after initial contact. In late-stage syphilis, tissue damage is profound and irreversible. The person suffers damage to the cardiovascular system, central nervous system, eyes, and skin, and death from the effects of the disease is likely.

Treatment
Depending on the stage, syphilis is treated with varying doses of Benzathine penicillin G. See Table 13-5 for protocol specifics.

People usually notice they have a pubic lice infestation when they suffer intense itching in the genital region. Prescription and OTC creams, lotions, and shampoos are usually effective in killing both the lice and their eggs, although some reports suggest that lice are becoming resistant to OTC treatments.[31]

Lice are not transmitted exclusively through sexual contact, but also by contact with bedsheets and clothes that may be contaminated. If you develop a pubic lice infestation, you must thoroughly treat yourself, your clothes, your sheets, and your furniture.

Vaginal Infections

Two common pathogens produce uncomfortable vaginal infections in women. The first is the yeast or fungus pathogen *Candida (Monilia) albicans,* which produces the yeast infection often called *thrush.* These organisms, commonly found in the vagina, seem to multiply rapidly when some unusual stressor (pregnancy, use of birth control pills or antibiotics, diabetes) affects a woman's body. This infection, now called vulvovaginal candidiasis (VVC),[28] is signaled by a white or cream-colored vaginal discharge that resembles cottage cheese. Vaginal itching and vulvar swelling are also commonly reported. Current treatment is based on the use of one of several prescription and OTC azole drugs.

Recently introduced nonprescription azole-based products offer effective home treatment. One should first consult with a physician before using these new products for the first time. (Men rarely report this monilial infection, although some may report mildly painful urination or a barely noticeable discharge at the urethral opening or beneath the foreskin of the penis.)

The protozoan Trichomonas vaginalis also produces a vaginal infection. This parasite can be transmitted through sexual intercourse or by contact with contaminated (often damp) objects, such as towels, clothing, or toilet seats, that may contain some vaginal discharge. In women, this infection, called *trichomoniasis,* or "trich," produces a foamy, yellow-green, foul-smelling discharge that may be accompanied by itching, swelling, and painful urination. Although topically applied treatments with limited effectiveness for trichomoniasis are available, only one highly effective oral medication is currently on the market.[28] Men infrequently contract trichomoniasis but may harbor the organisms without realizing it. They also should be treated to minimize reinfection of partners.[28]

The vagina is warm, dark, and moist, an ideal breeding environment for a variety of organisms. Unfortunately, some highly promoted commercial products seem to increase the incidence of vaginal infections. Among these are tight panty hose (without cotton panels), which tend to increase the vaginal temperature, and commercial vaginal douches, which can alter the acidic level of the vagina. Both of these products might promote infections. Women are advised to wipe from front to back after every bowel movement to reduce the opportunity for direct transmission of pathogenic agents from the rectum to the vagina. Avoiding public bathrooms when possible is also a good practice. Of course, if you notice any unusual discharge from the vagina, you should report this to your physician.

Cystitis and Urethritis

Cystitis, an infection of the urinary bladder, and urethritis, an infection of the urethra, occasionally can be caused by a sexually transmitted organism. Such infections can also be caused by the organisms that cause vaginitis and organisms found in the intestinal tract. A culture is required to identify the specific pathogen associated with a particular case of cystitis or urethritis. The symptoms are pain when urinating, the need to urinate frequently, a dull aching pain above the pubic bone, and the passing of blood-streaked urine.

Physicians can easily treat cystitis and urethritis with antibiotics when the specific organism has been identified. A newly introduced drug, Monurol, which requires only a single dose, has proved effective. Few complications result from infections that are treated promptly. If cystitis or urethritis is left untreated, the infectious agent could move upward in the urinary system and infect the ureters and kidneys. These upper-urinary-tract infections are more serious and require more extensive evaluation and aggressive treatment. Therefore one should obtain medical care immediately upon noticing symptoms.

Preventing cystitis and urethritis depends to some degree on the source of the infectious agent. One can generally reduce the incidence of infection by urinating completely (to fully empty the urinary bladder) and by drinking ample fluids to flush the urinary tract. Drinking cranberry juice has been found to reduce urinary tract infections.

Personal Applications

• What would your initial reaction be if you learned that someone close to you had a sexually transmitted disease?

Real Life
Real choices

- In what ways is HIV spread?
- What are some ways in which Chris Karasawa can deal with his employees' fear of working with John Travers?
- To what degree do you think hospital patients and health-care providers should be required to undergo HIV testing?

And Now, Your Choices . . .
- If John Travers were your classmate or coworker, how would you feel about him and behave toward him?
- If you were in John Travers's situation, how would you respond to the concerns of prospective coworkers?

Summary

- We have made progress in reducing the incidence of some forms of infectious disease, but other infectious conditions are becoming more common.
- A variety of pathogenic agents are responsible for infectious conditions.
- A chain of infection with six potential links characterizes every infectious condition.
- Infectious conditions progress through five distinct stages.
- One can acquire immunity for some diseases through both natural and artificial means. Children should be immunized according to a schedule.
- The immune system's response to infection relies on cellular and humoral elements.
- The common cold and influenza produce many similar symptoms but differ in their infectious agents, incubation period, prevention, and treatment.
- Tuberculosis and pneumonia are potentially fatal infections of the respiratory system.
- Mononucleosis and chronic fatigue syndrome are infections that produce chronic tiredness.
- Measles and mumps are childhood infections that can be harmful when contracted during adulthood.
- Lyme disease is a bacterial infection contracted through outdoor activities.

- Hantavirus pulmonary syndrome is caused by a virus carried by deer mice; human-to-human transmission has also been reported.
- Hepatitis B (serum hepatitis) is a bloodborne infectious condition that produces serious liver damage. Other varieties are hepatitis A, C, and D.
- HIV/AIDS is a widespread, incurable viral disease transmitted through sexual activity, through intravenous drug use, in infected blood products, or across the placenta during pregnancy.
- The definitive diagnosis of AIDS can be based on the presence of specific conditions or a reduced number of helper T cells.
- HIV and AIDS are currently best treated with triple-drug therapy using a protease inhibitor and two reverse-transcriptase inhibitors; an effective vaccine for prevention has not been developed.
- There are a variety of sexually transmitted conditions, many of which do not produce symptoms in most infected women and many infected men.
- Safer sex practices can reduce the risk of contracting STDs.

Review Questions

1. What are the agents responsible for the most familiar infectious conditions?
2. Describe the six links in the chain of infection.
3. What are the five stages that characterize the progression of infectious conditions?
4. What are the two principal components of the immune system, and how do they cooperate to protect the body from infectious agents and abnormal cells?
5. How are the common cold and influenza similar? How do they differ in their causative agents, incubation period, prevention, and treatment?

6. What symptoms make mononucleosis and chronic fatigue syndrome similar? What aspects of each are different?
7. Why are mumps and measles more serious conditions when they develop in adults?
8. Why is outdoor activity a risk factor for contracting Lyme disease?
9. How is hepatitis B transmitted, and which occupational group is at greatest risk of contracting this infection? How do forms A, C, and D compare with hepatitis B?

10. How is HIV transmitted? How are HIV/AIDS currently treated, and how effective is the treatment? What does the term *safer sex* mean?
11. What specific infectious diseases could be classified as STDs?
12. Why are women more often asymptomatic for STDs than men?
13. To what extent and in what manner can STD transmission be prevented?

References

1. Black J. *Microbiology: principles and applications.* 3rd ed. Englewood Cliffs, NJ: Prentice-Hall, 1996.
2. Hamann B. *Disease: identification, prevention and control.* Dubuque, IA: WCB/McGraw-Hill, 1994.
3. Saladin KS. *Anatomy & physiology: unity of form and function.* Dubuque, IA: WCB/McGraw-Hill, 1998.
4. Center for Biologics Evaluation and Research. *Product approval information-licensing action.* Food and Drug Administration, Sept. 3, 1998.
5. Glenn GM et al. Skin immunization made possible by cholera atoxin. *Nature* 1998; 391(6670):851.
6. Tacket CO et al. Immunogenicity in humans of a recombinant bacterial antigen delivered in a transgenic potato. *Nature Medicine* 1998; 4(5):607–9.
7. Wagner JE et al. Allogenic sibling umbilical cord blood transplantation in children with malignant and nonmalignant disease. *Lancet* 1995; 346:214–19.
8. Leukaemia Research Fund (United Kingdom). *Blood cell production.* 1997. http://www.leukaemia.demon.co.uk/bloodprd.htm
9. Gorman C. Good news for flu sufferers. *Time* 1998; 152(14):99.
10. Painter K. Report backs flu shots for kids. *Health: inside health and science* 1998 Nov 11. http://www.usatoday.com/life/health/general/lhegen051.htm
11. Manning A. TB cases in USA continue to drop. *USA Today* 1997 March 24:8D.
12. Cole ST et al. Deciphering the biology of *Mycobacterium tuberculosis* from the complete genome sequence. *Nature* 1998; 393(6685):537–44.
13. Musher DM. Pneumococcal outbreaks in nursing homes. *N Engl J Med* 1998; 338(26):1861–68.
14. National Institute of Allergy and Infectious Diseases (NIAID). *Chronic fatigue syndrome—etiological theories.* 1998. http://www.niaid.nih.gov/publication/cfs/etio.htm
15. *Summary of notifiable diseases—United States 1996.* http://www.cdc.gov/epo/mmwr/preview/mmwrhtml/00050719.htm
16. Crowly L. *Introduction to human disease.* 4th ed. Boston: Jones & Bartlett, 1996.
17. Fix AD, Strickland GT, Grant J. Tick bites and Lyme disease in an endemic setting: problematic use of serologic testing and prophylactic antibiotic therapy. *JAMA* 1998; 279(3):206–10.
18. Sternberg S. FDA approves Lyme disease vaccine. *USA Today* 1998 Dec 12:1A.
19. Update: Hantavirus infection—United States, 1993. *MMWR* 1993; 42:517–19, as reported in *JAMA* 1993; 270(4):429–32.
20. On El Niño's deadly tail: southwest fears a tiny killer's second attack. *USA Today* 1998 July 2:1D.
21. FDA approves AIDS drug for use against hepatitis B. *USA Today* 1998 Dec 12:4D.
22. FDA approves hepatitis C combination product. *FDA talk paper.* Dec 9, 1998. http://www.fda.gov/bbs/topics/ANSWERS/ANS00929.htm
23. Centers for Disease Control and Prevention. *HIV/AIDS surveillance report.* Midyear Edition 1998 June; 10(1).
24. Edwards S, Carne C. Oral sex and the transmission of viral STIs. *Sex Transm Infect.* 1998; 74(1):6–10.
25. Johns Hopkins AIDS Service. Jan 1999. http://www.Hopkins-aids.edu
26. Altman LK. FDA authorizes first full testing of HIV vaccine. *New York Times* 1998 June 4:A1.
27. Burstein GR et al. Incidence of *Chlamydia trachomatis* infections among inner-city adolescent females. *JAMA* 1998; 280(6):521–26.
28. 1998 Guidelines for treatment of sexually transmitted diseases. *MMWR* (suppl) 1997 Jan; 47(RR-1):1–116.
29. Hatcher R et al. *Contraceptive technology: 1998.* 17th ed. New York: Irvington, 1998.
30. Syphilis down. *USA Today.* 1997 May 28:1D.
31. Manning A. Head lice show signs of resisting usual treatments. *USA Today* 1997 April 29:5D.

Suggested Readings

Turkington C. *Hepatitis C: the silent killer.* Chicago: Contemporary Books, 1998. This book is intended particularly for persons recently diagnosed with hepatitis C and their loved ones. The author presents current information in an understandable manner regarding the cause, treatment, and management of this viral infection of the liver.

Vanderhood-Forschner K. *Everything you need to know about Lyme disease and other tick-borne disorders.* New York: John Wiley & Sons, 1997. Considered by many to be the strongest title on Lyme disease for the general reader, this book comes highly recommended. The author, herself a victim of Lyme disease, became an expert on tick-borne disease. As founder of the Lyme Disease Foundation, the author shares, in addition to disease-related information, an array of helpful insights regarding support groups, insurance companies, products, and sources of further information.

Marr L. *Sexually transmitted diseases: a physician tells you what you need to know.* Baltimore: John Hopkins University Press, 1998. Simple, understandable, and helpful information regarding the cause, treatment, and prevention of subsequent infections is presented by a physician experienced in the treatment of infectious conditions. The author addresses myths about many aspects of STD transmission and treatment.

Stine GJ. *Acquired immune deficiency syndrome: biological, medical, social, and legal issues.* 3rd ed. Saddle River, NJ: Prentice-Hall, 1998. Written by a highly respected geneticist, this book is the most acclaimed title available that focuses on HIV/AIDS. It provides comprehensive, balanced, and highly understandable coverage of the biological, medical, social, and legal aspects of this pandemic disease. The author answers questions honestly and on the basis of what is currently known (and now known) about the topic.

The Hot Zone: New Infectious Diseases Emerge from the Rain Forest

Just a generation ago, many scientists believed we were wiping out infectious disease. Armed with improved sanitation, better hygiene practices, antibiotics, and pesticides, humankind had malaria, cholera, and tuberculosis (TB) on the run and smallpox and polio well on the way to extinction.[1] In fact, infectious diseases were in decline until 1980,[2] but as we approach the next century, the tide is turning. Ebola, HIV, Marburg virus, Lassa fever, Legionnaires' disease, hantavirus, and hepatitis C are but a few of the more than thirty new pathogens researchers have identified in the last twenty years.[1]

Most of these diseases are emerging from the newly inhabited and exploited rain forests of Africa and South America. These areas form a climatic hot zone—a region of elevated temperatures circling the equator. The term *hot zone* has another meaning within the context of infectious disease: It is a military term that means "a place contaminated with a lethal and incurable virus."[3] Appropriately enough, Richard Preston chose *The Hot Zone* as the title of his bestselling novel based on the 1993 Ebola outbreak in Zaire.

New diseases are not the only problem—old diseases have not vanished as scientists had hoped. In fact, many diseases, such as tuberculosis and malaria, have returned in forms resistant to our vaccines and medicines. Despite our efforts, infectious disease remains the third leading cause of death in the United States and the number one cause of death worldwide.[4,5]

Why Are These New Infectious Diseases Taking Hold?

Previously unknown microbes have been evolving for thousands of years in animals and insects. They become threatening to humans only when conditions are right for transmission of the diseases from animals, including insects, to us. Quite a few conditions of modern life, such as global warming, drug resistance, overpopulation, and high-speed travel, make transmission all too easy.

Global climate change affects disease pathogens themselves, the insects that carry and transmit them, and ultimately us. Warmer temperatures are known to cause viruses to multiply more quickly in mosquitos and the mosquitos to expand their habitat range and bite more frequently, thus bringing new populations in contact with the disease and increasing the chance of infection. The more extreme weather conditions that accompany global warming further increase the odds of transmission of insect-borne diseases. Insects are more drought resistant than their predators, so droughts free the insects of some predation, thus increasing their numbers. Torrential rain also gives insects an advantage by providing more breeding places.[2] Warming also facilitates the spread of foodborne and waterborne disease. Warm oceans are more hospitable to cholera and toxic algae blooms that accumulate in fish and shellfish and then can infect humans who eat these animals. The extreme sensitivity of many diseases to climate change prompted the World Health Organization (WHO) of the United Nations to cite climatic change as one of the most important public health challenges of the upcoming century.[6]

Viruses and other microbes are naturally good at developing drug resistance. They have a high built-in mutation rate and reproduce rapidly.[7] A few organisms that survive drug treatment breed quickly, passing on their genes for resistance, and before long the original drug becomes useless.

Human reproduction is also a factor in the disease equation. Development associated with overpopulation puts people in contact with rare diseases. Deforestation and road and dam building encroach on remote ecosystems, exposing people to diseases that their immune systems can't recognize and fight. Urban areas have their own problems. Crowded cities allow infectious diseases to thrive, mainly by increasing the likelihood of spread by personal contact. Overburdened water supply and sanitation systems are also sources of disease in these areas.

Last, global travel allows people, and the organisms that they carry, to reach anywhere in the world in twenty-four hours. In many cases, this is shorter than the incubation time of the particular disease organism,[7] which enables the traveler to spread the organism far and wide before he or she even feels or appears sick.

Recent Global Epidemics

The Ebola virus struck in the African countries of Zaire and Sudan in 1976, and again in Sudan in 1979.[8] The source of Ebola in nature is unclear. Monkeys do become infected but die quickly, as do humans. To be an effective reservoir or source of disease, an animal must be able to tolerate the disease organism and therefore remain active and alive for a longer time in which the virus can be spread. For example, monkeys may be the source of human immunodeficiency virus (HIV) because they harbor a similar virus, simian immunodeficiency virus (SIV), but don't become sick. Of course, HIV/AIDS is a dangerous virus, but Ebola is more infective and runs a shorter disease course. As one author put it, "Ebola does in ten days what it takes AIDS ten years to accomplish."[3] This is terrible for the nine out of ten people infected with Ebola who die in a matter of days, but ironically by making its victims so sick so quickly, Ebola limits its own spread. Being deathly ill limits the social interactions of carriers. In 1995 Ebola revisited Zaire, but in Gabon in 1996 it was recognized and stopped before it could take hold.

Many other diseases also pose threats.[9] After a heat wave in 1988, mosquitos carrying dengue (pronounced "ding-ee") spread through Mexico. In 1991 an epidemic of cholera in South America killed 5,000 of the 500,000 people infected.[6] A record year for infectious disease occurred in 1993, possibly set into effect by weather patterns associated with El Niño, which warmed the waters in the tropical Pacific.[10] A year later, epidemic bubonic plague swept through India. In the summer of 1996, a dengue outbreak began in Latin America. By the time it ended, 140,000 people from Argentina to Texas had been infected, and 4,000 of those infected had died.[6]

Occurrence of New Infectious Diseases in the United States

As the 1996 dengue outbreak illustrates, infectious disease is not just a problem for developing countries. In 1989 an airborne strain of Ebola, which fortunately was not dangerous to humans, was brought to Virginia in Philippine crab-eating monkeys that were to be distributed to research labs across the United States.

Hantavirus became an American problem in 1993. Following an extremely rainy year that was good for vegetation, the rodent population exploded in the Four Corners area of New Mexico, Arizona, Colorado,

and Utah. The rodent population spread hantavirus to sixteen states. This virus killed half of the ninety-four people it infected.[10] More recently, the first case of hantavirus transmission between humans occurred in Argentina. Apparently eighteen people, including five physicians, contracted the disease after having contact with sick patients.[11]

The 1994 earthquake in Southern California provided more evidence to support the theory that new infectious diseases can spread to humans during environmental disturbances. The earthquake exposed a soil fungus that infected 200 people and killed 3.

Leading the Fight for Public Health

The United States leads the international health community with its premier monitoring and response services provided by the Centers for Disease Control and Prevention (CDC).[12] Of course, international cooperation is vital, but we have seen why disease vigilance is in our own interest as well. To move from the reactive system now in place to a predictive one, some specific goals must be met.[1] Rather than holding congressional hearings to point blame when a problem arises, we need to examine the infrastructure of the public health system itself.[7]

A global network of epidemiological field stations should be established to detect and characterize outbreaks early, both here and abroad. Insect carriers of disease need to be managed in a variety of ways, including but not solely relying on pesticides. Further, insecticides and pesticides must be developed that are both effective and environmentally safe. Safe food and water must be made available to everyone, and new antibiotics and vaccines need to be developed. These goals are hard to achieve, particularly in the face of episodes of armed conflict within and between countries, growing religious intolerance that becomes transformed into national disputes, and a global economy that continues to separate the affluent developed countries from those far less developed and affluent.

As we enter the new millennium, Americans may encounter the threat of emerging diseases associated with biological weapons and regional armed conflict.[13] This threat looms even larger when one realizes that some countries view these disease organisms as agents of war and are capable of using them as such. With about a dozen countries in possession or pursuit of biological weapons arsenals, the understanding of deadly pathogens becomes a matter of national security as well as global health.

For Discussion . . .

In your view, what is the most important step we can take to fight infectious disease? Do you think the United States does more than its share in monitoring these diseases? Do you know anyone who works in the public health field? If so, what does he or she do?

References

1. Lemonick MD; Guerrilla warfare. *Time* 1996; 148(14):58–62.
2. Hileman B. Warning of infectious disease threat issued. *Chemical and Engineering News* 1996; 74(4):9.
3. Tucker JB. Invaders from the rain forest. *Technology Review* 1995; 98(3):77–78.
4. Winker M, Flanagin A. Infectious diseases—a global approach to a global problem. *JAMA* 1996; 275(3):245–46.
5. Marwich C. Effective response to emerging diseases called an essential priority worldwide. *JAMA* 1995; 273(3):189–90.
6. Monastersky R. Health in the hot zone. *Science News* 1996; 149(14):218–19.
7. Lederberg J. Infectious disease: a threat to global health and security. *JAMA* 1996; 276(5):417–19.
8. Re-emergence of Ebola virus in Africa. *Emerg Infect Dis* 1995 July–Sept; 1(3):1–3.
9. Gubler DJ. Resurgent vector-borne diseases as a global health problem. *Emerg Infect Dis* 1998; 4(3):442–50.
10. Anon. Climate creates a hot zone. *Environment* 1996; 37(10):27.
11. Manning A. Humans pass on hantavirus in Argentina. *USA Today* 1997 June 17:ID.
12. Preventing emerging infectious diseases: a strategy for the 21st century: overview of the updated plan. *MMWR* (suppl) 1998; 47(15):1–14.
13. Nelan BW. America the vulnerable: a disaster is just waiting to happen if Iraq unleashes its poisons and germs. *Time* 1997; 150(22):50–51.

InfoLinks

www.who.ch/
www.cdc.gov/ncidod

MASTERING TASKS

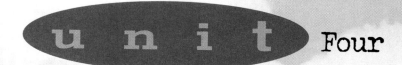

Preventing Diseases

Illness and major health problems influence the progress we make with respect to the five developmental tasks: identity, independence, responsibility, social skills, and intimacy. The reverse is also true. The progress we make regarding these developmental tasks has some bearing on our susceptibility to illness and our ability to recover from illness. Let us look more closely at each task.

Forming an Initial Adult Identity

Most of us probably go through life without really believing that we might one day become seriously ill. We prefer to imagine ourselves as always being free from major health problems. Our identity is based on a view of ourselves as being healthy. However, we encourage you to think occasionally about how your identity might be changed if you were to contract or develop a serious illness. What would the impact be on your view of yourself, your interactions with others, and your dreams for the future? We believe that such introspection is healthful, because it serves two purposes: it prepares us for the future and it allows us to appreciate the good health we have today.

Establishing Independence

As you move into and through adulthood, you will probably find yourself increasingly seeking ways of expressing your individualism, freedom, and independence. In turn, the collective society expects you to balance this independence with some realism.

You will be expected to manage your finances, make academic and career decisions, and select friends according to your own criteria. Most college students relish these new opportunities.

Developing an independent lifestyle also means that you will be gradually moving away from those people you have regularly turned to for advice and support. With respect to the content in this unit, this emerging independence means that you may be forced to start experiencing illnesses all by yourself. The years of having others care for all of your health needs may nearly be over. Thus, as an emerging independent adult, you must become familiar with many techniques regarding self-care, prevention, and access to the health-care system. Fortunately, you are the beneficiary of this growth process.

Assuming Responsibility

Nearly every day, we are being encouraged by health professionals to be active participants in the promotion of our health. We are asked to become more responsible for aspects of our health that we can control, such as our weight, alcohol and other drug use, fitness level, and dietary practices. Indeed, the collective society is losing patience with people who completely ignore the importance of living a healthful life.

Not only do irresponsible people hurt themselves, but they also have a significant impact on the lives of others. Those who, by their own actions, are frequently ill and absent from work, overuse group health insurance protection, and place great burdens on family and friends can reduce the quality

of life for everyone. Practicing preventive health measures enables you to be responsible to the collective society.

Developing Social Skills

The content in Chapters 10, 11, 12, and 13 provides a large stage for the practice and rehearsal of social skills. From the social involvement with friends who have a chronic health condition to the intimate discussions couples have concerning possible STD transmission, it is important to feel comfortable while communicating with others. Interacting with sick people, their families, and members of the health-care delivery system sometimes takes persistence and a good deal of tact. For most people, these social skills tend to develop with practice.

Developing Intimacy

Too frequently, chronic illness, such as heart disease, cancer, degenerative conditions, and infections, makes intimacy difficult because of frequent hospitalizations, reduced energy, and the effects of medications and treatment.

In contrast, though, a chronic illness can actually build a new dimension into an intimate relationship as it forces everyone to reassess their interactions with each other. For the ill person, there is greater reliance on the well partner. For the partner who is well, there is a greater-than-normal opportunity to express concern and give care. Although an illness can ultimately end a relationship, it can, for a while, enhance the quality of that very same relationship.

unit

Sexuality

Sexuality is an important part of our being. It colors the way we interact with the world around us and affects our goals, relationships, and roles in society.

1 Physical Dimension

Sexuality is closely related to the physical dimension of health. For example, our bodies mature at puberty, we respond to sexual arousal, we make choices about contraception and pregnancy, and we adjust our sexual behavior as we age. Sexual experiences and relationships can be very complex and demanding because they are fueled by energy and time. They are enhanced when the body is well maintained, rested, and relatively free from illness.

2 Emotional Dimension

One of the most stressful aspects of life is sexual intimacy. Feelings about your own sexual behavior can range from exhilaration to ambivalence to depression. Being comfortable with your sexuality comes from being guided by your core values, knowing how to express your sexual feelings openly, being able to set limits when appropriate, and understanding how to communicate effectively with your partner.

3 Social Dimension

Because sexuality often involves interaction with others, the development of social skills in this area is imperative. For many, dating is an excellent arena in which to establish specific social skills. As a relationship becomes more serious, communication skills will grow. These skills are important factors in the process of mate selection and marriage for those who choose this path.

4 Intellectual Dimension

As a relationship matures, opportunities abound for contemplation, analysis, and reflection. You may have to sort through your feelings, examine your values, and use lessons from past experiences as you take part in this process of introspection. You will also draw on your intellectual resources as you learn about reproductive anatomy, fertility, sexual response, contraception, and birth.

5 Spiritual Dimension

As an intimate relationship progresses, you may have to explore your feelings about your sense of morality, the appropriateness of premarital sex, or the value of fidelity in a marriage or other long-term committed relationship. Dating, courtship, and particularly marriage offer opportunities to enhance your spirituality by extending sympathy, support, and love to another person. Some people even find the sexual act itself to be a way of expressing their spirituality.

6 Occupational Dimension

Decisions about reproduction can have a significant effect on your occupational dimension of health. Women who are pregnant may have to work even when they are not feeling well. Then they must decide how much time to take off work after the child is born. They and their partners must also make difficult choices about long-term child care arrangements. The decisions they make will affect their occupational satisfaction and sense of fulfillment.

7 Environmental Dimension

Although your environmental health is not directly related to your sexuality, the dimensions of health are interconnected; taking care of the other dimensions of your health is likely to enhance your environmental health as well.

Exploring the Origins of Sexuality

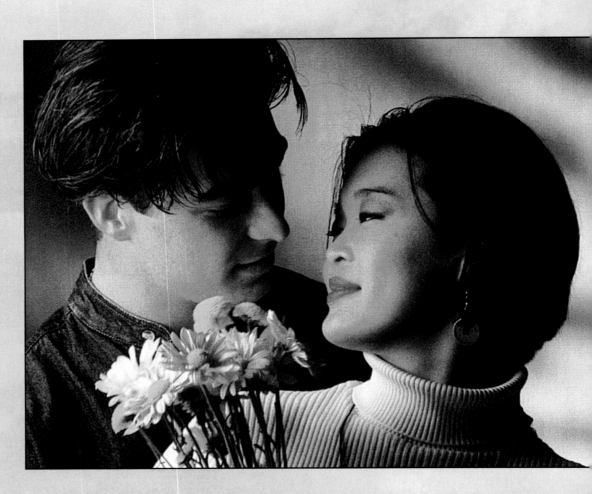

As we move beyond the year 2000, we have reached a better understanding of both the biological and psychosocial factors that contribute to the complex expression of our sexuality. As a society, we are now inclined to view human behavior in terms of a complex script written on the basis of both biology and conditioning.

Reflecting this understanding is the way in which we use the words *male* or *female* to refer to the biological roots of our sexuality and the words *man* or *woman* to refer to the psychosocial roots of our sexuality. In this chapter, we explore human sexuality as it relates to the dynamic interplay of the biological and psychosocial bases that form our masculinity or femininity.

HEALTHY PEOPLE: LOOKING AHEAD TO 2010

Key indicators of progress in areas related to sexuality include reducing the number of unintended pregnancies, increasing the age of initial sexual intercourse, increasing the rate of abstinence among young people who have already had sexual intercourse and increasing the use of effective contraception (including the use of methods that also reduce the risk of various sexually transmitted diseases) among sexually active young people.

Progress toward achieving the target goals in these areas has been mixed. Despite intensive efforts to curb early sexual exploration, the age of initial sexual intercourse continues to drop. However, some small gains have been made in promoting abstinence among girls who have already been sexually active. In addition, there has been a slight increase in the percentage of teenagers who use effective contraception.

As we near the turn of the century, college students have become especially interested in developing meaningful, safe relationships. Like generations of students in the past, many of today's college students are sexually active. With sexual health as one of the main focus areas of the *Healthy People 2010* framework, we can expect a variety of health objectives aimed at college students and other young adults.

Real Life
Real choices

- Name: Diana Schumacher Lutz and Jerry Lutz
- Age: 34 and 32
- Occupations: Diana, high school principal, Jerry, insurance broker

"Sugar and spice and everything nice . . ." "Snips and snails and puppy dog tails . . ." In these words from an old nursery rhyme, it isn't hard to figure out which phrase applies to girls and which to boys. Girls are supposed to be sweet, quiet, and nice; boys are expected to be frisky, adventurous, and scruffy.

That's exactly how things were in both Diana and Jerry Lutz's families when they were growing up in a small, conservative farm town in western Kansas. The girls wore dresses, did housework, and tended the garden while the boys cared for livestock, fished and hunted, and tinkered with old cars.

When Diana won a full scholarship to a prestigious out-of-state university, she entered a radically different world where many women wore jeans, majored in engineering, and left dishes in the sink, while men often baked bread, raised herbs,

and cleaned house—and where everyone felt free to do some, all, or none of these activities without regard to their traditional sex-based roles.

That's the way Diana wants to bring up her and Jerry's children: Jenny, 9, and Richard, 6. But Jerry is adamantly opposed to the idea of his son baking cakes and his daughter playing rugby. He's far less stern than his parents, but he still believes in the traditional sex roles with which both he and Diana grew up. He's proud of Jenny's school record but is uncomfortable with her enthusiastic talk of being an astronaut or an architect. First-grader Richard can already name more than 20 flowering plants and loves to help his mother in the garden, but Jerry tries to distract him by suggesting they practice batting or toss the football.

Diana and Jerry don't argue or contradict each other in front of the kids, but everyone's aware of the tension caused by their conflict over appropriate sex roles.

As you study this chapter, think about the issues that confront the Lutzes, and prepare yourself to answer the questions in **Your Turn** at the end of the chapter.

Biological Bases of Human Sexuality

Within a few seconds after the birth of a baby, someone (a doctor, nurse, or parent) emphatically labels the child: "It's a boy," or "It's a girl." For the parents and society as a whole, the child's biological sexuality is being displayed and identified. Another female or male enters the world.

Genetic Basis

At the moment of conception, a Y-bearing or an X-bearing sperm cell joins with the X-bearing ovum to establish the true basis of biological sexuality.[1] A fertilized ovum with sex chromosomes XX is biologically female, whereas a fertilized ovum bearing the XY sex chromosome is biologically male. Genetics forms the most basic level of an individual's biological sexuality.

Gonadal Basis

The gonadal basis for biological sexuality refers to the growing embryo's development of *gonads*. Male embryos develop testes about the seventh week after conception, and female embryos develop ovaries about the twelfth week after conception.

Structural Development

The development of male or female reproductive structures is initially determined by the presence or

absence of hormones produced by the developing testes—androgens and müllerian inhibiting substance (MIS). With these hormones present, the male embryo starts to develop male reproductive structures (penis, scrotum, vas deferens, seminal vesicles, prostate gland, and Cowper's glands).

Because the female embryo is not exposed to these male hormones, it develops the characteristic female reproductive structures: the uterus, fallopian tubes, vagina, labia, and clitoris.

Biological Sexuality and the Childhood Years

The growth and development of the child in terms of reproductive organs and physiological processes have traditionally been thought to be "latent" during the childhood years. However, a gradual degree of growth occurs in both girls and boys. The reproductive organs, however, will undergo faster growth at the onset of puberty and will achieve their adult size and capabilities shortly thereafter.

Puberty

The entry into puberty is a gradual maturing process for young girls and boys. For young girls, the onset of menstruation, called *menarche*, occurs around age thirteen but may come somewhat earlier or later.[2] Early menstrual cycles tend to be anovulatory (ovulation does not occur). Menarche is usually preceded by a growth spurt that includes the budding of breasts and the growth of pubic and underarm hair.[3]

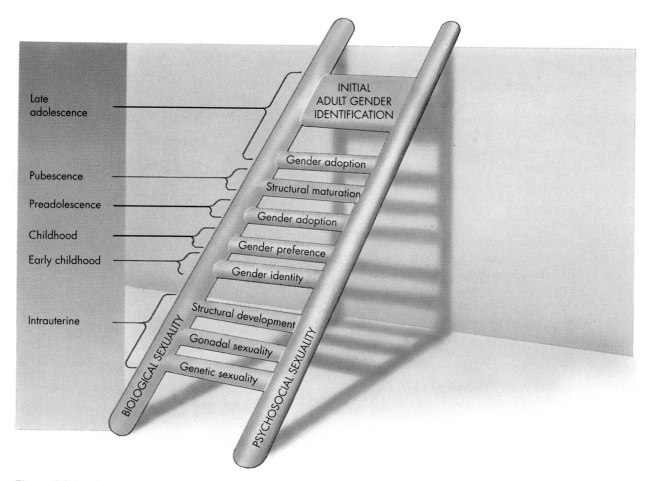

Figure 14-1 Our sexuality develops through biological and psychosocial stages.

Young males follow a similar pattern of maturation, including a growth spurt followed by a gradual sexual maturity. However, this process takes place about two years later than in young females. Genital enlargement, underarm and pubic hair growth, and a lowering of the voice commonly occur. The male's first ejaculation is generally experienced by the age of fourteen, most commonly through **nocturnal emission** or masturbation. For many young boys, fully mature sperm do not develop until about age fifteen.

Reproductive capability only gradually declines over the course of the adult years. In the woman, however, the onset of **menopause** signals a more direct turning off of the reproductive system than is the case for the male adult. By the early to mid-fifties, virtually all women have entered a postmenopausal period, but for men, relatively high-level **spermatogenesis** may continue for a decade or two.

The story of sexual maturation and reproductive maturity cannot, however, be solely focused on the changes that take place in the body. Now we will discuss the psychosocial processes that accompany the biological changes.

Personal Applications

• How would you describe your feelings about the changes in your body that took place during puberty?

Psychosocial Bases of Human Sexuality

If you visualized growth and development of sexuality as a ladder (Figure 14-1), one vertical rail of the ladder would represent our biological sexuality. Arising at various points along this rail would be rungs representing the sequential unfolding of the genetic, gonadal, and structural components.

---

nocturnal emission ejaculation that occurs during sleep; "wet dream."

menopause decline and eventual cessation of hormone production by the female reproductive system.

spermatogenesis (sper mat oh **jen** uh sis) process of sperm production.

Because humans, more so than any other life form, can rise above a life centered on reproduction, we have a second dimension or rail to our sexuality—our **psychosocial sexuality**. The reason we possess the ability to be more than reproductive beings is a question for the theologian or philosopher. We are considerably more complex than the functions determined by biology. The process that transforms a male into a man and a female into a woman begins at birth and continues to influence us throughout the course of our lives.

Gender Identity

Although expectant parents may prefer to have a child of one **gender** over the other, they frequently must wait until the birth of the baby to have their question answered. External genitals "cast the die," and femininity or masculinity begins to receive its traditional reinforcement by the parents and society in general. By the eighteenth month, typical children have both the language and the insight to correctly identify their gender. They have established a **gender identity**.[4] The first rung rising from the psychosocial rail of the ladder has been climbed.

Gender Preference

During the preschool years, children receive the second component of the scripting required for the full development of psychosocial sexuality—the preference for the gender to which they have been assigned. The process whereby **gender preference** is transmitted to the child is more than likely a less subtle form of the practices observed during the gender identity period (the first 18 months). Many parents begin to control the child's exposure to experiences traditionally reserved for children of the opposite gender. This is particularly true for boys; parents will stop play activities they perceive as being too feminine.

Attitudes toward gender roles have become more flexible in recent years. Many parents now allow their children to pursue the activities they enjoy, regardless of whether the activities were once considered strictly masculine, such as playing baseball or building a model airplane, or feminine, such as growing flowers or cooking.

Parents should not become alarmed if their children or teenagers experiment with their gender identity through their appearance or activities. Such experimentation is natural and a part of finding the gender identity that best fits them. Such children often become very secure in their gender identity as adults.

With the recent acceleration in the importance of competitive sports for women, many of the skills and experiences once reserved for boys are now being fostered in young girls. What effect, if any, this movement will have on the speed at which gender preference is reached will be a topic for further research.

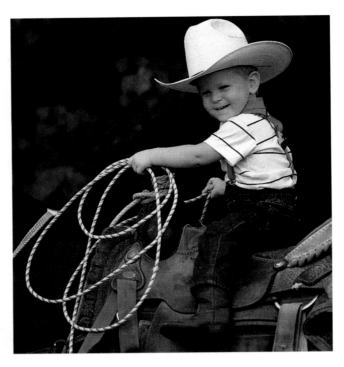

Parents and society reinforce gender identity by encouraging children to participate in traditionally masculine or feminine activities.

Personal Applications

• Other than biological differences, what do you think are the typical qualities of men? Of women? Why?

Gender Adoption

The process of reaching an initial adult gender identification requires a considerable period of time. The specific knowledge, attitudes, and behavior characteristic of adults must be observed, analyzed, and practiced. The process of acquiring and personalizing these "insights" about how men and women think, feel, and act is reflected by the term **gender adoption**, the first and third rungs below the initial adult gender identification rail of the ladder in Figure 14-1.

In addition to the construction of a personalized version of an adult sexual identity, it is important that the child and particularly the adolescent construct a gender schema for a member of the opposite gender. Clearly, the world of adulthood, with its involvement with intimacy, parenting, and employment, will require that men know women and women know men. Gender adoption provides an opportunity to begin this equally valuable "picture" of what the other gender is like.

Initial Adult Gender Identification

By the time young people have climbed all of the rungs of the sexuality ladder, they have arrived at the chronological point in the life cycle when they need to

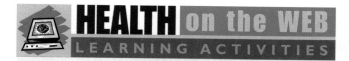

Learning About the Female Reproductive System

In this chapter, you are studying the female and male reproductive systems. To learn more about the external and internal female reproductive organs, go to http://body matters.com/ teachers/guide4.html#thef. Explore the interactive information, and read the list of questions and suggested answers. Did you learn anything surprising?

Understanding the Menstrual Cycle

Whether you're a man or a woman, knowing how the menstrual cycle works will help you understand pregnancy, contraception, menopause, and other issues. Go to http:// bodymatters.com to learn more about the menstrual cycle. Select a topic of interest to you, and read more about it. How can you put this knowledge to use now or later in your life?

Learning About the Male Reproductive System

For an in-depth review of the male reproductive system, go to www.msms.doe.k12.ms.us/biology/anatomy/reproductive/male.html. Read what each anatomical structure is responsible for, and click to view its function more clearly. How does this information help you understand sexual behavior?

For more activities, log on to our Online Learning Center at www.mhhe.com/hper/health/payne

construct an initial adult **gender identification**. You might notice that this label seems remarkably similar to the terminology used to describe one of the developmental tasks being used in this textbook. In fact, the task of forming an initial adult identity is closely related to developing an initial adult image of oneself as a man or a woman. Although most of us currently support the concept of "person" in many gender-neutral contexts (for some very valid reasons), we still must identify ourselves as either a man or a woman.

Androgyny: Sharing the Pluses

Over the last twenty years our society has increasingly accepted an image of a person who possesses both masculine and feminine qualities. This accepted image has taken years to develop because our society traditionally has reinforced rigid masculine roles for men and rigid feminine roles for women.

In the past, from the time a child was born, we assigned and reinforced only those roles and traits that were thought to be directly related to his or her biological gender. Boys were not allowed to cry, play with dolls, or help in the kitchen. Girls were not encouraged to become involved in sports; they were told to learn to sew, cook, and baby-sit. Men were encouraged to be strong, expressive, dominant, aggressive, and career oriented, whereas women were encouraged to be weak, shy, submissive, passive, and home oriented.

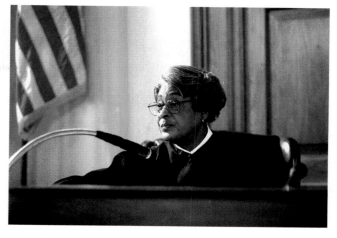

Many women have reached the highest levels in traditionally male professions, such as law, medicine, and business.

These traditional biases have resulted in some interesting phenomena related to career opportunities. Women were denied jobs requiring above-average physical strength, admittance into professional schools requiring high intellectual capacities, such as law, medicine, and business, and entry into most levels of military participation. Likewise, men were not encouraged to enter traditionally feminine careers, such as nursing, clerical work, and elementary school teaching.

For a variety of reasons, the traditional picture has changed. **Androgyny,** or the blending of both feminine and masculine qualities, is more clearly evident in our society now than ever before. Today it is more acceptable to see men involved in raising children (including changing diapers) and doing routine housework. On the other hand, it is also more acceptable to see women entering the workplace in jobs traditionally managed by men and participating in sports traditionally played by men. Men are not scoffed at when they are seen crying after a touching movie. Women are not laughed at

psychosocial sexuality   masculine and feminine aspects of sexuality.

gender   general term reflecting a biological basis of sexuality; the male gender or the female gender.

gender identity   recognition of one's gender.

gender preference   emotional and intellectual acceptance of one's own gender.

gender adoption   long process of learning the behavior that is traditional for one's gender.

gender identification   achievement of a personally satisfying interpretation of one's masculinity or femininity.

androgyny (an **droj** en ee)   the blending of both masculine and feminine qualities.

Personal Assessment

Respond to each of the following statements by selecting a numbered response (1–5) that most accurately reflects your feelings. Circle the number of your selection. At the end of the questionnaire, total these numbers for use in interpreting your responses.

1	Agree strongly
2	Agree moderately
3	Uncertain
4	Disagree moderately
5	Disagree strongly

Men and women have greater differences than they have similarities.	1	2	3	4	5
Homosexuality and bisexuality are immoral and unnatural.	1	2	3	4	5
Our society is too sexually oriented.	1	2	3	4	5
Pornography encourages sexual promiscuity.	1	2	3	4	5
Children know far too much about sex.	1	2	3	4	5
Education about sexuality is solely the responsibility of the family.	1	2	3	4	5
Dating begins far too early in our society.	1	2	3	4	5
Sexual intimacy before marriage leads to emotional stress and damage to one's reputation.	1	2	3	4	5
Sexual availability is far too frequently the reason people marry.	1	2	3	4	5
Reproduction is the most important reason for sexual intimacy during marriage.	1	2	3	4	5
Modern families are too small.	1	2	3	4	5
Family planning clinics should not receive public funds.	1	2	3	4	5
Contraception is the woman's responsibility.	1	2	3	4	5
Abortion is the murder of an innocent child.	1	2	3	4	5
Marriage has been weakened by the changing role of women in society.	1	2	3	4	5
Divorce is an unacceptable means of resolving marital difficulties.	1	2	3	4	5
Extramarital sexual intimacy will destroy a marriage.	1	2	3	4	5
Sexual abuse of a child does not generally occur unless the child encourages the adult.	1	2	3	4	5
Provocative behavior by the woman is a factor in almost every case of rape.	1	2	3	4	5
Reproduction is not a right but a privilege.	1	2	3	4	5

YOUR TOTAL POINTS _____

Interpretation

20–34 points	A very traditional attitude toward sexuality
35–54 points	A moderately traditional attitude toward sexuality
55–65 points	A rather ambivalent attitude toward sexuality
66–85 points	A moderately nontraditional attitude toward sexuality
86–100 points	A very nontraditional attitude toward sexuality

To Carry This Further . . .

Compare your results with those of a roommate or close friend. How do you think your parents would score on this assessment?

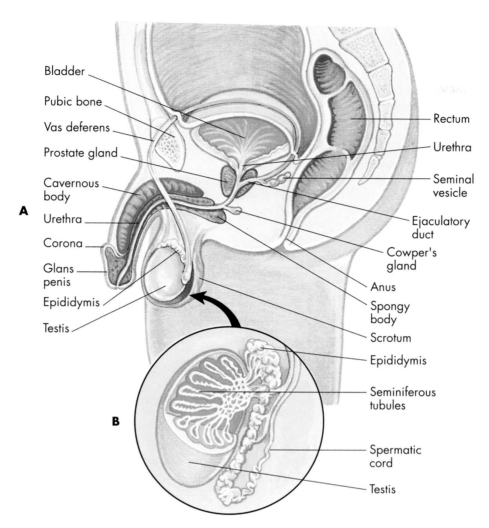

A

Bladder
Pubic bone
Vas deferens
Prostate gland
Cavernous body
Urethra
Corona
Glans penis
Epididymis
Testis

Rectum
Urethra
Seminal vesicle
Ejaculatory duct
Cowper's gland
Anus
Spongy body
Scrotum
Epididymis
Seminiferous tubules
Spermatic cord
Testis

B

Figure 14-2 **A,** Male reproductive structures, side view. The production and delivery of sperm, as well as the production of the sex hormone testosterone, is accomplished by the male reproductive structures. **B,** Cross section of a testis.

when they choose to assert themselves. The disposal of many sexual stereotypes has probably benefited our society immensely by relieving people of the pressure to be 100 percent "womanly" or 100 percent "macho."

Research data suggest that androgynous people are more flexible, have greater self-esteem, and show more social skills and motivation to achieve.[4] Complete the Personal Assessment on page 430 to explore your own attitudes about sexuality and sex roles. Then read the Topics for Today article on page 443.

Reproductive Systems

The most familiar aspects of biological sexuality are the structures that compose the reproductive systems. Each structure contributes in unique ways to the reproductive process. Thus with these structures, males have the ability to impregnate. Females have the ability to become pregnant, give birth, and nourish in-

fants through breastfeeding. In addition, many of these structures are associated with nonreproductive sexual behavior.

Male Reproductive System

The male reproductive system consists of external structures of genitals (the penis and scrotum) and internal structures (the testes, various passageways or ducts, seminal vesicles, the prostate gland, and the Cowper's glands) (Figure 14-2A).

Male newborn babies are routinely circumcised by all Muslims and Jews and also by some Christians in Egypt, the United States, and Canada. This routine practice has recently become a subject of debate. Many researchers argue that male circumcision should no longer be an automatic choice, but rather that parents should consider the pros and cons. See the Star Box on page 432 for a look at this debate.

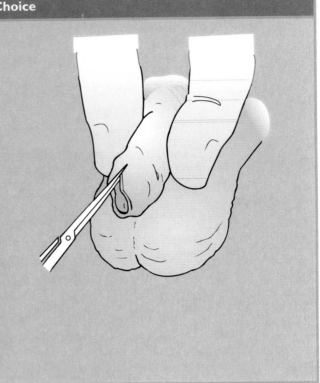

Male Circumcision: No Longer an Automatic Choice

Should newborn boys still be routinely circumcised? Researchers no longer think so. For example, a committee of the Canadian Paediatric Society recently studied the issue and concluded that newborns should not be routinely circumcised. The study compared the costs and complications of the procedure itself, the incidence of urinary tract infections, sexually transmitted diseases, and cancer of the penis in both circumcised and uncircumcised males, and of cervical cancer in their partners. The committee concluded that routine circumcision cannot be justified.[5] This recommendation echoes that of the American Academy of Pediatrics and the Canadian Paediatric Society.

Another study reported that the rate of penile cancer in fact is lower in circumcised men, but that this difference alone is not sufficient to justify routine circumcision. Other researchers are more vehement, calling circumcision the mutilation of healthy organs. If parents do decide on circumcision, it should be performed only by a trained surgeon in a medical institution, as 85 percent of complications and nearly all disastrous circumcisions are performed by traditional, but medically untrained, circumcisers.[6] In addition, the surgeon should have adequate training in pain relief for this treatment, in view of the overwhelming evidence that newborn circumcision is painful.[7] The parents, in consultation with their physician, should make the final decision.[8,9]

The Testes

The testes (also called gonads or testicles) are two egg-shaped bodies that lie within a saclike structure called the scrotum. During most of fetal development, the testes lie within the abdominal cavity. They descend into the scrotum during the last two months of fetal life.

The testes are housed in the scrotum because a temperature lower than the body core temperature is required for adequate sperm development. The walls of the scrotum are composed of contractile tissue and can draw the testes closer to the body during cold temperatures (and sexual arousal) and relax during warm temperatures. Scrotal contraction and relaxation allow a constant, productive temperature to be maintained in the testes.

A cross-sectional view of a single testis reveals an intricate network of structures called *seminiferous tubules* (Figure 14-2B). Within these 300 or so seminiferous tubules, the process of sperm production (spermatogenesis) takes place. Sperm cell development starts at about age eleven in boys and is influenced by the release of the hormone **ICSH (interstitial cell-stimulating hormone)** from the pituitary gland. ICSH does primarily what its name suggests: It stimulates specific cells (called *interstitial cells*) within the testes to begin producing the male sex hormone *testosterone.* Testosterone in turn is primarily responsible for the gradual development of the male secondary sex characteristics at the onset of puberty. By the time a boy is approximately fifteen years old, sufficient levels of testosterone exist so that the testes become capable of full spermatogenesis.

Before the age of about fifteen, most of the sperm cells produced in the testes are incapable of fertilization. The production of fully mature sperm (*spermatozoa*) is triggered by another hormone secreted by the brain's pituitary gland—**FSH (follicle-stimulating hormone)**. FSH influences the seminiferous tubules to begin producing spermatozoa capable of fertilization.

Ducts

Spermatogenesis takes place around the clock, with hundreds of millions of sperm cells produced daily. The sperm cells do not stay in the seminiferous tubules but rather are transferred through a system of ducts that lead into the epididymis. The epididymis is a tubular coil that attaches to the back side of each testicle. These collecting structures house the maturing sperm cells for two to three weeks. During this period the sperm finally become capable of motion, but they remain inactive until they mix with the secretions from the accessory glands (the seminal vesicles, prostate gland, and Cowper's glands).

Each epididymis leads into an eighteen-inch passageway known as the *vas deferens.* Sperm, moved along by the action of hairlike projections called *cilia,* can also remain in the vas deferens for an extended time without losing their ability to fertilize an egg.

Seminal Vesicles

The two vasa deferens extend into the abdominal cavity, where each meets with a *seminal vesicle*—the first of the three accessory structures or glands. Each seminal vesicle contributes a clear, alkaline fluid that nourishes the sperm cells with fructose and permits the sperm cells to be suspended in a movable medium. The fusion of a vas deferens with the seminal vesicle results in the formation of a passageway called the ejaculatory duct. Each ejaculatory duct is only about one inch long and empties into the final passageway for the sperm—the urethra.

Prostate Gland

This juncture takes place in an area surrounded by the second accessory gland—the *prostate gland.* The prostate gland secretes a milky fluid containing a variety of substances, including proteins, cholesterol, citric acid, calcium, buffering salts, and various enzymes. The prostate secretions further nourish the sperm cells and also raise the pH level, making the mixture quite alkaline. The alkalinity permits the sperm to have greater longevity as they are transported during ejaculation through the urethra, out of the penis, and into the highly acidic vagina.

Cowper's Glands

The third accessory gland, the Cowper's glands, serves primarily to lubricate the urethra with a clear, viscous mucus. These paired glands empty their small amounts of preejaculatory fluid during the arousal stage of the sexual response cycle. Alkaline in nature, this fluid also neutralizes the acidic level of the urethra. It is hypothesized that viable sperm cells can be suspended in this fluid and can enter the female reproductive tract before full ejaculation by the male.[3] This may account for many of the failures of the "withdrawal" method of contraception.

The sperm cells, when combined with secretions from the seminal vesicles and the prostate gland, form a sticky substance called **semen**. Interestingly, the microscopic sperm actually makes up less than 5 percent of the seminal fluid discharged at ejaculation. Contrary to popular belief, the paired seminal vesicles contribute about 60 percent of the semen volume, and the prostate gland adds about 30 percent.[10] Thus the fear of some men that a **vasectomy** will destroy their ability to ejaculate is completely unfounded (see Chapter 16).

During *emission* (the gathering of semen in the upper part of the urethra), a sphincter muscle at the base of the bladder contracts and inhibits semen from being pushed into the bladder and urine from being deposited into the urethra.[3] Thus semen and urine rarely intermingle, even though they leave the body through the same passageway.

Penis

Ejaculation takes place when the semen is forced out of the penis through the urethral opening. The involuntary, rhythmic muscle contractions that control ejaculation result in a series of pleasurable sensations known as *orgasm.*

The urethra lies on the underside of the penis and extends through one of three cylindrical chambers of erectile tissue (two *cavernous bodies* and one *spongy body*). Each of these three chambers provides the vascular space required for sufficient erection of the penis. When a male becomes sexually aroused, the areas become congested with blood (*vasocongestion*). After ejaculation or when a male is no longer sexually stimulated, these chambers release the blood into the general circulation and the penis returns to a **flaccid** state.

The *shaft* of the penis is covered by a thin layer of skin that is an extension of the skin that covers the scrotum. This loose layer of skin is sensitive to sexual stimulation and extends over the head of the penis, except in males who have been circumcised. The *glans* (or head) of the penis is the most sexually sensitive (to tactile stimulation) part of the male body. Nerve receptor sites are especially prominent along the *corona* (the ridge of the glans) and the *frenulum* (the thin tissue at the base of the glans).

Later in life, men begin to experience some changes in their reproductive system. The level of androgens, or male hormones, decreases with age, and the size of the prostate gland often increases. A deficiency of androgens has been found to cause health problems in older men, including a lack of strength or energy, changes in mood, osteoporosis, and a decrease in muscle mass.[11]

As a result, researchers are considering the benefits and risks of androgen replacement therapy in men, similar to the estrogen replacement therapy given to women. The benefits are an increase in bone

---

ICSH (interstitial cell-stimulating hormone) (in ter **stish** ul)   a gonadotropic hormone of the male required for the production of testosterone.

FSH (follicle-stimulating hormone)   a gonadotropic hormone required for initial development of ova (in the female) and sperm (in the male).

semen   a secretion containing sperm and nutrients discharged from the urethra at ejaculation.

vasectomy   a surgical procedure in which the vasa deferens are cut to prevent the passage of sperm from the testicles; the most common form of male sterilization.

flaccid (fla sid)   nonerect; the state of erectile tissue when vasocongestion is not occurring.

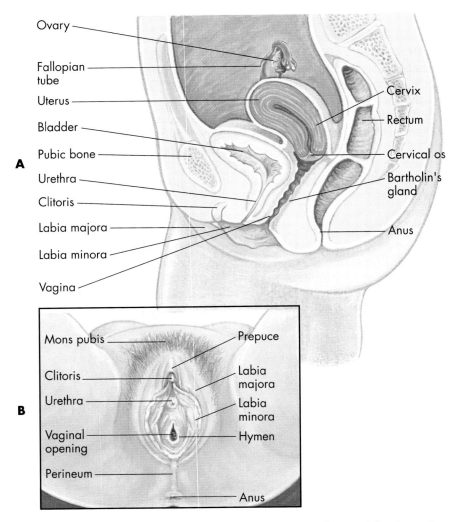

Figure 14-3 **A,** Female reproductive structures, side view. The formation of ova, production of the sex hormones estrogen and progesterone, and support for the developing fetus are functions of the structures of the female reproductive system. **B,** External view of the female genitals.

and muscle mass, improved muscular and cardiovascular function, improved sexual function, and an overall better sense of well-being. The possible risks include an increased incidence of prostate disease and cardiovascular disease.[11] More study is needed.

Female Reproductive System

The external structures (genitals) of the female reproductive system consist of the mons pubis, labia majora, labia minora, clitoris, and vestibule (Figure 14-3). Collectively these structures form the *vulva* or vulval area.

Mons Pubis

The mons pubis is the fatty covering over the pubic bone. The mons pubis (or mons veneris, "mound of Venus") is covered by pubic hair and is quite sensitive to sexual stimulation.

Labia Majora and Labia Minora

The *labia majora* are large longitudinal skin folds that cover the entrance to the vagina, whereas the *labia minora* are the smaller longitudinal skin folds that lie within the labia majora. These hairless skin folds of the labia minora join at the top to form the *prepuce*. The prepuce covers the glans of the *clitoris*, which is the most sexually sensitive part of the female body.

Clitoris

In terms of its tactile sensitivity, the clitoris is the most sensitive part of the female genitals. It contains a glans and a shaft, although the shaft is below the skin surface. It is composed of erectile tissue that can become engorged with blood. It is covered by skin folds (the clitoral prepuce) and can collect **smegma** beneath these tissue folds.[4]

Vestibule

The *vestibule* is the region enclosed by the labia minora. Evident here are the urethral opening and the entrance to the vagina (vaginal orifice). Also located at the vaginal opening are the *Bartholin's glands*, which secrete a minute amount of lubricating fluid during sexual excitement.

The hymen is a thin layer of tissue that stretches across the opening of the vagina. Once thought to be the only indication of virginity, the intact hymen rarely covers the vaginal opening entirely. Openings in the hymen are necessary for the discharge of menstrual fluid and vaginal secretions. Many hymens are stretched or torn to full opening by adolescent physical activity or by the insertion of tampons. In women whose hymens are not fully ruptured, the first act of sexual intercourse will generally accomplish this. Pain may accompany first intercourse in females with relatively intact hymens.

The internal reproductive structures of the female include the vagina, uterus, fallopian tubes, and ovaries.

Vagina

The *vagina* is the structure that forms a canal from the orifice, through the vestibule, to the uterine cervix. Normally the walls of the vagina are collapsed, except during sexual stimulation, when the vaginal walls widen and elongate to accommodate the erect penis. Only the outer third of the vagina is especially sensitive to sexual stimulation. In this location, vaginal tissues swell considerably to form the **orgasmic platform**. This platform constricts the vaginal opening and in effect "grips" the penis—regardless of its size.[4] Thus the belief that a woman receives considerably more sexual pleasure from men with large penises is not supported from an anatomical standpoint.

Uterus

The *uterus* (or *womb*) is approximately the size and shape of a small pear. This highly muscular organ is capable of undergoing a wide range of physical changes, as evidenced by its enlargement during pregnancy, its contraction during menstruation and labor, and its movement during the orgasmic phase of the female sexual response cycle. The primary function of the uterus is to provide a suitable environment for the possible implantation of a fertilized ovum, or egg. This implantation, should it occur, will take place in the innermost lining of the uterus—the *endometrium*. In the mature female, the endometrium undergoes cyclic changes as it prepares a new lining on a near-monthly basis.

The lower third of the uterus is called the *cervix*. The cervix extends slightly into the vagina. Sperm can enter the uterus through the cervical opening, or *cervical os*. Mucous glands in the cervix secrete a fluid that is thin and watery near the time of ovulation. Mucus

of this consistency apparently facilitates sperm passage into the uterus and deeper structures. However, cervical mucus is much thicker during portions of the menstrual cycle when pregnancy is improbable, and during pregnancy, to protect against bacterial agents and other substances that are especially dangerous to the developing fetus.

The upper two-thirds of the uterus is called the *corpus* or *body*. This is where the fertilized ovum generally implants into the uterus.

Fallopian Tubes

The upper portion of the uterus opens into *two fallopian tubes*, sometimes called oviducts or uterine tubes, each about four inches long. The fallopian tubes are each directed toward an ovary. They serve as a passageway for the ovum in its weeklong voyage toward the uterus. In most cases, conception takes place in the upper third of the fallopian tubes.

Ovaries

The ovaries are analogous to the testes in the male. Their function is to produce the ovum, or egg. Usually, one ovary produces and releases just one egg each month. Approximately the size and shape of an unshelled almond, an ovary produces viable ova in the process known as *oogenesis*.

The ovaries also produce the female sex hormones through the efforts of specific structures within the ovaries. These hormones play multiple roles in the development of female secondary sex characteristics, but their primary function is to prepare the endometrium of the uterus for possible implantation of a fertilized ovum. In the average healthy female, this preparation takes place about thirteen times a year for a period of about thirty-five years. At menopause, the ovaries shrink considerably and stop nearly all hormonal production.

Menstrual Cycle

Each month or so, the inner wall of the uterus prepares for a possible pregnancy. When a pregnancy does not occur (as is the case throughout most months of a woman's fertile years), this lining must be released and a new one prepared. The breakdown of this endometrial wall and the resultant discharge of blood and endometrial tissue is known as

---

smegma   cellular discharge that can accumulate beneath the clitoral hood and the foreskin of an uncircumcised penis.

orgasmic platform   expanded outer third of the vagina, which grips penis during sexual intercourse.

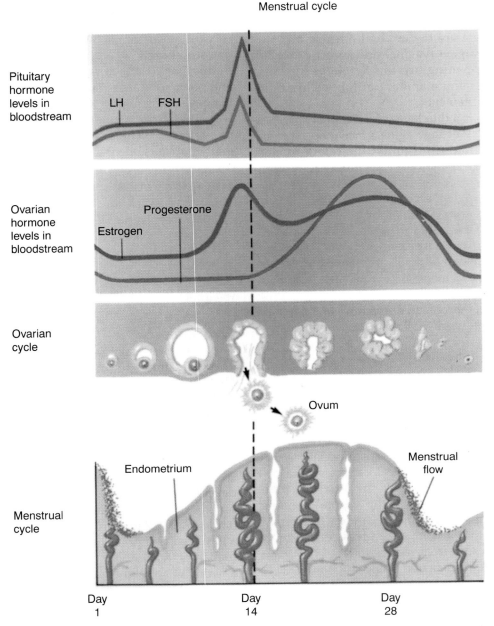

Menstrual cycle

Pituitary hormone levels in bloodstream

LH   FSH

Ovarian hormone levels in bloodstream

Progesterone

Estrogen

Ovarian cycle

Ovum

Menstrual cycle

Endometrium

Menstrual flow

Day 1   Day 14   Day 28

Figure 14-4   The menstrual cycle involves the development and release of an ovum, supported by hormones from the pituitary, and the buildup of the endometrium, supported by hormones from the ovary, for the purpose of establishing a pregnancy.

menstruation (or *menses*) (Figure 14-4). The cyclic timing of this is controlled by a woman's hormones.

Girls generally have their first menstrual cycle, the onset of which is called *menarche,* sometime between 12 and 14 years of age. Recently, doctors have noticed that girls have begun showing the first signs of puberty at an earlier age. At age 8, nearly half of African-American girls and 15 percent of white girls begin to show the first signs of puberty.[12] Researchers worry that the early onset may result from chemicals in the environment that mimic the action of estrogen. They cannot yet explain the racial disparity. Body

weight, nutrition, heredity, and overall health all affect menarche. After a girl first menstruates, her cycles may be anovulatory for a year or longer before a viable ovum is released during her cycle. She will then continue this cyclic activity until age 45 to 55.

This text refers to a menstrual cycle that lasts twenty-eight days. Be assured that few women display absolutely perfect twenty-eight day cycles. Most women fluctuate by a few days to a week or more around this twenty-eight-day pattern.

Your knowledge about the menstrual cycle is critical for your understanding of pregnancy, contra-

Endometriosis

Endometriosis is a condition in which endometrial tissue that normally lines the uterus is found growing within the pelvic cavity. Because the tissue remains sensitive to circulating hormones, it is the source of pain and discomfort during the latter half of the menstrual cycle. Endometriosis is most commonly found in younger women and is frequently related to infertility.

In addition to pain before and during menstruation, the symptoms of endometriosis include low back pain, pain during intercourse, and a variety of lower digestive tract symptoms, such as diarrhea and constipation. As with the general pain and discomfort of endometriosis, these symptoms are also more noticeable during the latter weeks of the cycle.

Treatment of endometriosis largely depends on its extent. Drugs to suppress ovulation, including birth control pills, may be helpful in mild cases. For more severe cases, surgical removal of the tissue or a hysterectomy may be necessary. For some women, endometriosis is suppressed during pregnancy and does not return after pregnancy.

ception, menopause, and issues related to the overall health and comfort of women (see the Star Box above for a discussion of endometriosis). Although seemingly complicated, each segment of the cycle can be studied separately for better understanding.

The menstrual cycle can be thought of as occurring in three segments or phases: the menstrual phase (lasting about one week), the proliferative phase (also lasting about one week), and the secretory phase (lasting about two weeks). Day 1 of this cycle starts with the first day of bleeding, or menstrual flow.

Menstrual Phase

The *menstrual phase* signals the woman that a pregnancy has not taken place and that her uterine lining is being sloughed off. During a five- to seven-day period, a woman will discharge about one-fourth to one-half cup of blood and tissue. (Only about one ounce of the menstrual flow is actual blood.) The menstrual flow is heaviest during the first days of this phase. Because the muscular uterus must contract to accomplish this tissue removal, some women have uncomfortable cramping during menstruation. Most women, however, report more pain and discomfort during the few days before the first day of bleeding. (See the discussion of menstrual pain on p. 438.)

Modern methods of absorbing menstrual flow include the use of internal tampons and external pads. Caution must be exercised by the user of tampons to prevent the possibility of toxic shock syndrome (TSS) (see Chapter 12). Because menstrual flow is a positive sign of good health, women are encouraged to be normally active during menstruation.

Proliferative Phase

The *proliferative phase* of the menstrual cycle starts about the time menstruation stops. Lasting about one week, this phase is first influenced by the release of FSH from the pituitary gland. FSH circulates in the bloodstream and directs the ovaries to start the process of maturing approximately twenty primary ovarian *follicles*. Thousands of primary egg follicles are present in each ovary at birth. These follicles resemble shells that house immature ova. As these follicles ripen under FSH influence, they release the hormone *estrogen*. Estrogen's primary function is to direct the endometrium to start the development of a thick, highly vascular wall. As FSH secretions are reduced, the pituitary gland prepares for the surge of the **luteinizing hormone (LH)** required to accomplish ovulation.[13]

Personal Applications

• To what extent do you think that knowledge about the menstrual cycle will be pertinent to you as you move through adulthood? (This question is for *both* men and women.)

In the days immediately before ovulation, one of the primary follicles (called the *graafian follicle*) matures fully. The other primary follicles degenerate and are absorbed by the body. The graafian follicle moves toward the surface of the ovary. When LH is released in massive quantities on about day 14, the graafian follicle bursts to release the fully mature ovum. The release of the ovum is called **ovulation**. Regardless of the overall length of a woman's cycle, ovulation occurs 14 days before her first day of menstrual flow.

The ovum is quickly captured by the fingerlike projections (*fimbriae*) of the fallopian tubes. In the upper third of the fallopian tubes, the ovum is capable of being fertilized in a twenty-four to thirty-six-hour period. If the ovum is not fertilized by a sperm cell, it will begin to degenerate and eventually be absorbed by the body.

Secretory Phase

After ovulation, the *secretory phase* of the menstrual cycle starts when the remnants of the graafian follicle restructure themselves into a **corpus luteum**. The

luteinizing hormone (LH) (loo ten eye zing) a gonadotropic hormone of the female required for fullest development and release of ova; ovulating hormone.

ovulation   the release of a mature egg from the ovary.

corpus luteum (kore pus **loo** tee um)   cellular remnant of the graafian follicle after the release of an ovum.

HEALTH ACTION GUIDE

Dealing with Menstrual Pain

The medical term is *dysmenorrhea,* but most women know it as menstrual cramps, and most women suffer from it at one time or another. Fortunately, the medical profession seems to be paying more attention to this problem, and various treatments are being studied. Currently, the most popular treatments still seem to be exercise and prostaglandin inhibitors.

The periodic cramps can occur before and during the menstrual phase, when the uterus must contract to remove the uterine lining. These contractions are produced by prostaglandin hormones normally found in the body. The problem occurs when the body produces an excess of one of the prostaglandin hormones, and the result is excessive cramping and pain. Thus prostaglandin-inhibiting medications can be used to reduce the body's production of prostaglandins and thereby reduce the intensity of cramping. Antiprostaglandin medications include ibuprofen, aspirin, and some prescription medications.

Before beginning treatment, however, the first step is to see a physician to rule out other causes of the dysmenorrhea. If other underlying causes are eliminated, consider the following treatment suggestions:

• Consume a well-balanced diet, with limited salt and sugar intake. Reduce spicy foods, and drink six to eight glasses of water per day.

• Consider taking aspirin, ibuprofen, other over-the-counter medications, or prescription medications, with your physician's guidance. Do not take aspirin if you are allergic to aspirin or have anemia, ulcers, or intestinal bleeding.
• Try taking a warm bath or placing a hot water bottle on your abdomen.

Try the following exercise routine that targets menstrual cramping.[14]

• Lie face up with the legs and knees bent; perform abdominal breathing about 10 times. Feel the abdomen slowly inflate and then slowly fall.
• Stand and hold the back of a chair; lift one heel off the floor, then the other. Repeat 20 times.
• Lie on your back; lift and bring your knees to your chin; repeat 10 times.

Other treatments currently being explored include herbal remedies, acupuncture,[15] transcutaneous electrical nerve stimulation,[16] and microwave diathermy.[17] In particular, several studies report relief through the use of a Chinese herb called Shakuyaku-kanzo-to.[18–20] Like several other medications, Shakuyaku-kanzo-to works by reducing the production of prostaglandins.[19]

---

corpus luteum remains inside the ovary, secreting estrogen and a fourth hormone called *progesterone.* Progesterone, which literally means "for pregnancy," continues to direct the endometrial buildup. If pregnancy occurs, the corpus luteum monitors progesterone and estrogen levels throughout the pregnancy. If pregnancy does not occur, high levels of progesterone signal the pituitary to stop the release of LH and the corpus luteum starts to disintegrate on about day 24. When estrogen and progesterone levels diminish significantly by day 28, the endometrium is discharged from the uterus and out the vagina. The secretory phase ends, and the cycle is complete.

Premenstrual Syndrome (PMS)

PMS is characterized by psychological symptoms, such as depression, lethargy, irritability, and aggressiveness, or somatic symptoms, such as headache, backache, asthma, acne, and epilepsy, that recur in the same phase of each menstrual cycle, followed by a symptom-free phase in each cycle. Some of the more frequently reported symptoms of PMS include tension, tender breasts, fainting, fatigue, abdominal cramps, and weight gain.

The cause of PMS appears to be hormonal. Perhaps a woman's body is insensitive to a normal level of progesterone, or her ovaries fail to produce a normal amount of progesterone. These reasons seem plausible because PMS-type symptoms do not occur

during pregnancy, during which natural progesterone levels are very high, and because women with PMS seem to feel much better after receiving high doses of natural progesterone in suppository form. When using oral contraceptives that supply synthetic progesterone at normal levels, many women report relief from some symptoms of PMS. However, the effectiveness of a common form of treatment, progesterone suppositories, is now being questioned. See the Health Action Guide above.

Until the effectiveness of progesterone has been fully researched, the medical community is unlikely to treat PMS through any approach other than a relatively conservative treatment of symptoms with the use of analgesic drugs (including prostaglandin inhibitors), diuretic drugs, dietary modifications (including restriction of caffeine and salt), vitamin B_6 therapy, exercise, and stress-reduction exercises. The exact nature of PMS has been further complicated by the classification of severe PMS as a mental disturbance by some segments of the American Psychiatric Association.

Fibrocystic Breast Condition

In some women, particularly those who have never been pregnant, stimulation of the breast tissues by estrogen and progesterone during the menstrual cycle results in an unusually high degree of secretory activity by the cells lining the ducts. The fluid released by

Hormone Therapy Can Reduce Symptoms of Menopause

You'll remember from Chapter 10, on the cardiovascular system, that hormone-replacement therapy is being used to reduce the risk of cardiovascular disease in many postmenopausal women.

Now researchers have found that hormone replacement therapy (HRT) can also reduce the symptoms of menopause in women who are undergoing this physiological change.

Although attitudes toward this normal change have evolved to the point where most women have positive or neutral attitudes toward menopause,[21] it is frequently accompanied by distressing physical and emotional symptoms.

Women undergoing menopause may suffer any of a variety of symptoms, including flushes, night sweats, vaginal dryness, and insomnia. Researchers have found that HRT can help to control these symptoms. The HRT can include a variety of estrogen and estrogen-progesterone regimens.

As always, women should use all possible nonpharmacologic methods before they consider a pharmacologic solution. Some of the nondrug techniques are exercise, paced breathing, and psychotherapy. In addition, women should stop smoking and maintain a healthy body weight to reduce their symptoms of menopause.

The decision to use hormone replacement therapy is complex. Although its benefits in reducing the symptoms of menopause are established, its other effects are still being studied.[22] Several large clinical trials, including the Women's Health Initiative (WHI) and the Heart and Estrogen Replacement Therapy Study (HERS) in the United States, are currently under way. These trials should answer many of the questions about HRT.

In addition, not all women are candidates for HRT. In particular, women who have a history of estrogen-dependent gynecologic tumors or breast cancer must be evaluated on an individual basis. Other women are unwilling to use this treatment for a variety of reasons, including reluctance to use hormones and fear of unknown risks. These women should compare the potential benefits with the potential risks and also consider the nonpharmacologic techniques.

---

the secretory lining finds its way into the fibrous connective tissue areas in the lower half of the breast, where in pocketlike cysts the fluid presses against neighboring tissues. Excessive secretory activity produces in many women a fibrocystic breast condition characterized by swollen, firm, or hardened tender breast tissue before menstruation.

Recently, researchers have begun to describe the importance of a healthy diet in preventing fibrocystic breast condition, in particular a low-fat diet. Because physicians cannot be certain whether fibroadenomas (benign breast cysts) will ever develop into a full-blown malignancy of the breast, some researchers still prefer to refer to this condition as precancerous, and use such terms as *proliferative breast disease*. Women with more extensive fibrocystic conditions can be treated with drugs that have a "calming" effect on progesterone production. Occasional draining of cysts can bring relief.

Menopause

For the vast majority of women in their late forties through their mid-fifties, a gradual decline in reproductive system function, called *menopause*, occurs. Menopause is a normal physiological process, not a disease process. It can, however, become a health concern for some middle-aged women who have unpleasant side effects resulting from this natural ending of ovum production and menstruation.

As ovarian function and hormone production diminish, the hypothalamus, ovaries, uterus, and other estrogen-sensitive tissues must adjust. The extent of menopause as a health problem is determined by the degree to which **hot flashes**, vaginal wall dry-

ness, depression and melancholy, breast changes, and the uncertainty of fertility are seen as problems.

Many of today's midlife women are likely to find menopause to be a relatively positive experience. The end of fertility, combined with children leaving home, makes the middle years a period of personal rediscovery for many women.

For women who are troubled by the changes brought about by menopause, physicians may prescribe **hormone replacement therapy (HRT)**. This can relieve many symptoms and offer benefits to help reduce the incidence of osteoporosis (see Chapters 4 and 5) and heart disease. The Star Box above takes a closer look at HRT.

Additional Aspects of Human Sexuality

Earlier in this chapter, we identified the biological and psychosocial bases of our sexuality. In this section we explore three additional aspects of our sexuality—reproductive, genital, and expressionistic—around which many of our important decisions in life

---

hot flashes temporary feelings of warmth experienced by women during and after menopause, caused by blood vessel dilation.

hormone replacement therapy (HRT) medically administered estrogen to replace estrogen lost as the result of menopause.

Learning
From Our Diversity

No Fear of Fifty: The New Model for Menopause

Just a generation ago, menopause was regarded almost as a dreaded disease by many women—not to mention the men who were married to them. It was seen not just as the end of fertility but as the loss of youth, attractiveness, femininity, sex appeal, and sexual enjoyment. Both women and their husbands dreaded the onset of hot flashes, mood swings, depression, and loss of sex drive that were commonly believed to be every woman's fate during premenopause. In the minds not just of middle-aged women but also of men and young people, the definition of menopause was "old."

That was then; this is now. With the first women of the baby boom generation now approaching menopause, it's a whole new story. The generation that said it would never get old is not taking menopause on the chin—instead, today's women are fighting back, with every weapon at their command. Regular exercise and stress reducers like meditation and yoga go a long way toward easing the emotional swings associated with menopause—and a balanced diet, rich in healthful sources of calcium, helps stabilize mood and prevent osteoporosis. For some women, estrogen replacement therapy (ERT) is helpful in alleviating unpleasant symptoms of menopause and in reducing bone loss; others opt not to use ERT and instead pursue treatments offered by alternative medicine, or simply let nature take its course.

Jane Fonda . . . Raquel Welch . . . Farrah Fawcett—these are just a few of the "new" 50-plus women who are treating menopause as a natural process instead of a disease. Rather than using menopause as an excuse to stop exercising and eating healthfully, these women and thousands of others see it as a compelling reason to stay fit.

With their children grown and gone, midlife women who have spent decades raising a family now find that they have time to themselves—and for themselves. Career women, whether they're mothers or not, have usually achieved their major goals or are in sight of them, and they no longer need to make an all-out push to scale the corporate or professional ladder. There's more time for friendships, for hobbies and interests, for travel, and for contemplating instead of competing. There's more time for the healthful, self-nuturing pursuits that help ease the transition into menopause. And there's more life to be lived than at any time in the past. No longer considered the figurative end of a woman's life, menopause now is increasingly regarded as a passage into the next stage, with all the challenges and rewards it offers.

Increasingly, physicians are rejecting the "menopause as disease" model in favor of a more positive approach that empowers women to manage this stage of their lives proactively instead of being overwhelmed or overmedicated by it. Women of the baby boom generation may be aging—but they're not doing it passively.

are made.* With these new perspectives in mind, you will be better able to see the complexity associated with our development as productive and satisfied beings.

Reproductive Sexuality

Of these three aspects of sexuality, *reproductive sexuality* reflects the most basic level of sexuality over which the adult must exercise discretion and display insight. Simply stated, reproductive sexuality is related to your knowledge of, desire for, and ability to participate in the act of *procreation*. Pregnancy, delivery, natural childbirth, breastfeeding, fertility control, and pregnancy termination are terms related to this dimension of sexuality. Demographic data indicate that most (but not all) of you will choose to be active in this dimension of your sexuality by becoming parents.

*We cite no specific source for the terms *reproductive sexuality*, *genital sexuality*, and *expressionistic sexuality*. They are labels we and our colleagues use in instructional units associated with human sexuality.

Genital Sexuality

Genital sexuality refers to the nonreproductive use of the reproductive organs. In comparison with the concept of reproductive sexuality, genital sexuality implies recreation and communication rather than procreation. The behaviors and meanings associated with the terms *orgasm, having sex, making love, oral-genital sex* and *sexual responsiveness* are genital in their orientation.

In the most positive sense, sexual experiences that are genitally oriented should be sensual, erotic, and stimulating and should give the individual a sense of release. Genital sexuality reflects our gift to ourselves and to our partners as well. However, many forms of genital sexuality may not be condoned by certain groups of people or religions.

Personal Applications

- Do you think a celibate lifestyle is possible or practical in the present time? Why or why not?
- What are your estimates of the percentages of men and women at your college who have had sexual intercourse?

For some, genital sexuality can be a volatile experience. Far too frequently a genitally centered sexual experience results in an unanticipated and unwanted pregnancy. In such circumstances the couple, or more often the female acting alone, is forced to make decisions that could significantly affect the future. An unexpected pregnancy, even for a relatively mature college person, may result in a series of compromises. In addition, the close association between genital sexuality and sexually transmitted diseases (including HIV infection) makes some sexual activities potentially dangerous.

For some people, genital sexuality becomes the mode of communication with which they feel most comfortable. In such cases, partners may know each other only in a very limited way. Growth in sexual technique may readily occur within the context of a genitally centered relationship, but a fully developed relationship will not be formed. Genitally based relationships are rarely elevated to a much higher level.

Expressionistic Sexuality

Expressionistic sexuality represents the most broadly based dimension of yourself as a man or woman. As the name implies, this is your expression of your current gender schema. Cognitively, *affectively*, and behaviorally, you are playing out your initial adult gender identification. The way you dress, the occupation you pursue, and the leisure activities you develop are all aspects of this dimension of your sexuality.

Expressionistic sexuality encompasses the reproductive and genital dimensions of your sexuality, but it is more. It is the sexuality that will serve you the most fully for the rest of your life. Most adults probably are conventional in their patterns of expressionistic sexuality, yet many people also express a variety of additional patterns (see Chapter 15).

Real Life
Real choices

Your Turn

- What is the term used to describe the blending of male and female qualities?
- Do you identify more strongly with Jerry or with Diana? Why?
- How do you think Diana and Jerry can resolve their conflict over appropriate sex roles for their children?

And Now, Your Choices . . .
- What were your parents' attitudes about sex roles when you were growing up? Were you comfortable with their treatment of you and your siblings in this respect?
- If you are now a parent or plan to have children, do you or will you use your parents' approach to sex roles, or something different? In each case, give reasons for your answer.

Summary

- The biological basis of human sexuality includes genetic, gonadal, and structural components.
- The structural basis of sexuality begins as the male and female reproductive structures develop in the growing embryo and fetus. Structural sexuality changes as one moves through adolescence and later life.
- The psychosocial basis of human sexuality includes gender identity, gender preference, gender adoption, and initial adult gender identification.
- Androgyny is the blending of feminine and masculine qualities; androgynous people are often more flexible, have greater self-esteem, and possess better social skills and motivation to achieve than people who maintain rigid gender roles.
- Circumcision of newborn males can no longer be automatically justified, and parents should make this decision in consultation with their physician.

- The male and female reproductive structures are external and internal. The complex functioning of these structures is controlled by hormones.
- The menstrual cycle's primary functions are to produce ova and to develop a supportive environment for the fetus in the uterus.
- Endometriosis is a condition in which endometrial tissue that normally lines the uterus grows within the pelvic cavity, causing pain before and during menstruation and often leading to infertility.
- Fibrocystic breast condition is characterized by swollen, firm, or hardened tender breast tissue before menstruation.
- Estrogen therapy has benefits in treating the symptoms of menopause and of PMS but may carry risks for some women.
- Androgen replacement therapy has significant benefits for some older men but requires further study before it can be widely prescribed.

- Reproductive sexuality is related to knowledge of, desire for, and ability to participate in the act of procreation.
- Genital sexuality refers to the nonreproductive use of the reproductive organs.

- Expressionistic sexuality is the cognitive, affective, and behavioral expression of your current gender schema.

Review Questions

1. Describe the following foundations of our biological sexuality: the genetic basis, the gonadal basis, and structural development.
2. Define and explain the following terms: gender identity, gender preference, gender adoption, and initial adult gender identification.
3. Define androgyny and explain its advantages.
4. Identify the major components of the male and female reproductive systems. Trace the passageways for sperm and ova.
5. Identify and describe the four main hormones that control the menstrual cycle.
6. What are some of the nonpharmacologic techniques for reducing the symptoms of PMS?
7. What are the symptoms of fibrocystic breast condition and endometriosis?
8. Name two circumstances in which estrogen replacement therapy might be prescribed for women.
9. What is expressionistic sexuality?

References

1. Thibodeau GA, Patton KT. *The human body in health and disease.* St. Louis: Mosby-Year Book, 1996.
2. Hyde JS. *Understanding human sexuality.* 5th ed. New York: McGraw-Hill, 1994.
3. Haas K, Haas A. *Understanding sexuality.* 3rd ed. St. Louis: Mosby, 1993.
4. Crooks R, Baur K. *Our sexuality.* 7th ed. Pacific Grove, CA: Brooks/Cole Publishing, 1998.
5. Anonymous. Neonatal circumcision revisited. Fetus and Newborn Committee, Canadian Paediatric Society (review) *Can Med Assoc J* 1996 March 15; 154(6):769–80.
6. Azdemir E. Significantly increased complication risks with mass circumcisions. *Br J Urol* 1997; 80(1):136–39.
7. Howard CR et al. Neonatal circumcision and pain relief: current training practices. *Pediatrics* 1998; 101 (3, part 1 of 2):423–28.
8. Tran PT, Giacomantonio M. Routine neonatal circumcision? (review). *Can Family Physician* 1996 Nov; 42:2201–04.
9. Laumann EO, Masi CM, Zuckerman EW. Circumcision in the United States. Prevalence, prophylactic effects, and sexual practice. *JAMA* 1997; 277(13):1052–57.
10. Thibodeau GA, Patton KT. *Structure and function of the body.* 10th ed. St. Louis: Mosby-Year Book, 1996.
11. Swedloss RS, Wang C. Androgen deficiency and aging in men (review), *West J Med* 1993 Nov; 159(50):579–85.
12. Health report. *Time* 1997 April 21:36.
13. Hatcher RA et al. *Contraceptive technology.* 17th ed. New York: Irvington Publishers, 1998.
14. *Exercise: dysmenorrhea exercise.* Beaverton, OR: Integrated BodyMind Information System, Integrated Medical Arts Group, 1998.
15. Tsenov D. The effect of acupuncture in dysmenorrhea. *Akush Ginekol (Sofiia)* 1996; 35(3):24–25.
16. Kaplan B et al. Transcutaneous electrical nerve stimulation (TENS) as a pain-relief device in obstetrics and gynecology. *Clin Exp Obstet Gynecol* 1997; 24(3):123–26.
17. Vance AR, Hayes SH, Spielholz NI. Microwave diathermy treatment for primary dysmenorrhea. *Phys Ther* 1996; 76(9):1003–8.
18. Kotani N et al. Analgesic effect of a herbal medicine for treatment of primary dysmenorrhea—a double-blind study. *Am J Chin Med* 1997; 25(2):205–12.
19. Imai A et al. Possible evidence that the herbal medicine shakuyaku-kanzo-to decreases prostaglandin levels through suppressing arachidonate turnover in endometrium. *J. Med* 1995; 26(3–4):163–74.
20. Shibata T et al. The effect of Shakuyaku-kanzo-to on prostaglandin production in human uterine myometrium. *Nippon Sanka Fujinka Gakkai Zasshi* 1996 May; 48(5):321–27.
21. Blumberg G et al. Women's attitudes towards menopause and hormone replacement therapy. *Int J Gynaecol Obstet* 1996; 54(3):271–77.
22. Johnson SR. Menopause and hormone replacement therapy. *Med Clin North Am* 1998; 82(2):297–320.

Suggested Readings

Choi P. *Female sexuality: psychology, biology, and social context.* Paramus, NJ: Prentice Hall, 1995. Contributors to this book challenge current scientific and popular beliefs about female sexuality. They explore topics such as sexual orientation and sexuality over the menstrual cycle.

Fausto-Sterling A. *Myths of gender: biological theories about women and men.* New York: Basic Books, 1992. A biologist examines biological, genetic, evolutionary, and psychological evidence and finds a lack of substance behind ideas about biologically based sex differences.

A Woman's Place: Reconsidering Gender Roles

In the 1996 film *Tin Cup*, Kevin Costner's golf-pro character stumps his bar buddies with the following riddle:

> A man is driving down the road with his son, and they get into an accident. Two ambulances arrive and take them to separate hospitals. When the son is wheeled into the operating room, the doctor looks at the boy and says, 'I can't operate on this boy—he's my son.' Who is the doctor?

Just as he's about to collect on his bet that no one can solve the riddle, Rene Russo enters the bar and says, "The doctor's a woman—she's the boy's mother."[1] This riddle illustrates how deeply gender stereotypes affect our decision making. You may have heard this riddle before, guessed the answer because of the focus of this chapter, or known the answer because you hold less rigid gender stereotypes than most people. Although Costner's character was enlightened enough to tell the riddle, he was still surprised when his next appointment for golf lessons—with a Dr. Griswald—turned out to be with Rene Russo's female psychologist character. We, too, may be aware of some of the gender stereotypes we hold but be unaware and somewhat guided by others.

A Pink- and Blue-Collar World

Women are entering male-dominated fields, such as politics, science, medicine, law, business, and blue-collar jobs, in increasing numbers. Men, too, are breaking into career fields not normally associated with their gender, becoming nurses, flight attendants, office administrators, and elementary school teachers.[2] Still, many career fields reveal a gender gap (see the table on the next page).

Although many career fields are dominated by men, more women than men are enrolled in U.S. colleges and universities. Collegiate women first found themselves in the majority in 1978, six years after Title IX legislation ended discriminatory admissions policies at most public colleges.[3] However, male and female students continue to be taught primarily by men.[4] And studies have shown that both male and

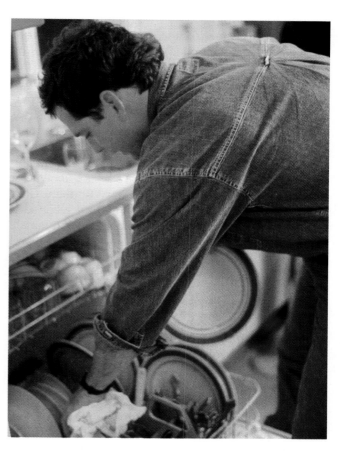

Marriage may be more satisfying for both partners when men and women take equal responsibility for household tasks and childrearing.

female faculty and students retain traditional stereotypes of men and women, even though they may view themselves individually outside the bounds of such stereotypes.[4]

As difficult as it may be for women pioneers in male-dominated fields, it may be even more difficult for men to enter traditionally female occupations. These areas traditionally pay less and are more likely to be part-time.[2] Men also struggle against a lack of flexibility in gender role behavior permitted by society.[5] Two-thirds of U.S. women report having been

Career Field	Percent Male[8]	Career Field	Percent Female[8]
Firefighters	97	Secretaries	98.7
Airplane pilots	96	Family child care	98.5
Civil engineers	92	Dental hygienists	98.4
Electrical engineers	89	Preschool and kindergarten teachers	98
Police officers	87	Registered nurses	94
Dentists	87	Elementary teachers	86
Physicists	85		
Doctors	79		
Lawyers	73		
Full-time university faculty[4]	73		

tomboys as young girls, a designation that is often popular with peers.[2] Yet the connotation of the word "sissy," sometimes applied to young boys, carries no such positive meaning.

The most challenging "feminine" fields for men to break into may not be career fields but interpersonal roles. Interpersonal and family relationships tend to be more successful and satisfying when there is an equitable gender stance. Despite the fact that women have traditionally been the homemakers and caregivers, that may not be the best arrangement for raising children. As First Lady Hillary Rodham Clinton says, "Children deserve the benefit of what society has traditionally considered to be male and female traits and skills to meet their physical, emotional, and intellectual needs and to offer them models for a range of human behaviors."[6]

Sex Role Pioneers

Since our society began reexamining its gender roles in the 1960s, many people have crossed over from their "assigned" roles into roles of the other gender, setting examples for young men and women to follow. For example, the field of government now boasts Attorney General Janet Reno and Secretary of State Madeleine Albright. Former senator Bob Dole was defeated in his run for president in the last presidential election, but his wife Elizabeth is being mentioned as potential candidate for a future presidential election. Likewise, Hillary Rodham Clinton has been considered a possible candidate to become the first president of the twenty-first century.

Men employed in traditionally "women's work," such as nursing, no longer elicit the same shock they once did. Unfortunately, when they assume these roles, men also take on the same disadvantages that women have long endured, including lower pay and less respect. Men who take time to help raise their families and assist in household duties also have made progress. For example, parental leave for both men and women has become a national issue, newspapers publish more stories on househusbands, and parenting magazines now target male as well as

female readers. Unfortunately, these men also face a public perception shaped by sitcom plots and long-held stereotypes.[7]

Sex Roles—Origins and Culture

Gender is but one facet of our complex identities. In addition to being male or female, we are members of racial, ethnic, religious, and class subsets of society. Of these, Freud remarked that "male or female is the first differentiation that you make when you meet another human being."[8] We actually find it difficult to relate to gender-ambiguous people, such as the Saturday Night Live character "Pat." As much as we take gender assignment for granted, it is actually a complicated combination of chromosomes, hormones, reproductive organs, and socialization to cultural norms.[2] Biology "makes the body for which cultures have expectations."[9] The body that biology gives us is changeable with modern techniques; the cultural component may be more fundamental. The same baby is treated differently based on the assumptions of the perceiver. If the baby is believed to be a boy, "he" is bounced, tossed, and roughhoused more. When the same child is thought to be a girl, "she" is talked to more.[5] One researcher asserts that "except at birth, physical body parts play an insignificant role in gender attribution."[8] It is our "cultural genitals," those that society ascribes as appropriate to our dress and behavior, that determine how others relate to us and what they expect from us.[8]

Identifying with one gender or another, and accepting the societal expectations that go along with that gender, does have some advantages. It helps us make sense of the world and gives us a feeling of belonging.[10]

Gender-Aware Therapy

As recently as the 1960s, gender roles were not studied. It was simply understood that men did masculine things and women did feminine things.[11] Recently, however, a new form of counseling, gender-aware therapy, seeks to help clients understand social concepts of gender and how such concepts limit the feelings, thoughts, and behavior of men and women, possibly contributing to the problems for which the individuals are seeking counseling.[12] Among the problems likely to be rooted in gender stereotyping are communication disorders, marital dissatisfaction, domestic violence, financial concerns, childrearing, eating disorders, substance abuse, and depression.[12]

Gender Identity Disorders

Gender itself, or more specifically a person's discomfort with his or her gender, can require counseling. Boys who have gender identity disorders are five times more likely to be referred for psychiatric help than girls.[9] If a person continues to be uncomfortable with his or her gender in adulthood, sex reassignment surgery is an option. "Transgenders," as they describe themselves, have become the newest group to demand equality.[13] Although only one state, Minnesota, has a law protecting transgenders from job and housing discrimination, several cities (including San Francisco, Seattle, and Evanston, Illinois) have passed similar legislation.

Androgyny

Rigid sex-role expectations can harm both individuals and society. The masculine bias in American society values qualities such as decisiveness, independence, and competitiveness. These characteristics are associated with self-esteem.[11] However, strict adherence to this role precludes having strong emotional support networks and thus may lead to loneliness, depression, or even physical health problems.[5]

Androgyny is the blending of masculine and feminine traits. Androgynous people are more flexible and are generally psychologically healthier. And groups with higher levels of androgyny tend to make more balanced decisions.[14] Thus it is in everyone's interest to accommodate and value a range of masculine and feminine traits in each person.

For Discussion . . .

Have you been told that you shouldn't or couldn't do something based on your gender? Did this affect your actions? Do you behave differently with your same-gender friends from how you do when you are with the opposite sex? What do you think of men and women who do not behave traditionally?

References

1. *Tin cup.* Warner Brothers, 1996.
2. Adler, LL. *International handbook on gender roles.* Westport, CT: Greenwood Press, 1993.
3. Compiled from Wire Services. Discrimination in education affects both male and female students on college campuses. St. Louis University, the *University News* Friday August 29, 1997.
4. Street S, Kromrey JD, Kimmelo E. University faculty gender roles perceptions. *Sex Roles: A Journal of Research* 1995; 32(5–6):407–23.
5. Beal, CR. *Boys and girls: the development of gender roles.* New York: McGraw-Hill, 1994.
6. Clinton HR. *It takes a village, and other lessons children teach us.* NY: Simon & Schuster, 1996.
7. Coltrane S. *Family man: fatherhood, housework, and gender equity.* NY: Oxford University Press, 1996.
8. Franke, KM. The central mistake of sex discrimination law: the disaggregation of sex from gender. *University of Pennsylvania Law Review* 1995; 144(1):1–99.
9. Frable DES. Gender, racial, ethnic, sexual, and class identities. *Annual Review of Psychology* 1997; 48:139–62.
10. Lott B. Politics or science? The question of gender sameness/difference. *American Psychologist* 1996; 51(2):155–56.
11. Burnett JW, Anderson WP, Heppner, PP. Gender roles and self-esteem: a consideration of environmental factors. *Journal of Counseling and Development* 1995; 73(3):323–26.
12. Good GE, Gilbert LA, Scher M. Gender aware therapy. *Journal of Counseling and Development* 1990; 68:376–80.
13. Cloud C. Trans across America. *Time* 1998; 152(3).
14. Kirchmeyer C. Gender roles and decision-making in demographically diverse groups: a case for reviving androgyny. *Sex Roles: A Journal of Research* 1996; 34(9–10):649–63.

InfoLinks
www.law.duke.edu/journals/djglp/
www.greatwomen.org

chapter

fifteen

Understanding Sexual Behavior and Relationships

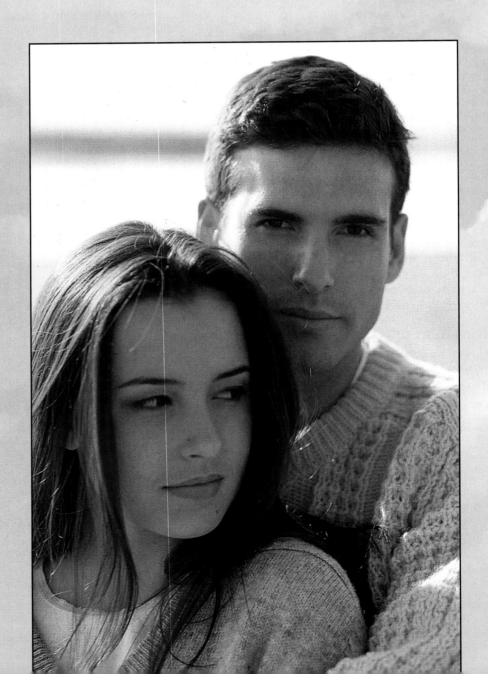

As we begin a new century and a new millennium, we have reached a greater understanding of the psychosocial factors that contribute to the complex expression of our sexuality. In this chapter, we explore human sexuality as it relates to the dynamic interplay of the psychosocial bases of sexual behavior and relationships.

We begin by examining the human sexual response pattern and types of sexual behavior. Then we take a look at the dating process, love, and a variety of relationships, such as friendship, marriage, and cohabitation. The chapter concludes with a discussion of sexual orientation and gender identity. Whether you choose to remain single or to form an intimate relationship, we think you will find these topics important and relevant to your own life.

HEALTHY PEOPLE: LOOKING AHEAD TO 2010

The *Healthy People 2010* document is not expected to focus particular attention on key indicators of progress in the areas of sexual behavior and relationships. No *Healthy People 2000* objectives specifically dealt with the quality of relationships and the ability to develop intimate relationships. No objectives were directed toward sexual performance, sexual satisfaction, or sexual dysfunction. (Although the *Healthy People 2010* document will address key indicators concerning contraception and pregnancy-related health issues, these will be discussed in Chapters 16 and 17.)

However, two pertinent areas examined in the *Healthy People 2000 Midcourse Review* were the areas of "age of initial sexual intercourse" and "unintended pregnancies" among adolescents and young adults. Progress toward achieving the target goals in these areas has not been good. Despite intensive efforts to curb early sexual exploration, the age of initial sexual intercourse continues to drop. Not surprisingly, we are moving away from the goal of fewer unintended pregnancies among adolescents. However, some small gains have been made in promoting abstinence among girls who have already been sexually active.

The pressure to be sexually active at earlier and earlier ages seems to have taken its toll, as increasing numbers of teenagers experience sexual intercourse at very young ages. This behavior can have a number of negative health consequences, including increases in unintended pregnancies and increases in the spread of sexually transmitted diseases. These are the physical offshoots of early sexual exploration. The mental and emotional consequences for both children and their families will add to the obstacles that some of our young people face.

The one positive gain reported in the *Healthy People 2000 Midcourse Review* concerned so-called "secondary virginity" (or secondary abstinence—the noncontinuation of intercourse after initial exploration). If we can continue to encourage youth to change their early, and perhaps risky, sexual behaviors, then not only will unintended pregnancies likely decline, but also youth can gain a more mature perspective on their sexual behavior and relationships. These perspectives will be beneficial as they move further into young adulthood.

Real Life
Real choices

I Love You, But . . . Running from the "M" Word

- Name: Kim Hendricks
- Age: 22
- Occupation: Law Student

"Love and marriage, love and marriage/Go together like a horse and carriage . . ." So went the lyrics to a popular song of the early 1950s, when most Americans still believed that true love always led to the exchange of vows to love, honor, and cherish till death do us part.

But although lifelong commitments offer comfort and security to many people, there are those, like Kim Hendricks, to whom weddings, rings, and promises are a cruel hoax. Her parents were divorced when she was in the first grade, and she and her older brothers not only had to deal with shuttling between two households but also had to adjust to a bewildering succession of new stepparents and siblings as their parents continued their pattern of marrying, divorcing, and remarrying. Every time, Kim recalls, she and her brothers heard the same refrain from a parent: "This is really the one, kids. This won't be like it was with Bob (or Irene). We're finally going to be a real family."

Despite these promises and each parent's good intentions, however, somehow the happy, stable, "forever" family scene never made it to real life. Kim's parents weren't promiscuous or abusive—they just kept repeating their old mistakes and dragging their children into each new "dream" marriage.

As a teenager, Kim enjoyed dating and the usual round of high school social activities; but no matter how much she liked and was attracted to a boy, she never wanted to get serious or talk about the future. When she was applying to colleges, she chose schools that were far from her hometown, which not only enabled her to get away from her parents' tangled lives but also made it easier to break up with her high school boyfriend.

Kim worked hard to obtain a scholarship during her undergraduate years. Now busy with her studies, Kim is very involved with the pressures and demands of law school, as well as occasionally tutoring students for extra income. She talks with her parents and brothers on the phone but rarely visits, always claiming to be too swamped at school. She's comfortable with her sexuality and twice has been in love, but at the first mention of a long-term commitment, she runs fast the other way rather than get tangled up in the sad chaos typical of her parents' marriage-go-round.

As you study this chapter, think about Kim's childhood experiences and resulting feelings, and prepare yourself to answer the questions in **Your Turn** at the end of the chapter.

The Human Sexual Response Pattern

Although history has many written and visual accounts of the human's ability to be sexually aroused, it was not until the pioneering work of Masters and Johnson[1] that the events associated with arousal were clinically documented. These researchers posed the following five questions, which gave direction to a series of studies involving the scientific evaluation of human sexual response.

Do the Sexual Responses of Men and Women Have a Predictable Pattern?

The answer to the first question posed by the researchers was an emphatic *yes*. A predictable sexual response pattern was identified;[1] it consists of an initial **excitement stage**, a **plateau stage**, an **orgasmic stage**, and a **resolution stage**. Each stage involves predictable changes in the structural characteristics and physiological function of reproductive and nonreproductive organs in both the male and female. These changes are shown in the Star Box on pages 450–451.

Is the Sexual Response Pattern Stimuli-Specific?

The research of Masters and Johnson[1] clearly established a *no* answer to the second question concerning stimuli specificity. Their findings demonstrated that several senses can supply the stimuli necessary for initiating the sexual response pattern. Although touching activities might initiate arousal in most people and maximize it for the vast majority of people, in both men and women, sight, smell, sound, and *vicariously formed stimuli* can also stimulate the same sexual arousal patterns.

What Differences Occur in the Sexual Response Pattern?

Differences between Men and Women

In response to the third question, several differences are observable when comparing the sexual response patterns of men and women:

- With the exception of some late adolescent males, the vast majority of men are not multiorgasmic. The **refractory phase** of the resolution stage prevents most men from experiencing more than one orgasm in a short time, even though sufficient stimulation is available.

- Women possess a **multiorgasmic capacity.** Masters and Johnson[1] found that as many as 10 percent to 30 percent of all female adults routinely experience multiple orgasms.
- Although they possess multiorgasmic potential, some 10 percent of all women are *anorgasmic*— that is, they never experience an orgasm.[1] For many anorgasmic women, orgasms can be experienced when masturbation, rather than **coitus,** provides the stimulation.
- When measured during coitus, men reach orgasm far more quickly than do women. However, when masturbation is the source of stimulation, women reach orgasm as quickly as men.[1]

More important than any of the differences pointed out is the finding that the sexual response patterns of men and women are far more alike than they are different. Not only do men and women experience the four basic stages of the response pattern, but they also have similar responses in specific areas, including the **erection** and *tumescence* of sexual structures; the appearance of a **sex flush;** the increase in cardiac output, blood pressure, and respiratory rate; and the occurrence of *rhythmic pelvic thrusting.*[1]

Differences among Subjects within a Same-Gender Group

When a group of subjects of the same gender was studied in an attempt to answer questions about similarities and differences in the sexual response pattern, Masters and Johnson noted considerable variation. Even when variables such as age, race, education, and general health were held constant, the extent and duration of virtually every stage of the response pattern varied.

Differences within the Same Individual

For a given person the nature of the sexual response pattern does not remain constant, even when observed over a relatively short period. A variety of internal and external factors can alter this pattern. The aging process, changes in general health status, levels of stress, altered environmental settings, use of alcohol and other drugs, and behavioral changes in a sexual partner can cause one's own sexual response pattern to change from one sexual experience to another.[2] Sexual performance difficulties and therapies are discussed in the Star Box on page 452.

What Are the Basic Physiological Mechanisms Underlying the Sexual Response Pattern?

The basic mechanisms in the fourth question posed by Masters and Johnson are now well recognized. One factor, *vasocongestion,* or the retention of blood or fluid

within a particular tissue, is critically important in the development of physiological changes that promote the sexual response pattern.[1] The presence of erectile tissue underlies the changes that can be noted in the penis, breasts, and scrotum of the male and the clitoris, breasts, and labia minora of the female.

A second mechanism now recognized as necessary for the development of the sexual response pattern is that of *myotonia,* or the buildup of neuromuscular tension within a variety of body structures.[3] At the end of the plateau stage of the response pattern, a sudden release of the accumulated neuromuscular tension gives rise to the rhythmic muscular contractions and pleasurable muscular spasms that constitute orgasm, as well as ejaculation in the male.

What Role Is Played by Specific Organs and Organ Systems Within the Sexual Response Pattern?

The fifth question posed by Masters and Johnson, which concerns the role played by specific organs and organ systems during each stage of the response pattern, can be readily answered by referring to the material presented in the following Star Box. As you study this box, remember that direct stimulation of the penis and either direct or indirect stimulation of the clitoris are the principal avenues toward orgasm. Also, intercourse represents only one activity that can lead to orgasmic pleasure.[4]

---

excitement stage   initial arousal stage of the sexual response pattern.

plateau stage   second stage of the sexual response pattern; a leveling off of arousal immediately before orgasm.

orgasmic stage   third stage of the sexual response pattern; the stage during which neuromuscular tension is released.

resolution stage   fourth stage of the sexual response pattern; the return of the body to a preexcitement state.

refractory phase   that portion of the male's resolution stage during which sexual arousal cannot occur.

multiorgasmic capacity   potential to have several orgasms within a single period of sexual arousal.

coitus (co ih tus)   penile-vaginal intercourse.

erection   the engorgement of erectile tissue with blood; characteristic of the penis, clitoris, nipples, labia minora, and scrotum.

sex flush   the reddish skin response that results from increasing sexual arousal.

Sexual Response Pattern

Unaroused Stage

Vas deferens
Bladder
Sphincteric band
Prostate gland
Urethral sphincter
Urethra
Penis
Scrotum
Testicle
Urethral bulb
Cowper's gland
Anus
Seminal vesicle

Uterus
Cervix
Vagina
Anus
Labia minora
Labia majora
Clitoris
Bartholin gland
Pubic bone
Bladder

Excitement Stage

Urethral opening dilates slightly
Partially aroused penis becomes erect
Testicles start to engorge and move closer to body
Scrotal skin thickens and tightens

Uterus enlarges and elevates
Clitoris enlarges in size
Labia majora flatten and separate
Labia minora swell and become darker
Inner two-thirds of vagina balloons and lengthens
Vaginal walls begin to lubricate

Plateau Stage

Glans enlarges and color deepens
Preejaculate fluid may be secreted from the Cowper's gland
Scrotal skin remains thick and tense
Testicles become completely engorged and elevated
Urethral bulb expands

Clitoris retracts under hood
Labia minora become even deeper in color
Outer third of vagina swells while narrowing the vagina to form orgasmic platform
Inner two-thirds of vagina expands to form a pool for semen

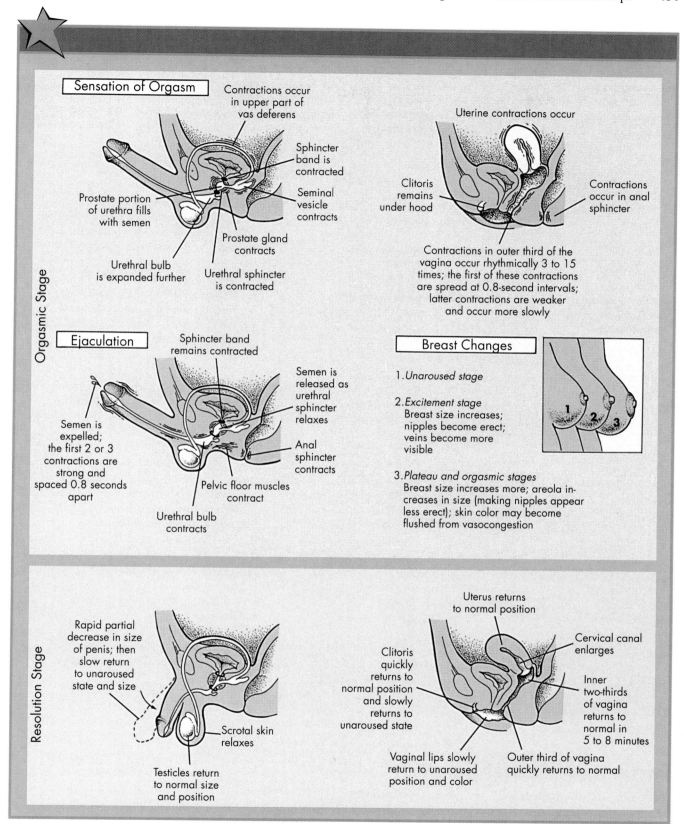

Orgasmic Stage

Sensation of Orgasm

Contractions occur in upper part of vas deferens

Sphincter band is contracted

Seminal vesicle contracts

Prostate portion of urethra fills with semen

Prostate gland contracts

Urethral bulb is expanded further

Urethral sphincter is contracted

Uterine contractions occur

Clitoris remains under hood

Contractions occur in anal sphincter

Contractions in outer third of the vagina occur rhythmically 3 to 15 times; the first of these contractions are spread at 0.8-second intervals; latter contractions are weaker and occur more slowly

Ejaculation

Sphincter band remains contracted

Semen is released as urethral sphincter relaxes

Semen is expelled; the first 2 or 3 contractions are strong and spaced 0.8 seconds apart

Anal sphincter contracts

Pelvic floor muscles contract

Urethral bulb contracts

Breast Changes

1. Unaroused stage

2. Excitement stage
Breast size increases; nipples become erect; veins become more visible

3. Plateau and orgasmic stages
Breast size increases more; areola increases in size (making nipples appear less erect); skin color may become flushed from vasocongestion

Resolution Stage

Rapid partial decrease in size of penis; then slow return to unaroused state and size

Scrotal skin relaxes

Testicles return to normal size and position

Uterus returns to normal position

Cervical canal enlarges

Clitoris quickly returns to normal position and slowly returns to unaroused state

Inner two-thirds of vagina returns to normal in 5 to 8 minutes

Vaginal lips slowly return to unaroused position and color

Outer third of vagina quickly returns to normal

Sexual Performance Difficulties and Therapies

For all of the predictability of the human sexual response pattern, many people find that at some point in their lives, they are no longer capable of responding sexually. The inability of a person to perform adequately is identified as a sexual difficulty or dysfunction. Sexual difficulties can have a negative influence on a person's sense of sexual satisfaction and on a partner's satisfaction. Fortunately, most sexual difficulties can be resolved through strategies that use individual, couple, or group counseling. Most sexual performance difficulties stem from psychogenic factors.

Difficulty	Possible Causes	Therapeutic Approaches
Women		
Orgasmic Difficulties Inability to have orgasm	Anxiety, fear, guilt, anger, poor self-concept; lack of knowledge about female responsiveness; inadequate sexual arousal; interpersonal problems with partner	Counseling to improve a couple's communication; educating a woman and her partner about female responsiveness; teaching a woman how to experience orgasm through masturbation
Vaginismus Painful, involuntary contractions of the vaginal muscles	Previous traumatic experiences with intercourse (rape, incest, uncaring partners); fear of pregnancy; religious prohibitions; anxiety about vaginal penetration of any kind (including tampons)	Counseling to alleviate psychogenic causes; gradual dilation of the vagina with woman's fingers or dilators; systematic desensitization exercises; relaxation training
Dyspareunia Painful intercourse	Insufficient sexual arousal; communication problems with partner; infections, inflammation; structural abnormalities; insufficient lubrication	Individual and couple counseling with a focus on relaxation and communication; medical strategies to reduce infections and structural abnormalities
Men		
Erectile Dysfunction Inability to achieve an erection (impotence)	Chronic diseases (including diabetes, vascular problems, and chemical dependencies); trauma; numerous psychogenic factors (including anxiety, guilt, fear, poor self-concept)	Medical intervention (including possible vascular surgery, drugs, or the use of penile implants); couple counseling using sensate focusing, pleasuring, and relaxation strategies
Rapid Ejaculation Ejaculating too quickly after penile penetration; premature ejaculation	Predominantly psychogenic in origin; a man's need to prove his sexual prowess; anxiety associated with previous sexual experiences	Counseling to free the man from the anxiety associated with rapid ejaculation; altering coital position, masturbation before intimacy; use of the squeeze technique as orgasm approaches
Dyspareunia Painful intercourse	Primarily physical in origin; inability of the penile foreskin to retract fully; urogenital tract infections; scar tissue in seminal passageways; insufficient lubrication	Medical care to reduce infection or repair damaged or abnormal tissue; additional lubrication

Patterns of Sexual Behavior

Although sex researchers may see sexual behavior in terms of the human sexual response pattern just described, most people are more interested in the observable dimensions of sexual behavior.

Celibacy

Celibacy can be defined as the self-imposed avoidance of sexual intimacy. Celibacy is synonymous with sexual abstinence. People could choose not to have a sexually intimate relationship for many reasons. For some, celibacy is part of a religious doctrine. Others might be afraid of contracting a sexually transmitted disease. For most, however, celibacy is preferred simply because it seems appropriate for them. Celibate people can certainly have deep, intimate relationships with other people—just not sexual relationships. Celibacy may be short term or last a lifetime, and no identified physical or psychological complications appear to result from a celibate lifestyle. For a look at the popularity of celibacy on college campuses, see the Star Box on page 464.

Masturbation

Throughout recorded history, **masturbation** has been a primary method of achieving sexual pleasure. Through masturbation, people can explore their sexual response patterns. Traditionally, some societies and religious groups have condemned this behavior based on the belief that intercourse is the only "right" sexual behavior. With sufficient lubrication, masturbation cannot do physical harm. Today masturbation is considered by most sex therapists and researchers to be a normal source of self-pleasure.

Fantasy and Erotic Dreams

The brain is the most sensual organ in the body. In fact, many sexuality experts classify **sexual fantasies** and **erotic dreams** as forms of sexual behavior. Particularly for people whose verbal ability is highly developed, the ability to create imaginary scenes enriches other forms of sexual behavior.

Sexual fantasies are generally found in association with some second type of sexual behavior. When occurring before intercourse or masturbation, fantasies prepare a person for the behavior that will follow. As an example, fantasies experienced while reading a book may focus your attention on sexual activity that will occur later in the day.

When fantasies occur with another form of sexual behavior, the second behavior may be greatly enhanced by the supportive fantasy. Both women and men fantasize during foreplay and intercourse. Masturbation and fantasizing are inseparable activities.

Erotic dreams occur during sleep in both men and women. The association between these dreams and ejaculation resulting in a nocturnal emission (wet dream) is readily recognized in men. In women, erotic dreams can lead not only to vaginal lubrication but to orgasm as well.

Shared Touching

Virtually the entire body can be an erogenous zone when sensual contact between partners is involved. A soft, light touch, a slight application of pressure, the brushing back of a partner's hair, and gentle massage are all forms of communication that heighten sexual arousal.

Genital Contact

Two important purposes can be identified for the practice of stimulating a partner's genitals. The first is the tactile component of **foreplay**. Genital contact, in the form of holding, rubbing, stroking, or caressing, heightens arousal to a level that allows for progression into intercourse.

The second role of genital contact is that of *mutual masturbation to orgasm*. Stimulation of the genitals so that both partners have orgasm is a form of sexual behavior practiced by many people, as well as by couples during the late stage of a pregnancy. For couples not desiring pregnancy, the risk of conception is virtually eliminated when this becomes the form of sexual intimacy practiced.

As is the case in other aspects of intimacy, genital stimulation is best enhanced when partners can talk about their needs, expectations, and reservations. Practice and communication can shape this form of contact into a pleasure-giving approach to sexual intimacy.

Oral-Genital Stimulation

Oral-genital stimulation brings together two of the body's most erogenous areas: the genitalia and the mouth. Couples who engage in oral sex consistently report that this form of intimacy is highly satisfactory. Some people have experimented with oral sex and found it unacceptable, and some have never experienced this form of sexual intimacy. Some couples prefer not to participate in oral sex because they consider it immoral (according to religious doctrine), illegal (which it is in some states), or unhygienic (because of a partner's unclean genitals). Some couples may refrain because of the mistaken belief that oral sex is a homosexual practice. Regardless of the reason, a person who does not consider oral sex to be pleasurable should not be coerced into this behavior.

Because oral-genital stimulation can involve an exchange of body fluids, the risk of disease transmission is real. Small tears of mouth or genital tissue may allow transmission of disease-causing pathogens. Only couples who are absolutely certain that they are free from all sexually transmitted diseases (including HIV infection) can practice unprotected oral sex. Couples in doubt should refrain from oral-genital sex or carefully use a condom (on the male) or a latex square to cover the female's vulval area. Increasingly, latex squares (dental dams) can be obtained from drug stores or

---

masturbation   self-stimulation of the genitals.

sexual fantasies   fantasies with sexual themes; sexual daydreams or imaginary events.

erotic dreams   dreams whose content elicits a sexual response.

foreplay   activities, often involving touching and caressing, that prepare individuals for sexual intercourse.

pharmacies. (Dentists may also provide you with dental dams, or you can make your own latex square by cutting a condom into an appropriate shape.)

Three basic forms of oral-genital stimulation are practiced by both heterosexual and homosexual couples.[4] **Fellatio,** in which the penis is sucked, licked, or kissed by the partner, is the most common of the three. **Cunnilingus,** in which the vulva of the female is kissed, licked, or penetrated by the partner's tongue, is only slightly less frequently practiced.

Mutual oral-genital stimulation, the third form of oral-genital stimulation, combines both fellatio and cunnilingus. When practiced by a heterosexual couple, the female partner performs fellatio on her partner while her male partner performs cunnilingus on her. Homosexual couples can practice mutual fellatio or cunnilingus.

Intercourse

Sexual intercourse (coitus) refers to the act of inserting the penis into the vagina. Intercourse is the sexual behavior that is most directly associated with **procreation.** For some, intercourse is the only natural and appropriate form of sexual intimacy.

The incidence and frequency of sexual intercourse is a much-studied topic. Information concerning the percentages of people who have engaged in intercourse is readily available in textbooks used in sexuality courses. Data concerning sexual intercourse among college students may be changing somewhat because of concerns about HIV infection and other STDs, but a reasonable estimate of the percentage of college students who engage in sexual intercourse is 65 percent to 80 percent.

These percentages reflect two important concepts about the sexual activity of college students. The first is that most college students are having intercourse. The second concept is that a large percentage (20% to 35%) of students are choosing to refrain from intercourse. Indeed, the belief that "everyone is doing it" may be a bit shortsighted. From a public health standpoint, we believe it is important to provide accurate health information to protect those who choose to have intercourse and to actively support a person's right to choose not to have intercourse.

Couples need to share their expectations concerning techniques and the desired frequency of intercourse. Even the "performance" factors, such as depth of penetration, nature of body movements, tempo of activity, and timing of orgasm are increasingly important to many couples. Issues concerning sexually transmitted diseases (including HIV infection) are also critically important for couples who are contemplating intercourse. These factors also need to be explored through open communication.

A variety of books (including textbooks) provide written and visually explicit information on intercourse positions. Four basic positions for intercourse—*man above, woman above, side by side,* and *rear entry*—each offer relative advantages and disadvantages.

Personal Applications

• If you are sexually active, what forms of sexual intimacy are most important to you and your partner? Do both of you feel comfortable expressing your sexual needs and preferences?

Sexuality and Aging

Students are often curious about how aging affects sexuality. This is understandable because we live in a society that idolizes youth and demands performance. Many younger people become anxious about growing older because of what they think will happen to their ability to express their sexuality. Interestingly, young adults are willing to accept other physical changes of aging (such as the slowing down of basal metabolism, reduced lung capacity, and even wrinkles) but not those changes related to sexuality.

Research shows that, although sexual activity does decline with age, the capacity to enjoy sex is not altered, and a significant proportion of elderly people remain sexually active.[5]

As with other aspects of aging, certain anatomical and physiological changes will be evident, but these changes do not necessarily reduce the ability to enjoy sexual activity.[2] Most experts in sexuality report that many older people remain interested in sexual activity. Furthermore, those who are exposed to regular sexual activity throughout a lifetime report being most satisfied with their sex lives as older adults.[3]

As people age, the likelihood of alterations in the male and female sexual response cycles increases. In the postmenopausal woman, vaginal lubrication commonly begins more slowly, and the amount of lubrication usually diminishes. However, clitoral sensitivity and nipple erection remain the same as in earlier years. The female capacity for multiple orgasms remains the same, although the number of contractions that occur at orgasm is typically reduced.

A recent study found that health problems are not the primary cause of a reduction in sexual activity in elderly women. Rather, the researchers concluded that women's body image, or perception of themselves as attractive or unattractive, was the greater influence on their sexuality.[6]

In the older man, physical changes are also evident. This is thought to be caused by the decrease in the production of testosterone between the ages of twenty and sixty years. After age sixty or so, testosterone levels remain relatively steady. Thus many men, despite a decrease in sperm production, remain fertile into their eighties.[3] Older men typically take longer to achieve an erection (however, they are able to maintain their erection longer before ejaculation), have fewer muscular contractions at orgasm, and ejaculate less forcefully than they once did. The volume of seminal fluid ejaculated is typically less than in earlier years, and its consistency is somewhat thinner. The resolution phase is usually longer in older men. In spite of these gradual changes, some elderly men engage in sexual intercourse with the same frequency as do much younger men.

A significant proportion of elderly people in nursing homes continue to be sexually active. Unfortunately, they face barriers such as a lack of privacy, chronic illness, lack of a willing partner, unsupportive attitudes of physicians and staff, feelings of unattractiveness, and a lack of knowledge about their own sexuality.[5]

Health care workers can help to remove these barriers by improving privacy, educating staff, arranging conjugal or home visits, encouraging several forms of sexual expression, and counseling interested patients.

Personal Applications

• How do you view sexuality among the elderly? Are you concerned about changes in your own sexuality as you age?

The Dating Process

A half-century ago, the events involved in a dating relationship were somewhat predictable. People met each other through their daily activities or groups of friends, and a formal request for a date was made. Ninety-nine times out of a hundred, the requestor was male and the invitee was female. After a period of formal and informal dates, the two made a commitment to steady dating or decided to "date around." If the relationship progressed, further commitments were made (for example, letter jackets, class rings, or other jewelry items were exchanged). After months or years of a committed relationship, the couple decided to get married. The man invariably asked for the woman's "hand" (after first receiving permission from her parents), and plans for a wedding ceremony were made.

Does this form of dating and mate selection exist as we approach the year 2000? For some couples, yes. The traditional way of dating and selecting a marriage partner works well for them. However, many young and midlife adults prefer a more flexible, less predictable format for dating and finding a person they might choose to marry. For example, more than ever, women are playing a more assertive role when it comes to initiating and establishing the ground rules for a relationship. Interestingly, a large number of our students do not even like to use the word *dating* because it connotes a formalized pattern of behavior followed by their parents and grandparents.

What do you think? Have you recognized this more flexible dating format? Has this less traditional pattern been beneficial to couples as they make critical decisions that will influence the rest of their lives?

Love

Love may be one of the most elusive yet widely recognized concepts that describe some level of emotional attachment to another. Haas and Haas[2] describe five forms of love, including erotic, friendship, devotional, parental, and altruistic love. Other behavioral scientists[3] have focused primarily on two types of love most closely associated with dating and mate selection: *passionate love* and *companionate love.*

Passionate love, also described as romantic love or **infatuation,** is a state of extreme absorption in another. It is characterized by intense feelings of tenderness, elation, anxiety, sexual desire, and ecstasy.[3] Often appearing early in a relationship, passionate love typically does not last very long. Passionate love is driven by the excitement of being closely involved with a person whose character is not fully known.

If a relationship progresses, passionate love is gradually replaced by companionate love. This type of love is a less intense emotion than passionate love. It is characterized by friendly affection and a deep attachment that is based on extensive familiarity with the loved one.[3] This love is enduring and capable of sustaining long-term mutual growth. Central to companionate love are feelings of empathy for, support of, and tolerance of the partner. Complete the Personal

---

fellatio (feh **lay** she oh)   oral stimulation of the penis.

cunnilingus (cun uh **ling** gus)   oral stimulation of the vulva or clitoris.

procreation   reproduction.

infatuation   an often shallow, intense attraction to another person.

Personal Assessment

This quiz will help test how compatible you and your partner's personalities are. You should each rate the truth of these 20 statements based on the following scale. Circle the number that reflects your feelings. Total your scores and check the interpretation following the quiz.

1   Never true
2   Sometimes true
3   Frequently true
4   Always true

Statement	1	2	3	4
We can communicate our innermost thoughts effectively.	1	2	3	4
We trust each other.	1	2	3	4
We agree on whose needs come first.	1	2	3	4
We have realistic expectations of each other and of ourselves.	1	2	3	4
Individual growth is important within our relationship.	1	2	3	4
We will go on as a couple even if our partner doesn't change.	1	2	3	4
Our personal problems are discussed with each other first.	1	2	3	4
We both do our best to compromise.	1	2	3	4
We usually fight fairly.	1	2	3	4
We try not to be rigid or unyielding.	1	2	3	4
We keep any needs to be "perfect" in proper perspective.	1	2	3	4
We can balance the desire to be sociable with the need to be alone.	1	2	3	4
We both make friends and keep them.	1	2	3	4
Neither of us stays down or up for long periods.	1	2	3	4
We can tolerate the other's mood without being affected by it.	1	2	3	4
We can deal with disappointment and disillusionment.	1	2	3	4
Both of us can tolerate failure.	1	2	3	4
We can both express anger appropriately.	1	2	3	4
We are both assertive when necessary.	1	2	3	4
We agree on how our personal surroundings are kept.	1	2	3	4

YOUR TOTAL POINTS _____

Interpretation

20–35 points   You and your partner seem quite incompatible. Professional help may open your lines of communication.

36–55 points   You probably need more awareness and compromise.

56–70 points   You are highly compatible. However, be aware of the areas where you can improve.

71–80 points   Your relationship is very fulfilling.

To Carry This Further . . .

Ask your partner to take this test, too. You may have a one-sided view of a "perfect" relationship. Even if you scored high on this assessment, be aware of areas where you can still improve.

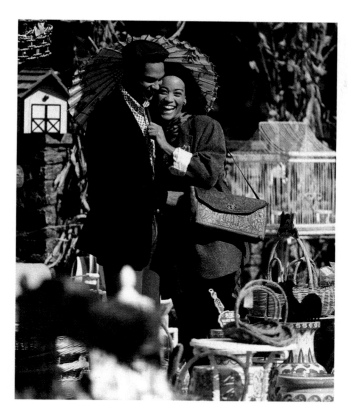

Companionate love is capable of sustaining mutual long-term growth.

Assessment on page 456 to determine whether you and your partner are truly compatible.

Friendship

One of the exciting aspects of college life is that you will probably meet many new people, some of whom will become your best friends. Because of your common experiences, it is likely that you will keep in contact with a few of these friends for a lifetime. Close attachments to other people can have an important influence on all of the dimensions of your health.

What is it that draws friends together? With the exception of physical intimacy, many of the same growth experiences seen in dating and mate selection are also seen in the development of friendships. Think about how you and your best friend developed the relationship you now have. You probably became friends when you shared similar interests and experiences. Your friendship progressed (and even faltered at times) through personal gains or losses. In all likelihood, you cared about each other and learned to share your deepest beliefs and feelings. You cemented your bond by turning your beliefs into behaviors.

Throughout the development of a deep friendship, the qualities of trust, tolerance, empathy, and support must be demonstrated. Otherwise the friendship can fall apart. You may have noticed that the

HEALTH ACTION GUIDE

Resolving Conflict

Here are some successful ways to manage conflict:

- Show mutual respect.
- Identify and resolve the real issue.
- Seek areas of agreement.
- Mutually participate in decision making.
- Be cooperative and specific.
- Focus on the present and future—not the past.
- Don't try to assign blame.
- Say what you are thinking and feeling.
- When talking, use sentences that begin with "I."
- Avoid using sentences that start with "You" or "Why."
- Set a time limit for discussing problems.
- Accept responsibility.
- Schedule time together.

InfoLinks

http://hometown.aol.com/uscccn/Conflict2000.index.html

qualities seen in a friendship are very similar to the qualities noted in the description of companionate love. In both cases, people develop deep attachments through extensive familiarity and understanding.

Intimacy

When most people hear the word **intimacy**, they immediately think about physical, sexual intimacy. However, sexuality experts and family therapists prefer to view intimacy more broadly, as any close, mutual, verbal or nonverbal behavior within a relationship. In this sense, intimate behavior can range from sharing deep feelings and experiences with a partner to sharing profound physical pleasures with a partner.

Intimacy is present in both love and friendship. You have likely shared intimate feelings with your closest friends, as well as with those you love. Intimacy helps us feel connected to others and allows us to feel the full measure of our own self-worth.

Marriage

Just as there is no single best way for two people to move through dating and mate selection, marriage is an equally variable undertaking. In marriage, two people join their lives in a way that affirms each as an individual and both as a legal pair. They are able to resolve conflict constructively (see the Health Action Guide above). However, for a large percentage of couples, the

---

intimacy   any close, mutual, verbal or nonverbal behavior within a relationship.

demands of marriage are too rigorous, confining, and demanding. They will find resolution for their dissatisfaction through divorce or extramarital affairs. For most, though, marriage will be an experience that alternates periods of happiness, productivity, and admiration with periods of frustration, unhappiness, and disillusionment with the partner. Each marriage is unique. The Health Action Guide below presents some advice for improving marriage.

As we move through the remainder of the 1990s, we see certain trends in marriage. The most obvious of these is the age at first marriage. Today men are waiting longer than ever to marry. Now the average age at first marriage for men is twenty-six years.[7] In addition, these new husbands are better educated than in the past and are more likely to be established in their careers. Women are also waiting longer to get married and tend to be more educated and career oriented. Recent statistics indicate that the average age at first marriage for women is twenty-four years.[7]

Gay and lesbian couples have begun working publicly for the right to marry, and the debate over same-sex marriage has reached the national level in recent years. When three gay couples were denied marriage licenses in Hawaii in 1990, they launched a legal fight to gain this right. See the Learning from Our Diversity box on page 459 for a closer look at this issue.

Marriage still appeals to most adults. Currently, 73 percent of adults aged eighteen and older are married, widowed, or divorced.[7] Thus about 27 percent of today's adults have not married. Within the last decade, the percentage of adults who have decided not to marry has nearly doubled. Singlehood and other alternatives to marriage are discussed later in this chapter.

Forms of Marriage

To describe the nature of marital relationships, we use the classic categories of marital relationships proposed by Cuber and Harroff.[8] These marriage types should not be viewed as either good or bad. Rather, you should recognize one simple reality: These marriages are routinely found and apparently meet the needs of the individuals involved. Some of the types of marriages we present began in their current form. Others, however, evolved into their present form, having once been a very different type of marital relationship.

HEALTH ACTION GUIDE

Improving Marriage

Few marital relationships are perfect. All marriages face occasional periods of strain or turmoil. Even marriages that do not exhibit major signs of distress can be improved, mostly through better communication. Marriage experts suggest that implementing some of these patterns can strengthen marriages:

- Problems that exist within the marriage should be brought into the open so that both partners become aware of the difficulties.
- Partners should balance the needs and expectations of each partner. They should make decisions jointly. Partners should support each other as much as they can. When one partner cannot actively support the other's goals, he or she should at least provide moral support and encouragement.
- Partners should establish realistic expectations. Partners should negotiate areas of disagreement. They should work together to determine how they will share resources.
- Participating in marriage counseling and marriage encounter groups can be helpful.

Beyond the patterns listed above, a sense of permanence helps sustain a marriage over the course of time. If the partners are convinced that their relationship can withstand difficult times, then they are more likely to take the time to make needed changes. Couples can develop a sense of permanence by implementing some of the patterns just described.

InfoLinks
www.competentcouples.com

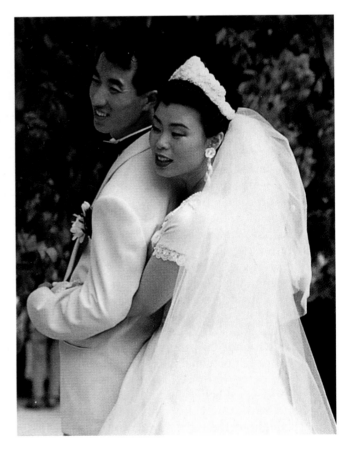

Recent statistics show that both men and women are waiting longer to get married.

Learning
From Our Diversity

The Debate Over Same-Sex Marriage

What is the definition of marriage? Must the marriage partners be a man and woman? Would same-sex marriages weaken our society?

If you haven't considered these questions before, you may begin to consider them shortly. A test case in Hawaii is bringing the issue to the public stage. Even if the Hawaii Supreme Court rules that gays do have the right to marry, the issue is expected to go to the U.S. Supreme Court, as other states attempt to pass laws refusing to recognize gay marriages performed in Hawaii.

"We want equal protection, not second-class citizenship," says Tracey Bennett, a lobbyist for the Hawaii Equal Rights Marriage Project. "The definition of family needs to be expanded," she says. To those who argue that gay marriage undermines the

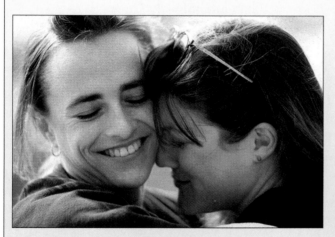

Legalization of same-sex marriage would grant gay couples a wide range of legal and economic rights.

family and thus weakens the foundation of our society, she answers, "Gays are not a problem for the family. We are loving people who want to be in the family of families."

Same-sex marriage would grant gays an array of legal and economic rights, including joint parental custody, insurance and health benefits, joint tax returns, alimony and child support, inheritance of property, hospital visitation rights, family leave, and a spouse's Social Security and retirement benefits.

Same-sex unions actually have been debated for many years. Some U.S. clergy were presiding over gay "marriages" in the 1980s, and several hundred companies now offer benefits to same-sex partners of employees. Gay publications debated the subject in the 1950s. In *Same-Sex Unions in Premodern Europe*, the late John Boswell, a Yale University historian, suggested that ancient marriage ceremonies provide evidence that Greeks and medieval Christians celebrated same-sex relationships.

The opposition is both religious and political. Opponents argue that Hawaii is just the first step in a national agenda toward same-sex marriage. "We can't have this redefinition of marriage," says the Rev. Marc Alexander, executive director of the Hawaii Catholic Council. "We've seen one social experiment after another deteriorate marriage and family. Marriage is a special relationship that deserves to be supported, benefited, and endorsed."

Six states have enacted laws to ban gay marriage. Another 32 have considered bans. President Clinton does not support gay marriages. Surprisingly, gays are winning some support among conservatives. "Isn't it wrong for the same right-wing activists who have descried gay **promiscuity** to now deny gay love and commitment?" asks conservative writer Bruce Bawer.

Some observers predict that this will be the greatest gay rights debate in history. Where do you stand on this issue? Should gay partners be granted the same legal right to marriage as heterosexual couples? Or do you believe legal marriage should be limited to its traditional definition of a union between opposite-sex partners?

Conflict-Habituated Marriage

"We fought on our first date, our honeymoon was a disaster, and we've disagreed on everything of importance ever since." This frank description of a marital relationship characterized by confrontation, disagreement, and perhaps physical abuse reflects a *conflict-habituated marriage*. The central theme of this type of marital relationship is conflict, and its continuous presence suggests that the partners are making no attempt at resolution. Couples in long-term conflict-habituated marriages simply agree to disagree.

Devitalized Marriage

In the same way a dying person is said to possess failing signs, a *devitalized marriage* has lost its signs of life.

Unlike the conflict-habituated marriage, which since its beginning was chronically impaired, the devitalized marriage was once a more active and satisfying marital relationship. However, the couple has lost its desire to keep the marriage dynamic.

The future of a devitalized marriage is difficult to predict. Some marriages of this type can be revitalized. Effective marriage counseling, a new job, or moving to a new community can rekindle a relationship. Other devitalized marriages are able to remain intact because

promiscuity	the practice of engaging in sexual intercourse indiscriminately or with many partners.

one or both partners find vitality through an extramarital relationship. Some devitalized marriages persist at low levels of involvement and commitment with little hope for improvement. We would not be surprised if, for those of you who have witnessed the dissolution of your own or your parents' marriage, devitalization was an important factor in its ending.

Passive-Congenial Marriage

Passive means a low level of commitment or involvement, and the word *congenial* suggests warmth and friendliness. When these two words are combined as they are in *passive-congenial marriage,* they describe perfectly the type of marital relationship sought by some couples.

For some of today's young professionals, the passive-congenial marriage offers a safe harbor from the rigors encountered in the competitive world of corporate business. Children may not be valued "commodities" in the passive-congenial marriage. The added financial and personal stressors related to child rearing could compromise an established lifestyle. You may be able to construct an image of a passive-congenial couple if you can picture two people meeting after work for a quiet dinner at a small restaurant, talking in muffled tones about their corporate battles, and planning their winter cruise.

Maintaining a passive-congenial marriage requires less time and energy than other forms of marriage. For two people who feel certain that their major contributions to society will be made through their efforts in the workplace, this marriage may be ideal. Certainly you may know many couples who are choosing this increasingly popular form of marriage.

Total Marriage

In the *total marriage,* little remains of the unique identities the two people had before their marriage took place. For reasons that are probably lost to the subconscious mind, two people possessing individual personalities use marriage to fuse their identities into one identity—the total pair.

The total marriage requires that the individual partners set aside all aspirations for individual growth and development. Decisions are not made with "me" or even "you" as the center of attention. Rather, energies are directed toward what is best for "us." Life outside of the marital relationship and partner's presence does not exist, at least figuratively speaking. Eventually outsiders, when speaking about these individuals, can no longer truly speak about the man or the woman but are limited to speaking about the couple.

Vital Marriage

The *vital marriage* is intended to serve as an arena for the growth of both the individuals and the pair. The partners focus on "my growth," "your growth," and "our growth." In a vital marriage, personal goals may at times be subordinated for the good of the partner or the paired relationship. Yet both the partners (and the children) know that those once-subordinated goals will assume top priority when this becomes possible and desirable. The relationship has equality of opportunity.

In describing the vital marriage, we must point out that this type of marital relationship is not perfect, nor is it appropriate for all couples. In today's complex society, the vital marriage may be especially difficult to maintain.

Personal Applications

• If you are married, which of these categories best describes your marriage? If you plan to marry, which kind of marriage do you hope to have, and why?

Divorce

Marriages, like many other kinds of interpersonal relationships, can end. Today, marriages—relationships begun with the intent of permanence "until death do us part"—end through divorce nearly as frequently as not.

Why should approximately half of marital relationships end? Unfortunately, marriage experts cannot provide one clear answer to this question. Rather, they suggest that divorce is a reflection of unfulfilled expectations for marriage on the part of one or both partners, including the following:

- The belief that marriage will ease your need to deal with your own faults and that your failures can be shared by your partner
- The belief that marriage will change faults that you know exist in your partner
- The belief that the high level of romance of your dating and courtship period will be continued through marriage
- The belief that marriage can provide you with an arena for the development of your personal power, and that once married, you will not need to compromise with your partner
- The belief that your marital partner will be successful in meeting all of your needs

If these expectations seem to be ones you anticipate through marriage, then you may find that disappointments will abound. To varying degrees, marriage is a partnership that requires much cooperation and compromise. Marriage can be complicated. Because of the high expectations that many people hold for marriage, the termination of marriage can be an emotionally difficult process to undertake (see the Health Action Guide on page 462).

The American attitude toward divorce has swung like a pendulum over the last century. Divorce has gone from being an embarrassing, painful ordeal, to a common, relatively simple legal procedure. More recently, some observers have begun to question the wisdom of no-fault divorce.

Our society is concerned about the well-being of children whose parents divorce. Different factors, however, influence the extent to which divorce affects children. Included among these factors are the gender and age of the children, custody arrangements, financial support, and the remarriage of one or both parents. Many children must adjust to accept their new status as a member of a blended family.

Personal Applications

• Has a divorce, either your own or that of someone close to you, affected your life? If so, how did you or the people involved cope with the divorce, accept the change in the relationship, and heal emotionally?

Alternatives to Marriage

Although most of you have experienced or will experience marriage, you certainly have alternatives to marriage. This section briefly explores singlehood, cohabitation, and single parenthood.

Singlehood

An alternative to marriage for adults is singlehood. For many people, being single is a lifestyle that affords the potential for pursuing intimacy, if desired, and provides an uncluttered path for independence

---

HEALTH ACTION GUIDE

Communication is Key to Relationships

The best-seller lists abound with books, like the *Men Are from Mars, Women Are from Venus* series, that stress the importance of communication. Other books tell couples how to strengthen their relationships, and religious groups offer marriage encounter weekends. Developing a healthy intimate relationship is tough work, and it's okay to seek help and advice. Besides book and counselors, look around for the couples you know who seem to be happy with each other, who have the kind of relationship you want.

You probably learned your current communication skills as a child in your family. In functional families, the children learn to have conversations, express their feelings, solve problems, and ask for what they want.

Unfortunately, not all families have these skills, so if you would like to strengthen your relationship, or better prepare yourself for a relationship, consider the following communication tips:

• Admit to your partner that solving a problem is difficult, and if you are scared, say so.
• Understand that disagreement is healthy, and arguing between any two human beings in a relationship is inevitable. The *way* you disagree can be healthy or destructive.
• Listen to your partner's expression of feelings, not only about the current issue, but also about your partner's background. For example, your partner may be upset about an issue such as overspending, but also carry an undercurrent of fear that developed in a childhood of financial uncertainty.
• Do not interrupt or apologize too quickly. This can be a way of cutting off your partner. Do not assume that you know what your partner is thinking or feeling. Even if you are right,

let your partner share his or her thoughts and feelings. Research has found that the act of listening actually is relaxing and reduces blood pressure.[9]
• Do not call your partner names or make broad, negative statements, even if you are very angry. Avoid broad indictments, such as "you always . . ." or "you are so . . ."
• Accept your partner's feelings and ideas. This does not necessarily mean you agree with them.
• Attempt to understand your partner's thoughts and feelings before you insist on being understood.
• If a discussion brings up intense feelings, and you have trouble sitting down and facing your partner, consider continuing the discussion during a brisk walk together.
• Sometimes you may be ready for a discussion, but your partner is not. But if your partner is never ready, you may have to reconsider his or her level of commitment.

Relationships do not always last forever, and some relationships are not worth trying to save. Warning signs or differences that may spell trouble for a relationship include:[10]

• Constant criticism or put-downs, even if presented in a joking manner.
• Unwillingness to talk about things that are important to either of you.
• Lack of willingness to socialize with others or reluctance to spend time alone with each other.
• Verbal or physical abuse. This is a clear sign that you should end the relationship.

InfoLinks
www.couples-place.com

HEALTH ACTION GUIDE

Coping with a Breakup

The end of a marriage or other long-term relationship is always a wrenching and painful experience. The following tips suggest both alternatives to breakup and ways to cope with it.

- Talk first. Try to deal effectively and directly with the conflicts. The old theory said that it was good for a couple to argue. However, anger can cause more anger and even lead to violence. Freely venting anger is as likely to damage a relationship as to improve it. Therefore, cool off first, then discuss issues fully and freely.

- Trial separation. Sometimes only a few weeks apart can convince a couple that it is better to work together than to go it totally alone. It is generally better to establish the rules of such a trial quite firmly. Will the individuals see others? What are the responsibilities if children are involved? There should also be a time limit, perhaps a month or two, after which the partners reunite and discuss their situation again.

- Obtain help. The services of a *qualified* counselor, psychologist, or psychiatrist may help a couple resolve their problems. Notice the emphasis on the word *qualified*. Some people who have little training or competence represent themselves as counselors. For this reason a couple should insist on verifying the counselor's training and licensing.

- Allow time for grief and healing. When a relationship ends, people are often tempted to immediately become as socially and sexually active as possible. This can be a way to express anger and relieve pain. But it can also cause frustration and despair. A better solution for many is to acknowledge the grief the breakup has caused and allow time for healing. Up to a year of continuing one's life and solidifying friendships typically helps the rejected partner establish a new equilibrium.

InfoLinks

www.cam.org/~jmauld/English/dateanal.html

and self-directedness. Other people, however, are single because of divorce, separation, death, or the absence of an opportunity to establish a partnership. The U.S. Bureau of the Census indicates that 41 percent of women and 37 percent of men over the age of eighteen are currently single.[7]

Single people can have many different living arrangements. Some single people live alone and choose not to share a household. Other arrangements for singles include cohabitation, periodic cohabitation, singlehood during the week and cohabitation on the weekends or during vacations, or the platonic sharing of a household with others. For young adults, large percentages of single men and women live with their parents.

Like living arrangements, the sexual intimacy patterns of singles are individually tailored. Some singles practice celibacy, others pursue heterosexual or homosexual intimate relationships in a **monoga-**mous pattern, and others have multiple partners. As in all interpersonal relationships, including marriage, the levels of commitment are as variable as the people involved.

Cohabitation

Cohabitation, or the sharing of living quarters by unmarried people, represents yet another alternative to marriage. According to the U.S. Bureau of the Census, the number of unmarried, opposite-gender couples living together climbed from 1.5 million couples in 1980 to more than 4 million in 1997.[7] Another 1.8 million lived with a partner of the same sex in 1997.

Although cohabitation may seem to imply a vision of sexual intimacy between male and female roommates, several forms of shared living arrangements can be viewed as cohabitation. For some couples, cohabitation is only a part-time arrangement for weekends, during summer vacation, or on a variable schedule. In addition, **platonic** cohabitation can exist when a couple shares living quarters but does so without establishing an intimate relationship. Close friends, people of retirement age, and homosexuals might all be included in a group called cohabitants.

The archetype of a cohabitation arrangement is the couple who has drifted into cohabitation as the result of a dating relationship that has progressed into sexual intimacy and occasional "overnighting." In the living arrangement that follows, both material possessions and emotional support are generally shared. A contractual relationship is only occasionally established. The partners are usually monogamous. Approximately half of cohabitation relationships will disband, and the people involved will depart with the feeling that they would cohabit again if it appeared desirable. Finally, cohabitation is neither more nor less likely to lead to marriage than is a more traditional dating relationship. It is, in fact, only an alternative to marriage.

Single Parenthood

Unmarried young women continue to become pregnant and then become single parents in this country. There is also a new and significantly different form of single parenthood: the planned entry into single parenthood by older, better educated people, the vast majority of whom are women.

In contrast to the teenaged girl who becomes a single parent through an unwed pregnancy, the more mature woman who desires single parenting has usually planned carefully for the experience. She has explored several important concerns, including questions regarding how she will become pregnant (with or without the knowledge of a male partner or through artificial insemination), the need for a father figure for the child, the effect of single parenting on her social life, and, of course, its effect on her career development. When these questions have been resolved, no legal barriers stand in the way of her becoming a single parent.

A very large number of women and a growing number of men are actively participating in single parenthood as a result of a divorce settlement or separation agreement involving sole or joint custody of children. More than a quarter of America's children now live with one parent.[11]

A few single parents have been awarded children through adoption. The likelihood of a single person's receiving a child is small, but more people have been successful recently in single-parent adoptions.

Personal Applications

• If you are not married, would permanent singlehood, cohabitation, or single parenthood be an option for you? If you reject these options, why do you feel they would not be appropriate for you?

Sexual Orientation

Sexual orientation refers to the direction in which people focus their sexual interests. People can be attracted to opposite-gender partners, same-gender partners, or partners of both genders.

Heterosexuality

Heterosexuality (or heterosexual orientation) refers to an attraction to opposite-gender partners. (*Heteros* is a Greek word that means "the other.") Throughout the world, this is the most common sexual orientation. For reasons related to species survival, heterosexuality has its most basic roots in the biological dimension of human sexuality. Beyond its biological roots, heterosexuality has significant cultural and religious support in virtually every country in the world. Most societies expect men to be attracted to women and women to be attracted to men. Worldwide, laws related to marriage, living arrangements, health benefits, child rearing, financial matters, sexual behavior, and inheritance generally support heterosexual relationships.

Homosexuality

Homosexuality (or homosexual orientation) refers to an attraction to same-gender partners. The term *homosexuality* comes from the Greek word *homos*, meaning "same." The word *homosexuality* may be used to apply to males or females. Frequently the word *gay* is used to refer to homosexual orientation in both males and females. *Lesbianism* is also used to refer to sexual attraction between females.

The distinctions among the three categories of sexual orientation are much less clear than their definitions might suggest. Most people probably fall somewhere along a continuum between exclusive heterosexuality and exclusive homosexuality. Kinsey in 1948 presented just such a continuum.[12]

Why does a given individual have a homosexual orientation? The question has no simple answer. (College human sexuality textbooks devote entire chapters to this topic.) In the mid-1990s, some research pointed to differences in the sizes of certain brain structures as a possible biological basis for homosexuality.[13] Other researchers propose genetic, environmental, hormonal, and other foundations for homosexuality. However, for sexual orientation in general, no single theory has emerged that fully explains this developmental process. Regardless of the reasons, however, homosexual individuals generally do not reverse to heterosexuality. Furthermore, most homosexuals report that no specific event "triggered" their homosexuality. Many homosexuals also say that they knew their orientations were different from other children as far back as their prepubertal years. Society's acceptance of homosexuality has become a subject of debate once again over the last few years.

The extent of homosexuality in our society is unclear. Gathering valid information of this kind is difficult. The extent of homosexual orientation is probably much greater than many heterosexuals realize. Furthermore, many people do not wish to reveal their homosexuality and thus prefer to remain "in the closet."

Although operational definitions of homosexuality may vary from researcher to researcher, Kinsey estimated that about 2 percent of American females and 4 percent of American males were exclusively homosexual.[12,14] More recent estimates place the overall combined figure of homosexuals at about 10 percent of the population.[3] Clearly the expression of same-gender attraction is not uncommon.

Personal Applications

• In comparison with a decade ago, are heterosexuals generally more comfortable or less comfortable with homosexuals in our society? Support your answer with specific examples.

---

monogamous (mo **nog** a mus) paired relationship with one partner.

cohabitation sharing of a residence by two unrelated, unmarried people; living together.

platonic close association between two people that does not include a sexual relationship.

Secondary Virginity

Do you feel that sex should happen automatically after three dates, or five dates, or two months? Do you think the women owes sex to her date if he takes her out to dinner? Do you believe that everyone else is doing it, and if you're not, there is something wrong with you?

Many college students have begun examining these attitudes and have decided that sex does not have to happen automatically, the woman never "owes" sex in return for a date, and certainly not everyone else is doing it. Some studies have shown that 40 percent to 50 percent of students are not sexually active.[15] Many students see the advantages of abstinence, also known as *secondary virginity*. Abstinence is defined as abstaining from genital, anal, or oral-genital intercourse.

College students today refrain from sex for many reasons. Among these are:

- They prefer to wait, for religious or moral reasons.
- They want to wait until there is a commitment in the relationship.
- They do not feel physically or emotionally ready for sex.
- They do not want to risk pregnancy.
- They do not want to risk sexually transmitted diseases, including incurable and potentially fatal ones.
- They do not feel they have the time or energy to establish a sexual relationship.

Some of the advantages of secondary virginity are:

- Abstinence eliminates the risk of pregnancy.
- Abstinence reduces the risk of HIV infection and STDs such as genital warts and herpes.
- Abstinence eliminates the expense of contraception.

- Abstinence allows two people to get to know each other in more than simply a sexual way.

Religious organizations such as True Love Waits have promoted abstinence in public campaigns, complete with pledge cards (promising to wait until the wedding night), pledge rings (not to come off until the wedding night), and rallies. Nearly a million pledge cards have been signed since the campaign was launched in 1993.[16] The campaign is attractive to many students because it allows sexually experienced students to declare born-again virginity.

College programs that encourage abstinence also offer a variety of ways to express love without having intercourse:[17]

- Eat ice cream cones together.
- Create a photo album of each other.
- Brush each other's hair.
- Do laundry together on Saturday morning.
- Send each other a secret love note in the campus newspaper.
- Have a picnic in the country.
- Go for a moonlit walk.
- Give a foot rub.
- Cook each other's favorite food.
- For those who do decide to be sexual, consider low-risk activities such as mutual masturbation.

Finally, consider that Isaac Newton, Martin Luther, Emily Dickinson, Beethoven, Sigmund Freud, Alfred Hitchcock, Henry David Thoreau, George Bernard Shaw, and Mother Teresa practiced abstinence for all or part of their lives. Even pop star Toni Braxton recently announced that she plans not have sex again until she is married.

Bisexuality

People whose preference for sexual partners includes both genders are referred to as *bisexuals.* Bisexuals may fall into one of three groups: those who are (1) genuinely attracted to both genders, (2) homosexual but also feel the need to behave heterosexually, or (3) aroused physically by the same gender but attracted emotionally to the opposite gender. Some people participate in a bisexual lifestyle for extended periods, whereas others move quickly to a more exclusive orientation. Little research has been conducted on bisexuality, and thus the size of the bisexual population is not accurately known.

A particularly pressing reason for learning more about the bisexual lifestyle is its relationship to the transmission of HIV infection. Next to intravenous drug users, bisexuals hold the greatest potential for extending HIV infection into the heterosexual population. Because the prevalence of bisexuality is unknown, the consistent use of safer sex practices becomes more important than ever.

Gender Identity

Unlike sexual orientation, which describes the gender to which an individual is attracted, *gender identity* describes an individual's self-image on a male-female scale, and how the individual presents this identity to others. Most adults are probably conventional in the gender identity they present to the world, but other forms of expression have recently become better known. Two of these forms are transsexualism and transvestism.

Transsexualism

Transsexualism describes the overwhelming conviction of individuals, typically males, that they are in fact the opposite of their biological gender. As they grow older, their discomfort with their gender increases, often until they turn to doctors for help. Some take feminizing hormones to develop a more feminine body, and some have their sex organs surgically altered so that they can live completely, and anatomically, as the opposite sex.

Transsexuals who complete the transition describe it as a liberation, a feeling of dropping a mask they had worn for many years. They then live the remainder of their lives in their new gender role.

For years, scientists have searched, without success, for measurable differences between most men and the ones who become transsexuals. Recently, however, investigators in the Netherlands, using autopsies of male-to-female transsexuals, reported that a tiny structure deep within a part of the brain that controls sexual function appears to be more like the type found in women than in men.[18]

This mismatch between brain and body could be found in the process by which embryos take on sex differences. All human embryos develop in the earliest stages of gestation along more or less feminine lines. Those destined to become males differentiate from the basic female pattern after a complex series of hormonal secretions. Miscues in this process could result in a female identity in the portion of the brain responsible for gender identity.

Transvestism

Public figures such as Dennis Rodman and RuPaul have turned a spotlight on cross-dressing, or transvestism. The term *transvestism* is typically used to describe a heterosexual male who, from time to time, dresses as a woman. The practice of transvestism can range from simple sexual gratification from the wearing of feminine clothing, to the expression of the feminine side of the individual's personality. Although many transvestites wish to express the feminine aspects of their personality, most are satisfied with their gender role and their biological gender. Many are married and may or may not have shared this aspect of their personality with their partner.

Years ago, psychologists attempted to cure cross-dressers, but today most have recognized that cross-dressing is lifelong and that they can obtain better results by teaching the cross-dresser to accept his feminine side.

One recent study found that typical cross-dressers are virtually indistinguishable from non-cross-dressing men in their personality traits, sexuality, and measures of psychological wellness.[19]

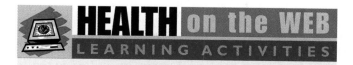

Understanding Patterns of Sexual Behavior

The Passions Sex Quiz is designed to help you compare your sexual behavior to the "norm" in the United States. However, keep in mind that a wide range of behavior, including celibacy, can be considered normal. Remember that no one is average across the spectrum of characteristics presented in the quiz. The quiz is personal, but your answers are strictly confidential. Go to www.thriveonline.com/sex/dyngames/gen/sex.quizldyngame.html, and complete the 14 items. When you are finished, click the *Submit* button to receive your personalized response.

Taking the Love Test

The Queendom website offers an interactive questionnaire consisting of 68 items drawn from current research on love. You can complete the test and review your results in less than an hour. You should take the test in private, and your answers are strictly confidential. When you submit your finished questionnaire, you will receive a report of how you scored and how to interpret your results. Check out the Love Test at www.queendom.com/test_frm.html.

Rating the Dating Process

Dating means different things to different people. For example, men and women may see it differently, and older and younger people might not agree. How do you see dating? Go to www.queendom.com/test_frm.html, and select *Date Test*. Do your ideas about the dating process seem traditional or more modern? Remember that there are no right answers here—just what seems right to you.

For more activities, log on to our Online Learning Center at www.mhhe.com/hper/health/payne

Real Life
Real choices

Your Turn

- Do you identify in any way with Kim Hendricks's feelings about commitment and marriage? Why or why not?
- How do you feel about the conviction expressed in the lyric "Love and marriage go together like a horse and carriage?"
- In what ways are your attitudes about commitment and marriage similar to and different from those of your parents?

And Now, Your Choices . . .
- Have you ever been in a relationship where one of you wanted to make a serious commitment and the other one didn't? If so, what was your position, why, and how did you handle the conflict?
- If you were in Kim's situation, would you try to change your attitude toward commitment and marriage, or would you deal with your feelings as she does, or in another way? Give reasons for your answer.

Summary

- Men and women share the four stages of sexual response: excitement, plateau, orgasm, and resolution.
- Several senses can supply the stimuli necessary for initiating the sexual response pattern.
- Some differences have been shown in the sexual response patterns of men and women.
- Two physiological mechanisms are critical to the sexual response pattern: vasocongestion, the retention of blood or fluid within a particular tissue, and myotonia, the buildup of neuromuscular tension.
- Direct stimulation of the penis and direct or indirect stimulation of the clitoris are the principle avenues toward orgasm.
- Celibacy is the self-imposed avoidance of sexual intimacy.
- Most sex therapists and researchers consider masturbation to be a normal source of self-pleasure.
- Shared touching, genital contact, oral-genital stimulation, and intercourse are common forms of sexual intimacy.
- Many older people remain interested in and continue to engage in sexual activities.
- Physiological changes may alter the way in which some older people perform sexually.
- The dating process has become more flexible and less formal and predictable during recent decades.
- Passionate love is gradually replaced by companionate love, which is characterized by deep affection and attachment.
- Friendship requires trust, tolerance, empathy, and support.
- Intimacy is any close, mutual, verbal or nonverbal behavior within a relationship.
- Forms of marriage include conflict-habituated marriage, devitalized marriage, passive-congenial marriage, total marriage, and vital marriage.
- Although most people marry at some time in their lives, there are alternatives to marriage, including singlehood, cohabitation, and single parenthood.
- Many people enter marriage with unrealistic expectations, including the idea that they will no longer have to deal with their own faults.
- Most marriages can be improved through better communication.
- The three sexual orientations are heterosexuality, homosexuality, and bisexuality.

Review Questions

1. What similarities and differences exist between the sexual response patterns of males and females?
2. Define celibacy, masturbation, sexual fantasies, erotic dreams, shared touching, genital contact, oral-genital stimulation, and sexual intercourse.
3. Approximately what percentage of today's college students report having had sexual intercourse?
4. What are some of the forms that intimacy can take?
5. Identify and describe the five forms of marriage presented in this chapter.
6. Approximately what percent of marriages end in divorce?
7. Discuss current trends in the areas of singlehood, cohabitation, and single parenthood.
8. What are some differences between passionate love and companionate love?
9. Explain the differences between heterosexuality, homosexuality, and bisexuality. How common are each of these sexual orientations in our society?

References

1. Masters W, Johnson V. *Human sexual response.* Boston: Little, Brown, 1966.
2. Haas K, Haas A. *Understanding sexuality.* 3rd ed. St. Louis: Mosby, 1993.
3. Crooks R, Baur K. *Our sexuality.* 7th ed. Pacific Grove, CA: Brooks/Cole Publishing, 1998.
4. Rathus SA, Nevid JS, Fichner-Rathus L. *Human sexuality in a world of discovery.* Needham Heights, MA: Allyn and Bacon, 1993.
5. Richardson JP, Lazur A. Sexuality in the nursing home patient (review). *Am Family Phys* 1995 Jan; 51(1):121–24.
6. Fooken I. Sexuality in the later years—the impact of health and body-image in a sample of older women. *Patient Ed Couns* 1994 July; 23(3):227–33.
7. U.S. Bureau of the Census. *Statistical abstract of the United States: 1997* 115th ed. Washington, DC: U.S. Government Printing Office, 1997.

8. Cuber J, Harroff P. *Sex and the significant Americans.* Baltimore: Penguin Books, 1965.
9. Ornstein R, Sobel D. *The healing brain: breakthrough discoveries about how the brain keeps us healthy.* New York: Guilford Press, 1991.
10. Woititz JG. *The intimacy struggle.* Deerfield Beach, FL: Health Communications, 1993.
11. U.S. Department of Commerce, Economics and Statistics Administration, Bureau of the Census. *Children with single parents—how they fare.* September 1997.
12. Pomeroy WB, Martin CE, Kinsey AC. *Sexual behavior in the human male.* Bloomington, IN: Indiana University Press, 1998.
13. Allen LS, Gorski RA. Sexual orientation and the size of the anterior commissure in the human brain. *Proc Nat Acad Sci USA* 1992; 89(15):7199–7202.
14. Staff of the Institute for Sex Research, Indiana University, Alfred C. Kinsey, et al. *Sexual behavior in the human female.* Bloomington, IN: Indiana University Press, 1998.
15. Barber-Murphy L. *Duke alcohol use and sexual behavior survey.* Durham, NC: Duke University, 1993.
16. True Love Waits. 1998. http://www.truelovewaits.com, Lifeway Christian Resources, Nashville, TN.
17. Smith LP. *101 ways to make love without doing it* (brochure). University of Pittsburgh at Bradford: Student Health Services, 1997.
18. Gorman C. Trapped in the body of a man? *Time* 1995 Nov 13: 94–95.
19. Brown GR et al. Personality characteristics and sexual functioning of 188 crossdressing men. *J Nervous Mental Dis* 1996 May; 184(5):265–73.
20. Gini A. Romance in the workplace. *Small Business Journal* 2(9), 1996.

Suggested Readings

DeAngelis B. *Ask Barbara: the 100 most-asked questions about love, sex, and relationships.* Dell Books, Random House, 1998. Barbara DeAngelis spotlights 100 intimate issues that often challenge couples in love and single people searching for the right partner. Questions include: How long should I wait for a commitment? Can you trust someone who cheated? Questions are organized by topic, and include love and intimacy, sex and physical affection, compatibility, commitment, communication, conflict, cheating, breaking up, and starting over.

Elliott L, Brantley C. *Sex on campus: the naked truth about the real sex lives of college students.* New York: Random House, 1997. This highly readable book reports the results of a survey of 20,000 current college students about their sex lives. Comparisons are presented to studies gathered over the last twenty years to show clear changes in sexual practices among this population. Also presented is useful information about human sexuality, reproduction, STDs, sexual problems, safer sex practices, and sex and drugs.

As We Go To PRESS

Office romances, once considered taboo, are on the rise, and employees are more open about their liaisons. More than 30 percent of employees report that they have been involved with a coworker at some time in their careers, according to a survey by the American Management Association. Companies have loosened their attitudes toward office romance, too.

As recently as ten years ago, many companies forbade dating among employees. The rationale was that office romances would breed tension, jealousy, and the appearance of favoritism. Many companies refused to hire married couples, and if two employees decided to marry, one of them would have to quit. These policies are changing simply to recognize reality. The average work week for both blue- and white-collar workers is now more than 50 hours, not counting commuting time.[20] Middle managers put in 58 to 65 hours a week. Many employees are thrown together on the road for days or weeks at a time. This leaves less time for recreation, as employees now spend much of their free time on domestic chores or simply recovering from exhaustion. So where

and when can employees find someone to meet, romance, and possibly marry? Where else but at work?

There are still some prohibitions to dating in the workplace:

• Most companies still strongly discourage or even prohibit managers and executives from dating their underlings. The differential in power still looks bad. The higher-up can look like he is abusing his power or sexually harassing the employee, and the underling can look like she is trying to sleep her way to the top. (The higher-up still is typically the man.) When these romances end, they can lead to lawsuits, damaged reputations, and possibly job loss for the participants.
• Some companies will separate couples, either by transferring one employee or by assigning one employee to a different supervisor, so that one partner does not report to the other.
• The "affair," in which one or both participants are married, is still considered inappropriate at most companies.

Virtual Love and Cybersex: How Far Should You Go on the Internet?

It's like a singles bar without the loud music. If you have a computer and a modem, you can gain access to the world's largest "meet market." From the comfort of your home, you can browse the Internet and meet people for conversation, friendship, romance, and even "sex" (such as it is in cyberspace). There is a cover charge, but you won't have to buy drinks to start up a conversation or get your toes smashed on the dance floor. You won't even have to worry about getting diseases (save for the occasional computer virus).

However, there are drawbacks when you enter this hangout. Can you be sure the person you're chatting with is all he or she seems to be? How can you be certain of a person's personality, age, or even his or her gender? And is there a safe way to meet a "cyber-friend" face-to-face? The Internet way of meeting people has its own built-in set of advantages—but inviting the world into your home has its dangers as well.

Today's Internet user can find a variety of potential conversation topics using a web browser and typing in various keywords. As the Internet grows, so does the number of websites and USENET discussion groups. Some people see this expansion as a source of entertainment. They think that the Internet is a fun and interesting way to meet people who share their interests. Others think that the Internet allows pornographers, pedophiles, and other deviants to perpetuate their behavior and prey on innocent children. Both groups are attempting to use the law either to keep the Internet as a haven for free speech or to clean it up and make it safer for children. This clash of ideals is creating a continual battle over the nature and character of the Internet.

Fun and Games on the Internet

The Internet is a large group of computer networks, both public and private, that connects millions of computer users in an estimated 150 countries. More than 70,000 private computer bulletin boards exist in the United States alone, and private commercial networks such as Prodigy, America Online, and CompuServe provide nearly 6 million subscribers worldwide with access to the Internet.[1] Although the Internet contains information about all facets of life, the sexually oriented sites are proving to be the most popular areas among the general public. For example, alt.sex, a USENET discussion group where people can chat in real time with other users, is the most often visited site on the Internet.[2] Brian Reid, director of the Network Systems Laboratory at Digital Equipment Corporation, reports that between 180,000 and 500,000 users drop in to this discussion group on a monthly basis.[3]

At websites, computer bulletin boards that usually include photographs, interested parties can find almost anything that conforms to their sexual desires. Many pictures of nude men and women like those found at most adult-oriented video stores and booksellers can be downloaded (placed on a user's computer disk or printed on his or her own printer).[1] However, other types of less common sexual images are also available at websites, including explicit images that many people find objectionable.

The Positive Side of the Internet

Despite the potentially offensive graphic images available on-line, the Internet does have several good points. One positive aspect is that people who are interested in meeting others can use the Internet as a sort of virtual pick-up bar without many of the unpleasant consequences. It gives people the freedom either to be themselves without fear of repercussions or to adopt a totally new persona. Best of all, cybersex participants don't have to worry about looking their best during a virtual date.[4] In cyberspace chat rooms, who you are (or who you pretend to be) becomes more important than what you look like. The growing popularity of the Internet as a meeting grounds is reflected in the mainstream movie *You've Got Mail,* in which characters played by Tom Hanks and Meg Ryan build a romance via the modem. New books now offer to guide you through an exploration of Internet relationships.[5,6]

Sexually oriented Internet sites can also be positive in the sense that they sometimes inspire creative impulses and prevent people from engaging in destructive behavior. Some sites house participatory novels in which users can create new realities for themselves and other participants.[7] In this respect, these sites are similar to fantasy game pages that house activities such as Dungeons & Dragons. People are able to cast off their old identities and create exciting new personas that are able to engage in sexual practices that the users themselves would never attempt in real life. Thus the Internet becomes a harmless outlet for sexual fantasies: the ultimate safe sex.

A third plus to using the Internet to meet people is that occasionally, people who use it do fall in "virtual love," choose to meet face-to-face, and end up developing a relationship or even getting married.[4] Although this is a rare occurrence, the chance that it could happen is enough to keep some people involved with Internet romances in the hope of finding a perfect cybermate who will be as good in person as they seem to be on-line.

Pitfalls of On-Line Sex

Although virtual sex has many points in its favor, it also has several negative aspects. One of the worst possible scenarios of on-line sex is discovering that the person with whom you have been pursuing a virtual relationship is not who he or she claims to be. This pitfall is particularly dangerous when one of the people in the relationship is a minor. In response to a recent on-line query, 130 female teenagers reported that they had posted erotic stories on a sexually oriented bulletin board and corresponded with adult men. In the stories, the teenagers pretended to be adults. Several of the teenagers also admitted that they had scheduled face-to-face meetings with these adult men without telling anyone.[8] Although none of the teenagers was harmed as a result of these meetings, the potential for danger was most certainly present. A recent case in which a 13-year-old girl from Kentucky ended up in Los Angeles after being lured there by her adult male Internet correspondent provides evidence to prove this point.[3] Additionally, several cases have been documented in which pedophiles used computer bulletin boards to contact children, learn their names and addresses, and set up meetings with them.

A second drawback to on-line sex is the considerable cost. Although chat rooms are sometimes free and websites have "visitor's passes" that allow sneak previews, most of the hard-core sexual activity is very expensive. Some chat rooms charge as much as $12 an hour for a conversation.[4] To get to the more explicit photographs and participatory novels on the Internet, a member's fee is required, which ranges anywhere from $19.95 for 6 months to $129.95 for a

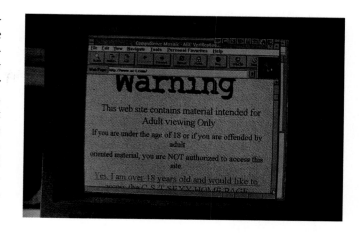

year. These fees are generally paid by credit card on-line. A digital video camera, which is necessary to create real-time pictures to transmit through a personal computer, costs at least $100. Upgrades to computer memory and equipment to handle more technologically advanced transmissions, such as video clips, can also be costly, running into the thousands of dollars.

A third potential problem is cybersex addiction. Some people become so involved with virtual reality that they find themselves uninterested in the real world. A librarian at a large college recently reported that many students have to be asked to log off the library's computers that have Internet connections. These students ignore library policy that limits their Internet use to 30 minutes. One student who was logged onto a sexually oriented chat room for almost 4 hours had to be threatened by campus police. As a result of these incidents, the college now blocks many sexually explicit sites and has disabled its computers' ability to download material.

Other observers proclaim that the problem is not addiction but simply time-wasting.[9] Nobody has trouble being away from the Internet when traveling or occupied with work, they say.

Avoiding Sex on the Internet

With all the publicity and notoriety surrounding sexually oriented Internet sites, many concerned parents want to ensure that their children do not have access to sexual material through their personal computers. Other people are offended by cybersex and do not want it coming into their homes for religious or moral reasons. For these people, several options exist. Parents can subscribe to an on-line service that blocks potentially offensive sites. Also, America Online and Prodigy have mechanisms available on their services to block access to areas that most parents would consider inappropriate for their children.[3] These mechanisms are available free of charge with subscription to the services.

A second option is to purchase a program that will block undesirable material. One such program, Surfwatch, will automatically block access to 1,000 sites and let you screen all user groups, websites, and other electronic avenues. The cost of this program is $49.95 plus a $5.95 monthly service fee. Other types of blocker programs include NetNanny, which lets parents monitor everything that passes through their computer, CyberPatrol, which offers controls similar to Surfwatch, and Time's Up, which lets parents set up time limits and appropriate times for their children to use the computer.

A third, decidedly low-tech option is the most obvious and also the most overlooked. Parents should watch what their children are doing while they are on-line and monitor all activities, perhaps by making computer use a family activity.[3] As columnist Michael J. Miller points out, much of the fear that children will accidentally stumble onto a sexually oriented site is unfounded. Unlike broadcast media, on the Internet, you must enter a specific address or follow a specific link to reach a sexually oriented site. While this is true for hard-core sites, many of which you have to pay for, some people put nude pictures of themselves on their home pages. It's easy to unknowingly stumble on such sites and get an unexpected eyeful. Parents who watch their kids will know exactly where the kids go during an on-line jaunt. Additionally, parents should teach their children some basic safety information, such as never to reveal their real name, address, or telephone number to people they meet on-line. Children should understand that even though they may have on-line friends, these people are really strangers that they know little about.[3,4,7,8]

The Telecommunications Competition and Deregulation Act

In February 1996 President Clinton signed into law the Telecommunications Competition and Deregulation Act, a law that contains a provision called the Telecommunications Decency Act to block indecency on-line. Anyone caught transmitting obscene, lewd, or indecent communications by any electronic means could be fined as much as $100,000 and sent to prison for as long as 2 years.[1,10,11] Civil libertarians and users of sexually oriented Internet sites oppose this law, stating that the First Amendment guarantees freedom of speech and that this freedom should include the Internet. They also believe that the law as written is too broad and confusing; it could be interpreted as banning any use of profanity or nudity on-line, including news reports, legal documents, literature, and even the Bible.[11]

Some parents and religious groups, on the other hand, applaud this new act. They feel it gives them more control over what kind of material is coming into their homes. They believe that this legislation is necessary to protect children from being exposed to pornography on-line. They also believe the law is good because it specifically targets material that is patently offensive and depicts graphic sexual activity.[11]

These same arguments swirl around the case of Jake Baker, a 20-year-old University of Michigan student. Baker was arrested by the FBI and indicted by a federal grand jury on charges of transmitting a threat to injure across state lines. He published a sexual fantasy story on an Internet chat room that involved the rape, torture, and murder of a young woman with the same name as one of his classmates. As clearly reprehensible as his actions seem to most people, one of the many others who argued that Baker's free speech had been violated further accused the University of Michigan of discouraging "free thought, articulate expression, and principled behavior."[12] These remarks illustrate what a wide variety of views people hold regarding Internet free speech and censorship issues.

A line has been drawn in the sand regarding sex on the Internet. Supporters of the new law are joining organizations such as Enough Is Enough, the National Coalition against Pornography, and the American Family Association Law Center. These groups work to defend traditional values and fight against increased pornography. Meanwhile, web search engines such as Yahoo protested the legislation by turning their web pages to black with white lettering for 48 hours to demonstrate "virtual mourning," and the American Civil Liberties Union filed a federal court complaint to block enforcement of the law.[11]

Using the Internet for sexual purposes can have both positive and negative consequences; therefore, people who do so should weigh all factors involved before they decide to enter the world of cybersex. Parents should be especially careful about what they allow to come into their homes via the personal computer. Although blocking methods and the new federal laws provide some protection from sexually oriented material, it is ultimately the individual's responsibility to choose and monitor what type of information comes up while surfing the Internet.

Personal Responsibility

Some people do not take this responsibility seriously enough. Many use work time to log onto sexually explicit Internet sites. On-line Penthouse was called up 1,000 times a month by employees at IBM, Apple, AT&T, NASA, and Hewlett-Packard. Compaq Computer recently dismissed 20 employees who had each logged over 1,000 hits on sexually explicit websites. They were dismissed for misuse of company resources.[13] Not only does this behavior result in a loss of productivity, it can also create a divisive and, in the worst cases, hostile work environment. In coming years, you can expect to see sexual harassment lawsuits involving lewd jokes on company computer bulletin boards, the use of explicit screen savers, and other on-screen and downloaded materials that use the work environment to target, exclude, and in other ways harass certain people in the workforce. If everyone assumed a little more personal responsibility, the call for cyberabstinence may fade.

For Discussion . . .

Have you or someone you know ever explored sexually oriented websites on the Internet? If so, was it a positive or a negative experience? Would you be willing to meet a virtual friend face-to-face? Do you support the new Telecommunications Indecency Act? Why or why not?

References

1. Lewis PH. Despite a new plan for cooling it off, cybersex stays hot. *New York Times* 1995 Mar 26:A1.
2. Nashawatz C. Where the wild things are: anonymous sex is back. *Entertainment Weekly* 1994 Sept 23.
3. Levy S, Stone B. No place for kids: a parents' guide to sex on the Net. *Newsweek* 1995 July 3.
4. Van de Leur G. Twilight zone of the id. *Time* 1995; (45)2.
5. Adamse M, Motta S. *Online friendship, chat room romance and cybersex.* Deerfield Beach, FL: Health Communications, 1996.
6. Levine D. *The joy of cybersex: a guide for creative lovers.* New York: Ballantine Books, 1998.
7. Machure B. MUDs and MUSHes and MOOs. *PC Magazine* 1995 Apr 30:10.
8. Bennahan DS. Lolitas on-line. *Harper's Bazaar* 1995 Sept: 3406.
9. Dvorak JC. Cybersex, addiction, and you. *PC Magazine Online* 1998 Oct 26.
10. Mezer M. A bad dream comes true in cyberspace. *Newsweek* 1996 Jan 8:2.
11. Wagner M. Tempers flare over web censorship. *Computerworld* 1996 Feb 12.
12. Wickens B. Going too far. *Maclean's* 1996; 108(9).
13. Gabriel T. New issue at work: on line sex sites. *The New York Times* 1996 June 27.

InfoLinks
www.socio.demon.co.uk/magazine/
magazine.html
www.cyberlaw.com

chapter
sixteen

Managing Your Fertility

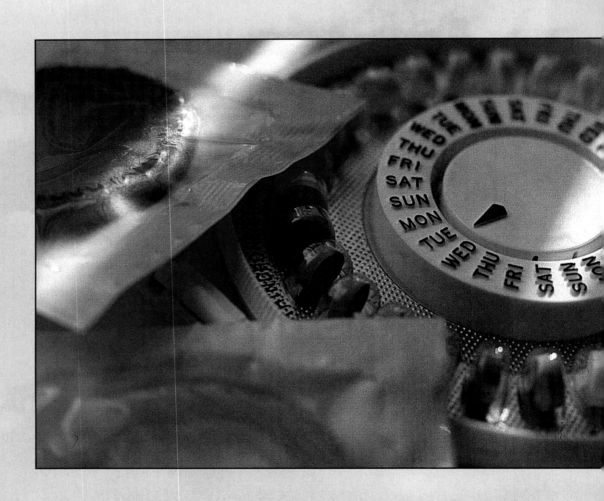

How you decide to control your fertility will have an important effect on your future. Your understanding of information and issues related to fertility control will help you make responsible decisions in this complex area.

For traditional-age students, these decisions may be fast approaching. Frequently, nontraditional students are parents who have had experiences that make them useful resources for other students in the class.

In the beginning of this chapter, we discuss the difference between birth control and contraception and introduce the concept of contraceptive effectiveness rates. We also take a look at why people use birth control. Then we discuss in detail the many birth control methods available today. The chapter concludes by examining the consequences of unintended pregnancy. We think the information presented in this chapter will be helpful as you make important decisions about managing your fertility.

HEALTHY PEOPLE: LOOKING AHEAD TO 2010

The *Healthy People 2010* objectives will undoubtedly include many important goals in the areas of family planning, fertility control, pregnancy, and childbirth. Data indicating our progress to date in these areas focus mainly on adolescents and teenagers, not college students. The *Healthy People 2000* objectives for these age groups include reducing pregnancy rates among adolescents, reducing the proportion of young people who have sexual intercourse, increasing the rate of abstinence among those who have already had intercourse, and increasing contraceptive use by sexually active adolescents and teens.

Progress toward achieving these objectives was mixed. The proportion of young people initiating

sexual activity by age 15 and by age 17 had increased. Some headway was made in promoting abstinence among girls who had already engaged in sexual intercourse. The only objective for which significant gains were reported was the increased use of contraceptives among teenagers.

The picture is more encouraging in the areas of pregnancy and childbirth. Data concerning pregnancy complications, infant mortality, prenatal care, breastfeeding, and cesarean delivery rates all indicated improvement by the late 1990s. We expect continued gains in these important areas as the specific objectives for *Healthy People 2010* are established.

The Morning After: Choice and Conflict

- Names: Laurie and Todd Lindemark
- Ages: 28 and 33
- Occupations: Laurie, symphony cellist
  Todd, architect

"Everything was so perfect—why couldn't it stay that way?"

To everyone who knows them, Laurie and Todd Lindemark seem to have a life that's about as close to perfect as it could be. That's what Laurie and Todd thought too, until a call from Laurie's gynecologist last week confirmed that, as she'd suspected, she's almost 4 weeks pregnant.

I can't be, she'd thought, as the phone slid from her nerveless fingers. Not now, not when I've just been asked to go on the symphony's European tour, not when Todd has just quit his job to start his own firm, not when we've just bought this condo . . . later, when we're settled, when we have more money saved, when we're ready to move to the suburbs . . . but not now.

It's been just 3 days since Laurie and Todd got the news, and it's been 72 hours of almost round-the-clock agonizing, debating, agreeing, we'll have the baby, we won't, we have to, we can't, until they're both wrung out, exhausted, incapable of making the hardest decision they may ever confront: whether to terminate their first pregnancy.

Like many couples, Laurie and Todd didn't plan to start a family until they'd become established in their professions and begun to build a stable financial base for their life together.

Their long years of study, work, and practice are finally beginning to produce results, and they'd just worked out a plan for accelerating the repayment of their student loans.

They've always been scrupulous about using birth control, and if their situation weren't so serious, it would almost be funny, because there was just one night after Don's party, that one extra glass of wine, that one time they left the package of condoms in the bedside table drawer.

Both Laurie and Todd are pro-choice and believe in a woman's right to reproductive freedom. Now that a formerly abstract issue has become reality, however, Todd tends to favor having the baby. He remembers the anguish of his sister and her husband when they decided to terminate their first pregnancy so they could both finish law school. Not only do they still mourn the loss of their unborn child, but they've spent the last 4 years unsuccessfully trying to have another.

Laurie leans more toward ending the pregnancy partly because she really feels unprepared to deal with the major changes to her body and her life. And also because she has a former college roommate who, in the same situation, chose to have the baby and is now the frazzled mother of a rambunctious 2-year-old. Her former roommate is light years away from the career she'd planned in cancer research.

As you study this chapter, think about the choice that confronts Laurie and Todd, and prepare yourself to answer the questions in **Your Turn** at the end of the chapter.

Birth Control Versus Contraception

Any discussion about the control of your **fertility** should start with an explanation of the subtle differences between the terms **birth control** and **contraception**. These terms reflect different perspectives about fertility control. *Birth control* is an umbrella term that refers to all of the procedures you might use to prevent the birth of a child. Birth control includes all available contraceptive measures, as well as sterilization, use of the intrauterine device (IUD), and abortion procedures.

Contraception is a much more specific term for any procedure used to prevent the fertilization of an ovum. Contraceptive measures vary widely in the mechanisms they use to accomplish this task. They also vary considerably in their method of use and their rate of success in preventing conception. A few examples of contraceptive methods are the use of condoms, oral contraceptives, spermicides, and diaphragms.

Beyond the methods mentioned, certain forms of sexual behavior not involving intercourse could be considered forms of contraception. For example, mutual masturbation by couples eliminates the possibility of pregnancy. This practice, as well as additional forms of sexual expression other than intercourse (such as kissing, touching, and massage), has been given the generic term **outercourse**. Outercourse protects against unplanned pregnancy, and may also significantly reduce the transmission of sexually transmitted diseases, including HIV infection.

Reasons for Choosing to Use Birth Control

People use birth control for many reasons. Many career-minded individuals carefully plan the timing and spacing of children to best provide for their children's financial support without sacrificing their job status. Others choose methods of birth control to ensure that they will never have children. Some use birth control methods to permit safe participation in a wide variety of sexual behaviors. Fear of contracting a sexually transmitted disease prompts some people to use particular forms of birth control.

Financial and legal considerations can be significant factors in the choice of certain birth control methods. Many people must of necessity take the cost of a method into account when selecting appropriate birth control. The cost of sterilization and abortion can prohibit some low-income people from choosing these alternatives, especially because federal funds do not support such procedures. A number of states have established statutes and policies that make contraceptive information and medical services relatively difficult to obtain.

Another important consideration in the use of birth control methods is the availability of professional services. An example of the effect of this factor may be the selection of birth control methods by college students. Some colleges and universities provide contraceptive services through their student health centers. Students enrolled in these schools have easy access to low-cost, comprehensive contraceptive services. Students enrolled in colleges that do not provide such complete services may find that access to accurate information and clinical services is difficult to obtain and that private professional services are expensive.

For many people, religious doctrine will be a factor in their selection of a birth control method. One example is the opposition of the Roman Catholic Church and other religious groups to the use of all forms of contraception other than natural family planning.

Theoretical Effectiveness Versus Use Effectiveness

People considering the use of a contraceptive method need to understand the difference between the two effectiveness rates given for each form of contraception. *Theoretical effectiveness* is a measure of a contraceptive method's ability to prevent a pregnancy when the method is used precisely as directed during every act of intercourse. *Use effectiveness*, however, refers to the effectiveness of a method in preventing conception when used by the general public. Use effectiveness rates take into account factors that lower effectiveness below that based on "perfect" use. Failure to follow proper instructions, illness of the user, forgetfulness, physician (or pharmacist) error, and a subconscious desire to experience risk or even pregnancy are a few of the factors that can lower the effectiveness of even the most theoretically effective contraceptive technique.

Effectiveness rates are often expressed as the percentage of women users of childbearing age who do not become pregnant while using the method for one year. For some methods the theoretical-effectiveness and use-effectiveness rates are vastly different; the theoretical rate is always higher than the use rate. Table 16-1 presents data concerning effectiveness rates, advantages, and disadvantages of many birth control methods.

Selecting Your Contraceptive Method

In this section, we discuss some of the many factors that should be important to you as you consider selecting a contraceptive method. Completing the Personal Assessment on page 478 will help you make this decision.

Those who wish to exercise a large measure of control over their fertility can consider the following:

- *It should be safe.*
- *It should be effective.*
- *It should be reliable.*
- *It should be reversible.*
- *It should be affordable.*
- *It should be easy to use.*
- *It should not interfere with sexual expression.*

Personal Applications

- What factors would be most important to you in selecting an appropriate contraceptive method?

Current Birth Control Methods

Abstinence

Abstinence as a form of birth control has gained attention recently on college campuses (see the Star Box on page 464). Abstinence is as close to 100 percent effective as possible. There have been isolated reports in medical literature of pregnancy without sexual intercourse, usually involving ejaculation by the male near the woman's vagina. Avoiding this situation should raise the effectiveness of abstinence to 100 percent.

Abstinence as a form of birth control has additional advantages in that it gives nearly 100 percent protection from sexually transmitted diseases, it is free, and it does not require a visit to a physician.

You can contract sexually transmitted diseases by other intercourse practices. A very common method is via oral sex with someone who has a fever

---

fertility   the ability to reproduce.

birth control   all of the methods and procedures that can prevent the birth of a child.

contraception   any method or procedure that prevents fertilization.

outercourse   sexual activity that does not involve intercourse.

Table 16-1   Effectiveness Rates of Birth Control for 100 Women during 1 Year of Use

| Method | Estimated Effectiveness | | Advantages | Disadvantages |
	Theoretical	Use		
No method (chance)	15%	15%	Inexpensive	Totally ineffective
Withdrawal	85%	75%–80%	No supplies or advance preparation needed; no side effects; men share responsibility for family planning. Inexpensive.	Interferes with coitus; may be difficult to use effectively; woman must trust man to withdraw as orgasm approaches.
Periodic abstinence Calendar Basal body temperature Cervical mucus method Symptothermal	90%–98%	75%–80%	No supplies needed; no side effects; men share responsibility for family planning; women learn about their bodies. Inexpensive.	Difficult to use, especially if menstrual cycles are irregular, as is common in young women; abstinence may be necessary for long periods; lengthy instruction and ongoing counseling may be needed.
Cervical cap	94%	82%	No health risks; helps protect against some STDs and cervical cancer. Cost: $150–$300, including office visit.	Limited availability.
Spermicide	97%–98%	75%–85%	No health risks; helps protect against some STDs; can be used with condoms to increase effectiveness considerably. Cost: $3–$8 per tube or package.	Must be inserted 5 to 30 minutes before coitus; effective for only 30 to 60 minutes; some women may find them awkward or embarrassing to use.
Diaphragm with spermicide	97%–98%	80%–90%	No health risks; helps protect against some STDs and cervical cancer. Cost: $150–$300, including office visit.	Must be inserted with jelly or foam before every act of coitus and left in place for at least 6 hours after coitus; must be fitted by health care personnel; some women may find it awkward or embarrassing to use; may be inconvenient to clean, store, and carry.
Male condom and male condom with spermicide	98% 99%	80%–90% 95%	Easy to use; easy to obtain; no health risks; very effective protection against some STDs; men share responsibility for family planning. Cost: condoms sometimes free, or $3–$10 per pack of 20; $3–$8 per tube or package of spermicide.	Must be put on just before coitus; some men and women complain of decreased sensation.

blister or cold sore. Any sexual contact with an infected person makes transmission of STDs possible.

Withdrawal

Withdrawal, or **coitus interruptus,** is the contraceptive practice in which the erect penis is removed from the vagina just before ejaculation of semen. Theoretically this procedure prevents sperm from entering the deeper structures of the female reproductive system. The use

effectiveness of this method, however, reflects how unsuccessful the method is in practice (see Table 16-1).

Strong evidence suggests that the clear preejaculate fluid that helps neutralize and lubricate the male urethra can contain *viable* (capable of fertilization) sperm.[1] This sperm can be deposited near the cervical opening before withdrawal. Thus the relatively low effectiveness. Furthermore, withdrawal does not protect users from the transmission of sexually transmit-

Table 16-1 *Continued*

Method	Estimated Effectiveness Theoretical	Use	Advantages	Disadvantages
Female condom	90%+	75%–79%	Relatively easy to use; no prescription required; polyurethane is stronger than latex; provides some STD protection; silicone-based lubrication provided; useful when male will not use a condom. Cost $2–$5 each.	Contraceptive effectiveness and STD protection not as high as with male condom; couples may be unfamiliar with a device that extends outside the vagina; more expensive than male condoms.
IUD	99%	95%–98%	Easy to use; highly effective in preventing pregnancy; does not interfere with coitus; repeated action not needed. Cost: $150–$500, including office visit.	May increase risk of pelvic inflammatory disease (PID) and infertility in women with more than one sexual partner; not usually recommended for women who have never had a child; must be inserted by health care personnel; may cause heavy bleeding and pain in some women.
Combined pill (Estrogen-progestin) Triphasic pill	99%	97%–98%	Easy to use; highly effective in preventing pregnancy; does not interfere with coitus; regulates menstrual cycle; reduces heavy bleeding and menstrual pain; helps protect against ovarian and endometrial cancer. Cost: $12–$30 per month.	Must be taken every day; requires medical examination and prescription; minor side effects such as nausea or menstrual spotting; possibility of circulatory problems, such as blood clotting, strokes, and hypertension, in a small percentage of users.
Minipill (progestin only)	99%+	96%–97%		
Depo-Provera	99%+	99%+	Easy to use; highly effective for 3-month period; continued use prevents menstruation. Cost: $30–$75 per shot.	Requires supervision by a physician; administered by injection; some women experience irregular menstrual spotting in early months of use.
Subdermal implants (progestin only)	99%+	99%+	Highly effective for 5-year period; helps prevent anemia and regulates menstrual cycle.	Requires minor surgery; some women experience irregular menstrual spotting. Cost: insertion, $450–$700; removal, $100–$300.
Tubal ligation	99%+	99%+	Permanent; removes fear of pregnancy.	Surgery-related risks; generally considered irreversible. Cost: $1,000–$2,500.
Vasectomy	99%+	99%+	Permanent; removes fear of pregnancy.	Generally considered irreversible. Cost: about $500.

ted diseases (STDs). It should never be considered a reliable contraceptive approach.

Periodic Abstinence

Four approaches are included in the birth control strategy called **periodic abstinence:** (1) the calendar method, (2) the basal body temperature (BBT) method, (3) the Billings cervical mucus method, and (4) the symptothermal method.[2] All four methods

coitus interruptus (withdrawal) (co ih tus in ter **rup** tus) a contraceptive practice in which the erect penis is removed from the vagina before ejaculation.

periodic abstinence birth control methods that rely on a couple's avoidance of intercourse during the ovulatory phase of a woman's menstrual cycle; also called fertility awareness or natural family planning.

Personal Assessment

To determine which birth control method would be best for you, answer the following questions, and check the interpretation below.

Do I:

	Yes	No
1. Need a contraceptive right away?	___	___
2. Want a contraceptive that can be used completely independent of sexual relations?	___	___
3. Need a contraceptive only once in a great while?	___	___
4. Want something with no harmful side effects?	___	___
5. Want to avoid going to the doctor?	___	___
6. Want something that will help protect against sexually transmitted diseases?	___	___
7. Have to be concerned about affordability?	___	___
8. Need to be virtually certain that pregnancy will not result?	___	___
9. Want to avoid pregnancy now but want to have a child sometime in the future?	___	___
10. Have any medical condition or lifestyle that may rule out some form of contraception?	___	___

Interpretation

If you have checked *Yes* to number:

1. Condoms and spermicides may be easily purchased without prescription in any pharmacy.
2. Sterilization, oral contraceptives, hormone implants or injections, cervical caps, and periodic abstinence techniques do not require that anything be done just before sexual relations.
3. Diaphragms, condoms, or spermicides can be used by people who have coitus only once in a while. Periodic abstinence techniques may also be appropriate but require a high degree of skill and motivation.
4. IUDs should be carefully discussed with your physician. Sometimes the use of oral contraceptives or hormone products results in some minor discomfort and may have harmful side effects.
5. Condoms and spermicides do not require a prescription from a physician.
6. Condoms and, to a lesser extent, spermicides and the other barrier methods may help protect against some sexually transmitted diseases. No method (except abstinence) can guarantee complete protection.
7. Be a wise consumer: check prices, ask pharmacists and physicians. The cost of sterilization is high, but there is no additional expense for a lifetime.
8. Sterilization provides near certainty. Oral contraceptives, hormone implants or injections, or a diaphragm-condom-spermicide combination also give a high measure of reliable protection. Periodic abstinence, withdrawal, and douche methods should be avoided. Outercourse may be a good alternative.
9. Although it is sometimes possible to reverse sterilization, it requires surgery and is more complex than simply stopping use of any of the other methods.
10. Smokers and people with a history of blood clots should probably not use oral contraceptives or other hormone approaches. Some people have an allergic reaction to a specific spermicide and should experiment with another brand. Some women cannot be fitted with a diaphragm or cervical cap because of the position of the uterus. The woman and her health care provider will then need to select another suitable means of contraception.

To Carry This Further . . .

There may be more than one method of birth control suitable for you. Always consider how a method you select can also help you avoid an STD. Study the methods suggested above, and consult Table 16-1 to determine what techniques may be most appropriate.

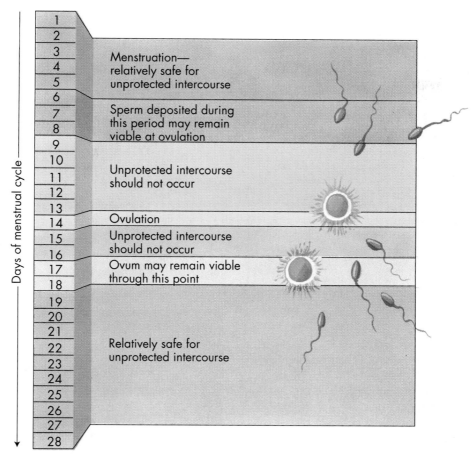

Figure 16-1 Periodic abstinence (fertility awareness or natural family planning) can combine use of the calendar, basal body temperature measurements, and Billings mucus techniques to identify the fertile period. Remember that most women's cycles are not consistently perfect 28-day cycles, as shown in most illustrations.

attempt to determine the time a woman ovulates. Figure 16-1 above shows a day-to-day fertility calendar used to calculate fertile periods. Most research indicates that an ovum is viable for only about twenty-four to thirty-six hours after its release from the ovary. (After they are inside the female reproductive tract, some sperm can survive up to a week.) When a woman can accurately determine when she ovulates, she must refrain from intercourse long enough for the ovum to begin to disintegrate. Fertility awareness, rhythm, natural birth control, and natural family planning are other terms for periodic abstinence. Remember that periodic abstinence methods *do not* provide protection against the spread of STDs, including HIV infection.

Periodic abstinence is the only method endorsed by the Roman Catholic Church. For some people who have deep concerns for the spiritual dimension of their health, selecting a method other than periodic abstinence may entail a serious compromise of beliefs.

The **calendar method** requires close examination of a woman's menstrual cycle for at least eight

cycles. Records are kept of the length (in days) of each cycle. A *cycle* is defined as the number of days from the first day of bleeding of one cycle to the first day of bleeding of the next cycle.

To determine the days she should abstain from intercourse, a woman should subtract eighteen from her shortest cycle; this is the first day she should abstain from intercourse. Then she should subtract eleven from her longest cycle; this is the last day she must abstain from intercourse (see the Health Action Guide on p. 480).[2]

The *basal body temperature method* requires a woman (for about three or four successive months) to take her body temperature every morning before she rises from bed. A finely calibrated thermometer, available in many drugstores, is used for this purpose. The theory behind this method is that there is a distinct

---

calendar method a form of periodic abstinence in which the variable lengths of a woman's menstrual cycle are used to calculate her fertile period.

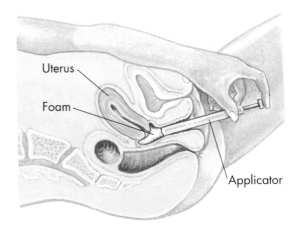

Figure 16-2   Spermicidal foams and suppositories are placed deep into the vagina in the region of the cervix no longer than 30 minutes before intercourse.

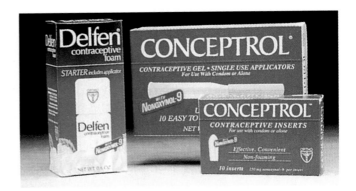

Vaginal spermicide.

correlation between body temperature and the process of ovulation. Just before ovulation, the body temperature supposedly dips and then rises about one degree Fahrenheit for the rest of the cycle. The woman is instructed to refrain from intercourse during the interval when the temperature change takes place.

Drawbacks of this procedure include the need for consistent, accurate temperature readings and the realization that all women's bodies are different. Some women may not fit the temperature pattern projection because of biochemical differences in their bodies. In addition, body temperature can fluctuate.

The *Billings cervical mucus method* is another periodic abstinence technique. Generally used with other periodic abstinence techniques, this method requires a woman to evaluate the daily mucous discharge from her cervix. Users of this method become familiar with the changes in both appearance (from clear to cloudy) and consistency (from watery to thick) of their cervical mucus throughout their cycles. Women are taught that the unsafe days are when the mucus becomes clear and is the consistency of raw egg whites. Such a technique of ovulation determination must be learned from a physician or family planning professional.

The *symptothermal method* of periodic abstinence combines the use of the BBT method and the cervical mucus method.[2] Thus, some family planning professionals consider the symptothermal method a combination of all of the periodic abstinence approaches.

Those who wish to practice one of these periodic abstinence methods should consult a professional to learn how to chart their menstrual cycle and detect the physical signs that help predict the "unsafe" days. Besides the lack of protection against STDs, the periodic abstinence methods have the following potential problems:

- Partner may be uncooperative.
- Couple may take risks during "unsafe" days.
- Record-keeping may be poor.
- Illness and lack of sleep can affect body temperature.
- Vaginal infections and douches change mucus.
- Method cannot be used with irregular periods or temperature patterns.

Vaginal Spermicides

Although they are not recommended as the primary form of fertility control, spermicidal agents are often recommended to be used with other forms of birth control. Alone, **spermicides** offer a reasonable amount of contraceptive protection for the woman who is sexually active on an *infrequent* basis. Spermicides containing nonoxynol-9 provide some protection (but *not full* protection) against STDs and HIV infection.

Modern spermicides are safe, reasonably effective, reversible forms of contraception that can be obtained without a physician's prescription; they can be purchased in most drugstores and in many supermarkets. Like condoms, spermicides are relatively inexpensive. When used together, spermicides and con-

Vaginal Contraceptive Film

A unique spermicide delivery system developed in England is vaginal contraceptive film (VCF). Vaginal contraceptive film is a sheet containing nonoxynol-9 that is inserted over the cervical opening. Shortly after insertion of the VCF, it dissolves into a gel-like material that clings to the cervical opening. The VCF can be inserted up to an hour before intercourse. Over the course of several hours, the material will be washed from the vagina in the normal vaginal secretions.

This spermicide is a nonprescription form of contraception that is as effective as other spermicidal foams and jellies. A box of twelve sheets costs about $7. Like other spermicidal agents, VCF may also help in minimizing the risk of some STDs and PID.

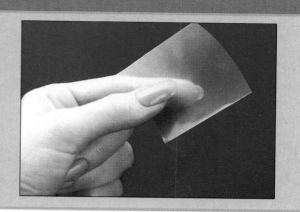

HEALTH ACTION GUIDE

Discussing Birth Control with Your Partner

How can two people feel comfortable enough with each other to discuss what they will do on their dates, where they will go, and even who will pay for the date, yet not feel comfortable enough to discuss birth control before engaging in sex? The simple fact is that if you don't feel you can discuss sex with your partner, you should consider whether you are intimate enough to have sex together.

If you believe there is even a chance you will engage in any kind of sex, or if you think your partner may pursue sex with you, you should be prepared and discuss the possibility before being swept along by the heat of an encounter. In addition, you and your partner will feel more comfortable about your relationship and your sexual activity if you first discuss your feelings about contraception, disease prevention, and pregnancy. Consider the following topics:

- First, the fact that you are discussing contraception together does not necessarily mean that you will engage in sex. In addition, you can discuss abstinence as a very effective form of contraception.
- Discussing contraception and disease prevention with your partner is not rude. It is simply common sense.
- Talking about contraception is a way of sharing responsibility and intimacy. It can bring you closer.
- Which type(s) of contraception will you use? See the section in this chapter on page 475, Selecting Your Contraception Method, for help in making your choices.

- If you feel unsure about how to broach the subject or are undecided about any of the issues, consider discussing the subject with a counselor or physician before you talk with your partner.
- Sort out your own feelings and understand all the alternatives, including their advantages and disadvantages, before you open the discussion.
- Pick the right occasion. Don't wait until you have begun sexual activity.
- Both partners have dignity and worth, and should be treated with dignity. If you and your boyfriend or girlfriend are discussing contraception and you have different views, you each have the right to your opinions. If necessary, you can agree to disagree.
- Listen carefully and ask questions. Speak honestly about your own feelings and beliefs.
- Who will pay for the contraceptive method? Will both partners share the cost?
- What will both of you do if the female partner becomes pregnant?

Have you discussed these issues in the past before initiating sex with a partner? Do you plan to discuss these issues in the future?

InfoLinks
www.arhp.org/success

doms provide a high degree of contraceptive protection and disease prevention.

Spermicides, which are available in foam, cream, paste, or film form, are made of water-soluble bases with a spermicidal chemical incorporated in the base. The base material is designed to liquefy at body temperature and distribute the spermicidal component in an even layer over the tissues of the upper vagina (Figure 16-2). The Star Box above describes a unique film type of spermicide.

Spermicides are not specific to sperm cells; they also attack other cells and thus may provide the woman with some additional protection against many STDs and **pelvic inflammatory disease (PID)**.

spermicides chemicals capable of killing sperm.

pelvic inflammatory disease (PID) a generalized infection of the pelvic cavity that results from the spread of an infection through a woman's reproductive structures.

However, when used alone, spermicides do not provide sufficient protection against most pathogens, including the virus that causes AIDS.

Condoms

Colored or natural, smooth or textured, straight or shaped, plain or reservoir-tipped, dry or lubricated—the condom is approaching an art form. Nevertheless, the familiar **condom** remains a safe, effective, reversible contraceptive device. All condoms manufactured in the United States must be approved by the FDA.

For couples who are highly motivated in their desire to prevent a pregnancy, the effectiveness of a condom can approach that of an oral contraceptive. A condom can be nearly 100 percent effective when used with contraceptive foam. Some lubricated condoms now also contain a spermicide. For couples who are less motivated or who use condoms on an irregular basis, the condom can be considerably less effective. This readily available and inexpensive method of contraception requires responsible use by both the man and woman if it is to achieve a high level of effectiveness (see the Health Action Guide below).

The condom offers a measure of protection against sexually transmitted diseases. For both the man and the woman, chlamydial infections, gonorrhea, HIV infection, and other STDs are less likely to be acquired when the condom is used. The condom should be used with a spermicide containing nonoxynol-9 to make it even more effective against the spread of STDs. Although advertisements suggest that condoms provide protection against the transmission of genital herpes, users of condoms must remember that this protection is limited to the penis and vagina—not to the surrounding genital region, where significant numbers of lesions are found. Like other barrier methods of contraception, the condom is a reasonable choice for couples who are motivated in their desire to prevent a pregnancy and who are willing to assume the level of responsibility required.

HEALTH ACTION GUIDE

Maximizing the Effectiveness of Condoms

These simple directions for using condoms correctly, in combination with your motivation and commitment to regular use, should provide you with reasonable protection:

- Keep a supply of condoms at hand. Condoms should be stored in a cool, dry place so that they are readily available at the time of intercourse. Condoms that are stored in wallets or automobile glove compartments may not be in satisfactory condition when they are used. Avoid temperature extremes. Check the condom package for the expiration date.
- Do not test a condom by inflating or stretching it. Handle it gently, and keep it away from sharp fingernails.
- For maximum effectiveness, put the condom on before genital contact. Either the man or the woman can put the condom in place. Early application is particularly important in the prevention of STDs. Early application also lessens the possibility of the release of preejaculate fluid into the vagina.
- Unroll the condom on the erect penis. For those using a condom without a reservoir tip, a half-inch space should be left to catch the ejaculate. To leave this space, pinch the tip of the condom as you roll it on the erect penis. Do not leave any air in the tip of the condom (see the accompanying illustration).
- Lubricate the condom if this has not already been done by the manufacturer. When doing this, be certain to use a water-soluble lubricant and not a petroleum-based product such as petroleum jelly. Petroleum can deteriorate the latex material. Other oil-based lubricants, such as mineral oil, baby oil, vegetable oil, shortening, and certain hand lotions, can quickly damage a condom. Use water-based lubricants only!
- After ejaculation, be certain that the condom does not become dislodged from the penis. Hold the rim of the condom firmly against the base of the penis during withdrawal. Do not allow the penis to become flaccid (soft) while still in the vagina.

- Inspect the condom for tears before throwing it away. If the condom is damaged in some way, immediately insert a spermicidal agent into the vagina.

InfoLinks
www.plannedparenthood.org/BIRTH-CONTROL/
condom.htm

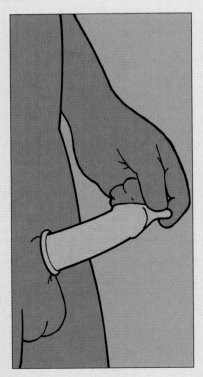

Pinch the end of the condom to leave one-half inch of space at the tip.

The Female Condom

In April 1993 the Wisconsin Pharmacal Company finally gained approval to market a female condom called Reality. This device consists of a soft, loose-fitting polyurethane sheath and two flexible rings (see photo). Reality is inserted like a tampon and lines the inner contours of the vagina. The device extends outside the vagina and covers the labia. Reality sells in three-packs for about $6.50.

Since then, other female condoms have been developed, including Lea's Shield and Femidon. Such devices are available in drugstores and supermarkets.

These devices typically are prelubricated and are intended for one-time use. Manufacturer's studies have shown that female condoms have fewer leaks and less slippage and dislodgement and provide less risk of exposure to semen than do male condoms. The polyurethane used is stronger and more resistant to oils than the latex membrane used for male condoms. Despite these claims, the FDA contends that male latex condoms provide greater contraceptive protection and protection from STDs than female condoms.[4] However, use of the female condom may help reduce women's risk of acquiring HIV, especially in relationships in which both partners are not monogamous.[5]

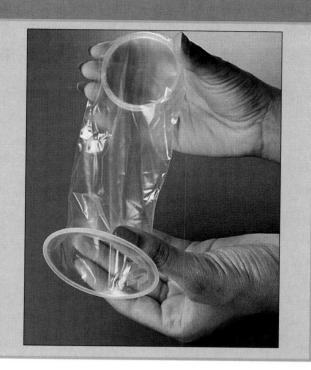

A newer alternative is the female condom (see the Star Box above for a discussion). This product is 79 percent to 95 percent effective.[3] Like the male condom, the female condom acts as a barrier to prevent the sperm from reaching the egg. The female condom also provides some protection against STDs and is easily available in drugstores and supermarkets.

Diaphragm

The **diaphragm** is a soft rubber cup with a springlike metal rim that rests in the top of the vagina. The diaphragm covers the cervical opening (Figure 16-3). During intercourse the diaphragm stays in place quite well and cannot usually be felt by either partner.

The diaphragm is always used with a spermicidal cream or jelly placed inside the cup and around the rim. When used properly with a spermicide, the diaphragm is a relatively effective contraceptive, and when combined with the man's use of a condom, its effectiveness is even greater. The diaphragm carries no major health risks, although it can increase the risk of a urinary tract infection. A single diaphragm can last several years.

Diaphragms must always be fitted and prescribed by a physician. The cost of obtaining a diaphragm and keeping a supply of spermicide may be higher than that of other methods. Also, the woman must have a high level of motivation to follow the instructions exactly.

Diaphragms and other vaginal barrier methods (such as the cervical cap) provide some protection

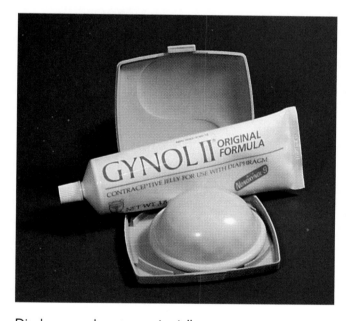

Diaphragm and contraceptive jelly.

against STDs, including gonorrhea and chlamydia, PID, and cervical cancer. However, the ability of diaphragms and other vaginal barrier methods to provide protection against HIV infection for either

condom a latex shield designed to cover the erect penis and retain semen upon ejaculation; "rubber."

diaphragm a soft rubber cup designed to cover the cervix.

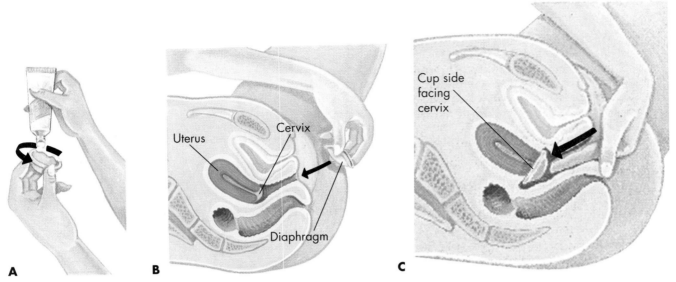

A **B** **C**

Figure 16-3 **A,** Spermicidal cream or jelly is placed into the diaphragm. **B,** The diaphragm is folded lengthwise and inserted into the vagina. **C,** The diaphragm is then placed against the cervix so that the cup portion containing the spermicide is facing the cervix. The outline of the cervix should be felt through the central part of the diaphragm.

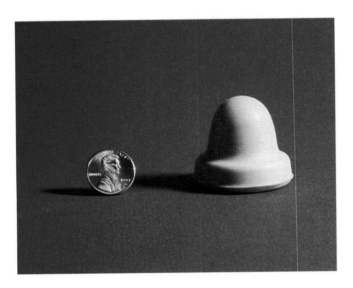

Cervical cap.

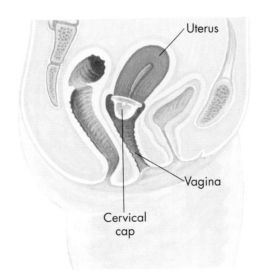

Figure 16-4 After the spermicidal cream or jelly is placed in the cervical cap, the cap is inserted into the vagina and placed against the cervix.

partner is not known. If you are concerned about possible HIV infection, either avoid sexual activity or use a latex condom and spermicide in combination.[4]

Cervical Cap

The **cervical cap** is a small, thimble-shaped device that fits over the entire cervix. Resembling a small diaphragm, the cervical cap is placed deeper than the diaphragm. The cap is held in place by suction rather than by pushing against anatomical structures (Figure 16-4). As with the diaphragm, the cervical cap is coated with spermicide and prevents the sperm from reaching the egg. The cap carries no major health risks and is nearly equal to the diaphragm in

effectiveness, although it can be slightly less effective for women who have already had a child.[3]

The cervical cap can be difficult for some women to use and may not fit all women. As with the diaphragm, a physician prescribes the cervical cap and shows the woman how to coat it with spermicide and use it.

Intrauterine Device

The modern **intrauterine device** is the most popular reversible contraceptive method in the world.[6] The IUD is a safe, effective method of birth control. Ex-

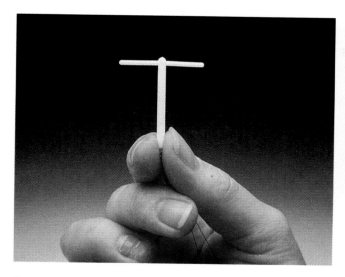

Progestasert IUD.

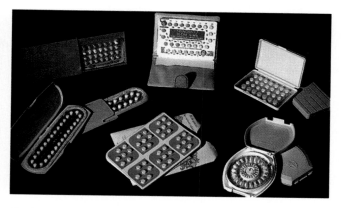

Oral contraceptives.

perts still do not understand how the IUD prevents pregnancy, but recent research suggests that IUDs may prevent conception, rather than prevent a fertilized ovum from implanting in the uterus as has been thought.[7] IUDs seem to affect the way the sperm or egg moves. The IUD might release substances that immobilize sperm, or the IUD might prompt the egg to move through the fallopian tube too fast to be fertilized. Research is ongoing.

Two types of IUDs are available in the United States: the Progestasert (a T-shaped IUD containing progestin) and the Copper T 380-A (ParaGard), a T-shaped IUD wrapped with copper wire. Copper IUDs may increase menstrual blood loss somewhat, but hormone-producing IUDs substantially reduce blood loss.

The Progestasert must be replaced every year, but the Copper T 380-A can remain in place for up to ten years. Only a skilled physician can prescribe and insert an IUD. Once inserted, an IUD is immediately effective. As with many other forms of contraception, IUDs do not offer protection against STDs, including the AIDS virus.

The IUD is inserted into the uterus by a trained clinician. Insertion is often scheduled during menstruation, when the opening of the cervix is softer and the woman is unlikely to be pregnant. Along with a physical examination, the physician will ask several questions about the woman's lifestyle, and she should be honest about her sex life, because the IUD is not for all women. Likewise, the woman should discuss her concerns openly. The IUD can be an acceptable form of contraception, especially for women who are in their middle to late reproductive years, unable to take birth control pills, in a stable, monogamous relationship, and not at risk for STDs.

Some women using IUDs experience increased menstrual bleeding and cramping. Two uncommon

but potentially serious side effects of IUD use are uterine perforation (in which the IUD imbeds itself into the uterine wall) and pelvic inflammatory disease (PID, a life-threatening infection of the abdominal cavity). However, in women in monogamous relationships, the risk of PID is low.[7] In addition, a study by the World Health Organization indicates that today's IUDs do not increase the risk of pelvic infection except in the early weeks after insertion.[8]

As Table 16-1 indicates, IUDs are very effective birth control devices, surpassed in effectiveness only by abstinence, sterilization, and oral (or implanted or injected) contraceptives.

Oral Contraceptives

Developed in the 1950s, the **oral contraceptive pill** provides the highest effectiveness rate of any single reversible contraceptive method used today. "The pill" is the method of choice for nearly 17 million users in the United States.[9]

Use of the pill requires a physician's examination and prescription. Because oral contraceptives are available in a wide range of formulas, follow-up examinations are important to ensure that a woman is receiving an effective dosage with as few side effects as possible. Matching the right prescription with the woman may require a few consultations.

All oral contraceptives contain synthetic (laboratory-made) hormones. The *combined pill* uses both synthetic estrogen and synthetic progesterone in each of

cervical cap a small, thimble-shaped device designed to fit over the cervix.

intrauterine device (IUD) a small, plastic, medicated or unmedicated device that prevents pregnancy when inserted in the uterus.

oral contraceptive pill a pill taken orally, composed of synthetic female hormones that prevent ovulation or implantation; "the pill."

Emergency Contraception

A "morning-after pill" is an emergency oral contraceptive a woman can take to reduce the possibility of pregnancy after unprotected intercourse. Many physicians and clinics have used the "pill" informally for this purpose for many years, and it has been used openly in Europe for more than a decade by a million women. Now, the U.S. Food and Drug Administration (FDA) has given its approval for the use of oral contraceptives up to three days after unprotected intercourse.

Emergency contraceptives currently available are high-dose estrogens, oral contraceptives, and Danazol. Some of these methods are plagued by side effects. Two recent studies published in the United Kingdom show RU 486, the drug best-known as a first-trimester abortion method, to be a very effective emergency contraceptive with fewer side effects than the current methods (see the Star Box on p. 490 for more information on RU 486). RU 486 may someday replace high doses of oral contraceptives as the method of choice for emergency contraception.

The use of emergency contraception draws opposition from some right-to-life advocates, who believe that life begins when the egg is fertilized, and who denounce any subsequent intervention. However, the emergency treatment actually can work in any of four stages in the female reproductive cycle. It can prevent ovulation, fertilization of the egg, or transportation of the egg to the uterus, and it can make the uterine lining inhospitable to implantation, says James Trussell, director of the Office of Population Research at Princeton University. In any individual, there is no way to determine at which stage pregnancy is prevented.

The use of emergency contraception in cases of rape or contraceptive failure is understandable. However, some clinic workers have expressed concern about the number of women who have used this emergency measure as a form of routine contraception. In addition, women engaging in unprotected sex may have been exposed to sexually transmitted diseases, including HIV.

twenty-one pills. In 1984 *triphasic pills* were introduced in the United States. In these pills the level of synthetic progesterone varies every seven days during the cycle.[2] Estrogen levels remain constant during the cycle. As with many forms of contraception, *oral contraceptives do not protect against the transmission of STDs, including HIV infection.* Also, the use of antibiotics may lower the pill's contraceptive effectiveness.

Oral contraceptives function in several ways. The estrogen in the pill tends to reduce ova development and ovulation. The progesterone in the pill helps reduce ovulation (by lowering the release of luteinizing hormone). The progesterone in the pill also causes the uterine wall to develop inadequately and helps thicken cervical mucus, thus making it difficult for sperm to enter the uterus. (For a discussion of emergency contraception, see the Star Box above.)

The physical changes produced by the oral contraceptive provide some beneficial side effects in women. Because the synthetic hormones are taken for twenty-one days and then are followed by **placebo pills** or no pills for seven days, the menstrual cycle becomes regulated. Even women who have irregular cycles immediately become "regular." Because the uterine lining is not developed to the extent seen in a non-pill-taking woman, the uterus is not forced to contract with the same amount of vigor. Thus menstrual cramping is reduced, and the resultant menstrual flow is diminished.

Research indicates that oral contraceptive use may provide protection against anemia, PID, non-cancerous breast tumors, recurrent ovarian cysts, ectopic pregnancy, endometrial cancer, osteoporosis (thinning of the bones), and cancer of the ovaries.[2] No conclusive evidence has been found that links oral contraceptive use to breast cancer. However, oral contraceptive use may be linked to a slight increase in cervical cancer risk.[2]

The negative side effects of the oral contraceptive pill can be divided into two general categories: (1) unpleasant and (2) potentially dangerous. The unpleasant side effects generally subside within two or three months for most women. A number of women report some or many of the following symptoms:

- Tenderness in breast tissue
- Nausea
- Mild headaches
- Slight, irregular spotting
- Weight gain
- Fluctuations in sex drive
- Mild depression
- More frequent vaginal infections

In many cases, a cause-and-effect relationship between these unpleasant side effects and the pill has never been proved, or the symptoms are so rare as to be clinically insignificant. Unfortunately, many women avoid this highly effective form of contraception because of the anecdotal stories they have heard about unpleasant symptoms.[10]

The potentially dangerous side effects of the oral contraceptive pill are most often seen in the cardiovascular system. Blood clotting, strokes, hypertension, and heart attack all seem to be associated with the estrogen component of the combined pill. When compared with nonusers, the risk of dying from cardiovascular complications is only slightly increased among healthy young oral contraceptive users. Nevertheless, the risks associated with pregnancy and childbirth are still much greater than those associated with oral contraceptive use.

There are some **contraindications** for the use of oral contraceptives. If you have a history of blood clotting, migraine headaches, liver disease, a heart condition, high blood pressure, obesity, diabetes, epilepsy, or anemia, or if you do not have regular menstrual cycles, the pill probably should not be your contraceptive choice. A thorough health history is important before a woman starts to take the pill.

Two additional contraindications are receiving considerable attention by the medical community. Cigarette smoking and advancing age are highly associated with an increased risk of potentially serious side effects. Increasing numbers of physicians are not prescribing oral contraceptives for their patients who smoke. The risk of cardiovascular-related deaths is greatly enhanced in women over age thirty-five. The risk is even higher in female smokers over thirty-five. The data are quite convincing.[2]

For the vast majority of women, however, the pill, when properly prescribed, is safe and effective. Careful scrutiny of one's health history and careful follow-up examinations when a problem is suspected are essential elements that can provide a margin of safety.

Personal Applications
• How well do you think college students understand that oral contraceptives do not protect against STDs, including HIV infection?

Minipills
Some women prefer not to use the combined oral contraceptive pill. Thus to avoid some of the potentially serious side effects of the combined pill, some physicians are prescribing **minipills.** These oral contraceptives contain no estrogen—only low-dose progesterone. The minipill seems to work by making an unsuitable environment for the transportation and implantation of the fertilized ovum. The effectiveness of the minipill is slightly lower than that of the combined pill. *Breakthrough bleeding* and **ectopic pregnancy** are more common in minipill users than in combined-pill users.

Injectable Contraceptives

For Women
In late 1992 the FDA approved a form of synthetic progesterone called Depo-Provera. This contraceptive is injectable and is 99 percent effective for three months. This hormone shot works by preventing the release of the egg, thickening the cervical mucus to keep the sperm from joining the egg, and preventing a fertilized egg from implanting in the uterus.

Like oral contraceptives, Depo-Provera has a variety of possible side effects and advantages. As with

the pill, the injectable hormone does not require any preparation just before intercourse, and it can reduce the severity of menstrual cramps.

The most common side effects of Depo-Provera are irregular bleeding and spotting followed by *amenorrhea* (the absence of periods).[11] In particular, new users of Depo-Provera report occasional breakthrough bleeding as the most common unpleasant side effect.[2] When the woman's body adjusts to the presence of this drug, breakthrough bleeding diminishes, and the most common side effect is amenorrhea. This is understandable, because the drug inhibits ovulation. Many women consider amenorrhea to be a desirable effect of Depo-Provera use. Unlike users of oral contraceptives and subdermal implants, whose fertility returns a few months after stopping their use, women who stop using Depo-Provera may experience infertility for a period of up to one year.[2]

For Men
Researchers are currently studying the use of *testosterone enanthate* as a male contraceptive. Studies have found that injections of this contraceptive are effective in inhibiting the production of sperm; however, it has a variety of side effects.[12] Researchers believe this method offers promise, and further studies are planned.

Subdermal Implants
In late 1990, subdermal implants (Norplant) were approved for use in the United States. This form of contraception uses six soft plastic rods filled with synthetic progesterone. Using a local anesthetic, a physician implants these rods just beneath the skin of the woman's upper or lower arm. The rods release low levels of the hormone for five years. (A second generation of implants will likely use a single rod and thus will be easier to implant.)

The most common side effects are irregular and often persistent menstrual bleeding and spotting. One study found, however, that women experienced less menstrual bleeding and more amenorrhea (cessation of menstrual periods) than IUD users.[13] Removal is technically more difficult and time-consuming than insertion. Norplant implants cost approximately $500

placebo pills (pla **see** bo) pills that contain no active ingredients.

contraindications factors that make the use of a drug inappropriate or dangerous for a particular person.

minipills low-dose progesterone oral contraceptives.

ectopic pregnancy a pregnancy in which the fertilized ovum implants at a site other than the uterus, typically in the fallopian tubes.

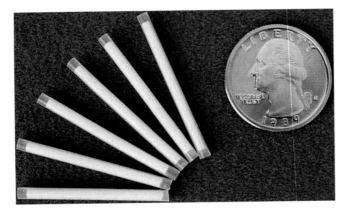

The Norplant subdermal implant.

to $600 for a five-year supply. Subdermal implants are an appropriate choice for women who prefer a contraceptive method that is convenient and does not require regular action by the woman. Studies have found implants to be a safe, effective, and acceptable form of contraception.[13,14]

Sterilization

All of the contraceptive mechanisms or methods already discussed have one quality in common: they are reversible. Although microsurgical techniques are providing medical breakthroughs, **sterilization** should still be considered an irreversible procedure.[15] When you decide to use sterilization, you no longer control your own fertility because you will no longer be able to produce offspring.

Therefore, couples considering sterilization procedures usually must undergo extensive discussions with a physician or family planning counselor to identify their true feelings about this finality. People must be aware of the possible changes in self-concept they might have after sterilization. If you are a man who equates fertility with masculinity, you may have trouble accepting your new status as a sterile man. If you are a woman who equates motherhood with femininity, you might have adjustment problems after sterilization. Some people later regret not being able to have children.

The male sterilization procedure is called a *vasectomy*. Accomplished with a local anesthetic in a physician's office, this twenty- to thirty-minute procedure consists of the surgical removal of a section of each vas deferens. After a small incision is made through the scrotum, the vas deferens is located and a small section removed. The remaining ends are either tied or *cauterized* (Figure 16-5A).

Immediately after a vasectomy, sperm may still be present in the vas deferens. A backup contraceptive is recommended until a physician microscopically examines a semen specimen. This examination usually occurs about six weeks after the surgery.

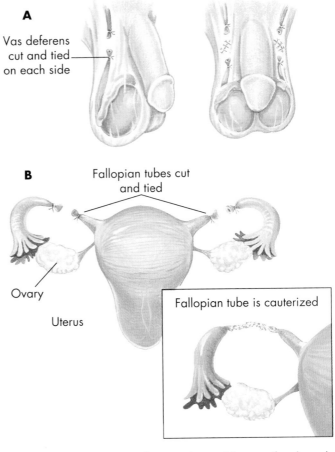

A
Vas deferens cut and tied on each side

B
Fallopian tubes cut and tied
Ovary
Uterus
Fallopian tube is cauterized

Figure 16-5 The most frequently used forms of male and female sterilization. **A,** Vasectomy. **B,** Tubal ligation.

After a vasectomy, men can still produce male sex hormones, get erections, have orgasms, and ejaculate. (Recall that sperm account for only a small portion of the semen.) Some men even report increased interest in sexual activity because their chances of impregnating a woman have been virtually eliminated.

What happens to the process of spermatogenesis within each testicle? Sperm cells are still being produced, but they are destroyed by specialized white blood cells called phagocytic leukocytes.

The future may hold a reversible form of vasectomy, as researchers experiment with injecting a plug-forming material into the vas deferens, with the intention that the plug could be removed at a later date if desired.[16]

The most common method of female sterilization is called *tubal ligation*. During this procedure, the fallopian tubes are cut and the ends tied back. Some physicians cauterize the tube ends to ensure complete sealing (Figure 16-5B). The fallopian tubes are usually reached through the abdominal wall. In a minilaparotomy, a small incision is made through the abdominal wall just below the navel. The resultant scar is small and is the basis for the term *band-aid surgery*.

Female sterilization requires about twenty to thirty minutes, with the patient under a local or general anesthetic. The use of a laparoscope has made female sterilization much simpler than in the past. The laparoscope is a small tube equipped with mirrors and lights. Inserted through a single incision, the laparoscope locates the fallopian tubes before they are cut, tied, or cauterized. When a laparoscope is used through an abdominal incision, the procedure is called a *laparoscopy.*

Women who are sterilized still produce female hormones, ovulate, and menstruate. However, the ovum cannot move down the fallopian tube. Within a day of its release, the ovum will start to disintegrate and be absorbed by the body. Freed of the possibility of becoming pregnant, many sterilized women report an increase in sex drive and activity.

Female sterilization is very effective, with failure rates of only 1 to 2 per 1,000 procedures. The complications tend to be few and minor, and there appear to be no serious long-term side effects. In addition, sterilization may provide some protection against ovarian cancer.[16]

Two other procedures produce sterilization in women. *Ovariectomy* (the surgical removal of the ovaries) and *hysterectomy* (the surgical removal of the uterus) accomplish sterilization. However, these procedures are used to remove diseased (cancerous, cystic, or hemorrhaging) organs and are not primarily considered sterilization techniques.

Personal Applications
• Will you or your partner someday undergo sterilization? If so, which of you will have the surgery?

Abortion

Regardless of the circumstances under which pregnancy occurs, women may now choose to terminate their pregnancies. No longer must women who do not want to be pregnant seek potentially dangerous, illegal abortions. On the basis of current technology and legality, women need never experience childbirth. The decision will be theirs to make.

Abortion is a highly controversial, personal decision—one that needs serious consideration by each woman. On the basis of the landmark 1973 U.S. Supreme Court case *Roe v. Wade,* the United States joined many of the world's most populated countries in legalizing abortion within the following guidelines:

1. For the first 3 months of pregnancy (first trimester), the decision to abort lies with the woman and her doctor. Most abortions are performed in the first trimester.

2. For the next 3 months of pregnancy (second trimester), state law may regulate the abortion procedure in ways that are reasonably related to maternal health.

3. For the last weeks of pregnancy (third trimester) when the fetus is judged capable of surviving if born, any state may regulate or even prohibit abortion except where abortion is necessary to preserve the life or health of the mother. If a pregnancy is terminated during the third trimester, a viable fetus would be considered a live birth and would not be allowed to die.

Each year, approximately 1.4 million women make the decision to terminate a pregnancy in the United States.[9] Thousands of additional women probably consider abortion but elect to continue their pregnancies.

Recently, the abortion rate has declined by 11 percent, from 27 to 24 abortions per 1,000 women annually. This drop parallels a decline in the rate of unintended pregnancy, which observers attribute to greater contraceptive use, including use by young women who become sexually active. Even so, about 49 percent of pregnancies among American women are unintended, and half of these are terminated by abortion.[17] Following are the abortion procedures currently available in the United States.

First-Trimester Abortion Procedures

Menstrual Extraction Also referred to as *menstrual regulation, menstrual induction,* and *preemptive abortion,* menstrual extraction is a process carried out between the fourth and sixth week after the last menstrual period (or in the days immediately after the first missed menstrual period). It is generally performed in a physician's office under a local anesthetic or *paracervical* anesthetic. A small plastic *cannula* is inserted through the undilated cervical canal into the cavity of the uterus. When the cannula is in position, a small amount of suction is applied by a hand-held syringe. By rotating and moving the cannula across the uterine wall, the physician can withdraw the endometrial tissue.

Vacuum Aspiration Induced abortions undertaken during the sixth through ninth weeks of pregnancy are generally performed through *vacuum aspiration* of the uterine contents. Vacuum aspiration is the most

---

sterilization generally permanent birth control techniques that surgically disrupt the normal passage of ova or sperm.

abortion induced premature termination of a pregnancy.

commonly performed abortion procedure. This procedure is similar to menstrual extraction. Unlike menstrual extraction, however, vacuum aspiration may require **dilation** of the cervical canal and the use of a local anesthetic. In this more advanced stage of pregnancy, a larger cannula must be inserted into the uterine cavity. This process can be performed by using metal dilators of increasingly larger sizes to open the canal. After aspiration by an electric vacuum pump, the uterine wall may also be scraped to confirm complete removal of the uterine contents.

Dilation and Curettage (D & C)   When a pregnancy is to be terminated during the ninth through fourteenth weeks, vacuum aspiration gives way to a somewhat similar procedure labeled **dilation and curettage,** or more familiarly, **D & C.** D & C usually requires a general anesthetic, not a local anesthetic.[2]

Like vacuum aspiration, the D & C involves the gradual enlargement of the cervical canal through the insertion of increasingly larger metal dilators. When the cervix has been dilated to a size sufficient to allow for the passage of a *curette,* the removal of the endometrial tissue can begin. The curette is a metal instrument resembling a spoon, with a cup-shaped cutting surface on its end. As the curette is drawn across the uterine wall, the soft endometrial tissue and fetal parts are scraped from the wall of the uterus. (The D & C is also used in the medical management of certain health conditions of the uterine wall, such as irregular bleeding or the buildup of endometrial tissue.)

As in the case of menstrual extraction, both vacuum aspiration and D & C are very safe procedures for the woman. The need to dilate the cervix more fully in a D & C increases the risk of cervical trauma and the possibility of perforation, but these risks are reported to be low. Bleeding, cramping, spotting, and infections present minimal controllable risks when procedures are performed by experienced clinicians.

Personal Applications
• Under what circumstances, if any, do you believe abortion is acceptable? Unacceptable?

The Abortion Pill   The Roussel-Uclaf company in Paris, France, produces a very controversial form of birth control, RU 486 (mifepristone). RU 486 is controversial because it is designed to induce an abortion. This drug is a pill that blocks the action of progesterone. When three 200-mg RU 486 pills are taken and followed forty-eight hours later by an injection (or vaginal suppository) of prostaglandin, menstruation begins, usually within five hours.

RU 486 Stirs Debate

Mifepristone, also known as RU 486 or the French abortion pill, was first synthesized in 1980. It is similar in structure to progesterone, which is essential in the establishment and maintenance of pregnancy. Because it is similar to progesterone, RU 486 can occupy the receptor sites for progesterone and displace it, thus preventing or terminating pregnancy.

Extensive trials over the last 10 years have shown that a single dose of RU 486 followed 48 hours later by a prostaglandin injection or suppository is an effective, safe abortion method.[19]

RU 486 is now used legally in France, China, and the United Kingdom. Because RU 486 has become an alternative to vacuum aspiration for the early termination of pregnancy, it has faced intense political, religious, and personal opposition in the United States. The Food and Drug Administration has declared RU 486 to be safe and effective.

The FDA has not yet approved the sale of mifepristone, but some clinics offer it in clinical trials, while other doctors and clinics use methotrexate, an anticancer drug now being used to induce abortion. One recent study found that the use of mifepristone and methotrexate to induce abortion has spread rapidly. Known as *medical abortion,* this procedure was used 4,300 times in the first half of 1997, more than in all of 1996.[20]

Research is focusing on the minimum effective dose of RU 486 with the fewest possible side effects. In addition, research is needed to determine the acceptability of this type of medical abortion to women in different cultures and societies.

Researchers also suggest that RU 486 has other medical uses, such as inducing labor in full-term pregnancy and in treating breast cancer and other diseases that affect women.

What do you think of the use of RU 486 in terminating a pregnancy?

In May 1994 Roussel-Uclaf agreed to give its patent rights to RU 486 to the Population Council, a New York-based international, nonprofit contraceptive research organization. This action paved the way for the Population Council to test this drug on U.S. women. If the testing indicates that RU 486 is as safe and effective as that found in the 150,000 women who have used the drug in Europe, then the FDA is likely to approve RU 486 as a prescription drug. See the Star Box above for a closer look at RU 486.

Multifetal Pregnancy Reduction (MFPR)   This technique is sometimes employed when women become pregnant with multiple fetuses (more than two) as a result of fertility treatments or techniques. MFPR is typically used to reduce the number of fetuses in order to reduce the risk of prematurity and to give the remaining fetuses a better chance of survival. Several methods have been used in the past, but the preferred method now seems to be the injection of

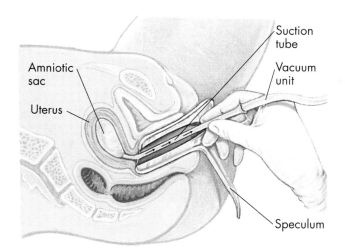

Figure 16-6 During dilation and evacuation, the cervix is dilated and the contents of the uterus are aspirated. This procedure is used to perform abortions during the second trimester.

potassium chloride into the fetal thorax to stop the heart.[18]

The emotional effects of this procedure are extremely distressing and complex, and couples facing this decision need thorough information, support, and counseling both before and after the procedure.

Second-Trimester Abortion Procedures

When a woman's pregnancy continues beyond the fourteenth week of gestation, termination becomes a more difficult matter. The procedures at this stage become more complicated and take longer to be completed, and complications become more common.

Dilation and Evacuation Vacuum aspiration and D & C can be combined in a procedure called *dilation and evacuation* (D & E) (Figure 16–6). D & E is a primary procedure for abortions between 13 and 15 weeks.[2]

Hypertonic Saline Procedure From the sixteenth week of gestation to the end of the second trimester, intrauterine injection of a strong salt solution into the amniotic sac is the procedure most frequently used. The administration of intrauterine **hypertonic saline solution** requires a skilled operator so that the needle used to introduce the salt solution enters the amniotic sac. When the needle is in place, some amniotic fluid is withdrawn, allowing the saline solution to be injected.

Some physicians support the saline procedure by dilating the cervix with *laminaria* or another dilatory product and administering the hormone oxytocin to stimulate uterine contractions. The onset of uterine contractions will expel the dehydrated uterine contents within twenty-four to thirty-six hours.

Prostaglandin Procedure The use of prostaglandin is the third type of abortion procedure used during the second trimester. Prostaglandins are hormonelike chemicals that have a variety of useful effects on human tissue. Produced naturally within the body, these substances influence the contractions of smooth muscle. Because the uterine wall is composed entirely of smooth muscle, it is particularly sensitive to the presence of prostaglandins. When prostaglandin is administered in sufficient quantity (through either a uterine intramuscular injection or a vaginal suppository), uterine contractions become strong enough to expel the fetal contents.

Third-Trimester Abortion Procedures

Should termination of a pregnancy be required in the latter weeks of the gestational period, a surgical procedure in which the fetus will be removed or a procedure in which the entire uterus is removed (hysterectomy) can be undertaken. As you can imagine, these procedures are more complicated and involve longer hospitalization, major abdominal surgery, and an extended period of recovery.

Antiabortion activists have targeted a late-term abortion procedure known medically as *intact dilation and extraction*. Abortion opponents have fought to persuade states and the U.S. Congress to ban this procedure. Since 1995, 28 states have passed legislation banning so-called partial-birth abortion, but many of these bans have been overturned in court, with several courts ruling that the bans were so broadly written that they prohibited other kinds of abortion. Congress twice passed a ban, but each time President Clinton vetoed it. Abortion-rights supporters oppose such bans on the grounds that they are an attempt to deny women's right to abortion. According to a recent study, intact dilation and extraction accounted for about 0.03 percent to 0.05 percent of the 1.4 million abortions in 1996, or about 363 such procedures.[20]

Personal Applications

• Can you identify locations at or near your college where professional family-planning services are available?

---

dilation gradual expansion of an opening or passageway, such as the cervix.

dilation and curettage (D & C) (kyoo re tahzh) a surgical procedure in which the cervical canal is dilated to allow the uterine wall to be scraped.

hypertonic saline solution a salt solution with a concentration higher than that found in human fluids.

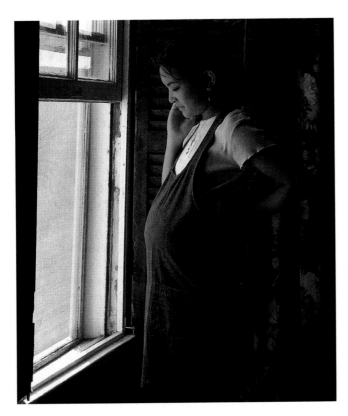

An unintended pregnancy often causes emotional and financial strain for the woman, the potential father, and their families.

Unintended Pregnancy

Each day, thousands of single women receive the news that they are pregnant.[21] For those who have been trying to have a child, this news is welcomed. For others, however, the news may not be so joyous. Even in ideal situations, an unintended pregnancy can cause emotional and financial strain for the woman, the potential father, and their families.

Important People in the Decision-Making Process

If the father-to-be or the potential grandparents were not there to hear the news with her, the woman faces the task of telling them she is pregnant. This is often a time of fear and uncertainty for the woman, and the way these people ultimately handle the news can be of critical importance to her.[22] A supportive family and father-to-be make later decision processes easier to deal with, whereas lack of support is sure to cause problems down the road.

The decisions of the potential father concerning the woman and an unplanned pregnancy are extremely important. He may abandon the woman altogether, which will make support from the woman's family even more critical. If he chooses to stay, more

decisions must be made. He may want to marry her. He may not want marriage but may still want to play an active role in supporting and rearing the child. He may want to play only a limited role. Whatever his decision, his role is a determining factor for decisions to be made later.

The families of both parents-to-be also play an important role in determining the outcome of the situation, especially when the potential parents are young. In many situations the families may be the primary source of financial and emotional support, and lack of this support may prove devastating.

Marriage

Traditionally, marriage has been the most socially acceptable alternative for pregnant women and their partners. In recent years, however, unwed motherhood has become more common and less stigmatized. Currently 30 percent of births in the United States are to unmarried women, and only 33 percent of teenage mothers are married.[22,24] Economic factors may play a role in determining whether a couple should get married when an unexpected pregnancy occurs. If the woman is financially secure or is receiving financial support from her family, she may find that single parenthood is the most desirable option. If income from both parents is necessary to support the child, marriage may prove to be the logical choice.

Abortion

Eventually the couple must make a decision about the fate of the child. The couple must decide to become parents, put the child up for adoption, or terminate the pregnancy. The decision to abort is often complicated and difficult and may depend on where the woman lives, her financial situation, and who is involved in the decision-making process with her. Couples also face moral, religious, and legal questions when making such a decision. If the woman's religious and moral beliefs are not compatible with those of her family or the father-to-be, these relationships may become greatly strained. The woman may also struggle with her own belief system and religious upbringing when making such a decision.

For younger girls, the decision may be further complicated by the law. Many states require parental consent before an abortion is performed for girls below a certain age. This may eliminate the abortion option for those girls who do not want their parents to know about their pregnancies or for girls whose parents refuse to give consent.[25]

Adoption

Putting the baby up for adoption may be an acceptable alternative for those women who reject abortion but do not wish to take on the responsibilities of

Learning
From Our Diversity

Improv Theatre: A Boost for Teen Moms' Self-Esteem

Teenage mothers, especially those from low-income homes or broken families, often suffer from low self-esteem. A program of Washington, D.C.'s Living Stage Theatre Company, Teen Mothers of Today, was created to help teenage mothers use their creativity to strengthen their self-esteem.[23] Using the art of improvisational theatre to effect social change, Living Stage strives to create theatre in which there is a direct connection between the art form and the lives of the company's participants and audience.

Launched in the early 1990s, the Teen Mothers of Today initiative focused on young mothers between the ages of 13 and 16 in Washington's African-American community. The participants initially demonstrated not only low self-esteem but also limited verbal and social skills, low aspirations, and poor physical health. They also, however, manifested some very positive characteristics: tenacity, determination, imagination, and unwavering love for their children.

In the early days of the intensive program, Living Stage presented the young women with creative challenges that allowed them to draw on their own life experiences for solutions. In the first performance, the group was presented with a familiar situation: A teenager is mistreated by a racist storekeeper and must decide whether or not to seek revenge for the insult to her dignity. The scene endings that the girls invented for this scenario showed their understanding of the problem and served to engage the group in developing the story. The teens eagerly joined in acting out the endings and were clearly enthusiastic about going further into the process.

Subsequently these young women were engaged in dialogue about world issues in many different forms. They were shown how to express their feelings through their bodies in human sculptures, through painting and other visual arts media, and through photography. Whatever the form being explored, the young women received consistent, sincere, positive feedback that helped them become more comfortable with expressing themselves.

Next, hypothetical situations were set up in which the participants became characters other than themselves and had to solve problems without resorting to violence. Most of these scenarios required resolving various family crises. The same girls who had experienced difficulty expressing their personal opinions now became active role players. As they dealt with these fictitious situations, the teens began transforming their own lives.

Think of someone you know who is a teenage mother living in a low-income, unstable, and possibly dangerous environment—or imagine what it would be like to be such a teenager. How do you think a person in this situation would benefit from a program like the Living Stage's Teen Mothers of Today?

---

child rearing. Many women may choose this option if they are not able to financially support a baby but also cannot consider aborting the child because of moral convictions. This option may eliminate the lifetime financial commitment but may be very difficult emotionally. The act of giving up a baby after carrying it to term can be heart-rending. The mother may have misgivings about the adoption for many years afterward. Many women who initially choose adoption for their child wind up changing their minds along the way, sometimes even after the baby is born. In recent years, several bitter court battles have been waged over such situations.

Parenthood

If the mother chooses the parenthood option, carrying the baby to term requires selfless devotion to its care. This often requires budgeting for the baby's needs well before it is born.[26] Most first-time parents do not realize the enormous costs that having a baby entails. The cost of giving birth varies widely among states. In recent years, the average total cost of hospital and physician charges for an uncomplicated vaginal delivery was $8,840 in New York, but less than half that amount in Arkansas. New York was the most expensive state in which to have a cesarean delivery, with an average cost of $13,700, whereas a cesarean birth in Oklahoma cost about $7,730.[23] Pediatrician bills during the first year of a child's life average $600 (assuming the child is healthy), and other necessities for the baby are even more expensive. For example, diapers can run between $500 and $700 a year during the pre-potty training days.[27] Clothes can cost as much as $1,000 the first year because the child grows so quickly. Feeding can cost as much as $2,000, depending on whether the mother is willing or able to breastfeed.[27]

The mother may have to make major changes in her lifestyle to keep the unborn child healthy. The mother should avoid drinking and smoking, which may be difficult for those women who are used to these activities.

Prenatal Care and Day Care

Prenatal care is necessary but can be expensive. For a typical, uncomplicated pregnancy, the average cost for adequate prenatal care is $500.[28] The cost of prenatal care can soar if there are any complications during the pregnancy.

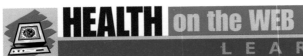

LEARNING ACTIVITIES

Selecting Your Contraceptive Method

People use birth control for many reasons. Career-minded men and women want to plan the timing and spacing of their children. Others want reliable birth control to ensure that they will never have children. Fear of contracting a sexually transmitted disease prompts some people to use particular forms of birth control. Go to www.fhi.org/fp/fpfaq/index.html and select *Frequently Asked Questions about Contraception* for help in selecting a contraceptive method if you are or may become sexually active.

Learning About the Pill

You can find more information about oral contraceptives on the web. An excellent resource for further birth control information is the Planned Parenthood website, www.igc.apc.org/ppfa/contraception/choices_main.html. Select *Birth Control Methods* and then select *Seven Myths about the Pill.* Did you have any mistaken beliefs about birth control pills?

Considering Abortion Rights

Understanding your values and beliefs is a good place to start in determining your views on political issues. Planned Parenthood believes in each person's right to manage his or her fertility, regardless of the individual's income, marital status, race, ethnicity, sexual orientation, age, national origin, or residence. Even if you don't agree with this position, you may find it helpful to learn about an opposing viewpoint. Go to Planned Parenthood's website at www.plannedparenthood.org, select *Pro-Choice,* and then select *Pro-Choice I.Q.* Read the questions, and answer each one honestly. How did this activity help you understand your own position, whether it's pro-choice or pro-life?

For more activities, log on to our Online Learning Center at www.mhhe.com/hper/health/payne

---

Women who decide to become parents must take steps to ensure that the baby will be cared for after it is born. The mother must arrange for day care if she hopes to work or continue with school. This can be a problem if no spouse or family member is able or willing to take care of the baby during times when the mother is gone. Many day care facilities do not care for newborns, and some require that the child be potty-trained before enrolling. Day care facilities can be expensive and often have waiting lists for admission.

More workplaces and schools now offer free or inexpensive day care services, but such programs are not found everywhere, and waiting lists cause delays as well. Some women are forced to take time off from school because of unintended pregnancy, and some leave altogether because of the financial hardships and physical strain of balancing school and parenthood. About half of all teenage mothers drop out of school.[21] Recent legislation has made it easier for new parents to take leave from work without penalty, but the law does not apply to all employers. As a result, some women are forced to leave jobs to care for their children.

Considering the Consequences

In the heat of passion, people often fail to think rationally about the potential outcomes of unprotected sex. Therefore, the time to prepare for the romantic moment is before you are in a position where you don't want to think about the possibility of an unintended result. If you choose to be sexually active, find a form of contraception that works for you and use it consistently.

Choosing to be celibate also is an option, and it is a form of contraception that can be 100 percent effective. Experts continue to debate the teaching of abstinence along with sex education for youngsters and teenagers.

> **Personal Applications**
>
> • What responsibility do you believe a man has to both the baby and the mother when he unintentionally fathers a child?

Real Life Real choices

Your Turn

- What do you think about Laurie and Todd Lindemark's reasons for (1) wanting and (2) not wanting to have an unplanned child?
- Can you think of any additional factors they might consider in trying to reach a decision?
- Have you been in a situation similar to the Lindemarks', or do you know anyone who has? If so, what was the decision, and what were the results?

And Now, Your Choices . . .

- If you are a man, try to decide how you would handle this situation in the best interests of yourself, your spouse, and your unborn child.
- If you are a woman, try to make the best decision for yourself, your spouse, and your unborn child.

Summary

- *Birth control* refers to all of the procedures that can prevent the birth of a child.
- *Contraception* refers to any procedure that prevents fertilization.
- Each birth control method has both a theoretical effectiveness rate and a use effectiveness rate. For some contraceptive approaches, these rates are similar (such as hormonal methods), and for others the rates are very different (such as condoms, diaphragms, and periodic abstinence).
- Many factors should be considered when deciding which contraceptive is best for you.
- Sterilization (vasectomy and tubal ligation) is usually considered an irreversible procedure.
- The birth control pill is safe and effective for the vast majority of women, but it does not protect against sexually transmitted diseases.
- Female condoms are currently available in drugstores without a prescription.

- The FDA is expected to give its final approval of RU 486, also known as the French abortion pill.
- Emergency contraception is safe and effective in preventing pregnancy after incidents of unprotected sex but should not be used repeatedly as a form of contraception.
- Currently, abortion remains a woman's choice under the guidelines of the 1973 *Roe v. Wade* decision and various state restrictions.
- Abortion procedures vary according to the stage of the pregnancy.
- Options for women who become pregnant unintentionally include marriage, abortion, adoption, and parenthood.
- An unplanned pregnancy also affects the potential father and the couple's families, who may also be involved in decision making.

Review Questions

1. Explain the difference between the terms *birth control* and *contraception*. Give examples of each.
2. Explain the difference between theoretical and use effectiveness rates. Which is always higher?
3. Identify some of the factors that should be given careful consideration when selecting a contraceptive method. Explain each factor.
4. What is periodic abstinence? Identify and describe each of the four approaches to this birth control strategy.
5. Describe how vaginal spermicides work and how effective they are as a contraceptive. How much protection do they offer against STDs?
6. What are the differences between the diaphragm and the cervical cap?

7. What are the potential complications of using an IUD?
8. How do minipills differ from the combined oral contraceptive? What is a morning-after pill?
9. How do subdermal implants (Norplant) differ from Depo-Provera?
10. Describe the various sterilization procedures.
11. Identify and describe the different abortion procedures that are used during each trimester of pregnancy.
12. Explain the options a woman has when she becomes pregnant unintentionally. What are the financial costs of pregnancy, childbirth, and parenthood, and what other difficulties will the potential mother or couple face?

References

1. Masters WH, Johnson VE, Kolodny RC. *Human sexuality.* 5th ed. New York: HarperCollins, 1995.
2. Hatcher RA et al. *Contraceptive technology.* 17th ed. New York: Irvington, 1998.
3. Planned Parenthood of America. *Your birth control choices.* PPFA Web Site. 1998. www.plannedparenthood.org
4. Goldberg MS. Choosing a contraceptive. *FDA Consumer* 1993; 27(7):18–25.
5. Sapire KE. The female condom (Femidon)—a study of user acceptability. *South African Med J* 1995 Oct; 85(10 Suppl):1081–84.
6. Vinker S et al. Follow-up of intrauterine contraceptive devices. *Harefuah* 1996 Nov 15; 131(10):391–93, 455, 456.
7. Adlind V. Modern intrauterine devices. *Baillieres Clin Obstet Gynaecol* 1996 Apr; 10(1):55–67.
8. Farley TMM et al. Intrauterine devices and pelvic inflammatory disease: an international study. *Lancet* 1992; 339(8796):785–88.
9. U.S. Bureau of the Census. *Statistical abstract of the United States: 1998.* 118th ed. Washington, DC: U.S. Government Printing Office, 1998.
10. Goldzieher JW: Oral contraceptive side effects: where's the beef? (review). *Contraception* 1995 Dec; 52(6):327–35.
11. Kaunitz AM. Long-acting contraceptive options. *Int J Fertil Menopausal Studies* 1996 Mar-Apr; 41(2):69–76.
12. Meriggiola MC. A combined regimen of cyproterone acetate and testosterone enanthate as a potentially

highly effective male contraceptive. *J Clin Endocrinol* 1996 Aug; 81(8):1018–23.

13. Noeroramana NP. A cohort study of Norplant implant: side effects and acceptance. *Adv. Contracep* 1995 June; 11(2):97–114.
14. Chetri M. Five-year evaluation of safety, efficacy, and acceptability of Norplant implants in Nepal. *Adv. Contracep* 1996 Sept; 12(3):187–99.
15. Kelly G. *Sexuality today: the human perspective.* 6th ed. New York: McGraw-Hill, 1998.
16. Wilson EW: Sterilization (review). *Baillieres Clin Obstet Gynaecol* 1996 Apr; 10(1):103–19.
17. Henshaw SK. Abortion incidence and services in the United States, 1995–1996. *Family Planning Perspectives* 1998; 30(6):263–70, 287.
18. Kuller JA, Chescheir NC, Cefalo RC. *Prenatal diagnosis and reproductive genetics.* St. Louis: Mosby-Year Book, 1996.
19. Baird D. Clinical use of mifepristone (RU 486). *Ann Med* 1993 Feb; 25(1):65–69.
20. New York Times Syndicate. Study estimates frequency of controversial abortion method. *Johns Hopkins Health Information: Intelihealth,* 1998. www.intelihealth.com
21. Book bags and baby bottles. *Scholastic Update* 1995 Mar; 127(11).
22. Bezduch-Moore SL. I was pregnant at 16. *Teen Magazine* 1995 Mar; 39(3).
23. Nelson J. Improvisational theatre helps teen mothers raise sights. *Children Today* 1993 Mar-April; 22(2):24.
24. Russell C. Why teen births boom. *American Demographics* 1995 Sept.
25. Thompson S. *Going all the way: teenage girls' tales of sex, romance, and pregnancy.* New York: Hill and Wang, 1995.
26. Foglino A. Single, pregnant, and struggling to stay in college. *Glamour* 1995 Nov; 232.
27. Winthrop A. How much does it cost to give birth? *American Baby* 1995 May; 14.
28. What price parenthood. *Town and Country Monthly* 1994 June; 148(5169).

Suggested Readings

Nofziger N, Kahan J, Dotzler E. *Signs of fertility: the personal science of natural birth control:* Deatsville, AL: MND Publishing, 1998. This reference book presents the physiological principles that underlie natural methods of birth control. It describes the natural signs of fertility, including basal temperature shift, changes in the cervical mucus, and cyclic changes in the cervix. It also presents a history of natural family planning and comparisons of birth control statistics.

Rodriguez-Armas O, Hedon B. *Clinical infertility and contraception:* Pearl River, NY: Parthenon Publishing Group, 1998. This reference text describes the clinical treatments for infertility and contraception that are recommended as standard care for all patients. Written by a team of specialists in reproductive medicine, the book presents a consensus on the way infertility should be treated and contraception managed near the end of the twentieth century.

Runkle A. *In good conscience: a practical, emotional, and spiritual guide to deciding whether to have an abortion:* San Francisco, CA: Jossey Bass Publishers, 1998. This book cuts through the religious and political rhetoric surrounding abortion and presents solid information in a compassionate tone for women who want to make this decision themselves.

Kluger-Bell K. *Unspeakable losses: understanding the experience of pregnancy loss, miscarriage, and abortion:* New York: WW Norton & Company, 1998. For those who have suffered a miscarriage or stillbirth, or who have elected to terminate a pregnancy, the experience has long been minimized, ignored, or shrouded in shame. The author presents in-depth stories from would-be parents who experienced such losses, discussing such issues as multifetal reductions (more common as fertilization procedures become more popular), the male experience of pregnancy loss, and how a woman can be pro-choice and still grieve over choosing abortion. She includes tools for moving through the grieving process, discussing losses, and helping loved ones who have experienced pregnancy loss.

As We Go To PRESS

In March 1999, a major announcement was made concerning the reintroduction of the Today Sponge. This extremely popular, safe and effective over-the-counter contraceptive device was taken off the market in 1995, when its manufacturer, Whitehall-Robins Healthcare decided not to upgrade the manufacturing plant where it made the sponge. A new company, Allendale Pharmaceuticals, Inc. purchased the rights to the Today Sponge and, as we go to press, was planning its market return in Fall 1999.

topics for Today

Childless by Choice: New Options for Women and Couples

Any aspect of reproduction is bound to be emotionally charged. Choosing not to reproduce is a subject that is rarely discussed openly.[1] Although there have been childless (some prefer the term *child-free*) women and couples throughout history, ours is one of the first generations of women who can bypass motherhood by their own will.[1] Safe, reliable contraception and paid employment have broadened possibilities for women, allowing them to choose motherhood without being absorbed by it or to reject motherhood for themselves and not be stigmatized by that choice.[2]

Making the Choice

Sterilization of males and females is the leading form of birth control. Forty-six percent of women ages 40 to 44 have been sterilized.[2] However, this procedure is more rare among younger women and those with no children. Many of these women rely on the second leading method of birth control, the oral contraceptive pill.[2]

At some point, the 42 percent of women who are in their childbearing years but have not yet given birth either become mothers or they don't.[3] For some this is a conscious choice. Others have children unthinkingly, or under pressure, while the rest continue to postpone having children until it is biologically too late. One-third of women who decide to remain childless do so before they marry.[4] Their future spouses rarely disagree with their choice, probably because these women have been leaning away from motherhood all along and tend to select men who agree with their choice or with whom childbearing would not be probable or in some cases possible. Marrying men who already have children or are unwilling or physically unable to have them removes some of the burden of choice from the woman.[1] Nine out of ten childless couples actively decide to remain so, whereas only two-thirds of parents make a deliberate decision to have children; the remaining one-third do so by default or accident.[4]

The rate of voluntary childlessness in this country is highest among Asian Americans and whites (7.7%) and American Indians (6%). African-

Americans have a 3% rate of voluntary childlessness, and the rate for Hispanic Americans is 1.6%.[4] Voluntary childlessness occurs among all socioeconomic groups rather than being the prerogative of privileged women, as once believed.[3]

The vast majority of women do become mothers by the age of 45. Since society views parenthood as natural, people rarely ask them why they had children. However, the opposite question is frequently asked of the minority of women who aren't mothers.

Why Women Choose Not to Be Mothers

One author sums up the complexity of the choice to remain childless in the following way: "A variety of factors make women psychologically receptive to considering the childless alternative, and then a combination of what happens to them and how they choose to live causes them ultimately to embrace it." So it is a combination of history, personality, and circumstance that leads some women to choose the unconventional life of a nonmother.

Characteristics of Childless Women and Couples

As a group, women who remain childless are typically firstborn or only children, untraditional, better educated, more cosmopolitan, less religious, and more likely to have a profession than mothers. They also tend to gravitate toward independent professions where they can be more in control of their working hours and conditions.[1] Nonmothers have the most education and best paid jobs of all American women.[3]

The wife in a childless marriage almost always works and frequently earns more money than her husband. Husbands in these unions tend to share more of the household responsibilities than men do when children are present.[1] These unconventional men and women have unconventional marriages as well. These couples may be older when they marry, and many have been married before. Differences in age, ethnicity, and social class between the partners are common.

Contrary to popular belief, nonmothers are not cold or selfish. They are deeply committed, nurturing, and generous, but on their own terms. They just prefer not to give up control of their lives to the unpredictability of child rearing. They also recognize that they can't put their own goals aside for a prolonged period of time without fostering resentment and anger. Nonmothers are so completely committed to whatever they undertake that they know they couldn't live up to their own standards of parenting and don't want to impose similar unrealistic expectations on a child.[1] For these women, the satisfaction of child rearing would not offset the costs.

The Role of Fathers

A woman without children has traditionally been called "barren," which implies an emptiness and causes others to question her femininity. No comparable term exists for a man without children, and no questions of his masculinity are raised.[1] Thus childlessness is a different prospect between the sexes, as is parenting. Many more men than women reject parenthood after the fact, which is evidenced by the soaring birthrate for single mothers.[3] Some women decide not to bring children into the world with partners who are less than totally committed to raising them.[4]

This concern is often valid. As it is, parenthood more commonly and more drastically alters a woman's life than a man's.[1] American fathers spend an average of 38 seconds a day with their babies, 26 minutes a day with preschoolers, and 16 minutes a day with school-aged children. Although many fathers do take an active role in caring for their children, half of all fathers have never changed a diaper and three-quarters take no responsibility for child care. The remainder of the responsibility for parenting usually falls to the mothers, for whom this extra burden can be emotionally draining.[4]

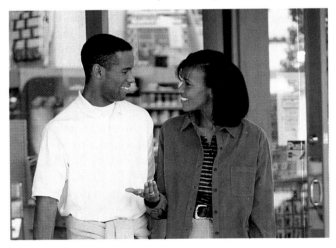

Choosing not to have children gives couples more time and money to pursue other interests, such as restoring a home.

Pros and Cons of a Childless Lifestyle

The following table is an abbreviated list of the pros and cons of choosing not to have children. These reasons are just examples, and there are many more on each side of the issue, many of which are uniquely personal. Also bear in mind that the same reasons that motivate some people to become parents cause others to avoid parenthood.[3]

Choosing a Childless Lifestyle

Pros	Cons
More time for travel and work	May have regrets in the future
Spontaneity remains possible	Feelings of selfishness may cause guilt
Uninterrupted privacy and intimacy	A new kind of intimacy may be missed
Easier to leave a bad relationship	Alone in old age
Don't contribute to overpopulation	No heirs
No worries of raising a child in today's dangerous world	No grandchildren for you or your parents
Less financial burden	Loss of friends your own age who are preoccupied with parenting

These advantages of the childless lifestyle are supported by a recent study that found that couples were happiest before their first baby arrived.[5] Their marital happiness then suffered a long drop as their children grew, reaching its lowest point during a child's teen years. The couples did not approach their pre-baby levels of satisfaction until their last child was on his or her own. Childless couples were found to be as happy as couples are before babies arrive, and, without the long cycle of child rearing, their happiness tended to stay at this high level over time.

Some people have babies for the wrong reasons, such as in an attempt to fix something in their lives. This is an impossibly large burden for a child. A baby can't revitalize an unhappy marriage, improve poor self-esteem, or lessen feelings of depression, frustration, or disappointment with work, friends, or family. Ultimately the desire to raise a child, not anxiety over your own past, present, or future, is the only good and fair reason to give birth. It is typical to approach this decision with avoidance, uncertainty, mixed emotions, and conflicting desires. The people who choose to remain childless will rethink their decision and reevaluate the pros and cons many times in their lives.[1]

Society's View

Although it is more acceptable now, voluntary childlessness is still viewed negatively in American society. Motherhood automatically brings status, structure, and a sense of purpose, whereas women who are childless by choice are often unfairly judged to be self-indulgent and immature. Instead of accepting childlessness as a personal choice, many people perceive it as a threat to society as a whole. The notion of remaining childless makes many people uneasy. Those who choose to remain childless often hear such prying questions and statements as:

- "Don't you think you're being selfish?"
- "You will be lonely when you're old."
- "You will change your mind after you have kids."
- "Do you dislike children?"
- "Don't you have any maternal instinct?"
- "Is it a physical problem?"

Parents of a childless couple may fear that the decision their child has made reflects poorly on their own parenting skills.[1] At family gatherings, childlessness is often spoken of in hushed tones, as if the woman or couple has a disease. With pity in their voices, they may whisper, "She doesn't [they don't] have any children."[1] They may add the word *yet* and tell stories of women in their 40s who have given birth, as if there is still hope for a cure.

But probably one of the most significant factors in determining how many children a couple has, if any, is religion and how strictly the couple practices it. Muslims, for example, have a higher fertility rate than non-Muslims, and Catholics have a higher fertility rate than Protestants or Jews.[2]

Living with the Decision

Historically, women were rewarded for producing male heirs to carry on the family name and daughters to take care of their parents in old age.[2] In today's society, a woman's earning ability, rather than her fertility, provides her security.[3]

The 22% of women born between 1956 and 1972 who will not bear children are in their own ways confronting what it has always meant to be born female.[2,6] While there have been notable childless women in history, their attitudes toward childlessness are unknown. Their personal stories, along with other feminine wisdom about whether or not to bear children, has been distorted, lost, or ignored.[3] This silence makes the decision all the more difficult.

Women who end up rejecting motherhood for themselves are not rejecting the institution of motherhood itself. On the contrary, they value it as something that requires special qualities and skills, rather than something just anyone can do. Those who choose not to take that course are different but not in any way defective as women.

For childless couples, friends replace the family as lifelines. Like-minded friends foster self-acceptance, while friends with children provide special bonding and involvement for the childless couple as special "aunts" and "uncles" or "adopted" neighbors to their children.[1]

Whether you decide to have children or not, the issue will probably never be completely resolved for you or anyone else. Nobody has it all. No one lives a life without limitations, and no one makes choices without loss. As long as you make a genuine, conscious choice for your own reasons, it won't be the wrong one.

For Discussion . . .

If you don't already have children, do you plan to become a parent one day? Why or why not? How do you view childless couples? Is there a person with no children of his or her own who was special to you during your childhood?

References

1. Safer J. *Beyond motherhood.* New York: Pocket Books, 1996.
2. Bartlett J. *Will you be a mother? Women who choose to say no.* New York: New York University Press, 1995.
3. Lisle L. *Without child: challenging the stigma of childlessness.* New York: Ballantine Books, 1996.
4. Lang SS. *Women without children: the reasons, the rewards, the regrets.* New York: Pharos Books, 1996.
5. Elias M. Couples in pre-kid, no-kid marriages happiest. *USA Today* 1997 March 12:1D.
6. Thomas IM. Childless by choice. *Hispanic* 1995; 8(4)50–52.

InfoLinks
www.cpc.unc.edu/pubs/paa_papers/1995/abma.html
www.globalideasbank.org/BI/BI-4.HTML

chapter
seventeen

Becoming
a Parent

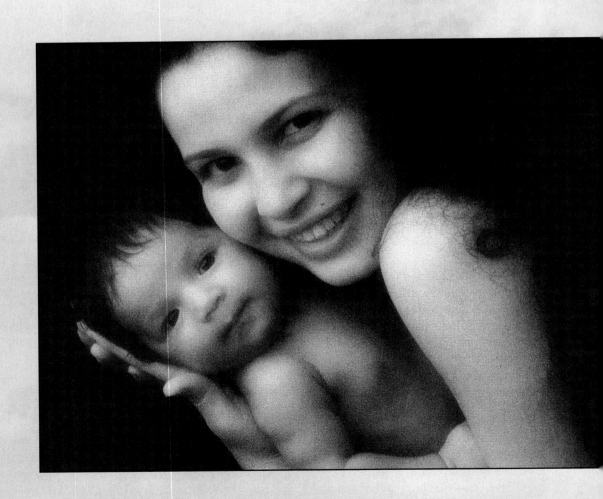

Although birth control is especially important for many young couples, most couples eventually want to have children and raise a family. In the past, couples had their children very quickly after either high school or college. Now the trend seems to be to wait longer before having children. Most likely, educational, economic, contraceptive, and occupational factors have laid the groundwork for this trend. To the relief of many people, medical research indicates that women over the age of thirty or thirty-five are quite capable of having healthy babies.

HEALTHY PEOPLE: LOOKING AHEAD TO 2010

As the *Healthy People 2010* document is drafted, some encouraging trends have been noted in the areas of pregnancy and childbirth, as well as some problems that the new objectives must address. One positive development is that more than half of the states have enacted legislation specifying that insurance must cover a minimum hospital stay for mothers and newborns after childbirth. Longer hospital stays are expected to reduce the incidence of jaundice and maternal infections. Another important step forward is the establishment of a toll-free number that connects callers to their state's maternal and child

health office for answers to questions about pregnancy, childbirth, and infant care.

The *Healthy People 2010* document will aim to reduce the persistent disparity in rates of infant mortality and low birth weight between black and white women of similar educational and social background. The objectives will also target the problem of tobacco, alcohol, marijuana, and cocaine use among pregnant women. Finally, goals will be set to increase the rate of breastfeeding and the proportion of women who receive early prenatal care.

Real Life
Real choices

- Names: Susan Williams-Johnson and Gary Johnson
- Ages: 36 and 35
- Occupations: Susan, investment banker
  Gary, plastic surgeon

"Us? Infertile? But that's impossible!"

When Susan and Gary Johnson learned that it would be extremely difficult or even impossible for them to conceive a child, they were as stunned as if they'd been told that the Earth had fallen off its axis. Married for 12 years, much of it devoted to education and training, they'd faithfully used birth control and planned to have their first child a year after Gary completed his residency in plastic surgery. Susan had intended to resign her position at a major bank and, a year after having a baby, to become an independent investment consultant. Through some long lean years together, a major focus of this couple had been on *not* having a baby until they were sure they were ready emotionally and financially to be parents.

Now they're ready—but nature, apparently, is not. After seemingly endless consultations and tests, a respected fertility specialist at Gary's hospital has told him and Susan that they belong to that small percentage of couples whose infertility has no detectable cause. She has explained to them the drug therapy, surgery, insemination, and fertilization procedures for which they may be candidates, but she has cautioned them that these procedures are likely to be time-consuming, expensive, and frustrating. And there is no guarantee of success. In addition to these procedures, the specialist has suggested that Gary and Susan also may want to consider other options, such as adoption or surrogate parenting.

Still reeling from news they never expected to hear, feeling that their lives and plans have been turned upside down, Gary and Susan know they have some difficult and painful decisions to make.

As you study this chapter, think about Gary and Susan's situation and choices, and prepare yourself to answer the questions in **Your Turn** at the end of the chapter.

Parenting Issues for Couples

Before deciding to have children, couples should frankly discuss the effects that pregnancy and a newborn child will have on their lives. In addition, anyone who is sexually active should consider these same issues, because very few contraceptive methods are 100 percent effective all the time, and pregnancy can result from nearly any act of intercourse. For those students contemplating single parenthood, we ask that you consider these issues as they relate to your particular situation and to excuse our consistent use of plural pronouns. In any event, couples should discuss some or all of the following basic considerations:

- What effect will pregnancy have on us individually and collectively?
- Why do we want to have a child?
- What effect will a child have on the images we have constructed for ourselves as adults?
- Can we afford to have a child and provide for its needs?
- How will the responsibilities related to raising a child be divided?
- How will a child affect our professional careers?
- Are we ready now to accept the extended responsibilities that can come with a new child?
- How will we rear our child in terms of religious training, discipline, and participation in activities?
- Are we ready to part with much of the freedom associated with late adolescence and the early young adult years?

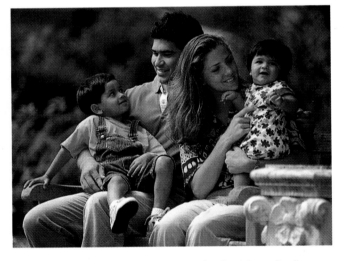

For many young couples, the rewards of raising a family outweigh the stress that inevitably accompanies parenthood.

- How will we handle the possibility of being awakened by 6 o'clock each morning for the next few years?
- What plans have we made in the event that our baby (or fetus) has a serious birth defect?
- Are we capable of handling the additional responsibilities associated with having a disabled child?
- Are we comfortable with the thought of bringing another child into an already overcrowded, violent, bigoted, and polluted world?

If these questions seem strikingly negative in tone, there is indeed a reason for this. We believe that all too

Learning
From Our Diversity

Pregnancy and Parenting After Forty

Women who become pregnant in their forties are not a new phenomenon. Many young people and baby boomers today were delivered by mothers who were 40 or more years old. What *is* new is women becoming pregnant for the first time at an age when many women begin menopause.

The reasons are several. Some couples may have tried to conceive for years and only succeeded when in their forties. Other women and couples delayed pregnancy in order to build their careers, travel, or become more financially secure. In addition, fertility technology, such as in vitro fertilization, microsurgery, and donor eggs or sperm have finally given many couples the baby they long wanted.

The trend of later childbearing began in the late 1970s, when better-educated baby-boom women began entering the work force. For women 40 to 44, the rate of first babies increased from 0.3 to 1.4 per 1,000, still a small percentage but a significant jump.[1]

The common belief that men can father babies well into middle age is supported not only by anecdotal evidence (such as Tony Randall, Larry King, and Anthony Quinn), but also recent research that shows that sperm function in older men does not differ significantly from that of younger men.[2]

Women traditionally were discouraged from becoming pregnant for the first time in their forties because of the health risks to the mother and the risk of birth defects for the baby. It is true that women 40 and older suffer more complications during childbirth, and the risk of having a baby with Down syndrome or another genetic abnormality increases as a mother ages.[1]

The chances of having a cesarean delivery are about 40 percent higher than a younger woman's.[3] The number of women with gestational diabetes and high blood pressure also was higher. Many had more difficulty with labor and delivered babies that were underweight or premature. In addition, the risk of fetal death is higher in women over 35 years old.[4]

Women who want to have a baby should use this information to prevent the problems, however, rather than let it discourage them from having a baby at all, researchers say.

Women who want to start families in their forties should consider the following points:

• Infertility can become a problem with age, but fertility drugs such as Clomid or treatments such as in vitro fertilization can help.
• The rate of miscarriage is higher among older women, so immediate prenatal care is vital.
• Early genetic testing can ease the fears about birth defects. Tests can reveal the presence of Down syndrome, Tay-Sachs disease, cystic fibrosis, and sickle-cell anemia.
• Cesarean sections are more common in older mothers.

On the plus side, another study recently reported that women who are able to give birth after age 40 (not including those who become pregnant through the use of fertility treatments) may be "slow to age" and live longer.[1] This can be good news to older moms who wonder whether they will have the energy to chase a toddler.

---

frequently the "nuts and bolts" issues related to childbearing and parenting are ignored or at least are placed on the back burner. Although it is important for future parents to consider how cute and cuddly a new baby will be, how holidays will be enhanced with a new child, and how pleased the grandparents will be, we consider these issues secondary to the serious realities of having a child enter your lives. Complete the Personal Assessment on page 504 to explore your feelings about parenting.

Being a Good Parent: What Children Need

You will recall from Maslow's hierarchy of needs, in Chapter 2, that human beings have needs for fulfill-

ment that begin with basic needs for food and comfort, through a need for belonging and love, to a striving for self-actualization and fulfillment.[5] Children have these same needs. They may go up and down the scale as some of the needs are met or denied. They grow as the child grows.

It is the parents' responsibility to meet all of these needs when the child is young and help the child learn to meet these needs as the child grows up. As with Maslow's pyramid, each level supports the next. These begin with the child's bodily needs.

Bodily Needs

Children need nutritious food, clean water and air, and a warm, dry place to sleep. Children and even infants feel enormous stress about having these needs met. Children can feel healthy about themselves if their parents meet these needs in a loving, caring way.

Children also should be taught that bowel movements and urinating are normal, healthy functions, and they should be toilet trained when they are ready.

Personal Assessment

Respond to each of the following items based on your own opinions about parenting. Circle the letters that best match your response.

SA   **Strongly agree**
A   **Agree**
U   **Undecided**
D   **Disagree**
SD   **Strongly disagree**

1. One cannot parent successfully without, at the same time, being a generally successful adult member of the community.   SA   A   U   D   SD
2. It is inappropriate to view parenting as a method of achieving immortality.   SA   A   U   D   SD
3. Parenting requires that one be willing to make major personal sacrifices for the benefit of the child.   SA   A   U   D   SD
4. Parenting adds a large measure of vitality to an adult's life.   SA   A   U   D   SD
5. Parenting demands greater creativity than any other adult pursuit.   SA   A   U   D   SD
6. A person who cannot comfortably make decisions for others should not consider parenting.   SA   A   U   D   SD
7. A family cannot exist in the absence of children.   SA   A   U   D   SD

To Carry This Further . . .

After completing this personal assessment, join three of your classmates in comparing and discussing your responses. What suggestions were made to help increase your awareness of all that parenting involves?

Need to Feel Safe and Secure

The greatest need in this category is for a decent place to live and protection from physical harm, along with a comfortable and safe place to sleep.

The biggest threat to a child's feeling of security often comes from a parent. Children are totally dependent on their parents, and they worry about whether the parent or parents will always be there for them. Parents also can help maintain their children's security by learning how to express their own anger or frustration in a healthy way without hurting their spouse or their children.

Need for Belonging and Love

Children need unconditional love—to know that they will always have a place in their family and their parents will always love them. Children learn how to love from their families, friends, and neighbors, but mostly from their parents. Children imitate the love, respect, and care the parents show for others.

Need for Self-Esteem

Self-esteem is respect for oneself. To develop self-esteem, children must receive unconditional support from their friends, family and especially parents. Parents can help their children develop self-esteem by praising them for their honesty, kindness, talent, hard

work, responsibility, and good decision making. Parents damage their children's self-esteem when they ridicule, abuse, shame, or hit them. Strong self-esteem enables children to become strong adults.

On the rare occasions when punishment is needed, it should be limited to the specific rule that was broken, should be brief, should not include the withdrawal of love, and should not inflict physical or emotional pain.

Need for Knowledge

Children need knowledge to be successful in life. Parents can best meet this need by setting a good example. Besides school, opportunities for learning include trips, hobbies, family projects, museums, hikes, camping trips, and concerts. Parents also should praise their children when they learn something new.

Need for Enrichment and Fulfillment

Like adults, children need to enrich their lives with beauty and harmony, and they need to develop and pursue their own goals. Examples of beauty and harmony can be found in music and art, nature, parents' spiritual beliefs, social customs, and loving relationships.

Parents can help their children pursue their goals by understanding that their children will not

---

HEALTH ACTION GUIDE

Fathers-to-be Need Understanding, Too

Expectant fathers have many of the same concerns as expectant mothers, and a few of their own, too. Although pregnancy was long considered only a woman's concern, the needs and feelings of fathers-to-be are now being recognized. Following are some of the common concerns and suggestions for handling them:[6]

- *Anxiety about mother's and baby's health.* These fears are common, even though the risks to both mother and baby are very small. Even so, you can reduce these fears by making sure the mother-to-be gets the best possible medical care, by shouldering more of the household chores, by reducing her stresses, by encouraging the mother to follow her prescribed diet, by making sure she abstains from alcohol, tobacco, and drugs, and by becoming familiar with the trouble signs.
- *Sympathy symptoms.* Expectant fathers can experience any or all of the symptoms their expectant partners experience, including morning sickness, mood swings, cramps, dizziness, appetite changes, and fatigue. Experts have suggested many theories to explain the sympathy symptoms, but they don't know for sure what causes them. You may want to consult with a physician to rule out an illness. Barring an illness, expectant fathers can deal with the problem by talking about what they are feeling, educating themselves about pregnancy, or taking a course in infant care.

- *Fear of sex.* In general, intercourse is not risky to the mother or baby in a normally progressing pregnancy. In fact, because both partners may need even more physical closeness and intimacy during pregnancy, intercourse can be very beneficial.
- *Feeling abandoned.* With all the attention society focuses on the mother-to-be, the expectant father can feel left out. The father can reduce this feeling by participating in all the classes and doctor visits with the mother, by giving up alcohol and tobacco with the mother during pregnancy, by learning everything possible about childbirth, and by talking about his feelings.
- *Moodiness.* Depression is common in both expectant mothers and fathers. Some remedies are to stay active, talk over your feelings with your partner, and make preparations for the baby. For depression that interferes with your life, seek professional help. Remember that the mother's mood swings are temporary.
- *Anxiety about delivery.* Some expectant fathers fear that they will faint or somehow fail their wives while watching the delivery. These things rarely happen. Once again, the best insurance against problems is to educate yourself, through books, through childbirth classes, and by talking with friends who have become parents.

InfoLinks

www.noah.cuny.edu/pregnancy/march_of_dimes/pre_preg.plan/dadbroch.html

want exactly what the parents want, and by encouraging their children to develop their talents and take responsible risks.

Pregnancy: An Extension of the Partnership

Pregnancy is a condition that requires a series of complex yet coordinated changes to occur in the female body. This chapter follows pregnancy from its beginning, at fertilization, to its conclusion, with labor and childbirth. Fathers-to-be share many of the joys and worries of pregnancy and childbirth. For a look at the concerns that expectant fathers may feel, see the Health Action Guide (on p. 505).

Physiological Obstacles and Aids to Fertilization

Many sexually active young people believe that they will become pregnant (or impregnate someone) only when they want to, despite their haphazard contraceptive practices. Because of this mistaken belief, many young people do not consistently use contraceptives. Young adults must remember that, to ensure the survival of our species, our bodies were designed to promote pregnancy. It is estimated that about 85 percent of sexually active women of childbearing age will become pregnant within one year if they do not use some form of contraception.[7]

With regard to pregnancy, each act of intercourse can be considered a game of physiological odds. Obstacles exist that may reduce a couple's chance of pregnancy, including the following.

Obstacles to Fertilization

1. *The acidic level of the vagina is destructive to sperm.* The low pH of the vagina will kill sperm that fail to enter the uterus quickly.
2. *The cervical mucus is thick during most of the menstrual cycle.* Sperm movement into the uterus is more difficult, except during the few days surrounding ovulation.
3. *The sperm must locate the cervical opening.* The cervical opening is small and may not be located by most sperm.
4. *Half of the sperm travel through the wrong fallopian tube.* Most commonly, only one ovum is released at ovulation. The two ovaries generally "take turns" each month. The sperm have no way of "knowing" which tube they should enter. Thus it is probable that half will travel through the wrong tube.
5. *The distance sperm must travel is relatively long compared with the tiny size of the sperm cells.*

Microscopic sperm must travel about seven or eight inches after they are inside the female.

6. *The sperm's travel is relatively "upstream."* The anatomical positioning of the female reproductive structures necessitates an "uphill" movement by the sperm.
7. *The contoured folds of the tubal walls trap many sperm.* These folds make it difficult for sperm to locate the egg. Many sperm are trapped in this maze.

There are also a variety of aids that tend to help sperm and egg cells join. Some of these are listed next.

Aids to Fertilization

1. *An astounding number of sperm are deposited during ejaculation.* Each ejaculation contains about a teaspoon of semen.[9] Within this quantity are between 200 and 500 million sperm cells. Even with large numbers of sperm killed in the vagina, millions are able to move to the deeper structures.
2. *Sperm are deposited near the cervical opening.* Ejaculation into the vagina by the penis places the sperm near the cervical opening.
3. *The male accessory glands help make the semen nonacidic.* The seminal vesicles, prostate gland, and Cowper's glands secrete fluids that provide an alkaline environment for the sperm. This environment helps sperm be better protected in the vagina until they can move into the deeper, more alkaline uterus and fallopian tubes.
4. *Uterine contractions aid sperm movement.* The rhythmic muscular contractions of the uterus tend to cause the sperm to move in the direction of the fallopian tubes.
5. *Sperm cells move rather quickly.* Despite their tiny size, sperm cells can move about one inch per hour. Powered by sugar solutions from the male accessory glands and the whiplike movements of their tails, sperm can reach the distant third of the fallopian tubes in less than eight hours as they swim in the direction of the descending ovum.
6. *After they are inside the fallopian tubes, sperm can live for days.* Some sperm may be viable for up to a week after reaching the comfortable, nonacidic environment of the fallopian tubes. Most sperm, however, will survive an average of forty-eight to seventy-two hours. Thus they can "wait in the wings" for the moment an ovum is released from the ovary (Figure 17-1).
7. *The cervical mucus is the consistency of raw egg whites at the time of ovulation.* This mucus allows for better passage of sperm through the cervical opening when the ovum is most capable of being fertilized.

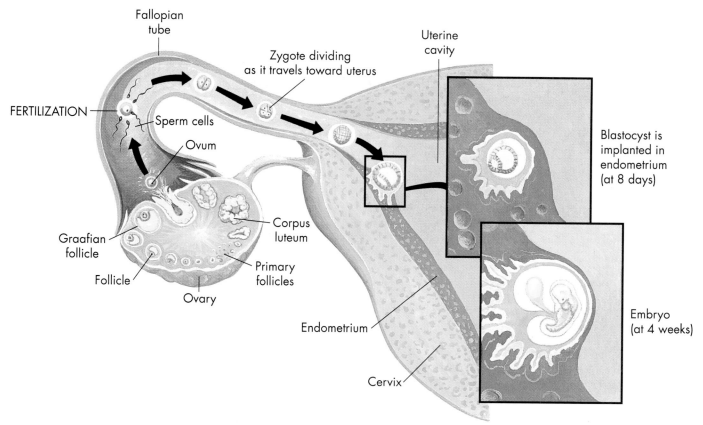

Fallopian tube

Zygote dividing as it travels toward uterus

Uterine cavity

FERTILIZATION

Sperm cells

Ovum

Graafian follicle

Follicle

Corpus luteum

Primary follicles

Ovary

Endometrium

Cervix

Blastocyst is implanted in endometrium (at 8 days)

Embryo (at 4 weeks)

Figure 17-1 After its release from the follicle, the ovum begins its weeklong journey down the fallopian tube. Fertilization generally occurs in the outermost third of the tube. Now fertilized, the ovum progresses toward the uterus, where it embeds itself in the endometrium. A pregnancy is established.

Signs of Pregnancy

Aside from pregnancy tests done in a professional laboratory, a woman can sometimes recognize early signs and symptoms. The signs of pregnancy have been divided into three categories.

Presumptive Signs of Pregnancy

Missed period after unprotected intercourse the previous month

Nausea on awakening or during the day (morning sickness)

Increase in size and tenderness of breasts

Darkening of the areolar tissue surrounding the nipples

Probable Signs of Pregnancy

Increase in the frequency of urination (the growing uterus presses against the bladder)

Increase in the size of the abdomen

Cervix becomes softer by the sixth week (detected by a pelvic examination by a clinician)

Positive pregnancy test (see the Star Box at right)

Home Pregnancy Tests

Using technology similar to that in the laboratory-based immune response tests, these pregnancy tests can be conducted in the privacy of one's home. Home pregnancy tests use a urine sample to identify the hormone human chorionic gonadotropin (HCG). The low cost and convenience make these tests attractive to many people.

Despite these advantages, home pregnancy tests are not nearly as accurate as laboratory-based ones. Manufacturers claim that the tests are 90 percent accurate, but research studies have found lower accuracy rates. Inaccuracies result not so much from the test itself but from the difficulties some people have in following directions and interpreting the results. The most common error stems from using the test kit too early in pregnancy, before the HCG can be detected.[7] Such an error (in this case, a false negative) could delay important prenatal care.

Most physicians will immediately order a more accurate test when a woman indicates she had a positive result on her home pregnancy test. This raises questions about duplication of health care costs. Nevertheless, the convenience and privacy provided by home tests continue to make them popular items for sexually active couples.

HEALTH ACTION GUIDE

Pregnancy Can Bring a Roller Coaster of Emotions

Expectant couples typically experience a roller coaster of emotional and physical changes. If they do not understand that these changes are normal, the woman may begin to doubt her emotional health, and the man may feel confused or angry. By knowing what to expect, couples can make the pregnancy a positive experience.

Every pregnancy is different, but many changes are common to all pregnancies. Each trimester carries its own set of changes.[8]

- **The first trimester** often begins only with the news that the woman is pregnant. Even if the pregnancy is planned, the partners may feel surprise or even shock. They may worry about their fitness as parents, worry about the timing of the pregnancy, fear that they will lose sight of their career goals, or worry that they cannot afford a child. The mother may have fears about the pregnancy and delivery. The physical symptoms of morning sickness often appear, including nausea, vomiting, and breast tenderness. These physical symptoms often vary in intensity, or some may be completely absent. Emotions often become unstable; the woman may feel depressed but may be unable to explain why. She may become tearful over apparently small causes. These emotional swings are believed to be caused by hormonal changes in the woman's body.

The man may feel confused or overwhelmed by these changes and may withdraw, just at the time when the woman feels she needs more support and affection. When both partners understand that these intense emotions are normal in pregnancy, they can accept them as a part of the process. Men typically experience many of the same emotional swings

as women, and they may need help and support in handling their feelings. See the Health Action Guide on page 505, "Fathers-to-be Need Understanding, Too," for some suggestions.

- **The second trimester** usually brings more tranquility, as morning sickness begins to ease and the risk of miscarriage declines. The expectant mother begins to feel the baby move (quickening), begins to wear maternity clothes, and typically has more energy. The couple may begin attending childbirth classes.
- **The third trimester** brings more anxiety about the delivery to come, along with pride in becoming parents. The obviously pregnant woman may find the public becoming more attentive to her (e.g., offering their seats, helping her carry items). She may appreciate this help, or may feel offended, as if people assume she is helpless. The woman's physical discomfort may increase along with the size of her abdomen. She may be unable to find a comfortable position for sleeping. She may feel unattractive to her mate, which can be soothed by cuddling and being held by her partner. She may be worried about how all her relationships will be affected by the new baby, and she may fear the pain of delivery.

Both partners can allay their fears by learning more about childbirth and preparing for the delivery. Thus most of the intense feelings and concerns that trouble expectant parents are a normal part of pregnancy and can be handled with the support of both partners, their families, and occasionally the help of physicians or other resources.

InfoLinks
www.childbirth.org

Positive Signs of Pregnancy

Determination of a fetal heartbeat

Feeling of the fetus moving (quickening)

Observation of the fetus by ultrasound or optical viewers

Personal Applications

- If you (or your partner) have ever been pregnant, which of the presumptive and probable signs of pregnancy did you notice first? How was a positive determination of pregnancy made?

Agents That Can Damage a Fetus

A large number of agents that come into contact with a pregnant woman can affect fetal development. Many of these (rubella and herpes viruses, tobacco smoke, alcohol, and virtually all other drugs) are discussed in other chapters of this text. The best advice for a pregnant woman is to maintain close contact with her obstetrician during pregnancy and to consider carefully the ingestion of any over-the-counter

(OTC) drug (including aspirin, caffeine, and antacids) that could harm the fetus.

Women should also avoid exposure to radiation during pregnancy. Such exposure, most commonly through excessive x-rays or radiation fallout from nuclear testing, can irreversibly damage fetal genetic structures. In addition, pregnant women should avoid Accutane, a drug prescribed for the treatment of acne that can severely damage the fetus.

Personal Applications

- If a woman should not smoke, drink, or use other drugs during pregnancy, should these limitations also be placed on the father? Why or why not?

Childbirth: The Labor of Delivery

Childbirth, or *parturition,* is one of the true peak life experiences for both men and women. Most of the time, childbirth is a wonderfully exciting venture into the unknown. For the parents, this intriguing experience can provide a stage for personal growth, maturity, and insight into a dynamic, complex world.

During the last few weeks of the third **trimester,** most fetuses will move deeper into the pelvic cavity in a process called *lightening.* During this movement, the fetus's body will rotate and the head will begin to engage more deeply into the mother's pelvic girdle. Many women will report that their babies have "dropped."

Another indication that parturition may be relatively near is the increased reporting of *Braxton Hicks contractions.* These uterine contractions, which are of mild intensity and often occur at irregular intervals, may be felt throughout a pregnancy. During the last few weeks of pregnancy (*gestation*), these mild contractions can occur more frequently and cause a woman to feel as if she is going into labor **(false labor).**

Labor begins when uterine contractions become more intense and occur at regular intervals. The birth of a child can be divided into three stages: (1) effacement and dilation of the cervix, (2) delivery of the fetus, and (3) expulsion of the placenta (Figure 17-2). For a woman having her first child, the birth process lasts an average of twelve to sixteen hours. The average length of labor for subsequent births is much shorter—from four to ten hours on the average. Labor is very unpredictable: Labors that last from one to twenty-four hours occur daily at most hospitals.

Stage One: Effacement and Dilation of the Cervix

In the first stage of labor the uterine contractions attempt to thin (*efface*) the normally thick cervical walls and to enlarge (*dilate*) the cervical opening. These contractions are directed by the release of prostaglandins and the hormone oxytocin into the circulating bloodstream. In women delivering their first babies, effacement will occur before dilation. In subsequent deliveries, effacement and dilation usually occur at the same time.

The first stage of labor is often the longest. The cervical opening must thin and dilate to a diameter of ten centimeters before the first stage of labor is considered complete.[10] Often this stage begins with the dislodging of the cervical mucous plug. The subsequent *bloody show* (mucous plug and a small amount of blood) at the vaginal opening may indicate that effacement and dilation have begun. Another indication of labor's onset may be the bursting or tearing of the fetal amniotic sac. "Breaking the bag of waters" refers to this phenomenon, which happens in various measures in expectant women.

The pain of the uterine contractions becomes more intense as the woman moves through this first stage of labor. As the cervical opening effaces and dilates from zero to three centimeters, many women report feeling happy, exhilarated, and confident. In the early phase of the first stage of labor, the contractions are relatively short (lasting from fifteen to sixty seconds) and the intervals between contractions range from twenty minutes to five minutes as labor progresses. However, these rest intervals will become shorter and the contractions more forceful when the woman's uterus contracts to dilate four to seven centimeters.

In this second phase of the first stage of labor, the contractions usually last about one minute each and the rest intervals drop from about five minutes to one minute over a period of five to nine hours.

The third phase of the first stage of labor is called *transition.* During transition, the uterus contracts to dilate the cervical opening to the full ten centimeters required for safe passage of the fetus out of the uterus and into the vagina (birth canal). This period of labor is often the most painful part of the entire birth process. Fortunately, it is also the shortest phase of most labors. Lasting between fifteen and thirty minutes, transition contractions often last sixty to ninety seconds each. The rest intervals between contractions are short and vary from thirty to sixty seconds.

An examination of the cervix by a nurse or physician will reveal whether full dilation of ten centimeters has occurred. Until the full ten-centimeter dilation, women are cautioned not to "push" the fetus during the contractions. Special breathing and concentration techniques help many women cope with the first stage of labor.

Stage Two: Delivery of the Fetus

When the mother's cervix is fully dilated, she enters the second stage of labor, the delivery of the fetus through the birth canal. Now the mother is encouraged to help push the baby out (with her abdominal muscles) during each contraction. In this second stage the uterine contractions are less forceful than during the transition phase of the first stage and may last sixty seconds each, with a one- to three-minute rest interval.

This second stage may last up to two hours in first births.[9] For subsequent births, this stage will usually be much shorter. When the baby's head is first seen at the vaginal opening, *crowning* is said to have taken place. Generally the back of the baby's head appears first. (Infants whose feet or buttocks are presented first are said to be delivered in a *breech position.*) After the head is delivered, the baby's body rotates upward to let the shoulders come through. The rest of the

trimester a 3-month period; human pregnancies encompass three trimesters.

false labor conditions that resemble the start of true labor; may include irregular uterine contractions, pressure, and discomfort in the lower abdomen.

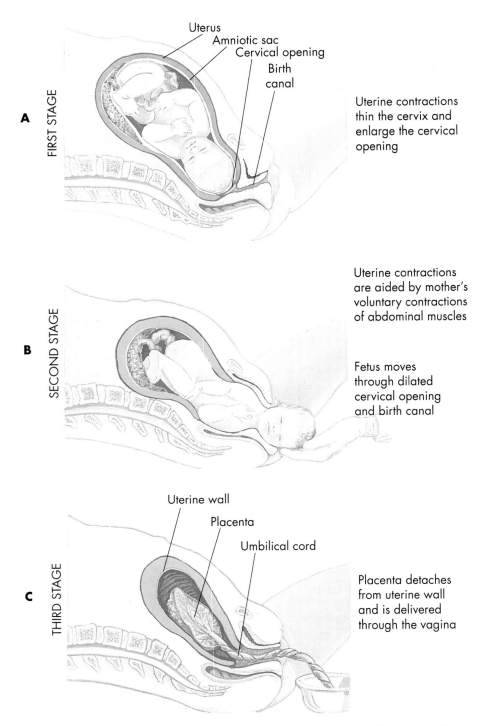

Figure 17-2 Labor, or childbirth, is a three-stage process. During effacement and dilation, the first stage **(A)**, the cervical canal is gradually opened by contractions of the uterine wall. The second stage **(B)**, delivery of the fetus, encompasses the actual delivery of the fetus from the uterus and through the birth canal. The delivery of the placenta, the third stage **(C),** empties the uterus, thus completing the process of childbirth.

body follows quite quickly. The second stage of labor ends when the fetus is fully expelled from the vagina. In the past, deliveries were often performed with an *episiotomy,* a surgical incision of the **perineum** intended to prevent lacerations (tearing) when the baby was delivered. (See the Star Box on p. 511).

Newly delivered babies often look "unusual." Their heads are often cone-shaped as a result of the compression of cranial bones that occurs during the delivery through the birth canal. Within a few days after birth, the newborn's head will assume a much more normal shape. Most babies (of all races) appear

HEALTH ACTION GUIDE

Guidelines for Successful Breastfeeding

Breastfeeding is a perfectly natural function, so every new mother should be able to do it instinctively, right? Well, not necessarily. Occasionally little problems occur, and reviewing some of the basic advice before beginning can make it a little smoother:[13]

- Begin as soon after birth as you can, when the baby's sucking instinct is strongest. Begin in the delivery room if possible.
- Don't allow the hospital's regulations or wishes to come between you and your baby. Arrange to room with your baby.
- When you are ready to begin, find a comfortable position.
- Position your baby facing your nipple.
- Support your breast with your free hand, gently tickle the baby's lips with your nipple, then let your baby take the initiative.
- Be sure the baby latches onto the areola as well as the nipple, or the baby will not compress the milk glands. This can cause soreness and cracking.
- Be sure the breast does not block the baby's nose.
- Watch the baby's cheek for the steady rhythm that indicates the baby is suckling.
- If your baby holds onto the breast after he or she has finished suckling, do not pull the nipple out abruptly to avoid injuring it. Instead, break the suction first by putting a finger into a corner of the baby's mouth or depressing the breast to admit some air.

InfoLinks
www.lalecheleague.org

bluish at first until they begin regular breathing. All babies are covered with a coating of *vernix,* a white, cheeselike substance that protects the skin.

Stage Three: Delivery of the Placenta

Usually within thirty minutes after the fetus is delivered, the uterus will again initiate a series of contractions to expel the placenta (or *afterbirth*). The placenta is examined by the attending physician to ensure that it was completely expelled. Torn remnants of the placenta could lead to dangerous hemorrhaging by the mother. Often the physician manually examines the uterus after the placenta has been delivered.

After the placenta has been delivered, the uterus continues with mild contractions to help control bleeding and start the gradual reduction of the uterus to its normal, nonpregnant size. This final aspect of the birth process is called **postpartum.** External abdominal massage of the lower abdomen seems to help the uterus contract, as does an infant's nursing at the mother's breast. For suggestions for successfully breastfeeding your baby, see the Health Action Guide on this page.

Personal Applications

- To what extent should fathers participate in the birth experience?

Cesarean Deliveries

A **cesarean delivery** (cesarean birth, C-section) is a procedure in which the fetus is surgically removed from the mother's uterus through the abdominal wall. This type of delivery, which is completed in up to an hour, can be performed with the mother having a regional or a general anesthetic.

Currently, 23 percent of all deliveries are by cesarean section.[14] The use of cesarean deliveries is questioned by some medical experts, although others point to the need for this kind of delivery when one or more of the following factors are present:

- The fetus is improperly positioned.
- The mother's pelvis is too small.

> **perineum**   in the female, the region between the vulva and the anus.
>
> **postpartum**   the period after the birth of a baby during which the uterus returns to its prepregnancy size.
>
> **cesarean delivery** (si **zare** ee an)   surgical removal of a fetus through the abdominal wall.

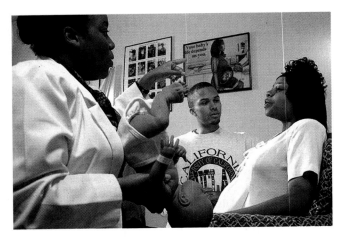

A nurse explains fetal rotation to expectant parents. A cesarean delivery may be required if the fetus is in a breech position.

- The fetus is especially large.
- The fetus shows signs of distress.
- The umbilical cord is compressed.
- The placenta is being delivered before the fetus.
- The mother's health is at risk.

Although a cesarean delivery is considered major surgery, most mothers cope well with the delivery and postsurgical and postpartum discomfort. The hospital stay is usually a few days longer than for a vaginal delivery. The mother can still nurse her child and may still be able to have vaginal deliveries with later children. More and more hospitals are allowing the father to be in the operating room during cesarean deliveries. Fortunately, research indicates that early **bonding** between child, mother, and father can still occur with cesarean deliveries. Cesarean deliveries are much more expensive than vaginal deliveries.

Complications in Pregnancy and Childbirth

Most women progress through pregnancy and delivery without complications, but once in a great while something goes wrong. Complications are usually the result of genetics, an environmental factor (such as the use of drugs or alcohol by the mother), or some combination of these. Pregnant women should remember that the following complications are unusual if they are consuming a healthy diet, avoiding agents that can damage a fetus, such as alcohol and drugs, and following their doctor's recommendations.

- *Ectopic pregnancy:* This is a pregnancy in which the embryo implants outside the uterus, most often in a fallopian tube. It can be serious and even life threatening, especially if not discovered early, but treatment can remove most of the risk for the mother while preserving future fertility.

- *Miscarriage:* Early miscarriage is very common, occurring in as many as 40 percent of conceptions, often passing unnoticed by the woman. It is usually related to a chromosomal abnormality or other problem in the fetus. Late miscarriage, on the other hand, is usually related to the mother's condition, her exposure to drugs or other toxins, or problems of the placenta.

- *Gestational diabetes:* This is a temporary condition in which the mother's body does not produce enough insulin to handle the increased blood sugar of pregnancy. Symptoms include unusual thirst, frequent urination, and fatigue. If treated, it is not a threat to the mother or baby.

- *Hyperemesis gravidarum:* This term literally means "excessive vomiting during pregnancy." This is a very unusual condition that is more serious than typical morning sickness. If untreated, it can result in malnutrition, dehydration, or damage to the fetus. It can be treated, however, with measures ranging from rest and antacids to hospitalization if necessary.

- *Preeclampsia (pregnancy-induced hypertension; toxemia):* This is a condition in which the woman's blood pressure becomes elevated during pregnancy; it occurs in one of every ten to twenty pregnancies, and if untreated, preeclampsia can be serious and even life threatening. Fortunately, physicians almost invariably identify the disease if the mother is receiving regular prenatal care, and a poor outcome is rare. Treatment depends on the severity of the disease and can include an immediate induction of labor or hospitalization of the mother until the fetus is sufficiently developed to survive outside the uterus.

- *Eclampsia:* The final stage of preeclampsia, this disease is very unusual when the mother is receiving regular prenatal care. Symptoms include convulsions and coma. Treatment includes preventing convulsions and inducing labor or performing a cesarean delivery as soon as possible.

- *Intrauterine growth retardation (IUGR):* This term is used to describe insufficient growth of the fetus, which can occur because of genetic factors, maternal disease, or fetal malnutrition. With regular prenatal care, this disease can be identified and reversed.

- *Premature rupture of the membranes (PROM):* Rupture of the chorionic membranes, often called "breaking of the water," can occur prematurely. Infection is a risk because the protective membrane has been broken. Doctors typically try to delay delivery as long as possible up to about thirty-seven weeks.

- *Premature labor:* Labor that begins after the fetus is considered viable and before term, at about thirty-seven weeks, is called *premature labor*. It carries a variety of risks, but in many cases premature labor can be halted, and the mother can carry the baby to term. Quick medical attention is paramount.
- *Fetal distress:* This term describes a category of fetal problems, in particular a lack of oxygen caused by any of a variety of factors. The treatment usually is immediate delivery, by cesarean if necessary.

Personal Applications

- Have you, your partner, or anyone close to you experienced a complication during pregnancy or delivery? If so, what was the outcome? Could the complication have been controlled or prevented?

Preconceptional Counseling

Prenatal diagnosis and counseling is one of the most beneficial advances in medical technology. Genetic counselors can provide timely, accurate, and complete information to patients, while maintaining the attitude that the patient's values should guide the decisions.

You should seek genetic counseling *before* attempting to conceive a child if you or your partner fall into any of the following categories:[15]

- History of multiple spontaneous abortions
- Consanguinity (partners are related by blood)
- Birth defect, possible genetic condition, neuromuscular or neurologic condition, or abnormalities of physical sexual development in the patient or families
- Ethnic background with increased risk of recessive genetic disease
- Maternal age of thirty-five or more years at delivery
- Paternal age of fifty-five or more years
- Positive maternal test for Down syndrome or trisomy 18
- Positive maternal test for an open neural tube defect
- Carrying a gene for a recessive disease that is more common in some ethnic populations
- Exposure to a known or suspected **teratogenic agent** (capable of causing birth abnormality)

The genetic counselor might use a variety of methods for gathering information about the couple,

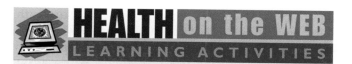

including DNA testing, other medical tests, medical records, family histories, and autopsy reports. When couples receive genetic counseling before conception and learn that they have a high risk of conceiving a child with birth defects, they then have a variety of options still open to them, such as artificial insemination by a donor, ovum donation, and adoption.

In addition, some couples can also reduce the risk of birth defects by changing their behavior or diet. For example, taking folate supplements has been shown to reduce the risk of neural tube defects. Abstaining from alcohol during pregnancy eliminates the risk of fetal alcohol syndrome. Stopping smoking reduces the risk of fetal intrauterine growth retardation, placental abruption (premature detachment of

---

bonding important initial recognition established between the newborn and those adults on whom the newborn will depend.

teratogenic agent any substance that is capable of causing birth defects.

the placenta from the uterine wall), and fetal death. Women with the disease phenylketonuria who eliminate phenylalanine from their diet before pregnancy drastically reduce the risk of mental retardation in their children.[15]

If you have already become pregnant, you still should work with your physician to identify risk factors in your first prenatal visit, to allow time for tests to be conducted and medical records to be reviewed. Tests commonly performed for those at risk are chorionic villus sampling (CVS) and amniocentesis.

In the second trimester, tests commonly performed include targeted ultrasound and screening for Down syndrome, trisomy 18, and open neural tube defects. Couples who learn of an increased risk through a second-trimester test tend to be significantly more anxious than those who learned of the risk earlier in the pregnancy. In general, couples should attempt to receive genetic counseling and testing while they still have the legal option to terminate the pregnancy.

Infertility

Most traditional-age college students are interested in preventing pregnancy. However, increasing numbers of other people are trying to do just the opposite: They are trying to become pregnant. It is estimated that about one in six couples has a problem with *infertility*. These couples wish to become pregnant but are unsuccessful.

Why are some couples infertile? The reasons are about evenly balanced between men and women. About 10 percent of infertility cases have no detectable cause. The most frequent male complication is insufficient sperm production and delivery.

Enhancing Fertility

A number of approaches can be used to increase sperm counts. Among the simple approaches are the application of periodic cold packs on the scrotum and the replacement of tight underwear with boxer shorts. When a structural problem reduces sperm production, surgery can be helpful. Opinion is divided concerning whether increased frequency of intercourse improves fertility. Most experts (reproductive endocrinologists) suggest that couples have intercourse at least a couple of times in the week preceding ovulation.

Artificial Insemination

Men can also collect (through masturbation) and save samples of their sperm to use in a procedure called *artificial insemination by partner*. Near the time of ovulation, the collected samples of sperm are deposited near the woman's cervical opening. In a related procedure called *artificial insemination by donor*, the sperm of

a donor are used. Donor semen is screened for the presence of pathogens, including the AIDS virus.

Surgical Remedies

Causes of infertility in women center mostly on obstructions in the reproductive tract and the inability to ovulate. The obstructions frequently result from tissue damage (scarring) caused by infections. Chlamydial and gonorrheal infections often produce fertility problems. In certain women the use of IUDs has produced infections and PID; both of these increase the chances of infertility. Other possible causes of structural abnormalities include scar tissue from previous surgery, fibroid tumors, polyps, and endometriosis. A variety of microsurgical techniques may correct some of these complications.

One of the most recent innovative procedures involves the use of **transcervical balloon tuboplasty.** In this procedure a series of balloon-tipped catheters are inserted through the uterus into the blocked fallopian tubes. After they are inflated, these balloon catheters help open the scarred passageways.

When a woman has ovulation difficulties, pinpointing the specific cause can be very difficult. Increasing age produces hormone fluctuations associated with lack of ovulation. Being significantly overweight or underweight also has a serious effect on fertility. However, in women of normal weight who are not approaching menopause, it appears that ovulation difficulties are caused by failure of synchronization between the hormones governing the menstrual cycle. Fertility drugs can help alter the menstrual cycle to produce ovulation. Clomiphene citrate (Clomid), in oral pill form, and injections of a mixture of luteinizing hormone (LH) and follicle-stimulating hormone (FSH) taken from the urine of menopausal women (Pergonal) are the most common fertility drugs available. Both are capable of producing multiple ova at ovulation (see the Topics for Today article on p. 519).

Reproductive Technology

For couples who are unable to conceive after drug therapy, surgery, and artificial insemination, the use of *in vitro fertilization and embryo transfer (IVF–ET)* is another option. This method is sometimes referred to as the "test tube" procedure. Costing up to $10,000 per attempt, IVF–ET consists of surgically retrieving fertilizable ova from the woman and combining them in a glass dish with sperm. After several days, the fertilized ova are transferred into the uterus.

A newer test tube procedure is called *gamete intrafallopian transfer (GIFT)*. Similar to IVF–ET, this procedure deposits a mixture of retrieved eggs and sperm directly into the fallopian tubes.

Fertilized ova (zygotes) can also be transferred from a laboratory dish into the fallopian tubes in a procedure called *zygote intrafallopian transfer (ZIFT)*. One advantage of this procedure is that the clinicians are certain that ova have been fertilized before the transfer to the fallopian tubes.

Surrogate Parenting

Surrogate parenting is another option that has been explored in the last decade, although the legal and ethical issues surrounding this method of conception have not been fully resolved. Surrogate parenting can take several forms. Typically, an infertile couple will make a contract with a woman (the surrogate parent), who will then be artificially inseminated with semen from the expectant father. In some instances the surrogate will receive an embryo from the donor parents. The surrogate carries the fetus to term and returns the newborn to the parents. In some cases, women have served as surrogates for their close relatives. Because of the concerns about true "ownership" of the baby, surrogate parenting may not be a particularly viable or legal option for many couples.

Options for Infertile Couples

The process of coping with infertility problems can be an emotionally stressful experience for a couple. Hours of waiting in physicians' offices, undergoing many examinations, scheduling intercourse, producing sperm samples, and undergoing surgical or drug treatments place multiple burdens on a couple. Knowing that other couples are able to conceive so effortlessly adds to the mental strain. Fortunately, support groups have been established to assist couples with infertility problems. Some of these groups are listed in the Star Box at right.

What can you do to reduce the chances of developing infertility problems? Certainly avoiding infections of the reproductive organs is one crucial factor. Barrier methods of contraception (condom, diaphragm) with a spermicide reportedly cut the risk of developing infertility in half. The use of an IUD should be carefully considered, and the risk from multiple partners should encourage responsible sexual activity. Men and women should be aware of the dangers from working around hazardous chemicals or using psychoactive drugs. Maintaining overall good health and having regular medical (and, for women, gynecological) checkups are also good ideas. Because infertility is linked with advancing age, couples may not want to indefinitely delay having children.

Adoption

For couples who have determined that biological childbirth is impossible, adoption offers an alternative. Adoptions peaked in the United States at 89,200 in 1970 and have fallen to about 50,000 a year today.

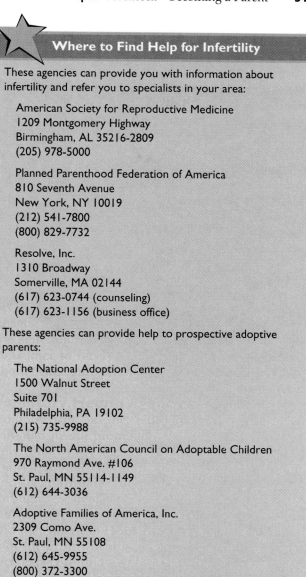

Where to Find Help for Infertility

These agencies can provide you with information about infertility and refer you to specialists in your area:

American Society for Reproductive Medicine
1209 Montgomery Highway
Birmingham, AL 35216-2809
(205) 978-5000

Planned Parenthood Federation of America
810 Seventh Avenue
New York, NY 10019
(212) 541-7800
(800) 829-7732

Resolve, Inc.
1310 Broadway
Somerville, MA 02144
(617) 623-0744 (counseling)
(617) 623-1156 (business office)

These agencies can provide help to prospective adoptive parents:

The National Adoption Center
1500 Walnut Street
Suite 701
Philadelphia, PA 19102
(215) 735-9988

The North American Council on Adoptable Children
970 Raymond Ave. #106
St. Paul, MN 55114-1149
(612) 644-3036

Adoptive Families of America, Inc.
2309 Como Ave.
St. Paul, MN 55108
(612) 645-9955
(800) 372-3300
Publishes OURS Magazine (Organization for United Response)

Adopted children currently represent about 2 percent of all children in the United States.

As the supply of adoptable infants has decreased, young women considering putting their babies up for adoption have gained new leverage. Couples determined to adopt a healthy infant have increasingly turned to independent adoptions arranged by a lawyer, or they may negotiate directly with the birth mother. Independent adoptions now surpass those arranged by social service agencies. For a look at the ethical and social issues surrounding adoption and other reproductive trends, see the Star Box on page 516.

transcervical balloon tuboplasty the use of inflatable balloon catheters to open blocked fallopian tubes; a procedure used for some women with fertility problems.

Reproduction Opens a Pandora's Box of Ethical Issues

Perhaps no area of health incites as many debates as reproduction. Throughout history, the intersection of reproduction and medical science has been an ethical battleground. Following are some of the issues currently being debated in the United States. Where do you stand on these issues?

- *Cloning.* Cloning hit the headlines in 1997 with the news that researchers in Scotland had successfully cloned a sheep named Dolly. In brief, the procedure works by inserting the complete nucleus of an adult cell into an unfertilized sheep egg. While the medical community debates the ethics of applying this technology to humans, governmental bodies have rushed to pass laws to make human cloning illegal.

- *In vitro fertilization (IVF).* Literally "in glass," in vitro fertilization is a process in which eggs are removed from the ovaries and mixed with sperm in vitro in the laboratory. The resulting embryos are transferred to the uterus. Issues include the use of IVF by postmenopausal women, IVF with donor eggs, medical risks to egg donors, and the practice of paying for donor eggs.

- *Prenatal testing.* The most common tests are amniocentesis and chorionic villus sampling. Advances in prenatal testing have led some observers to fear that fetuses will be aborted based on a diagnosis, such as Down syndrome, before the parents know what kind of life the child would really have. Others fear that a preference for boys might make abortion of female fetuses commonplace in the United States.

- *Preimplantation diagnosis.* Similar to prenatal testing, preimplantation diagnosis is the examination of embryos for genetic defects before they are implanted in the uterus. The technique has been used with couples at risk of having children with genetic diseases. Critics fear that this technique, like prenatal testing, can be abused and can reduce the variety that is essential to the survival of the species.

- *Artificial insemination.* Used since the 1880s, artificial insemination is the first known example of reproductive technology. One continuing issue is the control of artificial insemination by doctors or sperm banks, including a perceived inconsistency in the way women are approved for insemination. In addition, many religious authorities consider artificial insemination an assault on the dignity of marriage and the sanctity of the family. Finally, some observers would like to eliminate any payments to sperm donors to remove the appearance of payment for body parts or tissues.

- *Multifetal pregnancy reduction (MFPR).* In multifetal pregnancy reductions (see Chapter 16), one or more fetuses in a multiple pregnancy are terminated to give the surviving fetus(es) a better chance at reaching full term and surviving. Supporters argue that MFPR avoids the trauma of abortion, enables the parents to have their own child, and avoids the dangers of delivering multiple premature infants. Opponents argue that it is another form of abortion and thus is wrong.

- *Embryo freezing.* The growth in embryo freezing has led to the question of the disposal of unneeded embryos. Some experts have proposed that these surplus embryos be donated to other infertile couples to help them to form families.[16] This solution would lead to a variety of other questions, beginning with the question of whether such a donation would be a cell donation or an adoption.

- *Surrogate motherhood.* One of the most controversial responses to infertility, surrogacy has helped to spur the search for less questionable reproductive technologies. Between 1975 and 1990, about 4,500 children were born in the United States through surrogacy arrangements.[17] Opponents compare surrogacy with baby selling. Instances in which surrogate mothers have tried to regain custody of their children have generated enormous publicity. Many states have passed laws sharply limiting surrogacy arrangements.

- *Adoption.* One controversy currently swirling around adoption is the issue of the child's best interests versus parental rights, which some have warned approaches the level of class warfare, because the birth parents tend to be poor and single, and the adoptive parents tend to be middle class and married. Other issues are the right of the unwed father to veto the adoption of his child, and the ethics of interracial adoption.

- *Foster parenting.* As with adoption, the question of the child's best interests versus parental rights is a central issue with foster parenting. Critics argue that foster children languish in a limbo, drifting from foster home to foster home, because public agencies are unwilling to sever their ties to their biological parents.

Foster Parenting

The number of children in foster care who are waiting to be reunited with their biological parents or awaiting adoption has risen steadily since the mid-1980s. Experts attribute the rise to family problems caused by parental drug abuse, unemployment, alcoholism, and other difficulties. Currently about one-half million children a year spend time in foster homes.

Like adoption, foster parenting has presented a variety of ethical and legal issues, especially the debate between "the best interests of the child" and parental rights.

Personal Applications

- How far do you think couples should go in trying to achieve a pregnancy? If you wanted to have children and found out that you and your partner could not conceive, what options would you consider?

Real Life
Real choices

- What are the chief causes of (1) male and (2) female infertility?
- What procedures are used to correct causes of infertility and help women become pregnant?
- What is surrogate parenting, and what are the controversies that surround this issue?
- If you plan to have children, how important is it to you that they be the biological offspring of you and your spouse? Give reasons for your answer.

And Now, Your Choices . . .
- If you and your spouse, like Gary and Susan Johnson, very much wanted to have a child and found out in your late 30s that you had a serious fertility problem, what route would you choose: the available medical/surgical options, surrogate parenting, adoption, or another course of action (foster parenting, remaining childless)? Give reasons for your answer.

Summary

- Couples have many important issues to discuss before deciding to have children.
- Several physiological factors can be either aids or obstacles to fertilization.
- Women can often recognize the presumptive and probable signs of pregnancy; a physician can determine positive signs of pregnancy.
- Expectant fathers can experience many of the same symptoms and emotions as expectant mothers.
- Pregnant women, and women attempting to become pregnant, should avoid agents that can damage the fetus, including all drugs (prescription, over-the-counter, and illicit), tobacco smoke, and alcohol.

- Childbirth takes place in three distinct stages: effacement and dilation of the cervix, delivery of the fetus, and delivery of the placenta.
- Complications during pregnancy and delivery are varied and can be caused by genetics, environmental factors, or a combination of these.
- Genetic counselors can provide timely, accurate, and complete information to couples who are considering pregnancy.
- Regular prenatal care is vital and can help prevent or reverse complications of pregnancy.
- Infertility is an important concern for some couples. Various technologies are improving infertile couples' chances of having children.

Review Questions

1. What important issues should couples discuss before they decide to have children?
2. Identify the many needs children have as they grow and develop.
3. What are some obstacles and aids to fertilization presented in this chapter? Can you think of others?
4. What are the presumptive, probable, and positive signs of pregnancy?
5. Identify and describe the events that occur during each of the three stages of childbirth. Approximately how long is each stage?
6. Who should seek genetic counseling? How can the counselor assess the couple's risk of having a child with birth defects?
7. What is meant by the term preconceptional counseling?
8. List and describe several complications that can occur during pregnancy and delivery.
9. What can be done to reduce chances of infertility? Explain IVF-ET, GIFT, and ZIFT procedures.
10. What options does a couple have when they cannot conceive a child?

References

1. Blackburn B. Moms starting families in 40s test odds. *USA Today* 1997; Sept 24:14A.

2. Haidl G, Jung A, Schill WB. Aging and sperm function. *Hum Reprod* 1996; 11(3):558–60.

3. Later age pregnancy. Preparing for the happy, healthy event after 40. *Health Oasis,* Mayo Clinic, 1998. http://www.mayohealth.org/mayo/9708/htm/aged_p.htm

4. Fretts RC et al. Increased maternal age and risk of fetal death. *N Engl J Med* 1995; 333(15):953–57.

5. Knowles J. *How to be a good parent.* Planned Parenthood Federation of America, PPFA web site. September 1996. http://www.plannedparenthood.org/-guidesparents/

6. Eisenberg A. *What to expect when you're expecting.* 2nd ed. New York: Workman Publishing, 1996.

7. Hatcher RA et al. *Contraceptive technology.* 17th ed. New York: Irvington, 1998.

8. Emotions during pregnancy. *Iowa health book: obstetrics and gynecology.* Department of Nursing: Children's and Women's Services/OB-GYN Patient Education Committee, Virtual Hospital, 1997. http://www.vh.org/Patients/IHB/ObGyn/-Emotions.html

9. Hyde JS, Delamater JD. *Understanding human sexuality.* 6th ed. New York: McGraw-Hill, 1996.

10. Kelly GF: *Sexuality today: the human perspective.* 6th ed. New York: McGraw-Hill, 1998.

11. Lede RL, Belizan JM, Carroli G. Is routine use of episiotomy justified? (review). *Am J. Obstet Gynecol* 1996 May; 174(5):1399–1402.

12. Bansal RK et al. Is there a benefit to episiotomy at spontaneous vaginal delivery? A natural experiment. *Am J Obstet Gynecol* 1996 Oct; 174(4 pt 1):897–901.

13. La Leche League International. *When you breastfeed your baby: the first weeks.* Schaumburg, IL: La Leche League, 1993.

14. U.S. Bureau of the Census. *Statistical abstract of the United States: 1998.* 118th ed. Washington, D.C.: U.S. Government Printing Office, 1998.

15. Kuller JA, Chescheir NC, Cefalo RC. *Prenatal diagnosis and reproductive genetics.* St. Louis: Mosby-Year Book, 1996.

16. Robertston JA. Ethical and legal issues in human embryo donation (see comments)(review). *Fertil Steril* 1995 Nov; 64(5):885–94.

17. Phillips SC. Reproductive ethics. *CQ Researcher* 1994; Apr 8:301.

Suggested Readings

Engel B. *The parenthood decision: deciding whether you are ready and willing to become a parent.* New York: Doubleday, 1998. Deciding whether to become a parent is one of the biggest decisions you can make, yet many people become parents without giving the experience much thought, or even worse, with fantasies or unrealistic notions about parenthood. This book examines several issues facing potential parents, including: How can I know if the time is right? What are my real reasons for wanting a child? Are my motives questionable? Should I have a child at all? What if I want a child and my partner does not? Am I capable of being a good parent? Is my partner? What about money issues? The book leads readers through these issues with compassionate decision-making exercises.

Mungeam F, Gray J. *A guy's guide to pregnancy: preparing for pregnancy together.* Hillsboro, OR: Beyond Words Publishing, 1998. While women can find hundreds of pregnancy books aimed at women, men's concerns rarely get more than a mention. Designed to be guy-friendly, this book is divided into 40 chapters, one for each week of the pregnancy. It explains what happens at each stage of pregnancy, helping men to meet their own and their wives' needs throughout pregnancy and into parenthood.

Peck C, Wilkinson W, Kolkow-Garber H. *Parents at last: celebrating adoption and the new pathways to parenthood.* New York: Clarkson Potter, 1998. This book presents portraits of people who became parents through alternative means, including adoption, high-tech conception and birth, stepparenting, and foster parenting. Accompanying photos portray 32 families who persevered and succeeded in their quest to become a family.

Goldberg L, Brinkley G, Kukar J. *Pregnancy to parenthood: your personal step-by-step journey through the childbirth experience.* Garden City Park, NY: Avery Publishing Group, 1998. This book covers many of the latest developments in childbirth techniques and delivery environments, starting with the first day of pregnancy and continuing through the child's first year. Topics include relaxation exercises during pregnancy, birth positions and breathing techniques, physical changes during pregnancy, sex during pregnancy, the emotional aspects of pregnancy, nutrition, advice for the father, and breastfeeding.

Supertwins: The Boom in Multiple Births

During World War II their parents gave them patriotic names, such as Franklin, Delano, and Roosevelt, or Franklin D. (for Roosevelt) and Winnie C. (a girl named for Winston Churchill).[1] You may know them as Rachel, Richard, Rebecca, and Ryan or Courtney, Brittany, and Tiffany. They're supertwins—multiple-birth siblings such as triplets, quadruplets, quintuplets, and even sextuplets and more. From 1989 to 1993, an average of 1,057 sets of triplets, 241 sets of quads, and 32 sets of quints were born each year in the United States.[1] More recently, the McCaugheys of Iowa gave birth to septuplets on November 19, 1997. All of their septuplets are home and doing well. Nkem Chukwu and her husband Lyke Louis Udobi of Texas were not as lucky with their octuplets. One of the eight died shortly after delivery in 1998.

Such multiple births are controversial for several reasons, including the increased risk they bring to the mother and the fetuses.

The Good, the Bad, and the Unusual

A special type of bonding occurs among multiple-birth siblings that ranges from reading one another's moods to saving another's life, as in the case of twin

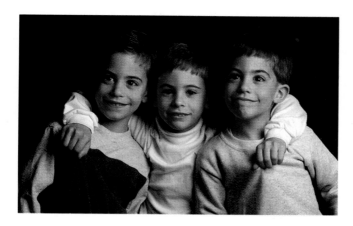

The increased use of fertility drugs and techniques has caused a boom in multiple births. More than 1,000 sets of triplets are born each year in the United States.

girls Brielle and Kyrie.[1,2] Kyrie, at 2 pounds 3 ounces, was doing well, but Brielle, the smaller twin, at 2 pounds, had had trouble breathing, an irregular heart rate, and a low blood oxygen level since birth. Then Brielle's condition suddenly became critical. The hospital staff tried every medical procedure they thought might help, to no avail. As a last resort, they put the girls in the same incubator, as some European hospitals do. Amazingly, Brielle's condition immediately improved and within minutes her blood oxygen level was the best it had been since birth. Studies have confirmed that double bedding of multiple-birth babies reduces the length of their hospital stay.[2]

On the darker side, sometimes multiple births, or the prospect of them, are exploited by parents. The Dionne quintuplets, now 60 years old, were the middle 5 of 13 children. When their father sold the rights to exhibit his daughters, the Ontario government made them wards of the state. But the government ended up exploiting them in a bizarre glass playground Quintland-type display, which attracted 10,000 visitors a month. When they were returned to their parents, they were made to feel guilty for their unusual birth and the ensuing familial discord.[3] The surviving quints have written a book about their experiences and have helped teach the world that multiples are not something to be exploited.

Recently, in England, a woman abused fertility drugs by taking them even though she was already fertile and ignoring her physician's instructions while on the drugs. She became pregnant with eight fetuses. She refused to undergo multifetal pregnancy reduction, which would have given the remaining fetuses a better chance of survival, because she had sold her story to a tabloid and would get more money for each baby born. All eight fetuses died at 19 weeks' gestation.[4]

Fertility Drugs and Techniques

Since the birth of the first "test tube baby" (conceived by in vitro fertilization) in 1978, the number of assisted pregnancies and multiple births has escalated. The use of fertility drugs and techniques that stimulate ovulation sometimes causes the release of multiple eggs per cycle.[1,5]

The infertility rate among married couples is 8.5 percent. While this rate has remained relatively constant in recent years, the number of couples seeking help for infertility has tripled.[6] Less than half of the couples who receive fertility treatment ever give birth, but one-fourth of those who *do* achieve a pregnancy give birth to more than one child.[1,6] This happens for a number of reasons. First, some fertility drugs are so strong that they cause multiple eggs to be released during one cycle. Second, some treatments are developed too quickly and are administered under too little supervision.[7] And third, fertility services are so competitive and lucrative ($67,000 to $114,000 per delivery[3]) that many clinics go to great lengths to increase the likelihood of pregnancy, such as implanting up to eight embryos in a woman's uterus. In the United Kingdom, a doctor can lose his or her license for implanting more than three embryos, but no such laws have been passed in the United States.[8] Usually, few or no embryos develop; if too many develop, however, multifetal pregnancy reduction is often suggested.[7] This abortion procedure is usually performed by injecting potassium chloride into the most accessible embryos to increase the odds of survival for the others.[9]

The whole process of fertility treatment has been described as an emotional roller coaster.[1] The parents often want children desperately but can't conceive naturally. The drugs and hormones women are given to promote pregnancy can cause great emotional distress. If a couple does achieve a pregnancy, exhilaration can turn to fear when they find out how many embryos are developing. Will they be able to care for that many children? What if some or all of the babies are sick, or die? Should some be aborted to give the others a better chance? Many fertility clinics do an unsatisfactory job of counseling couples about the likelihood of success and the risks associated with the procedures, so couples often must answer these tough questions without all the information they need.[7]

Medical Complications

After conception, the fertility specialist's job is finished. Everything that goes on during the course of pregnancy and delivery is in the hands of another physician, usually an obstetrician with a specialty in high-risk pregnancy. These physicians must discuss with the parents any risks and concerns that were not addressed earlier.[7]

Each additional fetus shaves roughly 3.5 weeks off the normal 40-week gestation period.[9] Prematurity brings with it a host of problems. The babies are about a third of the weight or less of single babies and much

more likely to be ill. The death rate before or soon after birth is 19 times higher for triplets than single babies.[1] From birth to 28 days, the death rate for multiples is still 7 times higher than for singles.[7] Surviving babies suffer higher rates of cerebral palsy and other neurological problems.[10]

Of course, multiple babies have longer hospital stays and are more likely to require intensive care during their stay than single babies. Although the issue of "drive-through" deliveries, in which mother and baby are released within 24 hours, has become a controversial topic lately, the average stay for a single baby is 4.6 days, compared with 8.2 days for twins and 34 days for triplets.[1,6] During their stays, 15 percent of single infants need intensive care, while 50 percent of twins and 75 percent of triplets, quads, and quints require this level of care.[6] Research has shown that most of the heavy use of medical resources in multiple births is due to lower gestational age and lower birth weight.[11]

Multiple births also increase the mother's need for care. The risks of cesarean delivery, anemia, hypertension, postpartum hemorrhage, and kidney failure are all greater in mothers of supertwins.[1,6] And this specialized care is extremely expensive: The estimated cost of a single birth is $9,850, compared with $37,950 for twins and $109,764 for triplets.[6] Hospital costs for quints can easily exceed half a million dollars.[1] If an insurance company covers this cost, we all pay in the form of increased premiums and deductibles. If they do not pay, it can spell financial ruin for the family. And these medical and financial complications all occur even before the newborns come home.

Public and Private Life

Parents of supertwins say the stress kicks in after about six months. Until then, they're busy just trying to meet their constant needs, which during the first three months involves feeding each of three to six babies seven to eight times per day.[1] Because of the stress of the babies' medical problems, financial strain, and pure exhaustion, child abuse is 2.5 to 9 times more likely in families with twins, compared with singles, and parents of supertwins are more likely to divorce.[1,7]

However, some people take it all in stride. One father of quintuplets regards the parenting of his five 3½ and one 7-month-old babies as character building. He's manufactured his own stairstep stroller, and he and his wife handle the 20 minutes of buckling, toy stowing, negotiating with the kids, and answering the questions of strangers whenever they go somewhere, with smiles on their faces.[1]

Some strangers beam at the sight of this unusual family, while others grimace and turn away. When people lightly tell their mother, "I'm glad it's you and not me," she answers in all seriousness, "Me too." The father sums up their situation this way: "Sure, it's a lifestyle change, but you take one day at a time, people help, and things work out."[1]

Family, friends, strangers, and even local and national companies do help out. Discounts on diapers and baby food, two years' worth of free formula, a night's stay at a local motel, discounts on vans, and money to start college funds are examples of public generosity to the families of quads and quints. But along with public generosity comes public nosiness. One family answered a knock on the door from a senior citizens' tour bus group that wanted the parents to wake up the kids for a picture. More commonly, strangers think they can touch the children or ask personal questions of the parents, such as "Are they natural?" and "So, have you had your tubes tied?" and so on.[1]

Two nonprofit support groups help families cope with the unique stressors that multiple-birth families face. The Triplet Connection, based in California, and Mothers of Supertwins (MOST), based in New York, were both founded in the 1980s by triplet moms to provide reliable, accessible information to the families of supertwins.[1] With the sincere help of most people and organizations like these, parents can increase the odds that the more will truly be the merrier.

For Discussion . . .

Do you know any sets of twins or supertwins? How are their lives and those of their parents different from other families? What would you do if you or your partner was pregnant with supertwins? Do you think society has an obligation to help support supertwin families?

References

1. Jackson DD. People say, you poor thing and I'm thinking I have four healthy kids. *Smithsonian* 1996; 27(6):30–39.
2. Sheehan N. A sister's helping hand. *Reader's Digest* 1996; 148(889):155–56.
3. Came B. A family tragedy. *Maclean's* 1994; 107:40–43.
4. Luscombe B. Eight at once is too many. *Time* 1996; 148(18):103.
5. Anonymous. Where are they now? *Time* 1996; 148(7):18.
6. Anonymous. The high cost of having some babies gets higher by the numbers. *Science News* 1994; 146(6):95.
7. Anonymous. And baby makes three or more: the ethics of fertility treatment are mainly a private matter. *The Economist* 1996; 340(7979):16.
8. Seligmann J. Fewer bundles of pain. Fertility doctors introduce reforms to reduce premature and multiple births. *Newsweek* 1996; 127(10):63.
9. Cowley G, Springen K. More is not merrier: when fertility drugs work too well. *Newsweek* 1996; 128(9):49.
10. Doyle P. The outcome of multiple pregnancy. *Hum Reprod* (11 Suppl) 1996; 4:110–17.
11. Ettner SL, Christiansen CL, Callahan TL, Hall JE. How low birth weight and gestational age contribute to increased inpatient costs for multiple births. *Inquiry* 1997–1998; 34(4):325–39.

InfoLinks
www.mostonline.org
www.nomotc.org

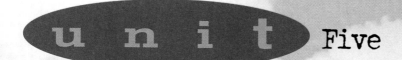

As you read through this unit, you probably saw connections between the nature of your own sexuality and the five developmental tasks: identity, independence, responsibility, social skills, and intimacy. If you are a traditional-age student, these connections were probably based on personal experiences or those you expect in the future. Nontraditional students may have reflected on their past or current experiences, as well as those of their children.

Forming an Initial Adult Identity

In your search to accomplish this particular developmental task, the same question is repeated: "Who am I?" As a young adult, or as an older person looking back on this period, you see yourself engaged in writing a script about who you are and who you will become in the near future. Certainly, this script will include information about your sexuality. We contend that to really know yourself, you must start to analyze the way you feel about aspects of your reproductive, genital, and expressionistic sexuality. Start asking yourself some important questions, such as: "What do I really want in a relationship?" "How much do I care about the feelings of my partner?" "Have I developed my personal code of ethics?" "Am I ready to become a parent?" "Am I happy with the way I express myself as a man or woman?" Answers to these kinds of questions will help you come to grips with your emerging adult identity.

Establishing Independence

For the majority of young adults, independence from the family encourages the freedom to live where you wish. This mobility provides the opportunity for experiences that allow you to achieve a fully developed adult gender identification. Living and working in new places and interacting with a variety of different individuals can help achieve this understanding of yourself. Being mobile allows you to see a wide range of masculine and feminine models. Some of these models you will appreciate more than others, yet we contend that you will learn something from them all. In much the same manner that college increases your pool of friends and presents alternative lifestyle experiences, your independence after college can further enhance this process.

Assuming Responsibility

Hand-in-hand with gaining independence goes the important task of increasing personal responsibility. In terms of a paired sexual relationship, how does one direct this responsibility? In our minds, the responsibility starts before the relationship begins. It is only beforehand that you have the opportunity to look carefully at intent regarding the sexual standards you will follow. You must ask yourself questions concerning personal standards and your ability to adhere to these standards. You must address questions concerning contraceptive effectiveness, the likelihood of STDs, and possible pregnancy. Ignoring these issues can lead to disappointment for yourself and frustration for others. Fortunately, many individuals want to share their responsibility with their partners.

Developing Social Skills

A discussion concerning paired sexual relationships and the development of social skills is very much like a description of the evolution of a friendship. In a growing friendship, new social skills are layered, level upon level. The evolving nature of the paired sexual relationship follows a similar pattern of growth and development in social skills.

A person engaged in dating relationships must develop insights, sensitivities, and responses that will be of value not only through courtship but more important, in marriage. Social skills particularly relevant to mate selection include the ability to form and assess perceptions, to recognize the reward system around which you and your partner operate, to express your values, and to act on those values with honesty and consistency.

Developing Intimacy

To many, the word *intimacy* is inseparable from *sexual*, and only direct physical contact involving coital behavior or some form of erotic contact is considered intimate. They do not consider perceptions of femininity and masculinity, how people see themselves, and how they share with others. This narrow perspective diminishes the larger role that sexuality plays in structuring our intimate relationships. As the mate selection model presented in this section explains, for a lifelong relationship to prosper, the partners must feel comfortable with their own identities. Doing so provides greater opportunities for success in the relationships that you enjoy.

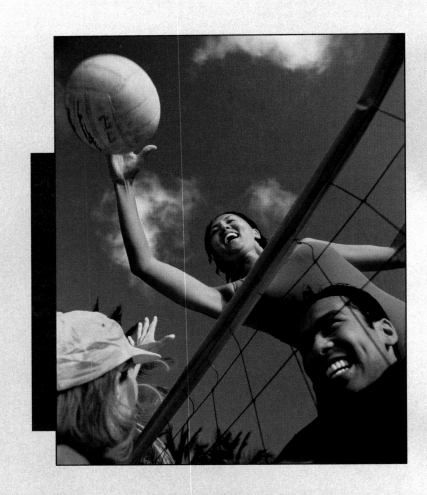

unit Six

Consumerism
and Environment

Unit Six includes chapters on consumer health, the environment, and safety. The decisions you make in each of these areas can have a profound effect on your well-being in each dimension of your health.

❶ Physical Dimension

The physical dimension of health is directly influenced by consumer decisions, such as the physician you choose. Similarly, the physical environment in which you live, work, and play has a measurable effect on your physical health. And, of course, it is crucial to learn how to protect yourself from physical harm caused by intentional or unintentional injury.

❷ Emotional Dimension

The effect of an overcrowded, highly industrialized society on your emotional health is often evident. Yet an even more powerful influence is the potential for violence or unintentional injury. Many people who are rape survivors or victims of other crimes feel fearful or angry for years afterward. Those who have behaved violently themselves may find that the knowledge of their actions erodes their emotional health.

❸ Social Dimension

Good health-care consumers are made, not born. The decisions you make about your health are shaped by many people. Your doctor, for example, may give you information about behavior change, or your insurance agent may offer you several managed care options from which to choose. Effective interaction with these professionals and many other people can help you meet your health-care needs.

❹ Intellectual Dimension

Understanding environmental issues and consumer options requires critical thinking skills. Isolating causes of environmental problems and devising workable solutions are complex tasks. In addition, you must be able to analyze a number of variables to make difficult decisions about your health.

❺ Spiritual Dimension

Nurturing our spirituality and caring for the environment are inextricably intertwined. As we search for solutions to complex environmental dilemmas, we must often make difficult decisions: Will we someday force people in developing countries to use contraception? Will we continue to protect endangered species? Will we enact bans on certain types of weapons, such as biological weapons and land mines? To build a better world for future generations may be the most serious challenge to our spiritual commitment to serve others.

❻ Occupational Dimension

Your occupational health can be enhanced by making sound decisions about your health care and personal safety. For example, choosing a health care provider who emphasizes prevention and positive behavior change will promote your overall well-being and minimize the number of days you are unable to work because of illness. In addition, avoiding intentional and unintentional injuries will allow you to perform at your peak.

❼ Environmental Dimension

Becoming a steward of the environment will enhance your health in all of its dimensions. We have devoted an entire chapter to examining environmental issues and discussing what you can do to protect the environment and ensure that it has only positive effects on your health.

Making Consumer Health-Care Decisions

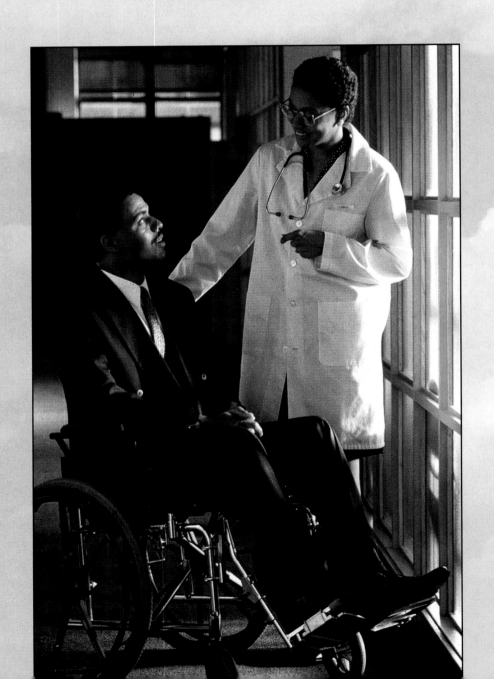

Health-care providers often evaluate you by criteria from their area of expertise. The nutritionist knows you by the food you eat. The physical fitness professional knows you by your body type and activity level. In the eyes of the expert in health consumerism, you are the product of the health information you believe, the health-influencing services you use, and the products you consume. When you make your decisions about health information, services, and products after careful study and consideration, your health will probably be improved. However, when your decisions lack insight, your health, as well as your pocketbook, may suffer.

HEALTHY PEOPLE: LOOKING AHEAD TO 2010

Access to primary medical services by virtually every member of the community is a cornerstone of health consumerism and was an important *Healthy People 2000* objective. The *Midcourse Review* reported that only limited progress had been made toward achieving this goal, and that it probably would not be met by 2000. The lack of agreement among federal legislators regarding a new national health-care system, changes in financing the present system, and the growing percentage of the population without health insurance were often cited as obstacles to achieving this objective.

As we move into the new century, *Healthy People 2010* will continue to advance health-care delivery goals. The elimination of health disparities is one of two main goals for the nation. Thus it is likely that access to primary care physicians, mental health services, maternal and child services, and a variety of community health promotion programs will take center stage.

Of all the chapters in your text, this one on health consumerism relates most closely to a major goal of *Healthy People 2010:* universal access to high-quality, affordable health-care services and safe, effective products. To accomplish this goal for all 270 million Americans, health-care providers likely will need to employ all of the development/delivery models described at the beginning of the text.

Real Life
Real choices

Migraine Headache: Is the Consumer Right?

- Name: Ellen Chang
- Age: 24
- Occupation: Graphic designer

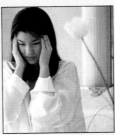

Flashing lights . . . pain like a steel vise tightening its grip on her skull . . . the agony of the slightest sound, the smallest movement. . . . Although she's experienced these symptoms for years, for Ellen Chang there's no such thing as "just another migraine." Each episode is excruciating, usually involving 2 or 3 days of lying motionless in a darkened room with the phone turned off, unable to eat, snatching moments of sleep, and praying that no one comes to the door.

Ellen's had migraine headaches about once a month since she began college, and she's pursued every mainstream medical option she could identify. She's had endless tests, including CAT scans, has consulted top neurologists, and has tried a pharmacy shelf full of prescription drugs. Sometimes she's achieved relief with a drug, but the temporary respite just isn't worth all the unpleasant side effects.

Ellen is an intelligent, talented graphic designer. She loves her work and is proud of her studio's excellent reputation among clients. Ellen enjoys a pleasant balance of work, friends, travel, and hobbies.

That is, she enjoys them when she's not totally incapacitated by a migraine headache. Tired of spending time and money in pursuit of traditional remedies that don't work, Ellen is now investigating a variety of alternative approaches to her problem. She's reading books about the Eastern-based philosophy of mind-body connection, about meditation, and about various botanical and herbal potions that have been used to treat migraine. Without telling her internist or neurologist, Ellen also has made appointments with an acupuncturist and a naturopath. If a cure for migraine exists, she's determined to find it, even if it's not sanctioned by the practitioners of Western medicine.

As you study this chapter, think about Ellen's migraine condition and her methods of dealing with it, and prepare yourself to answer the questions in **Your Turn** at the end of the chapter.

Health Information

The Informed Consumer

To be informed consumers, people must learn about services and products that can influence health. Practitioners, manufacturers, advertisers, and sales personnel use a variety of approaches to get people to buy these products or use these services. Because health is at stake when people "buy into" these messages, informed consumerism is important. Complete the Personal Assessment on page 529 to rate your own skills as a health-care consumer.

Sources of Information

Your sources of information on health topics are as diverse as the number of people you know, the number of publications you read, and the number of experts you see or hear. No single agency or profession regulates the quantity or quality of the health-related information you receive. In the next section, we look at many different sources of information. Readers will quickly recognize that all are familiar sources and that some provide more accurate and honest information than others.

Family and Friends

The accuracy of information you get from a friend or family member may be questionable. Too often the information your family and friends offer is based on "common knowledge" that is wrong. In addition, family members or friends may provide information they believe is in your best interest rather than facts that may have a more negative effect on you.

Unfortunately, some family members and friends today also might give biased health information because they are participating in a pyramid-type sales organization that sells health products. Some people might urge you to use a particular line of food supplements or vitamins or even ask you to join their sales team.

Advertisements and Commercials

Many people spend much of every day watching television, listening to the radio, and reading newspapers or magazines. Because many advertisements are health oriented, these are significant sources of information. The primary purpose of advertising, however, is to sell products or services. One newer example of this intertwining of health information with marketing is the "infomercial," in which a compensated studio audience watches a skillfully produced program that trumpets the benefits of a particular product or service.

In contrast to advertisements and commercials, the mass media routinely offer public service messages that give valuable health-related information.

Personal Assessment

Are You a Skilled Health Consumer?

Circle the selection that best describes your practice. Then total your points for an interpretation of your health consumer skills.

1   Never
2   Occasionally
3   Most of the time
4   All of the time

1. I read all warranties and then file them for safekeeping.   1   2   3   4
2. I read labels for information pertaining to the nutritional quality of food.   1   2   3   4
3. I practice comparative shopping and use unit pricing, when available.   1   2   3   4
4. I read health-related advertisements in a critical and careful manner.   1   2   3   4
5. I challenge all claims pertaining to secret cures or revolutionary new health devices.   1   2   3   4
6. I engage in appropriate medical self-care screening procedures.   1   2   3   4
7. I maintain a patient-provider relationship with a variety of health-care providers.   1   2   3   4
8. I inquire about the fees charged before using a health-care provider's services.   1   2   3   4
9. I maintain adequate health insurance coverage.   1   2   3   4
10. I consult reputable medical self-care books before seeing a physician.   1   2   3   4
11. I ask pertinent questions of health-care providers when I am uncertain about the information I have received.   1   2   3   4
12. I seek second opinions when the diagnosis of a condition or the recommended treatment seems questionable.   1   2   3   4
13. I follow directions pertaining to the use of prescription drugs, including continuing their use for the entire period prescribed.   1   2   3   4
14. I buy generic drugs when they are available.   1   2   3   4
15. I follow directions pertaining to the use of OTC drugs.   1   2   3   4
16. I maintain a well-supplied medicine cabinet.   1   2   3   4

YOUR TOTAL POINTS   _____

Interpretation

16–24 points   A very poorly skilled health consumer
25–40 points   An inadequately skilled health consumer
41–56 points   An adequately skilled health consumer
57–64 points   A highly skilled health consumer

To Carry This Further . . .

Could you ever have been the victim of consumer fraud? What will you need to do to be a skilled consumer?

Prozac 20 Mg Pulvule
Fluoxetine—Oral

USES: This medication is used to treat mental depression, obsessive-compulsive symptoms associated with Tourette's disorder, and in the treatment of bulimia nervosa.

HOW TO TAKE THIS MEDICATION: May be taken with food to prevent stomach upset.

Take this as prescribed. Try to take each dose at the same time(s) each day so you remember to routinely take it.

SIDE EFFECTS: May cause drowsiness or dizziness. Use caution performing tasks that require alertness.

Other side effects include heartburn, loss of appetite, headache, anxiety, flushing or sweating, change in sexual desire or ability. If these symptoms persist or become bothersome, inform your doctor.

Notify your doctor if you develop a rapid heart rate, difficulty breathing, difficulty urinating, a rash or hives while taking this medication.

PRECAUTIONS: Tell doctor if you had a recent heart attack or if you have a history of seizures; heart, liver, or kidney disease; or diabetes.

Fluoxetine may affect the amount of glucose (sugar) in your blood, so your dosage of diabetes medication may need to be adjusted when fluoxetine is started or discontinued.

Women who are pregnant, plan to become pregnant, or are breast-feeding should inform their doctors.

Avoid alcohol while taking this medication.

DRUG INTERACTIONS: Before taking fluoxetine, tell your doctor what prescription and nonprescription medications you are taking (or have taken in the last two weeks), especially tranquilizers, antidepressants (Buspar), MAO inhibitors (isocarboxazid or Marplan, phenelzine or Nardil, tranylcypromine or Parnate), lithium, tryptophan, medication for anxiety (tranquilizers like Valium), and medication for diabetes.

Do not take any nonprescription medication without consulting your doctor.

NOTES: Do not allow anyone else to take this medication.

MISSED DOSE: It is not necessary to make up the missed doses. Skip the missed dose and resume your usual dosing schedule. Do not "double up" the dose to catch up.

STORAGE: Store at room temperature between 59 and 86 degrees F (between 15 and 30 degrees C) away from moisture and sunlight. Do not store in the bathroom.

The information in this leaflet may be used as an education aid. This information does not cover all possible uses, actions, precautions, side effects, or interactions of this medicine. This information is not intended as medical advice for individual problems.

Copyright First Databank—The Hearst Corporation.

Figure 18-1 Prozac, a serotonin-specific antidepressant, is one of today's most frequently prescribed medications. Prozac has three labeled uses. In addition, physicians often prescribe it "off label" for other reasons, including smoking cessation. Pharmacies distribute patient information sheets like this one with each prescription they dispense.

Labels and Directions

Federal law requires that many consumer product labels, including all medications and many kinds of food (see Chapter 5), contain specific information. For example, when a pharmacist dispenses a prescription medication, he or she must give a detailed information sheet describing the drug along with the medication (Figure 18-1).

Many health-care providers and agencies give consumers detailed directions about their health problems. Generally, information from these sources is accurate and current and is given with the health of the consumer foremost in mind.

Folklore

Because it is passed down from generation to generation, folklore about health is the primary source of health-related information for some people.

The accuracy of health-related information obtained from family members, neighbors, and coworkers is difficult to evaluate. As a general rule, however, one should exercise caution relying on its scientific soundness. A blanket dismissal is not warranted,

however, because folk wisdom is occasionally supported by scientific evidence. In addition, the emotional support provided by the suppliers of this information could be the best medicine some people could receive.

Personal Applications

• How do you rate yourself as an informed consumer of health information, services, and products?

Testimonials

People strongly want to share information that has benefited them. Others may base their decisions on such testimonials. However, the exaggerated testimonials that accompany the sales pitches of the medical quack or the "satisfied" customers appearing in advertisements and on commercials and infomercials should never be interpreted as valid endorsements.

Mass Media

Health programming on cable television stations, stories in lifestyle sections of newspapers, health-care correspondents appearing on national network news shows, and the growing number of health-oriented magazines are sources of health information in the mass media.

Health-related information in the mass media is generally accurate, but it is sometimes presented so quickly or superficially that its usefulness is limited. The consumer who wants more complete coverage of a health topic might acquire it by subscribing to a cable channel devoted partly or entirely to health-related programming, such as *The Learning Channel*.

Practitioners

The health-care consumer also receives much information from individual health practitioners and their professional associations. In fact, today's health-care practitioner so clearly emphasizes patient education that finding one who does not offer some information to a patient would be difficult. Education improves patient **compliance** with health-care directives, which is important to the practitioner and the consumer.

Another important development in the trend toward patient education is the evolution of the hospital as an educational institution. Because the American Medical Association advocates patient education activities in hospitals, wellness centers, and other health facilities, it now refuses to endorse health products with its logo, which would create a conflict of interest.[1]

On-Line Computer Services

The development of computer technology in the last decade has opened new sources of health information. Today, more than 100 million Americans (out of 270 million) use on-line services.[2] By the end of 1997 nearly 40 percent of these people had accessed health-related information via the Web, particularly regarding women's health, cancer, and alternative remedies.[3] Clearly, the Internet offers expansive collections of information, including text and video, to people interested in health. However, this information is sometimes purveyed by quacks who wish to sell you a worthless product or service (see the Topics for Today article on p. 553). The health consumer must be wary of such misleading information.

Health Reference Publications

A substantial portion of all households own or subscribe to a health reference publication, such as the *Johns Hopkins Medical Handbook*,[4] the *Physicians' Desk Reference* (PDR),[5] or a newsletter such as *The Harvard Medical School Health Letter* or *The Johns Hopkins Medical Letter: Health After 50*. Some consumers also use personal computer programs and videocassettes featuring health-related information.

Reference Libraries

Public and university libraries continue to be popular sources of health-related information. One can consult with reference librarians and check out audiovisual collections and printed materials. More and more of these holdings can be accessed through the home computer.

Consumer Advocacy Groups

A variety of nonprofit consumer advocacy groups patrol the health-care marketplace (see the Star Box on p. 532). These groups produce and distribute information designed to help the consumer recognize questionable services and products. Large, well-organized groups, such as The National Consumers' League and Consumers Union, and smaller groups at the state and local levels champion the right of the consumer to receive valid and reliable information about health-care products and services.

Voluntary Health Agencies

Volunteerism and the traditional approach to health care and health promotion are virtually inseparable. Few countries besides the United States can boast so many national voluntary organizations, with state and local affiliates, dedicated to improving health through research, service, and public education. The American Cancer Society, the American Red Cross, and the American Heart Association all are voluntary (not-for-profit) health agencies. Consumers can, in fact, expect to find a voluntary health agency for virtually every health problem.

Government Agencies

Government agencies are also effective sources of information to the public. Through meetings and the release of information to the media, agencies such as the Food and Drug Administration, Federal Trade Commission, United States Postal Service, and Environmental Protection Agency publicize health issues. Government agencies also control the quality of information sent out to the buying public, particularly through labeling, advertising, and the distribution of information through the mail. The various divisions of the National Institutes of Health regularly release research findings and recommendations to clinical practices, which in turn reach the consumer through clinical practitioners.

---

compliance   willingness to follow the directions provided by another person.

Consumer Protection Agencies and Organizations

Federal Agencies

Office of Consumer Affairs, Food and Drug Administration
U.S. Department of Health and Human Services
5600 Fishers Lane
Rockville, MD 20857
(301) 443-5006

Federal Trade Commission
Consumer Inquiries
Public Reference Branch
6th Street and Pennsylvania Avenue
Washington, DC 20580
(202) 326-2222

Fraud Division
Chief Postal Inspector
U.S. Postal Service
475 L'Enfant Plaza
Washington, DC 20260
(202) 268-4299

Consumer Information Center
Department SC
Pueblo, CO 81009
(719) 948-3334

U.S. Consumer Product Safety Commission Hotline
Washington, DC
(800) 638-CPSC

Consumer Organizations

Consumers Union of the U.S., Inc.
101 Truman Avenue
Yonkers, NY 10703
(914) 378-2000

The National Consumers' League
1522 K Street, N.W.
Suite 406
Washington, DC 20005
(202) 639-8140

Professional Organizations

American Medical Association
535 N. Dearborn
Chicago, IL 60610
(312) 464-5000

American Hospital Association
840 N. Lake Shore Dr.
Chicago, IL 60611
(312) 280-6000

American Pharmaceutical Association
Health Education Center Service
2215 Constitution Avenue, NW
Washington, DC 20037
(202) 628-4410

Despite their best intentions, federal health agencies are often less effective than the public deserves. A variety of factors, including inadequate staff, poor administration, and lobbying by special interest groups, prevent these federal agencies from enforcing consumer-protection legislation. As a result, the public is left with a sense of false confidence in the consumer protection provided by the federal government.

State governments also distribute health-related information to the public. State agencies are primary sources of information, particularly in the areas of public health and environmental protection.

Qualified Health Educators

Health educators work in a variety of settings and offer their services to diverse groups. Community health educators work with virtually all of the agencies mentioned in this section; patient educators function in primary care settings; and school health educators are found at all educational levels. Health educators are increasingly being employed in a wide range of wellness-based programs in community, hospital, corporate, and school settings.

Health-Care Providers

The sources of health information just discussed can greatly help us make decisions as informed consumers. The choices we make about physicians, health services, and medical payment plans will reflect our commitment to remaining healthy and our trust in specific people who are trained in keeping us healthy. Refer to the Health Action Guides on page 533 for tips on choosing a physician and a hospital.

Why We Consult Health-Care Providers

Most of us seek care and advice from medical and health practitioners when we have a specific problem. A bad cold, a broken arm, or a newly discovered lump can motivate us to consult a health-care professional. Yet *diagnosis* and *treatment* are only two reasons that we might require the services of health-care providers.

We also might encounter health practitioners when we undergo *screening.* Screening is the examination of large numbers of people to discover particular

HEALTH ACTION GUIDE

Choosing a Physician

When choosing a physician, plan to obtain answers to the following questions during your initial visit:

- Obtain a description of the physician's medical background, such as education, residencies, and specialty areas.
- How does the physician keep up with new developments in the medical profession? Does the physician attend seminars and conferences, take courses, read medical journals, write articles, participate in professional organizations, or teach at a medical school?
- What are the normal office hours? What should be done if help is needed outside of normal office hours?
- What is included in a comprehensive physical examination?
- How does the physician feel about second and third opinions?
- With which hospitals is the physician affiliated in your area?
- With which specialists is the physician associated?
- What is the physician's fee schedule?

   Ask yourself the following questions after your visit:

- Was I comfortable with the physician's age, gender, race, and national origin?
- Was I comfortable with the physician's demeanor? Did I find communication with the physician to be understandable and reassuring? Were all my questions answered?
- Did the physician seem interested in having me as a patient?
- Are the physician's training and practice specialty in an area most closely associated with my present needs and concerns?
- Does the physician have staff privileges at a hospital I prefer?
- Does the physician's fee-for-service policy in any way exclude or limit my ability to receive necessary services?
- Did the physician take a complete medical history as a part of my initial visit? Did the physician address prevention, health promotion, or wellness during my visit?
- Did I at any time during my visit sense that the physician was unusually reluctant or eager to try new medical procedures or medications?
- When the physician is unavailable, are any colleagues on call 24 hours a day? Did I feel that telephone calls from me would be welcomed and returned in a reasonable time?

   If you have answered yes to most of these questions, you have found a physician with whom you should feel comfortable. If you have been using the services of a particular physician but are becoming dissatisfied, how could you resolve this dissatisfaction?

InfoLinks
www.coolware.com/health/medical_reporter/choosing.html

HEALTH ACTION GUIDE

Choosing a Hospital

Despite efforts in self-care and health promotion, most people will be hospitalized at some time in their lives. Serious threatening illnesses and rarer diseases are best treated in large research-oriented hospitals at major medical centers or regional teaching hospitals. Less serious illnesses or elective procedures can be accommodated in community hospitals. Regardless of the type of hospital, however, you should seek these characteristics:

- The hospital building should be neat, clean, and well maintained.
- The hospital should have recreational relaxation areas for patients, including outside areas.
- The public areas of the hospital (lobbies, snack bars, parking structures, and business areas) should be comfortable and clean.
- Visiting hours should be liberal, and children should be allowed some access.
- Accommodations should be available near the hospital for family and friends to stay overnight.
- Patients' meals should be carefully selected, attractively prepared, and efficiently served.
- Special meals should be provided when medically appropriate, and families should be assisted in postdischarge meal planning.
- Hospital rooms should be attractive, comfortable, and well situated for nursing services.
- Smoking by patients, staff, and visitors should be carefully controlled.

InfoLinks
www.healthscope.org/hs/choos_ho/index.htm

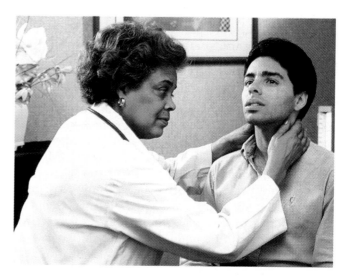

We often consult physicians for diagnosis and treatment of common ailments.

diseases or health characteristics. Your earliest experience with screening may have been in elementary school, where physicians, nurses, audiologists, and dentists sometimes examine all children for normal growth and development patterns. As an adult, you might use the services of health-care practitioners at a shopping center when you volunteer to be screened for hypertension or diabetes. Although screening should be considered much less precise than actual diagnosis, screening serves to identify people who should seek further medical examination.

Consultation is a fourth reason that knowledgeable consumers seek health-care providers. A consultation is the use of two or more professionals to deliberate a person's specific health problem or condition. Consultations are especially helpful when a physician requires the opinion of a specialist. Using an additional practitioner as a consultant can also help reassure patients who may have doubts about their own condition or about the abilities of their physician.

Prevention is a fifth reason we might seek a health-care provider. With the current emphasis on trying to stop problems before they begin, using health-care providers for prevention is becoming more common. People want information about how to prevent needless risks and promote their health, and they seek such advice from physicians, nurses, dentists, exercise physiologists, patient educators, and other health promotion specialists.

We also consult health practitioners for the general purpose of research. We might seek the service of a medical research scientist when we have a critical question in a relatively unexplored area. We also might require the help of a health-care provider in interpreting the results of conflicting research reports. We might encounter health-care practitioners if we volunteer to be a subject in an experiment in medical care, drug therapy, exercise physiology, or health education.

Physicians and Their Training

In every city and many smaller communities, the local telephone directory lists physicians in a variety of medical specialties. These health-care providers hold the academic degree of Doctor of Medicine (MD) or Doctor of Osteopathy (DO).

At one time, **allopathy** and **osteopathy** were clearly different health-care professions in terms of their healing philosophies and modes of practice. Today, however, MDs and DOs receive similar educations and engage in very similar forms of practice. Both can function as **primary-care physicians** or as board-certified specialists. Their differences are in the osteopathic physician's greater tendency to use manipulation in treating health problems. In addition, DOs perceive themselves as being more holistically oriented than MDs.

Medical and osteopathic physicians undergo a long training process. They usually take four years of initial undergraduate preparation with a heavy emphasis on the sciences—biology, chemistry, mathematics, anatomy, and physiology. Most undergraduate schools have preprofessional courses of study for students interested in medical or osteopathic schools.

After they are accepted into professional schools, students generally spend four or more years in intensive training that includes advanced study in the preclinical medical sciences and clinical practice. When they complete this phase of training, the students are awarded the MD or DO degree and then take the state medical license examination. Most newly licensed physicians complete an internship and residency at a hospital. Residency programs vary in length from three to four years. When they conclude their residency programs, physicians are granted board-eligible or board-certified status. The Star Box on page 535 describes several of the more familiar specialties. In addition to state and specialty board certification, comprehensive national certification is now in the trial phase.[6]

Alternative Practitioners

In addition to medical and osteopathic physicians, several other forms of health care offer alternatives within the large health-care market. Included within this group are chiropractic, acupuncture, homeopathy, naturopathy, herbalism, reflexology, and ayurveda.[7] Although the traditional medical community has long scoffed at these alternatives as ineffective and unscientific, many people use these forms of health care and believe strongly that they are as effective as (or more effective than) allopathic and osteopathic medicine. Following are brief descriptions of some of the more popular of these alternatives.

Chiropractic

This system is based on manual manipulation of the spine to correct misalignments. Recent studies have shown that **chiropractic** treatment of some types of low-back pain can be more effective than conventional care. With about 50,000 practitioners in the United States, chiropractic is the third-largest health profession, used by 15 to 20 million people. Some chiropractors are "straight," using only spinal manipulation, and others are "mixed," using other medical technologies, including food supplementation and massage.

Acupuncture

Acupuncture is, for Americans, the most familiar component of the 3,000-year-old Chinese medical system. This system is based on balancing the active and passive forces with the patient's body to strengthen the chi ("chee"), or life force. The system also employs herbs, food, massage, and exercise.

Medical Specialties

The American Board of Medical Specialties is a nonprofit organization that represents a variety of medical specialty boards.* Each board is composed of expert physicians already qualified in a particular field. These specialty boards evaluate physicians who wish to practice in a specific area of medicine. Some of the more common specialty areas consumers might encounter are:

Specialty	Scope of Practice
Allergy	Treatment of sensitivity disorders
Anesthesiology	Use of drugs to sedate or anesthetize
Cardiovascular surgery	Various forms of heart surgery
Dermatology	Skin diseases and disorders
Emergency medicine	Care of accident victims
Family practice	Broad-based family medical care
Geriatrics	Diseases and disorders of the elderly
Gynecology	Female reproductive health care
Internal medicine	Nonsurgical treatment of internal organ systems
Nephrology	Kidney diseases and disorders
Neurology	Diseases and disorders of the nervous system
Obstetrics	Prenatal care and child delivery
Oncology	Treatment of unusual growths and tumors
Ophthalmology	Disorders of the eye
Orthopedic surgery	Surgery for structural disorders of the bones and joints
Otolaryngology	Ear, nose, and throat problems
Pathology	Diagnosis of disease through the examination of body tissues
Pediatrics	Childhood health concerns
Psychiatry	Mental and emotional diseases or disorders
Radiology	Use of radiation to diagnose and treat diseases and injuries
Urological surgery	Surgery for urinary tract diseases and male reproductive dysfunctions

*Governed by these medical boards are 85 practice specialties.

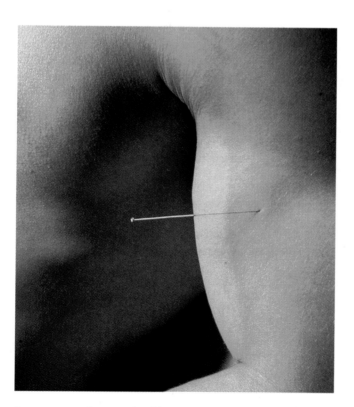

Acupuncture has received increasing acceptance within the Western medical community.

Acupuncturists place hair-thin needles at certain points in the body to stimulate the patient's chi. These points are said to correspond to different organs and bodily functions, and when stimulated, help the body's own defenses fight illness.

Of all the Chinese therapies, acupuncture is the most widely accepted in the West. Researchers have

allopathy (ah **lop** ah thee)   a system of medical practice in which specific remedies (often pharmaceutical agents) are used to produce effects different from those produced by a disease or injury.

osteopathy (os tee **op** ah thee)   a system of medical practice in which allopathic principles are combined with specific attention to postural mechanics of the body.

primary-care physician   the physician who sees a patient regularly, rather than a specialist, who sees the patient only for a specific condition or procedure.

chiropractic   manipulation of the vertebral column to relieve pressure and cure illness.

acupuncture   insertion of fine needles into the body to alter electroenergy fields and cure disease.

produced persuasive evidence of acupuncture's effectiveness as an anesthetic and as an antidote to chronic pain, migraines, dysmenorrhea, and osteoarthritis. In addition, some have suggested that acupuncture can help patients overcome addictions to alcohol, drugs, and tobacco. Other studies have shown that acupuncture is far more than a placebo and actually stimulates the body's opioid system.

Reflexology

Reflexology uses principles similar to those of acupuncture but focuses on treating certain disorders through massage of the soles of the feet.

Homeopathy

Widely accepted in Europe, **homeopathy** is the leading alternative therapy in France. Homeopathy uses infinitesimal doses of herbs, minerals, or even poisons to stimulate the body's curative powers. The theory on which homeopathy is based, the *law of similars,* contends that if large doses of a substance can cause a problem, tiny doses can trigger healing. A few small studies have shown homeopathy to be at least somewhat effective in treating hay fever, diarrhea, and flu symptoms, but members of the scientific community call the studies flawed or preliminary.[7]

Naturopathy

The core of naturopathic medicine is what Hippocrates called *medicatrix naturae,* or the healing power of nature. Proponents of **naturopathy** believe that when the mind and the body are in balance and receiving proper care, with a healthy diet, adequate rest, and minimal stress, the body's own vital forces are sufficient to fight off disease. Getting rid of an ailment is only the first step toward correcting the underlying imbalance that allowed the ailment to take hold, naturists believe. Correcting the imbalance might be as simple as rectifying a shortage of a particular nutrient, or as complex as reducing overlong work hours, strengthening a weakened immune system, and identifying an inability to digest certain foods.[7]

Naturopathy was popular in the nineteenth century and began a comeback in the 1970s in the Pacific Northwest, spurred by the back-to-nature themes of the counterculture. In some states, naturopaths are licensed, and health insurance plans must cover the treatment.

Herbalism

Herbalism may be the world's oldest and most widely used healing form. Herbalists make herbal brews for treating a variety of ills, such as depression, anxiety, and hypertension. In some cases, scientific research supports the herbalists' beliefs. For example, several studies have found St. John's wort to be more effective than a placebo in alleviating mild depression, and dozens of studies show that garlic reduces cholesterol and blood pressure. On the other hand, since some herbs can cause side effects, and no labeling requirements for safety and effectiveness exist, all herbal medications should be taken only under a professional health practitioner's guidance.

Ayurveda

Even older than Chinese medicine, India's **ayurveda** takes a preventive approach and focuses on the whole person. This system employs diet, tailored to the patient's constitutional type, or dosha; herbs; yoga and breathing exercises; meditation; massages; and purges, enemas, and aromatherapy. Practitioners of ayurveda report success in treating rheumatoid arthritis, headaches, and chronic sinusitis.

If you would like to consult a practitioner in one of the alternative disciplines but you don't know where to start, see the Health Action Guide on page 537 for some tips on choosing a provider in alternative medicine.

At the urging of many people in both the medical and alternative health-care fields, the National Institutes of Health requested federal funding to establish a scientific center for the study of alternative medical care ($50 million was granted for 1998).[8] Today the National Center for Complementary and Alternative Health assembles information about alternative approaches to medical care and provides a framework for well-controlled research into the effectiveness of each approach. Double-blind studies, so called because neither the participants nor the researchers know which treatment each participant is receiving, are being conducted. The first substantial recommendation regarding an alternative form of care was released in 1998. It concluded that acupuncture was safe and effective for controlling nausea and vomiting after surgery and chemotherapy, the nausea of pregnancy, and postoperative dental pain.[9]

Personal Applications

• Are there any types of providers mentioned in this chapter that you would not choose to consult? Explain your answer.

Restricted-Practice Health-Care Providers

We receive much of our health care from medical physicians. However, most of us also use the services of various health-care specialists who also have advanced graduate level training. Among these professionals are dentists, psychologists, podiatrists, and optometrists.

HEALTH ACTION GUIDE

Choosing the Best Alternative Practitioner for You

Perhaps you are one of the millions of people who feel that their doctors don't encourage them to ask questions, don't seek their opinion about their medical condition, or don't take a thorough medical history. Perhaps you want advice on improving your health rather than just a quick diagnosis and prescription.

For whatever reasons, millions of Americans are turning to alternative medical practitioners, such as doctors of naturopathy, Chinese medicine, or ayurveda. Unfortunately, the patient looking for these alternatives faces other problems: practitioners' training may be weak, they might not be licensed or covered by insurance, they are hard to find, and they usually are not permitted to prescribe drugs unless they also happen to be medical doctors.

This means that you must do some legwork to find a good provider who can meet your needs. According to one expert, writing in *Natural Health* magazine, you are most likely to find a good practitioner in these basic categories of health care: Ayurveda, Chinese medicine (including acupuncturists), chiropractic, holistic medicine, homeopathy, naturopathy, and osteopathy.

Within these broad categories, consider the following tips for finding the practitioner who is right for you:

- *Don't forget the family doctor.* Family-practice medicine is enjoying a surge in the United States, and many of these doctors tend to think holistically, although they might not advertise the fact. Andrew Weil, MD, a pioneer in alternative medicine, calls family-practice doctors the most open-minded and liberal of the medical specialists.
- *Find a doctor who believes in alternative therapies.* Your doctor's attitude toward the treatment can be just as important as your own. If your own physician agrees to give you herbal treatment only reluctantly, this can reduce your chance of success. Avoid those who are indifferent or overly skeptical about the treatment.

- *Give the treatment time.* Alternative therapies encourage the body to do its own healing. This often takes time. Seek a doctor who is confident in your self-healing ability, so you won't become discouraged if it takes some time.
- *Request natural healing.* Natural healing tends to change the internal conditions so that pathogens are less likely to gain a foothold; conventional medicine seeks to destroy the pathogen. Natural healing searches for the causes of symptoms, while conventional medicine treats symptoms. Natural healing usually uses nontoxic natural medicines, while conventional medicine uses powerful drugs. When you understand the differences, you can ask your doctor how he or she feels about natural approaches to healing.
- *Know your disease.* Find books that describe your conditions and offer alternative as well as conventional treatments. This way you can discuss your treatment with your doctor and create an effective treatment plan.
- *Treat yourself.* Don't overuse your health-care provider, whether conventional or alternative. For many conditions, you can be your own best doctor; of course, persistent or severe symptoms should send you to the doctor.
- *Learn whether the treatment is covered by insurance.* Coverage of alternative treatment differs sharply by state. Some insurance groups are beginning to pay for more alternative medicine, and HMOs are hiring some alternative specialists.
- *Talk to professional associations.* Most of the more established alternative fields have associations that can give you a list of providers. Use it as a start.
- *Get a brochure.* The doctor's literature can tell you a lot about his or her outlook and experience.
- *Interview the doctor.* Before making an appointment, talk with the doctor over the telephone. Then, in the doctor's office, take notes, even use a tape recorder, to make certain you understand. Watch for a doctor who is a good listener, a good communicator, and open-minded.

InfoLinks
http://altmed.od.nih.gov/

Dentists (Doctor of Dental Surgery, DDS) deal with a wide range of diseases and impairments of the teeth and oral cavity. Dentists undergo undergraduate predental programs that emphasize the sciences, followed by four additional years of study in dental school and, with increasing frequency, an internship program. State licensure examinations are required. As with physicians, dentists can also specialize by completing a postdoctoral master's degree in fields such as oral surgery, **orthodontics,** and **prosthodontics.** Dentists are also permitted to prescribe therapy programs (such as the treatment of temporomandibular joint [TMJ] dysfunction) and drugs that pertain to their practices (primarily analgesics and antibiotics).

Psychologists provide services to help patients understand behavior patterns or perceptions. More than forty states have certification or licensing laws that prohibit unqualified people from using the term

reflexology   massage applied to specific areas of the feet to treat illness and disease in other areas of the body.

homeopathy (hoe mee **op** ah thee)   the use of minute doses of herbs, minerals, or other substances to stimulate healing.

naturopathy (na chur **op** ah thee)   a system of treatment that avoids drugs and surgery and emphasizes the use of natural agents to correct underlying imbalances.

herbalism   an ancient form of healing in which herbal preparations are used to treat illness and disease.

ayurveda (ai yur **vey** da)   traditional Indian medicine based on herbal remedies.

orthodontics   a dental specialty that focuses on the proper alignment of the teeth.

prosthodontics   a dental specialty that focuses on the construction and fitting of artificial appliances to replace missing teeth.

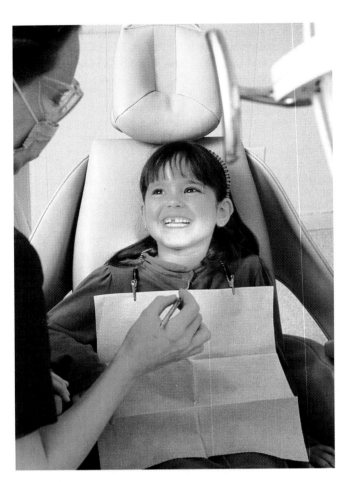

Dentists are one type of restricted-practice health-care provider.

psychologist. The consumer should examine a psychologist's credentials. Legitimate psychologists have received advanced graduate training (often leading to a PhD or EdD degree) in clinical, counseling, industrial, or educational psychology. Furthermore, these practitioners will have passed state certification examinations and, in many states, will have met further requirements that allow them to offer health services to the public. Psychologists may have special interests and credentials from professional societies in individual, group, family, or marriage counseling. Some are certified as sex therapists.

Unlike psychiatrists, who are medical physicians, psychologists cannot prescribe or dispense drugs. They may refer to or consult with medical physicians about clients who might benefit from drug therapy.

Podiatrists are highly trained clinicians who practice podiatric medicine, or care of the feet (and ankles). Although not MDs or DOs, doctors of podiatric medicine (DPM) treat a wide variety of conditions related to the feet, including corns, bunions, warts, bone spurs, hammertoes, fractures, diabetes-related conditions, athletic injuries, and structural abnormalities. Podiatrists perform surgery, prescribe

medications, and apply orthotics (supports or braces), splints, and corrective shoes for structural abnormalities of the feet.

Doctors of podiatric medicine follow an educational path similar to that taken by MDs and DOs, consisting of a four-year undergraduate preprofessional curriculum, four additional years of study in a podiatric medical school, and an optional residency of one or two years. Board-certified areas of specialization include surgery, orthopedics, and podiatric sports medicine. Hospital affiliation generally requires board certification in a specialized area.

Optometrists are eye specialists who primarily treat vision problems associated with **refractory errors.** They examine the eyes and prescribe glasses or contact lenses to correct visual disorders. Optometrists sometimes attempt to correct certain ocular muscle imbalances with specific exercise regimens. Optometrists must complete undergraduate training and additional years of coursework at one of sixteen accredited colleges of optometry in the United States or two Canadian colleges before taking a state licensing examination.

Opticians are technicians who manufacture and fit eyeglasses or contact lenses. Although they are rarely licensed by a state agency, they perform the important function of grinding lenses to the precise prescription designated by an optometrist or ophthalmologist (physicians who have specialized in vision care). To save money and time, many consumers take an optometrist's or ophthalmologist's prescription for glasses or contact lenses to optician-staffed retail stores that deal exclusively with eyewear products.

Nurse Professionals

Nurses constitute a large group of health professionals who practice in a variety of settings. Their responsibilities usually depend on their academic preparation. Registered nurses (RNs) are academically prepared at two levels: (1) the technical nurse, and (2) the professional nurse. The technical nurse is educated in a two-year associate degree program. The professional nurse receives four years of education and earns a bachelor's degree. Both technical and professional nurses must successfully complete state licensing examinations before they can practice as RNs.

Many professional nurses continue their education and earn master's and doctoral degrees in nursing or other health-related fields. Some professional nurses specialize in a clinical area (such as pediatrics, gerontology, public health, or school health) and become certified as *nurse practitioners.* Working under the supervision of physicians, nurse practitioners perform many of the diagnostic and treatment procedures performed by physicians. The ability of these highly trained nurses to function at this level gives communities additional primary-care providers and frees physicians to deal with more complex cases. With the expansion of managed care, the role of nurse practitioners is growing. This increases access to medical care and allows physicians to use their time more cost effectively.

Licensed practical nurses (LPNs) are trained in hospital-based programs that last twelve to eighteen months. Because of their brief training, LPNs' scope of practice is limited. Most LPN training programs are gradually being phased out.

Allied Health-Care Professionals

Our primary health-care providers are supported by a large group of allied health-care professionals, who are often responsible for highly technical services and procedures. These professionals include respiratory and inhalation therapists, radiological technologists, nuclear medicine technologists, pathology technicians, general medical technologists, operating room technicians, emergency medical technicians, registered nurse midwives, physical therapists, occupational therapists, cardiac rehabilitation therapists, dental technicians, physician assistants, and dental hygienists. Depending on the particular field, the training for these specialty support areas can take from one to five years of post–high school study. Programs include hospital-based training leading to a diploma through associate, bachelor's, and master's degrees. Most allied health-care professionals must also pass state or national licensing examinations.

Self-Care/Home Care

The emergence of the **self-care movement** suggests that many people are becoming more responsible for maintaining their health. They are developing the expertise to prevent or manage many types of illness, injuries, and conditions. They are learning to assess their health status and treat, monitor, and rehabilitate themselves in a manner that was once thought possible only through a physician or some other health-care specialist.

The benefits of this movement are that self-care can (1) reduce health-care costs, (2) provide effective care for particular conditions, (3) free physicians and other health-care specialists to spend time with other patients, and (4) increase interest in health-related activities.

Self-care is an appropriate alternative to professional care in three areas. First, self-care may be appropriate for certain acute conditions that have familiar symptoms and are limited in their duration and seriousness. Common colds and flu, many home injuries, sore throats, and nonallergic insect bites are often easily managed with self-care.

A second area in which self-care might be appropriate is therapy. For example, many people are now administering injections for allergies and migraine shots and continuing physical therapy programs in their homes. Asthma, diabetes, and hypertension are also conditions that can be managed or monitored with self-care.

A third area in which self-care has appropriate application is health promotion. Weight loss programs, physical conditioning activities, and stress-reduction programs are particularly well suited to self-care.

As the U.S. population ages, it is becoming increasingly common for family members to provide home care to elderly relatives. As the number of frail elderly people increases, home care can significantly reduce the need for institutional care. Home care also can be delivered by home health-care specialists. In fact, this form of care is proving so cost effective that some insurance programs, including **Medicare** and **Medicaid,** cover portions of the cost of home health care for seniors.

As professionally provided home health care for the elderly has boomed, a new industry has sprung up to provide home health-care services. This industry is so new, however, that regulation has lagged behind. Among the areas of concern are theft and patient abuse, unqualified caregivers, and billing fraud. The Health Care Financing Administration, which oversees Medicare and Medicaid, recently proposed new rules for home care providers. Although support for the reforms is strong, experts caution that in-home care is much more difficult to police, because the care is literally delivered behind closed doors.

A decision to provide home care, particularly for the elderly, is often made for admirable and understandable reasons, including love for the relative who needs care and the high cost of professional home care and institutional care. For the 22.4 million families who have made this decision,[10] providing home health care can be highly rewarding. It also can be very demanding, however, because of the needs and limitations of the person who requires care and the compromises the caregivers must make. Too often caregivers jeopardize their own health long before the recovery or death of the person for whom they are caring.

---

refractory errors incorrect patterns of light wave transmission through the structures of the eye.

self-care movement the trend toward individuals' taking increased responsibility for prevention or management of certain health conditions.

Medicare contributory governmental health insurance, primarily for people age 65 or older.

Medicaid noncontributory governmental health insurance for people receiving other types of public assistance.

People interested in practicing these forms of care must be skilled consumers. The self-care/home care marketplace is growing very rapidly and is expected to be a multibillion-dollar industry by the end of the decade. People who engage in self-care must bear the sometimes considerable expense of equipment, supplies, classes, and program membership. Providing home health care for others can involve not only financial but also physical and psychological costs. Among these unique "expenses" are factors such as physical fatigue, emotional strain, postponement of personal and family goals, loss of social contact, and even physical abuse of caregivers by those receiving care.

Personal Applications

• To what extent and in what ways have you engaged in self-care?

Health-Care Facilities

Most of us have a general idea of what a hospital is. However, all hospitals are not alike. They usually fall into one of three categories—private, public, or voluntary. *Private hospitals* (or proprietary hospitals) function as profit-making hospitals. They are not supported by tax monies and usually accept only clients who can pay all their expenses. Although there are some exceptions, these hospitals are generally smaller than tax-supported voluntary hospitals. Commonly owned by a group of business investors, a large hospital corporation, or a group of physicians, these hospitals sometimes limit their services to a few specific types of illnesses.

Public hospitals are supported primarily by tax dollars. They can be operated by government agencies at the state level (such as state mental hospitals) or at the federal level (such as the Veterans Administration Hospitals and various military service hospitals such as Walter Reed Army Hospital). Large county or city hospitals are frequently public hospitals. These hospitals routinely serve indigent segments of the population. They also function as *teaching hospitals.*

The most commonly recognized type of hospital is the *voluntary hospital.* Voluntary hospitals are maintained as nonprofit public institutions. Often supported by religious orders, fraternal groups, or charitable organizations, these hospitals usually offer a wider range of comprehensive services than do private hospitals or clinics. Voluntary hospitals are supported by patient fees (covered by health insurance), Medicare reimbursement, and Medicaid and public assistance reimbursement.

In the last decade, voluntary hospitals have expanded their scope of services. Today hospitals often operate *wellness centers*, stress centers, cardiac rehabilitation centers, chemical dependence programs, health education centers, and satellite centers for well-baby care and care for the homeless. It should be noted that an increasing number of voluntary hospitals are being sold and then re-opened as "for profit" institutions, reflecting the movement to managed health care.

Other health-care facilities include clinics (both private and tax-supported), nursing homes (most of which are private enterprises), and rehabilitation centers. Rehabilitation centers are often supported by charitable organizations devoted to the care of chronically ill or handicapped people, orthopedically injured people, or burn victims.

In recent years, many private, twenty-four-hour drop-in medical emergency and surgical centers have appeared. These clinics have their own professional staffs of physicians, nurses, and allied health professionals. They compete directly with larger hospital-based facilities. Some clinics specialize in women's health needs, including gynecological care, prenatal care, and childbirth services.

Patients' Institutional Rights

Regardless of the type of institution in which you are a patient, you have a variety of rights. These are intended to protect you from unnecessary harm and financial loss. The hospital too can expect your cooperation as a patient.

As a patient, you can expect the following from the institution:

- To be treated with respect and dignity
- To be afforded privacy and confidentiality consistent with federal and state laws, institutional policies, and the requirements of your insurance carrier
- To be provided services on request, as long as they are reasonable and consistent with appropriate care
- To be fully informed of the identity of the physicians and staff providing care
- To be kept fully updated about your condition, including its management and your prognosis for recovery
- For your concerns about the type and extent of care to be taken seriously

The institution can expect you, as a patient:

- To keep all appointments
- To provide all background information pertinent to your condition
- To treat hospital personnel with respect
- To ask questions and seek clarification about matters that affect you

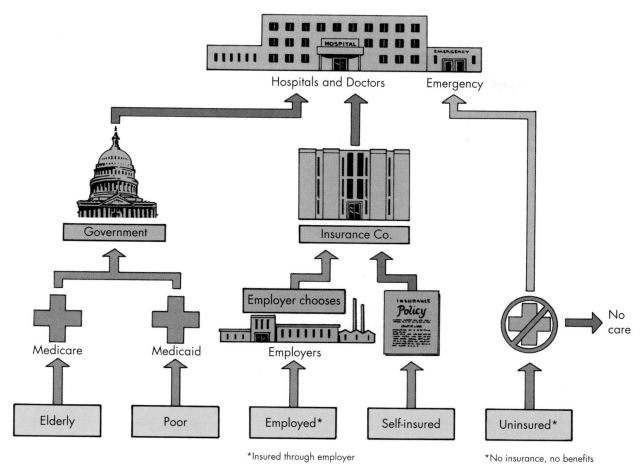

Figure 18-2   In the current U.S. health-care system, many layers of bureaucracy lie between people and their doctors.

- To follow the treatment prescribed by your physician
- To give information needed to ensure the fullest insurance coverage

As a patient, you may at any time:

- Refuse treatment
- Seek a second opinion
- Discharge yourself from the institution

Health-Care Costs and Reimbursement

As depicted in Figure 18-2, there are many avenues for receiving health care. However, being able to pay for quality health care is one of the greatest concerns of the American public. Using the latest available statistics (1996), 41.7 million Americans, or 15.6 percent of the population, lack health insurance, including 23 million dependent children.[11] Furthermore, Americans are less optimistic today about their ability to maintain adequate health insurance coverage, find

reasonably priced health care, and afford long-term homebound or nursing home care than ever before.[12] Unfortunately, the word *crisis* is appropriate to use when talking about our ability to afford high-quality health care today.

Cost is a basic concern about health care. It is estimated that in 1998 Americans spent $1.15 trillion on health care, and by 2007 this expenditure will increase to $2.13 trillion. Stated another way, in 1996 Americans incurred an average of $3,759 per person in health care–related costs. This amount is expected to increase to $5,000 per person by the year 2000. No developed country spends a greater percentage (13.5% in 1997) of its gross domestic product on health care than does America. Table 18-1 breaks down annual health-care expenditures in the United States.[13]

As a result of factors such as the high cost of modern medical technology, an emphasis on long life at any cost, the growing number of older people with chronic conditions that require expensive long-term care, and the AIDS epidemic, controlling the cost of medical care is one of the most complex problems facing the nation. Nevertheless, more than forty different

Table 18-1   Estimated Annual U.S. Health-Care Expenditures

Commodity	Amount (in billions)	
	2000	**2007**
Hospitals	$418	$649
Physicians	$253	$427
Nursing homes	$ 96	$148
Drugs/supplies	$125	$224
Dental care	$ 61	$ 95
Other	$ 16	$ 23

plans have been advanced since 1990 to respond to this problem. These range from only modest changes in the current system, to tax-credit strategies and mandatory employment-based insurance, to a federally controlled national health plan. Today government officials seem to be particularly interested in the role of Medicare in financing health care for older Americans. However, no single plan has yet caught the favor of the American public or the policymakers in Washington.

HMOs: Who Should Determine Coverage: Physicians or Administrators?

In the 1980s, when health maintenance organizations (HMOs) first appeared, they appealed strongly to businesses and their employees. They did so by providing broad-based health-care coverage that was more affordable than traditional health insurance because of the HMOs' focus on preventive medicine. As part of this effort, HMO administrators retained companies that monitored medical service costs and then formulated pricing guidelines for the reimbursement of providers.

Today HMOs are generally much larger, more centralized, and clearly focused on making a profit for their corporate investors. Many physicians employed by HMOs, and HMO members themselves, believe these organizations are now less concerned with making health care affordable and more interested in restricting services to enhance profits. Among these cost-cutting measures are classifying mastectomies as outpatient procedures; restricting the reasons for which women can receive hysterectomies; restricting the extent to which epidural pain medication can be administered during labor and delivery; and discharging new mothers and their babies within a day of birth (now, by law, no longer permitted). Physicians who work for HMOs strongly contend that these decisions restrict their ability to practice medicine in a manner that is safe and effective for their patients.

In your opinion, which should be the priority of HMOs: providing safe and effective medical care, or assuring stockholders of an adequate profit on their investment?

Health Insurance

Health insurance is a financial agreement between an insurance company and an individual or group for the payment of health costs. After paying a premium to an insurance company, the policyholder is covered for specific benefits. Each policy is different in its coverage of illnesses and injuries. Merely having an insurance policy does not mean that all health-care expenses will be covered. Most health insurance policies require various forms of payments by the policyholder, which includes deductible amounts, fixed indemnity benefits, coinsurance, and exclusions. In 1998 Americans spent $74.1 billion on private health insurance, and they are expected to spend $151.3 billion by 2007.[13]

A *deductible* amount is an established amount that the insuree must pay before the insurer reimburses for services. For example, a person or family may have to pay the first $200 of the year's medical expenses before insurance begins providing any coverage.

A policy with *fixed indemnity* benefits will pay only a specified amount for a particular procedure or service. If the policy pays only $1,000 for an appendectomy and the actual cost of the appendectomy was $1,500, then the policy owner will owe the health-care provider $500. A policy with full-service benefits, which pays the entire cost of a particular procedure or service, may be worth the extra cost.

Policies that have *coinsurance* features require that the policy owner and the insurance company share the costs of certain covered services, usually on a percentage basis. One standard coinsurance plan requires that the policyholder pay 20 percent of the costs above a deductible amount, and the company pays the remaining 80 percent.

An *exclusion* is a service or expense that is not covered by the policy. Elective or cosmetic surgery procedures, unusual treatment protocols, prescription drugs, and certain kinds of consultations are common exclusions. Illness and injuries that already exist at the time of purchase (preexisting conditions) are often excluded. In addition, injuries incurred during high-risk activities (ice hockey, hang gliding, mountain climbing, intramural sports) might not be covered by a policy.

Health insurance can be obtained through individual policies or group plans. Group health insurance plans usually offer the widest range of coverage at the lowest price and are often purchased cooperatively by companies and their employees. In 1994 American households spent $310.1 billion on private and group health insurance policies.[11] Fortunately, no employee is refused entry into a group insurance program. However, when employees leave the company, their previous group coverage will follow them for a prescribed period of time, usually 18 to 24 months. Today, as many large American companies lay off employees, the eventual loss of health insurance becomes a serious personal and family crisis.

Individual policies can be purchased by one person (or a family) from an insurance company. These policies are often much more expensive than group plans and may provide much less coverage. Still, people who do not have access to a group plan should attempt to secure individual policies, because the financial burdens resulting from a severe accident or illness that is not covered by some form of health insurance can be devastating. Many colleges and universities offer annually renewable health insurance policies that students can purchase. The Health Action Guide below gives the consumer some questions to consider before purchasing a health insurance policy.

HEALTH ACTION GUIDE

Selecting a Health Insurance Policy

Before you purchase a health insurance policy, ask yourself the following questions. The more questions you can answer with a yes, the more likely that the policy is right for you.

General Questions
- Do I really need an individual insurance policy?
- Am I already covered by a group insurance policy?
- Is the insurance company I am considering rated favorably by Best's Insurance Reports or my state insurance department?
- Have I compared health insurance policies from at least two other companies?
- Does this company have a "return rate" of 50 percent or more?
- Can I afford this insurance policy?
- Do I understand the factors that might raise the cost of this policy?

Specific Questions
- Do I clearly understand which health conditions are covered and which are not?
- Do I clearly understand whether I have fixed indemnity benefits or full-service benefits?
- Do I clearly understand the deductible amounts of this policy?
- Do I clearly understand when the major medical portion of this policy starts?
- Do I clearly understand all information in this policy that refers to exclusions and preexisting conditions?
- Do I clearly understand any disability provisions of this policy?
- Do I clearly understand all information concerning both cancellation and renewal of this policy?

InfoLinks
www.hiaa.org

Personal Applications
- Many insurance companies exclude certain kinds of illness (such as AIDS) from coverage and will not pay for the needed drugs. Who then should cover the cost? Under what circumstances do you think that expensive medications should be prescribed for terminally ill patients?

Health Maintenance Organizations

Health maintenance organizations (HMOs) are health-care delivery plans under which health-care providers agree to meet the covered medical needs of subscribers for a prepaid amount of money. For a fixed monthly fee, enrollees are given comprehensive health care with an emphasis on preventive health care. Enrollees receive their care from physicians, specialists, allied health professionals, and educators who are hired (group model) or contractually retained (network model) by the HMO.[12]

Managed care, and HMOs in particular, was a reaction to the sharply climbing costs of health care in the 1980s. Businesses, which paid a large portion of health-care costs through employee-benefit plans, complained that no one in the health-care loop had an incentive to control costs. Employers complained that consumers paid only a deductible and a small copayment, giving them little cause to question prices; doctors faced little financial oversight; and insurance companies merely rubber-stamped the bills.

When HMOs presented an alternative, employers began offering their workers incentives to select HMOs over traditional fee-for-service coverage, and thus attempted to rein in the runaway costs of health care. HMOs now cover nearly 70 million Americans.[14] In 1996 HMOs had an average cost per worker of $3,485, versus $3,850 for workers in a more traditional group health plan.

HMOs are usually the least expensive but most restrictive type of managed care. The premiums are 8 percent to 10 percent lower than traditional plans, they charge no deductibles or coinsurance payments, and copayments are $5 to $10 per visit. However, you are limited to using the doctors and hospitals in the HMO's network, and you must get approval for treatments and referrals.

In theory, HMOs were to be the ideal blend of medical care and health promotion. Today, however, many observers are concerned that too many HMOs are being too tightly controlled by a profit motive in which physicians are being paid to *not* refer patients to specialists or are prevented by "gag rules" from discussing certain treatment options with patients because of their costs to the HMOs.[15]

When operated in the manner consistent with how most members believe they should be operated, one of the advantages offered by HMOs is cost containment. Because most of the medical services with an HMO are centralized, there is little duplication of facilities, equipment, or support staff. Central filing of records gives all the HMO physicians access to a single client's file. This saves time, administrative costs, and the overlapping of care. HMOs also routinely use health-promotion activities.[12]

Other new approaches to reducing health costs are independent practice associations (IPAs) and preferred provider organizations (PPOs). An IPA is a modified form of an HMO that uses a group of doctors who offer prepaid services out of their own offices and not in a central HMO facility. IPAs are viewed as "HMOs without walls." A PPO is a group of private practitioners who sell their services at reduced rates to insurance companies. When a policyholder chooses a physician who is in that company's PPO network, the insurance company pays the entire physician's fee. When a policyholder selects a non-PPO physician, the insurance company pays only a portion of that physician's fee. Today, more than 63 percent of all employees are in some form of managed care program (HMO, IPA, or PPO).[16]

Government Insurance Plans

Created in 1965 by amendments to the Social Security Act, *Medicare* and *Medicaid* are types of governmental health insurance. Medicare provides health-care reimbursements primarily for people aged sixty-five years or older. Medicare is a contributory program—that is, through their working years, all employed citizens contribute a portion of their salaries (through Social Security taxes) to the Medicare fund. That amount currently is 1.45 percent of the Social Security taxes (FICA) paid on annual earnings.[17] When they reach age sixty-five, some of their health-care expenses are covered by Medicare. Regardless of their age, people who require kidney dialysis or transplants are covered by Medicare.

Medicare is actually composed of two parts. Medicare A is essentially a hospital insurance program. Part A pays for necessary hospital care (semiprivate room) after payment of the required deductible, for medically necessary inpatient care in a nursing home (skilled level care), and hospice care. In addition, it pays 80 percent of the cost of approved durable medical equipment, such as walkers, and for all units of blood used by an inpatient, after the first three units.[18] Medicare B is a voluntary program (for which the subscriber must pay a monthly fee, currently $45.50/month) that supplements Medicare A.[17] Medicare B provides regular medical insurance that covers a broad range of physicians' fees and other

health-care services. Physicians who "accept assignment" from Medicare agree to charge their elderly patients only the amount that Medicare will cover. Those who do not accept assignment may charge an amount up to 115 percent of the Medicare amount.[18] However, by doing so, they will be asking their elderly patients not only to pay the 20 percent copayment but an additional 15 percent as well. Consequently, many elderly will go only to physicians who accept assignment. Both Medicare plans are subject to yearly changes in coverages and administrative procedures.

One of the most recent attempts by Medicare at cost containment in the area of health care is the prospective pricing system established in 1984 by the federal government. Under this system, Medicare reimbursements to hospitals are based on 467 diagnosis-related groups (DRGs) rather than on the costs accrued by the hospitals. Each hospital stay is now assigned a DRG classification, and reimbursement to the hospital is based on that classification. This system encourages hospitals to deliver services at or below the DRG payment schedule.

President Clinton has proposed a multifaceted plan, using the nation's first budget surplus in decades, to "repair" Medicare for today's elderly and the baby boomers whose retirement is approaching.[19] Older Americans hope the "new Medicare" will give them a broader range of choices in health-care providers, reduce the amount of fraud and waste in current operations, and stimulate greater cooperation among physicians, hospitals, drug manufacturers, and recipients in cost containment. Whatever its form, the new Medicare likely will require recipients to pay a greater share of their health-care costs.

Medicaid is a noncontributory program for citizens who are receiving other types of public welfare assistance. It is designed to provide both Medicare deductibles and a variety of types of health-related coverage, including hospital, nursing home, physician, and home care. Unlike Medicare, Medicaid has no age requirements and is administered cooperatively through federal and state agencies. Medicaid is particularly important to older adults, because it covers nursing home care after eligibility has been established. In 1995, 20 percent of the entire Medicaid budget of $155 billion ($31 billion) was spent for nursing home care, principally for the elderly.[20]

Because of the bureaucracy currently surrounding these two government insurance programs, many private physicians and voluntary hospitals decline to accept Medicaid and Medicare patients. Thus observers wonder how the United States can provide proper health care to all of its citizens, including the aged, economically disadvantaged, and those whose life savings can be quickly depleted by a catastrophic illness.

Learning From Our Diversity

Immigrants in the Workplace: Reducing Hazards on the Job

For more than 200 years, America has been known as the "Land of Opportunity," where anyone who works hard can enjoy both material success and the freedom of living in a democracy. Indeed, millions of immigrants from all around the globe have poured into the United States, eager to work, learn, and build a better life for themselves and their families.

For many immigrants and refugees who come to America, however, the hard work they hope will be the path to the good life often puts them at risk for workplace-related illness and injury.

Immigrants who have little education and lack work and language skills often are forced to take jobs that are low paying, hazardous, or both. They sew for long hours in garment sweatshops, work with hazardous materials like asbestos or toxic chemicals without adequate protection, or labor in settings where they are targets of violent crime.

Although health and safety regulations offer protection, many immigrant and refugee workers are unaware of their existence or are too fearful of reprisals from employees or of deportation to alert the authorities to violations of the laws. And when these workers do become sick or injured, their problems are often compounded by lack of access to needed health care.

A prime location for sweatshops is New York City, where countless immigrants toil for long hours in conditions ranging from unsafe to hazardous. The New York State Department of Labor is trying to improve working conditions for garment workers by urging the manufacturers and their associations to police their own industry. The manufacturers themselves can benefit, because they're less assured of receiving the merchandise they've ordered when dealing with contractors who violate the health and safety laws.

In recent years, federal and state authorities have prosecuted a number of asbestos removal firms that used undocumented immigrants to work without training or the equipment needed to protect themselves and others from exposure. The dry cleaning industry, which draws a disproportionate number of immigrants, involves prolonged exposure to toxic solvents, including perchloroethylene (PCE), a potential human carcinogen. To help reduce this risk, the National Institute for Occupational Safety and Health has launched a pilot project to learn how best to get the message out to dry cleaners on how to reduce solvent exposure and other work-related health problems like burns and falls.

Clearly, all workplaces should be safe and healthy environments for their workers. Just as clearly, immigrants with low levels of skill and education must be protected from a host of workplace hazards that can cause illness, injury, and even death.

Which strategy do you think would be more likely to motivate a business with hazardous working conditions to improve those conditions: rewards for compliance, or penalties for noncompliance? Why?

Medicare Supplement Policies (Medigap)

Because Medicare A and Medicare B require deductibles and copayment by patients before Medicare begins payment, private companies offer insurance to cover these gaps in coverage. In the most basic "medigap" policies (policy version A), often sold via mass mailings, the patient is reimbursed for the deductible and copayment portions of the approved charges, as determined by the DRG (Medicare A) and approved physician fee (Medicare B). More expensive and more comprehensive supplement policies (policy versions B through J) pay for hospital care and equipment not covered by Medicare A and for physician fees that exceed the approved amount of coverage for Medicare B. The basic medigap policies and the more comprehensive policies that literally pay for everything not covered by Medicare differ greatly in cost.

Extended Care Insurance

With the aging of the population and the greater likelihood that nursing home care will be required (at about $35,000 per year), insurers have developed extended care policies. When purchased at an early age (by mid-50s), these policies are much more affordable than if purchased when a spouse or family member will soon require institutional care. However, not all older adults will need extensive nursing home care, so an extended care policy could be an unnecessary expenditure.

Access to Health Care

Getting and paying for medical care continues to be a problem for a substantial segment of the U.S. population. One recent study found that 31 percent of those surveyed had had at least one of three major problems in the last year: They lacked insurance, they could not get needed medical care, or they had difficulty paying medical bills.[21]

The problem does not hit just minorities and those with low income. About 41 million Americans, most of them middle class, have problems getting health care ranging from surgery to eyeglasses. This results from employers that do not offer insurance or that have reduced what is covered.[22]

The poor and minorities feel the problem even more. African-Americans, Hispanic Americans, and Native Americans have the worst health status of all Americans, yet they receive the fewest health-care services. For example, African-American men have a 45 percent higher incidence of lung cancer, and African-American women are three times more likely to die from cervical cancer than white women.[23] Proposals for health-care reform need to offer solutions to the cultural, geographic, and socioeconomic barriers that minorities face in receiving health care.

Health-Related Products

As you might imagine, prescription and over-the-counter (OTC) drugs constitute an important part of any discussion of health-related products.

Prescription Drugs

Caution: Federal law prohibits dispensing without prescription. This FDA warning appears on the labels of approximately three-fourths of all medications. Prescription drugs must be ordered for patients by a licensed practitioner. Because these compounds are legally controlled and may require special skills in their administration, our access to these drugs is limited. The Star Box at right lists classes of prescription drugs.

Although the *Physician's Desk Reference* lists more than 2,500 compounds that can be prescribed by a physician, only 200 drugs make up the bulk of the 2.8 million new prescriptions and refills dispensed by 50,000 pharmacies in 1998.[24] The most frequently prescribed drugs, by units dispensed, are Prilosec (acid reflux), Prozac (antidepressant), Zocor (cholesterol reducer), Epogen (RBC growth stimulator), and Zoloft (antidepressant). Collectively these five drugs generated sales of $8 billion in 1998.[24] Retail sales of prescription drugs were $102.5 billion, up 15 percent from 1996 sales.[25] Health-care dollars spent for prescription drugs account for 13 percent of the total health-care costs accrued by Americans.

Research and Development of New Drugs

As consumers of prescription drugs, you may be curious about the process by which drugs gain FDA approval. The rigor of this process may be the reason that only 100 new drugs were approved in 1997, up from 80 in 1996.[24]

The nation's pharmaceutical companies constantly explore the molecular structure of various chemical compounds in an attempt to discover important new compounds with desired types and levels of biological activity. When these new compounds are

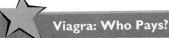

Viagra: Who Pays?

Viagra—the widely acclaimed anti-impotence drug developed for use by males—is prescribed by some physicians as an "off-label" adjunct to treat orgasmic dysfunction. Early clinical trials exploring the drug's safety and effectiveness in women are now under way. Based on minimal clinical testing, the drug appears to be effective in enhancing blood flow into genital structures, thus increasing vaginal lubrication, overall sexual arousal, and the likelihood of orgasm.

In spite of Viagra's proven and anticipated effectiveness as an aid to sexual performance, many people are asking who should pay for a drug that costs $8 to $12 a pill when the conditions it is being used to treat seem more "recreational" than medical. Some people who are opposed to paying for others' enhanced sexual performance believe that medical treatment for these conditions is not notably different from the treatment of male pattern baldness and the use of cosmetic surgery for facelifts, neither of which is generally covered by insurance. In contrast, many other people think the cost of Viagra should be reimbursed by group health insurance plans, HMOs, and even Medicaid. These supportive people believe that the enhancement of emotional well-being through improved sexual performance is a justifiable expenditure of health-care resources.

Where do you stand on this intriguing question?

identified, companies begin extensive in-house research with computer simulations and animal testing to determine whether clinical trials with humans are warranted. Of the 125,000 or more compounds under study each year, only a few thousand receive such extensive preclinical evaluation. Even fewer of these are then taken to the FDA to begin the evaluation process necessary to gain approval for further research with humans. When the FDA approves a drug for clinical trials, a pharmaceutical company can get a patent, which prevents the drug from being manufactured by other companies for the next seventeen years.

The $359 million price tag for bringing a new drug into the marketplace reflects this slow, careful process.[24] If the seven years of work needed to bring a new drug into the marketplace go well, a pharmaceutical company enjoys the remaining ten years of legally protected retail sales. Today new "fast-track" approval procedures at the FDA are progressively reducing the development period, particularly for desperately needed breakthrough drugs like those used to treat AIDS.[26]

Generic versus Brand-Name Drugs

When a new drug comes into the marketplace, it carries three names: its **chemical name**, its **generic name**, and its **brand name.** While the seventeen-year patent is in effect, no other drug with the same chemical formulation can be sold. When the patent expires, other

Dietary Supplements and the Self-Care Movement

Today some 60 million Americans are using an almost endless variety of vitamins, minerals, herbal products, hormones, and amino acids in a quest for improved health. Among the possible reasons for this trend are: the baby boomers are now in middle age and beginning to have concerns about illness and premature death; Americans increasingly view traditional Western medicine as impersonal; people are seeking an alternative to prescription medications; people want a greater sense of control over their own bodies. In 1997 Americans spent $12 billion on chemical compounds that are legally marketed under the name *dietary supplement*. These products are being consumed in record quantities, despite the fact that they are not subjected to research studies or FDA requirements for prescription medications. Like their European counterparts, major U.S. manufacturers of these products conduct research to ensure safety and effectiveness, but we know little about most of the 800 companies now in the marketplace, or the less reputable concerns that seek to profit from this trend.

On a more positive note, the traditional medical community increasingly is showing serious interest in tapping the health benefits of dietary supplements. A growing number of teaching hospitals are establishing departments of complementary medicine, and medical students are learning about the documented role food supplements can play in preventive medicine. Another reason for optimism is the entry of major international pharmaceutical companies into the research and development, clinical testing, and marketing of food supplements. Also contributing to the safer and more effective use of food supplements is the increasing availability of information based on credible research. Reputable professional journals are beginning to solicit and publish research related to food supplementation. In addition, the newly established National Center for Complementary and Alternative Medicine is funding well-designed research into a variety of areas, including food supplements. These studies will rapidly expand our understanding of the true role of food supplementation in the prevention and treatment of illness and the enhancement of human health.

The results of this research will provide valuable information to the 7.5 million users of St. John's wart, the 7.3 million who use echinacea, and the 10.8 million who take ginkgo biloba, as well as the millions who use other food supplements. Until then, however, these people should become studious consumers of supplements, knowing that they are participants in what is now a largely unregulated and potentially dangerous marketplace.

for brand-name drugs, as long as the prescribing physician approves.

In 1995 the *Physicians' Desk Reference—Generics* was first published. Like its companion publications for prescription and OTC drugs, *PDR—Generics* has been well received by both clinicians and the public.

Over-the-Counter Drugs

When people are asked when they last took some form of medication, for many the answer might be, "I took aspirin, or a cold pill, or a laxative this morning." In making this decision, people engaged in self-diagnosis, determined a course for their own treatment, self-administered their treatment, and freed a physician to serve people whose illnesses are more serious than theirs. None of this would have been possible without readily available, inexpensive, and effective OTC drugs.

While 2,500 prescription drugs are available, there are perhaps as many as 300,000 different OTC products, routinely classified into twenty-six different families. Like prescription drugs, nonprescription drugs are regulated by the FDA. However, for OTC drugs, the marketplace is a more powerful determinant of success.

The regulation of OTC drugs is based on a provision in a 1972 amendment to the 1938 Food, Drug, and Cosmetic Act. As a result of that action, OTC drugs were placed in three categories (I, II, and III) based on the safety and effectiveness of their active ingredient(s). Today, only category I OTC drugs that are safe, effective, and truthfully labeled are to be sold. The FDA's drug-classification process also allows some OTC drugs to be made stronger and some prescription drugs to become nonprescription drugs by reducing their strength through reformulation. In the latter case, 1995 marked the arrival in the OTC market of highly advertised heartburn remedies that were previously available only as prescription drugs. In 1996, Rogaine, the only FDA-approved treatment for male pattern baldness, was sold for the first time without a prescription.

The current labeling of OTC drugs is also set by the regulatory process. The labels must clearly state the type and quantity of active ingredients, alcohol content, side effects, instructions for appropriate use, warnings against inappropriate use, and the risks of using the product with other drugs (polydrug use).

companies can manufacture a drug of equivalent chemical composition and market it under the brand-name drug's original generic name. Because extensive research and development are unnecessary at this point, producing generic drugs is far less costly than developing the original brand-name drug. Nearly all states allow pharmacists to substitute generic drugs

chemical name name used to describe the molecular structure of a drug.

generic name common or nonproprietary name of a drug.

brand name specific patented name assigned to a drug by its manufacturer.

Unsubstantiated claims must be carefully avoided in advertisements for these products.

Health-Care Quackery and Consumer Fraud

A person who earns money by marketing inaccurate health information, unreliable health care, or ineffective health products is called a fraud, quack, or charlatan. **Consumer fraud** flourished with the old-fashioned medicine shows of the late 1880s. Unfortunately, consumer fraud still flourishes. You need look no further than large city newspapers to see questionable advertisements for disease cures and weight loss products. Quacks have found in health and illness the perfect avenues to make maximum gain with minimum effort.

When people are in poor health, they may be afraid of becoming disabled or dying. So powerful are their desires to live and avoid suffering that people are vulnerable to promises of health improvement and life-saving. Even though many people have great faith in their physicians, they also want access to experimental treatments or products touted as being superior to currently available therapies. When tempted by

the promise of help, people sometimes abandon traditional medical care. Of course, quacks recognize this vulnerability and present a variety of "reasons" to seek their help (see the Health Action Guide below).[27] Gullibility, blind faith, impatience, superstition, ignorance, or hostility toward professional expertise eventually carry the day. In spite of the best efforts of agencies at all levels, no branch of government can protect consumers from their own errors of judgment that so easily play into the hands of quacks and charlatans.

Regardless of the motivation that leads people into consumer fraud, the outcome is frequently the same. First, the consumer loses money. The services or products are grossly overpriced, and the consumers have little recourse to help them recover their money. Second, the consumers often feel disappointed, guilty, and angered by their own carelessness as consumers. Far too frequently, consumer fraud may lead to unnecessary suffering.

Personal Applications

- When you read a newspaper or magazine, do some health-related advertisements seem questionable to you? If so, which ones?

HEALTH ACTION GUIDE

Recognizing Quackery

"Duck" when you encounter these!

- Makes promises of quick, dramatic, simple, painless, or drugless treatment or cures
- Uses anecdotes, case histories, or testimonials to support claims
- Displays credentials or uses titles that might be confused with those of the scientific or medical community, such as Stan Smith, Ph.D. (in which the abbreviation stands for something other than Doctor of Philosophy)
- Claims a product or service treats or cures multiple or all illnesses and conditions
- States that this treatment or cure is either secret or not yet available in the United States
- States that medical doctors should not be trusted because they do more harm than good with their approaches to diagnosis and treatment
- Reports that most disease is due to a faulty diet and can be treated with nutritional supplements
- Promotes the use of hair analysis to diagnose illnesses or deficiencies
- Claims that "natural" products are superior to those sold in drugstores or dispensed by physicians
- Supports the "freedom of choice" concept that should allow you to try something even though it has not been proved safe and effective

InfoLinks
www.quackwatch.com

Becoming a Skilled Health-Care Consumer

After reading this discussion of health information, services, and products, you should be a wiser, more prepared consumer. However, information alone is not enough. Consider these six suggestions to help you become a more skilled, assertive consumer:

1. *Prepare yourself for consumerism.* In addition to this personal health course, your university may offer a course on consumerism. Libraries and bookstores offer trade books on a variety of consumer topics. Consumer protection agencies can guide you in some subjects. Government agencies also may help you in your choices.
2. *Comparison shop.* In our free-enterprise system, virtually every service or product can be duplicated on the open market. Very few items or services are one-of-a-kind. Take the time to study your choices before you purchase a product or service.
3. *Insist on formal contracts and dated receipts.* Under the consumer laws in most states, you have a limited time in which to void a contract. Formal documentation of your actions as a consumer will give you the maximum protection available.

4. *Obtain written instructions and warranties.* Be certain of the appropriate use of any product you purchase. If you use a product inappropriately, you might void its warranty. Be familiar with what you can reasonably anticipate from the products and services you buy. In addition, be aware that a written warranty supersedes any verbal assurances a salesperson might make.

5. *Put your complaints in writing.* A carefully constructed record of your complaints is vital. Accurate records of the names and addresses of all companies and people with whom you have done business will enable you to document your actions as a consumer.

6. *Press for resolution of your complaints.* As a consumer, you are entitled to effective products and services. If your consumer complaints are not resolved, you have legal recourse through the courts. You should not hesitate to assert your rights, not only for your own sake, but for consumers who might later become victims.

Consumerism is an active relationship between you and a provider. If the provider is competent and honest and you are an informed and active consumer, both of you will profit from the relationship. However, if the provider is not competent or honest, you can protect yourself by employing the preceding six suggestions.

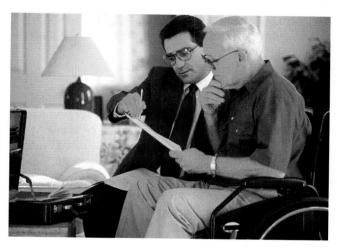

Comparison shopping is one way of becoming a wise consumer of health-care products and services, such as insurance policies.

Personal Applications

- Why do you think it is difficult to get people to seek preventive care even though it is usually less expensive than treatment services?

consumer fraud   marketing of unreliable and ineffective services, products, or information under the guise of curing disease or improving health; quackery.

Real Life
Real choices

Your Turn

- Do you experience migraine headaches or some other chronic physical condition that causes you intense pain? If so, how do you deal with it, and what are the results?
- Have you ever sought alternative forms of treatment for a chronic painful condition, or do you know anyone who has? If so, what were the results?
- Ellen Chang seems determined to explore alternative therapies for her migraine headaches. Based on what you have learned in this chapter, what are some cautions you can offer

her? What questions should she be asking about any practitioner she consults?

And Now, Your Choices . . .
- Would you consider using an alternative approach to treatment for a condition like Ellen's? Why or why not?
- If you did decide to seek alternative treatment, would you tell your regular physician? Why or why not?

Summary

- Sources of health information include family, friends, commercials, labels, and information supplied by health professionals.
- Physicians can be either Doctors of Medicine (MDs) or Doctors of Osteopathy (DOs). They receive similar training and engage in similar

forms of practice.
- Although alternative health-care providers, including chiropractors, naturopaths, and acupuncturists, meet the health-care needs of many people, systematic study of these forms of health care is only now under way.

- Restricted-practice health-care providers play important roles in meeting the health and wellness needs of the public.
- Nursing at all levels is a critical health-care profession.
- Self-care is often a viable approach to preventing illness and reducing the use of health-care providers.
- Our growing inability to afford health-care services has reached crisis proportions in the United States.
- More than 41 million Americans, not just the poor, have problems getting health care.
- Health insurance is critical to our ability to afford modern health-care services.

- HMOs provide an alternative way of receiving health-care services, although the influence of the profit motive in their operation is a concern.
- Medicare and Medicaid are governmental plans for paying for health-care services that could be significantly changed in our current quest for a balanced budget.
- The development of prescription medication is a long and expensive process for pharmaceutical manufacturers.
- Critical health consumerism, including avoiding health quackery, requires careful use of health-related information, products, and services.

Review Questions

1. Determine how you would test the accuracy of the health-related information you have received in your lifetime.
2. Identify and describe some sources of health-related information presented in this chapter. What factors should you consider when using these sources?
3. Describe the similarities between allopathic and osteopathic physicians. What is an alternative health-care practitioner? Give examples of the types of alternative practitioners.
4. What is the theory underlying acupuncture in particular and Chinese medicine in general?
5. Describe the services that are provided by the following limited health-care providers: dentists, psychologists, podiatrists, optometrists, and opticians. Identify several allied health-care professionals.

6. In what ways is the trend toward self-care evident? What are some reasons for the popularity of this movement?
7. What is health insurance? Explain the following terms relating to health insurance: deductible amount, fixed indemnity benefits, full-service benefits, coinsurance, exclusion, and preexisting condition.
8. What is a health maintenance organization? How do HMO plans reduce the costs of health care? What are IPAs and PPOs?
9. What do the chemical name, brand name, and generic name of a prescription drug represent? OTC drugs are approved for marketing on the basis of what two factors?
10. What is health-care quackery? What responsibilities have been given to the FDA? What can a consumer do to avoid consumer fraud?

References

1. Findlay S. AMA rethinks endorsing line of consumer goods. *USA Today* 1997 Aug 20:3A.
2. Weise E. Net use doubling every 100 days. U.S. Department of Commerce, *USA Today* 1998 April 16:1A.
3. Carey A, Cisqalitis G. A line on health information. Find/SVP, as reported in *USA Today* 1997 Nov 27:1D.
4. *The PDR family guide to prescription drugs.* Pittsburgh: Three Rivers Press, 1998.
5. Margolis S, Moses H., eds. *The Johns Hopkins medical handbook: the 100 major medical disorders for people over the age of 50.* New York: Random House, 1997.
6. Findlay S. AMA plan to accredit physicians. *USA Today* 1997 Nov 11:1D.
7. Griffin K, Butterer K. The new doctors of natural medicine. *Health* 1996 10(6):60.
8. *Appropriations bill establishes the National Center for Complementary and Alternative Medicine* (press release). Nov 3, 1998. http://altmed.od.nih.gov/nccam/news-events/press-release/10398shtml

9. *NIH panel issues consensus statement on acupuncture* (press release). Nov 5, 1997. http://www.nih.gov/news/pr/nov97/od.or.htm
10. Peterson K. More spending time caring for elders. National Alliance for Caregiving, as reported in *USA Today* 1997 March 18:1D.
11. U.S. Bureau of the Census. *Statistical abstract of the United States: 1998.* 118th ed. Washington, DC: U.S. Government Printing Office, 1998.
12. McKenzie JF, Pinger RR, Kotecki JE. *An introduction to community health.* 3rd ed. Sudbury, MA: Jones & Bartlett, 1999.
13. *National health expenditure amounts, and average annual increases.* Health Care Finance Administration. Sept 1998. http://www.gov/stats/NHE-Proj/tables/default.htm
14. U.S. Department of Health and Human Services, Group Health Association of America. CareData reports, Foster-Higgins. *USA Today* 1995 Oct 17:1D.

15. Gray P. Gagging the doctors. *Time* 1996 Jan; 8:50.
16. A variety of plans . . . and how to choose one. *AARP Bulletin* 1996 Nov 10.
17. Social Security Administration. *Social Security, SSI and Medicare update* (fact sheet). Jan 1999.
18. U.S. Department of Health and Human Services, Social Security Administration. SSA Pub. No. 05-10006, April 1997.
19. Clinton ignores impeachment, calls for Social Security reform. *CNN Website* Jan 19, 1999. http://www.cnn.com/allpolitics/stores/1999/01/19/s
20. Health Care Finance Administration. *USA Today* 1995 Sept 25:6A.
21. Painter K. Health care access, costs trouble many. *USA Today* 1996 Oct 23:6D.
22. Tangonan S. Health needs of middle class often unmet. *USA Today* 1996 May 6:1A.
23. Hartman HW, Reyes MC. Will health care reform give minorities a fair shake? *Hospital & Health Networks* 1994; 68(16):64.
24. Meyers B. Drugmakers have healthy outlook. IMS-America and Food & Drug Administration, as reported in *USA Today* 1998 July 20:3B.
25. *Industry facts.* National Association of Chain Drug Stores. Jan 1999. http://www.nacds.org/industry/fastfacts.html#retail
26. Wierenga DE, Eaton CR. *The drug development and approval process.* Office of Research and Development. Pharmaceutical Manufacturers Association, 1998. Philadelphia, PA.
27. Cornacchia HJ, Barrett S. *Consumer health: a guide to intelligent decisions.* 5th ed. St. Louis: Mosby, 1993.

Suggested Readings

Landis A. *Social Security: the inside story: an expert explains your rights and benefits.* Menlo Park, CA: Crisp Publishers, 1997. For many older adults, the complexities of Social Security can seem insurmountable. This book offers a comprehensive, current, and readable explanation of America's "safety net." The author explains the history of Social Security, as well as the program's current organizational framework and the various categories of benefits and special provisions. Tables and charts show how Social Security benefits are determined.

Brown D. (Visiting Nurse Association). *Caregiver's handbook: a complete guide to home health care.* New York: DK Publishing, 1998. This informative book covers virtually every aspect of providing home care to people with a variety of health problems. The author illustrates and describes equipment, supplies, and home care skills.

Rappaport K, ed. *Directory of schools for alternative and complementary health care.* Phoenix: Orxy Press, 1998. For people interested in pursuing training in the field of complementary health care, this book provides significant help in finding acceptable programs in the United States and Canada. The book presents a wide array of information, including names, locations, telephone and fax numbers, courses of study, admission requirements, costs, and accessibility to people with disabilities. Although programs are not ranked, background information is provided regarding accreditation, certification of graduates, and professional associations. A glossary of alternative medical terms appears at the end of the book.

Molony D. *The American Association of Oriental Medicine's complete guide to Chinese herbal medicine: how to treat illness and maintain wellness with Chinese herbal medicine.* New York: Berkeley Publishing, 1998. After reviewing the 4,000-year-old history of Chinese medicine and explaining the underlying principles associated with the role of herbs in promoting inner balance, the author details the efficacy and manner of use for 170 herbs, alone and in combination. The book includes a list of conditions that can be safely and effectively treated by herbs, a helpful glossary of terms, and the locations of reputable suppliers of medicinal herbs.

As We Go To PRESS

The FDA is preparing to approve the drug thalidomide to treat inflammation associated with leprosy. The drug may also prove useful in treating AIDS, rheumatoid arthritis, and several autoimmune disorders. Thalidomide first received the public's attention in North America and Europe nearly 35 years ago. The drug, which was then used as a sedative, caused severe birth defects when prescribed to pregnant women. Failure of limb buds to develop was routinely reported among the 12,000 babies exposed to the drug in utero. These children, many of whom have absent or malformed limbs, are now middle aged. They have been vocal in expessing their concern about the proposed return of a drug that so profoundly influenced their lives. Should thalidomide be approved, its use will be carefully restricted to patients unlikely to become pregnant while taking it.

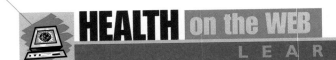

HEALTH on the WEB

Understanding the Benefits of Health Insurance

Who will pay your hospital bills if you have a serious accident or illness and must receive medical treatment? You purchase health insurance for the same reason you buy other kinds of insurance: to protect yourself financially. Go to www.healthtouch.com/level1/leaflets/115218/115218.htm to learn more about health insurance. Choose a topic of interest to you and read the information. What did you learn? Do you have the health insurance protection you may need?

Visiting a Virtual Medical Center

A new, interactive medical information service is available at http://mediconsult.com. Created by practicing physicians, this service offers confidential answers to your medical questions. This website is patient supported and was developed to educate the general public about various medical issues. Scroll down to *Current Poll* and answer the questions listed. Do you agree with the poll results? Why or why not?

Staying Informed About Your Medications

At the Healthtouch website you can find information about more than 7,000 prescription and over-the-counter medications, including common uses of a drug, proper ways to use the medicine, and possible side effects. Please note that it is advisable to discuss medication information with your pharmacist, doctor, or other health professional to find out how it applies to your particular case. Go to www.healthtouch.com/level1/p_dri.htm. To use the guide, enter the partial or complete name of the medicine in the space *Search for Match*. Be sure to enter the correct spelling.

For more activities, go to our Online Learning Center at www.mhhe.com/hper/health/payne

Separating Fact from Fiction: Using Health Information on the Internet

So you want to find some information on health. Maybe you have a paper due in this class. Maybe you need more information on a condition that you or a loved one has. Or maybe you simply want to take advantage of the latest information on fitness and nutrition to make healthful decisions. No matter what information you're looking for, you can probably find it on the Internet. But be wary as you search—a great deal of misinformation is also available, and it may be hard for the average consumer to separate health fact from health fiction.

You can be relatively certain that government sites and links contain reliable information. In fact, the U.S. Department of Health and Human Services has established a new site to provide consumer information. It can be accessed under Health/General Health or directly at www.healthfinder.gov. This site was launched in April 1997 by the U.S. Secretary of Health and Human Services, Donna Shalala, in response to a request by Vice President Al Gore to improve consumer access to federal health information on-line. As Healthfinder points out in its introductory paragraph, information alone can't take the place of health care you may need. But it can make you an informed partner in your own health care. This site leads you to selected on-line publications, databases, websites, support and self-help groups, government agencies, not-for-profit organizations, and universities that provide reliable health information to the public.[1]

Unfortunately, the government does not have the resources to filter out all false and misleading health-care information. Many people mistakenly believe that advertising claims must be true or advertisers would not be allowed to continue making them.[2] Not enough time, money, and regulators are available to assess the validity of each and every health claim. However, health-care professionals and consumer advocates can give us the tools we need to determine the reliability of health information for ourselves.

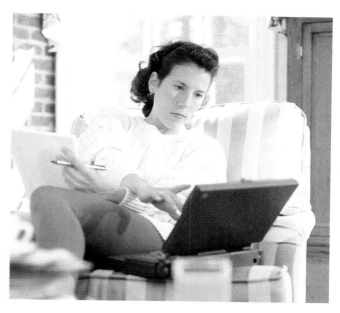

Using health information from reliable Internet sites can help you become an active participant in your own health care.

What Is Quackery and How Can You Spot It?

One prominent consumer advocate is Stephen Barrett, a retired physician and nationally renowned author (with 42 books to his credit).[3] In 1969 he founded the Lehigh Valley Committee against Health Fraud, which recently changed its name to Quackwatch.[4] Investigation of questionable claims, answering of inquiries, distribution of reliable publications, reporting of illegal marketing, and improvement of the overall quality of health information on the Internet are all tasks that this group takes on.

Quackery is more difficult to spot than most people think. Whereas fraud is deliberate deception and more easily recognized and corrected, quackery involves the use of methods that are not scientifically valid.[5] Information purveyed by quacks cannot be scientifically confirmed or denied, and this is where the problem arises. There is no way to separate the good from the bad or the harmful from the benign or helpful.

Anecdotes and Testimonials

Some alternative health-care methods have been accepted by the scientific community, having met reliable criteria for safety and effectiveness. Other methods are in the experimental stages. These methods are unproven but are based on plausible, rational principles and are undergoing responsible testing. But many other alternative health remedies are groundless and completely lack scientific rationale. Instead of scientific tests, people who promote these methods rely on anecdotes and testimonials to "prove" the effectiveness of their products. Perhaps you have noticed that claims of effectiveness are not found on the products themselves, but rather in brochures placed in conspicuous locations very near the products. This use of testimonials is unique to the dietary supplement market and reflects the virtual absence of regulatory power held by the FDA and FTC. Newly released FTC guidelines, however, will be helpful to consumers in this still under-regulated market.[6]

Intelligent Consumer Behavior

Americans waste $50 million to $150 million per year on bogus mail-order health remedies.[2] Many of these products are now available on the Internet. You can avoid wasting your money in this way by not buying any of these products without medical advice from your physician or other health-care professional. And don't be fooled by money back guarantees; they're usually as phony as the products that they back.

Be wary of characteristic quackery ploys.[7] Purveyors of quackery may say that they care about you, but their care, even if it were sincere, cannot make useless medicine work. These products are commonly touted as having no side effects. If this is true, then the product is too weak to have any effect at all. Quacks will encourage you to jump on the bandwagon of their time-tested remedy, as if popularity and market longevity are surrogates for effectiveness. When they do claim that their products are backed by scientific studies, these studies turn out to be untraceable, misinterpreted, irrelevant, nonexistent, or based on poorly designed research.[7]

The costs of buying into health-care quackery are more than financial. The psychological effects of disillusionment and the physical harm caused by the method itself or by abandoning more effective care are much worse.

HONcode Principles

Any reputable health information site on the Internet subscribes to the HONcode Principles. These principles are put forth and monitored by the Geneva-based Health On the Net Foundation and have arisen from input from webmasters and medical professionals in several countries.[8] According to these principles, any medical advice appearing at a site must meet the following requirements:

- It must be given by medically trained and qualified professionals unless a clear statement is made that the information comes from a non-medically qualified individual or organization.
- The information must be intended to support, not replace, the physician-patient relationship.
- Data relating to individual patients and visitors to a medical website are confidential.
- Site information must have clear references to source data and, where possible, specific links to that data.
- Claims related to the benefit or performance of a treatment, product, or service must be supported by appropriate, balanced evidence.
- The webmaster's e-mail address should be clearly displayed throughout the website.
- Commercial and noncommercial support and funding for the site should be clearly revealed.
- There must be a clear differentiation between advertising at the site and the original material created by the institution operating the site.

Be skeptical about any health information you find on the Internet that does not meet these criteria. Ask your physician whether the information is accurate, or move on to a more reliable site.

Assessing Health-Care Information

The Internet is a valuable health-care tool. Reliable information is supplied by government health agencies, research universities, hospitals, disease foundations, and other experts. However, not all health sites are reputable. As the saying goes, you can't believe everything you read, even if it's on the Internet. Anyone can create an on-line resource that looks professional. Ordinary people who believe they've been helped by a product, companies trying to sell products and services, and even cheats and quacks are all out there spouting their information. To protect yourself, you must be an informed consumer of information. To evaluate the credibility of an on-line source, ask yourself the following questions:

1. Who maintains the information?
2. Is it linked to other reputable sources of medical information?
3. When was it last updated?
4. Is it selling a product?

While the Internet cannot and should not replace visits with a physician, reliable information obtained on the net can make us more active partners in our own health care. It can give us information we can use to stay healthy and prevent disease. It can help us to ask our doctors the right questions and educate us so that we're not afraid to ask them. It can connect us to people who are experiencing the same things as we are. It can help us learn about our health, receive support from others, and make sound health-care decisions based on fact—not fiction.

For Discussion . . .

Which health-related sites have you visited on the Internet? Did you find them informative? reliable? fun? What could be done to improve the status of health information on the Internet?

References

1. U.S. Department of Health and Human Services. Healthfinder. 1997. http://www.healthfinder.gov
2. Barrett S. *Mail-order quackery.* 1996. http://www.quackwatch.com/01quackeryrelatedtopics/mailquack.htm
3. Barrett S. *About Dr. Barrett.* 1997. http://www.quackwatch.com/bio.html
4. Barrett S. *Mission statement.* 1997. http://www.quackwatch.com/00aboutquackwatch/mission.html
5. Barrett S. *Quackery: how should it be defined?* 1997. http://www.quackwatch.com/quackdof.html
6. Washington, DC: Federal Trade Commission. *Business guide for dietary supplement industry* (news release). Nov 18, 1998. http://www.ftc.gov/opa/1998/9811/dietary.htm
7. Barrett S, Herbert V. *More ploys that may fool you.* 1997. http://www.quackwatch.com/01quackeryrelatedtopics/oloys.html
8. Health on the New Foundation. *HONcode principles.* 1997. http://www.quackwatch.com/00aboutquackwatch/honcode.html

InfoLinks
www.hon.ch
www.nnlm.nlm.nih.gov/gmr/publish/eval.html

Caring for Our Environment

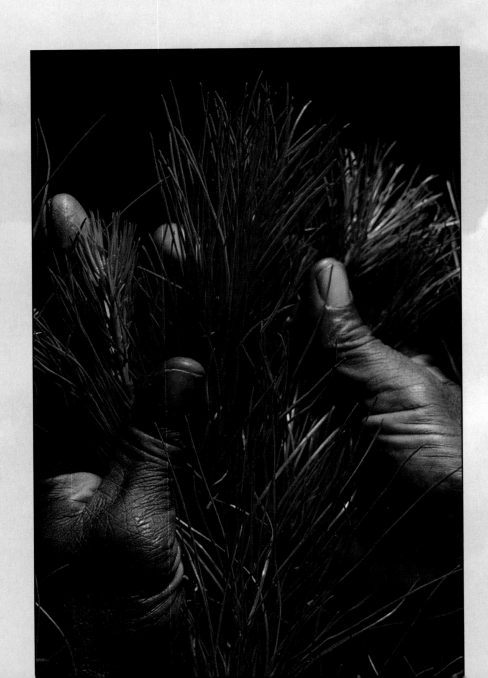

Throughout this book we have read about areas of health over which people have significant control. For example, people select the foods they eat, how much alcohol they consume, and how they manage the stressors in their lives. The study of the environment and its effect on health contrasts with the daily control people have over their own health. Perhaps because of the natural processes of life and death and the vital role of the environment, we tend to think that we cannot make decisions that affect our environment. This attitude, however, is changing.

HEALTHY PEOPLE: LOOKING AHEAD TO 2010

Progress was inconsistent in meeting the environmental objectives set forth in the *Healthy People 2000* document. However, substantial headway was made in promoting cleaner air. Few counties in the United States now exceed air pollution limits, although this could change if proposed new standards are approved.

Another environmental objective was to reduce the human exposure to solid waste contamination of water, air, and soil. Progress toward this goal was limited because of increased production of solid waste by American households. Some gains were made in establishing recycling programs and reducing levels of environmental carcinogens.

Healthy People 2010 will continue our national effort to improve the environment. One change being proposed for the new objectives is to redefine the home and workplace as "environments." Thus some maternal and child health goals, occupational health goals, and violence-related concerns could be considered environmental health objectives.

Because of the encompassing nature of the environment and the number of at-risk groups within the larger population, it is likely that virtually every approach to program development and implementation will be used in attempting to meet *Healthy People 2010* objectives in this area. A complicating factor is the need for various government agencies to deal with each other and with powerful special interest groups. Among all the objectives of *Healthy People 2010,* the environment clearly is the most complex in terms of predicting positive change. Unlike objectives related to more traditional health problems, it is unlikely that a single technological breakthrough will improve the health of the environment in all of its dimensions.

Real Life
Real choices

- Name: David Cloudwalker
- Age: 23
- Occupation: Medical student

"Save the Earth!" "Fight Pollution!" "Clean Air NOW!"

Slowing his beat-up VW bug to let a throng of student demonstrators cross the street, David Cloudwalker glances at the signs they carry and shakes his head. Four hundred years of abusing and exploiting the environment, and these people think all it takes to clean up the mess is signs and marches. How many of these kids, he wonders, know what it's like to pay every day of your life for the waste dump someone else has made of your native land?

David knows. A member of the Crow nation, he grew up with eight brothers and sisters in grinding poverty on the edge of an old mining town in Montana. Scarred hillsides and towering slagheaps stand in stark contrast to the craggy majesty of ancient mountains and the colorful profusion of native wildflowers. The clear cold stream where David's ancestors fished still gleams and sparkles . . . but with the rainbow hues of chemical waste from the nearby plastics plant. The vast blue bowl of western sky is streaked with black plumes from the factory's exhaust stacks, and the roar and crash of freight trains shatter the peaceful mountain night.

Like other families in Indian Hollow, the Cloudwalkers had no health insurance and little access to medical care. Sanitation facilities were crude and poorly maintained, and people always seemed to be passing the same disease-causing germs back and forth. David's father, a laborer at the plastics factory, died at the age of 36 of what the plant physician vaguely called "weak lungs." But George Cloudwalker never smoked, and as a young man he

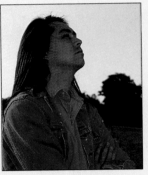

won every running competition at tribal gatherings. His weak lungs, David is sure, were the result of long-term exposure to the choking filth of the factory air. Two of David's brothers have worked at the plant since high school, and they always seem to be coughing or wiping watery eyes. And now a new generation of kids is coughing, sneezing, and getting gastrointestinal "bugs."

The lands of David's ancestors have been invaded not only by technology but also by tourists. The once abandoned mining town has been restored to attract summer visitors. The old brick and frame storefronts of the main street now display pricey western and Native American clothing, jewelry, and souvenirs. Costly cars with out-of-state license plates line the dusty streets, and synthetic country music thunders from speakers on the pavilion of a trendy line-dance spot.

David doesn't long to be a painted warrior or a daring buffalo hunter. He's working his way through one of the top medical schools in the country, and his goal is to become a neurosurgeon. But he's proud of his heritage, and he's both sad and angry about the heedless exploitation of our country's vast natural riches.

As you study this chapter, think about David's experiences as a Native American dealing with environmental damage, and prepare yourself to answer the questions in **Your Turn** at the end of the chapter.

Compared with the 1980s, when concerns about the environment focused on problems over which we had little direct responsibility or control (such as the ozone layer and nuclear accidents), the 1990s have been characterized by a focus on the individual and the home. Issues such as the disposal of municipal waste; the recycling of glass, plastic, and aluminum; the venting of radon gas from basements; and the reduction of water use show that people can act to support the environment (see the Health Action Guide on p. 559).

Environmental concerns also extend to developing countries as well. With the world population at 5.67 billion in 1994 and moving toward 10.8 billion in 2060 (with the greatest rate of increase in developing countries), the demands made on the environment are already substantial. As people continue to destroy tropical rain forests, the search for living space and natural resources continues unabated despite our knowledge of the damage of earlier decades. Complete the Personal Assessment on page 560 to see how well you are helping protect the Environment.

World Population Growth

Population growth affects not just our own homes and communities but the entire planet. Each year the world's population grows by 90 million people. By the middle of the next century, there could be 50 percent more people than there are today. By the year 2060, experts project that 10.8 billion people will be alive. In fact, in 1992 it was predicted that by the year 2000, more than half of the developing countries in the world may not be able to feed their populations from food grown on their own land.[1] As seen in North Korea, a large population in combination with natural disasters, limited technological resources for self-sufficiency, and government policies that restrict humanitarian assistance can lead to the most extreme human suffering.

To fully appreciate the impact of overpopulation, we can consider the variables used in population studies.[2] For example, the *doubling time* for population in developed countries is currently 148 years, and 41

HEALTH ACTION GUIDE

10 Things You Can Do to Improve the Environment

1. Visit and help support our national parks.
2. Recycle newspapers, glass, plastic, and aluminum.
3. Conserve energy and use energy-efficient lighting.
4. Keep tires properly inflated to improve gas mileage and extend tire life.
5. Plant trees.
6. Organize a Christmas tree recycling program in your community.
7. Find an alternative to chemical pesticides for your lawn.
8. Purchase only those brands of tuna marked "dolphin safe."
9. Organize a community group to clean up a local stream, highway, park, or beach.
10. Become a member of an environmental action group, such as the Environmental Defense Fund, the Nature Conservancy, or the Sierra Club.

InfoLinks

http://www.earthshare.org/earthshare/index.html

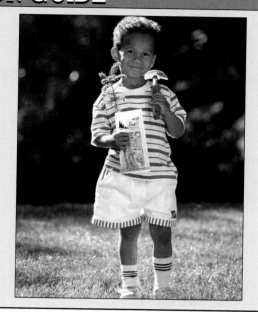

years for the world at large. Today, however, doubling times of less than 20 years exist in 14 countries and times of between 20 and 34 years in another 66 countries, virtually all of which are located in *underdeveloped* or *developing* areas of the world. A second important variable, *contraceptive prevalence rate,* reflecting access to and use of effective birth control, is 71 percent in developed countries and 55 percent for the world at large. In Sub-Saharan Africa, for example, 16 countries are deemed to be "critical," with rates of less than 34 percent, including 11 countries with rates of 10 percent or less and 7 countries with values of 5 percent or less.

Additional variables underscore the consequences of excessive population growth.[2] For example, the 1992 *gross national product per capita* (GNP) in developed countries was $17,640 (U.S. dollars) and $3,740 worldwide. In contrast, the GNP per capita was $800 (U.S. dollars) in developing countries—a level that is a direct effect of rapidly increasing populations within those countries. Another significant variable is the *percent of the population capable of being fed in the year 2000.* Using Asia as an example, seven countries are known to be incapable of feeding all of their population with a combination of domestic productivity and purchases made in the international market, while three countries are known to be at risk in this regard. Only five Asian countries for which data were available are known to be capable of meeting the food requirements of their population. Again, overpopulation is an important factor in the shaping of this demographic variable.

Although specific data are not available, additional overpopulation-influenced variables also are cause for concern:[2] crop land per capita, annual forest loss, threatened mammal species and threatened bird species per 10,000 square kilometers, commercial energy use per capita, carbon dioxide release per capita, annual water resources, people without safe drinking water, and people without sanitation services. Again, with only minor exceptions, experts report a consistently strong relationship between population growth and the inability to control fertility. Clearly, the complex and often controversial question of controlling the rate of population growth is a key variable in determining whether our environmental resources will be sufficient to meet the health-related needs of the population. Without the consistent use of effective fertility control, the disparity between developed countries and underdeveloped/developing countries will continue to widen. How (or if) this level of use will be achieved is a major unanswered question for the early decades of the new millennium.

Air Pollution

If you think that air pollution is a modern by-product of technology that has gone astray, remember that nature routinely pollutes the air. Sea salt, soil particles, ash, dust, soot, microbes, assorted trace elements, and plant pollens are consistently found in the air.

Pollution caused in part by humans also has a long history. From the fires that filled our ancestors' caves with choking smoke, through the "killer fogs"

Personal Assessment

How many ways can you help the environment? Give yourself 2 points for each of the following that you do regularly, 1 point for each that you do occasionally, and a 0 for those that you do not do. Total your points and compare your score with those that follow the assessment.

_____ 1. Promptly repair leaky faucets.

_____ 2. Use the microwave as often as possible rather than the stove or the oven.

_____ 3. Buy brands that come in minimal amounts of packaging.

_____ 4. Do not run excess water while washing dishes.

_____ 5. Use paper bags rather than plastic.

_____ 6. Use sponges or dishcloths for spills rather than paper towels.

_____ 7. Recycle newspapers rather than throw them out.

_____ 8. Snip six-pack rings.

_____ 9. Walk or bicycle rather than drive.

_____ 10. Purchase products in the larger sizes.

_____ 11. Preheat your oven for the minimal amount of time necessary.

_____ 12. Turn off water while brushing your teeth.

_____ 13. Do not use a trash compactor.

_____ 14. Eat fresh fruits and vegetables rather than processed foods.

_____ 15. Pull weeds by hand rather than spraying them with chemicals.

_____ 16. Carpool to work.

_____ 17. Limit garbage disposal use as much as possible.

_____ 18. Use canvas or cloth bags for shopping.

_____ 19. Sweep driveways and sidewalks rather than use a hose.

_____ 20. Recycle bottles and jars.

_____ 21. Pick up litter when you see it.

_____ 22. Make note pads out of used office stationery and paper.

_____ 23. Wear clothing that is right for the weather.

_____ 24. Use rechargeable batteries.

_____ 25. Clean the lint screen in the dryer after each load.

_____ 26. Put trash in only one bag (or the fewest needed).

_____ 27. Use refillable containers for household products (such as liquid hand soap).

_____ 28. Keep the water heater at the lowest level needed.

_____ 29. Open blinds and curtains during daylight periods during winter months.

_____ 30. Close blinds and curtains during periods of bright sunshine during summer months.

_____ 31. Turn off lights when you leave a room.

_____ 32. Take quick showers rather than leisurely baths.

_____ 33. Turn off stereos, radios, and televisions when leaving the house.

_____ 34. Turn off the water when washing the car and use a bucket when possible.

_____ 35. Place a brick or a plastic bottle of water inside the toilet storage tank.

_____ 36. Buy laundry detergents that are phosphate-free when other options are available.

_____ 37. Drink "ice water" from the refrigerator rather than run tap water to get it cooler.

_____ 38. Run the dishwasher only when full.

_____ 39. Use hairspray in nonaerosol bottles.

_____ 40. Clean and change filters on the furnace and air conditioner regularly.

_____ 41. Keep a reusable mug or cup at the office.

_____ 42. Purchase clothing that can be washed rather than only dry cleaned.

_____ 43. Wash clothing only when dirty.

_____ 44. Close the refrigerator door promptly.

_____ 45. Keep the car properly tuned.

_____ 46. Collect rain water for use in plants and gardens.

_____ 47. Donate outgrown clothing to nonprofit organizations.

_____ 48. Participate in organized cleanup days when they are held in your community.

_____ 49. Replace a conventional shower head with a water-conserving model.

_____ 50. Write elected officials to support environmental legislation.

Your total points   _____

Interpretation

90–100 points: Your conservation efforts are in the superior range. Keep up the excellent work!

80–89 points: You are clearly above average and should also be congratulated!

70–79 points: Although your score is average, your efforts at conserving the environment are important contributions to the total effort. Keep up the good work and look for additional ways to conserve.

60–69 points: Your score is passing but below average. Try to find more ways to help the environment. You have room for improvement.

59 and below: Time has not run out! You can still earn a passing grade but you need to follow the suggestions in this assessment and chapter to help the environment.

To Carry This Further . . .

Share these suggestions, or any others that you find useful, with family, friends, classmates, and other associates as a means of further helping our environment.

of nineteenth-century London, to the dust storms of the Great Depression, humans have contributed to air pollution. Today its effects can be seen in countries throughout the world. The five countries that produce the most airborne gases that contribute to global warming (the United States, the former USSR, Japan, China, and Brazil) are located in North America, Europe, Asia, and South America.

As we near the end of the century, the United States as well as the international community is attempting to implement policies and procedures to improve the quality of the air. In this country the Office of Air and Radiation of the U.S. Environmental Protection Agency (EPA) in 1997 proposed new air quality standards related to ozone (see p. 563) and particulate matter size (see p. 564).[3,4] Using several peer-reviewed studies as the basis of their recommendation, the EPA believes that, if implemented, the standards could improve the respiratory health of 40 million children and save the lives of 15,000 elderly or frail Americans. In addition, adults and children with asthma and other respiratory disorders would experience improvement, particularly during periods of activity and exercise.

Despite the anticipated benefits of adopting these regulations, opposition from Congress is likely to continue. The opposition is based largely on the cost of implementation and especially its impact on small businesses, which would be required to install expensive air cleaning technology to meet the standards. Environmentalists and health advocates now fear that the recently enacted Small Business Regulatory Environment and Fairness Act may result in a relaxation of the proposed guidelines.

The EPA also has proposed haze reduction regulations, that would apply to wilderness areas in or near our national parks and recreation areas.[5] The EPA believes these standards would reduce haze to a point where natural wonders could be viewed at clear and unobstructed levels enjoyed in earlier days. Again, congressional opposition based on cost may serve to soften or eliminate these guidelines.

At the international level, the United States in 1997 signed an international global warming treaty formulated in Kyoto, Japan.[6] Ratification in Congress appears doubtful because of the high costs of implementation for businesses in developed countries compared with the treaty's very light restrictions on underdeveloped nations.

Sources of Air Pollution

You probably know the sources of modern air pollutants. A leading source is the internal combustion engine. Automobiles, trucks, and buses release a variety of materials into the air, including carbon monoxide and hydrocarbons. (Americans run a billion errands daily by car.)[7] Industrial processes, domestic heating, refuse burning, and the use of pesticides and herbicides also contribute to our air pollution problem. In recent years, the massive deforestation of the tropical rain forest in the Amazon River basin of South America has contributed significant amounts of gaseous and particulate pollutants to the air.

Gaseous Pollutants

The pollutants dispersed into the air by the sources just identified are generally in the form of gases, including *carbon dioxide* and *carbon monoxide*. Carbon dioxide is the natural by-product of combustion and is produced whenever fuels are burned. Electricity production, car and truck emissions, and industry are the principal producers of carbon dioxide.

As first predicted well over a decade ago, the progressive increase in carbon dioxide appears to have produced a **greenhouse effect** (Figure 19-1). This effect has caused a slight but progressive warming of the earth's surface. An increase of only 1.5 degrees since 1860, resulting from increased trapping of industrial gases, has shifted the world's hydrologic cycles.[8] Today the atmosphere is more laden with moisture, and air circulation patterns have shifted, leading to greater extremes in all aspects of weather.

Whether these trends will continue into the next century is, of course, uncertain. Current attempts to reduce hydrocarbon emissions could be effective enough to begin moderating the temperature increase noted during this century.

Carbon monoxide, the colorless and odorless gas produced when fuels are burned incompletely, was discussed in the chapter on cardiovascular disease (see Chapter 10). Also occurring in gaseous form are methane, from decaying vegetation; the terpenes, produced by trees; and benzene and benzopyrene, which may cause cancer of the respiratory system.

Nitrogen and *sulfur* compounds are pollutants produced by a variety of industrial processes, including the burning of high-sulfur content fuels, especially coal. When nitrogen and sulfur oxides combine with moisture in the atmosphere, they are converted to nitric and sulfuric acids. The resulting **acid rain,** acid snow, and acid fog are responsible, for example, for the destruction of aquatic life and vegetation in the eastern United States and Canada.[9]

In urban areas located in cooler climates (or other cities during the winter months), sulfur oxides and particulate matter (from heating systems) combine with moisture to form a grayish haze, or **smog.** This gray-air smog contributes to respiratory problems that are common in these areas during the winter months. In warmer areas, or during the summer months in other areas, brown-air smog develops

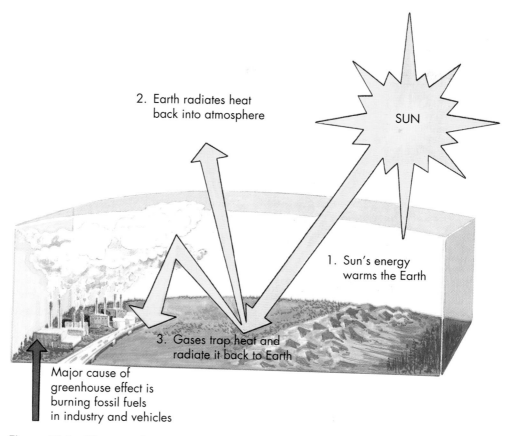

1. Sun's energy warms the Earth

2. Earth radiates heat back into atmosphere

SUN

3. Gases trap heat and radiate it back to Earth

Major cause of greenhouse effect is burning fossil fuels in industry and vehicles

Figure 19-1 The greenhouse effect.

when hydrocarbons and particulate matter from automobile exhaust interact in the presence of sunlight.[9] This photochemical smog produces ozone. Ozone is highly reactive to the human respiratory system, plants, and materials such as rubber. Regulations issued in 1998 required power plants in 22 states to reduce their nitrogen oxide emmisions; compliance should begin to reduce smog and acid rain-related damage in Eastern states.[10]

One method of reducing these gaseous pollutants is **telecommuting.** Recent advances in computer technology and communications technology are enabling more employees to work from home. Telecommuting also reduces vehicular wear and tear and reduces energy requirements and costs incurred by driving. It also reduces traffic on the roads in general.

Although telecommuting appears to have many environmental advantages, it may have drawbacks. As workers realize that they need not live near urban workplaces, many of these workers may move to more rural areas to improve their quality of life. These rural areas may not have the infrastructure to handle a massive influx of new residents.[11] Urban areas may face decay as citizens (and possibly businesses) leave cities. Forests and open land also may be destroyed as population expands in rural areas.[11]

Another environmental concern currently being studied is the destruction of the **ozone layer.** The ozone layer is important to humans because of its ability to absorb cancer-causing ultraviolet sunlight. Nitrous oxides and materials containing **chlorofluorocarbons (CFCs)** can destroy this protective ozone

greenhouse effect warming of the earth's surface that is produced when solar heat becomes trapped by layers of carbon dioxide and other gases.

acid rain rain that has a lower pH (more acidic) than that normally associated with rain.

smog air pollution made up of a combination of smoke, photochemical compounds, and fog.

telecommuting using recent advances in computer and telecommunications technology to work from an office at home, rather than commuting daily to an office in a central (usually urban) location.

ozone layer the layer of triatomic oxygen that surrounds the earth and filters much of the sun's radiation before it can reach the earth's surface.

chlorofluorocarbons (CFCs) gaseous chemical compounds that contain chlorine and fluorine.

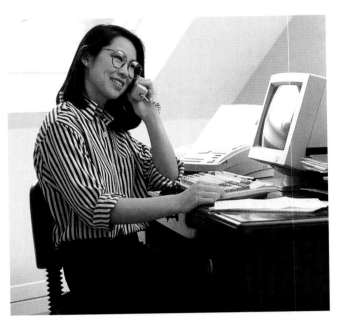

Telecommuting may be a partial answer to the problem of air pollution caused by auto emissions.

layer within the stratosphere. Nitrous oxides come from the burning of fossil fuels such as coal and gasoline. CFCs are used in air conditioners, many fast-food containers, insulation materials, and solvents.

Although changes in the ozone layer have been recognized for more than a decade, the deterioration is increasing in spite of international efforts to slow its pace. In a 1994 study, NASA reported that the annual thinning of the Antarctic ozone layer was about 9 million square miles, about the size of North America.[12] In 1998, for the first time, seasonal deterioration of this protective ozone layer extended slightly beyond the immediate Antarctic region. If the ozone layer continues to deteriorate, health dangers such as skin cancer, cataracts, snowblindness, and premature wrinkling of skin will continue to increase.

Personal Applications

• To what extent do your driving habits contribute to air pollution?

Particulate Pollutants

Many particulate pollutants exist, including both naturally occurring materials and particles derived from industrial processes, mining, agriculture, and, of course, tobacco smoke. Inhaling particulate matter can cause potentially fatal respiratory diseases, including those caused by quartz dust, asbestos fibers, and cotton fibers. Because of its widespread presence, asbestos is a particular concern. In 1989 the **Environ-**

mental Protection Agency (EPA) ordered asbestos use to be stopped by 1997 and current sources of asbestos to be removed from public buildings. In the latter regard, some people question whether the expense involved can be justified.

Trace mineral elements, including lead, nickel, iron, zinc, copper, and magnesium, are also among the particles polluting the air. Chronic **lead toxicity** is among the most serious health problems associated with this form of air pollution, although legislation requiring the use of unleaded gasoline has reduced the severity of this problem. However, even today, lead toxicity is disproportionately seen in children of low-income families, principally because of the lead-based paints found in older houses, heavy motor vehicle traffic on city streets, and the use of lead soldering in older plumbing systems. As a result, these children may bear lower IQs, attention disorders, and long-term learning disabilities. Children with high lead levels in their blood are also more likely to be impulsive, aggressive, and delinquent.[13]

Temperature Inversions

On a normal sunny day, radiant energy from the sun warms the ground and the air immediately above it. As this warmed air rises, it carries pollutants upward and disperses them into a larger, cooler air mass above. Cool air sinking to replace the rising warmed air minimizes the concentration of pollutants.

When high pressure settles over an area, warm air can be trapped immediately above the ground. Unable to rise, this trapped, warm, polluted air layer stagnates and produces a potentially health-threatening *subsidence inversion*.[9] (This is the inversion layer that meteorologists talk about on the evening news.)

A second form of thermal inversion, *radiation inversion*, is frequently seen during winter.[9] In the winter, late afternoon cooling of the ground causes a layer of cool air to develop under a higher, warmer layer of air. With the cool layer of air unable to rise, pollutants begin to accumulate near the ground and remain there until the next morning.

Indoor Air Pollution

Not all air pollution occurs outside. The health risks of indoor air pollution are a growing concern. Toxic materials, including cigarette smoke (see Chapter 9), asbestos, radon, formaldehyde, vinyl chloride, and cooking gases, can be found in buildings ranging from houses and apartments to huge office complexes and manufacturing plants.

Of all the indoor air pollutants, none is a greater concern than tobacco smoke. In December 1992 the EPA identified environmental tobacco smoke as a Group A (known human) carcinogen.[14] Gaining attention recently is formaldehyde, an indoor air pollutant that is thought to have a carcinogenic potential. A study of 55 home products, ranging from newly laid hardwood floors and fingernail hardener to latex paint and particleboard, demonstrated higher than expected levels of formaldehyde.[15]

Radon gas is a form of indoor air pollution whose role as a serious health risk is currently under investigation.[16] This radioactive gas enters buildings through a variety of routes (the water supply, block walls, slab joints, drains, even cracks in the floor) from underlying rock formations and stone building materials where it is found. Because radon gas can concentrate when air is stagnant, energy-efficient airtight homes, schoolrooms, and buildings are most affected. Radon buildup is a concern because of the relationship of radon exposure to lung cancer. A recent study involving radiation, of the same type and in equivalent amounts to that delivered by exposure to residential radon, failed to produce cancerous changes in the respiratory tracts of mice. The authors concluded that the estimated 21,800 cases of radon-induced lung cancer in humans might be somewhat overstated.[17]

Those who are concerned about the level of radon gas in their homes can purchase test kits (manufactured by some 200 companies and priced at $10 to $50) or have their homes tested by radon testing laboratories. Opponents of the "radon myth," however, suggest that these tests may generate false-positive rates greater than 90 percent.[16] Furthermore, repairing homes with high radon levels can be expensive, with some repairs costing as much as $30,000. One form of repair, the installation of a home ventilation system, may cost from $300 to $500.

Environmental tobacco smoke and radon gas join formaldehyde (from building material), vinyl chloride (from PVC plumbing), and other pollutants (including asbestos from insulation) to cause "sick building syndrome."[18] For people with respiratory illnesses and immune system hypersensitivities, as well as the elderly, home or work sites could be less healthy than was once thought. The Health Action Guide on this page describes ways to prevent indoor air pollution.

• Is your home protected from radon gas?

Health Implications

Because many health problems are complex, it is difficult to clearly assess the effects of air pollution on health. Age, gender, genetic predisposition, occupation, residency, and personal health practices complicate this assessment. Nevertheless, air pollution may severely aggravate health problems of elderly people, people who smoke or have respiratory conditions such as asthma, and people who must work in polluted air.

Water Pollution

Although water is the most abundant chemical compound on the earth's surface, maintaining a plentiful and usable supply is becoming increasingly difficult. Pollution, excessive use, and misuse are depriving people of the water they need to meet their daily needs (see Table 19-1). Observers estimate that 40 percent of the fresh water in the United States is unusable.[19]

HEALTH ACTION GUIDE

Preventing Indoor Air Pollution

To reduce the level of indoor pollution in your home, follow these simple steps. How many of these steps are you already performing?

• Hang dry-cleaned clothing outside to air out before hanging it in the closet.
• Clean humidifiers, and replace belts on a regular basis.
• Limit use of aerosol personal care products to the bare minimum.
• Store fuel for mowers, snow blowers, trimmers, and other gasoline-powered tools in an approved container in a well-ventilated area.
• Do not run the engine of a car in an attached garage or closed carport.
• Properly close containers of household cleaning products that are capable of emitting toxic fumes.
• Frequently ventilate rooms in which new carpet and drapes have been installed.
• Have fireplaces cleaned and inspected regularly.
• Eliminate cigarette smoking within the home.
• Properly discard unused paint, hobby supplies, herbicides, and pesticides regularly.
• Inspect gas appliances for proper ventilation.
• Use products that are as free as possible of asbestos and formaldehyde when remodeling.

InfoLinks
http://www.lungusa.org/learn/environment/index.html

Environmental Protection Agency (EPA) the federal agency charged with protecting natural resources and the quality of the environment.

lead toxicity a blood lead level above 25 micrograms/deciliter. (If adopted, the new standard will be 10 micrograms/deciliter.)

radon gas a naturally occurring radioactive gas produced by the decay of uranium.

Table 19-1 Home Water Use

Use	Gallons
Washing car	100
Taking a bath	36
Washing clothes	35 to 60
Washing dishes	10 to 30
Brushing teeth	10 to 20
Shaving	10 to 20
Watering the lawn	8/min
Taking a shower	7/min
Flushing the toilet	5 to 7
Leaky faucet	2/day

Yesterday's Pollution Problem

Like air pollution, water pollution is not solely a phenomenon of twentieth-century overpopulation or unchecked technology. Nature has, in fact, routinely polluted our surface and groundwater with minerals leached from the soil, acids produced by decaying vegetation, and the decomposition of animal products. In addition, people have polluted their own water supplies. Even today, people living in rural areas occasionally find that their feed lots, chicken coops, and septic tank systems polluted their water supplies.

Today's Pollution Problem

Today water sources are most often damaged by pollutants from agricultural, urban, and industrial sources. Most of these pollutants are either biological or chemical products, and many can be either removed from the water or brought within acceptable safety limits. For some pollutants, however, management technology has been only partially successful or is still being developed.

Sources of Water Pollution

Water pollution is not the result of only one type of pollutant; it has many sources.

Pathogens

Pathogenic agents, in the form of bacteria, viruses, and protozoa, enter the water supply through human and animal wastes. Communities with sewage treatment systems that combine sanitary and storm systems can, during heavy rain or snow melt, allow untreated sewage to rush through the processing plant. In addition, pathogenic organisms can enter the water supply when sewage is flushed from boats. Pathogenic agents are also introduced into the water supply from animal wastes at feed lots and at meat-processing facilities.

Sewage treatment plants and public health laboratories routinely test for the presence of pathogenic agents. Unfortunately, however, nearly one-fifth of

the U.S. population (50 million people) consumes undertreated water.[19] The presence of **coliform bacteria** in the water supply indicates contamination with human or animal feces. An unexpected example of this form of infection was seen during the summer of 1998 when water contaminated by dirty diapers infected patrons of highly popular water parks.[20]

Biological Imbalances

Aquatic plants tend to thrive in water rich in nitrates and phosphates. This leads to **eutrophication,** which can render a stream or lake unusable.[21]

During hot, dry summers, aquatic plants die in large numbers. Because the decay of vegetation requires aerobic bacterial action, the biochemical oxygen demand is high and much of the water's oxygen is used. In such conditions, fish may be killed in great numbers. **Putrefaction** of the dead fish further pollutes the water and also fouls the air.

Toxic Substances

Of the pollutants found in today's surface water and groundwater supply, perhaps none are of greater concern than toxic chemical substances. These chemical toxins, including metals and hydrocarbons, are dangerous because when in the surface water, they can enter the food chain. When they do, their concentration per unit of weight increases with each life form in the chain. By the time humans consume the fish that have fed on the contaminated lower forms of aquatic life, the toxic chemicals have been concentrated to dangerous levels.[21] In groundwater supplies, of course, toxic substances are consumed directly by humans in drinking water.

Among the important toxic substances is mercury in the form of methyl mercury. Derived from industrial wastes, methyl mercury is ingested and concentrated by shellfish and other fish. When humans eat these fish regularly, mercury levels increase to the point that hemoglobin and central nervous system function can be seriously damaged.

A variety of other metals have also been found in North American rivers, lakes, and groundwater sources. In the surface water, arsenic, cadmium, copper, lead, and silver can all enter the food chain. In many cases, one must consume only very small amounts of these metals before they become harmful.

Of the wide variety of agricultural products currently used on American and Canadian farms, pesticides and herbicides are among the most toxic. These agricultural products contain more than 1,800 different chemical compounds, adding a diverse array of chemicals to our water supply, as well as directly to the food that people eat. The level of herbicides in the water supply rises particularly rapidly during the summer.

Today experts are concerned that pesticides and herbicides contribute to the development of testicular

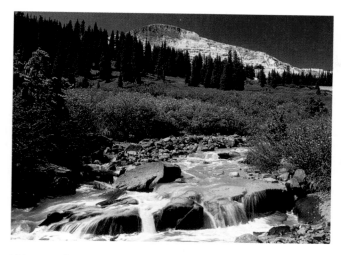

Water pollution harms the environment in both urban and rural areas. This stream is discolored by acid mine drainage.

cancer and reduced sperm production in men,[22] nervous system disorders in children, and breast cancer in women.

Among the most serious of the toxic chemicals found in our water are the chlorinated hydrocarbons, including DDT (dichlorodiphenyltrichloroethane), chlordane, and Kepone (chlordecone). Experts continue to study the **mutagenic, carcinogenic,** and **teratogenic** effects of these hydrocarbon products.

Polychlorinated biphenyls (PCBs) are another group of hydrocarbons found in the water supply that cause concern. PCBs are, on the basis of their chemical structure, very stable, heat-resistant compounds that have been used extensively in transformers and electrical capacitors. In many areas of the country, discarded electrical equipment has broken open and released PCBs into the surrounding water supply. In laboratory animals, PCBs produce liver and kidney damage, gastric and reproductive disorders, skin lesions, and tumors.[23] Researchers are studying people who have been exposed to high levels of PCBs in drinking water.

Chlorine, one of the most extensively used chemicals in industry, is now recognized as a widespread pollutant of the country's water supply, particularly in the Great Lakes. Experts believe that elevated levels of chlorine from chlorine-containing chemicals damage animals and could produce a variety of health problems in humans.

The Clean Water Act (1994) required the plastics, organic chemicals, pulp and paper processing, and wastewater management industries to replace chlorine with an acceptable substitute. Observers will closely monitor their progress in meeting the requirements.

Personal Applications

• How do your recreational activities contribute to water pollution?

Livestock Pollution

Another source of increasing concern is the contamination of surface and subsurface water supplies by animal manure. Rising levels of microbes and toxic residues are being reported in many areas of the country. In response, the Environmental Protection Agency and the Agriculture Department have issued new guidelines for safe containment and disposal of animal wastes; the guidelines are to be implemented by 2005 and 2008 for large- and small-scale producers, respectively.[24]

Other Sources

Three additional types of pollution that affect our water are important, although their effect on human health is not fully understood. The pollution from these sources harms aquatic life, damages the aesthetic value of our waterways, and reduces the recreational use of our rivers, lakes, and shores.

Oil spills include not only the severe spills resulting from tanker accidents but also spills that occur on inland waters and the seeping of crude oil from the ground. Any kind of oil spill can foul our water. Fish, aquatic plants, seabirds, and beaches can be damaged by both surface-oil film and tar masses that float below the surface or roll along the ocean bottom. The contamination of groundwater by inappropriately discarded oil-based products or by gasoline leaking from underground storage tanks is less noticeable but potentially harmful to human health.

Power plants that use water from lakes and rivers to cool their steam turbines cause thermal pollution. When this heated water is returned to its source, it can raise water temperatures significantly. As temperatures increase, the oxygen-carrying capacity of the water decreases and the balance of aquatic life forms is altered. In water that is raised only 10° C (18° F), entire species of fish can disappear and aquatic plants can proliferate out of control.

Finally, sediments in the form of sand, clay, and other soil constituents regularly reach waterway channels. Rivers, lakes, reservoirs, and oceans serve as

coliform bacteria   intestinal tract bacteria whose presence in a water supply indicates contamination by human or animal waste.

eutrophication   enrichment of a body of water with nutrients, which causes overabundant growth of plants.

putrefaction   decomposition of organic matter.

mutagenic   capable of causing genetic alterations in cells.

carcinogenic   related to the production of cancerous changes; a property of environmental agents, including drugs, that may stimulate the development of cancerous changes within cells.

teratogenic   capable of causing birth defects.

settling basins for these sediments. If we cannot return cleared land to vegetative cover, then dredging may be required to keep the waterways usable, although this is an expensive and relatively ineffective response.

Effects on Wetlands

We are losing wetlands through intentional drainage and through the dumping of debris. When we lose wetlands, countless species of fish, shellfish, birds, and marine mammals lose their habitat. By the end of this century, over half of the country's wetlands will have vanished.[25] On a more positive note, many people are making concerted efforts to reestablish wetlands throughout the country. Unfortunately, wetlands are being lost at the same time in other areas.

Health Implications

When water becomes polluted, its quality falls below acceptable standards for its intended use, and some aspects of our health are harmed (see the Health Action Guide below). Polluted water is associated with disease and illness, but it also distresses us emotionally, limits our social activities, and challenges us intellectually and spiritually to become more active stewards of our environment.

Land Pollution

Because we live, work, and play on land, we may have difficulty believing that land constitutes only about 30 percent of the earth's surface. The rest is, of course, water. The rivers, streams, marshes, and lakes found on our land surfaces make our inhabitable land seem even smaller. Uninhabitable land areas, such as

swamps, deserts, and mountain ranges, further reduce usable land. Our land is a precious commodity.

We can see the effects of our growing population on our limited land resources. However, the greatest threat to our land comes from the products our society discards: solid waste products and chemical waste products.

Solid Waste

Each year, Americans dispose of paper, newspaper, cardboard, clothing, yard waste, wood pallets, food waste, cafeteria waste, glass, metal, disposable tableware, plastics, and an endless variety of other types of municipal solid waste (MSW). Each American produces more than 4.3 pounds of MSW each year.[26]

Although MSW is an important problem, it makes up only a small amount of the solid waste discarded in this country. Agricultural, mining, and industrial wastes contribute much more to our solid waste problems. As an example, it is estimated that 800 million discarded tires can be found in mountainous piles around the country, with 100 million in Ohio alone.[27] Regardless of the source, solid waste requires some form of disposal. Traditionally, these forms have been the following:

Open dumping. Solid waste is compacted and dumped on a dump site. Open dumps are discouraged or illegal in many urban areas.

Sanitary landfill. Solid waste is compacted and buried in huge open pits. Each day, a layer of soil is pushed over the most recently dumped material to encourage decomposition, reduce unpleasant odors, and contain the material to keep it from being scattered.

Incineration. Solid waste can be incinerated. Several kinds of incinerators are used, including

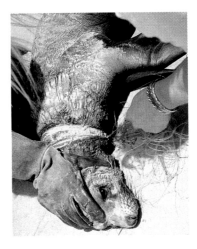

Carelessness can have a devastating effect on our natural world. Rescue workers are helping this California sea lion, which has had a fishing net wrapped tightly around its neck for months.

Learning
From Our Diversity

Stewardship of the Land: Tradition vs. Technology

Late 1998 marked the death of the Native American actor whose tear-stained face appeared in each of a series of public service commercials from the seventies and eighties urging heightened environmental awareness. The distress over the degradation of the environment so graphically depicted on his face was meant to remind us that this land had once been unspoiled and that a sacred relationship existed between it and the indigenous people who first occupied North America. Today, long after the commercials last appeared on television, we are again hearing of this enduring relationship. From Native Americans' rich oral history, we learn of their deep appreciation for the bounty of the land, their use of only that which was necessary for survival, and their willingness to protect and sustain that which was not. We also learn that the arrival of European settlers, their unchecked quest for expansion and use of

technology introduction of virulent diseases, and the eventual claim to Native American lands challenges and denigrates their tradition.

Today segments of the indigenous population seek the return of their ancestral lands through a variety of means, including the rescinding of treaties. Both within and outside this movement are persons who support its quest in part on the basis of an ecotopian vision—a belief that given time and fostering by the indigenous people, the environment eventually can return to its pristine state. For those who hold this view, no other alternative for environmental restoration would be so effective or so moral as the return of these lands. Others not only question the accuracy of the historical record regarding stewardship, but also question whether today's indigenous people could or would return to stewardship unencumbered by the demands and expectations of the twenty-first century. What do you think?

cement kilns, boilers and furnaces, and commercial incinerators.

Ocean dumping. When solid waste is close enough to the ocean, it can be collected, loaded into barges, and taken to offshore dump sites.

As consumers and environmentally concerned citizens, we need to commit to the three Rs: reduce, reuse, and recycle.

The first step is to find ways to reduce our use of materials that eventually pollute our environment. We need to become willing to make do with less, such as expecting less packaging material used with small consumer products.

Second, as concerned citizens, we all must learn to reuse as much as possible. Glass milk bottles that the dairy can reuse, as well as cloth diapers rather than the nondegradable disposable diapers, are examples of reuse.

Finally, we must recycle as much material as possible. **Recycling** will grow only as much as the demand and a market for recycled materials allows (Figure 19-2). The cost of recycling and a lack of markets for reclaimed materials often discourage municipalities and industries from practicing more recycling. Lack of time and interest, failure to understand how to recycle, messiness, and a lack of curbside pickup are also frequently mentioned as reasons for not recycling in the home. Recent experience has taught us, however, that Americans will recycle when they are given a system for collecting material.

When combined, the three Rs of reduction, reuse, and recycling could significantly reduce our need to dispose of costly toxic wastes.

Hazardous and Toxic Wastes

According to many environmental consumer group leaders, the quality of our lives is deteriorating, in part because of the unsafe disposal of hazardous chemicals from industrial and agricultural sources. This contention is based on the knowledge that each day this country produces 11 billion tons (5 billion metric tons) of solid waste, much of which is dangerously toxic in composition.[28] This waste, averaging nearly 4 pounds per person, is released into the air and water, buried in the land, sent through sewer systems, and stored in vulnerable forms in dump sites located in every state. The General Accounting Office estimates that 425,000 such sites exist; those with the highest toxic composition are classified as superfund sites. As of January 1999, 1,206 of these sites were listed by the EPA for eventual restoration, each at a cost of millions of dollars from the general revenues of the federal government.[29]

In addition, to their number, our hazardous wastes may be distributed unfairly. Poor and minority

> **recycling** the ability to convert disposable items into reusable materials.

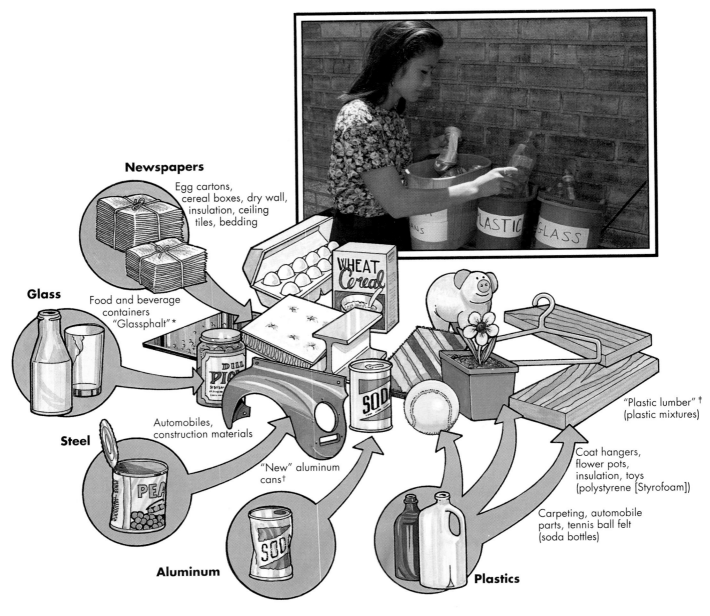

* A combination of glass and asphalt that makes an attractive roadway.
† 20 recycled aluminum cans can be made for the same amount of energy required to make one new can from ore.
‡ A durable construction material similar to wood that can be made into fence posts, decks, or park benches.

Figure 19-2 Many useful products can be made from recycled materials. The amount of material that is recycled depends on consumer demand for these products. Would you be willing to use an alternative product made from recycled components, such as a deck made of plastic lumber?

neighborhoods are often exposed to higher levels of toxic chemicals, such as hazardous waste sites, than more affluent neighborhoods.

Personal Applications

• If land reclaimed from a toxic waste dump site were very inexpensive, would you build a house there?

Pesticides

Since Rachel Carson wrote her now-classic book *Silent Spring* in 1962, the public has known the potential dangers associated with some **pesticides.** Although Carson's primary concern was the pesticide DDT, several other hazardous pesticides have since been removed from the marketplace. The EPA has restricted the use of other, less-hazardous pesticides. Farmers contend they need to use effective poisons to save their crops from insect destruction. However, ob-

The National Park Service: Managing Resources for the Enjoyment of All

With the development of Yellowstone National Park in 1872 and the establishment of the National Park Service in 1916, the United States began the systematic management of wilderness areas, national historic sites, and natural monuments for the use and enjoyment of all Americans. As stated in the original legislation, the purpose was "to conserve the scenery and the natural and historical objects and the wildlife therein and to provide for the enjoyment of the same in such manner and by such means as will leave them unimpaired for the enjoyment of future generations." Today the National Park Service manages 378 sites—covering 83 million acres—in 49 states, the District of Columbia, and five territories. The success of this pioneering effort to preserve the natural beauty, bountiful wildlife, and unique features of the public lands is reflected in efforts of more than 100 other nations to do the same.

Today the National Park Service (NPS) is using its expertise to support other versions of its approach to preserving the environment. Among these programs are the Federal Lands-to-Parks Program, in which excess federal lands, including decommissioned military bases, are being provided to state and local governments for use as wildlife and recreational areas; the Rivers, Trails, and Conservation Assistance Program, in which the NPS assists local governments and nonprofit organizations in efforts to enhance their own natural and recreational resources; and the Long Distance Trails Program, which envisions a series of trails that cross the entire country.

When these programs join the existing system of national parks, historic sites, and natural monuments, we will possess a legacy of environmental preservation and recreational opportunity for use well into the coming millennium.

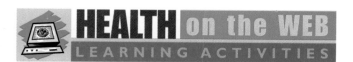

Taking a Virtual Nature Walk

Go to www.audubon.org/local/sanctuary/corkscrew/index.html to take a virtual nature walk of the National Audubon Society's Corkscrew Swamp Sanctuary. The sanctuary is near Naples, Florida and offers a refuge for owls, heron, deer, and even alligators and bears. It also contains an array of native plants, including orchids. You can explore the swamps, marshes, and forests of the sanctuary in cyberspace. Then do a keyword search to find a virtual nature tour in your part of the country.

Exploring World Population Growth

As the world's population approaches 6 billion people, the United Nations Population Fund is dedicated to studying the problem of overpopulation and finding solutions that accommodate diverse perspectives on the issue. In fact, the fund is committed to the idea that population is about people, not numbers. Go to www.unfpa.org and explore the population center, the FAQs link, and the AIDS clock. Then register to receive e-mail news updates about population issues.

Making a Habit of Recycling

As consumers and environmentally concerned citizens, we need to do more than simply control the disposal of solid waste so that it does not harm our health and that of our environment. We must also commit to the three Rs: reduce, reuse, and recycle. The Manitoba Product Stewardship Corporation (MPSC) has a website aimed solely at promoting recycling. Go to www.virtualrecycling.com/map.htm and complete a few of the many recycling quizzes that are offered. What steps can you take today to reduce, reuse, and recycle?

For more activities, log on to our Online Learning Center at www.mhhe.com/hper/health/payne

servers now are equally concerned about the effects of pesticides on food and water supplies, soil quality, animals, other insects, and humans. Recall (page 566) that pesticides (and herbicides) are increasingly present in surface and subsurface water supplies, thus exposing people who reside far beyond the point of application.

In addition, many consumers now are practicing "community-supported agriculture," an arrangement in which consumers contract directly with a farmer to buy his crops. The farmer gets a guaranteed income, and the consumers get a supply of fresh, typically organic, vegetables and fruits. See the Star Box on page 572 for a closer look at this trend.

Herbicides

Herbicides also contribute to the growing problem of water and soil pollution and to the contamination of the food chain. These weed-killing chemicals are sprayed onto plants and incorporated into the soil with plowing but are not totally taken up by the plant tissues they are intended to kill. The extent to which herbicides causes illness in humans is not fully known, although the potential appears to be significant.

Radiation

We have lived in the nuclear age since the end of World War II. With the threat of nuclear war receding, today our hopes for nuclear energy lie primarily in its enormous potential to reduce our dependence on fossil fuels as energy sources. In addition, nuclear energy can (and already does) improve our industrial and medical technology, as seen in the expanding use of radioactive materials in the diagnosis and treatment of various health disorders.

pesticides   agents used to destroy insects and other pests.

Community-Supported Agriculture Brings Organic Produce to Consumers

You could call community-supported agriculture (CSA) a grassroots trend toward healthier eating. In this arrangement, a group of ordinary consumers, anywhere from 4 to 400 "shareholders," contracts directly with a small farmer to buy his or her crop. The shareholders pay a portion of the farmer's budget, and in return, they get an array of fresh vegetables, fruits, herbs, and even flowers every week throughout the growing season.

The concept was born in Japan in 1965, when a group of women grew concerned with the amount of food being imported, and their loss of a connection to the land. They approached a farmer with their offer: We'll pay you for your supplies and labor, and you give us your crop. About 50,000 people now belong to these "teikei" (tay-kay) clubs. The idea spread to Western Europe in the 1970s and the United States in the mid-1980s. About 400 CSAs now operate in the United States.

Jill Agnew, of Sabattus, Maine, was the first CSA farmer in her state. Her Willow Pond Farm offers 35 kinds of vegetables along with fresh herbs and flowers. She has 70 shareholders, who pay $400 for a full share or $275 for a half share.

Her shareholders get more than food. Agnew also describes her more unusual vegetables in a newsletter, and on pickup days, she stays near the house and makes herself available to answer questions. She also holds a bean-threshing in the fall, and a jack-o-lantern "extravaganza" at Halloween. Her shareholders say the fresh-picked lettuce, corn, and tomatoes taste far better than anything that comes from a supermarket.

Of course, not all CSAs prosper, and not all shareholders are happy. Some shareholders complain that they must take whatever is offered each week, including food they don't like. In addition, arranging for the pickup can be difficult for some shareholders. If organic produce is available at a local co-op, some people consider the CSA to be too much hassle.

We really don't have proof that organic foods are more nutritious, admits gardening advocate Joan Gussow in *Health* magazine. The main argument for eating organically is the environment, she says. Buying produce from nearby organic farmers helps prevent more farmland from disappearing and

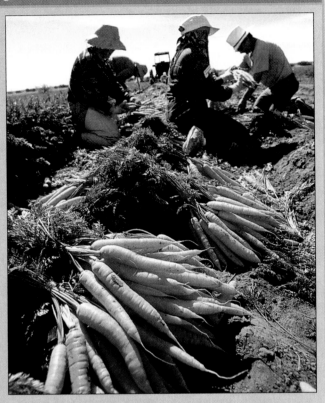

Community-supported agriculture (CSA) shareholders receive a weekly supply of seasonal fruits, vegetables, and herbs grown organically by a local farmer.

ensures that fewer chemicals taint the water supply and farm wildlife. Buying locally raised food also helps you feel like part of a complete community.

For a free list of CSAs in the United States and Canada, call the Biodynamic Farming and Gardening Association at (800) 516-7797. For the contact person and telephone number of the CSA nearest you, call Melody Newcombe, editor of the *Harvest Times*, at (914) 688-5030.

The two greatest concerns over nuclear energy are (1) the harmful health effects that come from daily exposure to radiation and (2) the potential for a nuclear accident of regional or global consequences. Some observers add a third concern, nuclear terrorism.

Fission, the decay of radioactive material, produces not only a great amount of energy but also **ionizing radiation.** We are exposed to various forms of ionizing radiation daily through natural radiation, including ultraviolet radiation and radioactive mineral deposits, and through synthetic radiation, including waste from nuclear reactors, industrial products, and x-ray examinations. Most of the exposures we get each day pose negligible health risks. Although clearly no kind of radiation

exposure is good for you, safe levels of exposure are difficult to determine.

Health Effects of Radiation Exposure

The health effects of radiation exposure depend on many factors, including the duration, type, dose of exposure, and individual sensitivity. Clearly, heavy exposure (as in a severe nuclear accident) can cause **radiation sickness** or immediate death. Lesser exposure can be very harmful as well. Particular concerns are the effects of radiation on egg and sperm production and on embryonic development, and dangerous or irreversible changes to the eyes and skin.

Avoidance of radiation exposure may be difficult to achieve, however, because of the need to safely collect, transport, and store the 36,826 metric tons of spent uranium fuel being stored in nuclear facilities around the country. As work progresses on a massive underground storage facility near Carlsbad, New Mexico, cement "dry casks"—containing waste deteriorate in aboveground storage facilities, while plans for their movement westward cause increasing concern in communities along proposed routes.[30]

Personal Applications

• How close to a nuclear power plant would you feel comfortable living?

Electromagnetic Radiation

What do water-bed heaters, electric razors, electric blankets, high-tension electrical transmission lines, and cellular telephones have in common? They all produce electromagnetic fields or electromagnetic waves that come close to the body or pass very near your home, as in the case of transmission lines.

Recently, some people have voiced fears that the electromagnetic fields generated by these familiar devices could cause cancer. Research using laboratory animals and studies comparing the incidence of cancer in people using these devices with those who do not have been inconclusive. A recent study of 138,905 utility workers who were exposed to electromagnetic fields through power lines did, however, show a higher-than-expected rate of death from brain cancer.[31]

Therefore, in light of this study and until we have more research on non-employment-related exposure, we should exercise some care in the use of appliances that generate radiation fields. For example, water-bed heaters should be turned on early to allow the bed to warm and then turned off after one goes to bed, cellular telephone calls should be kept short, and a morning shave should not last more than a few minutes.

Personal Applications

• The environmental focus of the 1990s has shifted from global concerns, such as the ozone layer, to local concerns, such as recycling. Will it now be possible to "think globally while acting locally"?

Nuclear Reactor Accidents and Waste Disposal

To generate the nuclear energy used to produce electrical energy, more than 100 nuclear power plants have been constructed in North America. Built mostly by utility companies, these nuclear power plants were designed to produce electrical energy in an efficient, economical, and safe manner. Critics claim that their safety and efficiency have not been documented.

These fears were reinforced on April 26, 1986, when the Chernobyl nuclear power plant in the then Soviet Union experienced a **meltdown.** Human error created a situation that allowed excessive heat to build up in the core of the nuclear reactor. The resultant explosion killed two people, hospitalized hundreds, and exposed hundreds of thousands of people to nuclear radiation. As a result of the Chernobyl accident, the Soviet government had to resettle 200,000 people at an estimated cost of $26 billion. Furthermore, a leading Soviet scientist estimated that 10,000 miners and soldiers died as a result of exposure to radiation received during cleanup operations after the accident. Families exposed to the explosion of the Chernobyl nuclear power plant are having children with genetic mutations at twice the rate of other families.

In the United States, residents downwind of the accident at Three Mile Island in 1979 suffered an increase in leukemia and lung cancer, according to a recent study. These people faced five times the risk of lung cancer and seven times the risk of leukemia.

Disposing of nuclear waste safely is another serious problem that has not been fully solved. The by-products of nuclear fission remain radioactive for many years. Although the current method of disposing of these wastes is to bury them, they could eventually leak into our environment, posing a serious threat.

Proponents of nuclear power maintain that not one person in the United States has died as the result of a power plant accident, and they remind us that our fossil fuel supply is limited. Supporters of the nuclear industry believe that a public commitment to establishing more nuclear reactors is important to the future of our country. Nearly 20 percent of our electrical energy is currently generated by nuclear power.

Another concern about nuclear power generation is what to do with reactors that have outlived their usefulness. By the year 2012 it is projected that nearly a dozen nuclear power plants will be closed and their reactors dismantled. These "spent" reactors could be buried in nuclear waste landfills, but more

---

ionizing radiation a form of radiation capable of releasing electrons from atoms.

radiation sickness an illness characterized by fatigue, nausea, weight loss, fever, bleeding from mouth and gums, hair loss, and immune deficiencies, caused by overexposure to ionizing radiation.

meltdown the overheating and eventual melting of the uranium fuel rods in the core of a nuclear reactor.

likely they will be sold to other countries that may or may not be able to operate them safely.[32]

Radiation Tests

In 1995 we learned that 16,000 American citizens (prisoners, children, mentally retarded people, pregnant women, and patients in public hospitals) were intentionally exposed to nuclear radiation between World War II and 1970. In 435 separate projects, of which about 10 percent are now known to have been excessively dangerous, radiation was used to determine how the human body functions and to develop the procedures that now make up nuclear medical technology. Concern arose in 1998 about the possibility of an estimated 75,000 cases of thyroid cancer in persons exposed to fallout during Cold War nuclear testing. This concern is being investigated, but experts have advised against wide-scale screening at this time.[33, 34]

Noise Pollution

Noise is an unwanted sound that can damage our overall health. In some cases a sound that is desirable, such as music, can function as a true noise because of the intensity of the sound. Today's world is characterized by sounds whose loudness and unrelenting presence are dangerous to our health. These intense sounds can reduce our hearing acuity, disrupt our emotional tranquility, infringe on our social interaction, and interrupt our concentration.

Noise-Induced Hearing Loss

Sound, or a wave of compressed air molecules moving in response to a pressure change, is characterized by two qualities—frequency and intensity. High intensity is primarily responsible for the loss of hearing experienced by many people living in noise-polluted environments. Sound intensity exceeding 80 to 85 decibels (1,200 to 4,800 cycles-per-second frequency) can damage hearing. The Star Box above shows sound intensity associated with several common environmental sound sources.

The interpretation of a sound (hearing) is a sophisticated and sensitive physiological process in which acoustical energy is converted to mechanical energy, then to hydraulic energy, and, finally, to electrochemical energy. Electrochemical energy is then transmitted by the acoustic nerve to the brain for interpretation. High-intensity sounds damage hearing by destroying special hair cells in the inner ear that convert hydraulic energy into electrochemical energy. Loud music, jet engine noise, vehicular traffic, and a wide variety of industrial noises can collapse these sensitive cells. Ironically, the cells that are damaged are those responsible for hearing the high-frequency sounds associated with normal conversation, not those that hear the damaging sound itself. Thus the environmental sources of noise

HEALTH ACTION GUIDE

Reducing Noise Pollution

You can support legislation and enforcement policies designed to reduce environmental noise pollution. But what else can you do to reduce noise pollution in your life? Following are a few recommended approaches:

- Limit your exposure to highly amplified music. The damage from occasional exposure to sound intensity between 110 and 120 decibels can be reversible. Daily exposure, however, will permanently damage hearing.
- Reduce the volume on your portable headset. If others can hear the music coming through your headset while you are wearing it, you should probably turn down the volume.
- Wear ear plugs (wax or soft plastic) and sound-absorbing ear muffs when using firearms or operating loud machinery.
- Keep your automobile, motorcycle, and lawn mower exhaust systems in good working order.
- Furnish your room, apartment, home, and office with sound-absorbing materials. Drapes, carpeting, and cork wall tiles are excellent for reducing both interior and exterior noises.
- Establish noise reduction as a criterion in choosing your residence. An apartment complex near a freeway or airport or property near an interstate highway may prove to be undesirable.

Because you have a lifetime of hearing ahead of you, efforts to reduce noise pollution deserve your participation and support.

InfoLinks
http://www.nonoise.org/

Organizations Related to Environmental Concerns

Federal Departments, Agencies, and Offices
Environmental Protection Agency, 401 M St. S.W., Washington, DC 20460; (202) 382-2090
Council of Environmental Quality, 722 Jackson Pl. N.W., Washington, DC 20503; (202) 395-5750
Department of Energy, Forrestal Bldg., 1000 Independence Ave. S.W., Washington, DC 20585; (202) 586-6210
Department of the Interior, Interior Bldg., 1849 C St. N.W., Washington, DC 20240; (202) 208-3100
National Oceanic and Atmospheric Administration, Rockville, MD 20852; (301) 443-8910
United States Fish and Wildlife Service, 1849 C Street, N.W., Washington, DC 20240; (202) 208-5634

National Organizations
National Wildlife Federation, 1400 16th St. N.W., Washington, DC 20036; (202) 797-6800 and (800) 432-6564
Sierra Club, 730 Polk St., San Francisco, CA 94109; (415) 776-2211
Cousteau Society, Inc., 870 Greenbriar Circle, Suite 402, Chesapeake, VA 23320 (804) 523-9335
Greenpeace USA, 1436 U Street, N.W., Washington, DC 20009; (202) 462-1177
The Wilderness Society, 900 17th Street, N.W., Washington, DC 20006; (202) 833-2300
The Nature Conservancy, 1815 N. Lynn St., Arlington, VA, 22209; (703) 841-5300
The Environmental Defense Fund, 257 Park Avenue South, New York, NY 10010; (800) 684-3322

Canadian Organization
Environment Canada, Ottawa, Ontario K1A OH3; (819) 997-1441

rob you of your ability to hear sound of a far greater value—the sound of the unamplified human voice.

The damage just described is initially reversible. However, the changes in the sensitive cells of the inner ear become permanent with continued exposure. The Health Action Guide above suggests ways to reduce noise pollution.

Noise as a Stressor

Besides damaging our hearing, noise has a recognized effect as a stressor. Indeed, the absence of noise (silence) and prolonged noise are both proven techniques to break the will of prisoners during war. Researchers have recently shifted their attention to the role of noise in the stress response, as presented in Chapter 3. In people stressed by unrelenting noise, elevated epinephrine levels contribute to hypertension and other stress-related health problems.

In Search of Balance

How often have you heard people yearn for a return to the "good old days"? They reminisce about times when people moved more slowly, cared more for their neighbors, and appreciated their natural resources. After listening to these nostalgic impressions,

Personal Applications

- Would you be willing to spend more for a lightbulb designed to burn for 20,000 hours, use little energy, and last several years than for a much less expensive incandescent bulb?

you could believe that our society was once almost idyllic—with little or no pollution, population concerns, or threats of nuclear accidents.

Certainly it is nice to dream, but our advancing technology and exploding worldwide population probably will not permit us to find such an ideal world. Instead, we need to find the appropriate balance between technological growth and environmental deterioration. Perhaps some of the organizations listed in the Star Box above can help us in our efforts.

We must learn to think beyond the present. With each choice we make we should consider its influence on our environmental systems (see the Star Box on p. 576). If we base our decisions solely on financial gain or personal convenience, we will commit a monumental disservice to our planet, our children, and future generations.

Your Role in Creating a Sustainable Environment

As we search for solutions to complex environmental problems, we may have to make some difficult decisions. For example, will people in developing countries be forced to use contraception or sterilization? Will we attempt to feed the world's hungry people? Will we continue to protect endangered species of plants and animals? Will we push more forcefully for nuclear disarmament? Can we commit ourselves to cleaning up all of our toxic waste sites? Answers to these complex questions about stewardship will probably be based on not only our knowledge but also our moral predispositions.

We can answer these sorts of complex questions by recognizing the value of a sustainable environment. We will develop this environment only when individuals and groups are willing to do the following:

• Evaluate their environment

• Become environmentally educated

• Choose a simpler, less consumption-oriented lifestyle

• Recognize the limitations of technology in solving problems

• Become involved in environmental protection activities

• Work with people on all sides of environmental issues

These suggestions might sound abstract for a person confronting a local environmental problem. However, each of these steps can be applied to a local situation with only limited modifications. The PCB soil contamination in Indiana, the nerve gas weapons storage in Kentucky, the toxic waste site cleanup in Missouri, and the transportation of nuclear waste materials in California and other states are local issues to which these steps can be applied. Are you sufficiently committed to a sustainable environment to practice these steps?

Real Life
Real choices

Your Turn

• What are the major sources of air and water pollution in the environment today?
• What are the sources of environmental pollution in David Cloudwalker's hometown?
• Do you think environmental damage falls more heavily on poor people and/or minorities? Why or why not?

And Now, Your Choices . . .
• If you had grown up in circumstances similar to David's, how would you react to student "clean air" demonstrators on your campus?
• If you were one of the demonstrators on David's campus, how would you respond to his observation that signs and marches won't clean up the mess in our environment?

Summary

• World population is increasing at an alarming rate and damaging the environment.
• Gases and solid pollutants contribute to air pollution and its associated health risks.
• Worldwide increases in carbon dioxide production could produce a greenhouse effect, leading to climatic warming and extreme weather conditions.
• Acid rain, acid fog, acid snow, and smog are caused by the release of gaseous and particulate pollutants into the air.
• Deterioration of the ozone layer could expose us to high levels of ultraviolet radiation and serious health problems.
• Particulate matter, including fibers and trace mineral elements, is found in the air.
• Temperature inversions increase the intensity of air pollution.
• Indoor air pollution is recognized as a serious threat to health, particularly from radon gas, which can easily accumulate in modern houses.

• Water pollution results from a variety of causes, including toxic chemicals and pathogens from human and animal wastes.
• Increased levels of pesticides and herbicides can be found in both surface water and groundwater.
• Chlorine from a variety of sources, including PCBs, can also be found in both surface water and groundwater.
• Municipal solid waste is a small but important component of all solid waste.
• Solid wastes are traditionally buried, dumped, or incinerated.
• Reduction, reuse, and recycling are important methods of reducing environmental pollution.
• Toxic wastes from both industry and agriculture are serious sources of land pollution.
• Eating more organic vegetables, such as found at a farmer's market or purchased through community-supported agriculture (CSA), is one way to reduce

the amount of pesticides and herbicides we consume and that are added to the environment.
- Pesticides and herbicides have been found to pollute land, in addition to water.
- Radiation, including ultraviolet and ionizing radiation from nuclear power plants, could produce serious health problems.

- Electromagnetic radiation may be associated with severe health problems, including brain cancer.
- Noise pollution can cause hearing loss, particularly the ability to hear the human voice.
- We must seek a balance between lifestyle and the health of the environment, not only for our generation but for those that will follow.

Review Questions

1. In what direction is the world population changing? What could be the effects of this change on the environment? How can we modify this rate of change?
2. What is the greenhouse effect? How does deforestation affect this process? What is the expected consequence of the greenhouse effect?
3. How are acid rain, acid fog, and acid snow produced? What and where is the damage they cause?
4. What is causing the deterioration of the ozone layer? What step has been taken to slow this process? What are the consequences of ozone layer deterioration?
5. What are the major particulate pollutants in our air? What is the principal risk associated with lead as a pollutant? What specific diseases are associated with particulate material in our air?
6. How are gray-air smog and brown-air smog formed? When and where is one form more likely to be seen than the other?
7. What air pollutant is classified as a Group A carcinogen? What other pollutants contribute to indoor air pollution? What risks are associated with radon gas?
8. What toxic chemicals are most often the sources of water pollution? What is the consequence of

having too little oxygen dissolved in water? What is thermal pollution? How do pesticides and herbicides enter both our water supply and soil? What is the principal source of the chlorine found in water?
9. What are two advantages of organic food? What is community-supported agriculture?
10. What are several forms of municipal solid waste? How much municipal solid waste does the typical person produce per day? How much do Americans produce in a year?
11. How do people most often dispose of solid wastes? Why are these techniques not acceptable?
12. What are the three Rs of better solid waste prevention?
13. What are the principal sources of radiation that concern us today? Which are natural sources of radiation, and which are the result of human intervention? What familiar appliances may be sources of electromagnetic fields?
14. How does noise pollution cause hearing loss? What are the most common sources of noise pollution?
15. For whom is a balance between a modern lifestyle and a healthful environment important?

References

1. The environment and population growth: decade for action. *Population Reports* Series 1992; M. 20(10):2–3.
2. Green CP. Environment & population (suppl). *Population Reports* Series 1992; M. 20(10).
3. *EPA's revised ozone standards.* (Fact sheet.) U.S. Environmental Protection Agency, Office of Air & Radiation, Office of Air Quality Planning & Standards, July 17, 1997.
4. *EPA's revised particulate matter standards.* (Fact sheet.) U.S. Environmental Protection Agency, Office of Air & Radiation, Office of Air Quality Planning & Standards, July 17, 1997.
5. *Proposed regional haze regulations for protection of visibility in national parks and wilderness areas.* (Fact sheet.) U.S. Environmental Protection Agency, Office of Air &

Radiation, Office of Air Quality Planning & Standards, July 18, 1997.
6. Watson T. U.S. signs international global warming treaty. *USA Today* 1998 Nov 13:19A.
7. *National personal transportation survey.* Washington, DC: Federal Highway Administration, Sept 1997.
8. Climatic Research Unit, University of East Anglia. As reported in *Newsweek* 1996 Jan 22.
9. Chiras D. *Environmental science: action for a sustainable future.* 4th ed. Redwood City, CA: Benjamin-Cummings, 1994.
10. EPA: 5 states in region must make plants cut nitrogen oxide. *EPA Environmental News Release.* No. 98-OPAA83, Sept 24, 1998.

11. Information superhighway: an environmental menace. *USA Today Magazine* 1995 Sept; 124(2604).
12. Ozone hole. *USA Today* 1994 Oct 7: 3A.
13. Needleman H et al. Bone lead levels and delinquent behavior. *JAMA* 1996; 275(5):363–69.
14. *Respiratory health effects of passive smoking: lung cancer and other diseases.* Office of Health and Environment, Office of Research and Development, U.S. Environmental Protection Agency, Dec 1992.
15. Kelly TJ, Smith DL, Satola J. Emission rates of formaldehyde from materials and consumer products found in California homes. *Environ Sci Technol* 1999; 33(1):81–88.
16. Cole L. *Element of risk: the politics of radon.* New York: Oxford University Press, 1994.
17. Miller RC et al. The oncogenic transforming potential of the passage of single particles through mammalian cell nuclei. *PNAS* 1999; 96(1):19–22.
18. Hedge A, Erickson W. *Sick building syndrome and office ergonomics: a targeted work environment.* Cornell University: Human Factors Laboratory, College of Human Ecology, Feb 24, 1998. http://www.news.cornell.edu/release/feb98/sickbuilding.ssl.html
19. Kanamine L. *40% of fresh water is unusable.* U.S. Environmental Protection Agency. As reported in *USA Today* 1994 April 21:1A.
20. Manning A. E. coli cases: 6 kids still hospitalized. *USA Today* 1998 June 26:4A.
21. Cunningham WP, Saigo B. *Environmental science: a global concern.* Dubuque, IA: WCB/McGraw-Hill, 1998.
22. Gray LE, Ostby J. Effects of pesticides and toxic substances on behavioral and morphological reproductive development: endocrine versus non-endocrine mechanisms. *Toxicol Ind Health* 1998; 14(1–2):159–84.
23. Miler GT. *Living in the environment: an introduction to environmental science.* 7th ed. Belmont, CA: International Thompson, 1992.
24. USDA, EPA announce joint strategy for animal feeding operations. *Headquarters press release.* U.S. Environmental Protection Agency, Sept 16, 1998. Draft copy available at: http://www.epa.gov/owm/afostrat.htm
25. Cunningham WP. *Understanding our environment.* Dubuque, IA: William C. Brown, 1994.
26. Franklin W, Franklin M. Putting the crusade into perspective: recycling and waste generation both are on the rise. *EPA Journal* 1992; 18(3):7.
27. Piling up. Scrap Tire Management Council. As reported in *USA Today* 1997 May 27:11A.
28. *Solid, toxic, and hazardous waste.* University of Miami (Ohio). Data supplied by the EPA. Jan 30, 1999. http://www.muohio.edu/~200cwis/200_121b/cs4_23.htm
29. *Final National Priorities List (NPL) sites.* Environmental Protection Agency. Jan 19, 1999. http://www.epa.gov/superfund/sites/nplfin.htm
30. *Nuclear fuel waste nationwide.* Nuclear Association of Regulatory Commissions, Nuclear Regulatory Commission, Dec 1998. http://www.nrc.gov/NRC/radwaste.html
31. Savitz DA, Loomis DP. Magnetic field exposure in relation to leukemia and brain cancer mortality among electric utility workers. *Am J Epidemiol* 1995; 141(2):123–28.
32. Hoversten P. Nuclear plant up for grabs in going-out-of-business sale. *USA Today* 1998 July 13.
33. *Exposure of the American people to Iodine-131 from Nevada atomic bomb tests: review of the National Cancer Institute report and public health implications.* National Academy of Sciences/National Academy of Engineering, National Academy Press, Sept 1998.
34. *Committee on thyroid screening related to Iodine-131 exposure* (report). Institute of Medicine, Board of Health Care Services, Sept 1998.

Suggested Readings

Tisdale ME, Booth B eds. *Beyond the national parks: a recreation guide to public lands in the west.* Washington, DC: Smithsonian Institution Press, 1998. Compiled by the Bureau of Land Management, this highly informative 400-page book describes in narrative and pictures regional areas of beauty and recreational potential. Detailed information is given about specific activities and seasonal weather conditions.

Freyfogle ET. *Bounded people, boundless lands: envisioning a new land ethic.* Washington, DC: Island Press, 1998. Far from a travel guide, Freyfogle's book represents a serious study of the legal, ethical, and moral dimensions of various environmental issues and the ways in which they interface with people's desire to live comfortably on this planet. The author uses his background as a legal scholar, and a case study approach, to shed light on the resolution of environmentally related concerns.

Benedick RE. *Ozone diplomacy: new directions in safeguarding the planet.* Cambridge, MA: Harvard University Press, 1998. In 1987 and again in 1990 when the international community met in Montreal to establish guidelines for dealing with pandemic environmental problems such as ozone depletion and global warming, the author presented the position of the United States. This book relates his view of the diplomacy and personalities that formulated the Montreal Protocol on Substances that Deplete the Ozone Layer. A fascinating aspect of the book is the interplay of environmental, legal, political, and economic variables in reaching an accord.

Spies JR. *Big cats & other animals: their beauty, dignity & survival.* Hollywood, FL: Lifetime Books, 1998. For the animal lover and the environmentalist, this beautifully photographed book depicts a variety of animals as they live both in captivity and in the wild. Because the author visually depicts his subjects in the context of their unique ecosystems, readers may better understand how imbalances in these systems affect these impressive animals.

topics for Today

Xeriscaping: Caring for Your Corner of the World

Project yourself a few years into the future to a time when you are a homeowner. You find yourself with the responsibility for a very hungry yard—it eats money from your pocket and time from your weekend. If you already have a house, you probably know this all too well. If you've only helped with outdoor chores occasionally and think that it's fun, just wait for the novelty to wear off. Granted, it *is* fun to spend time outside, but it shouldn't be all work and no play. You should have time left to enjoy your yard.

Xeriscaping is a way to reduce the amount of money and time you spend on your yard and do your part for the environment too. *Xeriscaping* means "dry landscaping."[1] In Xeriscaping, a trade name for "wildscaping" or "natural landscaping," excessive watering is unnecessary because the native plants used are adapted to the rainfall amounts of the region. Technologies that conserve water so that less goes to waste also reduce the overall need for water, contributing further to the "dry" concept.[2] In addition to a reduced water requirement, natural (indigenous) plants require less maintenance and attract local wildlife. To create such a landscape requires the use of drought-tolerant plant material, a water-conserving design, an overall reduction in turf, the effective use of mulches, and proper maintenance practices. Once the landscape is in place, a 30 percent to 50 percent reduction in household water use may be achieved.[1] As real estate development continues, what we do with our one-third acre corner of the world becomes increasingly important.

Why Is Xeriscaping Important?

It's important to understand our yards so that we can take steps to end the pesticide-fertilizer-irrigation cycle. Homeowners, in fact, use up to ten times more chemical pesticides per acre than farmers do. Quite a few problems are caused by pesticide overuse. First, some pests become resistant to a particular pesticide so that heavier and heavier applications or a more toxic chemical must be used to achieve the same kill rate. Second, when we destroy one pest we can't foresee what

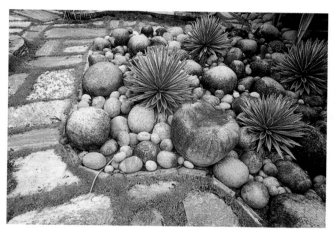

Xeriscaping uses native plants to reduce the need for water, pesticides, and fertilizer.

species will take its place, possibly leaving us worse off than with the original pest. Third, pesticides kill beneficial organisms in addition to the target species.[3]

The use of fertilizers is also a complicated issue. Fertilizers make the soil inhospitable for natural decomposers, such as earthworms and microbes. With fewer of these decomposers, nutrients are returned to the environment more slowly. More fertilizer is then needed to make up for the lack of naturally provided nutrients. Chemicals should be introduced only with great caution, since they weaken natural defenses and disrupt nutrient cycling.[3] Native plant species don't need chemical fertilizers, and natural insect predators reduce the need for pesticides.

Excessive fertilization, which causes the blades of grass to grow at the expense of the roots, also increases the need for irrigation.[3] For example, one-quarter of San Antonio's residential water supply is used for lawns and gardens, helping to drain the aquifer to levels low enough to threaten natural springs and endangered species, as well as future water supplies. Irrigation can cost the individual homeowner up to $50 a month.[4] Xeriscaping reduces outdoor water costs by up to 80 percent.[5] And by keeping your house warmer in the winter and cooler in the summer, it can trim 30 percent off your heating bill and 75 percent off your air conditioning bills.[6]

By using fewer chemicals and less water and energy, you can have a yard with many more plant and animal species, a variety of colors and shapes, seasonal beauty, and drought-resistant ground covering. The plants will do the work for you. For example, even the much-maligned dandelion has a function in nature's plan. The early-flowering dandelion is important to bees, who have spent the winter without pollen sources. In addition, its large taproot opens passageways in the soil and brings nutrients to the surface, fertilizing the lawn. Clover, only recently thought of as a weed, was a common part of lawns until a few decades ago. Clover's roots anchor the soil, which reduces soil erosion, and its white flowers provide food for bees. In addition, microorganisms that thrive on its roots can "fix" nitrogen (take it from the air and convert it to a form that plants can use).[3]

These and other plants are not naturally weeds. A weed is simply a plant that's growing someplace you don't want it to grow. Yes, weeds are just misunderstood plants. You may not be so eager to kill a weed if you understand its ecological role. According to this view, exotic plants that are not native to a given environment can be seen as weeds. This is especially true when exotic plants spread from private yards to parks and other natural areas, where they outcompete the local vegetation because they have no natural enemies.

Another benefit of Xeriscaping is that a yard planted with more than 50 percent native plant species provides food, water, and shelter for butterflies, songbirds, hummingbirds, and other animals, bringing your backyard to life with sight and sound.[7] The table below shows an example of a natural landscape in the San Antonio/Dallas, Texas, area. Keep in mind, though, that Xeriscaping can be used in almost any region of the country—this plan is just a sample.

The Traditional Lawn Reexamined

Although humankind's struggle to understand and control nature is ancient, the lawn itself did not originate until the eighteenth century in England and France. Grass was an important food for sheep and cattle in these regions, and these grazing animals or hand scythes were used to keep lawns in check until 1830, when Edwin Budding invented the first lawn mower. In 1901 the U.S. Congress allotted $17,000 to study the best native and foreign grass species for turfing lawns and pleasure grounds.[3] From these humble beginnings, a $25-billion-a-year lawn industry was born.

According to one environmental historian, the lawn industry is "part science, part aesthetics, part peer pressure, and increasingly part marketing."[3] The industry relies on technology, such as mowers, sod, seed, fertilizer, pesticides, herbicides, watering devices, and other tools, rather than on natural processes. An industrial or traditional lawn contributes to global warming by adding CO_2 to the atmosphere from fossil fuel–powered machinery and fossil energy used to pump water. The production of fertilizers and pesticides used to care for these lawns also contributes to global warming. Maintenance of a traditional lawn, then, upsets natural nutrient balance in the soil, inhibits growth of native plants, disturbs predator-prey relationships, and depletes groundwater. But what can one homeowner do?

Getting Started

The Texas Parks and Wildlife Department distributes information packets on using native plants in your yard to reduce resource consumption and offset habitat loss. If such packets aren't readily available in your area, you can find assistance with natural landscaping from botanical gardens, arboretums, native plant societies, county extension services, and other organizations.[6] You can reach the National Wildlife Federation's Backyard Wildlife Habitat Program at 1-800-822-9919. Some parks and recreation departments, colleges or universities, and commercial nurseries offer courses on Xeriscaping.

Xeriscaping requires a little thought and planning at the start, but you can return your yard to a natural state in stages over several months or years.[7] To start with, choose native plants that will thrive under the current conditions of your yard. Keep in mind which parts of the yard are sunny, shady, wet,

San Antonio/Dallas, Texas, Native Landscape Plan[7]

Nectar Source	Wildlife Area	Pond Area	Screening	Accessories
Clematis vine	American beautyberry	Buttonbush	Coral honeysuckle	Purple martin house
Lantana	Cherry laurel	Cardinal flower	Dwarf wax myrtle	Bat house
Mistflower	Mexican plum	Horsetail	Passion flower vine	
Scarlet sage	Persimmon	Louisiana iris		
Verbena	Swamp chestnut oak	Swamp lily		
		Halberd-leaf Hibiscus		

dry, and so on. Writing down your plan will help you stay organized. The seven steps outlined in the following box will help you get started:

> **7 Steps to Xeriscaping[6]**
> 1. Think about yard use, such as lawn games and children's play areas.
> 2. Improve the soil with organic matter, compost, or peat, which all hold moisture well.
> 3. Use turf only where needed; plant other ground cover elsewhere.
> 4. Select nursery-raised native plants, which are more likely to survive when transplanted.
> 5. Water the yard efficiently, setting sprinklers close to the ground; don't water the driveway or sidewalk.
> 6. Use organic mulches to help prevent weed growth and reduce erosion and water loss.
> 7. Watch for signs that watering is needed, rather than watering on a rigid schedule.

Bringing Your Neighbors on Board

You may encounter some resistance when you decide to return your yard to a natural state. For example, weed laws or ordinances may restrict the height of vegetation.[8] But there are legal precedents for granting variances from these laws to natural landscapers. Experts have determined that natural landscapes do not create fire hazards, are not health menaces, and do not depreciate property values.[9]

Because your yard is out of the ordinary, you might also hear objections from your neighbors. To make them more comfortable with your changes, you may want to border your planting areas to make them look more intentional. Putting up a sign that says something like "Susie's Nature Restoration" or "Bob's Butterfly Garden" adds legitimacy to your efforts, as does registering your site with the National Wildlife Federation's Backyard Wildlife Habitat Program or the National Institute for Urban Wildlife.[8]

Why go through all this trouble? Once established, your natural area will require less maintenance than a traditional lawn, which saves you time and money. A desire to experiment, enjoy wildlife, and be environmentally responsible are other reasons people take "the path less mowed."[3] And times are changing. In some American cities, nontraditional yards are more the rule than the exception. In Novato, California, homeowners are given cash incentives for reducing the amount of grass in their yard, and in Aurora, Colorado, an ordinance prohibits new residents from having more than half of their landscaped area in bluegrass. Any other turf must be a drought-resistant variety.

Think Globally, Act Locally

By caring for your yard, you can demonstrate your care for the planet. Even if you're not prepared to completely Xeriscape your yard, you can still do your part to conserve resources, reduce the amount of chemicals in the environment, and reduce waste.

Yard waste is the second largest component of the 160 million tons of solid waste produced each year. Grass clippings alone make up three-quarters of all yard waste. You can reduce this waste and benefit your yard by not bagging the clippings, leaving the cut grass to act as fertilizer. Keep the mower blade sharp enough to make clean cuts, which reduces the evaporation from the cuts. Cut the grass a little taller, since longer blades of grass shade the soil, reducing evaporation and decreasing root stress.

By understanding natural dynamics and updating the traditional lawn to fit our environmentally conscious times, all of us can feel more at home on this planet.

For Discussion . . .

Would you consider Xeriscaping your yard? To what extent? Do you know anyone who has a nontraditional yard? Have you asked them for a tour?

References

1. DeAguero A. *Xeriscaping.* Marriott Management Services. http://cagesun.nmsu.edu/AGRICULTURAL/wcc/xeri/index.html
2. Clinton B. Memorandum on environmentally beneficial landscaping. *Weekly Compilation of Presidential Documents* 1994; 30(17):16–17.
3. Bormann FH, Balmori D, Gebelle GT. *Redesigning the American lawn: a search for environmental harmony.* New Haven, CT: Yale University Press, 1993.
4. Zolfo S. A wilder San Antonio. *Audubon* 1996; 98(4):99–101.
5. Texans find xeriscaping can save on water, maintenance, money. *U.S. water news online.* Nov 1996. http://www.usawaternews.com/archive/96/conserv/textfin.html
6. Moffat A, Scheler M. *Energy-efficient and environmental landscaping.* 1994. http://www.ecodesign.bc.ca/res/eclib/ftx130.htm
7. *Planning your natural landscape.* Austin, TX: Texas Parks and Wildlife Department, 1996.
8. EPA. *Natural landscaping—Great Lakes Region.* 1996. Milwaukee, WI, Natural Landscapers, Ltd.
9. Rappaport B. Godmother of natural landscaping. *National Wildlife* 1996; 34(3):62.

chapter
twenty

Protecting
Your Safety

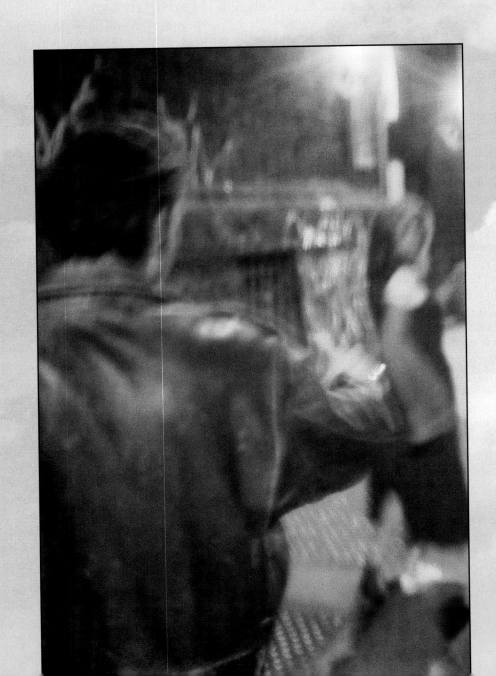

As recently as twenty years ago, the suspicious disappearance of a school-aged child or a domestic act of terrorism was virtually unheard of. In the late 1990s, several violent crimes have been the subject of intense media scrutiny and public outrage: the killings of reproductive health physician Dr. Barnett Slepian, designer Gianni Versace, and the Oklahoma City and Olympic Park bombings have received exhaustive press coverage. Several heinous sexual assaults and murders of children—Megan Kanka, JonBenet Ramsey, and Girl X in Chicago—have also generated much attention and angered the public. Most recently, multiple killings in public schools have shocked the nation.

HEALTHY PEOPLE: LOOKING AHEAD TO 2010

Like the *Healthy People 2000* objectives, the *Healthy People 2010* document will target goals in the two broad focus areas of violence and abusive behavior and unintentional injuries, the topics of this chapter. The mid-1990s assessment of progress in the area of violence indicated that the nation had moved closer to reaching only 3 of 18 objectives. First, suicide rates remained stable for the population as a whole, although suicide rates for young men were on the rise. Second, the incidence of rape and reported rape had declined. Third, fewer adolescents ages 14 to 17 were carrying weapons.

At mid-decade, the nation had lost ground in the areas of homicide, firearm-related deaths, assault injuries, and suicide attempts by adolescents. Public

health officials predicted that if the mid-1990s murder trends continued, the rate of firearm deaths would exceed the rate of traffic fatalities by 2003. Fortunately, it appears that homicide and firearm deaths have leveled off considerably.

The data concerning national health objectives in the area of safety were much more positive. Reports issued in the mid-1990s indicated progress toward achieving 14 of 16 objectives in the area of unintentional injuries. However, no gains had been made in reducing hip fractures among older adults and increasing the use of smoke detectors. We can expect continued progress toward achieving the safety objectives now being formulated for the *Healthy People 2010* document.

Real Life
Real choices

Date Rape: Shattered Trust

- **Names:** Debra Hemsath and Ron Mayer
- **Ages:** 19 and 20
- **Occupations:** College students

"I kept saying no, but he didn't stop. Even when I started screaming, he just wouldn't stop. It's not like I didn't want him to touch me—maybe I let things go too far—but I wasn't ready for sex yet, and I told him so." Trembling violently, her hands covered her face, gulping back tears, Debra Hemsath is recounting to a counselor in the student health center how an enjoyable evening with the man she'd been dating for 3 weeks turned into an emotional nightmare.

"We'd both had a lot of beers—way more than we'd had on other dates. I wasn't the only one who was in the mood—she was getting pretty hot and heavy herself. I mean, it wasn't like this was our first date, or some one night stand. I really liked her, and she knew it." Baffled, frustrated, alternating between anger and guilt, Ron Mayer is trying to explain to his closest friend how a pleasant interlude in his apartment turned into an accusation of date rape from a woman about whom he was beginning to feel pretty serious.

Between the enjoyable moments in Ron's dimly lit apartment and Debra's shattering accusation of rape there might lie a hundred misunderstandings, missed cues, false assumptions, and misinterpretations. Add in the emotional baggage each of them brought to the situation (family attitudes about sex, previous experiences in intimate relationships) plus Debra and Ron's affection for and attraction to each other, and the stage is set for the kind of collision that took place between these two students.

As you study this chapter, think about the factors that contributed to Debra and Ron's situation, and prepare yourself to answer the questions in **Your Turn** at the end of the chapter.

★ Gun Violence in Schools Threatens Kids' Safety

Despite studies that show that the nation's public schools are safer than they have been in decades, a recent rash of school shootings has made parents fear for their kids' safety. During a period of sixteen months in 1997 and 1998, 13 students and teachers were killed. The most highly publicized killings took place in Pearl, Mississippi (October 1997, where nine students were shot and two killed), West Paducah, Kentucky (December 1997, where eight students were shot and three killed), Jonesboro, Arkansas (March 1998, where fifteen people were shot and four students and a teacher were killed), and Springfield, Oregon (May 1998, where two students were killed).[14] Overall, school violence may be on the decline, but the magnitude of these isolated events has shocked the nation.

As this book goes to press, the most recent school shooting was in Carrollton, Georgia, on January 8, 1999. In this deadly incident, a teenage girl and her 17-year-old boyfriend were found wounded on the floor of a girls' bathroom. The girl died and the boy was critically wounded in what appeared to be a suicide pact. Police reported that a .22-caliber gun was used in the incident and that the gun had been stored under lock and key in the home of the girl's parents.

These killings appear to have some common characteristics. All of them were committed by boys, most of whom were under age 16. (In the Jonesboro shootings, an 11-year-old and a 13-year-old were charged.) The boys were frequently described as quiet loners who had only a few friends. Some of the boys were known to have had a history of torturing small animals. Most of the killers had indicated before the shootings (generally in indirect ways) that they were going to do something "bad" or something "big" to "get back at someone" or the school. In most cases the killings were carried in a random fashion with no particular victims in mind.

Why are these killings taking place? Experts point to a number of possibilities.[15] Some cite the easy accessibility of guns. The inability of some young people to distinguish between fantasy and reality is another possible cause. Some violence experts believe that in our culture, certain young

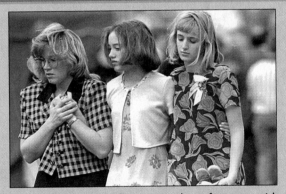

Three mourners console one another after graveside services for Natalie Brooks, one of the five victims of the Jonesboro, Arkansas, school shooting. (AP Photo/Chris Gardner)

people have not learned problem-solving skills or the skills required to control their anger in interpersonal disputes. When confronted with stressful situations, these young people act in violent ways because violence is what they have seen so frequently in their communities, on television, or in the movies.

How can these terrible tragedies be prevented? Not every incident can be averted; however, there may be some ways to reduce the occurrence of such acts of violence. Communities, parents, and schools need to talk with young people about violence and the many acceptable ways to cope with personal problems or stressful situations. We need to let young people know that there are places where they can talk with adults in a safe, non-threatening, nonjudgmental way.[15] Finally, everyone must learn to be more sensitive to the attitudes, feelings, and comments young people make. We must respond to (and report to appropriate officials) any warning signs or verbal hints that might foreshadow a violent incident. In this sense, we must believe that any such event could happen in our own community or in our schools.

Domestic violence directed at women and children seems to be increasing, and many people fear becoming a random victim of a homicide, robbery, or carjacking. Law enforcement officials contend that gang activities and hard-core drug involvement are significant factors that have led to violent behavior in our society.

Although violence may seem to be focused in urban areas, no community is completely safe. Even people who live in small towns and rural areas now must lock their doors and remain vigilant about protecting their safety. Crime on college campuses, much of which is a direct result of alcohol use, remains a threat. For tips on avoiding becoming a victim of a violent crime, see the Health Action Guide below.

For some students the content in this chapter may be the most important information in this textbook. Becoming a victim of violent behavior or sustaining an unintentional injury can harm your health as much (or more than) any of your own unhealthy behavior. The goal of this chapter is to help you understand the scope of violence and unintentional injury in our society and learn what you can do to avoid

becoming a victim. Complete the Personal Assessment on page 586 to see whether you are adequately protecting your own safety.

Reducing Risk Factors

Many factors influence your risk of suffering an injury or becoming a victim of crime. Some of these you cannot change. For example, the greatest percentage of violent crimes tend to be committed by, and suffered by, the young. This risk is multiplied for those who are young and African-American, and who live in an area with gang activity.

However, you *can* affect many of the other risk factors for injury or crime, as you will learn throughout this chapter. For example, alcohol plays a major role in driving, motorcycle, and boating accidents. You can reduce your risk of accidents by avoiding alcohol and drugs while you enjoy these activities. Likewise, boxes throughout this chapter will show you how to avoid becoming a victim of date rape, how to deal with a stalker, how to avoid accidents in your home and car, and more.

HEALTH ACTION GUIDE

Don't Be a Victim of Violent Crime

Do you know the steps you can take to avoid becoming a victim in your home, in your car, or at an ATM? Consider these tips:

At Your Home
• Do not hide an extra key in your mailbox, under your doormat, or anywhere around your house. Criminals know all the hiding places. If you must, leave an extra key with a trusted neighbor.
• If a service person or police officer rings your doorbell, examine their identification and call their office before allowing them entry.
• Use several timers set to turn on lights, stereo, and television at different times. Using a single timer to turn on everything at once tips off intruders that no one is home.
• As soon as you take possession of a new home, change the locks immediately. The expense may be minimal if the house has deadbolts, because they often can be simply rekeyed. If not, install deadbolts on all groundfloor doors, patio doors, and interior garage door.
• Join your community's neighborhood watch program.

In Your Car
• If your car breaks down, pull off the road and turn on your hazard lights. Hang a white cloth from a window or place a Send Help sign in your back window.
• Stay in your car with the doors locked and the windows rolled up. If someone approaches your car, do not get out, but ask the person to call the police for you. Do not open your hood for a stranger.

• If you feel threatened, blow your horn continuously to alert passersby.
• If someone bumps your car while you are driving, do not pull over if you do not feel entirely safe. Some criminals use this ploy to find a robbery victim. Drive to a busy, well-lit area or to a police station, then write down your insurance information and hand it out through a crack in the window.
• When you go shopping, park as close as possible to the mall entrance, or at least in a busy, well-lit area. Don't park next to tall vehicles that could block the view of your vehicle. Stay away from shrubbery that could hide an assailant. At night, ask a guard to walk you to your car.
• Check underneath, in the back seat, and behind your vehicle for intruders before getting into the vehicle.

At an ATM
• Use an ATM in a busy, indoor location, such as a supermarket, whenever possible.
• At a drive-up ATM, keep your doors locked and your windows rolled up as much as possible. Avoid going to ATMs after 9 P.M.
• Trust your instincts. If you do not feel safe near an ATM, do not use it.
• Do not lend out your ATM card, and do not tell anyone your personal identification number (PIN).
• Check your bank statement carefully each month, and promptly report any transactions you did not make.

InfoLinks
http://www.nra.org/rtbav/rtbvtips.html

Personal Assessment

This quiz will help you measure how well you manage your personal safety. For each item below, circle the number that reflects the frequency with which you do the safety activity. Then, add up your individual scores and check the interpretation at the end.

3 **I regularly do this**
2 **I sometimes do this**
I **I rarely do this**

1. I am aware of my surroundings and do not get lost.   3   2   I
2. I avoid locations in which my personal safety would be compromised.   3   2   I
3. I intentionally vary my daily routine (such as walking patterns to and from class, parking places, and jogging or biking routes) so that my whereabouts are not always predictable.   3   2   I
4. I walk across campus at night with other people.   3   2   I
5. I am careful about disclosing personal information (address, phone number, social security number, my daily schedule, etc.) to people I do not know.   3   2   I
6. I carefully monitor my alcohol intake at parties.   3   2   I
7. I watch carefully for dangerous weather conditions and know how to respond if necessary.   3   2   I
8. I do not keep a loaded gun in my home.   3   2   I
9. I know how I would handle myself if I were to be assaulted.   3   2   I
10. I maintain adequate insurance for my health and my property.   3   2   I
11. I keep emergency information numbers near my phone.   3   2   I
12. I keep my first aid skills up-to-date.   3   2   I
13. I use deadbolt locks on the doors of my home.   3   2   I
14. I use the safety locks on the windows at home.   3   2   I
15. I check the batteries used in my home smoke detector.   3   2   I
16. I have installed a carbon monoxide detector in my home.   3   2   I
17. I use adequate lighting in areas around my home and garage.   3   2   I
18. I have the electrical, heating, and cooling equipment in my home inspected regularly for safety and efficiency.   3   2   I
19. I use my car seatbelt.   3   2   I
20. I drive my car safely and defensively.   3   2   I
21. I keep my car in good mechanical order.   3   2   I
22. I keep my car doors locked.   3   2   I
23. I have a plan of action if my car should break down while I am driving it.   3   2   I
24. I use appropriate safety equipment, such as flotation devices, helmets, and elbow pads, in my recreational activities.   3   2   I
25. I can swim well enough to save myself in most situations.   3   2   I
26. I use suggestions for personal safety each day.   3   2   I

TOTAL POINTS _____

Interpretation

Your total may mean that:

72–78 points	You appear to carefully protect your personal safety.
65–71 points	You adequately protect many aspects of your personal safety.
58–64 points	You should consider improving some of your safety-related behaviors.
Below 58 points	You must consider improving some of your safety-related behaviors.

To Carry This Further . . .

Although no one can be completely safe from personal injury or possible random violence, there are ways to minimize the risks to your safety. Scoring high on this assessment will not guarantee your safety, but your likelihood for injury should remain relatively low. Scoring low on this assessment should encourage you to consider ways to make your life more safe. Refer to the text and this assessment to provide you with useful suggestions to enhance your personal safety. Which safety tips will you use today?

- To what extent are you concerned about your personal safety? Are you comfortable with your level of concern? Or do you think you need to pay more attention to your personal safety?

Intentional Injuries

Intentional injuries are injuries that are committed on purpose. With the exception of suicide (which is self-directed), intentional injuries reflect violence committed by one person acting against another person. Categories of intentional injuries include homicide, robbery, rape, suicide, assault, child abuse, partner abuse, and elder abuse. Each year in the United States, intentional injuries cause about 50,000 deaths. Violent crimes, such as murder, rape, robbery, and aggravated assault, victimize millions of other Americans each year.[1] Let's look at some of these violent crimes in more detail.

Homicide

Homicide, or murder, is the intentional killing of one person by another. Sadly, the United States leads the industrialized world in homicide rates. The 1996 murder rate, however, was 7.4 per 100,000 inhabitants. This reflected a 10 percent decline from the 1995 rate, the largest decrease in four years.[1]

Criminal justice experts are trying to pinpoint why U.S. homicide rates are dropping. No single answer has emerged, but some observers credit more intense policing efforts. In some communities, such as New York City, police have instituted a campaign against "quality of life" crimes, such as aggressive panhandling, graffiti, and public urination. Others credit the 1994 passage of the sweeping Federal Crime Bill; recent legislation, such as the Brady Law; and a variety of tough state laws, such as the "three strikes and you're out" provisions that mandate life sentences without parole for repeat violent offenders.

On the other hand, some attribute the declining crime rates to an improving economy, the fading of the crack wars, and the maturing of the baby boomers, rather than new policing tactics.

Some clear trends exist concerning homicides. The most vulnerable group of homicide victims is African-Americans, especially young male African-Americans. Homicide is the leading cause of death for male African-Americans aged fifteen to forty-four. African-American men have a one in twenty-one lifetime chance of becoming a victim of homicide.[2]

Another clear trend related to homicide is the extent to which illegal drug activity is related to homicide. A variety of research studies from large cities indicate that 25 percent to 50 percent of all homicides are drug related.[3] Most of these murders are related to activities involved in drug trafficking, including disputed drug transactions. In addition, high percentages of both homicide assailants and victims have drugs in their systems at the time of the homicide.[3]

Domestic Violence

Family life in the 1990s is a far cry from that portrayed in the popular 1950s and 1960s television shows like "The Donna Reed Show," "Father Knows Best," and "The Adventures of Ozzie and Harriet." The composition of families has changed considerably. In the 1950s a common family pattern included children being raised by both parents. Generally, the father was the income earner and the mother stayed at home and managed the growing family.

Today, family patterns are much more complex. Children are more frequently being raised in blended families headed by single parents. Since 1970 single-parent households have increased 112 percent, from 4 million to 8.9 million homes.[4] A much higher percentage of women are employed outside the home. Because of pressing family economic concerns, many children take care of themselves during after-school hours. Sociologists indicate that families, and the individuals in those families, are under more stress than ever.

Add to this precarious nature of the American family the factors of increased societal drug use, increased presence of handguns, and increased crime and violence.[5] What emerges is no surprise.

Partner Abuse

Partner abuse refers to violence committed against a domestic partner. Most often the victims are women, and a significant percentage of these women are spouses or former spouses of the assailant. Figures from the U.S. Department of Justice are frightening and reflect the magnitude of the problem of violence against women in the United States.[6] More than 2.5 million women are victims of some form of violence every year. Nearly two in three female victims of violent crimes are related to or know their attacker. About three out of four female victims resist the actions of their offenders either physically or verbally.[6]

---

intentional injuries   injuries that are purposely committed by a person.

homicide   the intentional killing of one person by another person.

partner abuse   violence committed against a domestic partner.

The most vulnerable female victims are African-American and Hispanic, live in large cities, are young and unmarried, and are from lower socioeconomic groups.[6] However, these trends do not mean that only women from these classifications are vulnerable to violent behavior. Women across all economic, racial, and age categories are potential victims.

One of the real difficulties related to domestic violence is the vast underreporting of this crime to law enforcement authorities. The U.S. Department of Justice estimates that about half of the victims of domestic violence do not report the crime to police. Too many victims view their violent situations as private or personal matters and not actual crimes. Despite painful injuries, many victims view the offenses against them as minor.[6]

Of course, it is easy to criticize the victims of domestic violence for not reporting the crimes committed against them, but this may be unfair. Why do women stay in these relationships? Many women who are injured may fear being killed if they report the crime. Women may also fear for the safety of their children. Women who receive economic support may fear being left with no financial resources.

However, help is available for victims of partner abuse. Most communities have family support or domestic violence hot lines that abused people can call for help. Communities are establishing shelters where abused women and their children can seek safety while their cases are being handled by the police or court officials. If you are being abused or know of someone who is the victim of domestic violence, do not hesitate to use the services of these local hot lines or shelters. Also, check the resources listed in the Health Reference Guide at the back of this text.

Child Abuse

Like many cases of partner abuse, **child abuse** tends to be a silent crime. Because many victims do not report their crimes, the incidence of child abuse is difficult to determine.

Children are abused in various ways. Physical abuse reflects physical injury, such as bruises, burns, abrasions, cuts, and fractures of the bones and skull. Sexual abuse includes acts that lead to sexual gratification of the abuser. Examples include fondling, touching, and various acts involved in rape, sodomy, and incest. Child neglect is also a form of child abuse and includes an extreme failure to provide children with adequate clothing, food, shelter, and medical attention. A strong case can also be made for psychological abuse as a form of child abuse. Certainly, children are scarred by family members and others who routinely damage their psychological development. Unfortunately, this form of abuse is especially difficult to identify and measure.[7]

The most frequent form of child abuse is neglect. The incidence of child neglect is approximately three times the incidence of physical abuse and about seven times the incidence of child sexual abuse. Each form of abuse can have devastating short- and long-term consequences for the child.

Research studies in the various areas of child abuse reveal some interesting trends. Abused children are much more likely than nonabused children to grow up to be child abusers themselves. It is also now understood that abused children are more likely to suffer from poor educational performance, increased health problems, and low levels of overall achievement. Abused children are significantly more likely than nonabused children to become involved in adult crime and violent criminal behavior.[7]

It is beyond the scope of this book to discuss in detail how to reduce child abuse. However, the violence directed against children can likely be lessened through a combination of early identification measures and violence prevention programs. Teachers, friends, relatives, social workers, counselors, psychologists, police, and the court system must not hesitate to intervene early in cases of suspected child abuse. The later the intervention, the more likely that the abuse will have worsened. When an individual has abused once, he or she is likely to do it again.

Violence prevention programs can help parents and caregivers learn how to resolve conflicts, improve communication, cope with anger, improve parenting skills, and challenge the view of violence presented in movies and television. These programs may help to stop violence before it begins to damage the lives of young children. Figure 20-1 provides simple alternatives parents can choose to avoid hitting a child.[8]

Elder Abuse

Among the nation's 35 million elderly people, 1.5 million are the victims of neglect and abuse. Particularly vulnerable are elderly women over the age of seventy-five years. More often than not, the abusers are the adult children of the victims.

Many elderly people are hit, kicked, attacked with knives, or denied food and medical care; others are robbed of their Social Security checks and automobiles. These crimes probably reflect a combination of factors, particularly the stress of caring for failing older people by middle-aged children who also face the additional demands of dependent children and careers. In many cases, the middle-aged children were themselves abused, or there may be a chemical dependence problem. The alternative, institutionalization, is so expensive that it is often not an option for either the abused or the abuser.

Although protective services are available, elder abuse is frequently unseen and unreported. In many

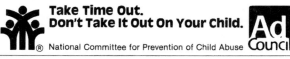

**12 alternatives
to lashing out at your child.**

The next time everyday pressures
build up to the point where
you feel like lashing out—STOP!
And try any of these simple alternatives.

You'll feel better . . . and so will your child.

1. Take a deep breath. And another. Then remember <u>you</u> are the adult . . .

2. Close your eyes and imagine you're hearing what your child is about to hear.

3. Press your lips together and count to 10. Or better yet, to 20.

4. Put your child in a time-out chair. (Remember the rule: one time-out minute for each year of age.)

5. Put yourself in a time-out chair. Think about why you are angry: Is it your child, or is your child simply a convenient target for your anger?

6. Phone a friend.

7. If someone can watch the children, go outside and take a walk.

8. Take a hot bath or splash cold water on your face.

9. Hug a pillow.

10. Turn on some music. Maybe even sing along.

11. Pick up a pencil and write down as many helpful words as you can think of. Save the list.

12. Write for parenting information: Parenting, Box 2866, Chicago, IL 60690.

**Take Time Out.
Don't Take It Out On Your Child.**

® National Committee for Prevention of Child Abuse — Ad Council

CHILD ABUSE PREVENTION CAMPAIGN
MAGAZINE AD NO. CA-2835-90—7" x 10"
Volunteer Agency: Lintas: Cambell-Ewald, Campaign Director: Beth M. Pritchard, S.C. Johnson & Son, Inc.

Figure 20-1 Alternatives to hitting your child.

cases, the elderly people themselves are afraid to report their children's behavior because of the fear of embarrassment that they were not good parents to their children. Regardless of the cause, however, elder abuse must be reported to the appropriate protective service so that the abuse can be stopped.

Gangs and Youth Violence

In the last twenty years, gangs and gang activities have been increasingly responsible for escalating violence and criminal activity. Before that time, gangs used fists, tire irons, and occasionally, cheap handguns ("Saturday night specials") as tools of enforcement. Now, gang members do not hesitate to use more lethal semiautomatic weapons.

Most, but not all, gangs arise from big city environments where many socially alienated, economically disadvantaged young people live. Convinced that society has no significant role for them, gang members can receive support from an association of peers that has well-defined lines of authority. Rituals

and membership initiation rites are important in gang socialization. Gangs often control territories within a city. Frequently, gangs are involved in criminal activities, the most common of which are illicit drug trafficking and robberies. In the late 1990s, gang-related murders and drive-by shootings, mostly related to drug dealing, contributed to the high death rate among young people and especially inner-city youth.

It is not only older male teenagers and young adults who are members of today's gangs. Law enforcement officials see younger people (ages twelve, thirteen, and fourteen) joining gangs. Some gangs have recently included young women as members, and some cities report a growing number of all-female gangs. Some female gangs are reported to be every bit as ruthless as the male gangs.

Attempting to control gang and youth violence is particularly expensive for communities. When you consider that for every gang-related homicide, there are about 100 nonfatal gang-related intentional injuries, it becomes obvious that gang violence is an expensive health care proposition. Furthermore, gang and youth violence takes an enormous financial and human toll on law enforcement, the judicial system, and corrections departments.

Fortunately, the recent decline in murders and other serious crimes also applies to gang-related crimes. Once again, some observers credit more aggressive police tactics for the decline. Others point to cities such as East St. Louis, Illinois, which experienced a 60 percent drop in murders between 1991 and 1996, a time when the community's police department could barely afford gas to run all of its police cars.[9] Thus, some say the drop in crime should be attributed to factors such as a stronger economy, the aging of the baby boomers out of the riskier age brackets, and the fading of the crack market.

At the same time that the crime rate is dropping for baby boomers, the violent crime rate among youths has been sharply increasing. Historically, younger teenagers rarely committed murders, but this has changed. Arrest rates show that fourteen- to seventeen-year-olds have surpassed eighteen- to twenty-four-year-olds in committing violent crimes.

Some of the tactics being used to meet this problem are the aggressive "quality of life" policing in some cities and President Clinton's COPS program (Community Oriented Policing Services) to hire new police officers and put them on foot patrols, where they become acquainted with residents. In Boston, a

child abuse harm that is committed against a child; usually referring to physical abuse, sexual abuse, or child neglect.

Learning
From Our Diversity

Reducing Youth Violence: California's Healthy Cities Program

The growing population of urban poor is a major contributor to violence in city neighborhoods—particularly in parts of the country where problems are exacerbated by conflicts among ethnic minorities. Increasingly, the escalating incidents of violence in urban areas involve young people. In California, a project called Healthy Cities has been operating for several years, and a number of participating cities are experiencing significant reductions in youth violence as the result of an intensive multifaceted effort to steer at-risk youth away from destructive behavior and toward positive attitudes and actions.[16]

The city of Oceanside launched a successful effort to curb graffiti, using the slogan "Community begins with me!" A Community Awareness Day was well attended, and the city made a video for elementary schools called "You Have No Right to Tag." Later, surveys conducted in Spanish and English among more than 200 neighborhood residents found there had been a 55 percent reduction in graffiti. Residents also reported increased participation in neighborhood watch and cleanup programs.

Cathedral City's initiative seeks to build self-esteem in troubled youth as a means of reducing incidents of graffiti vandalism, drug-related crime, and violence in schools. As part of this ef-

fort, students receive lessons in problem solving, conflict resolution, and other interpersonal skills. Other activities are leadership training, a call-in service for troubled youth who need support not available at home, and clubs and groups for at-risk kids.

The town of Vista also seeks to improve self-esteem among troubled youngsters in its mentoring program, Club Challenge. Each participant must sign a contract agreeing to increase school attendance by 20 percent, decrease detentions and suspensions by 50 percent, and participate in 18 productive community activities during the year. Activities may include feeding the homeless, cleaning parks and streams, attending a City Council meeting, or "shadowing" a mentor for a day.

Coachella's Bicycle Conversion Program provides at-risk youngsters with refurbished bikes in exchange for 10 hours of community service in litter removal, graffiti abatement, assisting senior citizens, and other activities. Like efforts in other cities, this one is aimed at reducing youth arrests, establishing positive youth activities, and decreasing graffiti and litter throughout the city.

California's Healthy Cities program provides an excellent model for other areas of the country that are plagued by the problem of youth violence among the urban poor. By offering young people positive options, guidance, and structure, these efforts go a long way toward turning troubled kids into productive citizens.[16]

---

campaign aimed at youth gangs offered summer jobs to gang members, combined with threats of federal prison sentences for gun violence. In a two-year period since that time, no youngsters under seventeen have been shot and killed in Boston.[9] Reducing gang and youth violence will be a continuing challenge for the nation as it moves through the year 2000.

Gun Violence

The tragic effect of gun violence has already been mentioned in a few sections of this chapter. Guns are being used more than ever in our society and in other parts of the world. More than 60 percent of the homicides and 55 percent of the suicides committed each year in the United States involve the use of guns. As previously mentioned, gun violence is a leading killer of teenagers and young men, especially African-American men, and the use of semiautomatic assault weapons by individuals and gang members is common. Accidental deaths of toddlers and young children from loaded handguns is another dimension of the violence attributable to guns in our society. In addition, guns are often used in **carjackings**.

The proliferation of firearm use has prompted serious discussions about the enactment of gun con-

trol laws. For years, gun control activists have been in direct battle with the National Rifle Association (NRA) and its congressional supporters. Gun control activists want fewer guns manufactured and greater controls over the sale and possession of handguns. Gun supporters believe that such controls are not necessary and that people (the criminals) are responsible for gun deaths, not simply the guns. This debate will certainly continue.

Personal Applications

• Has there been any gun violence at your college? Are you aware of any students carrying guns or other concealed weapons on your campus?

Bias and Hate Crimes

One sad aspect of any society is how some segments of the majority treat certain people in the minority. Nowhere is this more violently pronounced than in **bias and hate crimes.** These crimes are directed at individuals or groups of people solely because of a

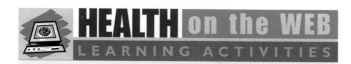

Understanding Domestic Violence

Many people have misconceptions about domestic violence and its effects on women and their families. Domestic violence is a complex issue that has no simple solution. But the first step toward preventing or stopping it is understanding it. Go to www.npcts.edu/uo/handson/domviol/domquiz.html and complete the Domestic Violence Quiz. How do you think our society should address this problem?

Preventing Rape and Sexual Assault

Rape and sexual assault are not crimes of passion, but crimes of hostility, aggression, and violence. Both men and women should learn about rape to develop an awareness of its causes and consequences. Go to www.netstuff.com/target/rape.htm and complete the Rape Quiz. What steps can you take to reduce the risk of rape, including date rape?

Learning CPR to Respond to Injuries

Cardiopulmonary resuscitation (CPR) is one of the most important measures that trained people can take when a seriously injured person needs immediate help. We encourage you to take an American Red Cross CPR class. To find out how much you know about CPR, go to www.learncpr.org/userquiz.html to complete a CPR Quiz. Did the quiz help persuade you to sign up for a training class?

For more activities, log on to our Online Learning Center at www.mhhe.com/hper/health/payne

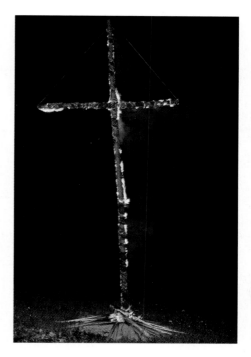

Racial minorities are often the targets of bias and hate crimes committed by white supremacist groups. More stringent laws have been enacted to make these crimes serious offenses.

racial, ethnic, religious, or other difference attributed to the victims. Victims are often verbally and physically attacked, their houses are spray painted with slurs, and many are forced to move from one neighborhood or community to another.

Typically, the offenders in bias or hate crimes are fringe elements of a larger society who believe that the mere presence of someone with a racial, ethnic, or religious difference is inherently bad for the community, state, or country. Examples of groups commonly known to commit bias and hate crimes in the United States are skinheads, the Ku Klux Klan, and other white supremacist groups. Increasingly, state and federal laws have been enacted to make bias and hate crimes serious offenses.

With a small but growing presence of neo-Nazi groups in Europe and clear evidence that ethnic cleansing took place in Kosovo, Bosnia, Serbia, Croatia, Rwanda, Iraq, and the former Soviet Union, bias and hate crimes are a worldwide problem. The recent push on college campuses to promote multicultural education and the celebration of diversity may help today's generation of college graduates understand the importance of tolerance and inclusion and avoid bigotry and exclusion.

Stalking

In recent years the crime of **stalking** has received considerable attention. Stalking refers to an assailant's planned efforts to pursue an intended victim. Most stalkers are male. (One notable exception was the convicted female stalker of talk show host David Letterman.) Many of these stalkers are excessively possessive or jealous and pursue people with whom they formerly had a relationship. Some stalkers pursue people with whom they have had only an imaginary relationship.

Some stalkers have served time in prison and have waited for years to "get back" at their victims. In some cases, stalkers go to great lengths to locate their intended victims and frequently know their daily whereabouts. Although not all stalkers plan to batter or kill their victims, their presence and potential for

carjacking a crime that involves a thief's attempt to steal a car while the owner is behind the wheel; carjackings are usually random and unpredictable, and frequently involve handguns.

bias and hate crimes criminal acts directed at a person or group solely because of a specific characteristic, such as race, religion, ethnic background, or political belief.

stalking a crime involving an assailant's planned efforts to pursue an intended victim.

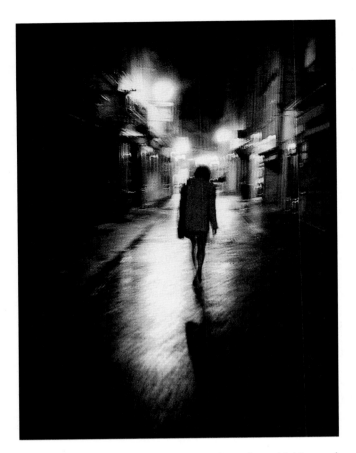

Preventing dangerous situations requires clear thinking and careful planning.

Dealing with a Stalker

Nearly every state has passed a law making stalking a crime in and of itself. Recently, however, women's groups, bar associations, and others have charged that local police departments are not actively enforcing the laws and that they do not intervene to help the victim until a violent or near-violent act has occurred.

So what can you do if you are being stalked? If someone continues to bother or intimidate you with phone calls, notes or letters, or unwanted gifts, take the following steps:

- Contact your local police immediately and fill out a report.

- Report the harassment to the telephone company and ask that they install call-tracing devices and tape recorders to gather evidence against the stalker.

- Keep a detailed record, with dates, times, and exact wording of all incidents or threats, including the number of telephone calls, letters, or other harassments.

- Save all letters, answering-machine tapes, and other evidence.

- Contact the local prosecutor and seek a court order prohibiting the stalker from any further contact. If the stalker violates the court order, press the prosecutor to take action, such as indicting the stalker.

- Keep the pressure on police to take the appropriate action.

- Law-enforcement officials urge against any contact with the stalker. Let the police, telephone company, postal investigators, and prosecutors handle the problem.

violence are enough to create an extremely frightening environment for the intended victim and family.

Fortunately, since 1990 virtually all states have enacted or tightened their laws related to stalking and have created stiff penalties for stalkers (see the Star Box). In many areas the criminal justice system is proactive in letting possible victims of stalking know, for example, when a particular prison inmate is going to be released. In other areas, citizens are banding together to provide support and protection for people who may be victims of stalkers.

If you think you are or someone you know is being stalked, contact the police (or a local crisis intervention hot line number) to report your case. See the Star Box for suggestions on handling a stalker.

Sexual Victimization

Ideally, sexual intimacy is a mutual, enjoyable form of communication between two people. Far too often, however, relationships are approached in an aggressive, hostile manner. These sexual aggressors always have a victim—someone who is physically or psychologically traumatized. *Sexual victimization* occurs in many forms and in a variety of settings. In this section we briefly look at sexual victimization as it occurs in rape and sexual assault, sexual abuse of children, sexual harassment, and the commercialization of sex.

Rape and Sexual Assault

As violence in our society increases, the incidence of *rape* and *sexual assault* correspondingly rises. The victims of these crimes fall into no single category. Survivors of rape and sexual assault include young and old, male and female. They can be mentally retarded people, prisoners, hospital patients, or college students. We are all potential victims, and self-protection is critical. Read the Star Box on page 593 to learn about the myths surrounding rape.

Sometimes a personal assault begins as a physical assault that may turn into a rape. Rape is generally considered a crime of sexual aggression in which the victim is forced to have sexual intercourse. Current thought concerning rape characterizes this behavior as a violent act that happens to be carried out through sexual contact. (See the Health Action Guides on rape prevention and help for the survivor.)

Myths about Rape

Despite the fact that we are all potential victims, many of us do not fully understand how vulnerable we are. Many people hold several myths (false assumptions) about rape, including the following:

- *Women are raped by strangers.* In approximately half of all reported rapes, the victim has some prior acquaintance with the rapist. Increasingly, women are being raped by husbands, dating partners, and relatives.

- *Rapes almost always occur in dark alleys or deserted places.* The opposite is true. Most rapes occur in or very near the victim's residence.

- *Rapists are easily identified by their demeanor or psychological profile.* Most experts indicate that rapists do not differ significantly from nonrapists.

- *The incidence of rape is overreported.* Estimates are that only one in five rapes is reported.

- *Rape happens only to people in low socioeconomic classes.* Rape occurs in all socioeconomic classes. Each person, male or female, young or old, is a potential victim.

- *There is a standard way to escape from a potential rape situation.* Each rape situation is different. No one method to avoid rape can work in every potential rape situation. Because of this, we encourage personal health classes to invite speakers from a local rape prevention services bureau to discuss approaches to rape prevention.

HEALTH ACTION GUIDE

Rape Prevention Guidelines

To prevent rape from occurring:

- Never forget that you could be a candidate for assault.
- Use approved campus security or escort services, especially at night.
- Think carefully about your patterns of movement to and from class or work. Alter your routes frequently.
- Walk briskly with a sense of purpose. Try not to walk alone at night.
- Dress so that the clothes you wear do not unnecessarily restrict your movement or make you more vulnerable.
- Always be aware of your surroundings. Look over your shoulder occasionally. Know where you are so that you won't get lost.
- Avoid getting into a car if you do not know the driver well.
- If you think you are being followed, look for a safe retreat. This might be a store, a fire or police station, or a group of people.
- Be especially cautious of first dates, blind dates, or people you meet at a party or bar who push to be alone with you.
- Let trusted friends know where you are and when you plan to return.
- Keep your car in good working order. Think beforehand how you would handle the situation should your car break down.
- Limit, and even avoid, alcohol to minimize the risk of rape.
- Trust your best instincts if you are assaulted. Each situation is different. Do what you can to protect your life.

InfoLinks
www.cs.utk.edu/~bartley/index/prevention/

Acquaintance and Date Rape

Sexual victimization can occur in relationships. *Acquaintance rape* refers to forced sexual intercourse between individuals who know each other. *Date rape* is a form of acquaintance rape that involves forced sexual intercourse by a dating partner. Studies on a number of campuses suggest that about 20 percent of college women report having experienced date rape. An even higher percentage of women report being kissed and touched against their will. Alcohol is frequently a significant contributing factor in these rape situations. (See Chapter 8 concerning alcohol's role in campus crime.) Some men have reported being psychologically coerced into intercourse by their female dating partners. In many cases the aggressive partner will display certain behaviors that can serve as warning signs (see the Health Action Guide on p. 595).

Psychologists believe that aside from the physical harm of date rape, a greater amount of emotional damage may occur. Such damage stems from the concept of broken trust. Date rape survivors feel particularly violated because the perpetrator was not a stranger; it was someone they initially trusted, at least to some degree. Once that trust has been broken, developing new relationships with other people becomes much more difficult for the date rape survivor.

Nearly all survivors of date rape seem to suffer from *posttraumatic stress syndrome.* They can have anxiety, sleeplessness, eating disorders, and nightmares. Guilt concerning their own behavior, self-esteem, and judgment of other people can be overwhelming, and the individual may require professional counseling. Indeed, all students should be aware of the risk of date rape.

Personal Applications

- Do you know of educational programs on your campus that have dealt with rape prevention? Where can you go on your campus to seek help for crises related to these issues?

Sexual Abuse of Children

One of the most tragic forms of sexual victimization is the sexual abuse of children. Children are especially vulnerable to sexual abuse because of their dependent relationships with parents, relatives, and caregivers (such as babysitters, teachers, and neighbors). Often, children are unable to readily understand the difference between appropriate and inappropriate physical contact. Abuse may range from blatant physical manipulation, including fondling, to oral sex, sodomy, and intercourse.

Because of the subordinate role of children in relationships involving adults, sexually abusive practices often go unreported. Sexual abuse can leave emotional scars that make it difficult to establish meaningful relationships later in life. For this reason, it is especially important for people to pay close attention to any information shared by children that could indicate a potentially abusive situation. Most states require that information concerning child abuse be reported to law enforcement officials.

Sexual Harassment

Sexual harassment consists of unwanted attention of a sexual nature that creates embarrassment or stress. Examples of sexual harassment include unwanted physical contact, excessive pressure for dates, sexually explicit humor, sexual innuendos or remarks, of-

HEALTH ACTION GUIDE

Help for the Rape Survivor

If you have been raped, seek help as soon as possible. The following procedures may be helpful.

- Call the police immediately to report the assault. Police can take you to the hospital and start gathering information that may help them apprehend the rapist. Fortunately, many police departments now use specially trained officers (many of whom are female) to work closely with rape survivors during all stages of the investigation.
- If you would rather not contact the police immediately, call a local rape crisis center. Operated generally on a twenty-four-hour hot line basis, these centers have trained counselors to help you evaluate your options, contact the police, escort you to the hospital, and provide aftercare counseling.
- Do not alter any potential evidence related to the rape. Do not change your clothes, douche, take a bath, or rearrange the scene of the crime. Wait until all the evidence has been gathered.
- Report all bruises, cuts, and scratches, even if they seem insignificant. Report any information about the attack as completely and accurately as possible.
- You will probably be given a thorough pelvic examination. You may have to ask for STD tests and a pregnancy test.
- Although it is unusual for a rape survivor's name to appear in the media, you might request that the police withhold your name as long as is legally possible.

InfoLinks
www.feminist.org

fers of job advancement based on sexual favors, and overt sexual assault. Unlike more overt forms of sexual victimization, sexual harassment may be applied in a subtle manner and can, in some cases, go unnoticed by coworkers and fellow students. Nevertheless, sexual harassment produces stress that cannot be resolved until the harasser is identified and forced to stop. Both men and women can be victims of sexual harassment.

Sexual harassment can occur in many settings, including employment and academic settings. On the college campus, harassment may be primarily in terms of the offer of sex for grades. If this happens to you, think carefully about the situation and document the specific times, events, and places where the harassment took place. Consult your college's policy concerning harassment. Next, you should report these events to the appropriate administrative officer (perhaps the affirmative action officer, dean of academic affairs, or dean of students). You may also want to discuss the situation with a staff member of the university counseling center.

If harassment occurs in the work environment, the victim should document the occurrences and report them to the appropriate management or personnel official. Reporting procedures will vary from setting to setting. Sexual harassment is a form of illegal sex discrimination and violates Title VII of the Civil Rights Act of 1964.

In 1986 the U.S. Supreme Court ruled that the creation of a "hostile environment" in a work setting was sufficient evidence to support the claim of sexual harassment. This action served as an impetus for thousands of women to step forward with sexual harassment allegations. Additionally, some men are also filing sexual harassment lawsuits against female supervisors.

Not surprisingly, this rising number of complaints has served as a wake-up call for employers. From university settings to factory production lines to corporate board rooms, employers are scrambling to make certain that employees are fully aware of actions that could lead to a sexual harassment lawsuit. Sexual harassment workshops and educational seminars on harassment are now common and serve to educate both men and women about this complex problem.

Violence and the Commercialization of Sex

It is beyond the scope of this book to explore whether sexual violence can be related to society's exploitation or commercialization of sex. However, sexually related products and messages are intentionally placed before the public to try to sway consumer decisions. Do you believe that there could be a connection between commercial products, such as violent pornography in films and magazines, and violence against women? Does prostitution lead directly to violence? Do sexually explicit "900" phone numbers or pornography on the Internet cause an increase in violent acts? Can the sexual messages in beer commercials lead to acquaintance rape? What do you think?

Campus Safety

Although many of the topics in this chapter are quite unsettling, students and faculty must continue to lead normal lives in the campus environment despite potential threats to our health. The first step in being able to function adequately is knowing about these potential threats. You have read about these threats in this section on intentional injuries; now you must think about how this information applies to your campus situation.

The campus environment is no longer immune to many of the social ills that plague our society. At one time the university campus was thought to be a safe haven from the real world. Now there is plenty of evidence to indicate that significant intentional and unintentional injuries can happen to anyone at any time on the college campus.

For this reason, you must make it a habit to think constructively about protecting your safety. In addition to the personal safety tips presented earlier in this section, remember to use the safety assistance resources available on your campus. One of these might be your use of university-approved escort services, especially in the evenings as you move from one campus location to another. Another resource is the campus security department (campus police). Typically, campus police have a twenty-four-hour emergency phone number. If you think you need help, do not hesitate to call this number. Campus security departments frequently offer short seminars on safety topics to student organizations or residence hall groups. Your counseling center on campus might also offer programs on rape prevention and personal protection.

If you are motivated to make your campus environment safer, you might wish to contact two organizations that specifically focus on campus crime. The first is Safe Campuses Now, a nonprofit student group that tracks legislation, provides educational seminars, and monitors community incidents involving students. For information about Safe Campuses Now, including how to start a chapter on your campus, call (706) 354-1115. Visit the web page for Safe Campuses Now (www.uga.edu\safe-campus). This organization is located at the University of Georgia. We encourage you to become active in making your campus a safer place to live.

HEALTH ACTION GUIDE

Avoiding Date Rape

The first step in avoiding date rape is to consider your partner's behaviors. Many, but not all, date rapists show one or more of the following behaviors: a disrespectful attitude toward you and others, lack of concern for your feelings, violence and hostility, obsessive jealousy, extreme competitiveness, a desire to dominate, and unnecessary physical roughness. Consider these behaviors as warning signs for possible problems in the future. Reevaluate your participation in the relationship. Following are some specific ways both men and women can avoid a date rape situation.

Men

- Know your sexual desires and limits. Communicate them clearly. Be aware of social pressures. It's okay not to "score."
- Being turned down when you ask for sex is not a rejection of you personally. Women who say no to sex are not rejecting the person; they are expressing their desire not to participate in a single act. Your desires may be beyond control, but your actions are within your control.
- Accept the woman's decision. "No" means "No." Don't read other meanings into the answer. Don't continue after you are told "No!"
- Don't assume that just because a woman dresses in a sexy manner and flirts that she wants to have sexual intercourse.
- Don't assume that previous permission for sexual contact applies to the current situation.

- Avoid excessive use of alcohol and drugs. Alcohol and other drugs interfere with clear thinking and effective communication.

Women

- Know your sexual desires and limits. Believe in your right to set those limits. If you are not sure, STOP and talk about it.
- Communicate your limits clearly. If someone starts to offend you, tell him so firmly and immediately. Polite approaches may be misunderstood or ignored. Say "No" when you mean "No."
- Be assertive. Often men interpret passivity as permission. Be direct and firm with someone who is sexually pressuring you.
- Be aware that your nonverbal actions send a message. If you dress in a sexy manner and flirt, some men may assume you want to have sex. This does not make your dress or behavior wrong, but it is important to be aware of a possible misunderstanding.
- Pay attention to what is happening around you. Watch the nonverbal clues. Do not put yourself into vulnerable situations.
- Trust your intuitions. If you feel you are being pressured into unwanted sex, you probably are.
- Avoid excessive use of alcohol and drugs. Alcohol and other drugs interfere with clear thinking and effective communication.

InfoLinks

www.lia.org/daterape.htm

Unintentional Injuries

Unintentional injuries are injuries that have occurred without anyone's intending that any harm be done. Common examples include injuries resulting from car crashes, falls, fires, drownings, firearm accidents, recreational accidents, and residential accidents. Each year, unintentional injuries account for more than 150,000 deaths and millions of nonfatal injuries.

Unintentional injuries are very expensive for our society, both from a financial standpoint and from a personal and family standpoint. Fortunately, to a large extent it is possible to avoid becoming a victim of an unintentional injury. By carefully considering the tips presented in the safety categories that follow, you will be protecting yourself from many preventable injuries.

Since this section of the chapter focuses on a selected number of safety categories, we encourage readers to consider some additional, related activities. For further information in the area of safety, consult a safety textbook (one of which is listed in the references for this chapter).[10] To review important points in the area of first aid skills, consult Appendix 1 in this text. Finally, we encourage you to take a first aid course from the American Red Cross. American Red Cross first aid courses incorporate a significant amount of safety prevention information along with the teaching of specific first aid skills.

Residential Safety

Many serious accidents and personal assaults occur in dorm rooms, apartments, and houses. As a responsible adult, you should make every reasonable effort to prevent these tragedies from happening. One good idea is to discuss some of the following points with your family or roommates and see what cooperative strategies you can implement:

- Fireproof your residence. Are all electrical appliances and heating and cooling systems in safe working order? Are flammable materials safely stored?
- Prepare a fire escape plan. Install smoke or heat detectors.
- Do not give personal information over the phone to a stranger.
- Use initials for first names on mailboxes and in phone books.
- Install a peephole and deadbolt locks on doors.
- If possible, avoid living in first floor apartments. Change locks when moving to a new place.
- Put locks on all windows.
- Require repair people or delivery people to show valid identification.
- Do not use an elevator if it is occupied by someone who makes you feel uneasy.
- Be cautious around garages, laundry rooms, and driveways (especially at night). Use lighting for prevention of assault.

Recreational Safety

The thrills we get from risk taking are an essential part of our recreational endeavors. But sometimes we can get into serious accidents because we fail to consider important recreational safety information. Do some of the following recommendations apply to you?

- Seek appropriate instruction for your intended activity. Few skill activities are as easy as they look.
- Make certain that your equipment is in excellent working order.
- Involve yourself gradually in an activity before attempting more complicated, dangerous skills.
- Enroll in an American Red Cross first aid course to enable you to cope with unexpected injuries.
- Remember that alcohol use greatly increases the likelihood that people will get hurt.
- Protect your eyes from injury (see the Health Action Guide on p. 597).
- Learn to swim. Most drowning victims are people who never intended to be in the water.
- Obey the laws related to your recreational pursuits. Many laws are directly related to the safety of the participants.
- Be aware of weather conditions. Many outdoor activities turn to tragedy with sudden shifts in the weather. Always prepare yourself for the worst possible weather.

Bicycle Safety

With a little common sense and a few precautions, bicycling can be a very safe and enjoyable aerobic activity. Remember these key points:

- Wear a helmet. More than any other precaution, wearing a helmet is paramount and can save your life.

HEALTH ACTION GUIDE

Protecting Your Eyes

More than a million people suffer eye injuries each year in the United States. Almost half of these accidents occur at home, and more than 90 percent of them could have been prevented. Keep these steps in mind for protecting your eyes:[17]

In the Home
- Make sure that all spray nozzles are directed away from you before you pull the handle.
- Read instructions carefully before using cleaning fluids, detergents, ammonia, or harsh chemicals. Wash your hands thoroughly after use.
- Use grease shields on frying pans to protect your eyes from splattering.
- Wear appropriate goggles to shield your eyes from fumes and splashes when using powerful chemicals.
- Use opaque goggles to avoid burns from sunlamps.

In the Workshop
- Think about the work you will be doing, and protect your eyes from flying fragments, fumes, dust particles, sparks, and splashing chemicals *before* you begin work.
- Read instructions carefully before using tools and chemicals, and follow precautions for their use.
- Protect yourself by wearing safety goggles.

Around Children
- Remember your child's age and responsibility level when you buy toys and games. Avoid projectile toys such as darts and pellet guns, which can hit the eye from a distance.
- Supervise children when they are playing with toys or games that can be dangerous.
- Teach children the correct way to handle items such as scissors and pencils.

In the Yard
- Keep everyone away when you use a lawnmower. Don't let anyone stand on the side or in front when you mow the lawn.
- Pick up rocks and stones before mowing. These objects can shoot out of the blades, rebound off curbs or walls, and cause severe injury to the eye.

- Make sure that pesticide spray-can nozzles are pointed away from your face.
- Avoid low-hanging branches.

Around the Car
- Sparks and fumes can ignite easily and explode. Battery acid can cause serious eye injuries.
- Put out all cigarettes and matches before opening the hood of the car. Use a flashlight, not a match or lighter, to look at the battery at night.
- Keep protective goggles next to your jumper cables and wear them.
- Wear protective goggles during auto body repairs when grinding metal or striking metal against metal.

When You Jump-Start a Car
- Make sure the cars are not touching each other.
- Make sure that the jumper-cable clamps never touch each other.
- Never lean over the battery when attaching cables.
- Attach the positive (red) cable to the positive terminal of the dead battery first; then attach the other end of the positive cable to the good battery. Attach the negative (black) cable to the negative terminal of the good battery, then attach the other end of the negative cable to a grounded area on the engine away from the negative terminal of the dead battery. *Never attach a cable to the negative terminal of the dead battery.*

In Sports
- Wear protective safety glasses, especially for sports such as tennis, racquetball, squash, baseball, and basketball.
- Wear protective caps, helmets, or face protectors when appropriate, especially for sports such as ice hockey.

Around Fireworks
All fireworks can be dangerous to people of all ages.
- Never allow children to ignite fireworks.
- Do not stand near others when lighting fireworks.

InfoLinks
www.elvex.com

- When cycling at night or when visibility is poor, wear brightly colored reflective clothing.
- Use hand signals so drivers around you know what you plan to do.
- Obey traffic signals just like any other vehicle on the road. You have a right to bicycle on the road, but you also have the same responsibilities as other vehicles. Don't run stop signs or red lights!
- Brake carefully, and use both hand brakes at the same time. Using only the front brake can send you over the handlebars, and using only the back brake can cause a skid. On long downhills or in wet weather, gently tap the brakes to retain control. Be especially careful in wet weather, when wet brake pads are not very helpful.

Boating Safety

Most boating deaths result from drowning, when the victim was not wearing a personal flotation device (PFD). Of the 613 boaters who drowned in 1994, 550 could have been saved if they had been wearing a PFD, according to the U.S. Coast Guard.

The other major cause of boating accidents and fatalities is "operator error," including (1) inattention, not looking in the direction in which one is moving, (2) carelessness, going out in bad weather or water conditions or while intoxicated, and (3) speeding. In

unintentional injuries   injuries that have occurred without anyone's intending that harm be done.

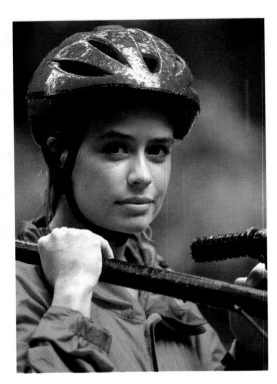

Wearing a helmet is an essential safety measure for cyclists.

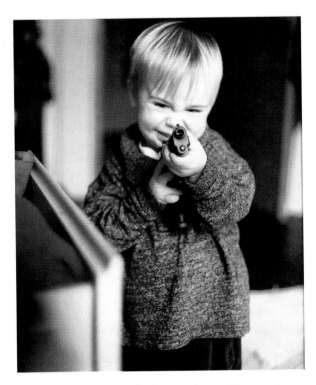

A toddler with a gun is a frightening image. Guns and ammunition should be stored separately in locked containers, and children should be taught that guns are not toys.

particular, intoxication is a factor in more than half of all boating accidents.[11] Too many casual boaters assume that rules of boating safety do not apply to them. Every boater should learn how to handle high winds, storms, whitecaps, rough waters, and heavy boat traffic. Most boat dealers can give you information about PFDs, "rules of the road," and Coast Guard safety regulations.

Even some experienced boaters tend to go too fast. Some modern watercraft tend to climb out of the water at higher speeds, and less hull in the water means less stability. With less stability, the boat tends to rock from side to side, and this rocking is a warning that you are about to lose control.

Firearm Safety

Each year over 11,000 Americans are murdered with guns and another 1,200 die in gun-related accidents.[2] Most murders are committed with handguns. (Shotguns and rifles tend to be more cumbersome than handguns and thus are not as frequently used in murders, accidents, or suicides.)

More than half of all murders result from quarrels and arguments between acquaintances or relatives. With many homeowners arming themselves with handguns for protection against intruders, it is not surprising that more than half of all gun accidents occur in the home. Children are frequently involved in gun accidents, often after they discover a gun they think is unloaded.

The United States leads the world in handgun homicides, with about 7,500 a year.[2] By comparison, only 75 people were murdered with handguns in 1994 in Britain. After 16 schoolchildren and their teacher were gunned down in Scotland in 1996, the British government proposed a ban on virtually all handguns. Such a proposal would face heavy opposition in the United States, from the National Rifle Association to the Clinton administration. In addition, there are already up to 230 million guns in civilian hands in the United States; 50 percent of homes have one, versus 5 percent in Britain.[12]

Handgun owners are reminded to adhere to the following safety rules:

- Make certain that you follow the gun possession laws in your state. Special permits may be required to carry a handgun.
- Make certain that your gun is in good mechanical order.
- If you are a novice, enroll in a gun safety course.
- Consider every gun to be a loaded gun, even if someone tells you it is unloaded.
- Never point a gun at an unintended target.
- Keep your finger off the trigger until you are ready to shoot.
- When moving with a handgun, keep the barrel pointed down.
- Load and unload your gun carefully.

⭐
Light Trucks and Sport Utility Vehicles: How Safe Are They?

In the United States, the hottest-selling vehicles at the turn of the millennium are light trucks, a category that includes sport utility vehicles (SUVs). In comparison to the average midsize sedan, these new "kings of the road" are heavier vehicles that have much stronger frames and more powerful engines. SUVs typically sit higher off the ground than cars. Often equipped with manual four-wheel drive transmissions and large tires, SUVs seem to be made to handle off-road terrain and adverse weather conditions.

Indeed, these vehicles may be safer than the typical midsize car. Recent studies have concluded that in crashes involving SUVs and cars (called "mismatch" accidents), people riding in cars are four times more likely to die than if they had been struck by another car. Stated another way, four in five of the people who die in mismatch accidents are occupants of cars.[18] Most of the damage relates to the laws of physics and, of course, the heavier vehicles usually fare better in mismatch crashes. Also, by riding higher than the typical car, SUVs' bumpers miss the side-impact beams of many cars and thus can easily crash through the weakest parts of most cars—the upper doors and window frame areas.

Critics of light trucks and SUVs are clamoring for the auto industry to reduce the weight of these vehicles and to make the bodies of SUVs more flexible, so they cannot damage cars as easily. Additionally, critics want SUVs to have more stringent fuel economy standards, uniform safety standards, and regulated bumper heights.[18]

Supporters of today's light trucks and SUVs point out that people purchase these vehicles in part because they are safer for their occupants. To redesign SUVs to make them lighter, less powerful, and lower to the ground would compromise important features that SUV customers want.

It will be interesting to see if there is an ultimate winner in this debate, or if a compromise can be reached. The success of the recently released Mercedes M-class (a lower-riding SUV specifically designed to help protect occupants of both vehicles in a crash) may have some influence on the future direction taken by SUV manufacturers.

- Store your gun and ammunition safely in separate locked containers. Use a trigger lock on your gun when not in use.
- Take target practice only at approved ranges.
- Never play with guns at parties. Never handle a gun when intoxicated.
- Educate children about gun safety and the potential dangers of gun use. Children must never believe that a gun is a toy.

Motor Vehicle Safety

The greatest number of accidental deaths in the United States occur on highways and streets. Young people are most likely to die from a motor vehicle accident. The following is a description of a prime candidate for such a death: a male, fifteen to twenty-four years of age, driving on a two-lane, rural road between the hours of 10 P.M. and 2 A.M. on a Saturday night.[10] If he has been drinking and is driving a subcompact car or motorcycle, the likelihood that he and his passengers will have a fatal accident is even more pronounced.

Motor vehicle accidents also cause disabling injuries. With nearly 2 million such injuries each year, all college students should be concerned about avoiding motor vehicle accidents. With this thought in mind, we offer some important safety tips for motor vehicle operators:

- Make certain that you are familiar with the traffic laws in your state.
- Do not operate an automobile or motorcycle unless it is in good mechanical order. Regularly inspect your brakes, lights, and exhaust system.

- Do not exceed the speed limit. Observe all traffic signs.
- Always wear safety belts, even on short trips. Require your passengers to buckle up. Always keep small children in child restraints.
- Never drink and drive. Avoid horseplay inside a car.
- Be certain that you can hear the traffic outside your car. Keep the car's music system at a reasonable decibel level.
- Give pedestrians the right-of-way.
- Drive defensively at all times. Do not challenge other drivers (see the Topics for Today article on p. 605). Refrain from drag racing.
- Look carefully before changing lanes.
- Be especially careful at intersections and railroad crossings.
- Carry a well-maintained first aid kit that includes flares or other signal devices.
- Drive even more carefully during bad weather.
- Do not drive when you have not had enough sleep (see Star Box on drowsy driving on p. 600).

Motorcycle Safety

Some emergency-room physicians call motorcycles "murder-cycles" because of their experience with motorcycle crash victims. The statistics support this grim view, with the death rate for motorcycles at 67.2 per 100,000 motorcycles, compared with a death rate for cars of 15.7 per 100,000.[13]

Drowsy Driving

Dean was driving home from college late on a moonlit Friday night. The summer night was crystal clear. The radio was playing loudly, there were few oncoming cars, and visibility was good. "I felt fine," Dean recalled later. "I was a little run down, but I wasn't sleepy at all. I was cruising along listening to tunes, and the next thing I knew I was surrounded by corn. The sound of the stalks hitting the car must have woken me up. It scared the hell out of me. I guess I fell asleep for a few seconds, but I don't know how it could have happened."

The Danger of Driving While Sleepy
Dean experienced a phenomenon that is too often ignored. Falling asleep at the wheel is something that no one thinks will happen to them, yet drowsy driving is estimated to cause up to 200,000 accidents per year on American roads.[19,20] Dean was lucky that he was not hurt or killed.

Sleepiness is a significant cause of traffic fatalities. Up to 3 percent of all yearly vehicular deaths in the United States can be attributed to driving while drowsy, yet Americans remain woefully uneducated about this problem.[19] Sleepiness undermines a person's ability to make sound decisions and reduces attention span considerably.[20] Any condition that impairs the judgment of drivers should be taken seriously. It has been estimated that 100 million Americans fail to get enough sleep and that up to 50 percent of all accident-related fatalities (not just driving fatalities) can be attributed to sleep deprivation.[21]

Tips to Avoid Drowsy Driving
Because of the stealthy manner in which sleep can overtake you, it is important to evaluate your condition before getting behind the wheel and also while you are on the road. It is also important to prevent regular sleep deprivation. We must reduce the risk of falling asleep while driving by using common sense. The following suggestions should help reduce your chances of driving while drowsy:[19]

- Get plenty of sleep. About 8 hours of sleep per night is desirable. If this is not practical, try to catch up on sleep when possible (take naps, sleep more on weekends, etc.).

- Take breaks while driving. Stop at least every 2 hours on long trips. If possible, avoid driving alone so the driving duties can be split. Don't eat heavy meals, and avoid too much caffeine.

- Stay alert. Talk, listen to the radio, sing, or do whatever you can to keep from drifting off. Don't let all of the passengers in the car sleep; having someone to converse with can help keep the driver alert.

- Don't get too comfortable. Getting too relaxed can promote dozing off. Avoid using cruise control. Reduce use of the heater, and keep the windows open when possible.

- Don't drink and drive. This is true anytime, but even a small amount of alcohol in the system can intensify the effects of fatigue on the body.

- If you feel yourself drifting off or you think you may be in danger of falling asleep, stop driving. Dozing off for a few seconds (a phenomenon known as *microsleep*) is a significant warning sign of fatigue. Don't try to fight through fatigue while driving. Pull off the road at a safe place and take a nap if you need to.

If you choose to ride a motorcycle, you can improve your chances of avoiding injury or death by following these suggestions:

- Most important of all, wear a helmet. A variety of studies have supported the effectiveness of helmets in preventing head injuries.[13] Warriors and athletes have worn helmets for centuries to protect themselves from head injuries. Modern examples include construction workers, football players, race car drivers, and military aircraft pilots.
- Wear boots, gloves, and heavy clothing to protect your skin from serious injury when you slide on pavement in a crash.
- Get proper training, such as the Motorcycle Safety Foundation course offered in some states.
- Your risk increases in wet weather. Consider whether a ride in the rain is necessary.
- Do not ride after taking medication that can affect your alertness or performance.
- Never ride after drinking alcohol or taking drugs. About half of motorcyclists killed in accidents had alcohol in their blood.

- Ride defensively. Remember that many drivers do not see you or may not give you the right-of-way you deserve.

Home Accident Prevention for Children and the Elderly

Approximately one person in ten is injured each year in a home accident. Children and the elderly spend significantly more hours each day in a home setting than do young adults and midlife people. These groups need more help to prevent accidents (see the Health Action Guide on p. 601). Here are some important tips to remember. Can you think of others?

For Everyone
- Be certain that you have adequate insurance protection.
- Install smoke detectors appropriately.
- Keep stairways clear of toys and debris. Install railings.
- Maintain electrical and heating equipment.
- Make certain that family members know how to get emergency help.

HEALTH ACTION GUIDE

Making Your Home Safe, Comfortable, and Secure

Entry
- Install a deadbolt lock on the front door and locks or bars on the windows.
- Add a peephole or small window in the front door.
- Trim bushes so burglars have no place to hide.
- Add lighting to the walkway and next to the front door.
- Get a large dog.

Bedroom and Nursery
- Install a smoke alarm and a carbon monoxide detector.
- Remove high threshold at doorway to avoid tripping.
- Humidifiers can be breeding grounds for bacteria; use them sparingly and follow the manufacturer's cleaning instructions.
- In the nursery, install pull-down shades or curtains instead of blinds with strings that could strangle a child.

Living Room
- Secure loose throw rugs or use ones with nonskid backing.
- Remove trailing wires where people walk.
- Cover unused electrical outlets if there are small children in the home.
- Provide additional lighting for reading, and install adjustable blinds to regulate glare.

Kitchen
- To avoid burns, move objects stored above the stove to another location.
- Install ceiling lighting and additional task lighting where food is prepared.
- Keep heavy objects on bottom shelves or countertops; store lightweight or seldom-used objects on top shelves.
- Promptly clean and store knives.
- Keep hot liquids such as coffee out of children's reach, and provide close supervision when the stove or other appliances are in use.
- To avoid foodborne illness, thoroughly clean surfaces that have come into contact with raw meat.

Bathroom
- A child can drown in standing water; keep the toilet lid down and the tub empty.
- Clean the shower, tub, sink, and toilet regularly to remove mold, mildew, and bacteria that can contribute to illness.
- Store medications in their original containers in a cool, dry place out of the reach of children.
- Add a bath mat or nonskid strips to the bottom of the tub.
- Add grab bars near the tub or shower and toilet, especially if there are elderly adults in the home.
- Keep a first aid kit stocked with bandages, first aid ointment, gauze, pain relievers, syrup of ipecac, and isotonic eyewash; include your physician's and a nearby emergency center's phone numbers.

Stairway
- Add a handrail for support.
- Remove all obstacles or stored items from stairs and landing.
- Repair or replace flooring material that is in poor condition.
- Add a light switch at the top of the stairs.
- If there is an elderly person in the home, add a contrasting color strip to the first and last steps to identify the change of level.

Fire Prevention Tips
- Install smoke detectors on every level of your home.
- Keep fire extinguishers handy in the kitchen, basement, and bedrooms.
- Have the chimney and fireplace cleaned by a professional when there is more than one-fourth inch of soot accumulation.
- Place space heaters at least 3 feet from beds, curtains, and other flammable objects.
- Don't overload electrical outlets, and position drapes so that they don't touch cords or outlets.
- Recycle or toss combustibles, such as newspapers, rags, old furniture, and chemicals.
- If you smoke, use caution with cigarettes and matches; never light up in bed.
- Plan escape routes and practice using them with your family.

InfoLinks
www.parentzone.com/parents/homesafty/index.htm

For Children
- Know all the ways to prevent accidental poisoning.
- Use toys that are appropriate for the age of the child.
- Never leave young children unattended, especially infants.
- Keep any hazardous items (guns, poisons, etc.) locked up.
- Keep small children away from kitchen stoves.

For the Elderly
- Protect from falls.
- Be certain that elderly people have a good understanding of the medications they may be taking. Know the side effects.
- Encourage elderly people to seek assistance for home repairs.
- Make certain that all door locks, lights, and safety equipment are in good working order.
- Refer to pages 588–589 for additional information related to the protection of older adults.

Personal Applications
- Read the preceding list and the Health Action Guide above, and then assess potential safety hazards in your own home. Do you see an accident waiting to happen? Is your home as secure as it could be against intruders?

Real Life
Real choices

- According to current thinking, is rape (1) a crime motivated by sexual desire or (2) a crime of violence that is carried out through sexual conduct?
- In some cases men have accused women of date rape. Whether you are male or female, do you believe this could be a valid claim? Why or why not?
- Have you ever been involved in a date rape situation, as either the aggressor or the victim? If so, how did you deal with the situation at the time? Afterward? What behaviors on your part and your partner's part do you think contributed to the situation?

And Now, Your Choices . . .

- Given what you know about rape in general and date rape in particular, what steps can you take to protect yourself from becoming involved in a situation like Debra and Ron's?
- If Ron or Debra were your friend, how do you think you could be most helpful to him or her in dealing with this experience?

Summary

- Everyone is a potential victim of violent crime.
- Each year in the United States, intentional injuries cause about 50,000 deaths and millions of additional nonfatal injuries.
- The national rate of serious crimes such as murder, rape, and robbery has been falling in recent years.
- Homicide is the leading cause of death for young male African-Americans. Handguns are the weapon of choice for homicides.
- About half of all homes in the United States have a gun, with a total of about 230 million guns.
- Because of factors related to family structure, increased drug use and crime, and the inability of people to resolve conflicts peacefully, domestic violence is on the rise.

- Forms of child abuse include physical abuse, sexual abuse, and child neglect. Child neglect is the most common form.
- Bicyclists and motorcyclists can best protect their safety by wearing a helmet.
- Bias and hate crimes, as well as the crime of stalking, are increasingly recognized as serious violent acts.
- Rape and sexual assault, acquaintance rape, date rape, and sexual harassment are forms of sexual victimization in which victims often are both physically and psychologically traumatized.
- Unintentional injuries are injuries that occur accidentally. The numbers of fatal and nonfatal unintentional injuries are exceedingly high.

Review Questions

1. Identify some of the categories of intentional injuries. How many people are affected each year by intentional injuries?
2. What are some of the most important facts concerning homicide in the United States? How are most homicides committed?
3. Identify changes in the traditional family structure that may be related to increased family stress and domestic violence. What additional factors also may be related to increased domestic violence?
4. What reasons might explain why so many women do not report domestic violence?
5. Aside from the immediate consequences of child abuse, what additional problems do many abused children face in the future?
6. List some examples of groups that are known to have committed bias or hate crimes.
7. Identify some general characteristics of a typical stalker.
8. Explain some of the myths associated with rape. How can date rape be prevented?
9. Identify some examples of behaviors that could be considered sexual harassment. Why are employers especially concerned about educating their employees about sexual harassment?
10. Identify some common examples of unintentional injuries. Point out three safety tips from each of the safety areas listed in this chapter.
11. Why do sport utility vehicles (SUVs) tend to fare better than a typical car in a "mismatch" crash?

References

1. *Health: United States, 1996–97 and injury chartbook.* DHHS pub. no. PHS 97-1232. Hyattsville, MD: National Center for Health Statistics, 1997.
2. *Firearm violence: in the nation.* Oklahoma City: Oklahoma State Department of Health, Jan 14, 1999. www.health.state.ok.us/program/injury/violence/firearmv.html
3. Bureau of Justice Statistics. *Drugs, crime, and the justice system: a national report.* U.S. Department of Justice, Washington, DC: U.S. Government Printing Office, Dec 1992.
4. U.S. Bureau of the Census. *Statistical abstract of the United States: 1996.* 116th ed. Washington, DC: U.S. Government Printing Office, 1996.
5. Bureau of Justice Statistics. *Guns and crime: handgun victimization, firearm self-defense, and firearm theft.* U.S. Department of Justice, Washington, DC: U.S. Government Printing Office, April 1994.
6. Bachman R. *Violence against women: a national crime victimization survey report.* U.S. Department of Justice, Washington, DC: U.S. Government Printing Office, Jan 1994.
7. Widom CS. The cycle of violence. *Research in brief.* National Institute of Justice, U.S. Department of Justice, Washington, DC: U.S. Government Printing Office, 1992.
8. National Committee for Prevention of Child Abuse. *12 alternatives to whacking your kid.* Chicago, undated pamphlet.
9. Glazer S. Declining crime rates. *CQ Researcher* 1997 April 4.
10. Bever DL. *Safety: a personal focus.* 4th ed. St. Louis: Mosby, 1996.
11. Acerrano A. Danger afloat. *Sports Afield* 1997 March: 49.
12. Witkin G. A very different gun culture. *U.S. News & World Report* 1996 Oct 28: 44.
13. Council on Scientific Affairs, American Medical Association. Helmets and preventing motorcycle- and bicycle-related injuries. *JAMA* 1994 Nov 16: 272(19):1535–38.
14. *Violence in U.S. schools: at least 13 killed in past months.* ABCNEWS and Starwave Corp., June 15, 1998. http://abcnews.com
15. *Why do teens kill?: explaining acts of brutality by youngsters.* ABCNEWS and Starwave Corp., May 24, 1998. http://abcnews.com
16. Reducing urban violence. *World Health* 1997 Jan-Feb; 49(1):36.
17. *Preventing eye injuries.* San Francisco: American Academy of Ophthalmology, 1993.
18. Baumgartner M. *Mismatch means death on the highway.* ABCNEWS and Starwave Corp., Sept. 26, 1998. http://archive.abcnews.go.com
19. Matson M. Forgotten menace on our highways. *Reader's Digest* 1994 June; 144(86).
20. Toufexis A. Drowsy America. *Time* 1990 Dec 17; 136(26).
21. Bennett G. Why you must get more sleep. *McCall's* 1994 Dec; 122(3).

Suggested Readings

Berry DB. *The domestic violence sourcebook: everything you need to know.* Lincolnwood, IL: Lowell House, 1998. This book provides a comprehensive examination of issues surrounding domestic violence. In individual chapters, the author discusses historical, psychological, social, family, and legal issues that pertain to domestic violence. Prevention and treatment are also viewed as critical issues. People who are affected by domestic violence will find this book useful, especially the current list of resources at the end of the book.

Goold GB. *First aid in the workplace: what to do in the first five minutes.* 2nd ed. Paramus, NJ, Prentice-Hall, 1998. This book covers all essential elements required by OSHA's current guidelines. It is designed for a 6- to 8-hour first aid course for people who have had little or no first aid training. Clear and concise information details basic first aid procedures for a number of injuries that might occur in the workplace. Photographs are used to illustrate specific skills.

Levy B. *In love and danger: a teen's guide to breaking free of abusive relationships* 2nd ed. Seattle: Seal Press Feminist Publications, 1998. The author indicates that one out of three high school and college students experiences some degree of violence in his or her dating relationships. This book is useful for anyone who might be involved in an abusive relationship, whether the abuse is emotional, physical, or sexual in nature. Readers learn how to differentiate between a healthy relationship and an addictive relationship. An important part of the book is the information that tells the reader how to get out of an abusive relationship successfully. A list of resources for help is provided.

Marques L, Carter L, Nelson M. *Child safety made easy.* Concord, CA: Screamin' Mimi Publications, 1998. Illustrated with cartoon characters, this humorous book presents hundreds of important safety tips for people who care for small children. The writing style is straightforward and doesn't burden the reader with detailed explanations. This book will be especially useful for first-time parents.

O'Shea T, Lalonde J. *Sexual harassment: a practical guide to the law, your rights, and your options for taking action.* New York: Griffin Trade Paperback, 1998. This book was written by two women who themselves have experienced sexual harassment at work. The authors explain the differences between the two types of sexual harassment: quid pro quo and the hostile work environment. Information is presented that helps readers learn what to do when they feel they are being harassed. A step-by-step plan tells readers how to keep records of incidents, confront the harasser, file a complaint, inform a supervisor, and get legal help.

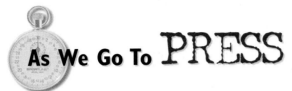

As We Go To PRESS

Two employees were recently injured during a shooting rampage at a Salt Lake City television station. A woman with a 9 mm pistol and a bag of bullets entered the downtown office building and began firing. One employee was critically injured by a shot to the head. Another was shot but not seriously injured before the woman was captured and disarmed by workers in the building. Do you think a violent incident could occur in your workplace? What can you do to protect yourself?

In other news as we go to press, early 1999 was a prosperous time for many Americans. As a result of corporate mergers and downsizing, however, increasing numbers of employees are receiving layoff notices. This trend has caused safety officials to become nervous about the possibility of increased workplace violence. Companies are scrambling to develop safety plans that may reduce the average 1,000 murders that take place on the job each year. Workplace homicide is the leading cause of on-the-job deaths for women employees and the second leading cause of workplace-related deaths for men.

Rage on the Road: The Danger of Aggressive Driving

The driver behind you is following so closely that you can't see his license plate in your rear view mirror. Or maybe the car in front of you is hogging the passing lane and won't even do the speed limit. Surprise! A driver in the next lane slips in front of you, without using a turn signal, into a space that is only a carlength because you slowed down so she wouldn't hit you. On another road, it's more of the same. Someone feels compelled to pull out in front of the last car in a line of traffic rather than wait a fraction of a second for the road to be clear. People run stop signs and stop lights that are long since yellow. At merges, drivers drag race until someone "chickens out" when the lane ends, rather than take turns. And there are those people who speed past the line of cars forming for an exit or lane closure and try to cut in at the front of the line. Add four-letter words, horn honking, and a couple of hand gestures and you have all of the elements of a daily commute. These rude and unthinking drivers set the stage for highway aggression and danger.

Motorists are aware of an increasing sense of aggression on America's congested highways. An unthinking act or no provocation at all can result in a deadly face-off with a complete stranger.[1] Over the last six years, aggressive drivers have killed 218 people and injured another 12,610, at a frequency that increases by about 7 percent each year.[2] This is just the tip of the iceberg. For every incident serious enough to result in a police report or newspaper story, hundreds or thousands of other incidents take place that are never reported. The problem has become so severe that, according to a National Highway Safety Administration report, the public is more concerned about aggressive drivers (40%) than drunk drivers (33%).[1]

During the average 22.4-minute commute[3] and on leisure excursions, millions of American drivers are conditioned to accept stupid, uncivilized driving. The hostile and aggressive behavior of the instigators and those who react to them reinforces the belief that belligerence works.[4] Of course, belligerence does not work—it only causes anger to escalate, which can result in accidents, property damage, injury, and death. Various weapons are used when traffic altercations become violent. Conventional weapons, such as firearms, knives, clubs, and tire irons, were used in 44 percent of reported violent traffic altercations. The vehicle itself became the weapon in 23 percent of the cases, and in 12 percent of the incidents the car and a conventional weapon were both used. In several unusual cases, pepper spray, eggs, golf clubs, and even a crossbow were involved.[2]

Characteristics of Aggressive Drivers

Although there is no profile *per se* of the typical aggressive driver, most aggressive drivers are men between the ages of 18 and 26. Many of these men are poorly educated, and some have criminal records or histories of violence and substance abuse, but hundreds of others are successful men and women, of all ages, with no such history.[2]

Between the sexes, men are angered most by police presence and slow driving, whereas illegal behavior and traffic obstructions tend to frustrate women. When all factors are added in, though, men and women do not differ in total driving anger scores.[5] Increasingly, women are acting on their anger. Only 4 percent of recorded aggressive driving incidents involved women drivers,[2] but during the last 15 years the number of fatal accidents involving women drivers has increased dramatically while men's risks have dropped.[6] Most of the increase for women has occurred because more women are on the road at riskier times, but women are also increasingly displaying the more aggressive driving tactics common among men.[6]

Individually, people generally think of themselves as better-than-average drivers. This holds true even among younger people, who consider themselves to be good drivers but their peers to be the worst drivers of any age group.[7] But perceptions and reality are not always identical. While some people are aware of their aggressive tendencies on the road, other people see themselves as innocent and the issue of aggressive driving as everyone else's problem. The truth is, we're all human and can let our emotions run away from us. Many professionals suggest that you tape-record your vocalizations in the car to become

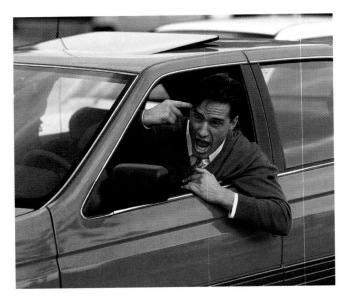

The stresses of home, work, and commuting, the anonymity of driving, and other factors can add up to rage on the road.

aware of and change your own negative and intense driving behavior.[8]

Causes of Aggressive Driving

Violent traffic disputes result not from single incidents but from personal attitudes and accumulated stress in motorists' lives. Specifically, drug use, domestic arguments or violence, racism, the desire to evade or attack police, and the everyday stresses of home, work, and commuting can lead to aggressive driving.[2] For the general population, the anonymity and physical excitement of driving, combined with a feeling of control and power and the ability to drive away, sow the seeds of aggression.[9] Some people drive to "win" rather than to arrive safely at their destination.[1] Adding to this climate are overpowered cars, driver's licenses that are easy to qualify for, and sporadically lax enforcement of traffic laws.[4]

Unfortunately, and perhaps tellingly, the people who spend the most time on the road are the least effective at dealing with its stressors. Long-distance commuters have higher blood pressure, less tolerance for frustration, and more frequent negative moods than short- or medium-distance commuters.[6] Carpooling, which only 13 percent of American drivers do,[3] not only saves gas and miles on the car, but it also lessens the negative effects of commuting, especially over long distances, for everybody in the carpool. Ride sharing has actually been shown to lower the blood pressure of those in carpools.[6]

Recent Incidents

The next time you say to yourself, "Who does this speed demon behind me think he is, Richard Petty?" you may be right. In 1996 race car driver Richard

Petty was fined $65 and assessed 4 points against his North Carolina driver's license for "bumping" a car that he was tailgating at over 70 mph.[10]

More recently, two New Jersey male drivers faced criminal charges in the death of a woman who was a passenger in one of the cars. In this road rage incident, one driver cut off the path of the other. A dangerous high-speed chase ensued. Eventually one of the cars veered off the road and crashed, killing the woman.[11]

In Orlando, Florida, a 21-year-old man was sentenced to 11 years in prison after being convicted of attempted murder in an August 1997 shooting. In this case of road rage, the convicted man shot and nearly killed a person who was pushing his stalled car off a main road. Apparently he was upset at being delayed by the stalled car.[12]

In January 1999, a 40-year-old truck driver stuck in a massive traffic jam reportedly took out his road rage against the car in front of him. The Tulsa, Oklahoma, trucker was arrested for ramming his rig ten times into the woman's nearby car. She eventually found a safe area and called police on her cell phone.[13]

Avoiding Aggressive Drivers

The best way to stay out of driving conflicts is not to be an aggressive driver yourself. You can do a number of things to reduce your stress and thus reduce the tendency toward aggression. First, allow plenty of time for your trip. We tend to overschedule our days and not allow enough time to get from one place to the next. Sure, under perfect conditions you could cover X number of miles in X amount of time, but weather, traffic, and road construction are facts of life. Not building extra travel time into our schedules causes us to run late when we encounter these variables and then get angry and possibly aggressive. Other ways to reduce stress are to listen to soothing music, improve the comfort of your vehicle, and probably most important, understand that you can't control the traffic—only your reaction to it.[2]

If traffic really pushes your buttons, you may want to avoid peak commuting hours. If your company doesn't have a flextime policy, you can go in a little earlier and leave a little later.[6] If you're still tempted to let another driver have it, imagine that you're being videotaped.[8] How would you react if the world were watching? Or imagine that the driver in the other car is someone you love—a spouse, parent, grandparent, sibling, or friend. How would you treat them? Practice driving courtesy and keep the following points in mind:

- Do not make obscene gestures.
- Use your horn sparingly.
- Do not block the passing lane.

- Do not switch lanes without signaling.
- Do not block the right-hand turn lane.
- Do not take more than one parking space.
- If you are not disabled, do not park in a space reserved for disabled people.
- Do not allow your door to hit the car parked next to you.
- Do not tailgate.
- If you travel slowly, pull over and allow traffic to pass.
- Avoid unnecessary use of high-beam headlights.
- Do not let the car phone distract you.
- Do not stop in the road to talk to a pedestrian or another driver.
- Do not inflict loud music on neighboring cars.[2]

Avoid engaging other drivers by following the limousine drivers' rule: Duty bound to protect their passengers, they do not make eye contact with other drivers.[1] If another driver is following you, don't drive home. Instead, drive to a public place, ideally a police station. This or using your cell phone to call for help is usually enough to scare off the offending driver.

Of course, it's hard not to respond when challenged. It may help to look at the other driver's mistakes and actions objectively and not take them personally.[2] Treat their poor behavior as their problem; don't make it yours. Remember how dangerous the situation can become.

It's not one driver's job to teach other drivers proper manners.[8] In all certainty, you won't be successful. Instead, try being extra nice to a fellow driver. Courtesy can be as contagious as aggression.

For Discussion . . .

What aspect of driving makes you the angriest? How do you handle the situation? Do you recognize any of your own bad driving habits in the list above? What can be done about the problem of aggressive driving?

References

1. Cook WJ. Mad driver's disease: a survival guide for handling highway nuts, from a recovering lunatic. *U.S. News and World Report* 1996; 121(19):74–76.
2. AAA Foundation. *Road rage on the rise.* 1997. http://webfirst.com/aaa
3. Anonymous. A nation of drivers. *U.S. News and World Report* 1996; 121(8):13.
4. Magliozzi TL. Cars, civilization and world peace. *Technology Review* 1994; 97(4):62–63.
5. Deffenbacher JL, Oetting ER, Lynch RS. Development of a driving anger scale. *Psychological Reports* 1994; 74(1):83–91.
6. Spilner M. Destress your commute. *Prevention* 1995; 47(3):60–62.
7. Guerin B. What do people think about the risks of driving? Implications for traffic safety interventions. *J App Soc Psychol* 1994; 24(11):994–1021.
8. James L, Nahl D. *Dr. Driving says.* 1997. http://www.aloha.net/%7Edyc
9. Thurber S. Don't drive under the influence of emotion. *Safety and Health* 1994; 150(1):66–68.
10. Toner R. He just hates running second. *The New York Times* 1996; 145(1):24.
11. Road rage race leads to charges. *Yahoo News.* Reuters Ltd., Jan 7, 1999. http://dailynews.yahoo.com
12. Road rage shooting sentence. *Yahoo News.* Reuters Ltd., Jan 6, 1999. http://dailynews.yahoo.com
13. Police hold trucker for road rage. *Yahoo News.* Reuters Ltd., Jan 6, 1999. http://dailynews.yahoo.com

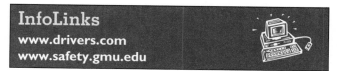

InfoLinks
www.drivers.com
www.safety.gmu.edu

MASTERING TASKS

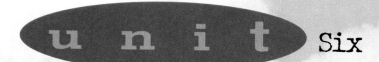

unit Six

Consumerism and Environment

Throughout Unit 6 we have explored the health-related issues of consumerism, the environment, and violence and safety. Now we relate these topics to the important developmental tasks of identity, independence, responsibility, social skills, and intimacy.

Forming an Initial Adult Identity

Whether we are able to admit it or not, we all want to find out "who we are." To develop the confidence to face the world and to contribute to its improvement require that we come to grips with personal strengths and limitations. Although it may be valuable to be able to understand and analyze others, it is much more significant that we discover, develop, and define our own identity. Examining attitudes and behaviors about health consumerism, the environment, and violence can help us learn about ourselves. In the area of self-care, we can examine how we value and manage health; we learn about ourselves as we consider how we take care of ourselves when we are ill. Are you a person who must always visit a doctor when ill, or are you able to cope reasonably well with self-limiting conditions? Are you a skilled consumer in purchasing prescriptions or over-the-counter medications? Honest answers to these kinds of questions will help you understand your unique identity.

Establishing Independence

Gaining a sense of independence can be a refreshing, exciting experience for most young adults. Relocation, employment, and new friendships will propel you into consumer involvement on a scale greater than that required while at home or in college.

Besides choosing new health care providers, you will independently obtain the insurance needed to pay for these services. Health insurance and disability insurance are critical investments you must make. Independence often brings with it new acquaintances who may attempt to push you into areas of consumerism for which you have no real need. Start preparing yourself now to live and work among people who will try to influence your consumer perspectives.

Assuming Responsibility

There is no area of responsibility more immediate than the responsibility you assume for your own safety. As violence escalates in our society, including on campuses, you must be increasingly responsible for your actions and your responses to the actions of others. Make a concerted effort to understand the environmental cues associated with personal safety and plan ahead in dealing with threatening situations.

Developing Social Skills

Regardless of whether we are involved in decisions related to our environment or our consumer choices, we frequently make these decisions with other individuals, companies, or agencies. Our social skills help us convey our needs, interpret directions, and voice concerns. Effective speaking, listening, writing, reading, and cooperation with others are the tools we need to refine as we work to improve our health or the health of others.

Sometimes in the areas of consumerism, environment, and safety, the social interactions we have with others may not always be pleasant. For example, voicing a complaint about a health-related product may require a face-to-face confrontation with a store manager. Speaking up at a public debate on a local environmental issue might be intimidating. Poise, tact, and a degree of assertiveness may be beneficial in both of these situations. Fortunately, these social skills can be developed and sharpened with practice.

Developing Intimacy

The development of intimacy suggests a certain quality in (or about) the environment in which interactions take place. Your physical environment should contribute to a safe, aesthetic, and supportive backdrop to life. In the absence of such an environment, intimacy as well as safety can be compromised by a variety of concerns. The environment in which you pursue intimacy must be safe from acts of violence. Victimization of a person by a partner, including harassment and rape, is the antithesis of all that is implied in intimacy.

Part of intimacy is openness and honesty. These qualities must also be present in the intimate relationships that we have with health care providers and others whom we trust to deliver products, services, and information required for lifelong health.

u
n
i
t

The Life Cycle

This last unit comprises a single chapter on a topic that inevitably affects each of us: dying and death. Traditional-age students may think that death will not touch their lives until they grow older. Yet many young people must face the reality of death much sooner, when a loved one is lost to gang violence, AIDS, suicide, an accident, or some other tragedy.

1 Physical Dimension

Unless we die suddenly, at a young age, most of us will enjoy years of good physical health before we begin a period of gradual decline. Eventually we may experience an extended period of failing health before dying of a chronic condition, such as heart disease. However, many people today experience their highest level of physical health late in life. An adequate activity level, weight management, smoking cessation, and moderation of alcohol use can increase the likelihood that an older adult will be able to enjoy good physical health well into his or her later years.

2 Emotional Dimension

The process of dying and death can be emotionally draining for both the dying person and his or her loved ones. The death of a spouse, close friend, or child, especially when it is unexpected, can be emotionally taxing. The grieving person may feel anger, sadness, regret, and a range of other complex emotions. Indeed, coping with death can be a great challenge to the emotional stability of even the healthiest person.

3 Social Dimension

The dying process and the event of a loved one's death offer opportunities for reaching out to others. In fact, many people who have had these experiences report that having a social support system was essential to maintaining their emotional balance during the ordeal. The families of people who are dying must also deal effectively with health-care professionals, funeral directors, and estate executors.

4 Intellectual Dimension

As in any other crisis, a strong intellect is a valuable resource during the dying and death process. Complex decisions about treatment options must be made. Loved ones may be left to sort out the finances of a family member who has died. These difficult situations require an ability to analyze many variables in order to make sound choices.

5 Spiritual Dimension

Confronting the reality of death requires drawing on spiritual resources. Those who have a strong religious faith may find comfort in their beliefs, while others may find that their faith is shaken by the experience. Those who are not religious may look for other ways to find meaning in the event.

6 Occupational Dimension

The dying process often unfolds slowly. A person who is terminally ill may have to continue working for months or even years before he or she becomes so ill that work is no longer possible. Clearly, such an illness can make work difficult. However, some people find that their job provides a welcome diversion as well as a social support network.

7 Environmental Dimension

Many people who are terminally ill or who have a loved one who is dying find that communion with nature and the environment is comforting and strengthens their spirituality as they move through the dying process.

chapter
twenty-one

Accepting Dying
and Death

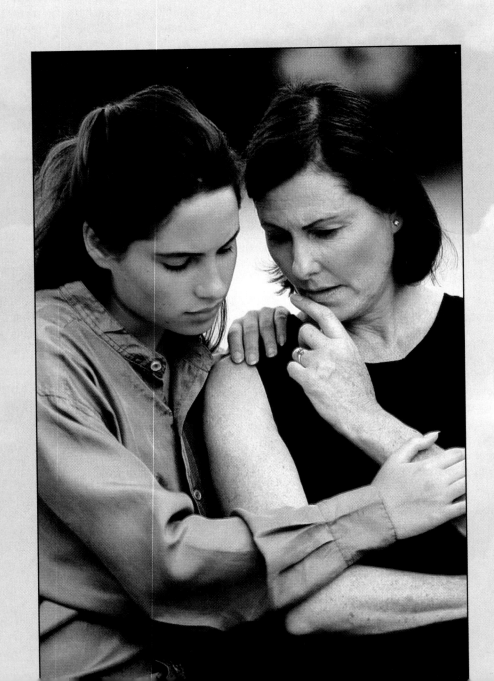

The primary goal of this chapter is to help people realize that accepting the reality of death can motivate us to live a more enjoyable, productive, and meaningful life. Each day in our lives becomes especially meaningful only after we have fully accepted the reality that someday we will die. We can then live each day to its fullest, as if it were our last day.

Our mortality gives us a framework from which to appreciate and conduct our lives. It should help us prioritize our activities so that we can accomplish our goals (in our academic work, our relationships with others, and our recreation) before we die. Quite simply, death gives us our only absolute reason for living.

HEALTHY PEOPLE: LOOKING AHEAD TO 2010

In the last decade, national health objectives have focused on increasing the life span and years of healthy life for Americans, reducing death rates from various diseases, and reducing infant mortality rates. With few exceptions, the nation has made steady progress toward reaching target goals for many of these objectives.

For the American population as a whole, life expectancy has increased rapidly, with the average life span now at nearly 76 years. However, among racial and ethnic minorities, these estimates of years of healthy life have been less encouraging. Despite the increase in life expectancy, declines in health-related quality of life measures have been troubling.

Real progress has been made in reducing death rates in other areas. For example, the number of

deaths caused by unintentional injuries has declined. A reduction in traffic fatalities, especially among young people, has been the most important factor in meeting this goal. The number of deaths caused by work-related injuries has also been reduced significantly.

With continual advances that preserve life and health, we expect the *Healthy People 2010* objectives to focus on additional ways the nation can reduce death rates and increase longevity. These objectives will be found in the target areas of chronic diseases, unintentional injuries, occupational health, and health services. Special efforts aimed at racial and ethnic minority populations will be an important priority.

Real Life
Real choices

- Name: Wendy DuBois
- Age: 21
- Occupation: Physical education student

EXIT 47B-SHORE POINTS reads the green and white sign just ahead on Wendy's right. The cloudless blue sky and brisk off-shore breeze promise another perfect beach day, but that's not where Wendy's going. Instead of joining the crawling knot of ocean-bound vehicles in the left lane of the exit ramp, Wendy whisks along the empty right lane, following the sign that says SOUTH SHORE MEDICAL CENTER.

No trace of the sparkling summer day follows Wendy through the whispering revolving door at the hospital's entrance. In here, she thinks, the weather is always the same: cool, dim, windless.

The west wing of the fifth floor is quiet this early July afternoon, and patients are sleeping or resting in many of the rooms Wendy passes. At the half-open door to Room 518 she pauses, feeling overwhelmed once again by the surge of conflicting emotions that wash over her every time she sees Jenny in this bed. As always, her impulse is to say, "Come on—let's get out of here," as if those words would magically cause the tubes and needles in Jenny's arms to vanish, the bruises to fade, the glow of health to return to her pale cheeks, the horror of the last several months to seep back into the black hole from which it emerged.

"Hey, Zebra!" As always, Jenny has sensed Wendy's presence without having seen her, and now she turns toward her best friend with the smile that even radiation and chemotherapy haven't dimmed. "Hey, Wing," Wendy replies, in a ritual that dates back to their days on the junior high field hockey team.

It seems like just last week that they were eager novices at the game they both grew to love. But it was almost 10 years ago, Wendy reflects. How fast the time has gone, how fast it's going now, how suddenly Jenny got sick, how soon she'll . . . "NO!" screams a voice inside Wendy. No—she isn't dying, she can't, I won't let her. But she's in pain, says another voice. She still laughs, banters with the nurses, is cheerful with me and with her family. But the shadow is over her; it's growing longer every day. I can't stand to let her go and I can't stand to see how hard she has to work to keep *us* from being afraid.

Fear is just one of the emotions Wendy feels as she helplessly watches her best friend lose ground every day to the ravages of leukemia. Terror, anguish, rage, and hope all do battle within her as she tries to accept the fact Jenny is dying. Sometimes Wendy sees the mute pleading in Jenny's eyes and knows her friend is weary and longing for release from pain, drugs, nausea, from other people's fears and expectations, from the effort it costs her to fight for one more day. For Wendy it seems impossible to choose between encouraging Jenny to hang on and acknowledging her need to let go, between talking about her recovery and dealing with her reality. I love you, Jenny, Wendy says silently. I want to help you do it your way.

As you study this chapter, think about Wendy's feelings as she tries to come to terms with Jenny's dying, and prepare yourself to answer the questions in **Your Turn** at the end of the chapter.

Dying in Today's Society

Since the 1920s, the way people experience death in this society has changed. Formerly, most people died in their own homes, surrounded by family and friends. Young children frequently lived in the same home with their aging grandparents and saw them grow older and eventually die. Death was seen as a natural extension of life. Children grew up with a keen sense of what death meant, both to the dying person and to the grieving survivors.

Times have indeed changed. Today about 70 percent of people die in hospitals, nursing homes, and extended care facilities, rather than in their own homes. The extended family is seldom at the bedside of the dying person.[1] Sometimes, frantic efforts are made to keep a dying person alive. Although medical technology has improved our lives, some people believe that it has reduced our ability to die with dignity. Many are convinced that our way of dying has become more artificial and less civilized than it used to be. The trend toward hospice care may be a positive response to this high-tech manner of dying (see p. 621).

Many families are forced to deal with death unexpectedly when a loved one dies in an accident or by violence. The emotions they feel are somewhat different from the ones normally evoked when a friend or relative dies of a disease or failing health in old age. See the Topics for Today article on page 631 for a look at the unique needs and concerns of these families.

Definitions of Death

Death was once easy to define. People were considered dead when a heartbeat could no longer be detected and when breathing ceased. Now, with the technological advances in medicine, especially emergency medicine, some patients who give every indication of being dead can be resuscitated. Critically ill people, even those in comas, can now be kept alive for years with many of their bodily functions maintained by medical devices, including feeding tubes and respirators.

Thus death can be a very difficult concept to define.[2] Many professional associations and ad hoc interdisciplinary committees have struggled with this problem and have developed criteria by which to establish death. Some of these criteria have been adopted by state legislatures, although there is certainly no consensus definition of death that all states embrace.

Clinical determinants of death measure bodily functions. Often judged by a physician, who can then sign a legal document called a *medical death certificate,* these clinical criteria include the following:

1. Lack of heartbeat and breathing.
2. Lack of central nervous system function, including all reflex activity and environmental responsiveness. This can often be confirmed by an **electroencephalograph** reading. If no brain wave activity is recorded after an initial measurement and a second measurement after twenty-four hours, the person is said to have undergone *brain death.*
3. The presence of **rigor mortis**, indicating that body tissues and organs are no longer functioning at the cellular level. This is sometimes called *cellular death.*

The legal determinants used by government officials are established by state law and often adhere closely to the clinical determinants just listed. A person is not legally dead until a physician, **coroner,** or health department officer has signed a death certificate.

Euthanasia

There are two types of euthanasia for desperately ill people: They are either intentionally put to death (**direct [active] euthanasia**) or allowed to die without being subjected to heroic lifesaving efforts (**indirect [passive] euthanasia**). Direct euthanasia is usually performed through the administration of large amounts of depressant drugs, which eventually causes all central nervous system function to stop. Although direct euthanasia is commonly practiced on house pets and laboratory animals, it is illegal for humans in the United States, Canada, and other developed countries. However, in 1992, the Netherlands became the first country to enact legislation that permits euthanasia under strict guidelines. See the Star Box above for a discussion of direct euthanasia.

Indirect euthanasia is increasingly occurring in a number of hospitals, nursing homes, and medical centers. Physicians who withhold heroic lifesaving techniques or drug therapy treatments or who disconnect life-support systems from terminally ill patients are practicing indirect euthanasia. Although some people still consider this form of euthanasia a type of murder, indirect euthanasia seems to be gaining legal and public

Direct Euthanasia and Dr. Kevorkian

Since 1990 Dr. Jack Kevorkian, a retired pathologist, has led a crusade for the legalization of physician-assisted suicide. Kevorkian reportedly has helped approximately 130 terminally ill patients end their lives. Until late 1998 Kevorkian typically provided delivery devices and drugs for patients who wished to die. The patients would then trigger the flow of lethal drugs themselves. Kevorkian had been acquitted in three trials in Michigan.

In November 1998 Kevorkian showed his opposition to a new Michigan law banning assisted suicide, which went into effect in September 1998, by giving the CBS news program "60 Minutes" a provocative videotape showing him performing direct euthanasia. The videotape appeared to show someone (allegedly Kevorkian) directly injecting Thomas Youk, a victim of Lou Gehrig's disease, with potassium chloride. This videotape of Youk's death was shown by CBS to approximately 15 million viewing households on November 22, 1998.[18]

Michigan prosecutors charged Kevorkian with murder, not assisted suicide. In March 1999, after a brief trial in which Kevorkian served as his own attorney, a jury convicted him of second degree murder. At the time of this writing, Kevorkian was awaiting sentencing in April. The 70-year-old Kevorkian could have received 10 to 25 years in prison. Do you know the final outcome of this landmark trial?

acceptance for people with certain terminal illnesses—near-death cancer patients, brain-dead accident victims, and hopelessly ill newborn babies. Examples of passive euthanasia that are familiar to hospital personnel include physicians' orders of "do not resuscitate" (DNR) and "comfort measures only" (CMO).

Personal Applications

• If you were determined to be in a persistent vegetative state, would you want your life support to be disconnected?

electroencephalograph an instrument that measures the electrical activity of the brain.

rigor mortis rigidity of the body that occurs after death.

coroner an elected legal official empowered to pronounce death and to determine the official cause of a suspicious or violent death.

direct (active) euthanasia the process of inducing death, often through the injection of lethal drugs.

indirect (passive) euthanasia the process of allowing a person to die by disconnecting life support systems or withholding lifesaving techniques.

Advance Medical Directives

Because some physicians and families have difficulty supporting indirect euthanasia, many people are starting to use legal documents called *advance medical directives*.[3] One of these medical directives is the living will (see the Star Box on p. 617). This is a document that confirms a dying person's desire to be allowed to die peacefully and with a measure of dignity if a time should arise when little hope exists for recovery from a terminal illness or severe injury. All fifty states and the District of Columbia have living will statutes. The living will requires that physicians or family members carry out a person's wishes to die naturally, without receiving life-sustaining treatments.[4] About 25 percent to 30 percent of U.S. citizens have signed living wills.[4]

A second important document that can assist terminally ill or incapacitated patients is the **medical power of attorney for health care** document. This legal document authorizes another person to make specific health-care decisions about treatment and care under specified circumstances, most commonly when patients are in long-term vegetative states and cannot communicate their medical wishes. This document helps tell hospitals and physicians which person will help make the critical medical decisions. Usually this person is a loving relative. Concerned people should complete both a living will and a medical power of attorney for health-care document.

Personal Applications

- Have you or any of your relatives prepared a living will or a durable power of attorney for health care document?

Emotional Stages of Dying

People who have a terminal illness undergo a process of self-adjustment. The stages in this process have helped form the basis for the modern movement of death education. Knowing these stages may help you understand how people adjust to other important losses in their lives.

Perhaps the most widely recognized name in the area of death education is Dr. Elisabeth Kübler-Ross. As a psychiatrist working closely with terminally ill patients at the University of Chicago's Billings Hospital, Kübler-Ross could observe the emotional reactions of dying people. In her classic book *On Death and Dying*, Kübler-Ross summarized the psychological stages that dying people often experience.[5]

- *Denial.* This is the stage of disbelief. Patients refuse to believe that they actually will die. Denial can serve as a temporary defense mechanism and can allow patients the time to accept their prognosis on their own terms.
- *Anger.* A common emotional reaction after denial is anger. Patients can feel as if they have been cheated. By expressing anger, patients can vent some of their fears, jealousies, anxieties, and frustrations. Patients often direct their anger at relatives, physicians and nurses, religious symbols, and normally healthy people.
- *Bargaining.* Terminally ill people follow the anger stage with a bargaining stage. Patients who desperately want to avoid their inevitable deaths attempt to strike bargains—often with God or a church leader. Some people undergo religious conversions. The goal is to buy time by promising to repent for past sins, to restructure and rededicate their lives, or to make a large financial contribution to a religious cause.
- *Depression.* When patients realize that, at best, bargaining can only postpone their fate, they may begin an unpredictable period of depression. In a sense, terminally ill people are grieving for their own anticipated death. They may become quite withdrawn and refuse to visit with close relatives and friends. Prolonged periods of silence or crying are normal components of this stage and should not be discouraged.
- *Acceptance.* During the acceptance stage, patients fully realize that they will die. Acceptance ensures a relative sense of peace for most dying people. Anger, resentment, and depression are usually gone. Kübler-Ross describes this stage as one without much feeling. Patients feel neither happy nor sad. Many are calm and introspective and prefer to be left either alone or with a few close relatives or friends.

The psychological stages of dying include two more important points. Just as each person's life is totally unique, so is each person's death. Unfolding deaths vary as much as do unfolding lives. Some people move through Kübler-Ross's stages of dying very predictably, but others do not. It is not uncommon for some dying people to avoid one or more of these stages entirely.

The second important point about Kübler-Ross's stages of dying is that the family members or friends of dying people often pass through similar stages as they observe their loved ones dying. When

---

medical power of attorney for health care   a legal document that designates who will make health-care decisions for people unable to do so for themselves.

The Living Will

The living will is a legally binding document in all 50 states and the District of Columbia. This document allows individuals to express their wishes about dying with dignity. When such a document has been drawn, families and physicians are better able to follow the wishes of people who are near death.

A living will instructs physicians to withhold or withdraw certain medical treatments or procedures that could postpone death if the patient has a terminal illness or is in a coma or a persistent vegetative state. Two physicians, one of whom is the attending physician, must determine and document that (1) the patient's cognitive functioning is substantially impaired and (2) there is no reasonable expectation of recovery.

Both federal and state laws govern the use of advance directives. The federal law, called the Patient Self-Determination Act, requires health-care facilities that receive Medicare and Medicaid funds to inform patients of their right to execute an advance directive.

Choice in Dying is a not-for-profit organization that developed the first living will in 1967. This organization provides advance directives, counsels patients and families, trains professionals, advocates right-to-die legislation, and offers a wide range of publications and services. At its website (http://www.choices.org), for a small fee you can download state-specific advance directive packages (see the illustration below for a sample generic living will). You can also learn about recent changes in state law that may necessitate executing a new living will. For specific questions, contact Choice in Dying at (800) 989-WILL.

Canadians can log into the Living Wills Registry (http://www.sentex.net), which offers information about living wills in Canada and explains the Power of Attorney for Personal Care (PAPC) document. This site also covers organ donation issues and tracks recent Canadian court cases related to right-to-die legislation.

INSTRUCTIONS	**Florida Living Will**
Print the date	Declaration made this _____ day of _____, 19
Print your name	____.
	I, _____, willfully
	and voluntarily make known my desire that my dying not be artificially prolonged under the circumstances set forth below, and I do hereby declare:
	If at any time I have a terminal condition and if my attending or treating physician and another consulting physician have determined that there is no medical probability of my recovery from such condition, I direct that life-prolonging procedures be withheld and withdrawn when the application of such procedures would serve only to prolong artificially the process of dying, and that I be permitted to die naturally with only the administration of medication or the performance of any medical procedure deemed necessary to provide me with comfort care or to alleviate pain.
	It is my intention that this declaration be honored by my family and physician as the final expression of my legal right to refuse medical or surgical treatment and to allow the consequences for such refusal.
	In the event that I have been determined to be unable to provide express and informed consent regarding the withholding, withdrawal, or continuation of life-prolonging procedures, I wish to designate, as my surrogate to carry out the provisions of this declaration:
Print the name, home address, and telephone number of your surrogate	Name: _____
	Address: _____
	_____ Zip Code: _____
	Phone: _____
© 1996 Choice In Dying, Inc.	

	I wish to designate the following person as my alternate surrogate, to carry out the provisions of this declaration should my surrogate be unwilling or unable to act on my behalf:
Print name, home address, and telephone number of your alternate surrogate	Name: _____
	Address: _____
	_____ Zip Code: _____
	Phone: _____
Add personal instructions (if any)	Additional instructions (optional):
	I understand the full importance of this declaration, and I am emotionally and mentally competent to make this declaration.
Sign the document	Signed: _____
Witnessing Procedure	Witness 1:
	Signed: _____
	Address: _____
Two witnesses must sign and print their addresses	Witness 2:
	Signed: _____
	Address: _____
© 1996 Choice In Dying, Inc.	Courtesy of Choice In Dying, Inc. 6/96 1036 80th Street, NW Washington, DC 20007 800-989-9455 Page 2

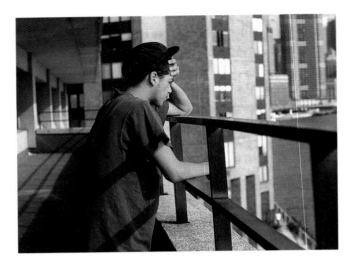

Family members and friends often experience emotions similar to those of the dying person.

informed that a close friend or relative is dying, many people also experience varying degrees of denial, anger, bargaining, depression, and acceptance. Because of this, as caring people we need to recognize that the emotional needs of the living must be fulfilled in ways that do not differ appreciably from those of the dying.[6]

Near-Death Experiences

Death ends our physical existence. Perhaps this is the ultimate connection between death and our physical dimension of health. Many people believe that, in a positive sense, death brings a sense of relief and comfort—two qualities one may need most when one is dying. The classic work of Raymond Moody,[7] who examined reports of people who had near-death experiences, suggests that we may have less to fear about dying than we have generally thought.

In a comprehensive study of more than 100 people who had near-death experiences, Kenneth Ring[8] reported that these people shared a core experience. This experience was composed of some or all of the following stages:

1. A sense of well-being and peace
2. An out-of-body experience in which the dying person floats above his or her body and witnesses the activities that are occurring
3. A movement into extreme blackness or darkness
4. A shaft of intense light that generally leads upward or lies in the distance
5. A decision to enter into the light

Central to this experience is the need to decide whether to move toward death or to return to the body that has been temporarily vacated.

Several studies, including surveys of recently resuscitated hospital patients and a nationwide poll of the general population, estimate that near-death experiences are reported by 30 percent to 40 percent of individuals who come close to death, or about 5 percent of the U.S. population.[9]

Experts do not agree whether near-death experiences are truly associated with death or more closely associated with the depersonalization that some people experience during particularly frightening situations. In a scientific sense, near-death experiences are impossible to prove. Science can neither verify nor deny the existence of out-of-body experiences.[1]

Regardless, for those who have had near-death experiences, simply knowing that death might not be such an unpleasant experience appears to be comforting. Most seem to have formed a new orientation toward living.[1]

Interacting with Dying People

Facing the impending death of a friend, relative, or loved one is a difficult experience. If you have yet to go through this situation, be assured that, as you grow older, your opportunities will increase. This is part of the reality of living.

Most counselors, physicians, nurses, and ministers who spend time with terminally ill people suggest that you display one quality when interacting with dying people: honesty. Just the thought of talking with a dying person may make you feel uncomfortable. (Most of us have had no training in this sort of thing.) Sometimes, to make ourselves feel less anxious or depressed, we may tend to deny that the person we are with is dying. Our words and nonverbal behavior reveal that we prefer not to face the truth. Our words become stilted as we gloss over the facts and merely attempt to cheer up both our dying friend and ourselves. This behavior is rarely beneficial or supportive—for either party.

As much as possible, we should attempt to be genuine and honest. We should not try to avoid crying if we feel the need to cry. At the same time, we can give dying people emotional support by allowing them to express their feelings openly. We should resist the temptation to try to pull someone out of the denial, anger, or depression. We should not feel obliged to talk constantly and to fill long pauses with idle talk. Sometimes nonverbal communication, including touching, may be much more appreciated than mere talk. Because our interactions with dying people help fulfill our needs, we too should express our emotions and concerns as openly as possible.

The Millennium and Mass Suicides

Every few years we seem to hear a shocking news report about a mass suicide of members of some cult. In the spring of 1997 police made the grisly discovery that 39 members of a group called Heaven's Gate had committed suicide together in southern California. Before this incident, David Koresh ended a long standoff with government authorities in Waco, Texas, by leading his followers to a fiery death.

As this textbook goes to press, the start of the new millennium is close at hand. This event is expected to prompt irrational violent behavior among groups around the world. The most prominent case at this time involves a doomsday sect called the Concerned Christians, a group of American Christians based in Colorado under the leadership of Monte Kim Miller. In October 1998 Miller prophesied that the city of Denver would suffer from apocalyptic destruction by an earthquake. Obviously this prophecy never materialized, and some 75 cult members later headed for Israel.[19]

Israel was a logical place for these cult members to gather, because Miller had said he would die in the streets of Jerusalem in December 1999 and then be resurrected three days later. Family members and experts on cult activity believed that Miller, age 44, had convinced the members of Concerned Christians that God speaks directly through him. They also believed that he had the power to convince his cult members that they must end their own lives on earth.[19]

In early January 1999 authorities in Israel arrested 14 of the cult members, accused them of plotting violence, and deported them. Israeli officials feared this group might cause chaos by committing a public bloodbath or by trying to destroy religious shrines, such as the Temple Mount in the Old City of Jerusalem. On January 9 the cult members returned to Denver, where they faced no criminal charges.[20]

It is unfortunate that concerns over mass suicides and terrorist activities will dampen some of the enthusiasm the world will experience as we move into the new millennium.

Talking with Children About Death

Because most children are curious about everything, we should not be surprised that they are also fascinated about death. From very young ages, children are exposed to death through mass media (see the Star Box about mass suicide, above), adult conversations ("Aunt Emily died today," "Uncle George is terminally ill"), and their discoveries (a dead bird, a crushed bug, a dead flower). The way children learn about death greatly affects their ability to recognize and accept their own mortality and to cope with the deaths of others.

Psychologists encourage parents and older friends to avoid shielding children from or misleading children about the reality of death. Young children need to realize that death is not temporary and is not like sleeping. Parents should make certain they understand children's questions about death before they give an answer. Most children want simple, direct answers to their questions, not long, detailed dissertations, which often confuse the issues. For example, when a four-year-old asks her father, "Why is Tommy's dog dead?" an appropriate answer might be, "Because he got very, very sick and his heart stopped beating." Getting involved in a long discussion about "doggy heaven" or the causes of specific canine diseases may not be necessary or appropriate.

When a child suffers the loss of a near relative, informing the child is a painful task. Adults are usually present when a near relative dies, but children in Western societies are unlikely to be present at the time of death. In the death of a parent, the surviving parent usually must tell the child. The surviving parent sometimes tells the child the news much later, and often in a misleading form.

For example, the surviving parent typically tells the child that the spouse has gone to heaven. For those who are devoutly religious, this fits in with the parent's own belief. For many others, however, this conflicts with the parent's belief and creates conflicts and mistaken ideas in the child. Unless they are told otherwise, children may believe that heaven is a place like any other, and that it is only a matter of time before the parent returns.

Another common tendency is to tell children that the deceased has "gone to sleep." Young children take things literally and may not understand this figure of speech. Such a report can cause a child to fear falling asleep. Other surviving parents hide their feelings of loss in an effort to shield their children from emotional pain or out of fear of the intensity of the children's emotions.

The two crucial pieces of information that the child must know eventually are that the dead parent will never return and that the body has been buried in the ground or burned to ashes.[10] Often parents will find that the schoolchild or adolescent has a greater capacity to face the truth than was supposed. Children should be given the truth, and the sympathy and support to bear it.

Parents should answer questions when they arise and always respond with openness and honesty. In this way, children can learn that death is a real part of life and that sad feelings are a normal part of accepting the death of a loved one.

Personal Applications

• How were issues of death handled in your family when you were growing up?

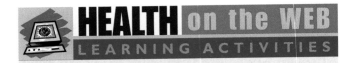

HEALTH on the WEB
LEARNING ACTIVITIES

Learning About Hospice Care

Hospice is an alternative approach to dying for terminally ill patients and their families. The goal of hospice care is to improve the quality of life of dying people and their loved ones. Visit the Hospice Net Inc. website at www.hospicenet.org and select *What Questions Should I Ask About Hospice Care?* Read through the frequently asked questions and their answers. What did you learn about hospice care?

Exploring Grief for a Public Figure

The expression of grief is a valuable process that gradually permits people to detach themselves from the deceased. When Princess Diana died in 1997, a public outpouring of grief occurred. Most people remember where they were when they heard Diana had died. Did her death affect you? Did you feel a sense of loss, as if someone you knew personally had died? Go to broadcast.web-point.com/wbzl/d98po.htm and complete the statements related to how you felt about Diana's death. Compare your results with those of others who have completed the survey.

Raising Your Awareness About Organ Donation

The Coalition on Donation is a not-for-profit alliance of local coalitions and national organizations that have joined forces to promote organ and tissue donation. The coalition has created national education and action campaign packets for distribution by its 50 local affiliates. The campaign stresses the importance of deciding to become an organ and tissue donor and the need to tell your family of your decision. Visit the Coalition on Donation website at www.shareyourlife.org. Select *Fact or Fiction?* to test your knowledge of organ donation.

For more activities, log on to our Online Learning Center at www.mhhe.com/hper/health/payne

Death of a Child

Adults face not only the death of their parents and friends but perhaps also the death of a child. Whether because of sudden infant death syndrome (SIDS), chronic illness, accident, or suicide, adults are sometimes forced to grieve the loss of someone who was "too young to die."

Parents and children are bound by physical and emotional ties like no other relationship. When the tragic death of a young child severs that bond, the pain and anguish the parents feel can be too much to bear. Getting through such a traumatic experience can be one of life's toughest challenges.

Miscarriage

Most pregnancies progress to full term and result in the birth of a healthy child. However, researchers now believe that about one-third of pregnancies end in miscarriage. Since accurate home-pregnancy tests were developed, many women began learning early in the first trimester that they are pregnant. Thus, rather than mistaking the miscarriage for a late heavy menstrual period, more women now know that their pregnancy has ended. Most then go through a grieving process.

In addition, other couples may learn of complications that lead them to choose an elective abortion, or the baby may die during birth or during infancy. Though most people know that such things can happen, many believe that such tragedies happen only to others. When they face the death or potential loss of a child, parents often find their beliefs shaken and their faith tested.[11]

Miscarriage can be especially difficult for the mother. She may think that something she did (or did not do) has caused the miscarriage. An exact cause of a miscarriage may never be determined, and the woman needs to be reassured that she did not cause any abnormalities in the fetus.[11]

A miscarriage can be painful and stressful for the woman. Physical symptoms may not occur when the baby dies but may be delayed for some time. Sometimes parents find out about a potentially fatal or severely debilitating problem with the fetus before the child is born. In these situations, the parents face the choice of continuing the pregnancy or terminating it. Hearing such a diagnosis, taking in all available information, and reaching a decision can be a traumatic experience. Parents must weigh many factors when making this decision, including their spiritual beliefs, potential suffering of the baby (if the long-term prognosis is poor), effects on the family of having a child with special needs, and financial considerations. If the couple decides to terminate the pregnancy (or if a continued pregnancy may result in miscarriage or stillbirth), the couple must be prepared for the sadness and trauma of parting with their baby.

Death During the Birthing Process

In some instances, the parents know beforehand that the baby has a poor chance of surviving through birth, so they have an opportunity to prepare for this occurrence. For others, however, the baby's death is totally unexpected. Parents who thought they would be bringing home a healthy baby end up dealing with the devastation of losing their child.

In the past, babies with lethal birth defects often were quickly taken away from their mothers, but today many parents are being given the option of spending time holding and saying good-bye to their baby, and medical personnel are encouraged to accommodate the parents and support their wishes in this regard.[12]

Losing a Baby After It Is Born

Even after a baby is delivered, there are health risks. The support of family and friends is especially important when a couple is trying to recover from the death of a child. Friends and co-workers can help by acknowledging the death of the child and offering support. Often people will not mention the baby because they think that the parents will become upset, but not talking about the baby can cause pain for the parents.[12] Showing up in person (as opposed to just calling or sending a card) to offer support can also help.[13]

Tactful language can also help prevent unpleasant feelings for the parents. If an unhealthy fetus is miscarried or aborted, sometimes people try to rationalize the loss for the parents by saying it was "nature's way" of preventing the birth of an imperfect child.[13] Such comments are not only insensitive, but they imply that the parents should be grateful that they lost the baby. Even seemingly innocent comments can cause pain in the wrong context.

Parents often want to hold on to the memory of the child. Such feelings are normal and do not mean that the parents are clinging to their grief or are neurotic.[12] Remembering the child can give a sense of meaning to parents' lives. Parents often do something constructive to help them remember their baby and get over the death. Putting together a scrapbook, donating the baby's clothes and toys to charity, writing memoirs, or setting up a place for remembrance can help the family keep memories of the baby.[12,13]

Eventually the grief should lose its intensity. It may flare up again around "anniversaries" (the baby's due date or birthday, the date of the baby's death), but gradually things should become bearable. The family will be forever changed by the experience. The death of a child can change the parents' value system, and their spiritual beliefs may be challenged as well.[12]

The Grieving Process

The way a baby dies can affect the grieving process. Whether the child is lost before birth (miscarriage, abortion), during birth (stillbirth, trauma), or in infancy (sudden infant death syndrome [SIDS], accident, birth defect) can affect how the parents deal with the loss. It can also can affect the way family and friends support the parents.

Coping with the death of a child gives adults a difficult period of adjustment, particularly when the death was unexpected. Experts agree that grieving adults, particularly the parents, should express their grief fully and proceed cautiously to return to normal routines. They can avoid many pitfalls. Adults who are grieving for dead children should do the following:

- Avoid trying to cope by using alcohol or drugs.
- Make no important life changes. Moving to a different home, relocating, or changing jobs usually doesn't help parents deal any better with the grief they are experiencing.

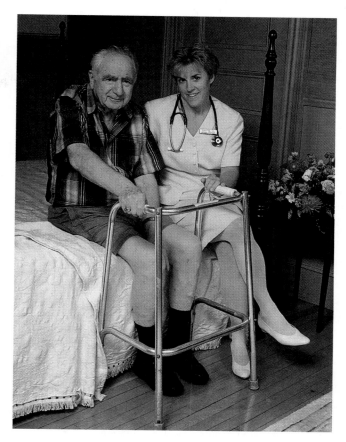

Hospice care allows terminally ill patients to spend their last days in a warm, homelike setting.

- Share their feelings with others. Grieving adults should share their feelings particularly with other adults who have experienced a similar loss. Group support is available in many communities.
- Avoid trying to erase the death. Giving away clothing and possessions that belonged to the child cannot erase the adult's memories of the child.
- Give themselves the time and space to grieve. On the anniversary of the child's death or on the child's birthday, family members should give themselves special time just for grieving.
- Don't attempt to replace the child. Do not quickly have another child or use the deceased child's name for another child.

For most adults, grief over the death of a child will require an extended time. Eventually, however, life can return to normal.

Hospice Care for the Terminally Ill

The thought of dying in a hospital ward, with spotless floors, pay television, and strict visiting hours,

Learning
From Our Diversity

Hospice: Spiritual Healing for the Dying

Once considered a radical approach to caring for people with terminal illness, the hospice movement has been experiencing increasing popularity in the United States over the past two decades. Founded in England by Dr. Cicely Saunders, the modern hospice movement seeks to provide comfort and relief of physical pain to the dying without seeking a cure or using heroic measures to sustain life. Whereas some patients choose to live in a hospice facility, the majority remain in their homes, where care is provided by family and friends under the guidance of hospice health-care professionals. Whether in a facility or at home, hospice patients have chosen to accept the reality of their terminal illness and to forgo medical care that is aimed at prolonging life or achieving a cure.[21]

In addition to physical pain relief, a less well known but equally important goal of hospice care is to alleviate "spiritual pain," which Cicely Saunders identifies as part of the "total pain" of dying. This is the pain of the whole person and is the overlapping of the physical, psychological, social, and spiritual. One physician experienced in hospice care identified these elements of spiritual pain: "the experiences of disconnection, disharmony, non-alignment, and disintegration."

Dr. Saunders recognized in the dying the presence of spiritual pain, and she directed the resources of hospice professionals to alleviate this special kind of distress. This pain is a combined fear of dying, guilt and regret about one's life, and sadness about the imminent separation from spouse, children, or friends. Such distress comes from the awareness that life is almost over and death is near. Although medical skills can help patients live longer and more comfortably with physical pain, spiritual pain can be more intense and last longer.

The "why" questions—such as "Why me?" and "Why now?"—are indicators of spiritual pain. The feelings expressed are despair, fear, guilt, failure, and hopelessness. Sometimes, according to one expert, listening is enough to bring about some spiritual peace and quiet, which he describes as "experiences such as connection, alignment, harmony, and meaningfulness."

Sometimes, he says, healing and spiritual peace and quiet just happen on their own. To realize that spiritual healing sometimes "just happens" is important because, even though those who care for the dying can help in healing, it is the dying who heal themselves. One caution he gives is that "our own personal answers" about life and our own religious beliefs should not be given in an effort to heal someone. Caregivers should always offer words of encouragement, he says; these words, along with the loving way that medical and nursing care is given, can, as Cicely Saunders says, reach the most hidden places in the person's spirit.

Have you known a dying person who chose to spend his or her last days in hospice care instead of a hospital? What is your impression of that person's experience with hospice? Which choice do you think you would make for yourself: hospice care or hospital?

leaves many people with a cold feeling. Perhaps this thought alone has helped encourage the concept of **hospice care.** Hospice care is an alternative approach to dying for terminally ill patients and their families. The goal of hospice care is to maximize the quality of life of dying people and their family members. Popularized in England during the 1960s, yet derived from a concept developed during the Middle Ages (where hospitable lodges took care of weary travelers), the hospice helps people die comfortably and with dignity by using one or more of the following strategies:

- *Pain control.* Dying people usually are not treated for their terminal disease; they are given appropriate drugs to keep them free from pain, alert, and in control of their faculties. Drug dependence is of little concern, and patients can receive pain medication when they feel they need it.
- *Family involvement.* Family members and friends are trained and encouraged to interact with the dying person and with each other. Family members often care for the dying person at home. If the hospice arrangement includes a

hospice ward in a hospital or a separate building (also called a hospice), the family members have no restrictions on visitation.
- *Multidisciplinary approach.* The hospice concept promotes a team approach. Specially trained physicians, nurses, social workers, counselors, and volunteers work with the patient and family to fulfill important needs. The needs of the family receive nearly the same priority as those of the patient.
- *Patient decisions.* Contrary to most hospital approaches, hospice programs encourage patients to make their own decisions. The patient decides when to eat, sleep, go for a walk, and just be alone. By maintaining a personal schedule, the patient is more apt to feel in control of his or her life, even as that life is slipping away.

Another way the hospice differs from the hospital approach is in the care given to the survivors. Even after the death of the patient, the family receives a significant amount of follow-up counseling. Helping families with their grief is an important role of the hospice team.

The number of hospices in the United States has climbed quickly to more than 2,400.[14] People seem to be convinced that the hospice system does work effectively. Part of this approval may be the cost factor. The cost of caring for a dying person in a hospice is usually less than the cost of full (inpatient) services provided by a hospital. Although insurance companies are delighted to see the lower cost of hospice care, many are still uncertain how to define hospice care. Thus not all insurance companies are fully reimbursing patients for their hospice care. Before you discuss the possibility of hospice care for members of your family, you should consider the extent of hospice coverage in your health insurance policy.

Personal Applications

• Will hospice care be an option you might choose someday?

Grief and the Resolution of Grief

The emotional feelings that people experience after the death of a friend or relative are collectively called *grief. Mourning* is the process of experiencing these emotional feelings in a culturally defined manner. See the Star Box at right for more information about the grieving process. The expression of grief is seen as a valuable process that gradually permits people to detach themselves from the deceased. Expressing grief, then, is a sign of good health.

Although people experience grief in remarkably different ways, most people have some of the following sensations and emotions:

• *Physical discomfort.* Shortly after the death of a loved one, grieving people display a similar pattern of physical discomfort. This discomfort is characterized by "sensations of somatic distress occurring in waves lasting from twenty minutes to an hour at a time, a feeling of tightness in the throat, choking with shortness of breath, need for sighing, and an empty feeling in the abdomen, lack of muscular power, and an intense subjective distress described as a tension or mental pain. The person soon learns that these waves of discomfort can be precipitated by visits, by mentioning the deceased, and by receiving sympathy."[15]
• *Sense of numbness.* Grieving people may feel as if they are numb or in a state of shock. They may deny the death of their loved one.
• *Feelings of detachment from others.* Grieving people see other people as being distant from

The Grieving Process

The grieving process consists of four phases, each of which varies in length and form in each individual. These phases are composed of the following:

1. *Internalization of the deceased person's image.* By forming an idealized mental picture of the dead person, the grieving person is freed from dealing too quickly with the reality of the death.
2. *Intellectualization of the death.* Mental processing of the death and the events leading up to its occurrence move the grieving person to a clear understanding that death has occurred.
3. *Emotional reconciliation.* During this third and often delayed phase, the grieving person allows conflicting feelings and thoughts to be expressed and eventually reconciled with the reality of the death.
4. *Behavioral reconciliation.* Finally, the grieving person can comfortably return to a life in which the death has been fully reconciled. The survivor reestablishes old routines and adopts new patterns of living where necessary. The grieving person has largely recovered.

The friends of a grieving person sometimes make the mistake of encouraging a return to normal behavior too quickly. When friends urge the grieving person to return to work right away, make new friends, or become involved in time-consuming projects, they may be preventing necessary grieving. It is not easy or desirable to forget about the fact that a spouse, friend, or child has recently died.

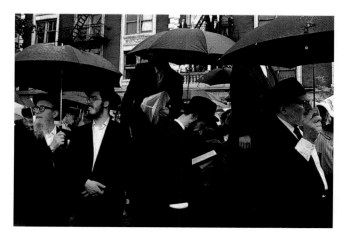

Mourning rituals are culturally defined; these Jewish men are attending the Brooklyn funeral of Lubavich Grand Rabbi Schneerson.

them, perhaps because the others cannot feel the loss. A person in grief can feel very lonely. This is a common response.

hospice care (hos pis)   an approach to caring for terminally ill patients that maximizes the quality of life and allows death with dignity.

- *Preoccupation with the image of the deceased.* The grieving person may not be able to complete daily tasks without constantly thinking about the deceased.
- *Guilt.* The survivor may be overwhelmed with guilt. Thoughts may center on how the deceased was neglected or ignored. Sensitive survivors feel guilt merely because they are still alive. Indeed, guilt is a common emotion.
- *Hostility.* Survivors may express feelings of loss and remorse through hostility, which they direct at other family members, physicians, lawyers, and others. Sometimes survivors may feel anger at the deceased person, perhaps at the suddenness of the death, at leaving the survivor to deal with problems, or at abandoning the survivor. Such a feeling may cause the survivor to feel guilty and ashamed. Survivors should know that such hostility can be a normal part of grieving.
- *Disruption in daily schedule.* Grieving people often find it difficult to complete daily routines. They can suffer from an anxious type of depression. Seemingly easy tasks take a great deal of effort. Starting new activities and relationships can be difficult. Social interaction skills can be lost.
- *Delayed grief.* In some people, the typical pattern of grief can be delayed for weeks, months, and even years.

HEALTH ACTION GUIDE

Helping the Bereaved

Leming and Dickinson[1] report that the peak time of grief begins in the week after a loved one's funeral. Realizing that there is no one guaranteed formula for helping the bereaved, friends and caregivers can help by performing some or all of the following:

- Make few demands on the bereaved person; allow him or her to grieve.
- Help with the household tasks.
- Recognize that the bereaved person may vent anguish and anger and that some of it may be directed at you.
- Recognize that the bereaved person has painful and difficult tasks to complete; mourning cannot be rushed or avoided.
- Do not be afraid to talk about the deceased person; this lets the bereaved know that you care for the deceased.
- Express your own genuine feelings of sadness, but avoid pity. Speak from the heart.
- Reassure bereaved people that the intensity of their emotions is very natural.
- Advise the bereaved to get additional help if you suspect continuing severe emotional or physical distress.
- Keep in regular contact with the bereaved; let him or her know you continue to care about them.

InfoLinks
http://bereavement.org

The grief process continues until the bereaved person can establish new relationships, feel comfortable with others, and look back on the life of the deceased person with positive feelings (see the Health Action Guide below). Although the duration of the grief resolution process varies with the emotional attachments one has to a deceased person, grief usually lasts from a few months to a year. One should seek professional help when grieving is characterized by unresolved guilt, extreme hostility, physical illness, significant depression, and a lack of other meaningful relationships. Trained counselors, physicians, and hospice workers can all play significant roles in helping people through grief.

Rituals of Death

Our society has established many rituals associated with death that help the survivors accept the reality of death, ease the pain associated with the grief process, and provide a safe disposal of the body. Our rituals give us the chance to formalize our good-byes to a person and to receive emotional support and strength from family members and friends. In recent years, more of our rituals seem to be celebrating the life of the deceased. In doing this, our rituals also reaffirm the value of our own lives.

Most of our funeral rituals take place in funeral homes, churches, and cemeteries. Funeral homes (or mortuaries) are business establishments that provide a variety of services to the families of dead people. The services are carried out by funeral directors, who are licensed by the state in which they operate. Most funeral directors are responsible for preparing the bodies for viewing, filing death certificates, preparing obituary notices, establishing calling hours, assisting in the preparation and details of the funeral, selecting a casket, transporting mourners to and from the cemetery, and counseling the family. Although licensing procedures vary from state to state, most new funeral directors must complete one year of college, one year of mortuary school, and one year of internship with a funeral home before taking a state licensing examination.

Full Funeral Services

An ethical funeral director will attempt to follow the wishes of the deceased's family and provide only the services requested by the family. Most families want traditional, **full funeral services.** Three significant components of the full funeral services are as follows.

Embalming

Embalming is the process of using formaldehyde-based fluids to replace the blood components. Embalming helps preserve the body and return it to a natural look. Embalming permits friends and family members to view the body without being subjected to the odors associated with tissue decomposition. Embalming is often an optional procedure, except when death results from specific communicable diseases or when body disposition (disposal) is delayed.

Calling Hours

Sometimes called a *wake* or *visiting hours,* this is an established time when friends and family members can gather in a room to share their emotions and common experiences about the dead person. Generally in the same room, the body will be in a casket, with the lid open or closed. Open caskets assist some people to confirm that death truly did occur. Some families prefer not to have any calling hours.

Funeral Service

Funeral services vary according to religious preference and the emotional needs of the survivors. Although some services are held in a church, most funeral services today take place in a funeral home, where a special room might serve as a chapel. Some services are held at the graveside. Families may also choose to have a simple memorial service within a few days after the funeral. Completing the Personal Assessment on page 626 will help you think about what kind of funeral arrangements you would prefer for yourself.

Disposition of the Body

Ground Burial   We dispose of bodies in one of four ways. Ground burial is the most common method. About 75 percent of all bodies undergo ground burial. The casket is almost always placed in a metal or concrete *vault* before being buried. The vault serves to further protect the body (a need only of the survivors) and to prevent collapse of ground because of the decaying of caskets. Most cemeteries require the use of a vault.

Entombment   A second type of disposition is *entombment.* Entombment refers to nonground burial, most often in structures called **mausoleums.** A mausoleum contains a series of shelves where caskets can be sealed in vaultlike spaces called **crypts.** Entombment also can take place in the floors, walls, or basements of buildings. For example, the bodies of many famous British religious, cultural, and government leaders are entombed in the crypts of Westminster Abbey in London.

Cremation   Cremation is a third type of body disposition. In the United States, 21 percent of all bodies are cremated.[16] This practice is increasing. Generally both the body and casket (or cardboard cremation box) are incinerated so that only the bone ash from the body remains. The body of an average adult produces

about five to seven pounds of bone ash. These ashes then are placed in containers called *urns,* and then buried, entombed, or scattered, if permitted by state law. The itemized crematory fee (from $200 to $500) is much less than ground burial. Some families choose to cremate after having full funeral services.[17]

Anatomical Donation   A fourth method of body disposition is anatomical donation. Separate organs (such as corneal tissue, kidneys, or the heart) can be donated to a medical school, research facility, or organ donor network. Certain states permit people to state on their driver's licenses that they wish to donate their organs. However, family consent (by next of kin) is also required at the time of death for organ or tissue donation to proceed. Recently, hospitals have been required by federal law to inform the family of a deceased person about organ donation at the time of his or her death. Thus anyone who wishes to donate organs at the time of death should discuss these wishes with his or her family as soon as possible so that family members will support the donation at the time of the individual's death.

The need for donor organs is much greater than our current supply (see the Star Box on p. 627). For some, the decision to donate body tissue and organs is rewarding and comforting. Organ donors understand that their small sacrifice can help give life or improve the quality of life for another person. In this sense, their death can mean life for others. To become an organ donor, you must fill out a uniform organ donor card like the one in Figure 21-1.

Some people choose to donate their entire body to medical science. Often this is done through prior arrangements with medical schools. Bodies still require embalming. After they are studied, the remains are often cremated and returned to the family, if requested. Just as with an organ donation, those who wish to donate their bodies should discuss their wishes with family members beforehand so that their wishes can be carried out at the time of death.

Personal Applications

• At your death, would you want your organs or body tissue donated to help another person? Are there any organs you would prefer not to donate?

---

full funeral services   all of the professional services provided by funeral directors.

mausoleum (moz oh **lee** um)   an above-ground structure, which frequently resembles a small stone house, into which caskets can be placed for disposition.

crypts   burial spaces in mausoleums or churches.

Personal Assessment

In line with this chapter's positive theme of the value of personal death awareness, here is a funeral service assessment that can help you examine your reactions and thoughts about the funeral arrangements you would prefer for yourself.

After answering each of the following questions, you might wish to discuss your responses with a friend or close relative.

1. Have you ever considered how you would like your body to be handled after your death?
   _____ Yes _____ No
2. Have you already made funeral prearrangements for yourself?
   _____ Yes _____ No
3. Have you considered a specific funeral home or mortuary to handle your arrangements?
   _____ Yes _____ No
4. If you were to die today, which of the following would you prefer?
   _____ Embalming _____ Ground burial
   _____ Cremation _____ Entombment
   _____ Donation to medical science
5. If you prefer to be cremated, what would you want done with your ashes?
   _____ Buried _____ Entombed
   _____ Scattered
   _____ Other; please specify _____
6. If your funeral plans involve a casket, which of the following ones would you prefer?
   _____ Plywood (cloth covered)
   _____ Hardwood (oak, cherry, mahogany, or maple)
   _____ Steel (sealer or nonsealer type)
   _____ Stainless steel
   _____ Copper or bronze
   _____ Other; please specify _____
7. How important would a funeral service be for you?
   _____ Very important
   _____ Somewhat important
   _____ Somewhat unimportant
   _____ Very unimportant
   _____ No opinion
8. What kind of funeral service would you want for yourself?
   _____ No service at all
   _____ Visitation (calling hours) the day before the funeral service; funeral held at church or funeral home

_____ Graveside service only (no visitation)
_____ Memorial service (after body disposition)
_____ Other; please specify _____

9. How many people would you want to attend your funeral service or memorial service?
   _____ I do not want a funeral or memorial service
   _____ 1–10 people
   _____ 11–25 people
   _____ 26–50 people
   _____ Over 51 people
   _____ I do not care how many people attend
10. What format would you prefer at your funeral service or memorial service? Select any of the following that you would like:

	Yes	No
Religious music	_____	_____
Nonreligious music	_____	_____
Clergy present	_____	_____
Flower arrangements	_____	_____
Family member eulogy	_____	_____
Eulogy by friend(s)	_____	_____
Open casket	_____	_____
Religious format	_____	_____
Other; please specify		

11. Using today's prices, how much would you expect to pay for your total funeral arrangements, including cemetery expenses (if applicable)?
   _____ Less than $4,500
   _____ Between $4,501 and $6,000
   _____ Between $6,001 and $7,500
   _____ Between $7,501 and $9,000
   _____ Above $9,000

To Carry This Further . . .

Which items had you not thought about before? Were you surprised at the arrangements you selected? Will you share your responses with anyone else? If so, whom?

Current Organ Donation Issues

Two key issues in current organ donation practices in the United States are: (1) the continued shortage of organ donors and (2) the threat of disease transmission in certain donated tissues or organs.

The shortage of organ donors is life threatening to the thousands of patients waiting for a kidney, heart, lung, liver, or pancreas or for skin or bone marrow tissue. Although donor cards are widely available and hospitals are now required by law to ask survivors promptly if they will donate the deceased's organs, only a small percentage of organs and tissues are collected.

Why has the donor system not been more effective? Here are some possible reasons. Many people do not prepare living wills; likewise, most people do not prepare a uniform organ donor card. Many survivors also prefer not to consider organ donation during the stressful aftermath of death. Some physicians and hospital staff workers may feel uncomfortable asking survivors about organ donation.

Beyond the psychological obstacles that surround organ donation are some very real difficulties in the administration of organ donation programs. Regulations at different organ banks may vary, as may state and local laws. These regulations may make it difficult for organ banks to prepare and transport tissues or organs from one location to another. In addition, a hospital's ability to instantly recognize a patient as a registered donor requires donor registries across the country to be more compatible with each other. Finally, organ donation networks must find better ways to encourage people to understand the urgent need to provide these "gifts of life."

The second problem facing organ donation reached the public's attention in the spring of 1991. Tissues transplanted into multiple people came from a donor who had died from AIDS. This oversight caused considerable public alarm but has resulted in more stringent screening of donor candidates, as well as more careful examination and handling of organs and tissues. These tighter procedures are encouraging news for the public. Clearly, everyone waiting for an organ donation deserves the opportunity to receive a healthy organ.

UNIFORM DONOR CARD

of _____
(print or type name of donor)
In the hope that I may help others, I hereby make this anatomical gift, if medically acceptable, to take effect upon my death. The words and marks below indicate my wishes:
I give: (a) _____ any needed organs or parts
(b) _____ only the following organs or parts
_____
(specify the organ(s), tissue(s), or part(s))
for the purposes of transplantation, therapy, medical research or education;
(c) _____ my body for anatomical study if needed.
Limitations or special wishes, if any: _____

Signed by the donor and the following two witnesses in the presence of each other:

Signature of Donor _____ Date of Birth of Donor _____
Date Signed _____ City and State _____
Witness _____ Witness _____
This is a legal document under the Anatomical Gift Act or similar laws.
☐ Yes, I have discussed my wishes with my family.
For further information consult your physician or

THE NATIONAL KIDNEY FOUNDATION
30 East 33rd Street   New York, NY 10016
08-21

Figure 21-1   Signing a uniform organ donor card allows you to donate your organs to a research facility, medical school, or organ donor network.

Costs

The full funeral services offered by a funeral home average $2,000 to $3,000, and other expenses must be added to this price. Casket prices vary significantly, with the average cost between $1,500 and $2,500. If the family chooses an especially fancy casket, then the costs could spiral up to $10,000 or more. Costs that extend beyond these expenses include (should one choose them) those shown in Table 21-1. When all of the expenses associated with a typical funeral are totaled, the average cost is between $5,500 and $7,000.

Table 21-1   Estimated Funeral Costs

Cemetery lot	$400–$1,200
Opening and closing of grave	$300–$800
Vault	$350–$1,000
Mausoleum space	$1,500–$5,000
Honorarium for minister	$75–$100
Organist and vocalists	$50–$75 each
Flowers over casket	$100+
Grave marker	$500–$1,500+
Beautician services	$75+

Regardless of the rituals you select for the handling of your body (or the body of someone in your care), most educators encourage people to prearrange their plans. Before you die, you can save your survivors a lot of misery by putting your wishes in writing. *Funeral prearrangements* relieve the survivors of many of the details that must be handled at the time of your death. You can gather much of the information for your obituary notice and your wishes for the disposition of your body. You can make prearrangements with a funeral director, family member, or attorney. Many individuals also prepay the costs of their funeral. By making arrangements before the need arises, you can improve your own peace of mind. Currently about 30 percent to 40 percent of funerals are preplanned and prepaid. In the 1960s nearly all funerals were planned by relatives at the time of a person's death.

Personal Preparation for Death

We hope that this chapter helps you discover some new perspectives about death and develop your own personal death awareness. Remember that the ultimate goal of death education is a positive one—to help you best use and enjoy your life. Becoming aware of the reality of your own mortality is a step in the right direction. Reading about the process of dying, grief resolution, and the rituals surrounding death can also help you imagine that someday you too will die.

You can prepare for the reality of your own death in some additional ways. Preparing a will, purchasing a life insurance policy, making funeral prearrangements, preparing a living will, volunteering in a hospice (see the Star Box at right), and considering an anatomical or organ donation (see the Health Action Guide at right) are measures that help you prepare for your own death. At the appropriate time, you might also wish to talk with family and friends about your own death. You may discover that an upbeat, positive discussion about death can help relieve some of your apprehensions and those of others around you.

Another suggestion to help you emotionally prepare for your own death is to prepare an *obituary notice* or **eulogy** for yourself. Include all the things you would like to have said about you and your life. Now compare your obituary notice and eulogy with the current direction your life seems to be taking. Are you doing the kinds of activities for which you want to be known? If so, great! If not, perhaps you will want to consider why your current direction does not reflect how you would like to be remembered. Should you make some changes to restructure your life's agenda in a more personally meaningful fashion?

Another suggestion to help make you aware of your own eventual death is to write your own **epitaph.**

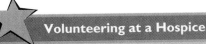

Volunteering at a Hospice

Whether you recently suffered the loss of a loved one or simply want to enrich your life, volunteering at a hospice can be a way to help others who are confronting death, and in so doing, gain courage and wisdom in dealing with death yourself.

Hospice care has grown from an alternative health-care movement to an accepted part of U.S. medical care. Especially as the U.S. population continues to age, hospices will play a greater role in caring for terminally ill patients.

A hospice is a residential community that provides palliative (symptom-relieving) care and supports the physical, social, and spiritual needs of patients at the end of life. As an alternative to the sterility and intensive life-saving environment of a hospital, the hospice gives terminally ill people an opportunity to deal with death in relative comfort and dignity.

As a hospice volunteer, you might act as a link between the professional staff and the family members who are suffering the impending loss of a loved one. You might help meet practical needs and, just as important, provide emotional support. Thus you could play a crucial role in the healing of the grieving family.

In one study, hospice volunteers were asked to describe their reasons for volunteering and their expectations. The typical response was that individuals volunteered out of a general desire to contribute to others, as well as a desire for interaction and personal growth. In many cases, the volunteers did not have predetermined expectations for the experience. Those who continued their service attributed their continuity to the support and sense of value they received from the staff and the residents.[22]

HEALTH ACTION GUIDE

Organ Donation

Donating organs is one of the most compassionate, responsible acts a person can perform. Only a few simple steps are required:

1. You must complete a uniform donor card. Obtain a card from a physician, a local hospital, or the nearest regional transplant or organ bank.
2. Print or type your name on the card.
3. Indicate which organs you wish to donate. You may also indicate your desire to donate all organs and tissues.
4. Sign your name in the presence of two witnesses, preferably your next of kin.
5. Fill in any additional information (such as date of birth, city and state in which the card is completed, and date the card is signed).
6. Tell others about your decision to donate. Some donor cards have detachable portions to give to your family.
7. Always carry your card with you.
8. If you have any questions, you can call the United Network for Organ Sharing (UNOS) at (800) 24-DONOR, or call (613) 727-1380 in Canada.

InfoLinks
www.asf.org

Before doing this, you might want to visit a cemetery. (Unfortunately, most of us visit cemeteries only when we are forced to do so.) Reading the epitaphs of others may help you develop your own epitaph.

You might increase your awareness of your own death by attempting to answer these questions in writing (because this pushes you beyond mere thinking): (1) If I had only one day to live, how would I spend it? (2) What one accomplishment would I like to make before I die? (3) After I am dead, what two or three things will people miss most about me? By answering these questions and accomplishing a few of the tasks suggested in this section, you will have a good start on accepting your own death and the value of life itself.

> ### Personal Applications
> • If you learned you were going to die tomorrow, what would you do today?

> **eulogy** a composition or speech that praises someone; often delivered at a funeral or memorial service.
>
> **epitaph** an inscription on a grave marker or monument.

Real Life
Real choices
Your Turn

• According to Elisabeth Kübler-Ross, what are the five psychological stages often experienced by both a dying person and his or her family and friends?
• Which of those stages do you think Jenny has gone through with respect to her own death? What about Wendy?
• Have you ever experienced the dying and death of a family member or close friend? If so, which of the five stages did the dying person go through? Which stages did you experience?

And Now, Your Choices . . .
• If your best friend had a terminal illness, how would you try to reconcile your feelings with your friend's needs?
• If you were terminally ill, how could your best friend be most helpful to you?

Summary

• Personal death awareness encourages you to live a meaningful life.
• Death is determined primarily by clinical and legal factors.
• Euthanasia can be performed through either direct or indirect measures.
• The most current advance medical directives are the living will and the medical power of attorney for health care. Both documents permit critically ill people (especially those who cannot communicate) to die with dignity.
• Denial, anger, bargaining, depression, and acceptance are the five classic psychological stages that dying people commonly experience, according to Kübler-Ross. Hospice care provides an alternative approach to dying for terminally ill people and their families.

• The expression of grief is a common response that can be expected when a friend or relative dies. The grief process can vary in intensity and duration.
• When a parent dies, a child needs support and the truth, especially two crucial pieces of information: that the dead parent will never return, and that the body has been buried in the ground or cremated.
• Volunteering in a hospice can give the opportunity to help others deal with the death of a loved one, and help the volunteer better accept his or her own eventual death.
• Death in our society is associated with many rituals to help survivors cope with the loss of a loved one and to ensure proper disposal of the body.

Review Questions

1. How does the experience of dying today differ from that in the early 1900s?

2. Identify and explain the clinical and legal determinants of death and identify who establishes each of them.

3. Explain the difference between direct and indirect euthanasia.
4. How does a living will differ from a medical power of attorney for health-care document? Why are these advance medical directives becoming increasingly popular?
5. Identify the five psychological stages that dying people tend to experience. Explain each stage.
6. Identify and explain the four strategies that form the basis of hospice care. What are the advantages of hospice care for the patient and the family?

7. Define the term *grief.* Identify and explain the sensations and emotions most people have when they experience grief. When does the grieving process end? How can adults cope with the death of a child? How can we assist grieving people?
8. What purposes do the rituals of death serve? What are the significant components of the full funeral service? What are the four ways in which bodies are disposed?
9. What activities can we undertake to become better aware of our own mortality?

References

1. Leming MR, Dickinson GE. *Understanding dying, death, and bereavement.* 3rd ed. Fort Worth, TX: Holt Rinehart & Winston, 1994.
2. Kastenbaum RJ. *Death, society, and human experience.* 6th ed. Boston: Allyn & Bacon, 1998.
3. Baer K. Death and dying: the final chapter. *Harvard Health Letter,* 1995; 20(4):1–3.
4. *Choice in dying.* Personal correspondence. Feb 10, 1998.
5. Kübler-Ross E. *On death and dying.* Reprint ed. New York: Collier Books, 1997.
6. Kübler-Ross E. *To live until we say goodbye.* Reprint ed. Paramus, NJ: Prentice-Hall, 1997.
7. Moody RA. *Life after life.* New York. Bantam Books, 1975.
8 Ring K. *Life at death: a scientific investigation of the near-death experience.* New York: Coward, McCann & Geoghegan, 1980.
9. Greyson B. Varieties of near-death experience. *Psychiatry* 1993 Nov; 56(4):390–99.
10. Fulton R, Bendikson R. *Death and identity.* 3rd ed. Philadelphia: Charles Press, 1994.
11. Pappas DJH, McCoy MC. Grief counseling. In Kuller JA et al, eds. *Prenatal diagnosis and reproductive genetics.* St. Louis: Mosby, 1996.
12. Cole D. When a child dies. *Parents' Magazine* 1994 Mar: 3.
13. Allison C. For Felicity. *Reader's Digest* 1993 Jan: 199.
14. National Hospice Organization, Arlington, VA, Jan 1999. http://www.nho.org
15. Lindemann E. Symptomology and management of acute grief. In Fulton et al, eds. *Death and dying: challenge and change.* Reading, MA: Addison-Wesley, 1978.
16. Raether H. Deaths and cremations: 1995, 1996, and beyond. *The Director* (National Funeral Directors Association) 1997; 69(11):77–81.
17. Bowman J (Licensed Funeral Director). Personal correspondence, Jan 11, 1999.
18. Kevorkian murder trial ordered. CBS Worldwide Corp., Dec 9, 1998. www.cbs.com
19. Dunn R. Millennium suicide sect found in Israel. *The Times of London* 1998 Nov 24. http://www.the-times.co.uk
20. Harrington M. Cult members deported from Israel arrive in Denver. *Reuters Ltd* 1999 Jan 10. http://nt.excite.com/news/r/990110/00news-cult
21. Carr W. Spiritual pain and healing in the hospice. *America* 1995 Aug 12; 173(4):26.
22. Murrant G, Strathdee SA. Motivations for service involvement at Casey House AIDS Hospice. *Hospice Journal* 1995; 10(3)27–38.

Suggested Readings

Despelder LA, Strickland AL. *The last dance: encountering death and dying.* 5th ed. Mountain View, CA: Mayfield Publishing, 1999. This college-level textbook covers all the topics relevant to a course in death and dying. *The Last Dance* is successful because it discusses the topics from a sociocultural perspective on death in America and the world. Now in its fifth edition, this fifteen-chapter book provides comprehensive, up-to-date information in an easy-to-read format.

Klein A. *The courage to laugh: humor, hope and healing in the face of death and dying.* New York: J.P. Tarcher, 1998. Klein is convinced that humor can help people face the end of life with dignity and compassion. While death itself is not funny, it does provide an opportunity for humorous thoughts and perspectives. Klein cleverly shows patients how to use humor to cope in difficult times. He gives readers permission to laugh when they may feel like crying. This book reflects poignant wisdom from children, parents, and healthcare workers. It is beneficial for patients, caregivers, family members, and friends.

Loving C. *My son, my sorrow: a mother's plea to Dr. Kevorkian.* Carrollton, TX: New Horizon Press, 1998. Carol Loving's 27-year-old son begged her to help him die as he developed increasingly serious complications from Lou Gehrig's disease. Confronting this dilemma, Loving turned to Dr. Kevorkian for assistance. This book illuminates one side of the debate about physician-assisted suicide.

topics for Today

No Time to Say Good-bye: Dealing with Accidental or Violent Death

Although we all know that death is inevitable, we somehow wish our loved ones could be exempt. If they must die, couldn't it happen peacefully during their sleep in old age? When people die in old age, the decline of their health is often gradual and the death not unexpected. Even when a younger person dies of a disease, family members usually have a chance to say good-bye. Family and friends of victims of violent death are cheated out of both of these conditions. Their loved ones are taken from them suddenly, sometimes under unknown circumstances and other times under circumstances known to be painfully cruel. The unexpected deaths of people who die by accident or by violence take a heavy toll on survivors.

Accidents

One kind of accident that touches sometimes hundreds of families at once is an airplane crash, such as the crash of Swissair Flight 111 into the waters of Peggy's Cove, Nova Scotia, on September 2, 1998,[1] the crash of ValuJet Flight 592 into the Florida Everglades on May 11, 1996, or the explosion of TWA Flight 800 as it left New York's JFK airport on July 17, 1996. Families of these victims are left with many questions. Their questions begin with, "Did my loved one get on that plane?" and progress to, "What happened?" as they try to imagine the last moments of the victim's life. From this uncertainty comes an urgency to have the victims' bodies found and identified.[2–4] Until the loved one is found, the survivors may continue to hope in vain that somehow the family member survived. The family may delay having a memorial service for the opposite reason—the hope that the loved one's remains can be found so that a proper funeral can take place instead. Recovery of the deceased person's personal belongings helps the grieving process: Having something tangible helps the family feel connected to their lost loved one as well as learn to let go.[4]

One man who lost both his wife and daughter in the ValuJet crash summed up the painful feelings of many survivors: "It will be a nightmare for a while

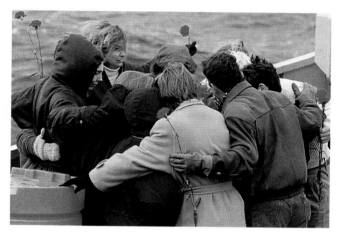

Relatives of victims of the crash of Swissair Flight 111 embrace during a ceremony at sea to remember their loved ones. The 11 family members, all from the United States, tossed red carnations into icy waters over the crash site. The jetliner crashed Sept. 2 off the Nova Scotia coast, killing all 229 people aboard. (AP Photo/CP, Andrew Vaughan)

and then not much better than that."[3] In a very personal way, he speaks of the grief, hysteria, and uneasy acceptance that victims' loved ones face. The loss of two adult daughters in a plane crash off a Boston runway all but destroyed one family. As one of their sisters later wrote, at first the family drank, stayed up all night, talked, danced, cried, and fought. They just couldn't stop moving; it was too lonely to sit still. They thought legal victory would bring revenge and revenge would bring healing, but they were wrong. The family did not seek counseling at the time, and their father lived out the rest of his life unable to find joy in his three living children or grandchildren.[5]

Two things that help families cope in this situation are prompt release of the passenger list and recovery and identification of the victims. This seems straightforward enough, but after one crash an unnamed airline buried unidentified victims in a mass grave without notifying the families.[3] During the crash investigation and the search for victims, families appreciate being briefed on new information before it is released to the media. When the investigation and search have been concluded, family and friends can receive help from associations of airline crash victims' loved ones. Besides supporting grieving relatives, these organizations lobby for stiffer safety standards and greater rights for crash victims' families.[2]

Fatal car accidents also take a terrible toll on the lives of victims' loved ones. Of these, hit-and-run accidents are especially hard to deal with. Because of the nature of the crime, both suspect and clues remain elusive. This robs the families of the solace of truth and the sad satisfaction of justice. They may return, again and again, to the site where their loved one fell, searching for information, or at least peace.[6]

One of the most heartbreaking types of accidents occurs when a family member unintentionally inflicts the harm. Bobby Crabtree lives with the fact that he accidentally shot and killed his 14-year-old daughter. He remembers, "My daddy always told me, 'Before you get a loaded gun out, you should be able to lay a hand on every member of your family.'"[7] When the sounds of an intruder came from his daughter's bedroom closet, Bobby went to get his gun. He could see his wife and mother-in-law on the couch, and he thought he could account for his daughter because she had called to say that she was spending the night at a friend's house. When he opened the closet door, his daughter and her friend jumped out at him as a prank, and he fired the gun reflexively. The family has not stayed in the house since that night. Bobby contemplated suicide but was afraid that if he took his own life he would not go to heaven, and what he wants most of all is to see his daughter again.[7]

Homicides

Many parents would agree that "every mother's nightmare is to see her child on either side of a gun."[8] Because of gang warfare, this nightmare is coming true for too many mothers. Lorna Hawkins lost two sons to street violence. One son was shot and killed when he was mistaken for someone else, and her other son was killed in a carjacking.[9] Carol Taylor's 17-year-old son was killed in a park on his way home from school.[10] And Marina Martinez grieves because she lost her son 11 years ago at Christmas time. He was a father of two who was caught in gang crossfire as he went to pick up a pizza for his kids.[11]

The pain never goes away, and some mothers even feel guilty for not having been able to protect their children from the violence.[10] In an effort to save other children from tragic deaths, these women organize and mobilize for peace. Mothers in one Los Angeles housing project, for example, hold love marches, peace barbeques, and candlelight vigils. They've even risked their own lives by forming a human wall between taunting rival gangs following a gang funeral. They are courageous because they see even greater risk in not acting.[8] Another organization, Women Against Gun Violence, channels the rage many victims' family members feel into a vehicle for change. They send sympathy letters to victims' families and work to limit the proliferation of guns and the frequency with which perpetrators walk free.[10]

When the slain loved one is a child, siblings under age 18 are often among the survivors. These siblings not only suffer the loss of a brother or sister, but they must also live with grieving parents. All too often the needs of these children are ignored. If their dead brother or sister is viewed as a criminal who earned his or her fate by being a gang member, the children may feel demeaned and isolated and may think they are being judged guilty by association. Even children without this added stress show significant symptoms of depression, anxiety, post-traumatic stress disorder, and psychosocial impairment after the murder of a sibling. Children who must deal with the murder of a schoolmate may respond with similar symptoms.[12]

Suicide

"Very few actions generate as much emotion in family members and friends as suicidal behavior," one writer comments, "[because] suicide is desertion in its worst form."[13] Ironically, those who commit suicide, who thought they didn't fit in and that nobody loved them, deeply wound the people they leave behind. High school freshman Alicia Hayes, age 15, and Amber Hernandez, age 14, took this way out. Although the incidents are not known to be related, a junior at their school had jumped from the same cliff with his girlfriend just months before the girls' double suicide. The counselors who responded to the death of the young man concentrated on helping members of his class deal with the tragedy. After Amber and Alicia killed themselves, the counselors identified other suicide risks and hospitalized some students for severe depression. Amber's father has a message for all parents: "Love your kids as much as you can," he urges, "because you never know what's going to happen."[14]

Living Again

Many bereaved family members become experts in and crusaders against the cause of their loved one's death,[2] whether it was an airplane crash, a car accident, or the result of street violence or suicide. They piece their lives back together in any way they can. For example, they may form a friendship with their widowed brother-in-law's new wife. Anniversaries of the loved one's death are painfully remembered, and milestones are noted, such as a younger child's birthday that makes him or her older than the deceased child had lived to be.[12]

One woman has learned to live again through forgiveness. Twelve years after her 19-year-old daughter was murdered, Gayle Blount wrote a letter of forgiveness to her daughter's killer on San Quinton's death row. She had lived much of the previous twelve years in grief and rage but through spirituality and religious teachings was able to turn her hatred into forgiveness. Once a week she now visits one of the seven death row inmates she has befriended. As part of a group called Murder Victims' Families for Reconciliation, she is an advocate against the death penalty.[15]

No matter how victims' loved ones decide to spend the rest of their lives, it is important that they learn how to go on living. Through community action, a spiritual awakening, or the support of family and friends, they must somehow find a way to say good-bye.

Grief Support Groups

People who have experienced tragic losses are often willing to help others who have suddenly lost family members or friends. Sometimes help is offered through the efforts of grief support groups, which are designed to provide a comprehensive support system for grieving people.

A good example of a grief support group is the Air Crash Support Network (ACSN), a national, nonprofit, nonpolitical, tax-exempt organization that aids the grieving process of people who have been involved with or affected by an air crash.[16] ACSN's mission is to provide emotional support for survivors, as well as information about organizations that can offer valuable resources. An important component of ACSN is the Volunteer Grief Mentoring and Referral Program, which links grieving survivors (via telephone and e-mail) with others who have experienced a similar tragic loss. The Air Crash Support Network can be reached toll-free by calling (877) ACSN-HELP or on the web at www.aircrashsupport.com.

Many of the resources found at the ACSN website can also be of value to people who are experiencing grief regardless of the cause. Among these resources are:

- The American Red Cross: (800) 435-7669 (www.redcross.org)
- The Salvation Army: (703) 684-5500 (www.salvationarmy.org)
- 1-800-LIFENET (www.800lifenet.com)
- Grief Net (www.griefnet.org)
- The Compassionate Friends: (630) 990-0010 (www.compassionatefriends.org)
- Rainbows International: (800) 266-3206 (www.rainbows.org)
- The Grief Recovery Helpline: (800) 445-4808
- Mothers Against Drunk Driving (www.madd.org)

For Discussion . . .

Have you been affected by the accidental or violent death of someone close to you? Are you able to share your feelings with others? Could you forgive someone who killed a member of your family? Do you think that the survivors discussed in this article are doing the right things to cope? What do you think you would do?

References

1. Swissair pilots may have turned off their flight recorders. CBS Newsworld Online. Jan 21, 1999. http://www.newsworld.cbc.ca
2. Kovaleski SF. For airline crash victims' families, strength is in associations. *The Washington Post* 1996; 119(360):A29.
3. Bragg R. Loved ones lost, perhaps never to be found. *The New York Times* 1996; 145:A1.
4. Kovaleski SF. For some victims' families the search for solace goes on. *The Washington Post* 1996; 119(252):A3.
5. Warren L. Surviving a crash. *The New York Times* 1996; 145:56.
6. Klein D. Sudden death on the streets. *Los Angeles Times* 1994 May 1:A1.
7. Voll D. The right to bear sorrow. *Esquire* 1995; 123(3):74–82.
8. Mohan G. Mothers rally to halt gang killing. *Los Angeles Times* 1995 Oct 8:B1.
9. Williams FB. Victims' families protest violence. *Los Angeles Times* 1995 Apr 24:B1.
10. Taylor CA, Mills K. Look at that gang member like he was your child. *Los Angeles Times* 1995 Mar 24:B7.
11. Perez MA. Decorations memorialize those who were murdered. *Los Angeles Times* 1996 Dec 12:A9.
12. Freeman LN, Shaffer D, Smith H. Neglected victims of homicide: the needs of young siblings of murder victims. *Am J Orthopsychiatry* 1996; 66(3):337–45.
13. Pahl JJ. The rippling effects of suicides. *USA Today (Magazine)* 1996; 125(2616):62–64.
14. Gleick E. Suicide's shadow. *Time* 1996; 148(5):40–42.
15. McCarthy C. Gayle Blount's journey. *The Washington Post* 1996; 119(312):A29.
16. Air Crash Support Newtwork. Jan 10, 1999. http://www.aircrashsupport.com

InfoLinks
www.cdc.gov/ncipc/ncipchm.htm
www.suicidology.org

appendix one
first aid

Accidents are the leading cause of death for people ages 1 to 37. Injuries sustained in accidents can often be tragic. They are grim reminders of our need to learn first aid skills and to practice preventive safety habits.

First aid knowledge and skills allow you to help people who are in need of immediate emergency care. They also can help you save yourself if you should become injured. We recommend that our students enroll in American Red Cross first aid and safety courses, which are available in local communities or through colleges or universities. In this appendix, we briefly present some information about common first aid emergencies. (Please note that our information is *not* a substitute for comprehensive American Red Cross first aid instruction.)

First Aid

- Keep a list of important phone numbers near your phone (your doctor, ambulance service, hospital, poison control center, police and fire departments).
- In case of serious injury or illness, call the appropriate emergency service immediately for help (if uncertain, call "911" or "0").

Specific Problem	What To Do
Asphyxiation Victim stops breathing and skin, lips, tongue, and fingernail beds turn bluish or gray.	Adult: Tip head back with one hand on forehead and other lifting the lower jaw near the chin. Look, listen, and feel for breathing. If not breathing, place your mouth over victim's mouth, pinch the nose, get a tight seal, and give 2 slow breaths. Recheck the breathing; if still not breathing, give breaths once every 5 seconds for an adult, once every 3 seconds for a child, once every 3 seconds for infants (do not exaggerate head tilt for babies).
Bleeding Victim bleeding severely can quickly go into shock and die within 1 or 2 minutes.	With the palm of your hand, apply firm, direct pressure to the wound with a clean dressing or pad. Elevate the body part if possible. Do not remove blood-soaked dressings; use additional layers, continue to apply pressure, and elevate the site.
Choking Accidental ingestion or inhalation of food or other objects causes suffocation that can quickly lead to death. There are over 3,000 deaths annually, mostly of infants, small children, and the elderly.	The procedure is easy to learn; however, the Heimlich maneuver must be learned from a qualified instructor. The procedure varies somewhat for infants, children, adults, pregnant women, and obese people.
Hyperventilation A situation in which a person breathes too rapidly; often the result of fear or anxiety; may cause confusion, shortness of breath, dizziness, or fainting. Intentional hyperventilation before an underwater swim is especially dangerous, since it may cause a swimmer to pass out in the water and drown.	Have the person relax and rest for a few minutes. Provide reassurance and a calming influence. Having the victim take a few breaths in a paper bag (not plastic) may be helpful. Do not permit swimmers to practice hyperventilation before attempting to swim.

continued

Specific Problem	What To Do
Bee Stings Not especially dangerous except for people who have developed an allergic hypersensitivity to a particular venom. Those who are not hypersensitive will experience swelling, redness, and pain. Hypersensitive people may develop extreme swelling, chest constriction, breathing difficulties, hives, and shock signs.	For nonsensitive people: Scrape stinger from skin and apply cold compresses or over-the-counter topical preparation for insect bites. For sensitive people: Get professional help immediately. Scrape the stinger from skin; position the person so that the stung body part is below the level of the heart; help administer prescribed medication (if available); apply cold compresses.
Poisoning Often poisoning can be prevented with adequate safety awareness. Children are frequent victims.	Call the poison control center immediately; follow the instructions provided. Keep syrup of ipecac on hand.
Shock A life-threatening depression of circulation, respiration, and temperature control, recognizable by a victim's cool, clammy, pale skin; weak and rapid pulse; shallow breathing; weakness; nausea; or unconsciousness.	Provide psychological reassurance. Keep victim calm and in a comfortable, reclining position; loosen tight clothing. Prevent loss of body heat; cover if necessary. Elevate legs 8 to 12 inches (if there are no head, neck, or back injuries, or possible broken bones involving the hips or legs). Do not give food or fluids. Seek further emergency assistance.
Burns Burns can cause severe tissue damage and lead to serious infection and shock.	Minor burns: immerse in cold water and then cover with sterile dressings; do not apply butter or grease to burns. Major burns: seek help immediately; cover affected area with large quantities of clean dressings or bandages; do not try to clean the burn area or break blisters. Chemical burns: flood the area with running water.
Broken Bones Fractures are a common result of car accidents, falls, and recreational accidents.	Do not move the victim unless absolutely necessary to prevent further injury. Immobilize the affected area. Give care for shock while waiting for further emergency assistance.

Epilepsy: Recognition and First Aid

Seizure Type	What It Looks Like	Often Mistaken For	What To Do	What Not To Do
Convulsive				
Generalized tonic-clonic (also called grand mal)	Sudden cry, fall, rigidity, followed by muscle jerks, frothy saliva on lips, shallow breathing or temporarily suspended breathing, bluish skin, possible loss of bladder or bowel control, usually last 2–5 minutes; normal breathing then starts again; there may be some confusion and/or fatigue, followed by return to full consciousness	Heart attack
Stroke
Unknown but life-threatening emergency	Look for medical identification
Protect from nearby hazards
Loosen ties or shirt collars
Place folded jacket under head
Turn on side to keep airway clear; reassure when consciousness returns
If single seizure lasted less than 10 minutes, ask if hospital evaluation wanted
If multiple seizures, or if one seizure lasts longer than 10 minutes, take to emergency room	Don't put any hard implement in the mouth
Don't try to hold tongue; it can't be swallowed
Don't try to give liquids during or just after seizure
Don't use oxygen unless there are symptoms of heart attack
Don't use artificial respiration unless breathing is absent after muscle jerks subside, or unless water has been inhaled
Don't restrain
Nonconvulsive				
	This category includes many different forms of seizures, ranging from temporary unawareness (petit mal) to brief, sudden, massive muscle jerks (myoclonic seizures)	Daydreaming, acting out, clumsiness, poor coordination, intoxication, random activity, mental illness, and many others	Usually no first aid necessary other than to provide reassurance and emotional support. Any nonconvulsive seizure that becomes convulsive should be managed as a convulsive seizure. Medical evaluation is recommended.	Do not shout at, restrain, expect verbal instructions to be obeyed, or grab a person having a nonconvulsive seizure (unless danger threatens)

appendix two
body systems

The Circulatory System

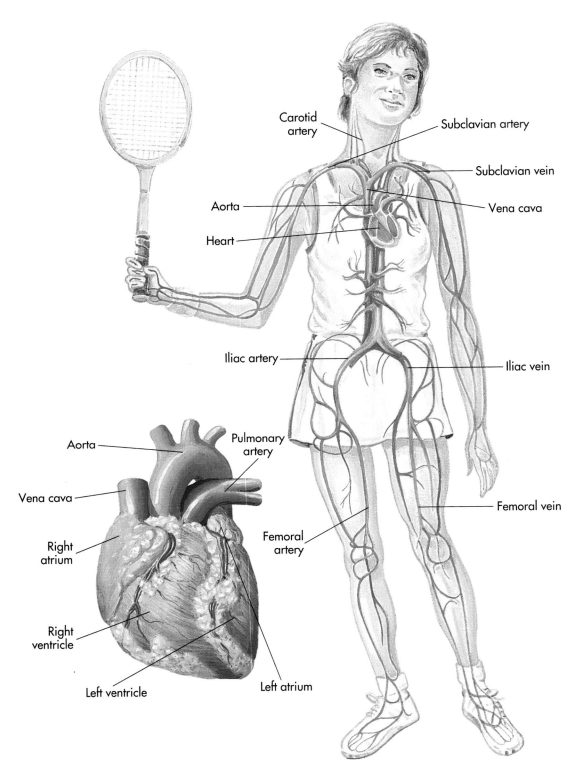

Carotid artery

Subclavian artery

Subclavian vein

Aorta

Vena cava

Heart

Iliac artery

Iliac vein

Aorta

Pulmonary artery

Vena cava

Right atrium

Femoral vein

Right ventricle

Femoral artery

Left ventricle

Left atrium

The Respiratory System

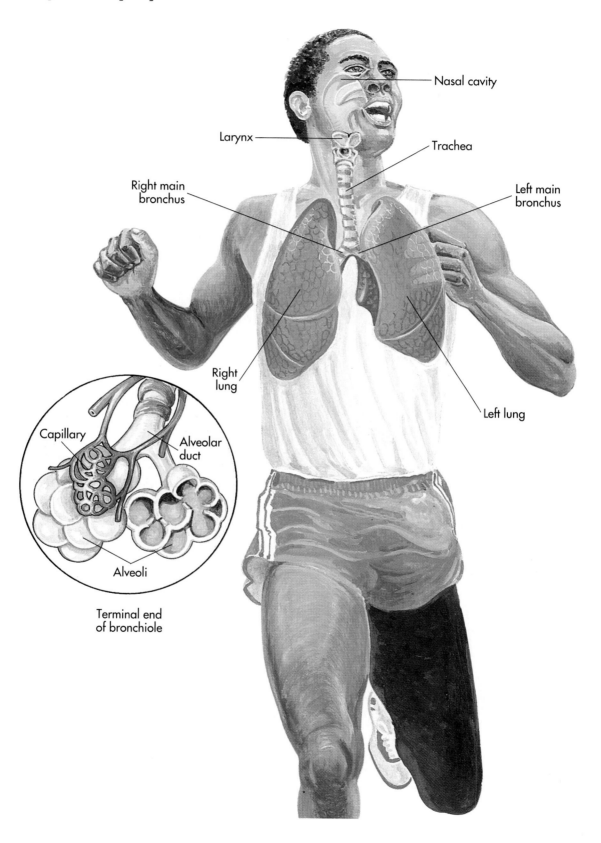

Nasal cavity

Larynx

Trachea

Right main bronchus

Left main bronchus

Capillary

Alveolar duct

Right lung

Left lung

Alveoli

Terminal end of bronchiole

The Muscular System

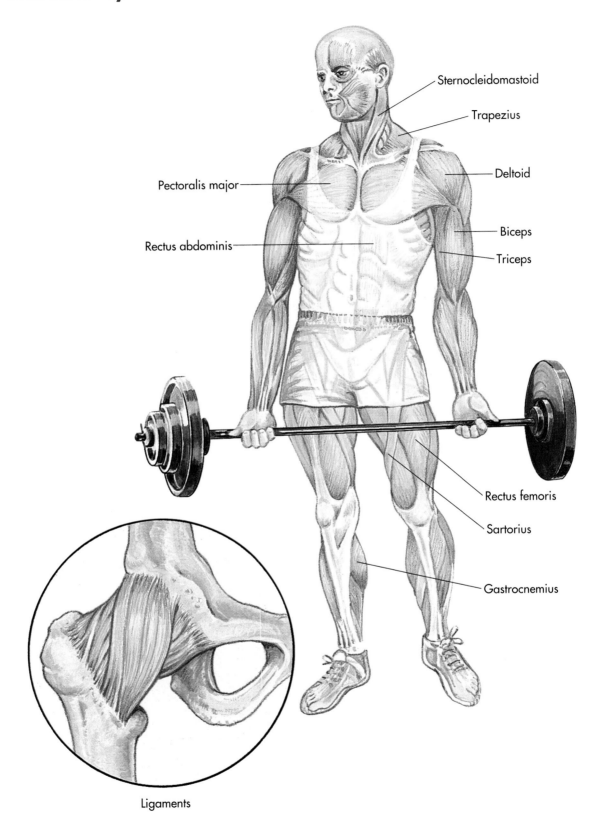

Sternocleidomastoid

Trapezius

Deltoid

Pectoralis major

Biceps

Rectus abdominis

Triceps

Rectus femoris

Sartorius

Gastrocnemius

Ligaments

The Skeletal System

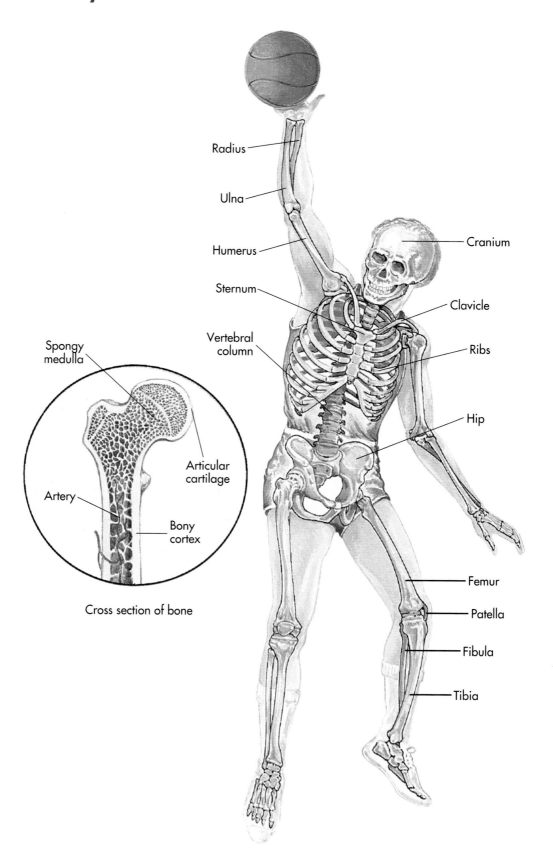

Radius

Ulna

Humerus

Sternum

Vertebral column

Cranium

Clavicle

Ribs

Hip

Femur

Patella

Fibula

Tibia

Spongy medulla

Articular cartilage

Artery

Bony cortex

Cross section of bone

The Nervous System

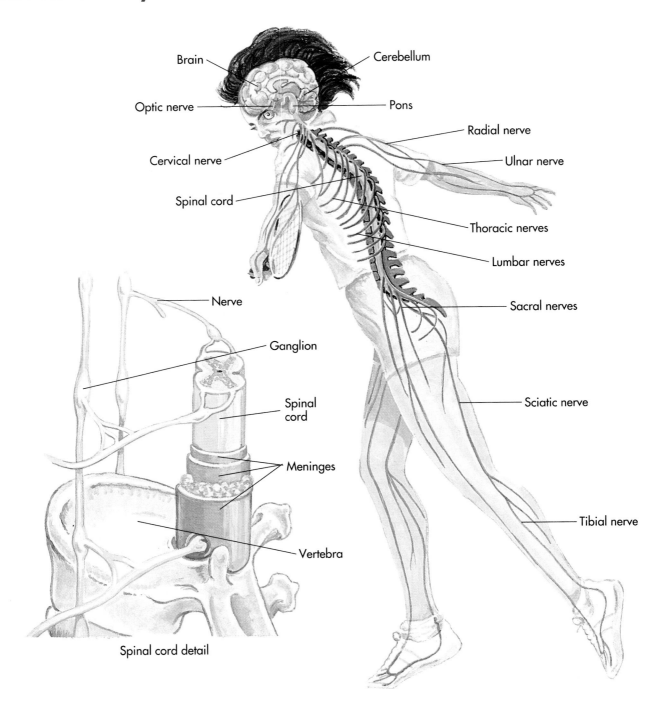

Brain

Cerebellum

Optic nerve

Pons

Radial nerve

Cervical nerve

Ulnar nerve

Spinal cord

Thoracic nerves

Lumbar nerves

Sacral nerves

Nerve

Ganglion

Spinal
cord

Meninges

Sciatic nerve

Vertebra

Tibial nerve

Spinal cord detail

The Digestive System

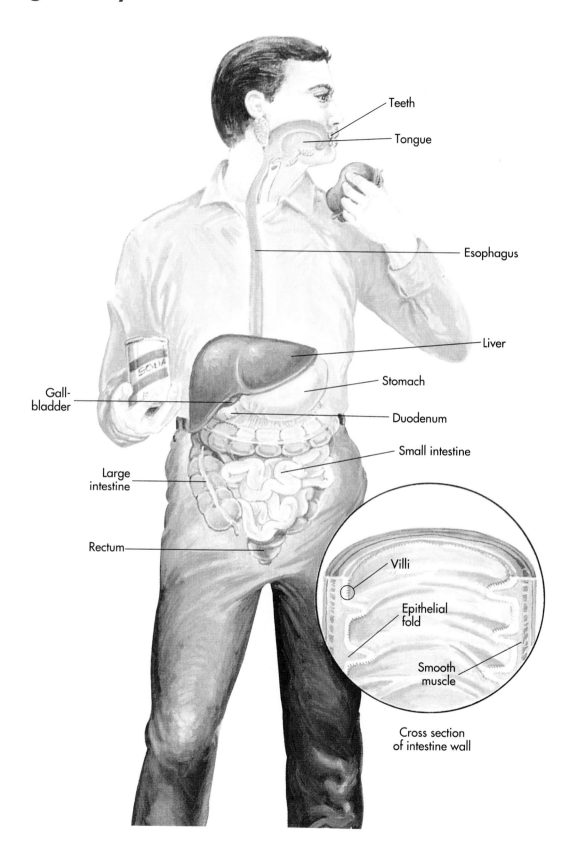

Teeth

Tongue

Esophagus

Liver

Stomach

Gall-
bladder

Duodenum

Small intestine

Large
intestine

Villi

Rectum

Epithelial
fold

Smooth
muscle

Cross section
of intestine wall

The Urinary System

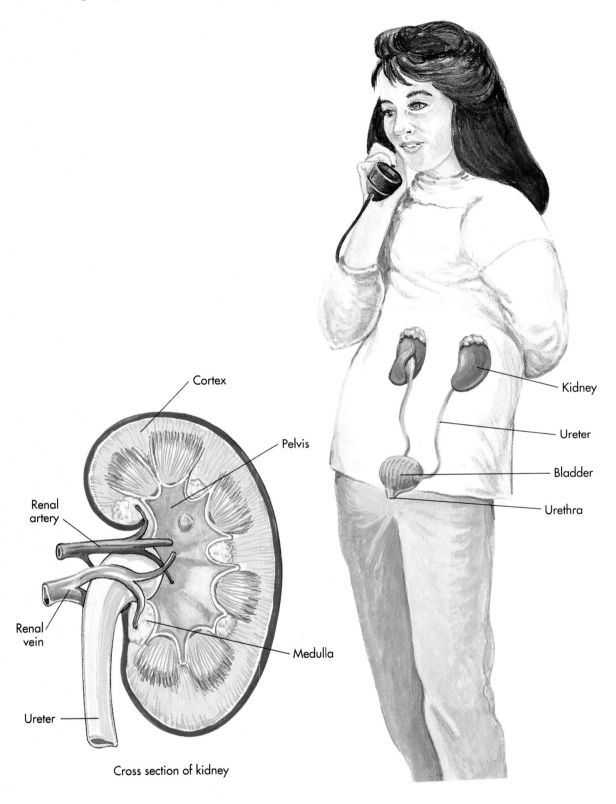

Cortex

Pelvis

Renal
artery

Renal
vein

Medulla

Ureter

Cross section of kidney

Kidney

Ureter

Bladder

Urethra

The Endocrine System

NOTE: Refer to Figures 14-2 and 14-3 for detailed anatomical illustrations of the reproductive systems.

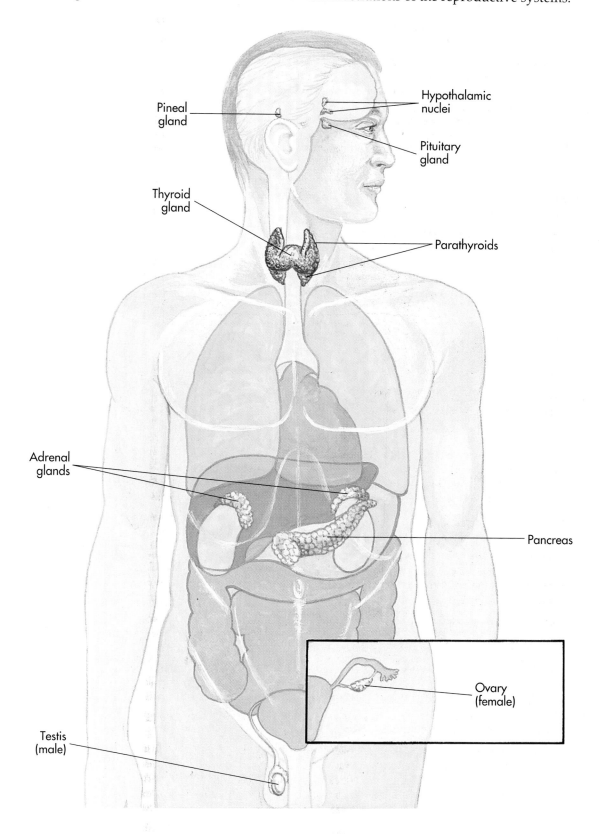

Pineal gland

Hypothalamic nuclei

Pituitary gland

Thyroid gland

Parathyroids

Adrenal glands

Pancreas

Ovary (female)

Testis (male)

appendix three
Canadian health

by Professor Don Morrow
The University of Western Ontario

Composed of 10 provinces and 2 territories, Canada is a huge geographic land mass with a relatively small population—some 30 million people. The population is mainly concentrated along the lower one-third of the country. Historically, relationships with its southern neighbor, the United States, have been good, although Canadians perceive themselves as distinctly different from Americans. The most obvious distinction is the bilingual nature of the country, English and French, with a significant concentration of the French-speaking population located in the province of Quebec. Unlike the United States, Canada has not experienced a major civil war. Still, escalating tensions over the potential for Quebec's separation from Canada's confederation to become a sovereign state have given rise to a great deal of discussion, reflection, and concern about nationhood and our current political structure. Clearly, the prospect of Quebec and succession threatens the integrity of Canada as a nation and as a society.

One unifying element in Canadian society has been its comprehensive program of national health insurance, in which coverage is provided to all citizens directly through government, without the involvement of insurance companies. The major responsibility for health care rests with the provinces, while the federal government has served as policymaker, along with assuming some direct health-care responsibilities for special populations such as Native Canadians, the two territories, and the military. The umbrella for Canadian health is a national health insurance program. The envy of many developed countries, this program represents a cost of about 10 percent of the gross domestic product; however, the expenses of maintaining the program have exceeded anyone's forecast. For example, in 1993 the total cost of the health-care system was some $55 billion, almost double the amount of just seven years earlier. Clearly, changes in concept, structure, and funding are needed if government is to continue offering any health-care system. This section outlines the history, nature, and future directions of health and health care in Canada. Further readings are listed at the end.

Historical Background

The first universal hospital insurance program in Canada was implemented in the province of Saskatchewan shortly after the end of World War II; by 1960 the other nine provinces had established similar programs, with federal legislation enacted for a national program in 1971 (Frankel et al. 1996; Pederson et al. 1994). In the early 1980s this federal, political infrastructure became the Canadian Health Promotion Directorate. Without question, the landmark federal initiative was the publication and dissemination in 1974 of the document titled *A New Perspective on the Health of Canadians*. The impact of this document nationally and internationally cannot be overstated. It received worldwide attention for its recasting of the concept of health toward what is now called *health promotion*. Whereas health traditionally had been equated with the health-care system, the *Perspective's* thrust was toward the broad concept of a *health field* that included all matters affecting health. This *health field concept* embraced four avenues or elements:

- health-care organization: the "system" of health care
- the environment
- lifestyle
- human biology

Such a concept was radical for the mid-1970s. It challenged the prevalent and ingrained equation that level of health equals quality of medicine. While applauding Canada's health-care system as "second to none in the world," the *New Perspective* underlined "ominous" counterforces threatening the standard of living, public health protection and advances in medical science; such counterforces as environmental pollution, city living, abuse of alcohol, tobacco and other drugs, eating patterns, and sedentary habits of indolence were identified for concern and action. In effect, the *Perspective* paper provided a whole new way of conceptualizing health as much broader than the traditional "medical model" of health and health care that had been so strongly focused on disease and illness.

The Health Field Concept

Careful to recognize that "the provision of personal health services to the general public is clearly a matter of provincial jurisdiction," the 1974 document highlighted the existence of national health problems that know no provincial boundaries and that arise from causes embedded in the social fabric of the nation as a whole (page 6). To convince health professionals and the public alike, the *New Perspective* showed that major causes of illness, defined as number of hospitalization days, were diseases of the cardiovascular system, followed by accidents and violence, then mental illness; in turn these were directly related to the interplay of the four elements identified as the health field concept. Thus, ill health was shown to be the direct result of self-imposed risks like drug abuse, poor diet and insufficient exercise as well as of careless driving, promiscuity, and so forth. Also tied to the health field concept were environmental problems such as urbanization, working conditions, rapid social change, and economic deprivation. The paradox so clearly illuminated in the *New Perspective* was that of lip-service agreement on the importance of research and prevention in health improvement, juxtaposed against the continued tendency to increase disproportionately the amount of money spent on existing illnesses and their treatment. The health field concept was characterized as comprehensive, as allowing for a workable system of analysis, and as bringing focus to neglected areas. The document's authors believed this reconfigured understanding of health would greatly assist in identifying factors that contribute to sickness/death and in determining actions that could improve the quality of health. In this regard the *New Perspective* offered 74 suggestions or proposals to analyze health-care issues and to develop more effective health-care policy.

Not only was the *New Perspective* document symbolic of major health reform, but it was also the first federal government articulation of a comprehensive and inclusive view of health that went far beyond the World Health Organization definition, "Health is a state of complete physical, mental, and social well-being and not merely the absence of disease and infirmity," so entrenched in health-care systems worldwide. In reality, however, this 1974 perspective was ahead of its time; and it presented a viewpoint that challenged the status quo as represented by the Canadian medical establishment, the country's health-care institutions, and the collective consciousness of Canadians themselves. It was just too easy to cling to the old equation of level of health = quality of medicine/health care. Moreover, economic prosperity and growth masked the significance of such threats to health as environmental and lifestyle factors. Further, it was widely held that the *New Perspective* was too narrow,

and that it intended to "blame the victim" for health problems. What was needed, critics said, was a more socially oriented view of health and health education, one that accounted more directly for environmental and social factors, to place health in context in Canadian society.

The Ottawa Charter

Major indicators of change were witnessed in the early 1980s. The city of Vancouver in British Columbia, Canada's westernmost province, hosted a "Shifting Medical Paradigm Conference" in 1980; formulated to usher in a shift from the medical, disease-prevention/treatment model, this conference represented more of a challenge to Western medical tradition, rather than offering any concrete concept of health promotion. Of somewhat greater impact was the Toronto-based 1984 conference, "Beyond Health Care," which stressed the need for transitions in public health policy to promote healthy cities and communities (Pederson et al. 1994). The most important piece of health legislation or reform was produced in 1986 when the *Ottawa Charter for Health Promotion* was created after a conference on health promotion hosted in Ottawa, the nation's capital. Spiraling health-care costs were the major force behind the reform initiatives that resulted in the *Charter*; however, individual and agency initiatives in the spirit of health reform complemented the federal document.

The *Charter* took bold and needed steps to move the concept of health away from the treatment of illnesses and the attendant technologies toward a concept and policy that truly focused on health. Instead of trying to change the definition of health—so sacred to many health professionals—the *Charter* used the concept of *health promotion,* or "the process of enabling people to increase control over, and to improve their health." Health in this sense was perceived as a resource for everyday life, not the goal or objective of living. This concept underscored the importance of quality of everyday life in the process of health in preference to the traditional statistical emphasis on longevity or illness. Health promotion was envisioned in this document as a process rather than as a set of risk factor outcomes or as the "social work of medicine" (Pederson et al. 1994). Health promotion was not merely presented as the responsibility of the health-care sector but as an arena of shared personal and social resources and decisions. The *Charter* identified the fundamental conditions and resources for health:

- peace
- shelter
- education
- food
- income

- stable economic system
- sustainable resources
- social justice
- equity

In short, this set of Maslow-like conditions reflected the multifaceted nature of the concept of health. Moreover, the *Charter* gained worldwide attention for its identification and explanation of strategies for change:

- Build healthy public policy.
- Create supportive environments.
- Strengthen community action.
- Develop personal skills.
- Reorient health services.

Set against the action orientations of *advocate, enable,* and *mediate,* the prerequisites for health and the strategies for change were aligned for a new conceptual and realistic vision of health and its promotion. Once again Canada played a leadership role in framing and operationalizing the concept of health promotion, just as it had in changing the medical perception of health care in 1974 via the *New Perspective* document.

A Framework for Health Promotion

The World Health Organization and Health and Welfare Canada were responsible for hosting the 1986 Ottawa conference and establishing an action-oriented *Charter* that challenged participating organizations, governments, and individuals to pursue a "health for all" goal for the year 2000 and beyond. In the same year, the federal Minister for Health and Welfare, Jake Epp, took the *Charter* out of the realm of abstract conceptualization by articulating and promoting a practical model to achieve the *Charter's* goal. It was called *A Framework for Health Promotion* and it is configured in the chart below.

Some explanation will be helpful. The *Framework* paper identified three major challenges that were not being addressed by current health policies and practices. First, disadvantaged groups had a significantly lower life expectancy, poorer health, and higher prevalence of disability than the average Canadian. Second, various forms of preventable diseases and injuries continued to undermine the health and quality of life of the citizenry. Third, the lack of support for chronically ill, disabled, or emotionally stressed people was pronounced and serious; improved coping mechanisms and support services were needed. Such challenges, the document stated, warranted mechanisms for relief. First, self-care, or the decisions and actions individuals take in the interests of their own health, was intrinsic to health promotion. Second, through mutual aid, people could help each other cope; and third, the creation of conditions and surroundings conducive to health was strongly recommended. These three strategies could be implemented in provinces, municipalities, and communities to enhance health.

The *Framework* received large-scale promotion and, like the 1974 federal document (*New Perspective*), it was criticized for being too vague in its strategies. Nonetheless, the *Framework* must be credited with targeting health promotion as the central focus of health reform and direction in Canada. Because health is constitutionally defined as a provincial concern, federal policy could serve only to stimulate, challenge, and frame new concepts and tactics for health. Together with the *Charter,* the *Framework* represented new commitments that both provoked and empowered changes in health in line with the World Health Organization's enabling definition of health promotion defined in the *Charter* and repeated above. If health promotion was to involve social responsibility, then the federal initiatives in 1986 did establish a new framework for health promotion. The challenge of "health for all" seems ambitious and lofty; however, if

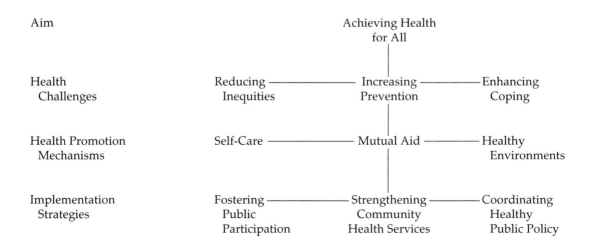

health can be perceived as an attitude and a process more than an end in itself, then the goal of health for all seems more realistic. Cost containment may well be an engine that drives health-care reform in Canada, yet reform is absolutely necessary, as is the reduction of health expenditures everywhere.

Current Provincial Perspectives

The acid test of any policy initiative is, of course, its implementation. In 1988 the Canadian Public Health Association, inspired by the three key strategies presented in the *Framework* model, created the Strengthening Community Health Program with a view toward focusing and applying health promotion at the community level. This program had its roots in the Ottawa *Charter* and might best be examined by considering a cross-Canada description of health promotion during the late 1980s and early 1990s. Most of the material discussed in this section is synthesized from Pederson's comprehensive book, *Health Promotion in Canada* (1994). The intent here is to provide a brief overview of the provincial and community responses to federal policy and strategy.

On the west coast, the province of British Columbia has been successful in inducing some 100 communities to join a vibrant "healthy community" movement inspired directly by the *Framework* document. Government initiatives in that province are directed toward recognizing, promoting, and linking community actions that reflect health promotion activities such as community health plans, conferences, surveys, and educational programs. By contrast, in neighboring Alberta, we see conflicting perspectives about health promotion that range from full commitment at one extreme to the notion that it represents an unaffordable luxury. Nevertheless, Alberta stresses changes related to promoting healthy lifestyles and addressing health determinants.

Saskatchewan, the first province to adopt a universal hospital insurance program, has a decades-old health action strategy of creating coalitions through which communities have been encouraged and supported in health promotion activities with dramatic success. In 1992, this province's government released a major health reform initiative, *A Saskatchewan Vision for Health*, which is based on two principles for action: the concept of wellness as the goal of health services; and community control of health service delivery. In the same year, the fourth prairie province, Manitoba, published its *Quality Health for Manitobans* paper to support health promotion for its 1 million inhabitants. Manitoba boasts seven strong healthy community projects based on a partners-for-health agreement between the government and the communities involved.

In central Canada, the most populous and arguably the most prosperous area of the country, responses to the *Charter* and the *Framework* are significantly different. The 10 million people in Ontario, have seen lengthy policy statements on the province's *Nurturing Health* documents, but very little in the way of developments at the community or grassroots level of health reform. Instead Ontario seems intent on the broad social view of health that is grounded in the determinants of health and the health-care system. Quebec's 7 million people (about 80% of whom are French speaking) and their governing bodies have given only token acknowledgment of federal initiatives in health promotion. The province has had very few "champions" of the concept of health promotion and very little political pressure for reform. As a unit, the Atlantic provinces are victims of inequity because they live in a distinctly poorer economic environment. Many of the communities in these four provinces are single-industry towns. As a result, change is slow and at best some of these provinces are just beginning to move toward the concept and practice of health promotion. Including the Yukon Territory, which is under direct federal health jurisdiction, it is evident that across Canada the contemporary trend is toward community or grassroots initiatives in health promotion. It will be helpful to examine the trends in health care as a means of viewing the community and provincial mores toward health reform in larger context.

Health Practices and Health Status

As we have seen in our review of provincial programs, health-care structures are rooted in the individual social ideologies of each province. Less evident is the effect of these programs on the actual health practices or health status of the Canadian population. If over $55 billion is currently spent on health care in Canada, it is useful to ascertain where the money is being spent in relation to health concepts, practices, and reform policies. In a recent publication, *The Sociology of Health and Health Care*, the authors point out that health-care expenditures in Canada consume a greater proportion of our gross national product than is the case in most other industrialized nations. This information is critical in discussing and understanding Canadian health. Just over one-third of total provincial budgets are expended on health, and by far the majority (75%) of that money goes to institutional and physician services, that is, for health care itself, not for prevention or programs for change (Sutherland and Fulton, 1990). Canadian life expectancy in general has increased, but the reasons for the increase have less to do with improvements in health care and more to do with positive changes in standard of living related to living conditions, nutrition and nutritional practices, and decreases in the rate of infant mortality. Frankel and other authors are careful to point out that increased life expectancy carries greater risks for decreases in the quality of life; for example, life expectancy does not automatically imply disability-free life expectancy. If social class is isolated, no matter which measure of socioeconomic status is used, higher income earners and people working in more prestigious jobs experience lower mortality rates and longer life expectancy even when the latter is adjusted for quality measures. Overall, changes in longevity among the Canadian population do not necessarily mean proportional changes in health status. The converse of this statement is equally instructive; in countries like Hungary and Finland, where life expectancy has decreased in spite of costly health-care systems, suicide and lifestyle risk have actually increased (Sutherland and Fulton, 1990). Thus, it is important to interpret longevity data in context with other measures or indicators of health and health status.

In this decade, cardiovascular diseases and cancer remain the most significant causes of death for both sexes from the age of 25 years onward (*Action Statement*). Mortality rates continue to be considerably higher for males than for females throughout the life span. The irony here is that females in Canada report higher rates of illness and higher rates of use of health services than do males (Frankel et al. 1996). Whether the latter tendency represents a cultural and/or gender difference in the approach to health behavior, it is a significant sex difference worthy of greater exploration and analysis. From a Canadian and a global perspective, it is critical to recognize the epidemic proportions of depression, anxiety, stress, loneliness, and insecurity (Sutherland and Fulton, 1990), all of which contribute to a decline in the quality of life and lifestyle—more evidence to underline the importance of health promotion that is beyond mere physical health or well-being.

Health workers make up about 8 percent of the Canadian labor force. Of that percentage, about three-quarters work in the nation's approximately 1,200 hospitals. The Canadian health-care system constitutes the largest social service sector in the country, and it is the third largest employer in the nation (Frankel et al. 1996). Sutherland and others contend that since the 1970s, Canada has had "too many physicians." This is a debatable point when the stature of physicians is so elevated in our society and when hospitals themselves serve as such powerful symbols of wealth and power. What is remarkable and worthy of reconsideration is the rejection of "alternative" forms of health practitioners like naturopaths, homeopaths, and practitioners of eastern forms

of medicine (acupuncture, for example). Also, in spite of community-based health policy reforms, the whole notion of community health centers is slow to gain acceptance by traditional medical personnel, who perceive them as threatening to their power and independence. The concept of community health-care centers is based on a team or shared approach to health delivery, which challenges the current top-down approach. Community health centers support a variety of health-care personnel only some of whom are medical doctors, in order to serve health consumers. To date, only the province of Quebec has achieved significant inroads in establishing such centers (Frankel et al. 1996), solid evidence that health promotion may be more of a factor in that province than its perceived lack of compliance with either the *Charter* or the strategies of the *Framework* documents.

Action Statement for Health Promotion

Lifestyle, special environments, age, sex, wealth, power, institutional dominance, biological factors, and a wide variety of other variables interact in Canada, as they do elsewhere in the world, to characterize the status of health in any given time period or social grouping. And still the mirage of the importance of the health-care system continues to overwhelm health-care reform and to monopolize human and economic resources. To renew efforts toward greater health promotion, with optimal health as a goal, the Canadian Public Health Association in 1996 recommitted itself to the strategies of the *Charter* and the *Framework*. In July of 1996, the association published a working paper called *Action Statement for Health Promotion in Canada,* with the following introductory comment:

> This *Action Statement* is the product of a two-year consultation process involving more than 1000 people. Participants in the process were mainly health professionals and volunteers who work to promote health. Other participants came from areas such as social services, education, recreation, environment and law enforcement. These people share the values and ways of working that define health promotion, even though they may not call themselves health promoters. Together we represent a community of shared purpose.

The Canadian Public Health Association is a group within the Population Health Directorate of the federal ministry, Health Canada. The *Action Statement* is a policy developed for provinces and health-care workers to consider and implement in local areas. Notice that paid professionals in the health-care industry, such as physicians and hospital personnel, are conspicuous by their absence in this process of formulating an action statement. Instead it is a grassroots commitment based on shared values with respect to the goals of health promotion. The wisdom or necessity of not using health professionals/workers in strategic policy is not the issue here; instead it is important to examine the direction of this proposal and then to look at examples of what has been happening recently in health promotion in the country.

The *Action Statement,* significantly, represents a recommitment to the framework established in the 1986 *Charter* as a viable approach to health promotion; 10 years after the charter was published, the *Action Statement* refines the document's focus to the mid-1990s. Noting global trends with respect to the escalation of poverty levels, rapidly increasing unemployment, and economic decisions and practices that threaten the environment and consolidate wealth and power in private corporations with few legal responsibilities to the common good, the *Action Statement* recommends that priorities be set to affirm and share the vision and values of health promotion. The statement also calls for the creation of alliances across and between different community and health sectors; honing knowledge, skills, and the capacity to improve health; emphasizing political commitment and the development of healthy public policies; working to ensure that health system reform truly promotes health both inside and outside the health-care system. Of major importance in this statement is the recognition that improving health is a vital component of human development. Instead of reiterating ill-health data, the *Action Statement* succinctly summarized the implications of that data in sifting out the following critical health determinants:

- healthy childhood development
- adequate incomes
- small gaps between the rich and poor
- absence of discrimination based on gender, culture, race, and sexual orientation
- lifelong learning opportunities
- healthy lifestyles
- meaningful work opportunities with some control over decision making
- social relationships that respect diversity
- freedom from violence or its threat
- freedom from exposure to infectious disease
- protection of humans from environmental hazard
- protection of the environment from human hazards

The *Action Statement* takes a refreshing approach to health status data by interpreting what it means to work toward health as a process with direction in-

stead of merely reporting the state of ill health. Further, the statement recognizes that health promotion has a firm values base. For example, of the six value statements given in the document, one stresses the value that individual liberties must be respected with a priority given to the common good, and another stresses that individuals must be treated with dignity and respect. Although these might seem like obvious commonsense principles, explicitly recognizing and stating them provides some validation for perceiving health in its fullest sense: physical, emotional, mental, and spiritual.

Also important, relative to this *Action Statement* is the learning gained from the 1986 commitment to health promotion. The document stresses that strategic principles must be understood in guiding the development and implementation of health promotion:

- Health promotion addresses health issues in social and environmental context.
- Health promotion supports a holistic approach to all aspects of healthy development.
- Health promotion requires a long-term perspective; time must be taken to create awareness and build understanding about health determinants.
- Health promotion supports a balance between centralized and decentralized decision making on policies affecting people.
- Health promotion is multisectional in that cooperation must be achieved between people and organizations to dovetail with program initiatives in the health sector.
- Health promotion draws on formal knowledge in the social, economic, political, medical, and environmental sciences and on personal experience.
- Health promotion emphasizes public accountability.

Apparently much has been learned about solidifying and implementing health promotion from a strategic perspective. In particular, it is recognized that, while change in health policy and behavior must come, it will come slowly; newer or "sexier" health initiatives are not the answer. Instead the *Action Statement* confirms health promotion from an empowerment perspective. Strategies require some concrete tactics for implementation, and the *Action Statement* supplies strong suggestions in that regard. Once again, the *Charter* is used as a springboard to reinvigorate specific thrusts in health promotion. With respect to advocating healthy public policy, the statement accurately highlights the shaping power of policies in determining how money, power, and material resources flow through institutions of health and thereby offer the determinants of health behavior and outcomes. During the past 10 years, the emphasis in policy making has been on support for creating and developing healthy lifestyles; more emphasis must now be placed on policies that create healthy living conditions and that give voice to society's least powerful groups. To that end, the *Action Statement* provides a comprehensive list of priorities and tactics for action in policy making.

Community Focus

Equally stressed in this 1996 document is the dominant and proven need to *strengthen communities* in the health promotion thrust. Because communities already share common space, identities, interests, and concerns through various agencies and activities, the *Action Statement* mentions several action priorities to provide community training opportunities, funding, support from/for community networks, and the development of evaluation methods for continued monitoring and improvement. The evidence is clear in Canada that changes in health promotion will not come from the institutionalized health-care sector. The provincial initiatives toward health promotion described earlier demonstrate that change in the area of health promotion works best at the community, grassroots level. Related to this fact is the third tactic identified in the *Action Statement*: the absolute necessity to *reform health systems.* The document narrows its focus to two specific objectives: to shift the emphasis from treating disease to improving health; and to increase the effectiveness and efficiency of the health-care system.

Both of these objectives form part of most provincial policy statements on health reform. Still, the reality of health system reform lags considerably behind the recognition that it is needed. Political debate and public attention tend to be focused on insured medical treatments and reducing the number of hospital beds; cuts in primary health care are widespread. For example, in Ontario, the *Toronto Daily Star* gave full-page coverage to the appointment of retired Queen's University former dean of medicine Duncan Sinclair to the chair of the province's Health Services Restructuring Committee (*TDS,* September 15, 1996). Sinclair's task, the article said, was to "shake up/down the Ontario hospital system" to rid the system of duplication and to "ensure there is a health care system for future generations." This is a prime example of praiseworthy reductions in cost but failure to address the broad determinants of health: closing hospitals is not the sole answer to health reform. Instead, according to the *Action Statement,* family- and community-based care must be improved with stronger health protection programs and access to client-centered primary health-care services. To achieve real benefits from and by

health promotion, the knowledge base about health determinants and regional health profiles must be increased and stronger alliances or coalitions must be fostered among different organizations that share the common goal of health promotion, and can effect real change in the broad determinants of health. Ultimately, as the *Action Statement* points out, if efforts to develop health promotion efforts in Canada are to succeed, they must be allied to similar efforts throughout the global community.

Current Initiatives and Future Directions

In Canada's health promotion survey in 1990, in which some 13,000 people across the country were interviewed regarding health status, practices, and beliefs, self-reports were compiled to assess the status of health promotion in the population. The respondents reported very little change in health status. The rich and the well educated were more likely to report good to excellent health status than those with less wealth and education. The same survey showed findings about social relationships, environmental health practices, personal health practices, alcohol and other drug use, nutritional practices, heart disease prevention, leisure time physical activity, cancer prevention practices, injury control and safety, sexual health, and dental health. The conclusion, once again, is that health education is absolutely critical as a catalyst for improvement in health behaviors.

Similarly, in 1991 Angus published an extensive "Review of Significant Health Care Commissions and Task Forces in Canada Since 1983–84," sponsored by the Canadian Medical Association. His finding? At the root of all of these commissions and reforms is the desire to rebalance and redirect the system in three important ways: toward greater emphasis on disease prevention and health promotion; toward community-based health-care alternatives; and toward greater accountability of the health-care system. Clearly, Canada has committed itself to the whole concept and implementation of health promotion. Is it working? This question is difficult to answer, because generalizations are impossible. The following section examines specific pockets of information and examples in an effort to find out if and how health promotion is being implemented in Canada.

The Implementation of Health Promotion

A positive sign of knowledge-based, applied research is the work of the Canadian Fitness and Lifestyle Research Institute (CFLRI). This organization's mission is to "enhance the well being of Canadians through research and communication of information about physically active lifestyles to the public and private sectors." The Institute seeks to understand active living by addressing fitness issues from the complementary perspectives of the health professions, the social and psychological sciences, and the physiological and biological sciences. In 1994 the CFLRI published its findings on "Health Promotion at Work: Results of the 1992 National Workplace Survey." The Institute recognized that because some 13 million Canadians are employed, the workplace is a very important environment and avenue for health promotion. Some 45,000 Canadian companies claim to have health promotion programs in place to varying degrees. The most popular lifestyle or health promotion intervention on the part of employees is in the realm of smoking cessation. Some 3,500 companies with 20 or more employees responded to the survey and provided information about such health determinants as stress, harassment, discrimination, financial uncertainty, conflicts at work, fatigue, and levels of physical activity. The survey data show that workplace health promotion efforts are increasing and expanding. Only businesses in Quebec were more likely to claim that health is the sole responsibility of the employee. Workplaces must continue to be targeted for health promotion and reform. Philosophically, however, such efforts run counter to the value system in a capitalist society. Capitalism is based on the values of material gain and inequality, reflected in most workplaces by the very fact of work and its goals. Health promotion, in contrast, is rooted in equality of opportunity and benefits as well as in the quality of everyday life rather than material ends or goals. This contradiction in values is one that must be resolved to functionally support and implement health promotion initiatives.

ParticipACTION

If data don't convince people—and the history of health data and ill-health data confirm that most people are not scared easily by statistical trends—then there must be alternatives to persuasion. In Canada, one of the most successful campaigns focused on healthy behavior has been ParticipACTION, a non-government movement to promote healthy lifestyles. Established in the early 1970s, this not-for-profit organization was initially commissioned by the federal government to campaign for improved fitness and lifestyle improvement. ParticipACTION's objective was to market physical fitness as one would market toothpaste or any other product. The organization used two key marketing strategies: (1) to employ modern marketing methods in advertising; and (2) to finance itself from the private sector, not the public purse. To implement the first strategy, the organization developed a four-cornered approach to marketing fitness: educate, motivate, remind, and provide solutions about/for physical fitness. The group leans heavily on private corporations to achieve its goals and is distinguished by its clever use of advertising. In its 30-year history, ParticipACTION has had to compete with service agencies and charities like the United Way for advertising time and space. Annual reviews of its efforts show impressive cost-benefit ratios for its advertising. It is difficult to open any newspaper today and not find some small ad or teasing clip provided by this organization, which is highly effective in targeting the population at the grassroots level.

ParticipACTION also publishes *Active Living,* a national magazine that provides resource information to educators, health professionals, fitness leaders, and others in the broad spectrum of health interests in Canada. This publication and the efforts of ParticipACTION to involve itself in wider aspects of health and behavior change and information exchange are clear indicators of health promotion at work.

Food Guides and Eating Patterns

A growing body of evidence suggests that symptoms and causes of ill health are directly attributable to eating choices and patterns. Canada has long been famed for its *Food Guide to Healthy Eating,* a simple, one-sheet "recipe" for appropriate daily food selection from the four main food groups. Heavy marketing emphasis is placed on low-fat foods, reducing portion sizes, focusing on "grazing" foods, and becoming better consumers by paying attention to food labels. The Heart and Stroke Foundation of Canada, long committed to decreasing the incidence and prevalence of these disorders, actively promotes *heart-smart* foods, and has supported the publication of a heart-healthy cookbook.

Another excellent example of promoting health through healthier eating is a highly successful recipe book called *Looneyspoons: Low-Fat Food Made Fun,* written by two sisters in Ontario. Using the teasing style employed in ParticipACTION campaigns, the book taps into the day-to-day experiences and interests of ordinary people. Chapter titles include, "If You Bake It, They Will Come," and, "Meatless in Seattle." Straightforward low-fat tasty recipes are presented with lighthearted comments like, "Low-fat eating is for those who are thick and tired of dieting," and "Dieting is the penalty for exceeding the feed limit." Even the recipe titles have flair and appeal: "Pita-the-Great," "Scalloping Gourmet," "Mission Shrimpossible," and "Veal of Fortune" are a few examples. Such an innovative approach to healthy behavior through nutritious eating is a solid and useful response to serious problems like obesity and anorexia nervosa, which so negatively affect the health and health costs of Canadians.

Wellness

Newspapers in Canada carry stories regularly about communities hosting "health fairs," local gatherings at which the public has easy access to health-care personnel, resources, and information. Similarly, educational curricula reflect growing trends toward teaching and learning about health. For example, the *Food Guide to Healthy Eating* is known to most elementary school children across Canada. In secondary schools, such as those in Ontario, the most senior course in physical education contains an entire, comprehensive section on "wellness" and "psychological and social development" related to a framework of holistic health education. Several universities have implemented wellness or well-being research; teaching and study centers patterned themselves after the phenomenally successful National Wellness Center in Stevens Point, Wisconsin, but with greater emphasis on the research component and mandate in postsecondary education.

Promoting Men's Health

In Canada, as in the United States and other Western Hemisphere countries, women are far more likely to seek help in matters of health than men—despite the fact that men have distinct health problems and earlier incidences of disease and premature death than do women. Part of the reason for this gender-based difference in response to health initiatives and reform lies in social conditioning; traditionally, men have been expected to be stoic, invulnerable, almost bulletproof in their day-to-day lives. Until recently, boys have been brought up to be self-reliant, to suppress "soft" emotions, and to "prove" their toughness through sports, hazardous jobs, war, and high-risk behaviors like workaholism, social isolation, and avoidance of intimacy. There are no clear answers to the dramatic difference in men's and women's responses to health promotion, but new approaches must be identified as the role of men in Canadian society continues to change.

A Regional Example

If health promotion is grounded in community-based programs and reform, then we must have evaluations and information bases for those communities. A comprehensive study, "Community Health and Well Being in Southwestern Ontario," recently was compiled to provide epidemiological information on the determinants of health and health status of the region,

a community of some 1.5 million people, or about 13 percent of the province's total population. Results of this study show that the region has significantly higher rates of mortality from heart attacks and other cardiovascular diseases and diabetes. Hospitalization rates are at least 10 percent higher for these same problems than in the rest of Ontario. The residents of this community smoke more, eat more fat, exercise less, and have more body fat than residents of Ontario as a whole—not surprising given the mortality and hospitalization findings presented above. The area has a higher proportion of seniors and residents aged 15 and over with less than a grade 9 education than do other parts of the province.

Significantly, the study found that the only factor that predicts life expectancy of a community is its poverty rate (not the number of hospital beds available or other traditional data); the higher the poverty level, the higher the rate of premature mortality. These findings are important for many reasons. First, they dramatically illustrate once again that health status does not equal health care. Further, they show that social environment, physical environment, and biological endowment (how well one chooses his/her parents!) all are determinants of health as is the individual's responses to those factors. Lifestyle factors, the study's authors stress, are not the sole or even the primary cause of poor health; rather, they are symptoms of a variety of social, psychological, and economic factors, perhaps the most important of which is low income. In fact, low income may be such a key health variable that it "may set off a domino effect on other health hazards." Community-based studies like this appear to contribute significantly to ongoing efforts toward health promotion and corresponding evaluation in Canada.

Summary

Health promotion is a slow process, but the changes occurring in health delivery and health behavior toward enhancement of quality lifestyles are rapid. The ability to diagnose symptoms from such sources as the Internet and its resources are a boon, as well as a challenge to traditional health procedures and forms of care. Clearly, changes in health cannot be the responsibility of government: individuals in communities must assume increasing responsibility for promoting health as a process, not a static end or achievable goal. In reality, health, like most forms of human behavior, is an attitude, one that is based on personal, social, and cultural values and practices. Until Canada or any other nation recognizes that fact, the achievement of true health will remain an elusive goal.

Sources and Further Reading

Action Statement for Health Promotion in Canada, Ottawa: Canadian Public Health Association, July, 1996.

Active Learning, September 1992, Volume 1, Number 4.

Alder, R., Vingilis, E., Mai, V., editors. London, Ontario: Middlesex-London Health Unit and the Faculty of Medicine, The University of Western Ontario, 1996.

Craig, C. L., Beaulieu, A., Cameron, C. *Health Promotion at Work: Results of the 1992 National Workplace Survey.* Ottawa: Canadian Fitness and Lifestyle Research Institute, 1994.

Crichton, A., Hsu, D., Tsand, S. *Canada's Health Care System: Its Funding and Organization.* Ottawa: Canadian Hospital Association, 1990.

Epp, J. *Achieving Health for All: A Framework for Health Promotion.* Ottawa: Health and Welfare Canada, 1986.

Frankel, G., Speechley, M., Wade, T. J. *The Sociology of Health and Health Care: A Canadian Perspective.* Toronto: Copp Clark Ltd., 1996.

Lazear, D. *Seven Ways of Knowing.* Palatine, IL: Skylight Publishing, 1991.

Ottawa Charter for Health Promotion. Ottawa: World Health Organization and Health and Welfare Canada, 1986.

Pederson, A., O'Neill, M., Rootman, I. *Health Promotion in Canada: Provincial, National and International Perspectives.* Toronto: W. B. Saunders Canada, 1994.

Podleski, J., Podleski, G. *Looneytoons: Low-Fat Food Made Fun.* Ottawa: Granet Publishing Inc., 1996.

Stephens, T., Fowler, G. D., editors. *Canada's Health Promotion Survey 1990: Technical Report.* Ottawa: Ministry of Supply and Services Canada, 1993.

Sutherland, R. W., Fulton, M. J. *Health Care in Canada: A Description and Analysis of Canadian Health Services.* Ottawa: The Health Group, 1990.

Chapter 1

Targeting Risk Reduction

InfoLink: www.cdc.gov/nccdphp/nccdhome.htm

National Center for Chronic Disease Prevention and Health Promotion Website

This site is a service of the National Center for Chronic Disease Prevention and Health Promotion, Centers for Disease Control and Prevention, U.S. Department of Health and Human Services. The mission of the NCCDP includes preventing death and disability from chronic diseases and promoting healthy personal behaviors. To learn more about risk behaviors that influence your health, visit this site.

Topics for Today Religious Diversity on Campus: A Different Kind of School Spirit

The Institute on Religion and Public Life

This site has the monthly publication *First Things* available for reading. *First Things* is published by the Institute on Religion and Public Life, an interreligious, nonpartisan research and education institute whose purpose is to advance a religiously informed public philosophy for the ordering of society. RPL also sponsors a number of other activities.

www.firstthings.com

Minnesota Cultural Diversity Center

The mission of the MCDC is (1) to promote multicultural understanding through educational programs of communication, ethnic events, and cultural learning, (2) to provide multiple resources to individuals, corporations, and community, nonprofit, government, educational organizations needing assistance in the areas of cultural diversity, and (3) to enhance the understanding of diversity as a means for all of us to prosper together.

www.mcdc.org

Chapter 2

Health Action Guide

Fostering Your Emotional Growth

InfoLink: www.mhsource.com/healthieryou.html

Mental Health InfoSource Healthier You Website

Healthier You is a virtual reference guide for the informed mental health consumer. It includes information on disorders, articles and information written specifically for the consumer, a mental health directory, and a list of worldwide web links arranged by topic.

Health Action Guide

Understanding Your Mental Health Rights

InfoLink: www.bazelon.org

Bazelon Center for Mental Health Law Website

The Judge David L. Bazelon Center for Mental Health Law is a nonprofit legal advocacy organization based in Washington, D.C. Their advocacy is based on the principle that every individual is entitled to choice and dignity. For many people with mental disabilities, this means something as basic as having a decent place to live, supportive services, and equality of opportunity.

Health Action Guide

Resources for Help with Depression

InfoLink: http://depression.cmhc.com

Mental Health Net Website

Mental Health Net has a very simple goal, to provide you with an easy-to-use, friendly resource in which to access all the mental health topics on the Internet. The link listed provides you with a wealth of information on-line about depression.

Topics for Today Lending a Helping Hand: Becoming a Volunteer

ImpactOnline and VirtualVolunteering

Many people actively search for volunteer opportunities they can complete via home or work computers, because of time constraints, personal preference, a disability, or a home-based obligation that prevents them from volunteering on-site. Virtual volunteering allows anyone to contribute time and expertise to not-for-profit organizations, schools, government offices and other agencies that utilize volunteer services, without leaving his or her home or office.

www.impactonline.org/vv

Hearts and Minds

Through their website, upcoming magazine and national publicity efforts, Hearts and Minds works to reach people nationwide (and all over the world). They motivate people to get involved, showing how to make volunteering and donations more effective.

www.heartsandminds.org/home.htm

Chapter 3

Health Action Guide
Coping with Test Anxiety
InfoLink: www.collegeview.com/student/step1.html

College View Publishing Website—
No More Test Anxiety
The material at this site is from *No More Test Anxiety,* an excellent book by Ed Newman, designed to help students better deal with the stress of taking tests and thereby improve scores.

Health Action Guide
Dealing with Work-Related Stress
InfoLink: www.hyperstress.com

The Institute for Stress Management
The Institute for Stress Management website offers products and free services guaranteed to provide specific, practical, result-producing ways to gain more control in your life and experience more enjoyment through stress management and Master Life Planning programs and techniques. You can also download free reports, articles, bulletin board posters, and bookmarks.

Topics for Today Going It Alone: Managing the Stress of Single Parenthood

Parents Place Website
ParentsPlace.com is a website where parents of all types connect, communicate, and celebrate the adventures of child rearing. Through our bulletin boards and chats, members share insights and lend a supportive ear. After all, parents are the best resource for other parents. At ParentsPlace.com, you can find information about women's health, child development, daily pet peeves, schoolwork, discipline issues, and current family-related politics.

www.parentsplace.com

Parenthood Website
Parenthoodweb.com is a website where parents can go and ask a panel of parenting/childcare experts questions or read the experts' answers to other ParenthoodWeb visitor questions.

www.parenthoodweb.com

Chapter 4

Health Action Guide
Tips to Help You Stick to Your Exercise Program
InfoLink: http://primusweb.com/fitnesspartner

Fitness Partner Connection Jumpsite Website
The mission of the Fitness Partner Connection Jumpsite website is to provide quality fitness, health- and nutrition-related information, and education across the globe. The Jumpsite is a noncommercial labor of love. It is their intent to wholeheartedly contribute to the awareness and momentum of the health and fitness movement by providing resources and support that will cultivate happy, healthy, and fit lifestyles.

Health Action Guide
How to Calculate Your Target Heart Rate
InfoLink: www.fitnesslink.com

FitnessLink Website
This site has information for exercise enthusiasts, fitness professionals, and individuals new to fitness. FitnessLink provides the resources you need to get fit and stay fit. The latest fitness news is updated daily, so check out this valuable fitness resource.

Health Action Guide
Activities to Promote Sound Sleep
InfoLink: www.sleepnet.com

SleepNet Website
One of SleepNet's goals is to link all the sleep information located on the Internet. As new sites become available they will be linked here. The Sandman's guide offers many different paths to find information and links. Sleep links and research links are rated and reviewed. In addition, sleep forums provide a place for everyone to read and post messages, questions, or responses.

Health Action Guide
Exercise Danger Signs
InfoLink: www.acsm.org/sportsmed/index.htm

American College of Sports Medicine Website
The American College of Sports Medicine (ACSM) is the largest, most respected sports medicine and exercise science organization in the world. ACSM promotes and integrates scientific research, education, and practical applications of sports medicine and exercise science to maintain and enhance physical performance, fitness, health, and quality of life. Information for athletes to those people chronically diseased or physically challenged is included on this site. ACSM continues to look for and find better methods to allow everyone to live longer and more productively. Healthier people make a healthier society.

Topics for Today Extreme Sports: Living on the Edge

Adventure Sports Website
If having the wind in your face and your heart in your throat is what makes you feel alive, then the Adventure Sports website is the place for you. A section titled Team Adventure makes it easy for you to find outfitters and tour guides for your next outdoor adventure. You can also access event calendars and download applications right here. Finally, if you are new to a sport or are trying to learn more about the sport, you'll find what you need to get started at this site.

www.adventuresports.com

ESPN Extreme Sports
Ongoing headline news about extreme sports from mountain biking to climbing can be found at the website of ESPN Sports, Inc.

http://espn.go.com/extreme/index.html

Chapter 5
Health Action Guide
Tips for Reducing the Fat Content of Meals
InfoLink: www.cspinet.org

Center for Science in the Public Interest Website
The Center for Science in the Public Interest (CSPI) is a nonprofit education and advocacy organization that focuses on improving the safety and nutritional quality of our food supply. CSPI seeks to promote health through educating the public about nutrition; it represents citizens' interests before legislative, regulatory, and judicial bodies; and it works to ensure that advances in science are used for the public's good.

Health Action Guide
USDA's Safety Tips for the Proper Handling of Meat
InfoLink: www.usda.gov/cnpp

Center for Nutrition Policy and Promotion
Website of the Food and Drug Administration
First and foremost, FDA is a public health agency, charged with protecting American consumers by enforcing the Federal Food, Drug, and Cosmetic Act and several related public health laws. The Food and Drug Administration touches the lives of virtually every American every day—it is the FDA's job to see that the food we eat is safe and wholesome and that radiation-emitting products such as microwave ovens will not harm us.

Health Action Guide
Tips for Eating on the Run
InfoLink: www.ag.uiuc.edu/~food-lab/nat

The Nutrition Analysis Tool Website
The Department of Food Science and Human Nutrition at the University of Illinois has developed an on-line Nutrition Analysis Tool (NAT). The NAT is a web-based program that allows anyone to analyze the foods they eat for various different nutrients. This tool is completely free and quite easy to use.

Health Action Guide
Making Healthful Restaurant Choices
InfoLink: www.navigator.tufts.edu
Center on Nutrition Communication, School of Nutrition Science and Policy, Tufts University Website
The Tufts University Nutrition Navigator is the first on-line rating and review guide that solves the two major problems web users have when seeking nutrition information: how to quickly find information best suited to their needs and whether to trust the information they find there.

Health Action Guide
Dietary Recommendations
InfoLink: www.nal.usda.gov/fnic/Dietary/dgreport.html

United States Department of Agriculture's Dietary Guidelines for Americans Website
The entire Report of the Dietary Guidelines Advisory Committee on the Dietary Guidelines for Americans is found at this link.

Health Action Guide
Making Healthful Food Choices
InfoLink: www.nal.usda.gov/fnic

Food and Nutrition Information Center Website
The Food and Nutrition Information Center (FNIC) is one of several information centers at the National Agricultural Library, part of the United States Department of Agriculture's Research Service. You can access all of FNIC's resource lists and databases, as well as many other food and nutrition related links from this site.

Topics for Today Meals Without Meat: Following a Semivegetarian Diet

The Vegetarian Society of the United Kingdom
The Vegetarian Society is working toward its vision of a future where the vegetarian diet is acknowledged as the norm. Many people think vegetarianism is a trendy new fad, but in reality it has a long history. Visit this site to learn more about vegetarian diets.

www.vegsoc.org/index1.html

Cornell University Vegetarian Diet Pyramid
To offer a healthful alternative to the 1992 USDA Food Guide Pyramid, which combines some animal and plant foods together in a single group, Cornell and Harvard university researchers have teamed up with other experts to assist the nonprofit foundation Oldways Preservation and Exchange Trust in unveiling an official Vegetarian Diet Pyramid. The Vegetarian Diet Pyramid emphasizes a wide base of foods to be eaten at every meal.

www.dol.net/~rave/cornellveg.html

Chapter 6
Health Action Guide
Changing Your Eating Patterns
InfoLink: http://dmi-www.mc.duke.edu/dfc/home.html

Duke University Diet and Fitness Center Website
The Duke University Diet and Fitness Center (DFC) helps people live healthier, fuller lives through weight loss and lifestyle change. The DFC program is a lifestyle, not a diet. It is based on sound scientific principles and experience, not the latest fad. Their team of health professionals use evaluation, education, experience, and encouragement. They work with their participants to help them plan and practice new strategies and healthier habits for life.

Health Action Guide
Choosing a Diet Book
InfoLink: www.shapeup.org/library/index.html

Shape Up America! Library Website
Shape Up America! is a high-profile national initiative to promote healthy weight and increased physical activity in America, involving a broad-based coalition of industry, medical/health, nutrition, physical fitness, and related organizations and experts. The Shape Up America! library contains all the documents they have published or

released, including news releases, annual reports, and most importantly, educational materials.

Health Action Guide
Evaluating a Weight Loss Program
InfoLink: www.shapeup.org

Shape Up America! Website
Shape Up America! announces its new support center. Visit their website if you want to learn more about the barriers to successful weight management and some practical solutions to help you overcome them. Their website is designed to provide you with the latest information about safe weight management, healthy eating, and physical fitness.

Health Action Guide
Weight Management
InfoLink: www.weight.com

Objective Medical Information on Obesity at Michael Myers, M.D., Website
The purpose of this site is to provide objective medical information on obesity, eating disorders, and associated medical conditions in a noncommercial environment where any editorial comment is appropriately noted. The author of this site is a practicing physician, and a member of the North American Association for the Study of Obesity.

Topics for Today Are You a Victim of Portion Distortion? Learning to Control Serving Sizes

Overeater's Anonymous
Overeaters Anonymous (OA) is a program based upon the 12 steps of Alcoholics Anonymous. Today, it is a growing organization that has meetings on every continent. It treats the food and weight problem not as a lack of will power or a moral defect but as a disease that can be arrested. This 12-step program offers a recovery for the physical, emotional, and spiritual aspects of compulsive eating.

http://recovery.hiwaay.net

Calorie Control Council
This website represents the low-calorie and reduced-fat food and beverage industry, and provides a wealth of information related to low-calorie foods. Moreover, this site includes a calorie counter calculator.

www.caloriecontrol.org

Chapter 7
Health Action Guide
Preventing Drug Use
InfoLink: www.doorway.org

The Doorway—A Center for Drug Prevention
Covering prevention, education, intervention, and recovery, this is a very user-friendly site loaded with information and links. Lots of strategies and resources are presented, making this a must for checking out drug prevention topics.

Topics for Today Caffeine: America's Most Popular Drug

Majestic Coffee and Tea, Inc.
This site contains a wealth of information on the history of coffee, the coffee plant, coffee plant diseases, coffee history, a glossary of coffee terms, and many other information topics related to coffee.

www.gardfoods.com/coffee/index.htm

Caffeine and the Cyclist
A few years ago the well-known exercise physiologist, David Costill, published the results of his research on caffeine and the physical performance of long-distance runners. This research has resulted in the faddish use of caffeine among some and a generally positive impression of caffeine that is not completely warranted. While caffeine may still be a fad among runners, it has a long history of use among European cyclists. Read about this important research at this site.

www.roble.com/marquis/caffeine

Chapter 8
Health Action Guide
Acute Alcohol Intoxication
InfoLink: www.ncadd.org

National Council on Alcoholism and Drug Dependency Website
Responsible drinking is covered on links found on the site of the National Council on Alcoholism and Drug Dependency. This comprehensive site contains a number of materials and links to education and prevention resources.

Health Action Guide
Guidelines for Hosting a Party Responsibly
InfoLink: www.madd.org

Mothers Against Drunk Driving (MADD)
For great practical advice on hosting a safe, fun party, log on to this site. Get tips for hosting a college party or an office party, and find out what you can do to make sure your guests enjoy themselves while keeping their drinking under control. The site even offers recipes for refreshing nonalcoholic beverages. You can also read the list of myths and facts about alcohol and driving and learn how to spot a drunk driver on the road.

Health Action Guide
Tips to Help You Keep Drinking Under Control
InfoLink: www.bacchusgamma.org

BACCHUS and GAMMA Peer Education Network Website
This comprehensive site contains an overwhelming set of links to related topics. A thorough discussion of symptoms is included. Besides in-depth discussions of intervention programs, a wealth of information is available on education and prevention programs.

Topics for Today Success in a Bottle? A Look at Alcohol Advertising

Alcohol and Advertising

This is an extremely useful research tool for students provided by the Addiction Research Foundation of Canada. It lists more than 80 books and articles on the subject of alcohol advertising, as well as additional bibliographic and Internet resources.

www.arf.org/isd/bib/advert.html

Alcohol Problems and Solutions

This comprehensive website by David Hanson, Professor and Research at the State University of New York, provides an impressive amount of information related to alcohol and advertising.

www2.potsdam.edu/alcohol-info

Chapter 9
Health Action Guide
Smokeless Tobacco Use
InfoLink: www.kidsource.com/index.html

Kidsource

This site is an excellent source for in-depth and timely education and health-care information that will make a difference in the lives of parents and their children. You will find information on smokeless tobacco use by teens and programs that will help educate youth about the negative effects of use of smokeless tobacco.

Health Action Guide
Countdown to Quit Day: A Plan for Smoking Cessation
InfoLink: http://kickbutt.org

The Kickbutt Action Center Website

The Kickbutt website was developed by Washington DOC (Doctors Ought to Care) on behalf of the tobacco control community. The goal of Kickbutt is to link different tobacco control groups, improve access to vital information, and provide communities with the necessary tools to work for change. This site has very good information on how to quit smoking.

Health Action Guide
Avoiding Weight Gain When You Stop Smoking
InfoLink: www.ash.org/papers/h3.htm

Smoking Cessation and Weight Gain

This is a very good site that looks not only at nicotine addiction, but at various aspects of quitting smoking. These aspects include reasons for quitting and a great section on smoking cessation and avoiding weight gain.

Topics for Today Smoking Among Women: Troubling Trends

Current Issues in Smoking and Reproductive Health

This site includes multilinked topics covering smoking's relationship to and effect on birth control, hormones, reproduction, pregnancy, and cancer. Education and prevention are also addressed. Links include articles, studies, and programs, making this a handy site for exploring the topic of smoking and reproduction.

www.arhp.org/clinical/index.html

Women and Heart Disease

This American Heart Association site is a great one to examine the effects of smoking on the heart. Its discussion of treatable and nontreatable risk factors complements a set of fast links to related topics of other smoking-related diseases, effects of smoking on children, smoking among minorities groups, and a host of other interesting and important topics.

www.amhrt.org/heart/womensheart.html

Chapter 10
Health Action Guide
Recognizing Signs of a Heart Attack
InfoLink: www.columbia-utah.com/heartattack.html

Recognizing Heart Attacks

This site informs the user on what heart attack symptoms are and what action to take if a person shows signs of a heart attack.

Health Action Guide
Monitoring Your Cholesterol
InfoLink: www.amhrt.org

American Heart Association—Cholesterol Levels

This sometimes confusing topic is made clear at the Heart Association's site. Definitions of terms help the layperson become conversant on the topic of cholesterol. The site also identifies ways to monitor one's cholesterol level. A large number of links to related topics make this an excellent research site.

Health Action Guide
Recognizing Warning Signs of Stroke
InfoLink: www.amhrt.org

Stroke: Prevention, Treatment, and Recovery

Select this site for a clear presentation of the symptoms and warning signs of stroke. The site links quickly to many related topics, including sections on available tests, treatments, and effects.

Topics for Today Hypertension in African-Americans: Targeting Prevention

Woman's Health

An excellent resource on women's health is found at Woman's Health Hot Line. This site is an independent, commercial-free newsletter created by medical author, professional speaker, and founder of National Women's Heart Health. You will find information related to women and heart disease at this site.

www.libov.com

Women's Heart Institute

The Women's Heart Institute is dedicated to the prevention, evaluation, diagnosis, and treatment of heart and blood vessel disease in women. It is located in Beverly Hills, California with the Cardiovascular Medical Group of Southern California. This site is an excellent resource for gathering information related to women and heart disease.

www.womensheartinstitute.com

Chapter 11

Health Action Guide
Cancer-Related Checkups
InfoLink: www.cancer.org

American Cancer Society—Guidelines for Cancer-Related Checkups Website

Most cancer types are covered in this clearly written site. Major cancer groups require specific types of examinations for early detection and prevention, and this site covers them in detail.

Health Action Guide
Breast Self-Examination
InfoLink: www.mskcc.org/pd.htm

Memorial Sloan-Kettering Cancer Center's Website

This exceptional site on cancer has a specific information on breast cancer. The site includes documents links finding the tumor early, treatment for breast cancer, what causes breast cancer, life after breast cancer, and how to do breast self-examination.

Health Action Guide
Testicular Self-Examination
InfoLink: www.mskcc.org/document/WICTEST.htm

Memorial Sloan-Kettering Cancer Center's Website

This exceptional site on cancer has specific information on testicular cancer. The site includes documents links to finding the tumor early, treatment for testicular cancer, what causes testicular cancer, life after testicular cancer, and most importantly, how to do testicular self-examination.

Health Action Guide
How to Look for Melanoma
InfoLink: www.asds-net.org/scfactsheet.html

The American Society for Dermatologic Surgery

This excellent site has specific information on skin cancer. Skin cancer is the uncontrollable growth of abnormal cells in a layer of the skin. It attacks one out of every seven Americans each year, making it the most prevalent form of cancer. However, 90 percent of all skin cancers can be cured if detected and treated in time. Go to this site to learn more about skin cancer.

Topics for Today Cancer and Genetic Testing: Answers Raise New Questions

Human Genome Project

Begun in 1990, the U.S. Human Genome Project is a 15-year effort coordinated by the U.S. Department of Energy and the National Institutes of Health to identify all the estimated 80,000 genes in human DNA, and determine the sequences of the 3 billion chemical bases that make up human DNA, store this information in databases, and develop tools for data analysis. It is believed that many cancers will be able to be detected and treated much earlier by knowing all the genes in the human DNA.

www.ornl.gov/TechResources/Human_Genome/ home.html

Frederick Cancer Research and Development Center

The business of the Frederick Cancer Research and Development Center (FCRDC) is science. At this site you will find links to the home pages for all the various research programs located at the FCRDC. Nearly 100 investigators direct research efforts at FCRDC. You will be able to browse their investigator listings by choosing any cancer topic you want.

www.ncifcrf.gov

Chapter 12

Health Action Guide
Tips for Controlling Exercise-Induced Asthma
InfoLink: www.mdnet.de/asthma

Asthma Information Center Website

This site is one of the largest resources of asthma information on the web. The information is intended for physicians, pharmacists, journalists, researchers, and other health-care professionals as well as for patients and parents of children with asthma. The main focus is on education.

Health Action Guide
Managing Inflammatory Bowel Disease
InfoLink:
http://members.aol.com/bospol/homepage/crohns.htm

Crohn's Disease Resource Center Website

This site provides information about Crohn's disease with pointers to books, articles, and other Internet resources. It's a guide to the most important Crohn's disease related resources.

Topics for Today Managing Chronic Pain: New Treatments Offer Solutions for Sufferers

The National Chronic Pain Outreach Association Website

The National Chronic Pain Outreach Association (NCPOA) publishes the quarterly newsletter, *Lifeline*. NCPOA also serves as a clearinghouse of information on any kind of chronic pain. They also maintain a list of support groups in many areas, have reprints of materials on all aspects of chronic pain, and can help in setting up a local support group.

http://neurosurgery.mgh.harvard.edu/ncpainoa.htm

American Pain Society

The American Pain Society (APS) is a multidisciplinary educational and scientific organization dedicated to serving people in pain. The society was founded in 1978 as a national chapter of the International Association for the Study of Pain (IASP), and now includes more than 3,200 physicians, nurses, psychologists, dentists, scientists, pharmacologists, therapists and social workers who research and treat pain and advocate for patients with pain. This site is an excellent source of information.

www.ampainsoc.org

Chapter 13
Health Action Guide
Reducing Your Risk of Contracting HIV
InfoLink: www.caps.ucsf.edu/FSindex.html

HIV Prevention Fact Sheet
This set of links from the University of California at San Francisco provides a great jumping-off point to research a wide range of HIV-risk reduction practices and techniques. Heterosexual, homosexual, youth, and IV drug-abuse issues are just some of the related topics covered bilingually.

Health Action Guide
Talking with Your Partner about Herpes
InfoLink: www.herpeszone.com/MainMenu.htm

Herpes Zone
This site contains a comprehensive set of links related to information on herpes. Coping with herpes, management of herpes, and living with herpes are some of the related topics covered at this site.

Topics for Today The Hot Zone: New Infectious Diseases Emerge from the Rain Forest

World Health Organization Website
The World Health Organization's home page provides many key links to important topics related to AIDS, Ebola, and monitoring, tracking, and research of these diseases.

www.who.ch

Emerging Infectious Diseases Resource Links
This CDC website offers the best groups of links to every possible subject related to infectious diseases—their origins, symptoms, and effects. Prevention strategies, bibliographies, and a comprehensive list of organizations dealing with infectious diseases may be found, with direct links to each.

www.cdc.gov/ncido

Chapter 14
Topics for Today A Woman's Place: Reconsidering Gender Roles

Duke Journal of Gender Law and Policy
The *Duke Journal of Gender Law & Policy* publishes one symposium issue per year relating to conferences hosted by the *Journal* at the Duke University School of Law and the Terry Sanford Institute of Public Policy at Duke University, Durham, North Carolina. There are many interest-

ing and important articles related to gender and law that are available to read from this on-line journal.

www.law.duke.edu/journals/djglp

National Women's Hall of Fame
In 1969, a group of women and men of Seneca Falls, New York, created the National Women's Hall of Fame, believing that the contribution of American women deserved a permanent home in the small village where it all began. The Hall is home to exhibits, artifacts of historical interest, a research library, and office. The National Women's Hall of Fame, a national membership organization, holds as its mission: "To honor in perpetuity these women, citizens of the United States of America whose contributions to the arts, athletics, business, education, government, the humanities, philanthropy, and science, have been the greatest value for the development of their country." Visit this site to read about some of the women honored.

www.greatwomen.org

Chapter 15
Health Action Guide
Coping with a Breakup
InfoLink: www.cam.org/~jmauld/English/dateanal.html

The Dating Patterns Analyzer Website
The Dating Patterns Analyzer evaluates your relationships and tells you what really makes you happy. There is no right or wrong answers to the questions posed. For example, some people like to talk, others value silence; some people like to climb mountains, others prefer to watch; some people like to laugh, others are more serious. Just answer each item as honestly as you can.

Health Action Guide
Resolving Conflict
InfoLink:
http://hometown.aol.com/uscccn/Conflict2000.index.html

Conflict Resolution 2000+ Website
A wide range of topics dealing with conflict resolution is covered at this site. Especially useful are the many links to resources for users interested in developing programs, learning in greater depth, or researching highly particularized conflicts.

Health Action Guide
Improving Marriage
InfoLink: www.competentcouples.com

Competent Couples Website
Competent Couples, created by Dr. Steven J. Isenberg, a Boston-area licensed psychologist with over 23 years experience as a couples and marital therapist, is a results-oriented series of psychoeducational programs that provide married and unmarried couples with powerful skills for creating loving, deeply satisfying, and enduring partnerships. The goal of the programs is to provide couples with the wisdom and know-how for building a relationship of profound connection, one that greatly increases intimacy

while honoring and supporting individuality. Visit this site to learn more about improving your relationship.

Health Action Guide
Communicating with Your Partner
InfoLink: www.couples-place.com

The Couples Place Website
The Couples Place site is a meeting place for people, both married and unmarried, who are thoughtful about committed couple relationships and wish to make their own a vital and growing success.

Topics for Today Virtual Love and Cybersex: How Far Should You Go on the Internet?

www.socio.demon.co.uk/magazine/magazine.html
www.cyberlaw.com

Chapter 16
Health Action Guide
Determining Your Cycle
InfoLink:

Health Action Guide
Discussing Birth Control with Your Partner
InfoLink: www.arhp.org/success

Successful Contraception
This site provides an interactive program to help you choose the birth control method that's right for you. Complete a questionnaire to get a profile of birth control options that appear best suited for you, based on your medical history and your lifestyle. There are many different kinds of birth control methods or contraceptives. No one contraceptive is right for every person and this is why it is important to find out what fits your body and needs. Even if you are not currently having sex, it is always a good idea to think ahead about birth control. It is important to discuss information you find on this and any other related website with your doctor or other health-care provider. This website is intended for informational purposes only.

Health Action Guide
Maximizing the Effective of Condoms
InfoLink: www.plannedparenthood.org/BIRTH-CONTROL/condom.htm

Planned Parenthood
A wide range of topics dealing with condoms is covered at this site. Especially useful are the many links to resources for users interested in learning about such topics, how to use condoms, putting on a condom, taking off a condom, benefits of condom use, disadvantages of the condom, side effects of condoms, and HIV-risk comparisons.

Topics for Today Childless by Choice: New Options for Women and Couples

Single Parents Association Voluntary Childlessness Research Among U.S. Women
An excellent academic study of recent trends in voluntary childlessness, this site has links to demographic and sta-

tistical information of great value for the person researching the topic. The site includes graphs and tables.

www.cpc.unc.edu/pubs/paa_papers/1995/abma.html

Childless by Choice
Childless by Choice is a national network for people without children that provides support, humor, and social commentary for people who have chosen not to raise children. The quarterly newsletter gives practical tips and humorous insights into the childless lifestyle. Articles discuss the social, environmental, political, and personal aspects of remaining child-free. Go to this site to read some of these articles.

www.globalideasbank.org/BI/BI-4.HTML

Chapter 17
Health Action Guide
Fathers-to-Be Need Understanding
InfoLink: www.noah.cuny.edu/pregnancy/march_of_dimes/ pre_preg.plan/dadbroch.html

A Guide for Expectant Fathers Website
You've just found out that you're going to be a father. It's an exciting but confusing time. How do you deal with all the different emotions you feel? The suggestions listed on this site will help you deal with these feelings and prepare for fatherhood.

Health Action Guide
Dealing with Your Emotions During Pregnancy and After Giving Birth
InfoLink: www.childbirth.org

Childbirth Website
The Childbirth website is dedicated to educating consumers about the best possible care that is essential to a healthy pregnancy. You will learn a tremendous amount from the many links related to information and education.

Health Action Guide
Guidelines for Successful Breastfeeding
InfoLink: www.lalecheleague.org

La Leche League International Website
La Leche League International is an international, nonprofit, nonsectarian organization dedicated to providing education, information, support, and encouragement to women who want to breastfeed. This site provides many links to breastfeeding.

Topics for Today Supertwins: The Boom in Multiple Births

Mothers of Supertwins
Mothers of Supertwins (MOST) is an international nonprofit support network of families with triplets and more. MOST provides information, resources, empathy, and good humor during pregnancy, infancy, toddlerhood, and school age. Go to this site to learn more.

www.mostonline.org

National Organization of Mothers of Twins Clubs, Inc.

The National Organization of Mothers of Twins Clubs (NOMOTC) was organized in 1960 primarily for the purpose of educating the parents, researchers, educators, and general public about the special aspects of child development for children of multiple birth and their families. Visit this site to learn about some of the membership benefits.

www.nomotc.org

Chapter 18

Health Action Guide

Choosing a Physician

InfoLink: www.coolware.com/health/medical_reporter/choosing.html

How to Choose and Get Maximum Milage from Your Primary Care Doctor

This well-written page not only clarifies for the user the right questions to ask to determine who your primary care physician should be but it also goes into detail on suggestions for building and maintaining a good relationship with the doctor.

Health Action Guide

Choosing a Hospital

InfoLink: www.healthscope.org/hs/choos_ho/ index.htm

HealthScope: Choosing a Hospital

Excellent links to important resources, such as health services, hospitals, and health plans, complements the materials that clearly guide the user through the complexities of hospital choice. The site links as well to important related topics, such as types of hospitals and choosing a nursing home.

Health Action Guide

Choosing the Best Alternative Practitioner for You

InfoLink: http://altmed.od.nih.gov

Alternative Practitioners and Medicine

This subsite of the National Institutes of Health provides an interface program to explore resources and information for consumers on selecting alternative medical practitioners.

Health Action Guide

Selecting a Health Insurance Policy

InfoLink: www.hiaa.org

Health Insurance Association of America

The vision of HIAA is a society of healthy individuals and communities. They have articulated goals to meet this vision for the country. Visit their website to learn more about these goals and other issues related to health insurance.

Health Action Guide

Recognizing Quackery

InfoLink: www.quackwatch.com

Quackwatch

What is quackery? How does it harm us? Tips for avoiding quackery, recognizing questionable products and services, and many other topics are covered in depth at this premier site, which includes helpful links to related information.

Topics for Today Separating Fact from Fiction: Using Health Information on the Internet

Health on the Net

Health on the Net, an international initiative, is a nonprofit organization, headquartered in Geneva, Switzerland. The Foundation is dedicated to realizing the benefits of the Internet and related technologies in the fields of medicine and health care. The purpose of the Foundation is to advance the development and application of new information technologies, notably in the fields of health and medicine. Visit their site to find out what this organization considers to be valid and reliable health-related worldwide websites.

www.hon.ch

Tips on Evaluating Web Resources

With the number of health-related websites growing daily, identifying web resources that provide accurate, reliable medical information is more difficult. This site provides some tips to help you develop your own evaluation criteria.

www.nnlm.nlm.nih.gov/gmr/publish/eval.html

Chapter 19

Health Action Guide

InfoLink:

Topics for Today Xeriscaping: Caring for Your Corner of the World

In Harmony

Though commercially oriented, this site is good for links to useful related topics, such as the benefits of organic landscaping. This site uses visuals well to illustrate techniques and results.

www.inharmony.com

Natural Resources Defense Council

The Natural Resources Defense Council's purpose is to safeguard the earth, its people, its plants and animals, and the natural systems on which all life depends. The Natural Resources Defense Council has many links to a wealth of information on the environment and its conservation.

www.nrdc.org

Chapter 20

Health Action Guide

Preventing Workplace Violence

InfoLink: http://noworkviolence.com/

Workplace Violence Research Institute

The Workplace Violence Research Institute (WVRI) is a full-service provider in workplace violence prevention programs: Consulting, Training, Incident Prevention, Crisis Response, and Program Maintenance. The WVRI is comprised of acknowledged experts in this specialized field and able to bring unique expertise to the business community, industry, and public agencies. Visit this site to learn more about preventing workplace violence.

Health Action Guide
Rape Prevention Guidelines
InfoLink: www.cs.utk.edu/~bartley/index/prevention

"Friends" Raping Friends— Could It Happen to You?
An outstanding site for research and resource, this page, a link from the Sexual Assault Information Page, covers in great depth the topic of how date rape occurs, what warning signs to watch for, and strategies to avoid date rape.

Health Action Guide
Help for the Rape Survivor
InfoLink: www.feminist.org

Feminist Internet Gateway
A vast range of well-indexed resources for rape victims is available and directly linked to this site. In addition, it includes related topics, such as resources for men, government papers, and general information pages.

Health Action Guide
Avoiding Date Rape
InfoLink: www.lia.org/daterape.htm

Avoiding Date Rape
This website provides very valuable information on healthy and unhealthy relationships, statistics related to date rape, and, most important, preventive steps to reduce your risk of date rape.

Health Action Guide
Protecting Your Eyes
InfoLink: www.elvex.com

Eye Safety Equipment Website
This site shows a fine line of high-performance safety products made by Elvex. This company specializes in face protection, eye protection, and laser eye protection products. The company's mission is to develop the most functional, effective, and user-acceptable safety products for the markets that we serve. Visit this website to see the latest in eye protection.

Health Action Guide
Making Your Home Safe, Comfortable, and Secure
InfoLink: www.parentzone.com/parents/homesafty/index.htm

ParentZone: Home Safety Website
The ParentZone site Home Safety section has many excellent articles on babyproofing the kitchen, bathroom, and nursery, bike safety, and more. Check out this site to discover ways to make your home safer for you and your family.

Topics for Today Rage on the Road: The Danger of Aggressive Driving

Traffic Safety Information
A series of articles on road rage and its effects and signs appears as a link at this comprehensive driving safety site. Articles address various factors of aggressive and violent driving, while the home page itself has links to related topics.

www.drivers.com

Promoting Awareness of Community Traffic Safety
The goal of this traffic program is to promote transportation safety in the Commonwealth of Virginia by evaluating transportation safety activities, identifying problems, developing safety programs, coordinating and facilitating action, thereby achieving effective, integrated transportation safety programs in partnership with individuals, local, state, and national organizations. This site includes many links related to aggressive driving.

www.safety.gmu.edu

Chapter 21
Health Action Guide
Helping the Bereaved
InfoLink: http://bereavement.org

The Bereavement Education Center
With special sections on teen grief and many links to resources for the bereaved, this is a great site for research on the topic of grief and bereavement.

Health Action Guide
Organ Donation
InfoLink: www.asf.org

American Share Foundation
This is the home of the Internet's largest transplant and organ donation related site, and it contains all the essential facts the user needs to know, including links to many related topics.

Topics for Today No Time to Say Goodbye: Dealing with Accidental or Violent Death

National Center for Injury Prevention and Control
The Injury Mortality Data available on this CDC website provide tabulations of the total numbers of deaths and the death rates per 100,000 population for major and other selected external causes of death from injury, by race, sex, and age groupings. National data on injury mortality are from 1979 through 1996 and will allow you to assess short-term trends in numbers of deaths and death rates due to injuries. This data provides us with a slice of reality regarding one of the most common death occurrences in the United States today.

www.cdc.gov/ncipc/ncipchm.htm

American Association of Suicidology
The American Association of Suicidology is a nonprofit organization dedicated to the understanding and prevention of suicide. The website includes some excellent information for survivors of suicide.

www.suicidology.org

A

abortion induced premature termination of a pregnancy.

absorption passage of nutrients or alcohol through the walls of the stomach or intestinal tract into the bloodstream.

abuse any use of a legal or an illicit drug that is detrimental to health.

acid-base balance acidity-alkalinity of body fluids.

acid rain rain that has a lower pH (more acidic) than that normally associated with rain.

ACOAs (Adult Children of Alcoholics) grown children who were raised in a family with one or more alcoholic parents.

acquaintance rape forced sexual intercourse between individuals who know each other.

acquired immunity (AI) major component of the immune system associated with the formation of antibodies and specialized blood cells that are capable of destroying pathogens.

ACTH adrenocorticotropic hormone.

activity requirement Calories required for daily physical work.

activity theory theory of aging that suggests that the elderly must (and desire to) remain in familiar and/or new areas of involvement.

acupuncture insertion of fine needles into the body to alter electroenergy fields and cure disease.

acute begins abruptly and subsides after a short period.

acute alcohol intoxication potentially fatal elevation of blood alcohol concentration, often resulting from heavy, rapid consumption of large amounts of alcohol.

acute rhinitis the common cold; the sudden onset of nasal inflammation.

adaptive thermogenesis body's response to inadequate or excessive calorie intake by adjusting the basal metabolic rate.

addiction term used interchangeably with physical dependence.

additive effect combined (but not exaggerated) effect produced by the concurrent use of two or more drugs.

adipose tissue tissue comprised of fibrous strands around which specialized cells designed to store liquefied fat are arranged.

adrenal cortex outer cell layers of the adrenal glands; cells of the cortex on stimulation by ACTH, produce corticoids.

adrenal glands paired triangular endocrine glands located at the top of each kidney; site of epinephrine and corticoid production.

adrenaline common name for epinephrine.

adrenocorticotropic hormone (ACTH) hormone produced in the pituitary gland and transmitted to the cortex of the adrenal glands; stimulates production and release of corticoids.

aerobic energy production body's production of energy when the respiratory and circulatory systems are able to process and transport sufficient amounts of oxygen to muscle cells.

affective pertaining to beliefs, values, and predispositions.

agent causal pathogen of a particular disease.

AIDS Acquired Immunodeficiency Syndrome; viral-based destruction of the immune system leading to illness and death from a variety of factors, including opportunistic infections.

alcoholism a primary, chronic disease with genetic, psychosocial, and environmental factors influencing its development and manifestations.

allergens environmental substances to which persons may be hypersensitive; allergens function as antigens.

allopathy system of medical practice in which specific remedies are used to produce effects different from those produced by a disease or injury.

alveoli thin, saclike terminal ends of the airways; the site at which gases are exchanged between the blood and inhaled air.

Alzheimer's disease gradual development of memory loss, confusion, and loss of reasoning; can eventually lead to total intellectual incapacitation, brain degeneration, and death.

amino acids "building blocks" of protein; manufactured by the body or obtained from dietary sources.

amotivational syndrome behavioral patterns characterized by widespread apathy toward productive activities.

anabolic steroids drugs that function like testosterone to produce increases in weight, strength, endurance, and aggressiveness.

anaerobic energy production body's production of energy when needed amounts of oxygen are not readily available.

analgesic drugs drugs that reduce the sensation of pain.

anaphylactic shock life-threatening congestion of the airways resulting from hypersensitivity to a foreign protein.

androgens male sex hormones.

androgyny the blending of both masculine and feminine qualities.

anemia condition reflecting abnormally low levels of hemoglobin.

anesthetics drugs capable of blocking pain sensations.

aneurysm a ballooning or outpouching on a weakened area of an artery.

angina pectoris chest pain that results from impaired blood supply to the heart muscle.

angiogenesis factor chemical messenger released by tumor cells that stimulates the development of additional capillaries into the tumor.

angioplasty surgical insertion of a balloon-tipped catheter into the coronary artery to open areas of narrowing.

anorexia nervosa disorder of emotional origin in which appetite and hunger are suppressed, and marked weight loss occurs.

anovulatory not ovulating; refers to a time period when the ovaries fail to release an ovum.

antagonistic effect effect produced when one drug reduces or offsets the effects of a second drug.

antibodies chemical compounds produced by the immune system to destroy antigens and their toxins.

antigens disease-producing microorganisms or foreign substances that on entering the body trigger an immune response.

aortic valve valve that controls the blood flow into the aorta from the left ventricle of the heart.

arrhythmias irregularities of the heart's normal rhythm or beating pattern.

arteriosclerosis calcification within the artery's wall that makes the vessel less elastic, more brittle, and more susceptible to bursting; hardening of the arteries.

artificial insemination depositing of sperm in the female reproductive tract in an attempt to impregnate; sperm may be those of the partner or of a donor.

artificially acquired immunity (AAI) type of acquired immunity resulting from the body's response to pathogens introduced into the body through immunizations.

asbestos fibrous material found in insulation and many other building materials; asbestosis.

asphyxiation death resulting from lack of oxygen to the brain.

atherosclerosis buildup of plaque on the inner wall of arteries.

attention deficit disorder (ADD) above-normal physical movement; often accompanied by an inability to concentrate on a specified task; also called hyperactivity.

audiologists health-care professionals trained to assess auditory function.

auditory acuity clarity or sharpness at which a particular sound can be heard.

authentic self positive self-identity that underlies the individual's more temporary mood identities; the most basic self-concept.

autoimmune immune response against the cells of a person's own body.

autoimmune disorders a variety of conditions reflecting tissue destruction by the body's own immune system.

autosomes non-sex chromosomes; 44 of the 46 chromosomes in a normal human cell; all chromosomes other than the two sex chromosomes (xx or xy); body chromosomes.

axon portion of a neuron that conducts electrical impulses to the dendrites of adjacent neurons; neurons typically have one axon.

ayurveda traditional Indian medicine based on herbal remedies.

AZT (azidothymidine) the first drug approved for use in the treatment of AIDS, capable of reducing symptoms and possibly extending life expectancy of the HIV-infected person.

B

balanced diet diet featuring food selections from each food group.

ballistic stretching a "bouncing" form of stretching in which a muscle group is lengthened repetitively to produce multiple, quick, forceful stretches.

bariatrician physician who specializes in the study and treatment of obesity.

basal cells foundation cells that underlie the epithelial cells.

basal metabolic rate (BMR) the amount of energy (in Calories) your body requires to maintain basic functions.

behavior modification behavioral therapy designed to change the learned behavior of an individual.

being needs needs associated with actualization and spiritual growth.

benign noncancerous; tumors that do not spread.

bestiality alternate term for zoophilia.

beta blockers drugs that prevent overactivity of the heart, which results in angina pectoris.

bias and hate crimes criminal acts directed at a person or group solely because of a specific characteristic such as race, religion, ethnic background, or political belief.

binge drinking consuming five or more alcoholic drinks during one drinking occasion.

biochemical oxygen demand index of water pollution based on the rate and extent that organic matter uses dissolved oxygen from a sample of water.

biofeedback self-monitoring of physiological processes as they occur within the body.

biological sexuality male and female aspects of sexuality.

biological toxins poisons produced by microorganisms during the course of an infectious disease.

biologically available term used to describe the ability of a particular material to be used by the body.

bipolar disorder clinical condition in which an individual's mood alternates between periods of excitement and depression; manic-depressive state.

birth control all of the procedures that can prevent the birth of a child.

birthing rooms hospital facilities that serve as both a labor and a delivery room.

bisexual a sexual orientation in which there is an attraction to same-sex and opposite-sex partners.

blackout temporary state of amnesia experienced by an alcoholic; an inability to remember events that occur during a period of alcohol use.

blood alcohol concentration (BAC) percentage of alcohol in a measured quantity of blood.

blood analysis chemical analysis of various substances in the blood; helpful in identifying possible disturbances in the body.

bodybuilding sports activity in which the participants train their bodies to reach desired goals of muscular size, symmetry, and proportion.

body fat analysis determination of the percentage of body tissue composed of fat.

body image subjective perception of how one's body appears.

body mass index (BMI) numerical expression of body weight based on height and weight.

bonding important, initial recognition established between the newborn and those adults on whom the newborn will depend.

bradycardia an unusually slow heart rate—less than 60 beats/minute.

brain death the absence of brain wave activity after an initial measurement followed by a second measurement 24 hours later.

brand name specific name assigned to a drug by its manufacturer.

Braxton Hicks contractions false labor contractions; mild and/or irregular spacing.

breakthrough bleeding midcycle uterine bleeding; spotting.

breast augmentation enlarging breasts for cosmetic purposes.

breech position birth position in which the baby's feet or buttocks are presented first.

bulimarexia binge eating followed by purging the body of the food.

bulimia disorder of emotional origin in which binge eating patterns are established; usually accompanied by purging.

C

caffeinism chronic, heavy consumption of caffeine.

calcium channel blockers drugs that prevent arterial spasms; used in the long-term management of angina pectoris.

calendar method form of periodic abstinence in which the variable lengths of a woman's menstrual cycle are used to calculate her fertile period.

calipers device to measure the thickness of a skinfold from which percent body fat can be calculated.

caloric balance caloric input equals caloric output; weight remains constant.

Calories units of heat (energy); specifically, 1 Calorie equals the heat required to raise 1 kilogram of water 1° C.

cannula hollow metal or plastic tube through which materials can be aspirated.

carbohydrates chemical compounds comprising sugar or saccharide units; the body's primary source of energy.

carbon monoxide (CO) gaseous compound that can reduce the ability of red blood cells to carry oxygen.

carcinogen an agent that stimulates the development of cancer.

carcinoma in situ cancer at its site of origin.

cardiac pertaining to the heart.

cardiac muscle specialized, smooth muscle tissue that forms the middle (muscular) layer of the heart wall.

cardiogram a tracing of heart and lung function from a cardiograph machine.

cardiorespiratory endurance ability of the heart, lungs, and blood vessels to process and transport oxygen required by muscle cells so that they can sustain aerobic energy production.

cardiovascular pertaining to the heart (cardio) and blood vessels (vascular).

carjacking a crime that involves a thief's attempt to steal a car while the owner is behind the wheel; carjackings are usually random, unpredictable, and frequently involve handguns.

catabolism metabolic process of breaking down tissue for the purpose of releasing bonding energy.

CAT scan computerized axial tomography; x-ray procedure designed to visualize structures within the body that would not normally be seen through conventional x-ray procedures.

cauterize to apply a small electrical current and permanently close a tube or vessel; to burn.

celibacy the practice of being sexually abstinent.

cell-mediated immunity form of acquired immunity that uses specialized white blood cells to destroy specific antigens that enter the body.

cellular cohesiveness tendency of normal cells to "stick together" rather than to move independently throughout the body.

central nervous system the brain and spinal cord.

cereal germ highly nutritious portions of the cereal grain, often removed during milling.

cerebral cortex outer covering of the brain; site of intellectual functioning.

cerebral hemorrhage bleeding from the cerebral arteries within the brain.

cerebrovascular accident stroke; brain tissue damage resulting from impaired circulation within the blood vessels in the brain.

cerebrovascular occlusions blockages to arteries supplying blood to the cerebral cortex of the brain; strokes.

cervical cap small, thimble-shaped contraceptive device designed to fit over the cervix.

cesarean delivery surgically assisted birth of a fetus through the abdominal wall.

chemical name name used to describe the molecular structure of a drug.

chemoprevention cancer prevention based on the selection of foods whose nutrient composition is thought to protect the body from certain forms of cancer.

child abuse harm that is committed against a child; usually referring to physical abuse, sexual abuse, or child neglect.

chippers a small percentage of smokers who can smoke a few cigarettes on a daily basis without becoming dependent.

chiropractic manipulation of the vertebral column to relieve pressure and cure illness.

chlamydia the most prevalent sexually transmitted disease; caused by a nongonococcal bacterium.

chlorofluorocarbons (CFCs) gaseous compounds that contain chlorine and fluorine.

cholesterol a primary form of fat found in the blood; lipid material manufactured within the body, as well as derived through dietary sources.

chorionic villi fingerlike extensions of the fetal portion of the placenta; these extensions carry fetal blood supply close to the maternal blood supply.

chorionic villi sampling (CVS) microscopic examination of the cells of the chorionic villi; process for identifying genetic defects earlier than can be done with amniocentesis.

chronic develops slowly and persists for a long period.

chronic bronchitis persistent inflammation and infection of the smaller airways within the lungs.

chronic fatigue syndrome (CFS) illness that causes severe exhaustion, fatigue, aches, and depression; mostly affects women in their thirties and forties.

cilia small, hairlike structures that extend from cells that line the air passages.

cirrhosis pathological changes to the liver resulting from chronic, heavy alcohol consumption; a frequent cause of death among heavy alcohol users.

clinical stage stage of an infectious disease at which symptoms are most fully expressed; acute stage.

clitoris small shaft of erectile tissue located in front of the vaginal opening; the female homolog of the male penis.

cochlea small, snail-shaped organ of the inner ear in which the energy of sound is converted into electrical energy for transmission to the brain.

codependence a strong, unconscious attraction to a chemically dependent person; codependent persons may exhibit behaviors that include both denial and enabling.

coenzyme   vitamin-based organic compound that assists a particular enzyme in performing its role in regulating biochemical reactions.

cohabitation   sharing of a residence by two unrelated, unmarried people; living together.

coitus   penile-vaginal intercourse.

coitus interruptus (withdrawal)   a contraceptive practice in which the erect penis is removed from the vagina before ejaculation.

cold turkey   immediate, total discontinuation of use of a drug; associated withdrawal discomfort.

coliform bacteria   intestinal tract bacteria; presence in a water supply suggests contamination by human or animal waste.

collateral circulation   newly developed blood vessels that by-pass an area of blockage; the development of additional blood vessels to more fully supply an area of tissue.

colonoscopy   visual inspection of the entire colon using a fiber optic scope.

colostomy   surgically created opening on the abdominal wall for the elimination of body wastes.

comorbidity   two or more diagnosed chronic health problems that occur at the same time in an individual.

companionate love   friendly affection and deep attachment, based on extensive familiarity with another person.

complex carbohydrates   carbohydrates composed of long molecular chains containing many saccharide units; starches.

compliance   willingness to follow the directions provided by another person.

compulsion   compelling emotional desire to engage in a particular behavior.

condom   latex shield designed to cover the erect penis and retain semen upon ejaculation; "rubber."

conflict-habituated marriage   marriage characterized by unending conflict and disagreement.

confrontation   an approach to convince drug-dependent people to enter treatment.

congestive heart failure   inability of the heart to pump out all the blood that returns to it; can lead to

dangerous fluid accumulations in lungs and soft tissues.

consumer fraud   marketing of unreliable and ineffective services, products, or information under the guise of curing disease or improving health; quackery.

contact inhibition   ability of a tissue, on reaching its mature size, to suppress additional growth.

contraception   any procedure that prevents fertilization.

contraceptive sponge   soft, spongy disk containing a spermicide that is moistened and inserted over the cervical area.

contraindications   factors that make the use of a drug inappropriate or dangerous for a particular person.

cooldown   stretching and walking after exercise.

coronary arteries   vessels that supply oxygenated blood to heart muscle.

coronary artery bypass surgery   surgical procedure designed to improve blood flow to the heart by providing alternate routes for blood to take around points of blockage.

coroner   an elected official empowered to pronounce death and to determine the official cause of a suspicious or violent death.

corpus luteum   cellular remnant of the graafian follicle after the release of an ovum.

corticoids   hormones generated by the adrenal cortex; corticoids influence the body's control of glucose, protein, and fat metabolism.

CPR   cardiopulmonary resuscitation; first aid procedure designed to restore breathing and heart function.

crack   a crystalline form of cocaine that is smoked; has an instantaneous effect and is highly dependence producing.

creativity   innovative ability; insightful capacity to solve problems; ability to move beyond analytical or logical approaches to experiences.

cross-tolerance   transfer of tolerance from one drug to another within the same general category.

crosstraining   use of more than one aerobic activity to achieve cardiovascular fitness.

crowning   first appearance of the fetal head at the vaginal opening.

cruciferous vegetables   vegetables that have flowers with four leaves in the pattern of a cross.

cryobiology   the science of freezing living tissue.

cryonics   an unproven technology in which dead bodies are frozen in hopes of preserving tissues until disease cures are found.

crypts   burial locations generally underneath churches.

crystal methamphetamine   a highly purified, smokable type of methamphetamine in crystalline form; also called "ice" or "crystal meth."

cunnilingus   oral stimulation of the vulva or clitoris.

cyanosis   blueness to the skin and nail beds reflecting incomplete oxygenation of the blood.

cystitis   infection of the urinary bladder.

D

date rape   a form of acquaintance rape that involves forced sexual intercourse by a dating partner.

deficiency needs   survival requirements; needs associated with normal function as a physical being.

degenerative   a generalized breakdown of structure or function of tissue in association with a disease process.

dehydration   abnormal depletion of fluids from the body; severe dehydration can lead to death.

delirium tremens (DTs)   uncontrollable shaking associated with withdrawal from heavy alcohol use.

dementia   loss of cognitive or intellectual function; associated with structural deterioration of the brain.

dendrite   portion of a neuron that receives electrical stimuli from adjacent neurons; neurons typically have several such branches or extensions.

denial   in this case, the failure to acknowledge that alcohol or drug use seriously affects one's life.

dependence   general term that reflects the need to keep consuming a drug for psychological or physical reasons, or both.

depressants   the psychoactive drugs that reduce the function of the central nervous system.

depression   an emotional state characterized by exaggerated feelings of sadness, melancholy, dejection, worthlessness, emptiness, and hopelessness that are inappropriate and out of proportion to reality.

designated driver a person who abstains or carefully limits alcohol consumption to be able to safely transport other people who have been drinking.

designer drugs drugs that chemically resemble drugs on the FDA Schedule I.

desirable weight weight range deemed appropriate for persons of a specific sex, age, and frame size.

devitalized marriage marriage that lacks the vitality or dynamic nature it once possessed.

diagnosis-related groups (DRGs) prospective billing categories established by the federal government for Medicare reimbursements to hospitals for patients' hospitalization.

diaphragm soft, rubber vaginal cup designed to cover the cervix.

diastolic pressure blood pressure against blood vessel walls when the heart relaxes.

dietary cholesterol cholesterol obtained from food sources.

diffusion movement of a substance across a membrane from an area of greater concentration to an area of lesser concentration.

dilation gradual expansion of an opening or passageway.

dilation and curettage (D & C) surgical procedure in which the cervical canal is dilated to allow the uterine wall to be scraped.

dilation and evacuation (D & E) surgical procedure using cervical dilation and vacuum aspiration to remove uterine wall material and fetal parts.

direct (active) euthanasia process of inducing death, often through the injection of a lethal drug.

disaccharides sugars composed of two monosaccharide units; sucrose, lactose, and maltose.

disengagement theory theory of aging that suggests that society slowly withdraws from the elderly and they in turn slowly withdraw from society.

dissonance feeling of uncertainty that occurs when a person believes two equally attractive but opposite ideas.

distillation production of alcohol by the vaporization and condensation of plant material; the process that produces liquor.

distress stress that diminishes the quality of life; commonly associated with disease, illness, and maladaptation.

diuresis the excessive loss of fluid through urination tissue.

double-blind study research protocol in which neither the researcher nor the subject is aware of whether a drug being tested is in an active or placebo version.

doubling mitotic reproductive division undertaken by cells of a particular tissue.

diuretic drugs drugs that aid the body in removing excess fluid.

dose related drug-related response pattern that changes according to the amount of a drug within the body.

drug synergism enhancement of a drug's effect as a result of the presence of additional drugs within the system.

durable power of attorney for health care a legal document that designates who will make health-care decisions for persons unable to do so for themselves.

duration length of time one needs to exercise at the target heart rate to produce the training effect.

dynamic in a state of change; health is dynamic because it can change from day to day.

E

ECG pattern electrocardiograph; an instrument to measure and record the electrical activity within the heart.

echocardiography procedure that uses high-frequency sound waves to visualize the structure and function of the heart.

ectopic pregnancy a pregnancy wherein the fertilized ovum implants at a site other than the uterus, typically in the fallopian tube.

EEG patterns patterns reflecting the type and extent of electrical activity occurring in the cerebral cortex of the brain.

effacement a thinning and pulling back of the cervical opening to allow movement of the fetus from the uterus, into the vagina.

electrical impedence method to test for the percentage of body fat using an electrical current.

electroencephalogram instrument that measures the electrical activity of the brain.

electrolyte balance proper concentration of various minerals within the blood and body fluids.

embolism potentially fatal condition in which a circulating blood clot lodges itself in a smaller vessel.

embryonic stage stage of human development from the second through the eighth week of pregnancy.

emotional health subjective value-oriented responses to changing situations reflected in feelings of joy, anger, compassion, sympathy, and frustration.

empowerment process in which people gain increasing measures of control over their health.

empty calories Calories obtained from foods that lack most other important nutrients.

enabling in this case, the inadvertent support that some people provide to alcohol or drug users.

endocrine system ductless glands that secrete one or more chemical messengers (hormones) into the bloodstream.

endometriosis growth of endometrial tissue into pelvic areas outside the uterus.

endometrium innermost lining of the uterus, broken down and discharged during menstruation.

enriched process of returning to foods some of the nutritional elements (B vitamins and iron) removed during processing.

Environmental Protection Agency (EPA) federal agency charged with the protection of natural resources and the quality of the environment.

environmental tobacco smoke tobacco smoke that is diluted and stays within a common source of air.

enzymes organic substances that control the rate of physiological reactions but are not altered in the process.

epidemic rapid spread of a disease among a large number of individuals within a given area or population.

epinephrine powerful adrenal hormone whose presence in the bloodstream prepares the body for maximal energy production and skeletal muscle response.

episiotomy a surgical procedure to enlarge the vaginal opening before giving birth.

epitaph inscription on a grave marker or monument.

erection the engorgement of erectile tissue with blood; characteristic of the penis, clitoris, nipples, labia minora, and scrotum.

erotic dreams dreams whose content elicits a sexual response.

essential amino acids nine amino acids that can be obtained only from dietary sources.

essential hypertension hypertension (high blood pressure) resulting from chronic widespread constriction of arterioles.

estrogen ovarian hormone that initiates the development of the uterine lining.

eulogy composition or speech that praises someone; often delivered at a funeral or memorial service.

eustress stress that adds a positive, enhancing dimension to the quality of life.

eutrophication enrichment of a body of water with nutrients, which causes overabundant growth of plants.

excitement stage initial arousal stage of the sexual response pattern.

exhibitionism exposure of one's genitals for the purpose of shocking other persons.

exocrine glands glands whose secretions leave through ducts in order to reach their intended sights of action; ducted glands.

expectorants drugs that help bring mucus and phlegm up from the respiratory system.

expressionistic sexuality complete expression of one's personally defined concept of sexuality.

F

faith the purposes and meanings that underlie an individual's hopes and dreams.

fallopian tubes paired tubes that allow passage of ova from the ovaries to the uterus; the oviducts.

false labor conditions that tend to resemble the start of true labor; may include irregular uterine contractions, pressure, and discomfort in the lower abdomen.

false negative in this case, a test result that indicates "no pregnancy" when, in fact, there is a pregnancy.

false positive in this case, a test result that indicates "pregnancy" when, in fact, there is no pregnancy.

fast foods convenience foods; foods featured in a variety of restaurants, including hamburgers, pizza, and tacos.

fast-twitch (FT) fibers type of muscle cells especially suited for anaerobic activities.

fat density percentage of a food's total calories that are derived from fat; above 30% reflects higher fat density.

fat soluble capable of being dissolved in fats or lipids.

fatty acid acid component that in combination with glycerol forms the dietary fat molecule.

FDA Schedule I list comprising drugs that hold a high potential for abuse but have no medical use.

fecundity the ability to produce offspring.

fellatio oral stimulation of the penis.

femininity behavioral expressions traditionally observed in females.

fermentation chemical process whereby plant products are converted into alcohol by the action of yeast on carbohydrates.

fertility ability to reproduce.

fertilization the union of ovum and sperm resulting in a fertilized egg; conception.

fetal alcohol syndrome characteristic birth defects noted in the children of some women who consume alcohol during their pregnancies.

fetal stage stage of human development from the end of the eighth week of gestation until the time of birth.

fetishism choice of a body part or inanimate object as a source of sexual excitement.

fiber cellulose-based plant material that cannot be digested; found in cereal, fruits, and vegetables.

fight-or-flight response the reaction to a stressor by confrontation or avoidance.

fistula a break or opening through the adjoining walls of two organs; example: rectal-vaginal fistula.

flaccid nonerect; the state of erectile tissue when vasocongestion is not occurring.

flashback unpredictable return of a psychedelic trip.

flexibility ability of joints to function through an intended range of motion.

folacin folic acid; a vitamin of the B-complex group; used in the treatment of nutritional anemia; necessary for neural tube closure.

follicle-stimulating hormone (FSH) gonadotrophic hormone required for initial development of ova (in the female) and sperm (in the male).

food additives chemical compounds that are intentionally or unintentionally added to our food supply.

food supplements nutrients taken in addition to those obtained through the diet; includes powdered protein, vitamins, and mineral extracts.

foreplay activities, often involving touching and caressing, that prepare individuals for sexual intercourse.

formaldehyde chemical found in many common building materials and home furnishings.

fraternal twins twins resulting when two separate ova are fertilized by different sperm.

freebase altered form of cocaine that can be smoked.

frequency (1) number of times per week one should exercise to achieve a training effect. (2) rate at which a sound source vibrates, measured in cycles per second.

fructose monosaccharide that provides a source of simple sugar; fruits and berries.

full funeral services all of the professional services provided by funeral directors.

G

gait pattern of walking.

gamete intrafallopian transfer (GIFT) retrieved ovum and partner's sperm are positioned in the fallopian tube for fertilization and subsequent movement into the uterus for implantation.

gaseous phase portion of tobacco smoke containing carbon monoxide and many other physiologically active gaseous compounds.

gateway drugs easily obtained legal or illegal drugs (alcohol, tobacco, marijuana) whose use may precede the use of less common illegal drugs.

gender general term reflecting a biological basis of sexuality; the male gender or the female gender.

gender adoption lengthy process of learning the behaviors that are traditional for one's gender.

gender identification achievement of a personally satisfying interpretation of one's masculinity or femininity.

gender identity recognition of one's gender.

gender preference emotional and intellectual acceptance for the gender that one is.

gender scheme a mental image of the cognitive, affective, and performance characteristics appropriate to a particular gender; a mental picture of being a man or a woman.

general adaptation syndrome sequenced physiological response to the presence of a stressor; the alarm, resistance, and exhaustion stages of the stress response.

generativity midlife developmental task; repaying society for its support through contributions associated with parenting, creativity, and occupation.

gene replacement therapy experimental procedure in which a healthy gene is incorporated into a virus in anticipation that the virus will introduce the gene into a cell containing a faulty version of that gene.

generic name common or nonproprietary name of a drug.

genetic counseling medical counseling regarding the transmission and management of inherited conditions.

genetic predisposition inherited tendency to develop a disease if necessary environmental factors exist.

genital sexuality sexuality that is centered in the recreational use of reproductive structures; the sexuality that encompasses sexual performance and eroticism.

glucose blood sugar; the body's primary source of energy.

goblet cells cells within the epithelial lining of the airways that produce the mucus required for cleaning the airways.

gonads male or female sex glands; testes produce sperm and ovaries produce ova (eggs).

greenhouse effect warming of the earth's surface that is produced when solar heat becomes trapped by layers of carbon dioxide and other gases.

grief the emotional feelings associated with death.

H

habituation term used interchangeably with psychological dependence.

hallucinogens psychoactive drugs capable of producing hallucinations (distortions of reality).

hardiness the capacity to respond to change quickly and effectively.

hashish resins collected from the flowering tops of marijuana plants.

hate crimes see bias crimes.

health maintenance organizations (HMOs) groups that supply prepaid comprehensive health care with an emphasis on prevention.

health promotion movement in which knowledge, practices, and values are transmitted to people for use in lengthening their lives, reducing the incidence of illness, and feeling better.

healthy body weight weight range based on waist and hip measurements and reflecting an acceptable, healthy amount of fat within the central body cavity.

heart catheterization procedure wherein a thin catheter is introduced through an arm or leg artery into the coronary circulation to visualize areas of blockage.

heart-lung machine device that oxygenates and circulates blood during bypass surgery.

hemorrhaging bleeding; often implies profuse bleeding.

herbalism the use of plants and plant parts for the cure and prevention of illness.

herbicides chemical agents used to destroy unwanted plants and weeds.

heterosexual a sexual orientation in which there is an attraction to opposite-sex partners.

high-risk health behaviors behavioral patterns known or expected of contributing to increased chances of illness and premature death.

HIV human immunodeficiency virus.

holistic health a view of health in terms of its physical, emotional, social, intellectual, and spiritual makeup.

homeopathy a form of health care that employs medications containing extremely small amounts of bioactive ingredients.

homicide the intentional killing of one person by another.

homosexual a sexual orientation in which there is an attraction to same-sex partners.

hormone replacement therapy medically administered estrogen to replace estrogen lost as the result of menopause.

hospice care approach to caring for terminally ill patients that maximizes

the quality of life and allows death with dignity.

host negligence a legal term that reflects the failure of a host to provide reasonable care and safety for persons visiting the host's residence or business.

hot flashes temporary feeling of warmth experienced by women during and following menopause; caused by blood vessel dilation.

human chorionic gonadotropin (HCG) gonadotropic hormone that maintains the ovaries' production of progesterone during pregnancy.

human genome the total genetic constitution of the human; every gene on each of the cell's 46 chromosomes.

Human Genome Project an international project in which geneticists are attempting to identify all genes on each chromosome.

human papilloma virus (HPV) sexually transmitted virus, some of which are capable of causing precancerous changes in the cervix; causative agent for genital warts.

humoral immunity form of acquired immunity that uses antibodies to counter specific antigens that enter the body.

hurry sickness excessive time dependence; seen in persons whose lives are geared to rigid schedules and high achievement aspirations.

hydrocephalus condition seen in infants who lack the ability to control cerebral-spinal fluid production, thus resulting in an excess accumulation of fluid within the skull; "water head."

hydrostatic weighing weighing the body while it is submerged in water.

hypercellular obesity form of obesity seen in individuals who possess an abnormally large number of fat cells.

hyperglycemia elevated blood glucose levels; an important indicator of diabetes mellitus.

hyperparathyroidism condition reflecting the overactive production of parathyroid hormone by the parathyroid glands.

hypertonic saline solution salt solution with a concentration higher than that found in human fluids.

hypertropic obesity form of obesity in which fat cells are enlarged, but not excessive in number.

hypervitaminosis excessive accumulation of vitamins within the body; associated with the fat-soluble vitamins.

hypochondriasis neurotic conviction that one is ill or afflicted with a particular disease.

hypoglycemia an abnormally low level of blood glucose; associated with excessive insulin use (diabetes), excess levels of physical activity, or as a clinical condition in its own right.

hypothalamus portion of the midbrain that provides a connection between the cerebral cortex and the pituitary gland.

hypothyroidism condition in which the thyroid gland produces an insufficient amount of its hormone, thyroxin.

hypoxia oxygenation deprivation at the cellular level.

hysterectomy surgical removal of the uterus.

I

identical twins twins resulting when only one ovum is fertilized but divides into two zygotes early in its development.

immune system system of cellular and chemical elements that protect the body from invading pathogens and foreign materials.

immunizations laboratory-prepared pathogens that are introduced into the body for the purpose of stimulating the body's immune system.

incest marriage or coitus (sexual intercourse) between closely related individuals.

incubation stage time required for a pathogen to multiply significantly enough for signs and symptoms to appear.

independent practice association (IPA) a modified HMO in which a group of physicians provide prepaid health care, but not from a central location within an HMO.

indirect (passive) euthanasia process of allowing a person to die by disconnecting life support systems or withholding lifesaving techniques.

indulgence strong emotional desire to engage in a particular behavior solely for one's own enjoyment or benefit.

infatuation an often shallow, intense attraction to another person.

inferior vena cava large vein that returns blood from lower body regions to the right atrium of the heart.

infertility inability of a male to impregnate, or of a female to become pregnant.

inhalants psychoactive drugs that enter the body through inhalation.

inhibitions inner controls that prevent a person's engaging in certain types of behavior.

insoluble fibers that can absorb water from the intestinal tract.

insulin pancreatic hormone required by the body for the effective metabolism of glucose.

insulin-dependent diabetes mellitus (type 1) form of diabetes in which the body can no longer produce insulin.

intensity (1) level of effort put into an activity. (2) strength or loudness of a particular sound, measured in decibels.

intentional injuries injuries that are purposefully committed by a person.

interstitial cells specialized cells within the testicles that on stimulation by ICSH produce the male sex hormone testosterone.

interstitial cell stimulating hormone (ICSH) a gonadotropic hormone of the male required for the production of testosterone.

intimacy any close, mutual verbal or nonverbal behavior within a relationship.

intrauterine device (IUD) small, plastic, medicated or unmedicated device that when inserted in the uterus prevents continued pregnancy.

introspective looking inward to examine one's feelings and beliefs.

in vivo fertilization and embryo transfer (IVF-ET) fertilization in the laboratory of an ovum taken from the woman with subsequent return of the developing embryo into the woman's uterus.

ionizing radiation form of radiation capable of releasing electrons from atoms.

isokinetic exercises muscular strength training exercises that use machines to provide variable resistances throughout the full range of motion.

isometric exercises muscular strength training exercises that use a resistance so great that the resistance object cannot be moved.

J

junk foods foods that contribute little healthful nutrition other than providing additional calories; includes foods that fit the "fats, oils, and sweets" food group.

K

kwashiorkor protein deficiency disease associated with early weaning of children and a diet lacking complete protein.

L

labia majora the larger, more external skinfolds that surround the vaginal opening.

labia minora the smaller skinfolds immediately adjacent to the vaginal opening.

lactating breastfeeding; nursing.

lactator female who is producing breast milk.

lactovegetarian diet vegetarian diet that includes the consumption of milk and dairy products.

laminaria plugs made of seaweed that on exposure to moisture expand and dilate the cervix into which they have been placed.

lead toxicity blood lead level above 25 micrograms/deciliter. (If adopted, the new standard will be 10 micrograms/deciliter.)

legumes peas and beans; plant sources high in the essential amino acids.

lesbianism female homosexuality.

life cycle artificial segmenting of the life span; each segment represents a developmental period.

lightening movement of fetus deeper into the pelvic cavity before the onset of the birth process.

lipogenesis process whereby the body develops (and fills) adipose cells.

lipoprotein proteinlike structure in the bloodstream to which circulating blood fats attach; various lipoprotein profiles are associated with cardiovascular disease.

liposuction vacuum aspiration used to remove fat cells.

living will document confirming a person's desire to be allowed to die peacefully and with a measure of dignity in cases of terminal illness or major injury.

low tar and nicotine brands cigarettes containing 15 mg of tar or less.

lumpectomy the removal of only a breast lump in comparison to the surgical removal of the entire breast.

luteinizing hormone (LH) a gonadotropic hormone of the female required for fullest development and release of ova; ovulating hormone.

Lyme disease bacterial infection transmitted by deer ticks.

M

macrobiotic diet vegetarian diet composed almost entirely of brown rice.

macrocytic anemia form of anemia in which large red blood cells predominate, but in which total red blood cell count is depressed.

macronutrients minerals needed in relatively high amounts.

mainstream smoke the smoke inhaled and then exhaled by a smoker.

maltose disaccharide derived from germinating cereals and lactose (the carbohydrate found in human and animal milk).

mammogram x-ray examination of the breast.

masculinity behavioral expressions traditionally observed in males.

masochism sexual excitement while being injured or humiliated.

mastectomy removal of breast tissue.

mastery when applied to growth within the young adult segment of the life cycle, mastery implies becoming more self-aware, independent, responsible, socially interactive, and capable of intimacy.

masturbation self-stimulation of the genitals.

maternal supportive tissues general term referring to the development of the placenta and other tissues specifically associated with pregnancy.

mausoleum aboveground structure into which caskets can be placed for disposition; frequently resembles a small stone house.

maximum heart rate maximum number of times the heart can beat per minute.

Medicaid noncontributory governmental health insurance for persons receiving other types of public assistance.

Medicare contributory governmental health insurance, primarily for persons 65 years of age or older.

meltdown the overheating and eventual melting of the uranium fuel rods in the core of a nuclear reactor.

memorial service form of funeral service in which the body or casket often is not present.

menarche time of a female's first menstrual period (cycle).

menopause decline and eventual cessation of hormone production by the female reproductive system.

menstrual extraction procedure using vacuum aspiration to remove uterine wall material within 2 weeks following a missed menstrual period.

menstrual phase phase of the menstrual cycle during which the broken-down lining of the uterus (endometrium) is discharged from the body.

menstruate to undergo cyclic buildup and destruction of the uterine wall.

metabolic rate rate or intensity at which the body produces energy.

metastasis spread of cancerous cells from their site of origin to other areas of the body.

micronutrients minerals needed in relatively small amounts.

midlife period between 45 and 65 years of age.

midlife crisis period of emotional upheaval noted among some midlife persons as they struggle with the finality of death and the nature of their past and future accomplishments.

minerals chemical elements that serve as structural elements within body tissue or participate in physiological processes.

minipills low-dose progesterone oral contraceptives.

misuse inappropriate use of legal drugs intended to be medications.

mitral (bicuspid) valve two-cusp valve that regulates blood flow between the left atrium and the left ventricle of the heart.

monogamous paired relationship with one partner.

mononuclear leukocytes large white blood cells that have only one nucleus.

mononucleosis ("mono") viral infection characterized by weakness, fatigue, swollen glands, and low-grade fever.

monosaccharides simple sugars; carbohydrate compounds of one saccharide unit.

monounsaturated fats fats made of compounds in which one hydrogen-bonding position remains to be filled; semisolid at room temperature;

derived primarily from peanut and olive oils.

morning-after pill high-dose combination oral contraceptive sometimes prescribed to terminate a possible pregnancy.

motorized scraper a motor-driven cutter that shaves off plaque deposits from inside artery walls.

mourning culturally defined manner of expressing grief.

mucus clear, sticky material produced by specialized cells within the mucous membranes of the body; mucus traps much of the suspended particulate matter within tobacco smoke.

MRI scan magnetic resonance imaging; an imaging procedure that uses a powerful magnet to generate an image of body tissue.

Müllerian inhibiting substance a hormone produced by the developing testes that helps prevent the development of female reproductive structures.

multifactorial an interplay of many factors.

multiorgasmic capacity potential to have several orgasms within a single period of sexual arousal.

murmur atypical heart sound that suggests a backwashing of blood into a chamber of the heart from which it has just left.

muscular endurance ability of a muscle or muscle group to function over time; supported by the respiratory and circulatory systems.

muscular strength ability to contract skeletal muscles to engage in work; the contractile force that a muscle can exert.

mutagenic capable of promoting genetic alterations in cells.

myelin white, fatty, insulating material that surrounds the axons of many nerve cells.

myocardial infarction heart attack; the death of heart muscle as a result of a blockage in one of the coronary arteries.

myotonia buildup of a neuromuscular tonus.

N

narcolepsy sleep-related disorder in which a person has a recurrent, overwhelming, and uncontrollable desire to sleep.

narcotics opiates; psychoactive drugs derived from the oriental poppy plant; narcotics relieve pain and induce sleep.

naturally acquired immunity (NAI) type of acquired immunity resulting from the body's response to naturally occurring pathogens.

naturopathy an approach to the cure and prevention of illness through the use of "natural" elements such as water, air, sunshine, and human touch.

necrosis cell death.

needle biopsy procedure minor surgical procedure in which a needle is inserted into an anesthetized portion of tissue and a sample of that tissue is removed for microscopic examination.

negative dependence behavior behavior that can not only create psychological dependence but can also harm structure and function.

nerve blockers drugs that can stop the flow of electrical impulses through nerves which have been injected.

neural tube the embryonic forerunner of the brain and spinal cord; failure of the neural tube to close results in a condition called spina bifida.

neuritic plaques characteristic changes to brain tissue found in association with Alzheimer's disease.

neurofibrillary tangles characteristic changes to brain tissue found in association with Alzheimer's disease.

neuromuscular tonus level of nervous tension within the muscle.

neuron nerve cell; the structural unit of the nervous system.

neurotransmitters chemical messengers released by neurons that permit electrical impulses to be transferred from one nerve cell to another.

nicotine physiologically active, dependence-producing drug found in tobacco.

nitroglycerin a blood vessel dilator used by some cardiac patients to relieve angina.

nocturnal emission ejaculation that occurs during sleep; "wet dream."

nodes in this case, the electrical centers found in cardiac muscle.

nomogram graphic means for finding an unknown value.

nonessential amino acids the eleven amino acids the body can make itself.

non-insulin-dependent diabetes mellitus (type 2) form of diabetes in which the body fails to recognize the presence of its own insulin.

nonoxynol-9 a spermicide commonly used with contraceptive devices.

nontraditional students administrative term used by colleges and universities for students who, for whatever reason, are pursuing undergraduate work at an age other than that associated with traditional college years (18–22).

norepinephrine adrenalin-like neurotransmitter produced within the nervous system.

nurse practitioners registered nurses who have taken specialized training in one or more clinical areas and are able to engage in limited diagnosis and treatment of illness.

nutrient density quantity of selected nutrients in 1000 calories of food.

nutrients elements in food that are required for energy, growth, repair, and the regulation of body processes.

O

obesity condition in which a person's excess fat accumulation results in a body weight that exceeds desirable weight by 20% or more.

obituary notice biographical sketch that appears in a newspaper shortly after a person's death.

obsessive-compulsive disorder psychological disorder in which a person engages in a rigidly defined but largely unnecessary behavior in a highly repetitive manner; OCD.

oncogenes genes that are believed to activate the development of cancer.

oogenesis production of ova in a biologically mature female.

oral contraceptive pill pill taken orally, composed of synthetic female hormones that prevent ovulation or implantation; "the pill."

orgasmic platform expanded outer third of the vagina that during the plateau phase of the sexual response grips the penis.

orgasmic stage third stage of the sexual response pattern; the stage during which neuromuscular tension is released.

orthodontics dental specialty that focuses on the proper alignment of the teeth.

osteoarthritis arthritis that develops with age.

osteopathy system of medical practice that combines allopathic principles with specific attention to postural mechanics of the body.

osteoporosis loss of calcium from the bone seen primarily in postmenopausal women.

outercourse sexual behaviors that do not involve intercourse.

ovary female reproductive structure that produces ova and the female gonadal sex hormones estrogen and progesterone.

overload principle principle whereby a person gradually increases the resistance load that must be moved or lifted; also applies to other types of fitness training.

overweight condition in which a person's excess fat accumulation results in a body weight that exceeds desirable weight by 1% to 19%.

ovolactovegetarian diet diet that excludes the use of all meat but does allow the consumption of eggs and dairy products.

ovulation the release of a mature egg from the ovary.

oxidation the burning of fuel within the cells; process that removes alcohol from the bloodstream.

oxygen debt period of time and amount of oxygen needed to reestabish the muscle's ability to engage in aerobic energy production following a period of anaerobic activity.

ozone layer layer of triatomic oxygen that surrounds the Earth and filters much of the sun's radiation before it can reach the Earth's surface.

P

pacemaker sinoatrial or SA node; an area of cells within the heart that controls its electrical activity.

palliative measure taken to reduce pain and discomfort but not to cure a disease.

pandemic spread of a disease process over a wide geographic area.

panic attack mood disorder characterized by sudden unexpected feelings of fear.

Pap smear screening procedure in which cells removed from the cervix are examined for pre-cancerous changes.

paracervical anesthetic anesthetic injected into tissues surrounding the cervical opening.

particulate phase portion of tobacco smoke composed of small suspended particles.

particulate pollutants class of air pollutants composed of small solid particles and liquid droplets.

partner abuse violence committed against a domestic partner.

parturition childbirth.

passionate love state of extreme absorption in another; tenderness, elation, anxiety, sexual desire, and ecstacy.

passive-congenial marriage marriage that primarily supports the outside interests of the partners.

passively acquired immunity (PAI) temporary immunity achieved by providing antibodies to a person exposed to a particular pathogen.

passive smoking inhalation of air that is heavily contaminated with tobacco smoke.

pathogen disease-causing agent.

patient education health education delivered in a hospital or health-care setting.

pedophilia sexual contact with children as a source of sexual excitement.

pelvic inflammatory disease (PID) acute or chronic infections of the peritoneum or lining of the abdominopelvic cavity; associated with a variety of symptoms and a potential cause of sterility; generalized infection of the pelvic cavity that results from the spread of an infection through a woman's reproductive structures.

perineum tissues that comprise the floor of the pelvic cavity.

periodic abstinence birth control methods that rely on a couple's avoidance of intercourse during the ovulatory phase of a woman's menstrual cycle; also called fertility awareness or natural family planning.

periodontal disease destruction to soft tissue and bone that surround the teeth.

peripheral artery disease (PAD) damage resulting from restricted blood flow to the extremities, especially the legs and feet.

peritonitis inflammation of the peritoneum or lining of the abdominopelvic cavity.

personality the distinctive and unique emotional characteristics of a person.

personality deterioration a general term reflecting noticeable changes in a person's familiar personality.

pesticide agent used to destroy pests.

phenol chemical found in tobacco smoke thought to inactivate the cilia lining air passages.

phenylpropanolamine (PPA) active chemical compound found in many over-the-counter diet products.

physical dependence need to continue using a drug to maintain normal body function and to avoid withdrawal illness; also called addiction.

pituitary gland "master gland" of the endocrine system; the wide variety of hormones produced by the pituitary are sent to structures throughout the body.

placebo pills pills that contain no active ingredients.

placenta structure through which oxygen, nutrients, metabolic wastes, and drugs (including alcohol) pass from the bloodstream of the mother into the bloodstream of the developing fetus.

plateau stage second stage of the sexual response pattern; a leveling off of arousal immediately before orgasm.

platelet adhesiveness tendency of platelets to clump together, thus enhancing speed at which the blood clots.

platonic close association between two people that does not include a sexual relationship.

podiatrists specialists who treat a variety of ailments of the feet.

polychlorinated biphenyls (PCBs) class of chlorinated organic compounds similar to the herbicide DDT.

polyneuropathy gradual destruction of nervous system functioning resulting from influence of alcohol on nerves.

polysaccharide complex carbohydrate; a compound of a long chain of glucose units; found primarily in vegetables, fruits, and grains.

polyunsaturated fats fats composed of compounds in which multiple hydrogen-bonding positions remain open; these fats are liquids at room temperature; derived from a variety of vegetable sources.

positive caloric balance caloric intake greater than caloric expenditure.

postpartum period of time after the birth of a baby during which the uterus returns to its prepregnancy size.

potentiated effect phenomenon whereby the use of one drug intensifies the effect of a second drug.

preferred provider organization (PPO) a group of physicians who market their professional services to an insurance company at predetermined fees.

premenstrual syndrome (PMS) a collection of physical and psychological signs and symptoms that recur in the same phase of the menstrual cycle, typically in the week before menstruation begins.

preventive medicine a form of medical care in which risk-factor reduction is undertaken in order to prevent the occurrence of illness.

primary care physician (PCP) the physician who sees a patient on a regular basis, rather than a specialist who sees the patient only for a specific condition or procedure.

primary prevention intervention (such as education) designed to prevent a particular behavioral pattern from ever developing.

private hospitals profit-making hospitals; proprietary hospitals.

problem drinking alcohol use pattern in which a drinker's behavior creates personal difficulties or difficulties for other persons.

procreation reproduction.

prodromal stage stage of an infectious disease process in which only general symptoms appear.

progesterone ovarian hormone that continues the development of the uterine wall that was initiated by estrogen.

progressive resistance exercises muscular strength training exercises that use traditional barbells and dumbbells with fixed resistance.

proliferative phase first half of the menstrual cycle.

promiscuity frequent indiscriminate sexual activity, often involving multiple partners over time.

proof twice the percentage of alcohol by volume in a beverage; 100 proof alcohol is 50% alcohol.

prophylactic mastectomy surgical removal of the healthy breast in order to prevent the development of breast cancer at a later time.

prophylactic oophorectomy surgical removal of the healthy ovaries in order to prevent the development of ovarian cancer at a later time.

prospective pricing system system of establishing in advance the reimbursement rates for health services.

prostaglandin inhibitors drugs that block the production of prostaglandins, thus eliminating the hormonal stimulation of smooth muscles.

prostaglandin intrauterine injection an injection of hormonelike chemicals into the uterine wall that causes uterine muscles to contract and expel fetal contents.

prostaglandins chemical substances that stimulate smooth muscle contractions.

prostate-specific antigen (PSA) test blood test to determine the presence of an immune response to antigens associated with pre-cancerous changes in the prostate.

prosthodontics dental specialty that focuses on the construction and fitting of artificial appliances to replace missing teeth.

proteins compounds composed of chains of amino acids; primary components of muscle and connective tissue.

proto-oncogenes normal regulatory genes that hold the potential of becoming cancer-causing oncogenes.

psychiatrist physician with speciality training in the diagnosis and treatment of psychological disorders.

psychoactive drug any substance capable of altering one's feelings, moods, or perceptions.

psychological dependence need to consume a drug for emotional reasons; also called habituation.

psychological health functional application of psychic traits, such as language, memory, perceptual processes, awareness states, and mind-body interaction.

psychologist non-physician clinician trained in the diagnosis and non-medical management of psychological disorders.

psychosocial sexuality masculine and feminine aspects of sexuality.

psychosomatic disorders physical illness of the body generated by the effects of stress.

puberty achievement of reproductive ability.

public hospitals hospitals operated by governmental agencies and supported by tax dollars.

pulmonary pertaining to the lungs and breathing.

pulmonary emphysema irreversible disease process in which the alveoli are destroyed.

pulmonary valve valve that controls the flow of blood into the pulmonary arteries from the right ventricle of the heart.

purging use of vomiting or laxatives to remove undigested food from the body.

putrefaction decomposition of organic matter.

Q

quackery marketing of unreliable and ineffective services, products, or information under the guise of curing disease or improving health.

R

radiation sickness illness characterized by fatigue, nausea, weight loss, fever, bleeding from mouth and gums, hair loss, and immune deficiencies, resulting from overexposure to ionizing radiation.

radionucleotide imaging a medical imaging procedure in which injected radioactive material allows a gamma ray camera to visually display the structure and function of an organ.

radon gas a naturally occurring radioactive gas released from underground rock formations.

range of motion distance through which a joint can be moved; measured in degrees.

rape an act of violence against another person wherein that person is forced to engage in sexual activities.

rapid eye movement (REM) sleep dream stage of sleep characterized by twitching movements of the eyes beneath the eyelids.

raves all-night dancing parties where electronically mixed music is often combined with video and laser light shows.

rebound effect excessive congestion that results from the overuse of nosedrops and sprays.

recessive inheritance pattern genetic characteristic whose expression requires the inheritance of the trait (recessive gene) from both biological parents.

recovery stage stage of an infectious disease at which the body's immune system has overcome the infectious agent and recovery is under way; convalescence stage.

recycling ability to convert disposable items into reusable materials.

reflexology massage applied to specific areas of the feet in order to treat illness and disease in other areas of the body.

refractory errors abnormal bending of light as it passes.

refractory phase that portion of the male's resolution stage during which sexual arousal cannot occur.

regulatory genes genes within the cell that control cellular replication or doubling.

rehabilitation return of function to a previous level.

relaxation training the use of various techniques to produce a state of relaxation.

remediation development of alternative forms of function to replace those which had been lost or were poorly developed.

repair gene gene intended to repair DNA, the cells' genetic blueprint, following mutational change.

reproductive sexuality sexuality that is centered in the structural, functional, and behavioral aspects of reproduction.

resolution stage fourth stage of the sexual response pattern; the return of the body to a preexcitement state.

retinal hemorrhage uncontrolled bleeding from arteries within the eye's retina.

rheumatic heart disease chronic damage to the heart (especially heart valves) resulting from the streptococcal infection within the heart; a complication associated with rheumatic fever.

rheumatoid arthritis the result of autoimmune deterioration of the joints.

rigor mortis rigidity of the body that occurs after death.

risk factor behavioral pattern or biomedical index (such as blood pressure) associated with a high probability of developing a particular illness.

role of health mission of health within a person's life cycle.

rubella German (or 3-day) measles.

rubeola red or common measles.

S

sadism sexual excitement achieved while inflicting injury or humiliation on another person.

sadomasochism combination of sadism and masochism into one sexual activity.

salt sensitive description of people who overreact to the presence of sodium by retaining fluid, and thus experience an increase in blood pressure.

satiety a feeling of no longer being hungry; a diminished desire to eat.

saturated fats fats that are difficult for the body to use; these are fats in solid form at room temperature; primarily animal fats.

sclerotic changes thickening or hardening of tissues.

screenings relatively superficial evaluations designed to identify deviations from normal.

secondary bacterial infection bacterial infection that develops as a consequence of a primary infection.

secondary prevention procedures, such as drug testing, to identify early drug use so that it can be stopped or prevented from becoming more extensive.

secretory cells specialized cells within the breast that will, on stimulation, produce milk.

secular recovery programs recovery programs based on a person's self-reliance and self-determination, and not upon the recognition of a higher power.

sediments fine particles of soil that are washed into a body of water, become suspended, and eventually settle to the bottom.

self-actualization highest level of personality development; self-actualized persons recognize their roles in life and use personal strengths to reach their fullest potential.

self-antigen body cells that lack the surface characteristics needed to prevent destruction by the body's own immune system.

self-care movement trend toward individuals taking increased responsibility for prevention or management of certain health conditions.

self-concept perception or mental picture of oneself.

self-esteem the quality of feeling good about yourself and your abilities; self-acceptance.

semen secretion containing sperm and other nutrients discharged from the male urethra at ejaculation.

semivegetarianism dietary pattern in which a limited amount of lean meat is included in an otherwise vegetarian diet.

sensory modalities vision, hearing, taste, touch, and smell; pathways for stimuli to register within the body.

serum lipid analysis analysis of fat substances in the bloodstream; includes cholesterol and triglyceride measurements.

set point genetically programmed range of body weight.

seven dimensions of health major areas of health in which specific strengths or limitations will be found: physical, emotional, social, intellectual, spiritual, occupational, and environmental.

sex chromosomes two of the cell's 46 chromosomes that in combination impact maleness (xy) or femaleness (xx).

sex flush reddish skin response that results from increasing sexual arousal.

sex reassignment operation surgical procedure designed to remove the external genitalia and replace them with genitalia appropriate to the opposite sex.

sexual fantasies fantasies with sexual themes; sexual daydreams or imaginary events.

sexual harassment unwanted attention of a sexual nature that creates embarrassment or stress.

sexuality the quality of being sexual; can be viewed from many biological and psychosocial perspectives.

sexual orientation the sex to which one is attracted.

sexual victimization sexual abuse of children, family members, or subordinates by a person in a position of power.

sexually transmitted diseases (STDs) infectious diseases that are spread primarily through intimate sexual contact.

shaft body of the penis.

shingles viral infection affecting the nerve endings of the skin.

shock profound collapse of many vital body functions; evident during acute alcohol intoxication and other serious health emergencies.

sidestream smoke the smoke that comes from the burning end of a cigarette, pipe, or cigar.

singlehood the state of not being married.

skinfold measurement measurement to determine the thickness of the fat layer that lies immediately beneath the skin.

sleep apnea a condition in which abnormalities in the structure of the airways lead to periods of greatly restricted air flow during sleeping, resulting in reduced levels of blood oxygen and placing greater strain on the heart to maintain adequate tissue oxygenation.

sliding scale method of payment by which patient fees are scaled according to income levels.

slow-twitch (ST) fibers type of muscle cell specially suited for aerobic activities.

slow wave (SW) sleep stage of sleep characterized by minimal dream activity.

smegma cellular discharge that can accumulate beneath the clitoral hood and the foreskin of an uncircumcized penis.

smog air pollution composed of a combination of smoke, photochemical compounds, and fog.

smokeless tobacco tobacco products (chewing tobacco and snuff) that are chewed or sucked rather than smoked.

snuff finely shredded smokeless tobacco; used for dipping.

sodomy penile-anal intercourse.

soluble fiber that turns to a gel within the intestinal tract and then binds to liver bile that has cholesterol attached; may be valuable in lowering blood cholesterol levels.

sonogram images of internal structures produced by high-frequency sound waves; also called ultrasound and ultrasonography.

specificity training concept that fitness components can be increased for very specific tasks or functions.

spermatogenesis process of sperm production.

spermicides chemicals capable of killing sperm.

stalking a crime involving an assailant's planned efforts to pursue an intended victim.

starch   complex carbohydrate; a polysaccharide; a compound of long-chain glucose units.

static stretching   the slow lengthening of a muscle group to an extended level of stretch; followed by holding the extended position for a recommended time period.

sterilization   generally permanent birth control techniques that surgically disrupt the normal passage of ova or sperm.

stewardship   acceptance of responsibility for the wise use and protection of the earth's natural resources.

stillborn   baby that is dead at the time of birth.

stimulants   psychoactive drugs that stimulate the function of the central nervous system.

stress   physiological and psychological state of disruption caused by the presence of an unanticipated, disruptive, or stimulating event.

stressors   factors or events, real or imagined, that elicit a response of stress.

stress test   examination and analysis of heart-lung function while the body is undergoing physical exercise; generally accomplished when the client walks or runs on a treadmill device while being monitored by a cardiograph.

subcutaneous fat   fat layer immediately beneath the skin.

subdermal implants   contraceptive devices that consist of surgically implanted rods containing synthetic progesterone.

sucrose   a disaccharide; table sugar.

sudden cardiac death   immediate death resulting from a sudden change in the rhythm of the heart.

superfund $12 billion fund to be used in cleaning-up selected toxic waste sites; EPA controlled.

superior vena cava   body's largest vein; the vessel that brings blood from the upper body regions back to the right atrium of the heart.

suppressor gene   gene intended to monitor cell regulatory activity and stop faulty regulatory activity.

surrogate parenting   one of several arrangements in which a woman becomes pregnant and gives birth for an infertile couple.

sustainable environment   an environment capable of supporting habitation; made possible by the efforts of individuals, organizations, and all levels of government.

sympto-thermal method   method of periodic abstinence that combines the basal body temperature method and the cervical mucus method.

synapse   location at which an electrical impulse from one neuron is transmitted to an adjacent neuron; synaptic junction.

synergistic drug effect   heightened, exaggerated effect produced by the concurrent use of two or more drugs.

synesthesia   perceptual process in which a stimulus produces a response from a different sensory modality.

systemic   throughout the body.

systolic pressure   blood pressure against blood vessel walls when the heart contracts.

T

tachycardia   above normal heart rate; "racing" heart rate.

tar   particulate phase of tobacco smoke with nicotine and water removed.

target heart rate (THR)   number of times per minute that the heart must contract to produce a training effect.

teaching hospital   hospital in which preprofessional students and graduates receive clinical experience.

telecommuting   utilization of computerized equipment in order to work from home.

temperament   personality traits that may be genetically conditioned, such as shyness and aggressiveness.

teratogenic   capable of producing birth defects.

tertiary prevention   prevention of continued drug use through incarceration or drug rehabilitation program participation.

testes   male reproductive structures that produce sperm and the sex hormone testosterone.

testosterone   male sex hormone that stimulates tissue development.

thermic effect   the energy the body requires for the digestion, absorption, and transportation of food.

thorax   the chest; portion of the torso above the diaphragm and within the rib cage.

thrombi   stationary blood clots.

titration   a particular level of a drug within the body.

tolerance   an acquired reaction to a drug; continued intake of the same dose has diminishing effects.

total marriage   marriage in which the needs and goals of each partner are assigned a lower priority for the good of the partnership.

total person   holistic view of the person, incorporating the dynamic interplay of physical, emotional, social, intellectual, spiritual, and occupational factors.

toxic shock syndrome   potentially fatal condition resulting from the proliferation of certain bacteria in the vagina, which enter the general blood circulation.

trace elements   minerals whose presence in the body occurs in very small amounts; micronutrient elements.

training effect   significant positive effect that exercise has on the heart, lungs, and blood vessels.

transcenders   self-actualized people who have achieved a quality of being ordinarily associated with higher levels of spiritual growth.

transcervical balloon tuboplasty   the use of inflatable balloon catheters to open blocked fallopian tubes; a procedure used for some women with fertility problems.

transient ischemic attack (TIA)   strokelike symptoms caused by temporary spasm of cerebral blood vessels.

transition   the third and last phase of the first stage of labor; full dilation of the cervix.

transsexualism   the profound rejection of the gender to which the individual has been born.

transvestism   recurrent, persistent cross-dressing as a source of sexual excitement.

tricuspid valve   three-cusp (leaf) valve that regulates blood flow between the right atrium and the right ventricle of the heart.

triglycerides   fats made up of glycerol units, each having three fatty acid molecules; high blood levels are associated with increased risk of cardiovascular disease.

triphasic pills   oral contraceptives in which the progesterone levels vary every seven days during the cycle while the estrogen levels remain constant.

trimester three-month period of time; human pregnancies encompass three trimesters.

tropical oils oils extracted from coconut, palm, and palm kernel that contain much higher levels of saturated fat than other vegetable oils.

tubal ligation sterilization procedure in which the fallopian tubes are cut and the ends tied back or cauterized.

tumescence state of being swollen or enlarged.

tumor mass of cells; may be cancerous (malignant) or noncancerous (benign).

twelve steps programs recovery programs based on the twelve steps to recovery used by Alcoholics Anonymous.

type I alcoholism inherited predisposition supported by environmental factors favoring alcoholism.

type II alcoholism male-limited alcoholism; an inherited form of alcoholism passed from father to son.

U

ultralow tar and nicotine brands cigarettes containing less than 6 mg of tar.

ultrasound high-frequency sound waves used to create an image of internal body structures or to elevate the internal temperature of cancer cells, thus killing the cells.

unbalanced diet diet lacking adequate representation from each of the food groups.

underweight condition in which body weight is below desirable weight.

unintentional injuries injuries that occur without anyone intending that any harm be done.

unipolar disorder clinical label for depression.

urethra passageway through which urine leaves the urinary bladder.

urethritis infection of the urethra.

uterine perforation penetration of a foreign object through the uterine wall.

V

vacuum aspiration abortion procedure in which the cervix is dilated and vacuum pressure is used to remove the uterine contents.

vaginal contraceptive film (VCF) spermicide-impregnated film that clings to the cervical opening.

variant different from the statistical average.

vas deferens (pl. vasa deferentia) passageway through which sperm move from the epididymis to the ejaculatory duct.

vascular system body's blood vessels; arteries, arterioles, capillaries, venules, and veins.

vasectomy surgical procedure in which the vasa deferentia are cut to prevent the passage of sperm from the testicles; the most common form of male sterilization.

vasocongestion retention of blood within a particular tissue.

vasodilators drugs that relax muscles in the walls of blood vessels (especially the arterioles); these drugs allow blood vessels to dilate (widen).

vegan vegetarian diet vegetarian diet that excludes the use of all animal products, including eggs and dairy products.

vegetarian diet relies on plant sources for nutrients needed by the body.

vicariously formed stimuli erotic stimuli that originate in one's imagination.

virulent capable of causing disease.

vital marriage marriage in which the needs and goals of the individual, as well as the needs of the marital union, are given top priority.

vitamins organic compounds that facilitate the action of enzymes.

voluntary hospitals nonprofit hospitals operated by a variety of organizations, including religious orders and fraternal groups.

voyeurism watching others undressing or engaging in sexual activities.

vulval tissues tissues surrounding the vaginal opening.

W

waist-to-hip ratio (WHR) see *healthy body weight.*

wake an established time for people to view the body of a dead person; the calling hours.

warm-up physical and mental preparation for exercise.

water soluble capable of being dissolved in water.

wellness a broadly based term used to describe a highly developed level of health.

wellness centers units within hospitals or clinics that provide a wide range of rehabilitation, disease prevention, and health enhancement programs.

whole-grain flour flour made from grain that has received only minimal processing (milling); flour containing many nutrients lost in more highly processed flour.

will legal document that describes how a person wishes his or her estate to be disposed of after death.

willed death a death in which a person gives up the desire to live and merely waits to die.

withdrawal illness uncomfortable, perhaps toxic response of the body as it attempts to maintain homeostasis in the absence of a drug; also called abstinence syndrome.

work movement of mass over distance.

Y

yeast single-cell plant responsible for the fermentation of plant products.

young adult years segment of the life cycle from ages 18 to 22; a transitional period between adolescence and adulthood.

yo-yo syndrome the repeated weight loss, followed by weight gain, experienced by many dieters.

Z

zero tolerance laws laws that severely restrict the right to drive for underage drinkers who have been convicted of driving under *any* influence of alcohol.

zoophilia sexual contact with animals as a preferred source of sexual excitement; bestiality.

Exam Prep

Chapter 1   Shaping Your Health

Multiple Choice

_____ 1. What health strategy involves following specific eating plans or exercise programs?
A. Health screenings
B. Education activities
C. Behavior change
D. Regimentation

_____ 2. Why is it necessary to formulate an initial adult identity?
A. So you can answer the question, "Who am I?"
B. To have a productive and satisfying life
C. To help you move through other stages of development
D. All of the above

_____ 3. Which developmental task involves using your own resources to follow a particular path?
A. Forming an initial adult identity
B. Assuming responsibility
C. Establishing independence
D. Developing social skills

_____ 4. Which of the following statements is false?
A. The deeper the emotional relationships a person has, the better.
B. Maintaining and improving your health is an important responsibility.
C. The need to interact socially will at times negatively influence your health.
D. Developing social skills can help you gain independence from your family.

_____ 5. What is _generativity?_
A. The process of generating wealth and status in midlife
B. The process of repaying society for its past support
C. The negative attitude one generation holds for another
D. None of the above

_____ 6. Which of the following are tasks for older adulthood?
A. Accepting the physical decline of aging
B. Maintaining high levels of physical function
C. Establishing a sense of integrity
D. All of the above

_____ 7. Which of the following is _not_ a dimension of health?
A. Transitional dimension of health
B. Emotional dimension of health
C. Holistic dimension of health
D. Both A and C

_____ 8. Which dimension of health do some professionals believe to be at the "core of wellness"?
A. Emotional
B. Spiritual
C. Social
D. Intellectual

_____ 9. Why is the occupational dimension of health important?
A. Because you won't be happy unless you make a lot of money after graduation
B. Because both external and internal rewards from work affect your happiness
C. Because when people feel good about their work, they are more likely to live a healthier lifestyle
D. Both B and C

_____ 10. Which of the following is a strategy for changing your behavior?
A. Make a personal contract to accomplish your goals.
B. Go it alone; it is better not to involve family or friends.
C. Don't reward yourself until you reach the final outcome.
D. Don't let any obstacles occur or you will fail.

_____ 11. Holistic health encompasses not only physical, social, and mental aspects, but also two additional components:
A. Genetic and educational
B. Metaphysical and sensory
C. Reproductive and financial
D. Intellectual and spiritual

_____ 12. All of the following are developmental tasks of young adulthood except
A. obtaining employment.
B. building wealth.
C. establishing independence.
D. forming an initial adult identity.

_____ 13. All of the following are developmental tasks of midlife adults except
A. repaying society for its support.
B. reassessing the goals of young adulthood.
C. pursuing pleasure rather than career goals.
D. coming to terms with the inevitability of death.

_____ 14. The leading cause of death in the United States is
A. AIDS.
B. homicide.
C. lung cancer.
D. major cardiovascular disease.

_____ 15. The developmental tasks of elderly adults include
A. establishing a sense of integrity.
B. maintaining a high level of physical functioning.
C. accepting the decline of aging.
D. all of the above.

Critical Thinking

1. What is health?

2. What does the term *wellness* mean?

3. How does *empowerment* affect overall health and well-being?

4. Which dimension of your health would you like to improve, and why?

5. How do you plan to successfully complete your developmental tasks?

Chapter 2   Achieving Psychological Wellness

Multiple Choice

_____ 1. Emotionally well people
A. experience the full range of human emotions but are not overcome by them.
B. are concerned only with their own well-being.
C. set goals far and above what they can realistically accomplish.
D. trust only those who have proven their worth.

_____ 2. What factors are capable of shaping self-esteem?
A. Warm and supportive physical contact
B. Religious indoctrination leading to guilt
C. Failure to be successful in early undertakings
D. All of the above

_____ 3. What three traits show a person's _hardiness_?
A. Success, direction, and ability
B. Commitment, control, and challenge
C. Commitment, self-control, and self-esteem
D. None of the above

_____ 4. Which of the following statements _most_ accurately describes adults in midlife?
A. Most experience a period of yearning for their youth called a _midlife crisis_.
B. Most experience a multitude of problems that fill them with melancholy and despair.
C. Most have less to think about than when they were younger.
D. Most see themselves as being in the prime of life.

_____ 5. Which of the following factors affects the quality of life of older adults?
A. Sexual intimacy
B. Marital status
C. Economic status
D. All of the above

_____ 6. What type of depression may occur after the death of a spouse or some other period of difficulty?
A. Primary depression
B. Reactive depression
C. Chemically induced depression
D. None of the above

_____ 7. Which is the _most_ mature form of conflict resolution?
A. Dialogue
B. Submission
C. Persuasion
D. Aggression

_____ 8. What is the first step toward taking a proactive approach to life?
A. Undertaking new experiences
B. Taking risks
C. Constructing mental pictures
D. None of the above

_____ 9. Which of the following are motivational needs defined by Maslow?
A. Physiological needs
B. Economic needs
C. Sexual needs
D. Material needs

_____ 10. Which of the following statements describes creative individuals?
A. They are intuitive and open to new experiences.
B. They are less interested in detail than in meaning and implications.
C. They are flexible.
D. All of the above describe them.

_____ 11. All of the following are positive steps in improving self-esteem except
A. setting and reaching realistic goals.
B. recognizing and correcting faults in others.
C. maintaining satisfying group relationships.
D. forming and maintaining a relationship with a mentor.

_____ 12. According to Maslow, transcenders have all of the following qualities except they
A. tend to accumulate substantial wealth and power.
B. have more peak or creative experiences.
C. are innovators who are attracted to mystery and the unknown.
D. tend to accept others with an unconditional positive regard.

_____ 13. _Anxiety_ is defined as
A. fear related to a specific task.
B. jealousy in response to successes of others.
C. unfocused worry or excessive concern.
D. a physical reaction to a personal failure.

_____ 14. A depression that occurs suddenly, within a two-week period, without an apparent external cause, is called
A. reactive depression.
B. dysthymic depression.
C. primary depression.
D. secondary depression.

_____ 15. Panic attacks can include all of the following symptoms except
A. rapid heart rate and chest pain.
B. feelings of increased focus and control.
C. choking and shortness of breath.
D. feelings of numbness and depersonalization.

Critical Thinking

1. What is meant by a "normal range of emotions"?

2. What are some ways to overcome feelings of loneliness and shyness?

3. What are the warning signs of suicide, and how should they be treated?

4. What is the four-step process that allows one to control the outcomes of experiences and learn about one's emotional resources?

5. How do faith and spirituality affect emotional well-being?

Chapter 3   Coping with Stress

Multiple Choice

_____ 1. An event that produces stress is called a
   A. response.
   B. stressor.
   C. type B factor.
   D. none of the above.

_____ 2. Positive stress is called
   A. eustress.
   B. distress.
   C. type R stress.
   D. none of the above.

_____ 3. Which of the following is _not_ a stage in Selye's general adaptation syndrome model?
   A. Alarm reaction stage
   B. Relaxation stage
   C. Resistance stage
   D. Exhaustion stage

_____ 4. Which part of the body is responsible for the interconnection between the nervous system and the endocrine system?
   A. Hypothalamus
   B. Pituitary gland
   C. Adrenal gland
   D. None of the above

_____ 5. When the body perceives stress, several responses are produced by the epinephrine (adrenaline) and corticoids that are released. Which of the following is an expected response?
   A. Decreased cardiac and pulmonary function
   B. Increased digestive activity
   C. Decreased fat use
   D. Altered immune system response

_____ 6. PMR, or progressive muscular relaxation, is
   A. a procedure of alternately contracting and relaxing muscle groups.
   B. a correct way of breathing, by relaxing the diaphragm.
   C. an Eastern relaxation technique that employs a mantra.
   D. a form of self-hypnosis that costs $250 to $400 to learn.

_____ 7. Which of the following diseases have some origin in unresolved stress?
   A. Irritable bowel syndrome
   B. Allergies
   C. Asthma
   D. All of the above

_____ 8. Which of the following personality traits fosters high levels of stress?
   A. Self-confidence and practicality
   B. Anger and cynicism
   C. Both A and B
   D. Neither A nor B

_____ 9. Stress is best described as
   A. something completely beyond your control.
   B. the leading cause of cynicism.
   C. a physical and emotional response to change.
   D. a realistic and positive outlook on life.

_____ 10. What body systems play the principal role in preparing the body to respond to stressors?
   A. Circulatory system and lymphatic system
   B. Nervous system and endocrine system
   C. Muscular system and nervous system
   D. Circulatory system and nervous system

_____ 11. When epinephrine is released by the adrenal glands, all of the following reactions can be expected except
   A. increased metabolic rate.
   B. decreased salivation.
   C. increased appetite.
   D. increased sweating.

_____ 12. All of the following are stress-management techniques except
   A. biomass.
   B. relaxation response.
   C. progressive muscular relaxation.
   D. self-hypnosis.

_____ 13. The following attitude can help one develop a realistic approach to life and stress:
   A. Do not trust anyone.
   B. Move away from negative thought patterns.
   C. Expect the worst.
   D. Limit the number of relationships you maintain.

_____ 14. The _metabolic rate_ is defined as the
   A. rate at which the body produces energy.
   B. heart rate.
   C. number of respirations per minute.
   D. rate at which the brain produces alpha waves.

Critical Thinking

1. What is stress? Give an example of a stressful situation and how the person might feel.

2. Can stress be positive? Give an example.

3. What physiological reactions does stress cause in the body?

4. How can repeated stress, if not dealt with properly, affect long-term health?

5. What are some healthy ways to deal with stress? Which would you choose to adopt, and why?

Chapter 4   Staying Physically Fit

Multiple Choice

_____ 1. Which of the following is *not* a benefit of physical fitness?
   A. The person can engage in various tasks and leisure activities.
   B. Body systems function efficiently to resist disease.
   C. Body systems are healthy enough to respond to emergency (threatening) situations.
   D. All of the above are benefits.

_____ 2. Which of the following areas of physical fitness do exercise physiologists say is *most* important?
   A. Muscular strength
   B. Muscular endurance
   C. Cardiorespiratory endurance
   D. Flexibility

_____ 3. Anaerobic, or oxygen-deprived, energy production is the result of
   A. low-intensity activity.
   B. short-duration activities that quickly cause muscle fatigue.
   C. activities such as walking, distance jogging, and bicycle touring.
   D. none of the above.

_____ 4. Which of the following types of training exercises are based on the *overload principle*?
   A. Isometric exercises
   B. Progressive resistance exercises
   C. Isokinetic exercises
   D. All of the above

_____ 5. Of the following statements, which accurately describes flexibility?
   A. It is relatively the same throughout your body.
   B. Not every joint in your body is equally flexible.
   C. Nothing alters the flexibility of a particular joint.
   D. Gender and age do not affect flexibility.

_____ 6. Which of the following statements is *true* about aging?
   A. Aging is predictable and the same for every person.
   B. The greatest change is in areas of the simplest function.
   C. Change often occurs suddenly and without warning.
   D. Two people of the same age may experience deterioration of different body systems.

_____ 7. The American College of Sports Medicine recommends five significant areas to emphasize in improving cardiorespiratory fitness. Which of these is *not* one of the areas?
   A. Mode of activity
   B. Frequency of training
   C. Intensity of training
   D. Popularity of training

_____ 8. What is target heart rate (THR)?
   A. An intensity level of 60% to 90% of maximum heart rate
   B. An intensity level of 70% to 100% of maximum heart rate
   C. The maximum number of times your heart should contract each minute to give your respiratory system a conditioning affect
   D. The rate at which you become so fatigued that you must stop exercising

_____ 9. What are the three basic parts of a good training session?
   A. Running, weight lifting, stretching
   B. Warm-up, workout, cooldown
   C. Warm-up, stretching, cooldown
   D. Mental warm-up, socialize, workout

_____ 10. Which of these is an abnormal warning sign during or after exercise?
   A. A delay of more than one hour in your body's return to a fully relaxed, comfortable state after exercise
   B. Difficulty sleeping
   C. Noticeable breathing difficulties or chest pains
   D. All of the above

_____ 11. Osteoporosis is found primarily in which of the following groups?
   A. World-class female athletes
   B. Malnourished babies
   C. Late middle-aged women
   D. Adolescent boys

_____ 12. Which of the following is *not* an activity that will improve cardiovascular fitness?
   A. Rollerblading
   B. Rowing
   C. Bowling
   D. Brisk walking

_____ 13. The American College of Sports Medicine recommends that you exercise how many times per week?
   A. Every day
   B. Once
   C. Twice
   D. Three to five times

_____ 14. Which of the following is *not* a potential side effect of steroid use?
   A. Aggressive, psychotic episodes
   B. Liver complications
   C. Thinning of the blood
   D. Cancer

_____ 15. Which of the following are some appropriate exercises for pregnant women?
   A. Walking, weight lifting, running
   B. Rollerblading, ice skating, hiking
   C. Golf, bowling, fishing
   D. Swimming, yoga, tai chi

Critical Thinking

1. What are the components of a well-designed fitness program for adults?

2. How serious is low back pain, and what should a person do to alleviate or prevent it?

3. Explain what steps you would take to develop a cardiorespiratory fitness program, incorporating all five areas recommended by the American College of Sports Medicine.

4. Describe some of the newest trends in physical activity (such as rollerblading, water exercise, or "street jam"). Which most appeals to you, and why?

5. Why is steroid use dangerous?

Chapter 5   Understanding Nutrition and Your Diet

Multiple Choice

_____ 1. What three nutrients provide the body with calories (energy)?
   A. Sugar, amino acids, and supplements
   B. Carbohydrates, fats, and proteins
   C. Tropical oils, food additives, and carbohydrates
   D. None of the above

_____ 2. Which of the following statements accurately describes carbohydrates?
   A. They occur in two forms only, depending on the number of proteins that make up the molecule.
   B. About 20% of our calories come from carbohydrates.
   C. Carbohydrates are combinations of sugar units, or saccharides.
   D. Each gram of carbohydrate contains 400 calories.

_____ 3. Which of the following statements is *false*?
   A. Fats are important nutrients in our diets.
   B. Fats make it impossible for our bodies to absorb vitamins A, D, E, and K.
   C. Fat insulates our bodies, helping us retain heat.
   D. Most of the fat we eat is "hidden" in food.

_____ 4. What are vitamins?
   A. Inorganic materials necessary for tissue repair and disease prevention
   B. Pills that can be taken each morning to give the body energy all day
   C. Organic compounds that are required in small amounts for normal growth, reproduction, and maintenance of health
   D. Nutrients that provide more than half our body weight

_____ 5. Which of the following nutrients could the body not live without for more than a week?
   A. Minerals   C. Vitamins
   B. Fiber   D. Water

_____ 6. Which of the following is a recommendation based on the USDA Food Guide Pyramid?
   A. Adults should eat two to four servings from the fruit group each day.
   B. Three to five servings from the vegetable group each day are recommended for an adult.
   C. Adults should consume two to three servings from the milk, yogurt, and cheese group each day.
   D. All of the above are recommendations.

_____ 7. What are phytochemicals?
   A. Physiologically active components that function as antioxidants and may deactivate carcinogens
   B. The additives used in foods that preserve freshness or improve flavor, color, or texture

   C. The chemicals used to enrich breads and cereals
   D. None of the above

_____ 8. What kind of vegetarian eats milk products but not eggs?
   A. Ovolactovegetarian
   B. Macrobiotic vegetarian
   C. Lactovegetarian
   D. Vegan vegetarian

_____ 9. What factors may influence nutritional changes as a person ages?
   A. Changes to the structure and function of the body resulting from age
   B. The progressive lowering of the body's basal metabolism
   C. Both A and B
   D. Neither A nor B

_____ 10. Which of the following is a suggested step toward increasing the worldwide availability of food?
   A. Increase the yield of land under cultivation.
   B. Increase the amount of land under cultivation.
   C. Use water more efficiently for the production of food.
   D. All of the above are suggested.

_____ 11. Which types of oils tend to be higher in the more healthy polyunsaturated fats?
   A. Safflower oil, sunflower oil, and corn oil
   B. Coconut oil, palm oil, and palm kernel oil
   C. Animal-based fats
   D. Hydrogenated vegetable oils

_____ 12. High-cholesterol foods include all of the following except
   A. shellfish.   C. peanut butter.
   B. whole milk.   D. animal fat.

_____ 13. Which of the following statements about minerals is *false*?
   A. Minerals are inorganic materials that make up about 5% of the body.
   B. Minerals function primarily as structural compounds.
   C. The body can synthesize some minerals through exposure to the sun.
   D. Minerals can be classified into major minerals and minor minerals.

_____ 14. All of the following are sources of dietary fiber except
   A. cereals.   C. vegetables.
   B. fruits.   D. dairy products.

_____ 15. A large group of food-based physiologically active compounds thought to be able to deactivate carcinogens are known as
   A. soluble fibers.   C. free radicals.
   B. metabolites.   D. phytochemicals.

Critical Thinking

1. Based on your assessment of your current diet, are you getting all the nutrients you need? In which areas do you need to improve?

2. What role does cholesterol play in the diet?

3. Explain the difference between *water-soluble* and *fat-soluble* vitamins and the characteristics of each.

4. Would you consider becoming a vegetarian? Why or why not?

5. What is *nutrient density?* Why is it important to consider this concept when making food choices?

Chapter 6   Maintaining a Healthy Weight

Multiple Choice

_____ 1. Which weight-measurement technique precisely measures relative amounts of fat and lean body mass by comparing underwater weight with out-of-water weight?
A. Skinfold measurements
B. Body mass index (BMI)
C. Electrical impedance
D. Hydrostatic weighing

_____ 2. Which may be the simplest method of determining a person's amount of body fat?
A. Appearance
B. Height-weight tables
C. Body mass index (BMI)
D. Waist-to-hip ratio

_____ 3. What influences obesity?
A. Environment
B. Genetics
C. Both environment and genetics
D. None of the above

_____ 4. Which area(s) within the hypothalamus tell the body when it should begin and end food consumption?
A. Feeding and satiety centers
B. Central nervous system (CNS)
C. Thyroid and pituitary glands
D. None of the above

_____ 5. Which of the following statements describes "brown fat"?
A. It is located in small amounts in the upper back between the shoulder blades.
B. There is renewed interest in the study of it.
C. It burns calories as heat incorporating them into compounds that are stored in fat cells.
D. All of the above describe it.

_____ 6. Which of Sheldon's three body types is characterized by a tall, slender build?
A. Ectomorph
B. Mesomorph
C. Endomorph
D. None of the above

_____ 7. What is hypercellular obesity?
A. The increase of fat cells as a result of being overfed in infancy or substantially gaining weight in childhood or adolescence
B. A condition in which fat cells increase in size as a result of long-term positive caloric balance in adulthood
C. Excessive fat around the waist, which can contribute to the onset of diabetes mellitus
D. None of the above

_____ 8. What would most experts cite as the *most* important reason for the widespread problem of obesity?
A. Family dietary practices
B. Endocrine influence
C. Infant feeding patterns
D. Inactivity

_____ 9. What is the basal metabolic rate (BMR)?
A. The rate of caloric intake to caloric output
B. The minimum amount of energy the body requires to carry on all vital functions
C. The rate of a food's thermic output
D. None of the above

_____ 10. Which weight-management technique involves the use of pharmaceuticals?
A. Balanced diets supported by portion control
B. Fad diets
C. Hunger/satiety-influencing products
D. Self-help weight-reduction programs

_____ 11. At what point is overweightness considered to be obesity?
A. 10% above ideal or desirable weight.
B. 20% above ideal or desirable weight.
C. 30% above ideal or desirable weight.
D. 40% above ideal or desirable weight.

_____ 12. Recent estimates indicate that the following proportion of people are obese in the United States:
A. One-tenth
B. One-fifth
C. One-quarter
D. One-third

_____ 13. Which type of fat accumulation is associated with the development of more serious health problems?
A. High cellulose accumulation
B. Central body cavity obesity
C. Thigh and hip fat accumulation
D. Lower body obesity

_____ 14. All of the following are methods of determining obesity except
A. body mass index.
B. body profile matching.
C. electrical impedance.
D. appearance.

_____ 15. All of the following are effective methods of weight control except
A. fad diets.
B. self-help weight-reduction programs.
C. balanced diet supported by portion control.
D. controlled fasting.

Critical Thinking

1. What factors influence your body image and self-concept?

2. What steps might you take to successfully control your weight throughout your lifetime?

3. Why is dieting alone not a good technique for achieving and maintaining weight loss?

4. Why is it said that, "If you don't want to develop an eating disorder, don't diet?" How should a person be treated for anorexia and bulimia?

5. What does it mean to exercise or eat compulsively?

Chapter 7   Living Drug-Free

Multiple Choice

_____ 1. Which of these is an aspect of addictive behavior?
A. Denial
B. Compulsion
C. Loss of control
D. All of the above

_____ 2. What kind of drugs alter the user's feelings, behaviors, or moods?
A. Antioxidants
B. Over-the-counter drugs
C. Psychoactive drugs
D. Steroids

_____ 3. Which type of dependence creates _full_ withdrawal symptoms when the drug use is stopped?
A. Psychological
B. Physical
C. Cross-tolerant
D. None of the above

_____ 4. What are neurotransmitters?
A. Chemical messengers that transmit electrical impulses
B. Proteins that carry the chemicals in drugs directly to the brain
C. Hallucinogenic drugs that are currently popular with college students
D. None of the above

_____ 5. How do psychotrophic drugs "work"?
A. By blocking the production of a neurotransmitter
B. By forcing the continued release of a neurotransmitter
C. Either A or B
D. Neither A nor B

_____ 6. Which type of psychoactive drug _excites_ the activity of the central nervous system (CNS)?
A. Inhalants
B. Hallucinogens
C. Narcotics
D. None of the above

_____ 7. What is "crack"?
A. Powdered cocaine that is alkalized in benzene or ether and smoked through a water pipe
B. A small, rocklike crystalline material made from cocaine hydrochloride and baking soda
C. A white powder that is snorted in "lines" through a rolled dollar bill or tube
D. A pure form of methamphetamine that looks like rock candy

_____ 8. What type of psychoactive drug _slows down_ the function of the central nervous system (CNS)?
A. Inhalants
B. Hallucinogens
C. Cannabis
D. Depressants

_____ 9. What is THC?
A. A hallucinogen derived from the peyote cactus plant
B. A drug popular in the 1960s
C. The active ingredient in marijuana
D. A new "designer" drug

_____ 10. Which drugs are among the most dependence-producing?
A. Inhalants
B. Hallucinogens
C. Depressants
D. Narcotics

_____ 11. What is "primary prevention" as it applies to drug use?
A. Preventing drug production before the drugs can be grown or synthesized
B. Preventing drug use before it begins
C. Preventing drugs from entering the United States
D. Preventing recovering drug users from having a relapse

_____ 12. Those living with a person who has a drug problem may themselves become
A. addicted to the drug.
B. immune to the problem.
C. stronger.
D. codependent.

_____ 13. A person can be said to be addicted when
A. body cells have become reliant on the drug.
B. the individual craves the drug.
C. the person suffers a drug overdose.
D. the person neglects the necessities of daily living.

_____ 14. All of the following are stimulants except
A. caffeine.
B. amphetamines.
C. mescaline.
D. cocaine.

_____ 15. All of the following are hallucinogens except
A. phencyclidine.
B. psilocybin.
C. peyote.
D. LSD.

Critical Thinking

1. What is the difference between drug *misuse* and drug *abuse?*

2. How has cocaine use affected poor urban areas?

3. What are possible long-term effects of marijuana use?

4. What is a synergistic effect, and why is it dangerous?

5. What do you think about the legalization of drugs and about drug testing?

Chapter 8   Using Alcohol Responsibly

Multiple Choice

_____ 1. What is binge drinking?
   A. The practice of drinking and then purging
   B. A harmless activity popular among college students
   C. The practice of consuming five or more drinks in a row, at least once in the previous two-week period
   D. The practice of consuming two drinks in a row, at least once a day

_____ 2. What is the alcohol content of a bottle of 140-proof gin?
   A. 140% alcohol per fluid ounce
   B. 70% alcohol per fluid ounce
   C. 14% alcohol per fluid ounce
   D. 1.4% alcohol per fluid ounce

_____ 3. What type of drug is alcohol?
   A. Stimulant
   B. Hallucinogen
   C. Depressant
   D. Narcotic

_____ 4. What should be done with people who become unconscious as a result of alcohol consumption?
   A. They should be given a cold shower to wake them up.
   B. They should be made to drink coffee.
   C. They should be taken to bed and left undisturbed for several hours.
   D. They should be placed on their side and monitored frequently.

_____ 5. Which of the following leading causes of accidental death has connections to alcohol use?
   A. Motor vehicle collisions
   B. Falls
   C. Drownings
   D. All of the above

_____ 6. Which of the following is a good guideline to follow for responsibly hosting a party?
   A. Make alcohol the primary entertainment, especially with a keg or other popular way to serve alcohol.
   B. Ridicule those who are afraid to drink.
   C. If friends say they are just fine to drive home even though they have been drinking, let them go.
   D. None of the above are good guidelines.

_____ 7. Which of the following groups does not promote responsible party hosting?
   A. AA
   B. MADD
   C. BACCHUS
   D. SADD

_____ 8. What is the main difference between problem drinking and alcoholism?
   A. Problem drinkers stay away from hard liquor.
   B. Alcoholic drinkers usually don't engage in binge drinking.
   C. Alcoholism involves a physical addiction to alcohol.
   D. Problem drinking is easier to detect.

_____ 9. Which support group appeals to the children of alcoholics?
   A. Al-Anon
   B. Antabuse
   C. Alateen
   D. MADD

_____ 10. Which new drug, approved by the FDA in 1995, is being used to treat alcoholism?
   A. Naltrexone
   B. Antabuse
   C. Heroin
   D. Maltodextrine

_____ 11. Which of the following does not affect the absorption of alcohol from the stomach?
   A. Use of birth control pills
   B. Presence of food
   C. Gender
   D. Quality of the liquor

_____ 12. The likelihood of being involved in a fatal collision is how many times higher for a drunk (0.10% BAC) driver?
   A. 1.5 times higher
   B. Twice as high
   C. Eight times as high

_____ 13. Alcoholism can dramatically affect which member(s) of the alcoholic's family?
   A. Spouse
   B. Children
   C. Parents
   D. All of the above

_____ 14. Which of the following is a common trait of adult children of alcoholics?
   A. Have difficulty identifying normal behavior
   B. Tend to be able to drink alcohol without being affected by it
   C. Have difficulty with intimate relationships
   D. A and C

_____ 15. Alcohol use is reported in what percentage of homicides?
   A. 15%
   B. 40%
   C. 67%
   D. 90%

Critical Thinking

1. In spite of their similarities to alcoholic beverages, why do non-alcoholic beverages fail to sell as well?

2. What physiological differences in women make them more susceptible to the effects of alcohol?

3. What are the possible effects of drinking alcohol while pregnant?

4. What role does alcohol use play in violent crime, family violence, and suicide?

5. Explain *denial, enabling,* and *codependence* as they occur with alcoholism.

Chapter 9   Rejecting Tobacco Use

Multiple Choice

_____ 1. Which factor *most* affects a person's decision to smoke?
   A. Gender
   B. Age
   C. Education
   D. Race

_____ 2. What are psychosocial factors of tobacco dependence?
   A. Manipulation
   B. Advertising
   C. Modeling
   D. Both A and C

_____ 3. On which consumer group is the FDA focusing its education efforts to discourage initial tobacco use?
   A. Women
   B. African-American men who attend predominately black universities
   C. Teens
   D. Older adults who began smoking before health risks were known

_____ 4. Which phase of tobacco use includes nicotine, water, and a variety of powerful chemical compounds known collectively as *tar*?
   A. Active phase
   B. Particulate phase
   C. Gaseous phase
   D. Nicotine phase

_____ 5. What signals the beginning of lung cancer?
   A. Changes in the basal cell layer resulting from constant irritation by the tar accumulating in the airways
   B. An inability to breathe normally
   C. A "smoker's cough"
   D. Mucus swept up to the throat by cilia, where it is swallowed and removed through the digestive system

_____ 6. What is COLD?
   A. Chronic obstructive lung disease
   B. A chronic disease in which air flow in and out of the lungs becomes progressively limited
   C. A disease state made up of chronic bronchitis and pulmonary emphysema
   D. All of the above

_____ 7. Which of the following statements is *false*?
   A. Women who smoke are strongly urged not to use oral contraceptives.
   B. Chewing tobacco and snuff generate blood levels of nicotine in amounts equivalent to those seen in cigarette smokers.
   C. Contrary to some claims, secondhand smoke is not a serious health threat.
   D. Children of parents who smoke are twice as likely to develop bronchitis or pneumonia during the first year of life.

_____ 8. Which of the following statements is *true*?
   A. Chewing tobacco is a safe alternative to smoking.
   B. Sidestream smoke makes up only 15% of our exposure to involuntary smoking.
   C. Spouses of smokers may have a 30% greater risk of lung cancer.
   D. The only effective way to quit smoking is to go "cold turkey."

_____ 9. Which is more effective as a means of quitting smoking?
   A. Nicotine-containing chewing gum
   B. Transdermal patch
   C. Neither A nor B
   D. A and B are equally effective

_____ 10. What is the main debate concerning smoking today?
   A. The validity of health warnings
   B. The rights of the nonsmoker vs. the rights of the smoker
   C. The rights of young adults to buy cigarettes
   D. None of the above

_____ 11. Dependence on tobacco is more easily established than dependence on
   A. alcohol.
   B. heroin.
   C. cocaine.
   D. all of the above.

_____ 12. What percentage of adult smokers have tried at least once to quit smoking?
   A. 25%
   B. 55%
   C. 70%
   D. 80%

_____ 13. The most damaging component found in the gaseous phase of tobacco smoke is
   A. carbon monoxide.
   B. ammonia.
   C. acetone.
   D. acetaldehyde.

_____ 14. A two-pack-a-day smoker can expect to die how much earlier than a nonsmoker?
   A. 2 to 4 years
   B. 5 to 6 years
   C. 7 to 8 years
   D. Cannot be estimated

_____ 15. Which of the following statement(s) about smoking and pregnancy is (are) *true*?
   A. The fetus of a mother who smokes is exposed to carbon monoxide and nicotine.
   B. Children born to mothers who smoked during pregnancy have lower birth weights.
   C. The fetus of a smoking mother is more likely to be stillborn, miscarried, or born prematurely.
   D. All of the above are true.

Critical Thinking

1. What advertising tactics do tobacco companies use to offset the potential decline in sales resulting from reports of health risks?

2. In what ways is tobacco addictive?

3. How does smoking adversely affect health?

4. Why should a pregnant or breastfeeding woman refrain from smoking?

5. Do you think smoking should continue to be banned from public places? Why or why not?

Chapter 10   Reducing Your Risk of Cardiovascular Disease

Multiple Choice

_____ 1. Why has the rate of death caused by cardiovascular disease declined?
   A. Changing lifestyles in the United States
   B. Medical advances in diagnosis and treatment
   C. A breakthrough new drug
   D. Both A and B

_____ 2. What is the nation's number-one "killer"?
   A. AIDS
   B. Lung disease
   C. Cancer
   D. Cardiovascular disease

_____ 3. Which of the following is a function of the blood?
   A. Regulation of the water content of body cells and fluids
   B. Transportation of nutrients, oxygen, wastes, and hormones
   C. Buffering to help maintain appropriate pH balance
   D. All of the above

_____ 4. Which of the following are three cardiovascular risk factors that cannot be changed?
   A. Age, gender, body composition
   B. Heredity, weight, glandular production
   C. Age, heredity, metabolism
   D. None of the above

_____ 5. Which of the following is a risk factor that can be changed?
   A. Cigarette/tobacco use
   B. Physical inactivity
   C. High blood pressure
   D. All of the above

_____ 6. Which disease predisposes people to developing heart disease?
   A. Cancer
   B. Epilepsy
   C. Diabetes
   D. Multiple sclerosis

_____ 7. Which form of cardiovascular disease involves damage to the vessels that supply blood to the heart muscle?
   A. Hypertension
   B. Stroke
   C. Coronary heart disease
   D. Congenital heart disease

_____ 8. What is cholesterol?
   A. The oil used to fry food
   B. A soft, fatlike material manufactured by the body
   C. A material necessary for production of blood
   D. None of the above

_____ 9. What is hypertension?
   A. A consistently elevated blood pressure
   B. Stress on arterial walls resulting from plaque buildup
   C. The tendency of blood to clot
   D. Abnormally low blood pressure

_____ 10. What is the name of the cardiovascular disease that begins as a streptococcal infection of the throat?
   A. Peripheral artery disease
   B. Rheumatic heart disease
   C. Phlebitis
   D. Congestive heart failure

_____ 11. What is one of the ways women differ from men in their symptoms of a heart attack?
   A. Women often experience more shortness of breath and nausea.
   B. Women often experience abdominal pain and fatigue with chest pain.
   C. Women are more likely to recognize their symptoms as a heart attack.
   D. Women are more likely to experience dizziness and intense thirst.

_____ 12. What is the heart attack risk of smokers compared with that of nonsmokers?
   A. Smokers have about the same risk of heart attack.
   B. Smokers have a slightly elevated risk of heart attack.
   C. Smokers have more than twice the risk of heart attack.
   D. None of the above describe the risk.

_____ 13. Which of the following is _not_ a risk resulting from obesity?
   A. Increased risk of cirrhosis of the liver
   B. Increased risk of heart disease
   C. Increased risk of stroke
   D. Increased risk of developing diabetes

_____ 14. What is one of the beneficial effects of estrogen that may be lost at menopause, leading physicians to prescribe estrogen-replacement therapy?
   A. Estrogen can help women maintain a beneficial profile of blood fats.
   B. Estrogen can strengthen the heart muscle, giving women a higher cardiovascular fitness level.
   C. A high level of estrogen can reduce the craving for nicotine in women who smoke.
   D. Estrogen can help women build more lean muscle mass.

_____ 15. The average adult has how much blood circulating in his or her circulatory system?
   A. 8 pints
   B. 12 pints
   C. 2 quarts
   D. 6 quarts

Critical Thinking

1. What components make up the cardiovascular system? How does the system work?

2. Do you exhibit any risk factors for cardiovascular disease? What steps can you take to change them, if they can be changed?

3. What is the difference between HDLs and LDLs?

4. How can hypertension be prevented?

5. What are the different causes of stroke?

Chapter 11   Living with Cancer

Multiple Choice

_____ 1. What happens to cells that leads to cancer?
   A. Their appearance may change.
   B. Their level of self-regulation is diminished.
   C. Neither A nor B.
   D. Both A and B.

_____ 2. What are proto-oncogenes?
   A. Genes that repair damaged cells
   B. Genes that suppress the immune system
   C. Genes that have the potential to become cancerous
   D. Abnormal genes

_____ 3. What is the Human Genome Project?
   A. The testing of new cancer-fighting drugs
   B. A scientific study of genes
   C. A secret military project that exposed World War II troops to carcinogens
   D. The study of cancer-producing viruses

_____ 4. Which type of cancer is found in the blood and blood-forming tissues?
   A. Lymphoma
   B. Neuroblastoma
   C. Carcinoma
   D. Leukemia

_____ 5. In women, what is the most common site in the body for the development of cancer?
   A. Breast
   B. Uterus
   C. Lung
   D. Skin

_____ 6. Which test greatly improves the chances of preventing cervical cancer?
   A. Mammography
   B. MRI
   C. Pap test
   D. Biopsy

_____ 7. Which type of cancer is referred to as the "silent" cancer because of its vague symptoms?
   A. Ovarian
   B. Prostate
   C. Vaginal
   D. Lung

_____ 8. Which traditional method of cancer treatment has had many successful advances in recent years?
   A. Surgery
   B. Chiropractic manipulation
   C. Chemotherapy
   D. Radiation

_____ 9. Cancer cells can produce an enzyme that blocks the cellular biological clock that informs normal cells that it is time to die. This enzyme is
   A. telomerase.
   B. dismutase.
   C. deaminase.
   D. glucosidase.

_____ 10. A cancer found most often in people who have had extensive sun exposure, particularly a deep, penetrating sunburn, is
   A. adenocarcinoma.
   B. sarcoma.
   C. neuroblastoma.
   D. basal cell carcinoma.

_____ 11. The most important step you can take to prevent lung cancer is to
   A. eat a healthy diet.
   B. avoid unnecessary radiation.
   C. exercise regularly.
   D. quit smoking and avoid environmental smoke.

_____ 12. Risk factors for cervical cancer include all of the following except
   A. history of infertility.
   B. early age at first intercourse.
   C. cigarette smoking.
   D. family history of breast cancer.

_____ 13. How many men currently die each year of prostate cancer in the United States?
   A. About 2,000
   B. About 14,000
   C. About 42,000
   D. About 120,000

_____ 14. You can reduce your risk of skin cancer by
   A. using a sunscreen with an SPF of 15 or greater.
   B. wearing a hat to protect your face.
   C. limiting outdoor activities from 11 A.M. to 2 P.M.
   D. doing all of the above.

_____ 15. An alternative cancer treatment that seeks to balance the flow of active and passive energy in the body is
   A. acupuncture.
   B. homeopathy.
   C. ayurveda.
   D. naturopathy.

Critical Thinking

1. What social and environmental factors contribute to the onset of cancer?

2. What steps can women take to prevent cancer or to detect the early stages of cancer?

3. What steps can men take to prevent cancer or to detect the early stages of cancer?

4. What are the seven warning signs of cancer?

5. What do you know about alternative forms of cancer therapy? Would you consider any of these for yourself?

Chapter 12   Managing Chronic Conditions

Multiple Choice

_____ 1. A condition found in males in which one Y chromosome is combined with two X chromosomes is called
  A. Down syndrome.
  B. SIADH.
  C. Klinefelter's syndrome.
  D. Reye's syndrome.

_____ 2. Tay-Sachs disease is caused by
  A. sickling of blood cells, reducing their oxygen-carrying ability.
  B. genetic inability to manufacture an enzyme needed to break down fat.
  C. impaired ability of the pancreas to produce digestive enzymes.
  D. additional chromosome number 21.

_____ 3. Duchenne muscular dystrophy affects primarily
  A. adult males.
  B. adult females.
  C. young male children.
  D. both elderly adult males and females.

_____ 4. Conditions that are present at birth are described as being
  A. congenital.
  B. genetic.
  C. metabolic.
  D. degenerative.

_____ 5. A possible cause of cleft lip and cleft palate is
  A. alcohol use during pregnancy.
  B. smoking during pregnancy.
  C. use of certain medications during pregnancy.
  D. all of the above.

_____ 6. Spina bifida is caused by
  A. incomplete development of the digestive tract.
  B. incomplete closure of the neural tube.
  C. failure of the body to react to thyroid hormone.
  D. failure of the lower leg and foot to develop normally.

_____ 7. A possible factor in developing non-insulin-dependent diabetes mellitus is
  A. obesity.
  B. stress.
  C. genetic predisposition.
  D. all of the above.

_____ 8. Lactose intolerance is caused by
  A. infant malnutrition.
  B. low blood sugar.
  C. low blood insulin levels.
  D. loss of ability to produce the enzyme lactase.

_____ 9. Which chronic disease most often appears in early adulthood and continues intermittently for the next 20 to 25 years?
  A. Diabetes mellitus
  B. Lupus
  C. Multiple sclerosis
  D. Asthma

_____ 10. Which type of asthma is caused by stress or as a consequence of frequent respiratory tract infections?
  A. Extrinsic
  B. Intrinsic
  C. EIA
  D. Childhood-onset asthma

_____ 11. Extrinsic asthma attacks may be triggered by
  A. cigarette smoke.
  B. certain foods or drugs.
  C. exercise.
  D. all of the above.

_____ 12. Parkinson's disease is known as a(n)
  A. autoimmune disorder.
  B. psychosomatic disease.
  C. neurological disorder.
  D. metabolic disorder.

_____ 13. Which of the following possible method(s) of preventing Alzheimer's disease are researchers currently studying?
  A. Use of ibuprofen to reduce inflammation of cells damaged by the disease
  B. Use of hormone-replacement therapy in postmenopausal women
  C. Use of trace-element supplements to reverse cell damage
  D. Both A and B

_____ 14. An abnormal lateral curvature of the spine is called
  A. patent foramen ovale.
  B. spina bifida.
  C. scoliosis.
  D. talipes.

_____ 15. Alzheimer's disease is caused by a gradual loss of the brain's ability to produce
  A. phenylalanine.
  B. lactase.
  C. acetylcholine.
  D. ketone bodies.

Critical Thinking

1. What are the differences and similarities between insulin-dependent and non-insulin-dependent diabetes?

2. Do you know anyone who drank alcohol, smoked, or took illegal drugs while pregnant? What are the possible effects of these practices?

3. Would you be willing to change your diet, exercise habits, and other lifestyle choices to reduce your risk of developing a chronic disease?

4. Has anyone in your family been affected by Alzheimer's disease? If so, how was the disease managed?

5. What are the four categories of chronic disease presented in this chapter? Describe each.

Chapter 13 Preventing Infectious Disease Transmission

Multiple Choice

_____ 1. What is a pathogen?
  A. A disease-causing agent
  B. A virus, bacterium, or fungus
  C. Neither A nor B
  D. Both A and B

_____ 2. What is the function of a reservoir in the chain of infection?
  A. To cause disease
  B. To offer a favorable environment in which an infectious agent can thrive
  C. To act as a portal of exit
  D. To transmit the agent from person to person

_____ 3. Which term describes insects, animals, or birds that carry diseases from human to human?
  A. Vectors
  B. Pathogens
  C. Reservoirs
  D. Agents

_____ 4. During which of the following stages of infection is the infected person _most_ contagious?
  A. Prodromal stage
  B. Clinical stage
  C. Decline stage
  D. Incubation stage

_____ 5. Which type of immunity is the result of vaccination or immunization?
  A. Naturally acquired immunity
  B. Artificially acquired immunity
  C. Passively acquired immunity
  D. None of the above

_____ 6. Which viral infection has mental fatigue and depression as side effects?
  A. Influenza
  B. Common cold
  C. Mononucleosis
  D. Mumps

_____ 7. What is chronic fatigue syndrome (CFS)?
  A. A mononucleosis-like condition most commonly seen in women in their thirties and forties.
  B. A condition that may be linked to neurally mediated hypotension.
  C. A condition that may be a psychological disorder.
  D. All of the above.

_____ 8. How is Lyme disease transmitted?
  A. Through droplet spread
  B. Through fecal-oral spread
  C. Through vector transmission
  D. Through direct transmission

_____ 9. Which sexually transmitted disease occurs as blisterlike lesions on the genitals or lips?
  A. Herpes simplex
  B. Gonorrhea
  C. Syphilis
  D. Human papillomavirus

_____ 10. Of the following STDs, which has no cure?
  A. Vaginal infections
  B. Cystitis and urethritis
  C. Herpes simplex
  D. Gonorrhea

_____ 11. AIDS is caused by which of the following viruses?
  A. HBV
  B. Ebola virus
  C. HIV
  D. Rotavirus

_____ 12. Antibiotics can be effective against
  A. viruses.
  B. bacteria.
  C. both viruses and bacteria.
  D. neither viruses nor bacteria.

_____ 13. A new treatment to slow the progression of AIDS involves the use of
  A. doxycycline.
  B. HIV vaccine.
  C. ampicillin.
  D. protease inhibitors.

_____ 14. Which of the following is caused by an autoimmune attack on healthy cells in one's own body?
  A. Chronic fatigue syndrome
  B. Osteoarthritis
  C. Rheumatoid arthritis
  D. Chickenpox

_____ 15. The smallest pathogen, a nonliving particle of genetic material surrounded by a protein coat, is a
  A. virus.
  B. fungus.
  C. protozoan.
  D. bacterium.

Critical Thinking

1. What are the two main components to the body's protective defense? How do they work?

2. Why do the elderly and people with additional health complications need to take extra precautions to avoid contracting influenza?

3. Why should people, especially college students, pay close attention to their immunization history?

4. What precautions should women take when using tampons to avoid toxic shock syndrome?

5. How is AIDS transmitted, and what precautions can be taken to avoid contracting it?

Chapter 14   Exploring the Origins of Sexuality

Multiple Choice

_____ 1. Which basis for biological sexuality refers to the growing embryo's development of gonads?
  A. Genetic
  B. Gonadal
  C. Structural
  D. None of the above

_____ 2. At which age are typical children able to correctly identify their gender?
  A. 4 years
  B. 2 years
  C. 18 months
  D. 6 months

_____ 3. What part of the testis produces sperm?
  A. Seminiferous tubules
  B. Scrotum
  C. Epididymis
  D. Interstitial cells

_____ 4. Which is the most sensitive part of the female body?
  A. Mons pubis
  B. Vagina
  C. Clitoris
  D. Prepuce

_____ 5. During which phase of the menstrual cycle does ovulation occur?
  A. Menstrual
  B. Proliferative
  C. Secretory
  D. None of the above

_____ 6. Which phase of the sexual response pattern prevents men from having multiple orgasms?
  A. Excitement
  B. Plateau
  C. Orgasmic
  D. Refractory

_____ 7. Why are the testes housed in the scrotum, outside the body?
  A. To reduce the distance the sperm must travel in their attempt to fertilize the egg
  B. To increase the male's sexual responsiveness
  C. To reduce the risk of injury
  D. Because spermatogenesis requires a lower temperature than the body core temperature

_____ 8. The production of sperm cells in boys is influenced by the release of what hormone?
  A. Follicle-stimulating hormone
  B. Interstitial-cell stimulating hormone
  C. Progesterone
  D. Luteinizing hormone

_____ 9. A lack of androgens in older men can result in all of the following except
  A. lack of energy.
  B. osteoporosis.
  C. baldness.
  D. changes in mood.

_____ 10. The lower third of the uterus is called the
  A. vagina.
  B. cervix.
  C. endometrium.
  D. clitoris.

_____ 11. What term describes the blending of traditionally male and female qualities within an individual?
  A. Homosexuality
  B. Bisexuality
  C. Androgyny
  D. Asexuality

_____ 12. How often does a healthy woman typically ovulate in her lifetime?
  A. 11 times a year for 30 years
  B. 12 times a year for 40 years
  C. 13 times a year for 20 years
  D. 13 times a year for 35 years

_____ 13. What is endometriosis?
  A. Condition that typically affects postmenupausal women; characterized by brittle, weak bones.
  B. Condition in which tissue that normally lines the uterus is found growing within the pelvic cavity.
  C. Condition that typically affects women who have delivered multiple babies.
  D. Condition in which a fertilized ovum implants in the fallopian tube rather than the uterus.

_____ 14. Which of the following statements about male circumcision is _true_?
  A. Routine male circumcision cannot be justified.
  B. Male circumcision reduces the incidence of prostate cancer.
  C. Male circumcision has a long tradition and should not be questioned.
  D. Male circumcision dramatically improves the reproductive health of men who undergo it.

_____ 15. Most sexual performance difficulties stem from
  A. physiological problems.
  B. psychogenic causes.
  C. poor diet.
  D. lack of experience.

Critical Thinking

1. How do biological and psychosocial factors contribute to the complex expression of our sexuality?

2. How has a blending of feminine and masculine qualities benefited society?

3. Why might the "withdrawal" method of contraception not work?

4. What changes, both physiological and psychological, might menopause create in a woman's life?

5. What effect does the aging process have on the sexual response pattern?

Chapter 15   Understanding Sexual Behavior and Relationships

Multiple Choice

_____ 1. Which of the following statements about the effects of aging on sexuality is *true*?
  A. Male production of testosterone increases steadily from age 20 to 60.
  B. The elderly in nursing homes enjoy a more satisfying sex life than others.
  C. Sexual desire typically disappears entirely by age 70.
  D. The capacity to enjoy sex is not altered.

_____ 2. What percentage of women routinely experience multiple orgasms?
  A. 2% to 5%
  B. 5% to 10%
  C. 10% to 30%
  D. 30% to 60%

_____ 3. What is the current view of masturbation among sex therapists and researchers?
  A. Masturbation is a sign of emotional immaturity.
  B. Masturbation should not be necessary when one is in a committed, intimate relationship.
  C. Masturbation is a harmless, normal source of self-pleasure.
  D. Masturbation is an unhealthy form of sexual expression.

_____ 4. Which of the following statements about marriage is *true*?
  A. Frustration and disillusionment are signs that one has married the wrong person.
  B. People tend to marry at an earlier age than in years past.
  C. A typical marriage has periods of happiness and unhappiness.
  D. Marriage tends to resolve one's personality problems and issues.

_____ 5. Which type of marriage is characterized by a loss of the signs of life?
  A. The conflict-habituated marriage
  B. The passive-congenial marriage
  C. The total marriage
  D. The devitalized marriage

_____ 6. Which of the following is *not* an alternative to marriage?
  A. Cohabitation
  B. Military service
  C. Singlehood
  D. Single parenthood

_____ 7. Which of the following statements is *not* true about celibacy?
  A. Celibate people may have intimate relationships without sex.
  B. It is defined as the self-imposed avoidance of sexual contact.
  C. Psychological complications often result from a celibate lifestyle.
  D. All are true.

_____ 8. Which type of oral-genital stimulation involves kissing and licking a woman's vulva?
  A. Foreplay
  B. Fellatio
  C. Cunnilingus
  D. None of the above

_____ 9. Which type of love is enduring and capable of sustaining long-term mutual growth?
  A. Infatuation
  B. Passionate love
  C. Companionate love
  D. Devotional love

_____ 10. Which of the following statements about cohabitation is *not* true?
  A. It is an alternative to marriage.
  B. It can sometimes exist between people sharing a platonic relationship.
  C. Approximately half of all cohabiting couples will disband.
  D. Couples who cohabit are more likely to get married than those in a more traditional relationship.

_____ 11. Recent estimates place the incidence of homosexuality in America at what percentage of the population?
  A. 5%
  B. 10%
  C. 18%
  D. 22%

_____ 12. Which of the following is *not* an appropriate technique for resolving conflict?
  A. Be specific in assigning blame for mistakes
  B. Identify and resolve the real issue
  C. Seek areas of agreement
  D. Say what you are thinking and feeling

_____ 13. Most marriages can be improved through
  A. molding your partner's behavior to meet your expectations.
  B. the unrestrained expression of anger.
  C. periodic affairs.
  D. better communication.

_____ 14. The debate over same-sex marriage is being explored in a test case in the state of
  A. Massachusetts.
  B. Texas.
  C. Hawaii.
  D. California.

_____ 15. Which of the following legal concepts is currently being reconsidered?
  A. No-fault divorce
  B. Common-law marriage
  C. Community property
  D. Joint custody

Critical Thinking

1. If you wish to marry someday, what type of marriage do you wish to have? If you are already married, how could you improve your marriage?

2. What are your attitudes and expectations toward dating? What do you expect from a date?

3. What is your relationship history? How do you think you could improve it?

4. How do you define intimacy?

5. What is your sexual orientation? What is your attitude toward those who differ from you in their sexual orientation or gender expression?

Chapter 16   Managing Your Fertility

Multiple Choice

_____ 1. Which form of birth control *does not* prevent STDs?
   A. Withdrawal
   B. Calendar method
   C. IUD
   D. All of the above

_____ 2. Which two forms of birth control, when used together, provide a high degree of contraceptive protection *and* disease control?
   A. IUD and spermicides
   B. Spermicides and condoms
   C. Calendar method and spermicides
   D. Oral contraceptives and spermicides

_____ 3. Which of the following statements about oral contraceptives is *false?*
   A. The use of antibiotics lowers oral contraceptive effectiveness.
   B. They regulate a woman's menstrual cycle.
   C. The user may experience more frequent vaginal infections, weight gain, mild headaches, and mild depression.
   D. They are useful in the prevention of STDs.

_____ 4. What are "minipills"?
   A. Smaller versions of the regular oral contraceptives that can be swallowed more easily
   B. The placebo pills taken between cycles
   C. Oral contraceptives that contain no estrogen—only low-dose progesterone
   D. Less expensive versions of the pill

_____ 5. What is Depo-Provera?
   A. An injectable contraceptive
   B. A subdermal implant contraceptive
   C. A type of diaphragm
   D. A brand of oral contraceptive

_____ 6. Which type of abortion is performed in the earliest stages of the first trimester?
   A. Menstrual extraction
   B. Dilation and curettage
   C. Dilation and evacuation
   D. Hypertonic saline procedure

_____ 7. What is RU 486?
   A. A drug that replaces estrogen in postmenopausal women
   B. The process of using prostaglandin to influence muscle contractions that expel uterine contents
   C. A hypertonic saline solution
   D. A drug that blocks the action of progesterone, thus producing an early abortion

_____ 8. What is the first thing a parent should do on arriving home?
   A. Collapse in front of the television
   B. Hug or hold his or her young children for at least a few minutes
   C. Begin making dinner
   D. Encourage children to do their chores

_____ 9. A procedure used to open blocked fallopian tubes is
   A. tubal ligation.
   B. transcervical balloon tuboplasty.
   C. preeclampsia.
   D. hypertonic saline procedure.

_____ 10. The following are all contraindications to taking oral contraceptives except
   A. a history of regular menstrual cycles.
   B. high blood pressure.
   C. a history of blood clotting.
   D. cigarette smoking.

_____ 11. All of the following are relatively effective forms of birth control except
   A. diaphragm.
   B. withdrawal.
   C. condom.
   D. IUD.

_____ 12. About how many abortions are performed in the United States each year?
   A. 600,000
   B. 1 million
   C. 1.5 million
   D. 3.5 million

_____ 13. How is female sterilization typically performed?
   A. The fallopian tubes are cut, tied, or cauterized.
   B. The ovaries are removed.
   C. The clitoris is excised.
   D. The uterus is removed.

_____ 14. What is the most common error in the use of home pregnancy test kits?
   A. Using test kits too frequently
   B. Using the test too late to detect the pregnancy
   C. Using the test while under the influence of alcohol or drugs
   D. Using the test too early to detect the pregnancy

_____ 15. What do young people say is the type of training that would *most* help them abstain from sexual activity?
   A. Refusal training
   B. Reproductive biology
   C. Instruction in birth control
   D. Literacy training

Critical Thinking

1. What factors should you consider when choosing a method of birth control?

2. Which of the available methods of birth control would you be most likely to use, if you needed to?

3. What are the guidelines set forth under *Roe v. Wade,* the landmark 1973 Supreme Court case?

4. What serious questions should one consider before deciding to have children?

5. What role do you expect your partner to play in birth control?

Chapter 17   Becoming a Parent

Multiple Choice

_____ 1. Which of the following is an obstacle to pregnancy?
  A. 200 to 500 million sperm cells are deposited in each ejaculation.
  B. Sperm cells are capable of moving quickly.
  C. The acidic level of the vagina is destructive to sperm.
  D. Once inside the fallopian tubes, sperm can live for days.

_____ 2. Which of the following agents can damage a fetus?
  A. Tobacco smoke
  B. Alcohol
  C. Radiation
  D. All of the above

_____ 3. What percentage of deliveries are currently performed through cesarean section?
  A. 5%
  B. 50%
  C. 16%
  D. 23%

_____ 4. All of the following are potential complications of pregnancy except:
  A. osteoporosis.
  B. gestational diabetes.
  C. preeclampsia.
  D. miscarriage.

_____ 5. A couple should seek genetic counseling if which of the following factors are present?
  A. Maternal age of 35 years or greater
  B. History of adoption in maternal or paternal families
  C. History of spontaneous abortions
  D. A and C

_____ 6. The following are all methods a man can use to increase his fertility except to
  A. take folate supplements.
  B. periodically apply cold packs to the scrotum.
  C. wear boxer shorts.
  D. have surgery to repair a structural problem.

_____ 7. Which type of artificial fertilization involves transferring fertilized ova from a laboratory dish into the fallopian tubes?
  A. In vitro fertilization and embryo transfer (IVF-ET)
  B. Gamete intrafallopian transfer (GIFT)
  C. Zygote intrafallopian transfer (ZIFT)
  D. Surrogate parenting

_____ 8. All of the following are risks during pregnancy and childbirth in developing countries except
  A. eclampsia.
  B. hemorrhage.
  C. infection.
  D. diabetes.

_____ 9. All of the following are stages of childbirth except
  A. delivery of the placenta.
  B. inversion of the fetus.
  C. effacement and dilation.
  D. delivery of the fetus.

_____ 10. An incision made in a woman's perineum to keep it from tearing during delivery is a(n)
  A. salpingostomy.
  B. thoracotomy.
  C. episiotomy.
  D. vagotomy.

_____ 11. All of the following are ways to ensure a healthy pregnancy except:
  A. Do not assume conception has occurred until proven by a reliable test.
  B. Take folate or other supplements as directed by a physician.
  C. Exercise as prescribed.
  D. Maintain an appropriate weight.

_____ 12. Fathers-to-be can reduce their own anxiety and concern through which of the following methods?
  A. Educate themselves about pregnancy
  B. Take a course in infant care
  C. Talk with their partner about what they are feeling
  D. All of the above

_____ 13. The process of removing an ovum, fertilizing it, then replacing it in the mother's uterus is called
  A. embryo freezing.
  B. gamete intrafallopian transfer (GIFT).
  C. artificial insemination.
  D. in vitro fertilization.

_____ 14. In women of normal weight who are not approaching menopause, ovulation difficulties are most often caused by
  A. failure to consume an adequate diet.
  B. failure of synchronization between the hormones governing the menstrual cycle.
  C. lack of exercise.
  D. exposure to agents that can damage the reproductive organs.

_____ 15. Adopted children currently represent what percentage of children in the United States?
  A. 2%
  B. 5%
  C. 10%
  D. 15%

Critical Thinking

1. Name three methods of reproductive technology. What do you think are the ethical issues of these methods?

2. Have you ever used a home-pregnancy test? If so, did you follow the directions carefully?

3. Do you think cloning of humans should be illegal?

4. If you had a child, would you want the baby to breast-feed?

5. Describe the birth process from beginning to end.

Chapter 18   Making Consumer Health-Care Decisions

Multiple Choice

_____ 1. Which of the following statements is *false*?
   A. The accuracy of health information from friends and family members may be questionable.
   B. The mass media routinely supply public service messages that give valuable health-related information.
   C. Never trust the labels and directions on prescription medication; it is usually misleading and intended to make you buy more of the product.
   D. Folk wisdom is sometimes supported by scientific evidence.

_____ 2. Which of the following most effectively distributes its health-related information by mail?
   A. On-line computer services
   B. Voluntary health agencies
   C. Government agencies
   D. Qualified health educators

_____ 3. What is the difference between allopathy and osteopathy?
   A. Osteopaths engage in quackery.
   B. Allopathic physicians are board-certified; osteopaths are not.
   C. Osteopaths perceive themselves as being more holistic.
   D. Only osteopaths function as primary care physicians.

_____ 4. Which type of health-care professional provides services related to understanding behavior patterns or perceptions but does not dispense drugs?
   A. Dentist
   B. Psychiatrist
   C. Podiatrist
   D. Psychologist

_____ 5. What does an optician do?
   A. Specializes in vision problems caused by refractory errors
   B. Writes prescriptions for eyewear products
   C. Grinds lenses according to a precise prescription
   D. Specializes in vision care with a base in general medicine

_____ 6. What type of nursing position is helping to provide communities with additional primary care providers?
   A. Nurse practitioner
   B. Registered nurse
   C. Licensed practical nurse
   D. Technical nurse

_____ 7. The established amount that the insured must pay before the insurer reimburses for services is
   A. fixed indemnity.
   B. coinsurance.
   C. deductible.
   D. exclusion.

_____ 8. What are Medicare and Medicaid?
   A. Preferred provider organizations (PPOs)
   B. Independent practice associations (IPAs)
   C. Health maintenance organizations (HMOs)
   D. Forms of governmental insurance

_____ 9. Which is the *most* frequently prescribed drug in the United States?
   A. Prozac (for depression)
   B. Vasotec (for high blood pressure)
   C. Mevacor (for high cholesterol)
   D. Zantac (for ulcers)

_____ 10. Which of the following is a sign of quackery?
   A. Makes promises of quick, dramatic, painless, or drugless treatment
   B. Claims a product provides treatment for multiple illnesses
   C. States that the treatment is secret or not yet available in this country
   D. All of the above

_____ 11. Which of the following alternative forms of medicine is based on balancing the active and passive forces of the patient's body to strengthen the chi ("chee"), or life force?
   A. Homeopathy
   B. Herbalism
   C. Acupuncture
   D. Ayurveda

_____ 12. The average cost of spending a year in a nursing home is
   A. $12,000.
   B. $20,000.
   C. $26,000.
   D. $32,000.

_____ 13. All of the following are techniques for becoming a more skilled consumer except
   A. reading books to educate yourself.
   B. putting complaints in writing.
   C. not questioning your caregiver's recommendations.
   D. comparison shopping.

_____ 14. Approximately how many people in the United States do not have health insurance coverage?
   A. 37 million
   B. 800,000
   C. 12 million
   D. 4 million

Critical Thinking

1. What are some of the pros and cons of obtaining health information from the mass media?

2. What are some sources of health information available to you?

3. What are some alternative health-care practices? Would you be willing to try them?

4. How can self-care benefit both individuals and the health-care industry?

5. What are the advantages and disadvantages of HMOs?

Chapter 19   Caring for Our Environment

Multiple Choice

_____ 1. Each year, the population of the world grows by
  A. 90 million people.
  B. 90,000 people.
  C. 90%.
  D. 90 billion people.

_____ 2. What is the leading source of air pollution?
  A. Kuwait oil fires
  B. Chemical production plants
  C. Internal combustion engines
  D. Coal-fired power plants

_____ 3. What has caused the greenhouse effect?
  A. A progressive increase in carbon dioxide in the atmosphere
  B. A hole in the ozone layer
  C. A slight warming of the earth's surface
  D. All of the above

_____ 4. What substances produce acid rain when they combine with moisture in the atmosphere?
  A. Coal and hydrogen
  B. Hydrocarbons and particulate matter
  C. Chlorofluorocarbons
  D. Nitrogen and sulfur

_____ 5. Which type of pollution disproportionately affects children of low-income families?
  A. Radon gas
  B. Lead
  C. Subsidence inversion
  D. Radiation inversion

_____ 6. What is eutrophication?
  A. A biological imbalance that causes fish to die in great numbers from lack of oxygen
  B. The overabundance of aquatic plants that results when water is rich in nitrates and phosphates
  C. Both A and B
  D. Neither A nor B

_____ 7. Which of the following is a hydrocarbon found in the water supply that has been linked to cancer?
  A. Chlorine
  B. PCB
  C. DDT
  D. EPA

_____ 8. Which of the following sources of water pollution comes from power plants?
  A. Oil spills
  B. Thermal pollution
  C. Sediments
  D. None of the above

_____ 9. Which type of solid waste disposal is discouraged or illegal in many urban areas?
  A. Ocean dumping
  B. Incineration
  C. Sanitary landfill
  D. Open dumping

_____ 10. Which of the following devices generates electromagnetic fields?
  A. Water bed heater
  B. Electric razor
  C. Cellular phone
  D. All of the above

_____ 11. All of the following are synthetic sources of radiation except
  A. dental x-ray examinations.
  B. medical diagnostic procedures.
  C. waste from nuclear reactors.
  D. mineral deposits.

_____ 12. A pollutant that is capable of producing birth defects is said to be
  A. mutagenic.
  B. carcinogenic.
  C. systemic.
  D. teratogenic.

_____ 13. Sound is measured according to its
  A. proximity and dynamics.
  B. frequency and intensity.
  C. bass and treble.
  D. energy and duration.

_____ 14. An arrangement in which individuals contract directly with a farmer to buy his or her crop is known as
  A. organic farming.
  B. agricultural price supports.
  C. community-supported agriculture.
  D. co-op farming.

_____ 15. How much of the earth's surface is inhabitable land?
  A. About 50%
  B. About 40%
  C. About 35%
  D. About 30%

Critical Thinking

1. How do different types of air pollution adversely affect us?

2. Why are metals, such as mercury, arsenic, and copper, particularly dangerous when they pollute our water supply?

3. What factors have kept recycling from being fully adopted in so many areas?

4. What are some concerns about nuclear energy?

5. What steps can you take to improve our environment and reduce your exposure to harmful environmental pollutants?

Chapter 20   Protecting Your Safety

Multiple Choice

_____ 1. Which form of violence received national attention because of the deaths in 1994 of Nicole Brown Simpson and Ronald Goldman?
   A. Child abuse
   B. Carjacking
   C. Domestic violence
   D. Elder abuse

_____ 2. Who is most often a victim of partner abuse?
   A. Prostitutes
   B. Teenage girls
   C. Spouses or former spouses of the assailant
   D. Men

_____ 3. Which form of child abuse occurs most frequently?
   A. Neglect
   B. Physical abuse
   C. Psychological abuse
   D. Sexual abuse

_____ 4. What may be the "single greatest crime problem in America today"?
   A. Youth violence
   B. Hate crimes
   C. Bank robberies
   D. Organized crime

_____ 5. Aside from the physical harm of rape, what other effects may occur?
   A. Posttraumatic stress syndrome
   B. Guilt
   C. Emotional damage resulting from "broken trust"
   D. All of the above

_____ 6. Which of the following constitutes sexual harassment?
   A. Excessive pressure for dates
   B. Sexually explicit humor
   C. Unwanted physical contact
   D. All of the above

_____ 7. Which of the following can help increase safety around your home?
   A. Make sure your name is spelled correctly in the phone book.
   B. Try to live in apartments on the first floor.
   C. Require repair people to show valid identification.
   D. Leave windows unlocked in case you need to leave in a hurry.

_____ 8. Over half of all murders result from
   A. random crime.
   B. domestic abuse.
   C. arguments between acquaintances or relatives.
   D. none of the above.

_____ 9. Which of the following profiles is a _most_ likely candidate for death by motor vehicle accident?
   A. Male, 55–65 years of age, driving in rainy conditions on a weekend afternoon
   B. Female, 35–45 years of age, driving on a freeway with the noise of children playing in the back seat
   C. Female, 65–75 years of age, driving in rush-hour traffic
   D. Male, 15–25 years of age, driving on a two-lane rural road on a Saturday night

_____ 10. Which of the following resources will help improve your safety on campus?
   A. University-approved escorts
   B. Campus security departments
   C. Campus counseling center
   D. All of the above

_____ 11. Studies on college campuses report that what percentage of college women have experienced date rape?
   A. 20%
   B. 15%
   C. 10%
   D. 7%

_____ 12. Which of the following steps can best help prevent injury when bicycling?
   A. Bicycle with a group
   B. Bicycle against, rather than with, the flow of traffic
   C. Carry water and food
   D. Wear a helmet

_____ 13. Most boating deaths can be prevented by
   A. avoiding crowded waterways.
   B. refraining from water skiing and parasailing.
   C. wearing a personal flotation device (PFD).
   D. regularly maintaining the engine and hull of the boat.

_____ 14. The United States leads the world in handgun homicides, with _____ per year.
   A. 5,000
   B. 8,500
   C. 15,000
   D. 22,000

_____ 15. All of the following are methods to avoid drowsy driving except
   A. taking frequent breaks.
   B. singing or talking.
   C. eating a big meal for energy.
   D. opening the window.

Critical Thinking

1. What factors may have contributed to a drop in U.S. homicide rates?

2. How should suspected child abuse be properly handled?

3. What is rape? What is acquaintance rape? What is date rape?

4. How can you increase your personal safety?

5. What steps can you take to protect children and the elderly?

Chapter 21   Accepting Dying and Death

Multiple Choice

_____ 1. Which of the following is a criterion by which death may be determined?
A. Lack of heartbeat and breathing
B. Lack of central nervous system function
C. Presence of rigor mortis
D. All of the above

_____ 2. Which type of euthanasia is illegal in the United States?
A. Direct euthanasia
B. Indirect euthanasia
C. Both A and B
D. Neither A nor B

_____ 3. What does the physician's order "DNR" mean?
A. Death not recorded
B. Do not resuscitate
C. Do not release
D. Do not recognize

_____ 4. What psychological stage for dying people serves as the earliest temporary defense mechanism?
A. Denial
B. Anger
C. Bargaining
D. None of the above

_____ 5. Which of the following describes the appropriate way to act toward someone who is dying?
A. Refrain from crying so as not to upset them.
B. Remain optimistic even when there is no hope for recovery.
C. Try to be genuine and honest.
D. Try to distract the person from talking about death.

_____ 6. Adults coping with the death of a child should
A. have another child and name that child after the deceased.
B. move to a different home for a change of environment.
C. give themselves time and space to grieve.
D. do all of the above.

_____ 7. Which of the following is _not_ a normal, healthy expression of grief over the loss of a loved one?
A. Physical discomfort
B. Sense of numbness
C. Guilt
D. Extreme hostility

_____ 8. How long do periods of grief usually last?
A. A few weeks
B. 2 to 5 years
C. A few months to a year
D. 10 years or more

_____ 9. What is a wake?
A. An established time for friends and family to share emotions and experiences about the deceased
B. A formaldehyde-based fluid used to replace blood components during embalming
C. A container for ashes from cremation
D. None of the above

_____ 10. Which of the following is the word for a notice of death printed in a newspaper?
A. Eulogy
B. Epitaph
C. Obituary
D. None of the above

_____ 11. When a child loses a loved one to death, the child should be
A. told that the loved one has "gone to sleep."
B. told the truth and given the support needed to bear it.
C. protected until he or she is old enough to understand the truth.
D. spared seeing the parent cry or otherwise experience grief.

_____ 12. Hospices differ from hospitals in which of the following ways?
A. A hospice can combat the disease more aggressively.
B. A hospice can better help people die in comfort and with dignity.
C. A hospice can provide more experimental treatments for the patient's condition.
D. A hospice prevents the patient from making decisions about treatment.

_____ 13. You can prepare for your own death in which of the following ways?
A. Volunteering in a hospice
B. Purchasing life insurance
C. Preparing a will
D. All of the above

_____ 14. You can make certain your wishes for organ donation are carried out by
A. placing your organ donation card in a safe deposit box for permanent storage.
B. telling your attorney.
C. signing your organ donation card in the presence of two witnesses, preferably your next of kin.
D. keeping your wishes private.

_____ 15. A mausoleum is a(n)
A. aboveground structure into which caskets can be placed.
B. burial location generally underneath a church.
C. inscription on a grave marker or monument.
D. speech about the deceased, often delivered at a funeral or memorial.

Critical Thinking

1. What are living wills and durable power of attorney documents? Why would it be prudent to have these documents?

2. How do the emotional stages of dying described by Elisabeth Kübler-Ross affect those close to the dying person?

3. Describe what might occur during an out-of-body experience.

4. How does a hospice differ from a traditional hospital in the care of the terminally ill?

5. How do death rituals help people deal with death?

Answers

Chapter 1

1. C
2. D
3. C
4. A
5. B
6. D
7. D
8. B
9. D
10. A
11. D
12. B
13. C
14. D
15. D

Chapter 2

1. A
2. D
3. B
4. D
5. D
6. B
7. A
8. C
9. A
10. D
11. B
12. A
13. C
14. C
15. B

Chapter 3

1. B
2. A
3. B
4. A
5. D
6. A
7. D
8. B
9. C
10. B
11. C
12. A
13. B
14. A

Chapter 4

1. D
2. C
3. B
4. D
5. B
6. D
7. D
8. C
9. B
10. D
11. C
12. C
13. D
14. C
15. D

Chapter 5

1. B
2. C
3. B
4. C
5. D
6. D
7. A
8. C
9. C
10. D
11. A
12. C
13. C
14. D
15. D

Chapter 6

1. D
2. A
3. C
4. A
5. D
6. A
7. A
8. D
9. B
10. C
11. B
12. D
13. B
14. B
15. A

Chapter 7

1. D
2. C
3. B
4. A
5. C
6. D
7. B
8. D
9. C
10. D
11. B
12. D
13. A
14. C
15. A

Chapter 8

1. C
2. B
3. C
4. D
5. D
6. D
7. A
8. C
9. C
10. A
11. D
12. C
13. D
14. D
15. C

Chapter 9

1. C
2. D
3. C
4. B
5. A
6. D
7. C
8. C
9. A
10. B
11. D
12. D
13. A
14. C
15. D

Chapter 10

1. D
2. D
3. D
4. D
5. D
6. C
7. C
8. B
9. A
10. B
11. B
12. C
13. A
14. A
15. D

Chapter 11

1. D
2. C
3. B
4. D
5. A
6. C
7. A
8. D
9. A
10. D
11. D
12. D
13. C
14. D
15. A

Chapter 12

1. C
2. B
3. A
4. A
5. D
6. B
7. D
8. D
9. C
10. B
11. D
12. C
13. D
14. C
15. C

Chapter 13

1. D
2. B
3. A
4. A
5. B
6. C
7. D
8. C
9. A
10. C
11. C
12. B
13. D
14. C
15. A

Chapter 14

1. B
2. C
3. A
4. C
5. B
6. D
7. D
8. B
9. C
10. B
11. C
12. D
13. B
14. A
15. B

Chapter 15

1. D
2. C
3. C
4. C
5. D
6. B
7. C
8. C
9. C
10. D
11. B
12. A
13. D
14. C
15. A

Chapter 16

1. D
2. B
3. D
4. C
5. A
6. A
7. D
8. B
9. B
10. A
11. B
12. C
13. A
14. D
15. A

Chapter 17

1. A
2. C
3. A
4. D
5. B
6. B
7. B
8. B
9. D
10. C
11. A
12. D
13. D
14. B
15. A

Chapter 18

1. C
2. C
3. C
4. D
5. C
6. A
7. C
8. D
9. D
10. D
11. C
12. D
13. C
14. A

Chapter 19

1. A
2. C
3. A
4. D
5. B
6. B
7. B
8. B
9. D
10. D
11. D
12. D
13. B
14. C
15. D

Chapter 20

1. C
2. C
3. A
4. A
5. D
6. D
7. C
8. C
9. D
10. D
11. A
12. D
13. D
14. C
15. C

Chapter 21

1. D
2. A
3. B
4. A
5. C
6. C
7. D
8. C
9. A
10. C
11. B
12. B
13. D
14. C
15. A

credits

Illustrations

Chapter 1

Table 1-1, From U.S. Bureau of the Census: *Statistical Abstract of the United States: 1997,* 117th ed Washington, DC: U.S. Government Printing Office, 1997.

Chapter 2

p. 31 (Personal Assessment), Adapted from the *Study Guide for Psychology Applied to Modern Life: Adjustment in the 90s* by W. Weiten and M. Sosulski. Copyright © 1994, 1991, 1986, 1983 Brooks/Cole Publishing Company, Pacific Grove, CA 93950, a division of International Thomson Publishing Inc. By permission of the publisher; **p. 41 (Star Box),** From Blumenthal SJ: Suicide; a guide to risk factors: assessment and treatment of suicidal patients. *Medical Clinics of North America* 72:937–971, 1988; **Figure 2-1,** "HIERARCHY OF NEEDS" from MOTIVATION AND PERSONALITY, 3rd ed. By ABRAHAM H. MASLOW. Revised by Robert Frager, James Fadiman, Cynthia McReynolds, and Ruth Cox. Copyright © 1970 by Abraham Maslow. Reprinted by permission of Addison Wesley.

Chapter 3

p. 57 (Personal Assessment), Modified from Holmes TH and Rahe RH: The social adjustment rating scale, *Journal of Psychosomatic Research,* 11:213–218, 1967; **p. 58 (Personal Assessment),** Modified by an inventory developed by Rosellen Bohlen, University of Scranton.

Chapter 4

Table 4-1, From Prentice, WE: *Fitness for college and life,* ed 5, New York, McGraw Hill, p. 319; **pp. 90–91 (Personal Assessment),** Data from the National Fitness Foundation; **pp. 99–100 (Star Box),** Copyright 1986, *USA Today.*

Chapter 5

Tables 5-2, 5-4, 5-5, 5-6, and 5-7, From Wardlaw G, Insel P: *Perspectives in nutrition,* ed 3, St. Louis, 1996, Mosby; **Tables 5-3A & 5-3B,** Modified from Food and Nutrition Board, National Research Council: *Recommended dietary allowances,* ed 10, Washington, DC, 1989, National Academy of Sciences; **Table 5-8,** US Department of Health and Human Services, Public Health Service, *The Surgeon General's report on nutrition and health,* Washington, DC, 1988, US Government Printing Office; **Figure 5-2,** US Department of Agriculture/US Department of Health and Human Services, August, 1992; **Figures 5-3 and 5-4,** From Wardlaw G, Insel P: *Perspectives in nutrition,* ed 3, St. Louis, 1996, Mosby; **Figure 5-5,** National Dairy Council, Rosemont, IL; **pp. 118–119 (Personal Assessment),** From *Nutrition for a healthy life,* courtesy of Marcy Leeds; **p. 133 (Personal Assessment),** Data on four food groups from Guthrie H: *Introductory nutrition,* ed 7, St. Louis, 1989, Mosby; **p. 143 (Health Guide, left),** US Department of Health and Human Services, Public Health Service, *The Surgeon General's report on nutrition and health,* Washington, DC, 1988, US Government Printing Office; **p. 143 (Health Guide, right),** © 1986, American Diabetic Association. *Health Food Choices,* used with permission.

Chapter 6

Figure 6-1, Modified from George A. Bray; **Table 6-1,** From Wardlaw G, Insel P, and Seyler M: *Contemporary nutrition: issues and insights,* ed 2, St. Louis, 1994, Mosby; **Table 6-2,** US Department of Agriculture; **Table 6-4,** Based on data from Bannister EW and Brown SR: The relative energy requirements of physical activity. In HB Falls, editor: *Exercise physiology,* New York, 1968; **Table 6-5,** Adapted from Guthrie H: *Introductory nutrition,* ed 7, St. Louis, 1989, Mosby-Year Book, pp. 226–227; **p. 173 (Personal Assessment),** Modified from Foreyt J, and Goodrick GK: Living without dieting, Houston: Harrison Publishing.

Chapter 7

Figure 7-1, Source: National Institute on Drug Abuse, 1990 survey; **Figure 7-2,** Source: American Management Association Survey; **Table 7-1,** Modified from the Muncie Star © 1987; **Table 7-2,** Caffeine data obtained from Consumers Union, Food and Drug Administration, National Coffee Association, National Soft Drink Association, and Physicians' Desk Reference for Non-Prescription Drugs. Reprinted from *Caffeine and endurance performance* by permission of the Gatorade Sports Science Institute, Chicago, IL.

Chapter 8

Table 8-1, US Department of Health and Human Services: Alcohol and health: fourth special report to the US Congress, Washington, DC, 1981, DHS Pub No ADM 81–1080; **Table 8-2,** Source: Wyngardner JB and Smith LH: Signs of intoxication at various BACs, *Cecil Textbook of Medicine,* Philadelphia, 1988, WB Saunders; **p. 248 (Health Guide),** Modified from a brochure of the Indiana Alcohol Countermeasure Program; **p. 252 (Star Box),** Modified from Woititz JG: *Adult children of alcoholics,* Pompano Beach, FL, 1983, Health Communications, Inc. In Pinger R, Payne W, Hahn D, Hahn E: *Drugs: issues for today,* St. Louis, 1991, Mosby; **p. 250 (Personal Assessment),** From *Are You Troubled By Someone's Drinking?,* © 1980, by Al-Anon Family Group headquarters, Inc. Reprinted by permission of Al-Anon Family Group Headquarters, Inc.

Chapter 9

p. 266 (Star Box), American Lung Association, *Lung Disease Data 1996,* New York, NY, 1997; **Table 9-1,** American Public Health Association; **p. 264 (Personal Assessment),** Reproduced with permission of the American Cancer Society.

Chapter 10

Figure 10-1, Data from American Heart Association, 1997 Heart and Stroke Facts; **p. 302 (Personal Assessment),** From Howard E: *Health risks,* Tucson, 1986, Body Press; **p. 307 (Health Guide),** Data from American Heart Association, 1988 Heart Facts.

Chapter 11

Figure 11-1, National Cancer Institute: *Horizons of cancer research,* NIH Pub No 90–3011, © 1989; **Figure 11-2,** Reprinted with permission of the American Cancer Society, Inc.; **p. 345 (Health Guide),** American Academy of Dermatology; **p. 331 (Health Guide),** Reprinted with permission of the American Cancer Society, Inc.

Chapter 12

p. 362 (Star Box), Reprinted with permission from the University of California at Berkeley, *Wellness Letter,* © Health Letter Associates, 1996, 1997. To order a one year subscription, call 800-829-9170; **p. 369 (Star Box),** Reprinted with permission from the University of California at Berkeley, *Wellness Letter,* © Health Letter Associates, 1996, 1997. To order a one year subscription, call 800-829-9170; **p. 373 (Star Box), p. 375 (Health Action Guide),** courtesy of Allergy and Asthma Network, Mothers of Asthmatics, Inc.; **p. 375 (Health Action Guide),** Reprinted with permission from the University of California at Berkeley, *Wellness Letter,* © Health Letter Associates, 1996, 1997. To order a one year subscription, call 800-829-9170; **p. 379 (Star Box),** by Mitzi Baker, reprinted with permission from HEALTH, © 1996.

Chapter 13

Table 13-2, p. 410 (Personal Assessment), Centers for Disease Control and Prevention; **Table 13-3,** Courtesy of the National Institute of Allergy and Infectious Diseases.

Chapter 15

p. 456 (Personal Assessment), Modified from *USA Today.*

Chapter 16

Table 16-1, Modified from Lisken L, et al: Youth in the 1980s; social and health concern, Population Reports, Series M, No 9, Population Information Program, Johns Hopkins University, November–December 1985; **p. 478 (Personal Assessment),** Adapted from Haas K and Haas A: *Understanding sexuality,* ed 3, St. Louis, 1993, Mosby.

Chapter 18

Figure 18-2, Data from SAMSHA News, Vol 1, #4, p. 3; **Figure 18-1,** First Databank, The Hearst Corp.; **p. 533 (Health Guide),** Source: Pell AR; *Making the most of Medicare,* DCI Publishing, 1990, in *in-sync,* Erie, PA, Spring, 1994, Erie Insurance Group.

Chapter 19

Figure 19-1, World Resources, 1988–1989; **Table 19-1,** Source: Water Pollution Control Federation; **p. 560 (Personal Assessment),** Modified from *Being green: some tips on how to help the earth,* Scripps Howard News Service; **p. 571 (Health Guide),** From McGrath M, Dadd DL: *Nontoxic, Natural, and Earthwise,* Los Angeles, 1990, Jeremy P. Tarcher.

Chapter 20

Figure 20-1, Courtesy of the National Committee to Prevent Child Abuse, Chicago; **p. 595 (Health Guide),** From the American College Health Association; **p. 597 (Health Guide),** Reprinted with the permission of the American Academy of Ophthalmology, *Preventing Eye Injuries.*

Chapter 21

Figure 21-1, The National Kidney Foundation Uniform Donor Card is reprinted with permission from the National Kidney Foundation, Inc. Copyright 1970, 1991, New York, NY; **p. 617 (Star Box),** Reprinted by permission of Choice In Dying, formerly Concern for Dying/Society for the Right to Die, 200 Varick Street, New York, NY 10014, (212) 366–5540; **p. 626 (Personal Assessment),** Courtesy Bowman, Meeks Mortuary, Muncie, IN.

Photos

All photos supplied by FPG International, unless otherwise noted.

Chapter 2

p. 28, CLG Photographic, Inc.; p. 35, Dr. Graham Hatcher; p. 38, Stewart Halperin; p. 50, Humane Society.

Chapter 3

p. 56, Dr. Graham Hatcher.

Chapter 4

pp. 90–91, 100, Stewart Halperin.

Chapter 8

p. 234, CLG Photographic, Inc.; p. 244, George Steinmetz; p. 247, Mothers Against Drunk Driving.

Chapter 12

p. 364, Custom Medical Stock Photo.

Chapter 13

p. 411, Phototake; p. 412, Custom Medical Stock Photo.

Chapter 15

p. 458, Stewart Halperin.

Chapter 19

p. 569, CLG Photographics, Inc.

Chapter 21

p. 631, Associated Press.

Social workers, role of, 44
Socioeconomic status
  and access to health care, 545–546
  and hypertension, 321–322
Sodium, functions/sources/
  deficiency information, 127
Solid waste, 568–569
  forms of, 568–569
Soluble fiber, sources of, 129
Special Olympics, 83
Spermatogenesis, 427, 432
Spermicides, 480–482
Spina bifida
  causes of, 365
  prevention of, 365
Spirituality
  as dimension of health, 16
  and emotional health, 35–36
  and hospice care, 622
  issues with as stressor, 60
Sports
  body building, 97
  extreme sports, 109–110
  performance enhancing drugs, 98,
    101–102, 108
Sports drinks, 97
Sports injuries, 104–106
  prevention of, 104
  types of injuries, 105–106
Stalking, 591–592
  self-protection guidelines, 592
Static stretching, 86
Sterilization, 488–489
  for female, 488–489
  for male, 488
Stimulant drugs, 211–217
  amphetamines, 213–214
  caffeine, 212–213, 229–231
  cocaine, 215–217
  crystal methamphetamine,
    214–215
  methamphetamine, 228
  Ritalin, 215
Strength training, 84–85, 93–94
  bodybuilding, popularity of, 97
  goal of, 84, 93
  isokinetic exercises, 85, 93
  isometric exercises, 84
  overload principle, 84, 85
  progressive resistance exercises, 85
Stress
  assessment of, 57–58
  and cardiovascular disease, 306, 322
  of college students, 56, 59–61
  definition of, 54, 55
  distress, 55, 56
  eustress, 55
  and illness, 56, 65–66
  individual responses to, 54
  and minorities, 55
  and personality traits, 66
Stress management, 67–70
  biofeedback, 69
  diaphragmatic breathing, 67–68
  exercise, 69
  meditation, 68–69
  progressive muscle relaxation, 67
  quieting, 67
  and realistic life perspective, 69–70
  relaxation response, 67
  self-hypnosis, 67
  for work-related stress, 68
  yoga, 67
Stressors
  definition of, 54, 55
  intensity, impact of, 66–67
  noise as, 575
  of single parent, 74–76
Stress response, 62–65
  alarm stage, 62
  and brain, 62–64
  and endocrine system, 64
  epinephrine, physiological effects
    of, 64–65

exhaustion stage, 62
fight-or-flight response, 62, 64–65
general adaptation syndrome, 62
resistance stage, 62
Stretching
  ballistic stretching, 86
  static stretching, 86
Stroke, 313–315
  cerebral aneurysm, 314
  cerebral hemorrhage, 314
  cerebrovascular occlusions,
    313–314
  diagnosis of, 314
  transient ischemic attack (TIA),
    314, 315
  treatment of, 314–315
  warning signs of, 314
Students Against Destructive
  Decisions (SADD), 247
Subculture, and drug abuse, 210
Subdermal implants, birth control,
  487–488
Sudden cardiac death, nature of, 275
Sugar
  and carbohydrates, 114–115
  hidden sugars in foods, 115
  limiting in diet, 141
Suicide, 40–41
  and alcohol abuse, 246
  mass suicides, 619
  prevention of, 41
  survivors, counseling for, 632
  warning signs, 41
Sulfur, functions/sources/deficiency
  information, 128
Sun exposure
  protection, 106, 344
  and skin cancer, 344
Supermasculinity, 359
Support groups, grief-oriented, 633
Supportive therapy, elements of, 45
Surgery
  cancer treatment, 346
  for coronary artery disease, 310
  for infertility, 514
  for weight loss, 179–180
Surrogate parenting, 515
  ethical issues, 516
Symptothermal method, birth
  control, 480
Synergistic effect, drugs, 222, 223, 247
Syphilis, 408–409, 412–413
  stages of, 413
Systemic lupus erythematosus, 376
  management of, 376
  signs of, 376
Systolic blood pressure, 312, 313

Tachycardia, 316, 317
Talipes, 364
Tamoxifen, 333, 337
Tampon use, and toxic shock
  syndrome, 401–402, 437, 446
Tar, in tobacco smoke, 273
Target heart rate (THR)
  calculation of, 93
  meaning of, 92, 93
Taxol, 340
Tay-Sachs disease, 361
  characteristics of, 361
  prevention of, 361
Telecommunications Decency Act, 470
Telecommuting, and environmental
  preservation, 563
Temperament, and personality, 30
Temperature inversions, 564
Tennis elbow, 106
Tension headaches, 65
Teratogenic agent, 513, 567
  meaning of, 341
Tertiary prevention, of drug use, 202
Test anxiety, coping with, 59
Testes, 432
Testicles, self-examination, 341, 342

Testicular cancer, 341–342
  early detection, 341
  forms of, 341
  prevention of, 341
  risk factors, 341
  treatment of, 341–342
Tetanus, 395
Thermic effect of food, 172
Thiamin, functions/sources/
  deficiency information, 124
Thorax, 299
Time management, 59–60
  tips for, 59–60
Titration, 268
  meaning of, 267
Tobacco. See also Cigarette smoking
  chemicals of, 272–273
  smokeless tobacco, 280–281
Tolerance, drug abuse, 204–205
Toxic shock syndrome, 401–402
  signs of, 402
  and tampon manufacturing, 446
Toxic substances, water pollution,
  566–567
Toxic waste, 569–570
TPA
  benefits for women, 304
  stroke, 314–315
Trace elements
  functions of, 125
  listing of, 126–127
Tranquilizers, types of, 217
Transcervical balloon tuboplasty, 514
Transdermal patches, for smoking
  cessation, 283
Trans-fatty acids, 116
Transient ischemic attack (TIA),
  314, 315
Transsexualism, 464–465
Transvestism, 465
Trichomoniasis, 414
Tropical areas, new diseases from,
  418–419
Tropical oils, fat content of, 116, 117
Tubal ligation, 488–489
Tuberculosis, 398–399
  drug-resistant type, 398
Tumors, benign tumors, 328, 329
Turner's syndrome, 359
Type A personality, 66

Unbalanced diet, meaning of, 147
Underweight, 185
  weight gain tips, 185
Unintentional injuries, 596
Universities, religious diversity on,
  22–23
Urethritis, 414
Urinary tract infection, 414
Uterine cancer, 338–339
  early detection, 339
  risk factors, 338–339
  treatment, 339
Uterus, 435

Vacuum aspiration, 489–490
Vagina, 435
Vaginal cancer, 339
  and DES exposure, 339
  early detection, 339
Vaginal infections, 407–408, 414
  candida infection, 414
  trichomonas infection, 414
Vaginismus, 452
Valium, 217
Vascular system, 298–299
  operation of, 298–300
Vasectomy, 433, 488
Vasodilators, 312
Vegan vegetarian diet, 146–147
Vegetables, 131–132
  cruciferous vegetables, 131–132
  greens, health benefits of, 169
  nutrients in, 131

recommended daily servings,
  131, 132
Vegetarian diets, 145–147, 152–154
  benefits of, 152–153
  dietary concerns, 146–147, 152–153
  lactovegetarian diet, 146
  ovolactovegetarina diet, 145–146
  ovovegetarian diet, 146
  semivegetarianism, 145, 153–154
  vegan vegetarian diet, 146–147
Verbal communication, 32–33
  listening, 33
Vestibule, 435
Viagra, insurance coverage issue, 546
Violence
  and alcohol abuse, 245–246
  domestic violence, 587–589
  gangs, 589–590
  gun violence, 590
  gun violence in schools, 584
  hate crime, 590–591
  homicide, 587
  intentional injuries, 587
  self-protection guidelines, 585
  sexual victimization, 592–595
  stalking, 591–592
  unintentional injuries. See
    Accidents
  violent death, dealing with, 632
Virginity, reasons for, 464
Virulent, meaning of, 390, 391
Visualization, 36–38
  steps in, 36–38
Vitamin A, functions/sources/
  deficiency information, 122
Vitamin B$_6$, functions/sources/
  deficiency information, 125
Vitamin B$_{12}$,
  functions/sources/deficiency
    information, 125
  and vegetarian diet, 152
Vitamin C
  fruit servings, 130–131
  functions/sources/deficiency
    information, 125
  increasing intake, 144
  and iron absorption, 144
Vitamin D
  functions/sources/deficiency
    information, 122
  and vegetarian diet, 152–153
Vitamin E, functions/sources/
  deficiency information, 122
Vitamin K, functions/sources/
  deficiency information, 122
Vitamins, 121–124
  fat-soluble vitamins, 121–122
  functions of, 121
  overuse, 121
  recommended dietary allowances,
    122–123
  supplements, recommended
    use, 124
  water-soluble vitamins, 121,
    123–124
Volunteers, 49–50
  diversity among, 49–50
  hospice volunteers, 628
  motives of, 49
  opportunities for, 50

Waist-to-hip ratio, 160–162
Warm-up, pre-exercise, 94
Warts, genital, 411
Water
  dehydration, signs of, 127
  functions of, 127
  importance as nutrient, 129
  recommended intake, 129
Water-borne illness, prevention
  guidelines, 568
Water pollution, 565–568
  effects on wetlands, 568
  and eutrophication, 566